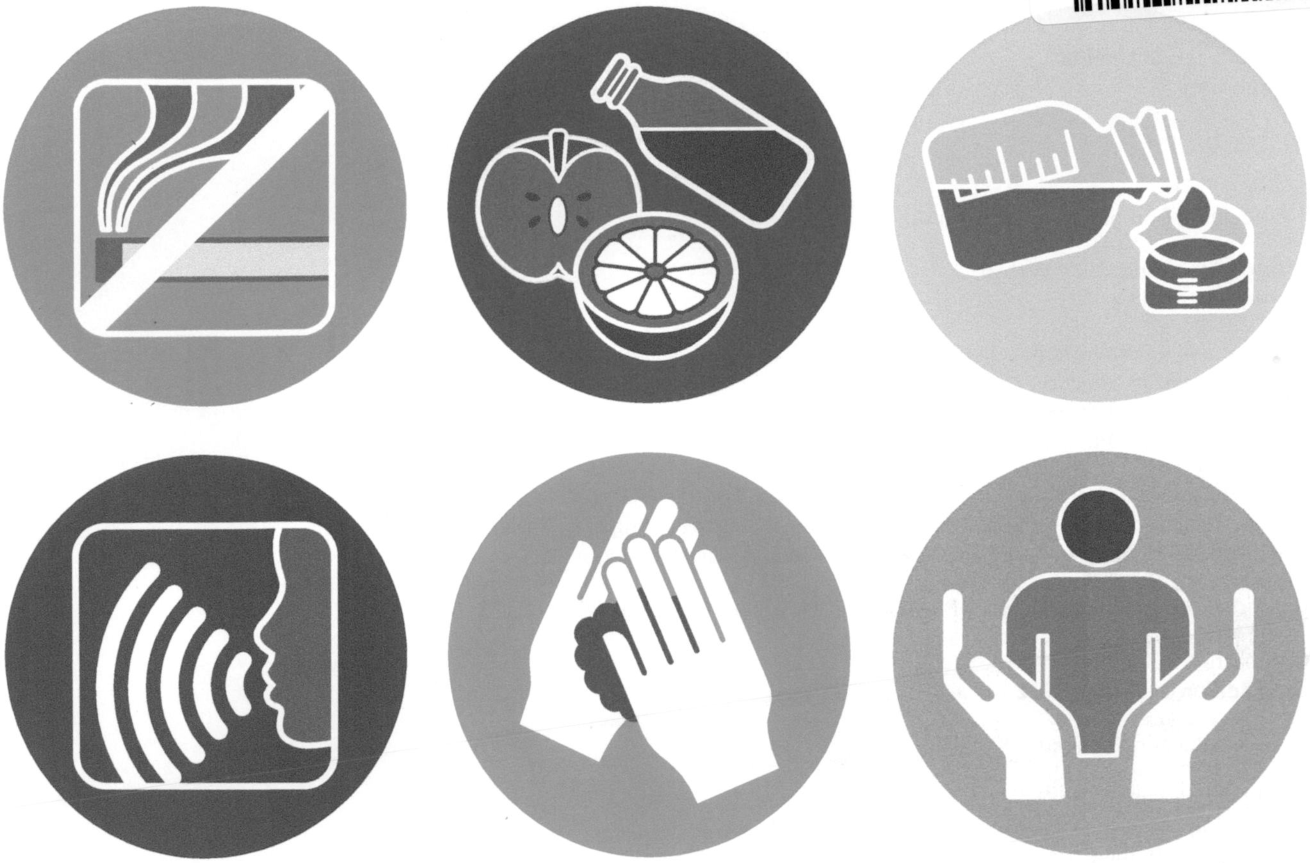

Second Edition

Fundamentals of NURSING

Concepts, process and practice

Barbara **Kozier** Glenora **Erb** Audrey **Berman** Shirlee **Snyder**
Sharon **Harvey** Heulwen **Morgan-Samuel**

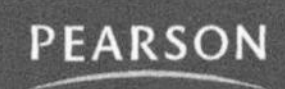

Harlow, England • London • New York • Boston • San Francisco • Toronto • Sydney • Singapore • Hong Kong
Tokyo • Seoul • Taipei • New Delhi • Cape Town • Madrid • Mexico City • Amsterdam • Munich • Paris • Milan

Pearson Education Limited
Edinburgh Gate
Harlow
Essex CM20 2JE
England

and Associated Companies throughout the world

Visit us on the World Wide Web at:
www.pearson.com.uk

Authorized adaptation from the United States edition, entitled *Fundamentals of Nursing: Concepts, Process, and Practice*, 7th Edition, ISBN: 0130455296 by Kozier, Barbara; Erb, Glenora; Berman, Audrey J.; Snyder, Shirlee; published by Pearson Education, Inc, publishing as Prentice Hall, Copyright © 2004.

First adaptation edition published by PEARSON EDUCATION LTD, Copyright © 2008

First published 2008
Second Edition published 2012

ISBN: 978-0-273-73908-1

British Library Cataloguing-in-Publication Data
A catalogue record for this book is available from the British Library

Library of Congress Cataloging-in-Publication Data
Fundamentals of nursing : concepts, process, and practce / Barbara Kozier . . .
[et al.]. -- 2nd ed.
p. ; cm.
"Authorized adaptation from the United States edition" of: Kozier & Erb's fundamentals of nursing / Barbara Kozier . . . [et al.]. 9th ed. c2012.
Includes bibliographical references and index.
ISBN 978-0-273-73908-1 (pbk.)
1. Nursing. I. Kozier, Barbara. II. Kozier & Erb's fundamentals of nursing / Audrey Berman . . . [et al.].
[DNLM: 1. Nursing Process. 2. Nursing Care. 3. Nursing Theory. WY 100]
RT41.F8813 2012c
610.73--dc23

2011027679

10 9 8 7 6 5 4 3 2
15 14 13

Typeset in 9.5/12pt Minion by 35
Printed and bound by Ashford Colour Press Ltd

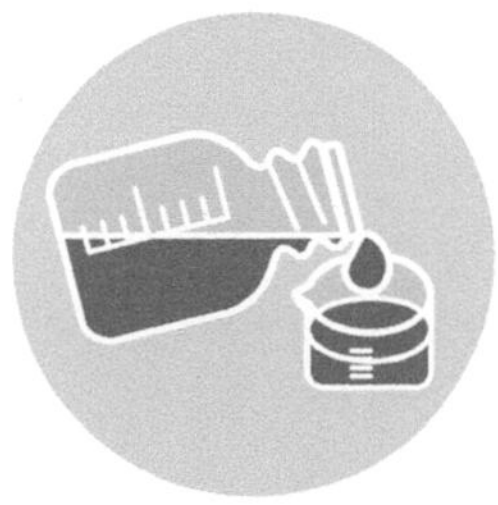
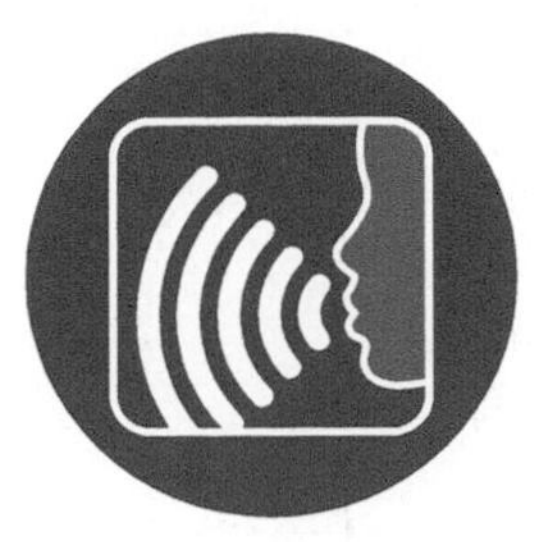
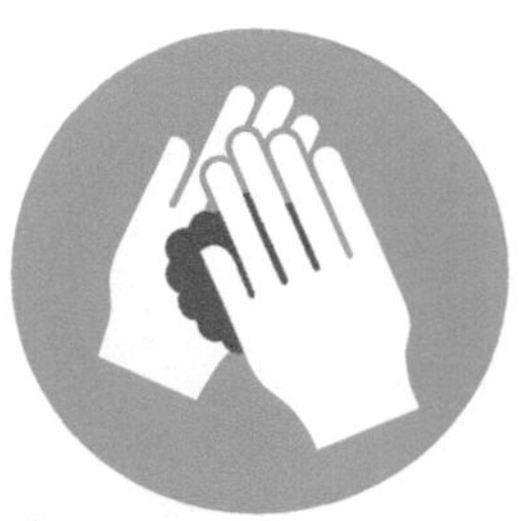

BRIEF CONTENTS

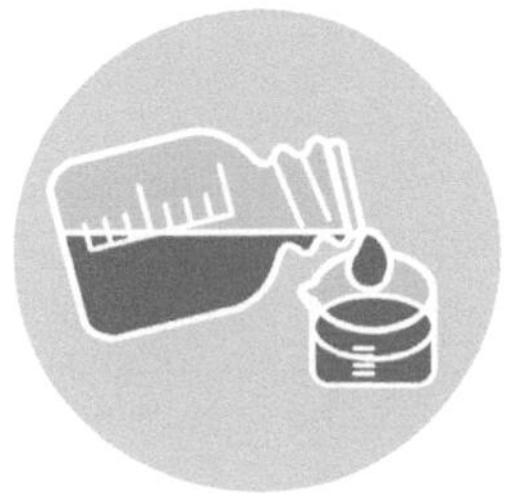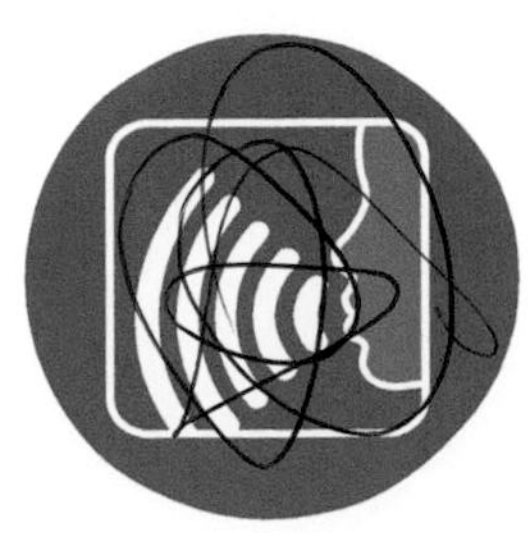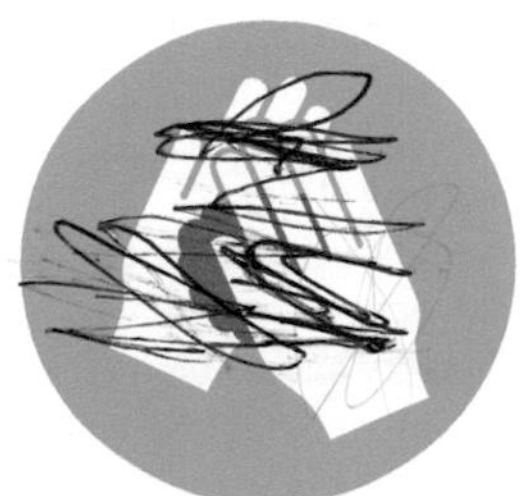

CONTENTS

SUPPORTING RESOURCES

Visit the *Fundamentals of Nursing*, Second Edition **MyNursingKit** at **www.pearsoned.co.uk/kozier** to find valuable online resources.

Companion Website for students

- Diagnostic Tests to confirm your understanding
- Interactive Scenario Simulations allowing you to practise skills safely and to confirm your knowledge and abilities
- Skills Videos
- An integrated customisable eText
- Useful Websites for further research
- Additional Short Answer Case Studies
- Flashcards to test your knowledge
- A fully searchable glossary

For instructors

- MyTest assessment testbank of questions
- PowerPoint slides of the key diagrams from the text

Also: MyNursingKit provides the following features:

- Search tool to help locate specific items of content
- E-mail results and profile tools to send results of quizzes to instructors
- Online help and support to assist with website usage and troubleshooting

For more information please contact your local Pearson Education sales representative or visit **www.pearsoned.co.uk/Kozier**

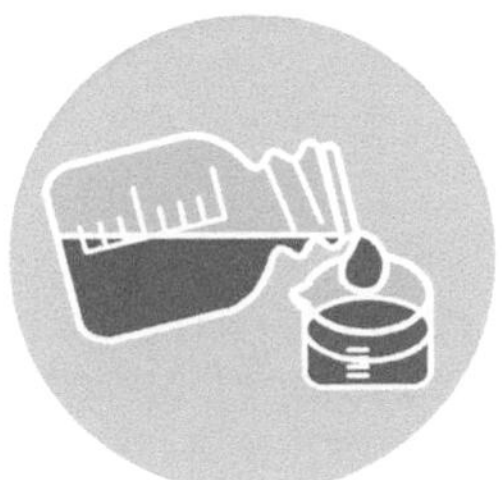
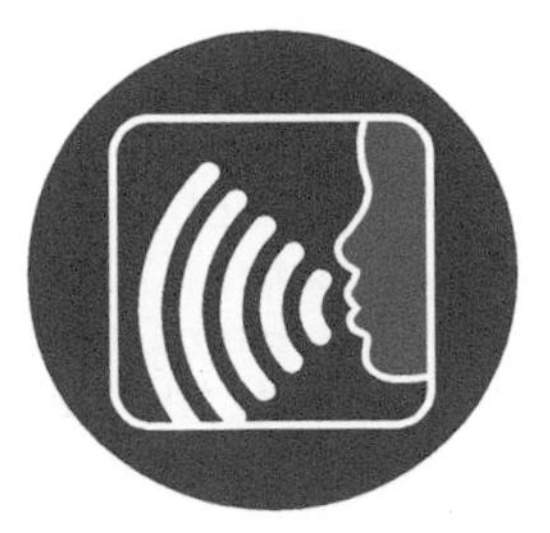
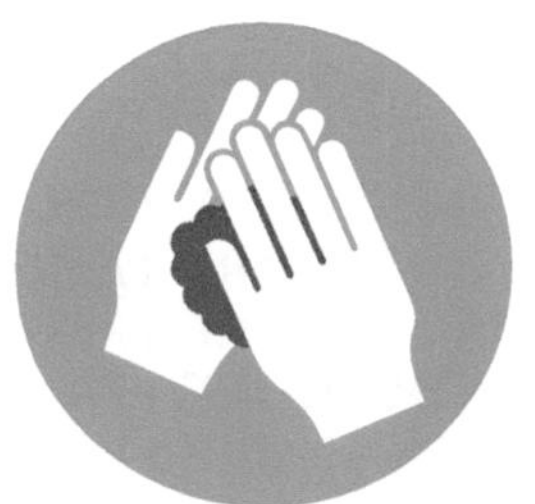

LIST OF PROCEDURES

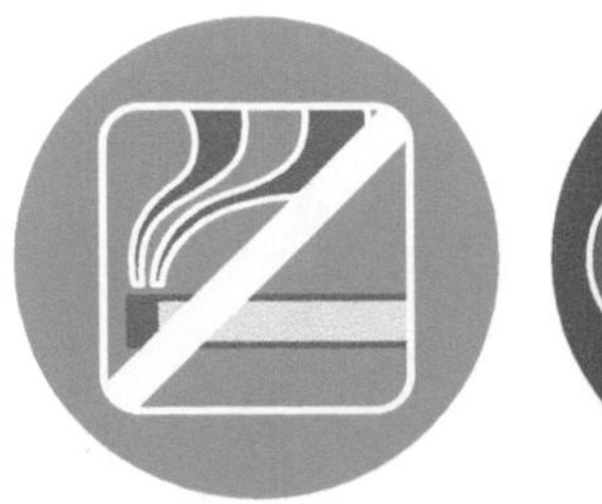
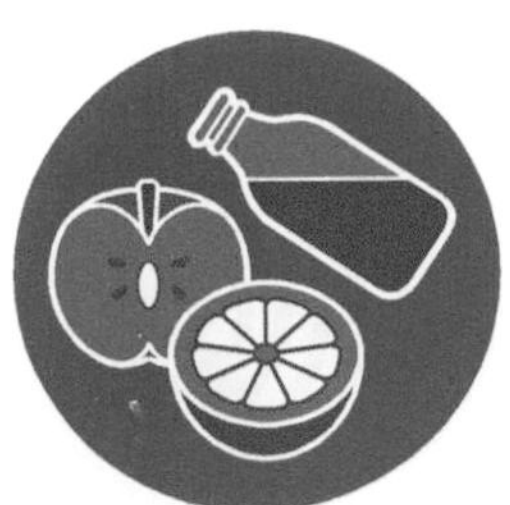
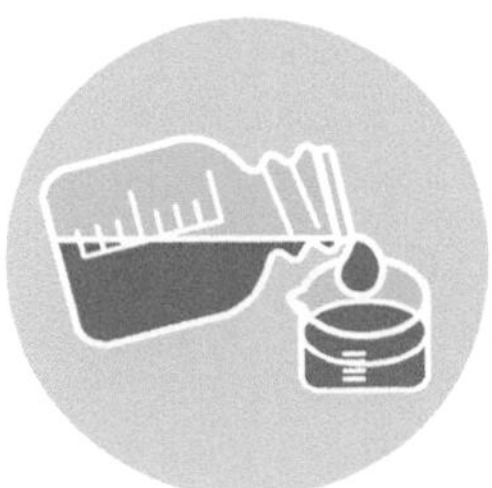
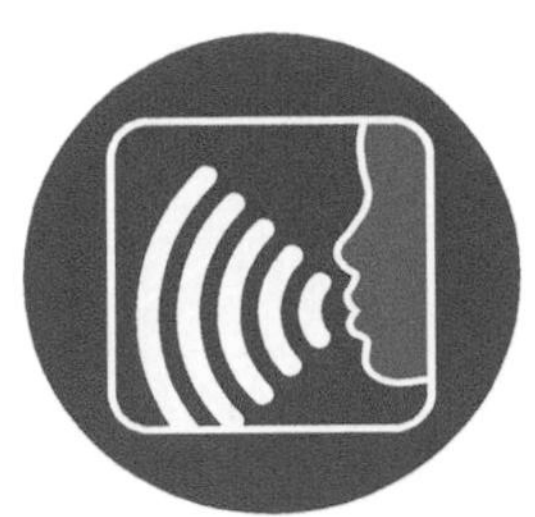
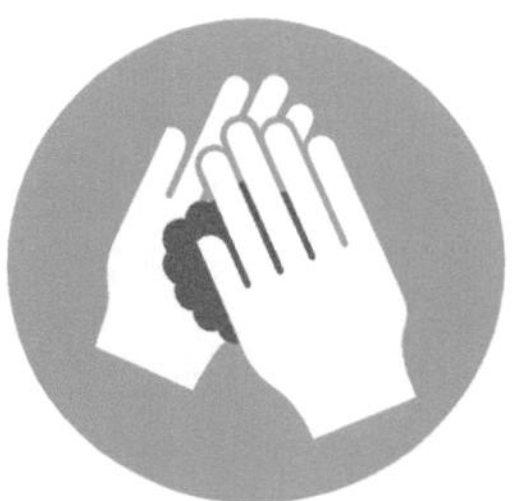

PREFACE

INTRODUCTION

Nursing is a difficult concept to define despite the fact that thousands of people experience nursing in some shape or form. We all know it's important, yet it's a concept that is often misunderstood. However, according to the Royal College of Nursing (RCN, 2003) the *purpose* of nursing is easier to define and the RCN identifies six key purposes: 'to promote and maintain health, to care for people when their health is compromised, to assist recovery, to facilitate independence, to meet needs and to improve/maintain well-being/quality of life'.

However you define nursing, it involves a number of key components; evidence-based decision making, competent clinical skills, efficient management, teaching, effective use of advancing technology and effective interpersonal skills, but ultimately it involves working with individuals, groups and families to improve the quality of life. All of which will be discussed in this book.

THE AIM OF THIS BOOK

The aim of this book is to explore the underpinning knowledge required to care for an individual whether they are an adult or child, have physical or mental health problems, or learning disabilities.

The text aims to be:

- *Current and evidence-based*: up-to-date references have been used to support current nursing practices.
- *Comprehensive* in its coverage of the significant concepts within nursing.
- *Practical and clinically based*: clinical procedures are clearly explained using step-by-step guides with illustrations.
- *European* in the examples used.

WHO SHOULD USE THIS BOOK?

This book has been designed as a study guide to support adult, child, learning disability and mental health student nurses at undergraduate level. However, students on other programmes such as Access to Health and Social Care may also find this book useful. The book has been written in line with the current *Standards for pre-registration nurse education* (NMC, 2010) and the Essential Skills Clusters (NMC, 2010).

NEW FOR THIS EDITION

Although we have aimed to stay true to the first edition of this book, a number of changes have been made.

- The book has been visually redesigned to emphasise key features.
- All chapters have been completely updated to match current standards and codes of practice.
- Each chapter begins with a case study and links with the critical reflection at the end of the chapter.
- There are new pedagogical features such as learning activities and a comprehensive Glossary.

Further chapters have been added in line with the latest *Standards for pre-registration nurse education* (NMC, 2010) and new child health and learning disabilities chapters are now included. Finally, we have developed a supporting website called **MyNursingKit**. This resource is designed to diagnose your knowledge and understanding of the subject and present further activities and support in an engaging and interactive manner.

References

NMC (2010) *Standards for pre-registration nurse education*, London: Nursing and Midwifery Council.

RCN (2003) *Defining nursing*, London: Royal College of Nursing.

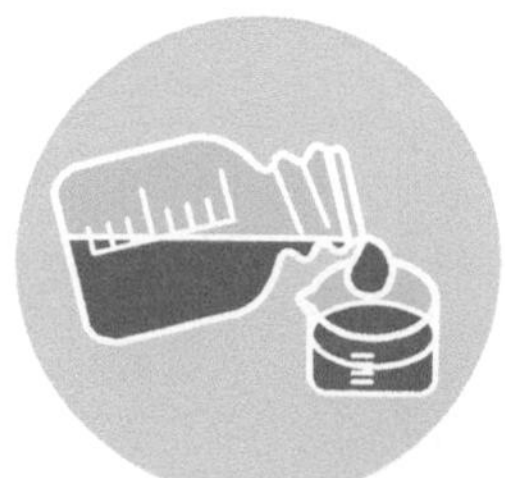
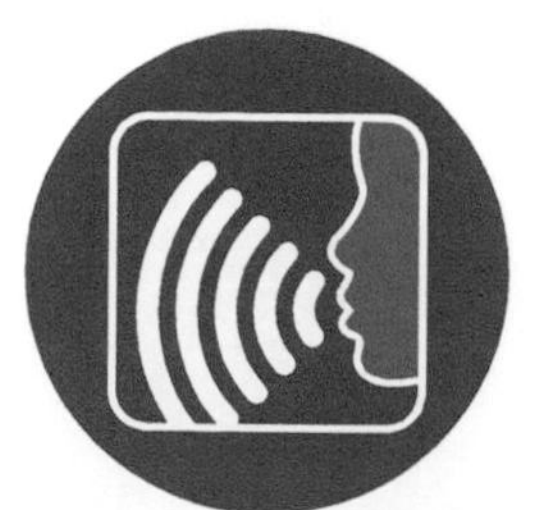
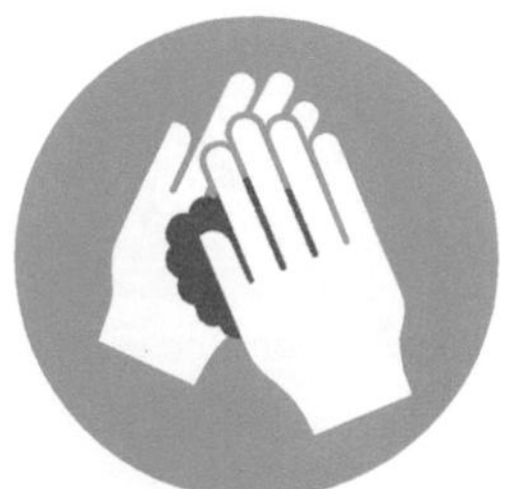

GUIDED TOUR OF THE BOOK

LEARNING OUTCOMES

After completing this chapter, you will be able to:

- Identify types and categories of pain according to location, aetiology and duration.
- Differentiate pain threshold from pain tolerance.
- Describe the four processes involved in nociception and how pain interventions can work during each process.
- Outline the gate control theory and its application to nursing care.
- Identify subjective and objective data to collect and analyse when assessing pain.
- Identify barriers to effective pain management.
- Describe pharmacological interventions for pain.
- Describe the World Health Organization's ladder step approach to cancer pain.
- Identify rationales for using various analgesic delivery routes.

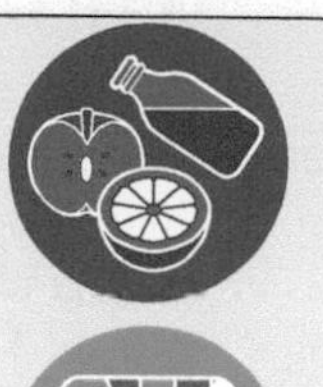

Learning Outcomes – set your objectives when reading the chapter.

Essential Skills Clusters – Links to the appropriate Essential Skills Clusters within the latest NMC standards are included at the start of each chapter.

After reading this chapter you will be able to reflect on the nursing role in providing healthcare, the way care is organised and the ethical and moral issues to be considered when providing care. It relates to Essential Skills Clusters (NMC, 2010) 1, 3, 4, 5, 6, 9, 10, 11, 18, 34, 35, 36. As appropriate for each progression point.

CASE STUDY

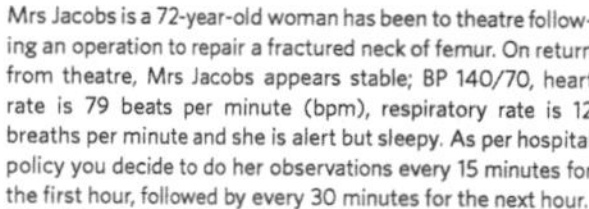

Mrs Jacobs is a 72-year-old woman has been to theatre following an operation to repair a fractured neck of femur. On return from theatre, Mrs Jacobs appears stable; BP 140/70, heart rate is 79 beats per minute (bpm), respiratory rate is 12 breaths per minute and she is alert but sleepy. As per hospital policy you decide to do her observations every 15 minutes for the first hour, followed by every 30 minutes for the next hour.

When you return to Mrs Jacobs to do her second set of observations you note that she is less responsive, only responding when you tell her to open her eyes, her BP is 100/70, heart rate is 115 bpm, and her respiratory rate is 22 breaths per minute. You decide to Fast bleep Mrs Jacobs' medical team. While you are waiting for the doctors to arrive you note that Mrs Jacobs becomes unresponsive.

Case Studies – can be used for your own personal reflection or group discussion. They are short, current, and illustrate the issues raised in the chapter. Hints and suggested answers are provided in the Critical Reflection feature at the end of each chapter.

Activities – can be used to help consolidate learning and further thinking. Suggested answers are provided at the end of each chapter.

ACTIVITY 17-1

Fred Bassett is an 82-year-old gentleman who lives alone. He has been a smoker for 60 years and has poor lower limb circulation. He visits the luncheon club once a week but needs the help of a carer as he has poor eyesight and mobility. His carer noticed that he was limping and, on questioning, she was advised that Fred had cut his toenails the previous evening and that, while he was unsure, he thought that he had cut too low and that his toenail bed had bled. Consider the care and reflect on the advice and support that a nurse would give Fred.

RESEARCH NOTE

Effects of Education and Experience on Nurses' Value of Ulcer Prevention

Using a qualitative research report, Samuriwo (2010) used the data from semi-structured interviews of 16 nurses in one NHS trust and university to determine the value that nurses place on pressure ulcer prevention. The findings of the study showed how the participants underwent a transition from placing low value on pressure ulcer prevention to high value based on their experience of caring for patients with pressure ulcers rather than the education they receive on pressure ulcer prevention. Caring for patients with pressure ulcers allowed the nurses to re-evaluate the care that they delivered.

From Samuriwo, R. (2010) Effects of education and experience on nurses' value of ulcer prevention, *British Journal of Nursing*, 19(20 supplement), S8–S18.

Research Notes – consider current research on a particular subject and serve as an illustration of research used in evidence-based practice.

Practice Guidelines - contain instant-access summaries of clinical dos and don'ts.

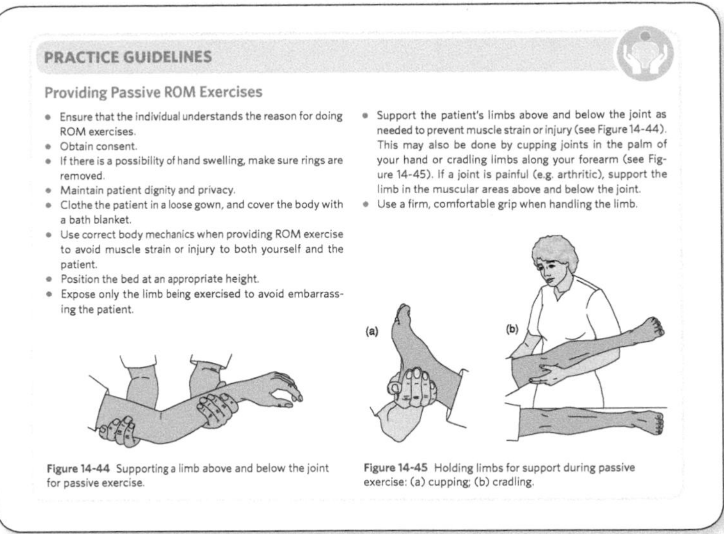

PRACTICE GUIDELINES

Providing Passive ROM Exercises

- Ensure that the individual understands the reason for doing ROM exercises.
- Obtain consent.
- If there is a possibility of hand swelling, make sure rings are removed.
- Maintain patient dignity and privacy.
- Clothe the patient in a loose gown, and cover the body with a bath blanket.
- Use correct body mechanics when providing ROM exercise to avoid muscle strain or injury to both yourself and the patient.
- Position the bed at an appropriate height.
- Expose only the limb being exercised to avoid embarrassing the patient.
- Support the patient's limbs above and below the joint as needed to prevent muscle strain or injury (see Figure 14-44). This may also be done by cupping joints in the palm of your hand or cradling limbs along your forearm (see Figure 14-45). If a joint is painful (e.g. arthritic), support the limb in the muscular areas above and below the joint.
- Use a firm, comfortable grip when handling the limb.

(a) (b)

Figure 14-44 Supporting a limb above and below the joint for passive exercise.

Figure 14-45 Holding limbs for support during passive exercise: (a) cupping; (b) cradling.

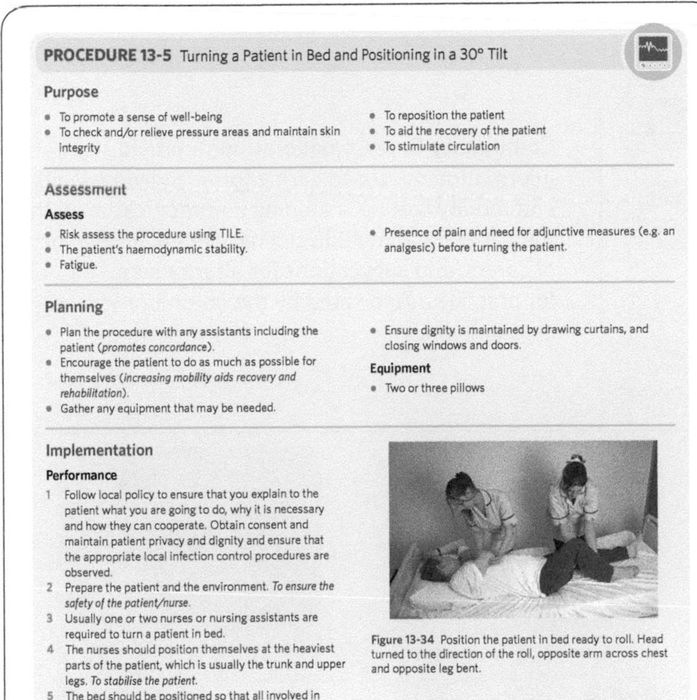

PROCEDURE 13-5 Turning a Patient in Bed and Positioning in a 30° Tilt

Purpose

- To promote a sense of well-being
- To check and/or relieve pressure areas and maintain skin integrity
- To reposition the patient
- To aid the recovery of the patient
- To stimulate circulation

Assessment

Assess

- Risk assess the procedure using TILE.
- The patient's haemodynamic stability.
- Fatigue.
- Presence of pain and need for adjunctive measures (e.g. an analgesic) before turning the patient.

Planning

- Plan the procedure with any assistants including the patient (*promotes concordance*).
- Encourage the patient to do as much as possible for themselves (*increasing mobility aids recovery and rehabilitation*).
- Gather any equipment that may be needed.
- Ensure dignity is maintained by drawing curtains, and closing windows and doors.

Equipment

- Two or three pillows

Implementation

Performance

1 Follow local policy to ensure that you explain to the patient what you are going to do, why it is necessary and how they can cooperate. Obtain consent and maintain patient privacy and dignity and ensure that the appropriate local infection control procedures are observed.
2 Prepare the patient and the environment. *To ensure the safety of the patient/nurse.*
3 Usually one or two nurses or nursing assistants are required to turn a patient in bed.
4 The nurses should position themselves at the heaviest parts of the patient, which is usually the trunk and upper legs. *To stabilise the patient.*
5 The bed should be positioned so that all involved in moving the patient are comfortable. *To promote safe working practices.*
6 Position the patient to aid moving (see Figure 13-34).
7 The nurse closest to the patient's head should place one hand on the patient's shoulder and one on their hip. While the other nurse should place one hand on the patient's hip and the other should be used to guide the legs over. No pressure should be applied to the knee joint as this can cause injury to the patient.

Figure 13-34 Position the patient in bed ready to roll. Head turned to the direction of the roll, opposite arm across chest and opposite leg bent.

8 When ready to move the patient the team leader should say 'Ready, steady, roll'. The nurses will then roll the patient. *To promote patient concordance.*
9 Once over on their side, pillows can be placed behind the patient and between the patient's knees. *To stabilise the patient.*
10 The patient should then be rested back onto the pillows.
11 The same process can be used for changing sheets and checking pressure areas.

Evaluation

- Note the patient's tolerance of the procedure (e.g. respiratory rate and effort, pulse rate, behaviour, cooperation).
- Document procedure and findings in the nursing notes.

Step-by-Step Procedures - are included in all clinical chapters. Clinical procedures are discussed using a step-by-step approach. Rationale is provided for aspects within the procedures based on current clinical evidence.

Clinical Alerts - are used in clinical chapters to highlight particular areas of practice that need to be taken into account when caring for an individual or group.

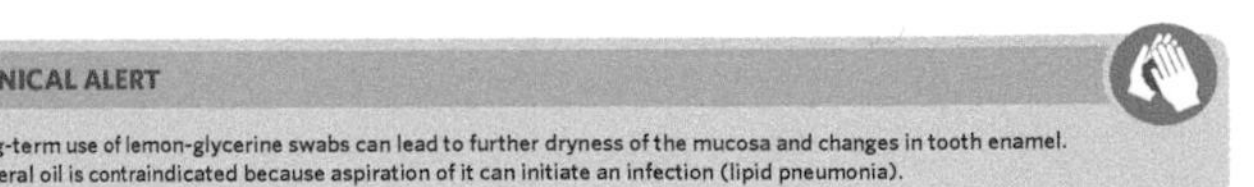

CLINICAL ALERT

Long-term use of lemon-glycerine swabs can lead to further dryness of the mucosa and changes in tooth enamel. Mineral oil is contraindicated because aspiration of it can initiate an infection (lipid pneumonia).

TEACHING: COMMUNITY CARE

Environmental Management

- Discuss injury-proofing the home to prevent the possibility of further tissue injury (e.g. use of padding, handrails, removal of hazards).
- Explore ways to control the environmental temperature and airflow (especially if the patient has an airborne pathogen).
- Determine the advisability of visitors and family members in proximity to the patient.
- Describe ways to manipulate the bed, the room and other household facilities.

Infection Control

- Teach proper hand washing and related hygienic measures to all family members.
- Discuss food hygiene and cleaning.
- Ensure access to and proper use of gloves and other

Infection Protection

- Teach the patient and family members the signs and symptoms of infection, and when to contact a healthcare provider.
- Teach the patient and family members how to avoid infections.
- Suggest techniques for safe food preservation and preparation.
- Emphasise the need for proper immunisations of all family members.

Wound Care (if appropriate)

- Teach the patient and family the signs of wound healing and of wound infection.
- Explain the proper technique for changing the dressing and disposing of the soiled one

Teaching Care - discuss particular issues relating to teaching individuals or groups.

LIFESPAN CONSIDERATIONS

Administering Otic Medications

Infants/Children

- Obtain assistance to ensure that the infant or young child doesn't make any sudden movements. This prevents accidental injury due to sudden movement during the procedure. The infant or child could sit in parent or carer's lap.
- For a child older than three, pull the pinna upward and backward similar to the procedure with an adult (see Figure 23-51). In infants and children under three, because the ear canal is directed upward and backward, the pinna should be pulled gently down and back (see Figure 23-53).

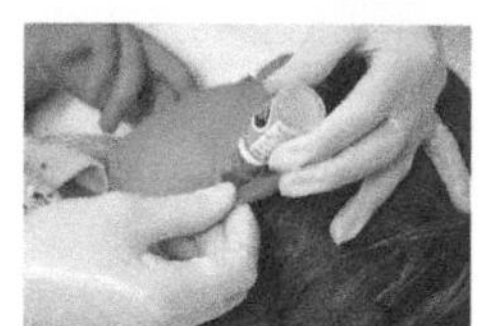

Figure 23-53 Straightening the ear canal of a child by pulling the pinna down and back.

Lifespan Considerations - highlight alternatives to practice when caring for infants, children and/or older adults.

COMMUNITY CARE CONSIDERATIONS

Hygiene

Patient and Environment

- *Self-care abilities for hygiene:* Assess the patient's ability to bathe, to manage the temperature of water and flow from taps, to dress and undress, to groom and to use the toilet.
- *Self-care aids required:* Determine if there is a need for a bath/shower seat (see Figure 17-1), a hand shower, a non-skid surface or mat in the bath or shower, hand bars on the sides of the bath (see Figure 17-2), or a raised toilet seat.
- *Facilities:* Check for the presence of laundry facilities and running water.
- *Mechanical barriers:* Note furniture obstructing access to the bathroom and toilet, or a doorway too narrow for a wheelchair.
- *Education needs:* Assess whether the caregiver needs instruction in how to assist the patient in and out of the bath, on and off the toilet, and so on.
- *Family role changes and coping:* Assess effects of patient's illness on financial status, parenting, spousal roles, sexuality and social roles.

Community

Explore resources that will provide assistance with bathing, laundry and foot care (e.g. home healthcare, podiatrist).

- Consult a social worker as needed to coordinate placement of a patient unable to remain in the home or to identify community resources that will help the patient stay in the home.

Community Care Considerations - provide information related to caring for an individual in the community setting, including communication with the patient and multidisciplinary team, involvement of carers, and suggestions for alternatives for practice as indicated by the community environment.

Photographs - bring the theory to life, showing you what you can expect to see in a clinical setting.

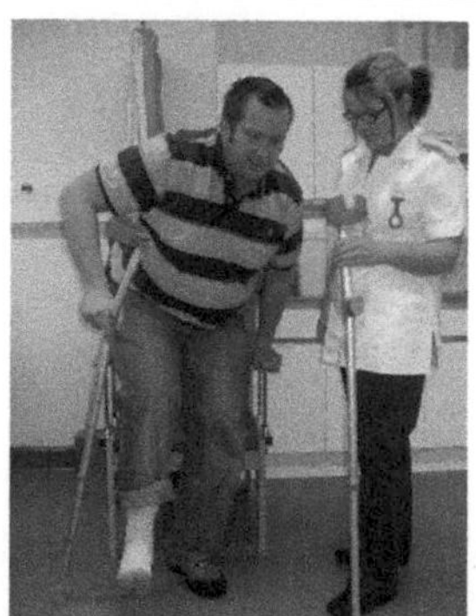

Figure 14-56 A patient using crutches getting into a chair.

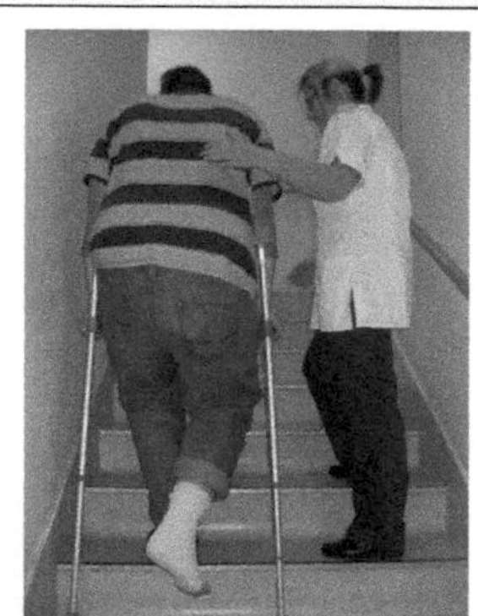

Figure 14-57 Climbing stairs: placing weight on the crutches while first moving the unaffected leg onto a step.

CRITICAL REFLECTION

There have been several opportunities within the chapter to reflect on some of the personal hygiene practices discussed within the chapter. The case study on page 493 highlights the difficulties of maintaining these standards when accidents happen that are life changing and impede on the individual's ability to maintain their own standards. Personal hygiene encompasses all areas that affect the individual in your care and, upon reflecting on this chapter and your experience in clinical practice, you should consider the issues raised within the chapter, explore, discuss and reflect on how your practice has changed in light of the information gained and how this would improve patient care, especially in relation to Joseph and his family. Points to consider are:

- Managing and organising care
- Caring and empathy
- Respect and dignity
- Physiological, psychological and psychosocial
- Communication
- Breathing
- Eating and drinking
- Personal hygiene
- Sleeping
- Sexuality
- Mobility
- Work and play
- Family support

Critical Reflections - are linked to the case study presented at the beginning of the chapter. They allow you to reflect on the case study and think more critically about the issues raised.

Assesment Interview - A practical feature that provides a detailed set of suitable questions for use when assessing patients.

ASSESSMENT INTERVIEW

Oxygenation

Current Respiratory Problems

- Have you noticed any changes in your breathing pattern (e.g. shortness of breath, difficulty in breathing, need to be in upright position to breathe, or rapid and shallow breathing)?
- If so, which of your activities might cause these symptom(s) to occur?
- How many pillows do you use to sleep at night?

History of Respiratory Disease

- Have you had colds, allergies, asthma, tuberculosis, bronchitis, pneumonia or emphysema?
- How frequently have these occurred? How long did they last? And how were they treated?

- Does the cough occur during certain activity or at certain times of the day?

Description of Sputum

- Do you produce any sputum?
- When is the sputum produced?
- What is the amount, colour, thickness, odour?
- Is it ever tinged with blood?

Presence of Chest Pain

- Do you experience any pain with breathing or activity?
- Where is the pain located?
- Describe the pain. How does it feel?
- Does it occur when you breathe in or out?

CHAPTER HIGHLIGHTS

- Surgery is a unique experience that creates stress that requires the patient to make necessary physical and psychological changes.
- There are three phases: pre-operative, intra-operative and post-operative.
- Surgical procedures are categorised by degree of urgency, purpose and degree of risk.
- Factors such as age, general health, nutritional status, medication use and mental status affect a patient's risk during surgery.
- Patients must agree to surgery and sign an informed consent.
- Pre-operative physical and psychological assessment can provide important information for planning pre-operative and post-operative care.
- The overall goal of nursing care during the pre-operative phase is to prepare the patient mentally and physically for surgery.
- Maintaining the patient's safety is the overall goal of nursing care during the intra-operative phase.
- Anaesthesia may be general or local.
- Positioning of the patient during surgery is important to reduce the risk of tissue and nerve damage.
- Immediate post-anaesthetic care focuses on assessment and monitoring parameters to prevent complications from anaesthesia or surgery.
- Initial and ongoing assessment of the post-operative patient includes level of consciousness, vital signs, oxygen saturation, skin colour and temperature, comfort, fluid balance, dressings, drains and tubes.
- The overall goals of nursing care during the post-operative period are to promote comfort and healing, restore the highest possible level of wellness, and prevent associated risks such as infection or respiratory and cardiovascular complications.

Chapter Highlights - summarise the main ideas discussed in the chapter. Ideal for reference and quick revision.

Activity Answers - Suggested answers and hints to the Activities spread throughout the chapter are included to help you confirm your understanding.

ACTIVITY ANSWERS

ACTIVITY 25-1 The patient's PAR score is 8. The correct course of action would be to fast bleep the patient's SHO/SpR and monitor the patient.

ACTIVITY 25-2 The ratio of compressions to ventilations is 30:2. Compressions should be performed at a rate of at least 100 per minute at a depth of 5–6cm. Inspiratory time of ventilations should be 1 second with enough volume given to produce normal chest rise. Ideally we would want to maintain a clear airway and allow for effective ventilations through tracheal intubation and use of a bag valve device.

ACTIVITY 25-3 Asystole does not require defibrillation as there is no electrical activity within the heart to organise. Therefore, the management of this patient would be CPR and trying to find out the cause of the arrest by going through the 4Hs and 4Ts. Adrenaline can be given every 3–5 minutes and electrolyte would be resolved by administering appropriate drugs, e.g. calcium.

REFERENCES

Brawley, E.C. (2002) 'Bathing environments: How to improve the bathing experience', *Alzheimer's Care Quarterly*, 3(1), 38–41.
British Contact Lens ...
Lomborg, K. and Kirkevold, M. (2005) 'Curtailing: Handling the complexity of body care in people hospitalized with severe ...

FURTHER RESOURCES

Essential Reading

Dimond, B. (2008) *Legal aspects of nursing* (5th edn), Harlow: Pearson.

Griffith, R. and Tengnah, C. (2010) *Legal and professional issues in nursing* (2nd edn), Exeter: Learning Matters.

Further Reading and Websites

To keep up to date with changes in health law the following is recommended:

www.bailii.org.uk: British and Irish Legal Information Institute, which provides free access to law reports from the UK courts.

www.dh.org.uk: outlines government policy on health in England.

www.dh.gov.uk: the Department of Health has good information on consent including model consent forms.

www.justice.gov.uk: the Ministry of Justice site gives detailed legal guidance on the Mental Capacity Act 2005.

Health Act 1999 Schedule 3 paragragh 8 available at www.statutelaw.gov.uk/content.aspx?...parentActiveTextDocId...activetextdocid

Nurses Midwives and Health Visitors Act 1997 at www.opsi.gov.uk/acts/acts1997/ukpga_19970024_en_1

Nursing and Midwifery Order 2001 www.opsi.gov.uk/si/si2002/20020253.htm

Data Protection Act 1998 (commencement no 2) Order 2008 available at www.legislation.gov.uk

References/Further Resources - are included to demonstrate the evidence base behind each chapter and to promote further study and research.

Glossary - A list of key terms and definitions, highlighted in the text, is included for quick reference.

GLOSSARY

Abduction The movement of a body part away from the midline.

Accountability The obligation of being answerable for one's actions and omissions.

Acetylcholine A *neurotransmitter* associated with attention, memory and sleep.

Acid Any chemical compound that, when dissolved in water, gives a solution with a hydrogen ion activity greater than in pure water, i.e. a pH less than 7.0.

Acidosis Abnormally high acidity (excess hydrogen-ion concentration) of the blood and other body tissues.

Acid-base balance The normal equilibrium between acids and alkalis within the body.

Anankastic Any behaviour relating to a compulsion. Generally refers to behaviours in OCD or when responding to voices in schizophrenia.

Anhedonia An inability to experience pleasure. A symptom of depression and one of the negative symptoms of schizophrenia.

Anorexia A physical disorder, resulting in inability to eat or a loss of appetite. Often confused with *anorexia nervosa*.

Anorexia Nervosa A psychological disorder characterised by an aversion to, or avoidance of, food.

Anoxia A condition in which tissues are severely or totally deprived of oxygen.

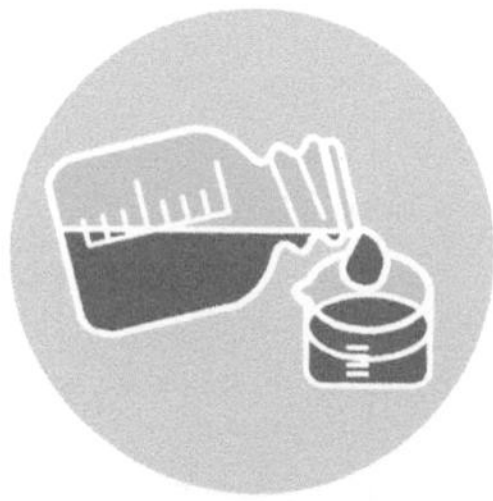
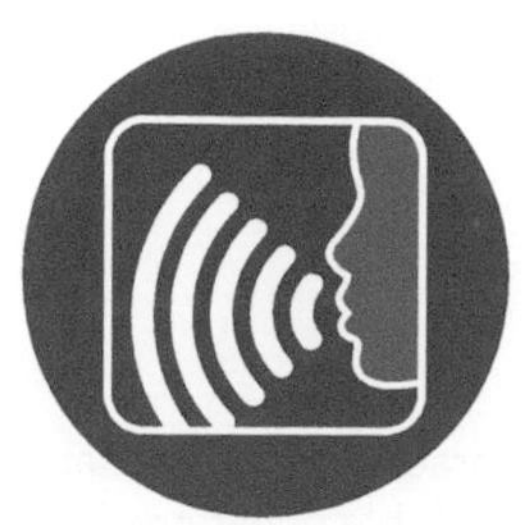
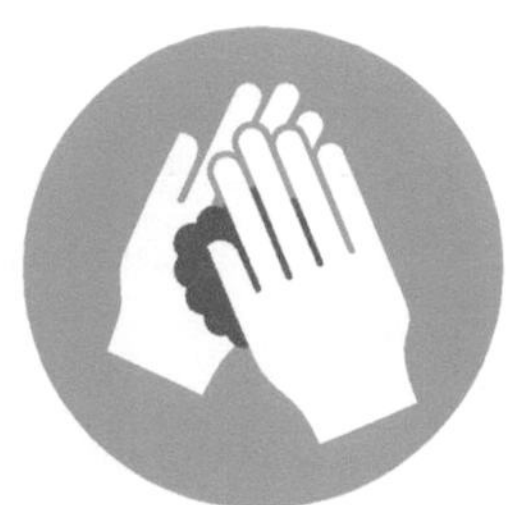

GUIDED TOUR OF PEARSON mynursingkit™

Diagnostic Tests - Self-test questions are included for each chapter so that you can assess your knowledge and understanding as you progress through your course. Review your test performance in the gradebook.

Home ▶ Student Resources ▶ Chapter 11: Infection control ▶ Pre Test

Pre-Test

Try the self-assessment questions below to test your knowledge of this chapter. Once you have completed the test, click on 'Submit Answers for Grading'

This activity contains 15 questions.

1. **What can health care workers do to prevent the transmission of infection?**

- ☐ Always use gloves
- ☐ Wash their hands after patient contact
- ☐ Wash their hands before patient contact
- ☐ Wear clean uniforms every day

2. **Some micro-organisms found in the human body are beneficial.**

- ○ True
- ○ False

Asepsis is the absence of ______ causing organisms.

David has just come into A&E and presented himself with breathing difficulties. You begin by asking him about his symptoms. Watch the video below and then decide what you should do next:

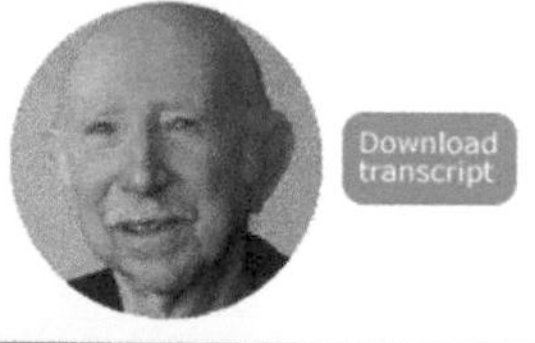

Download transcript

00:00 -02:21

Decide what you want to do next by choosing an option below:

- ☐ **Option 1:** You decide to consult David's notes.
- ☐ **Option 2:** You decide to listen to

Interactive Scenario Simulations - These realistic case studies allow you to practise skills safely in an interactive way. Make decisions and take courses of action just as you would in practice.

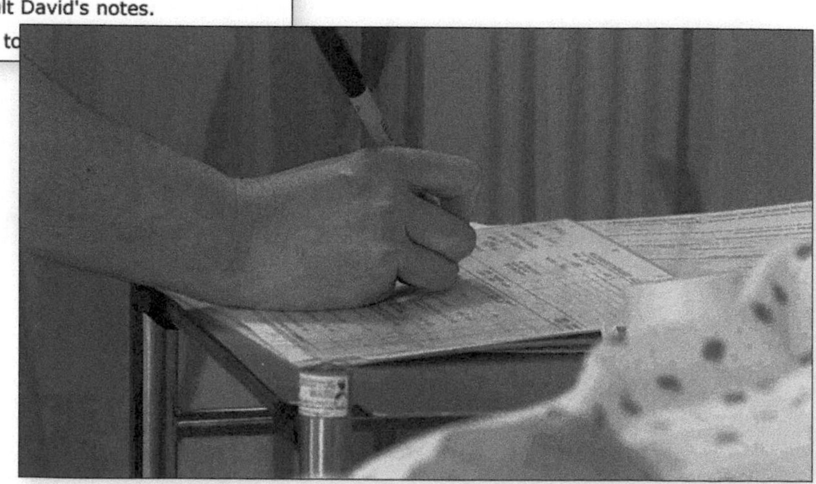

Skills Videos - Demonstration videos for core skills are included for review. Each is performed by experts in clinical skills teaching.

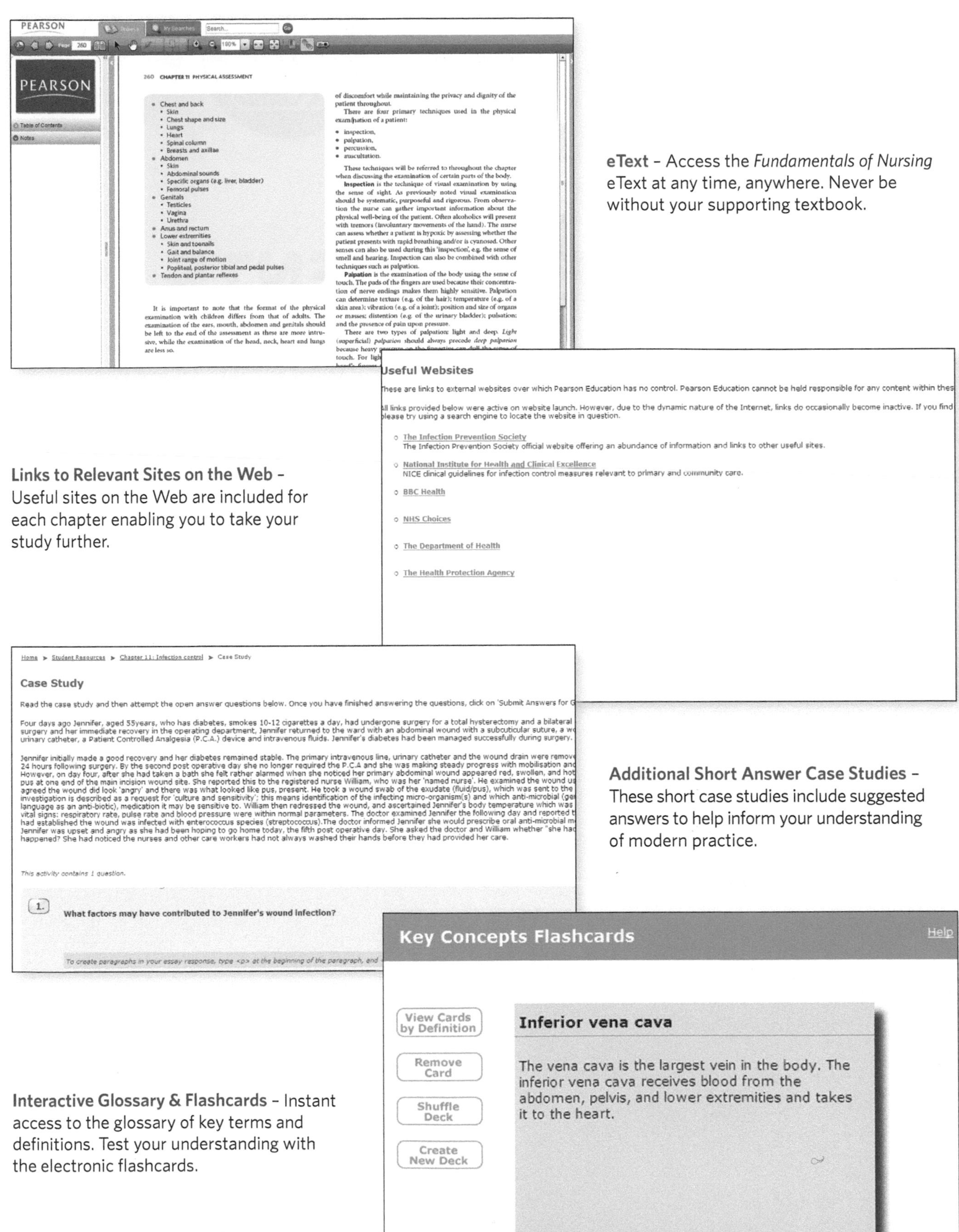
PEARSON
260 CHAPTER 11 PHYSICAL ASSESSMENT
Useful Websites
These are links to external websites over which Pearson Education has no control. Pearson Education cannot be held responsible for any content within thes
All links provided below were active on website launch. However, due to the dynamic nature of the Internet, links do occasionally become inactive. If you find
please try using a search engine to locate the website in question.
The Infection Prevention Society
The Infection Prevention Society official website offering an abundance of information and links to other useful sites.
National Institute for Health and Clinical Excellence
NICE clinical guidelines for infection control measures relevant to primary and community care.
BBC Health
NHS Choices
The Department of Health
The Health Protection Agency
Home ▸ Student Resources ▸ Chapter 11: Infection control ▸ Case Study
Case Study
This activity contains 1 question.
1. What factors may have contributed to Jennifer's wound infection?
Key Concepts Flashcards
Help
View Cards by Definition
Remove Card
Shuffle Deck
Create New Deck
Inferior vena cava
The vena cava is the largest vein in the body. The inferior vena cava receives blood from the abdomen, pelvis, and lower extremities and takes it to the heart.
Flip Card Over

eText - Access the *Fundamentals of Nursing* eText at any time, anywhere. Never be without your supporting textbook.

Links to Relevant Sites on the Web - Useful sites on the Web are included for each chapter enabling you to take your study further.

Additional Short Answer Case Studies - These short case studies include suggested answers to help inform your understanding of modern practice.

Interactive Glossary & Flashcards - Instant access to the glossary of key terms and definitions. Test your understanding with the electronic flashcards.

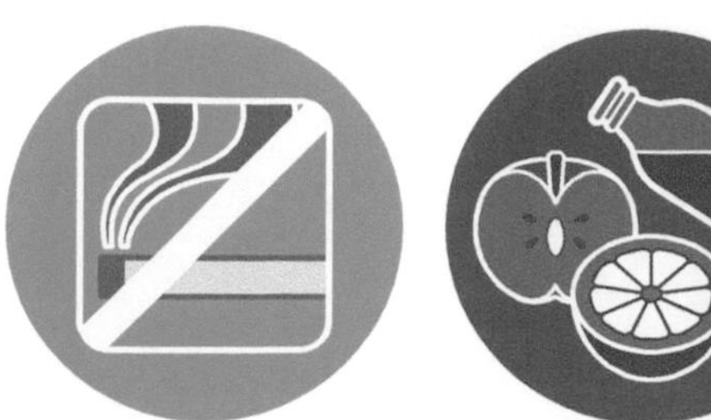
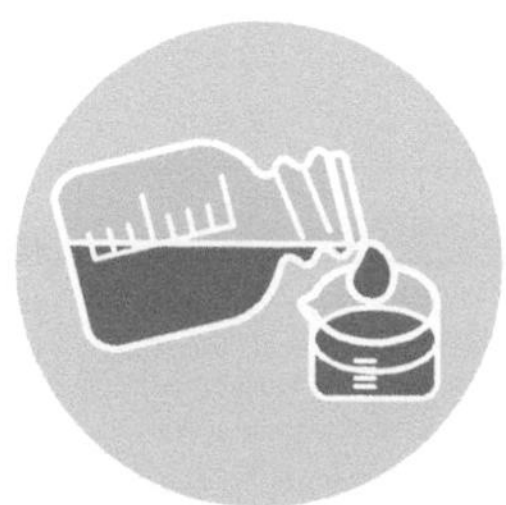
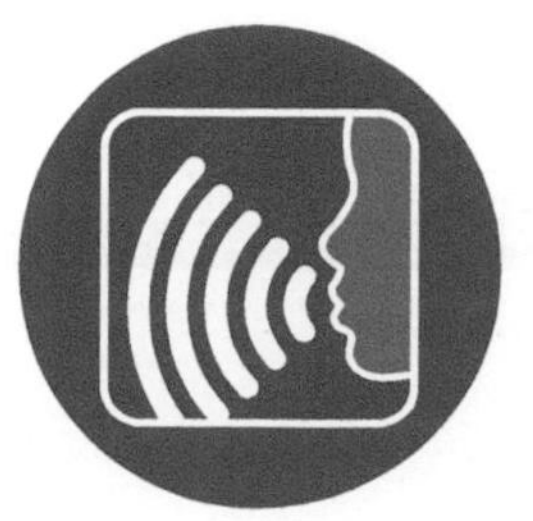
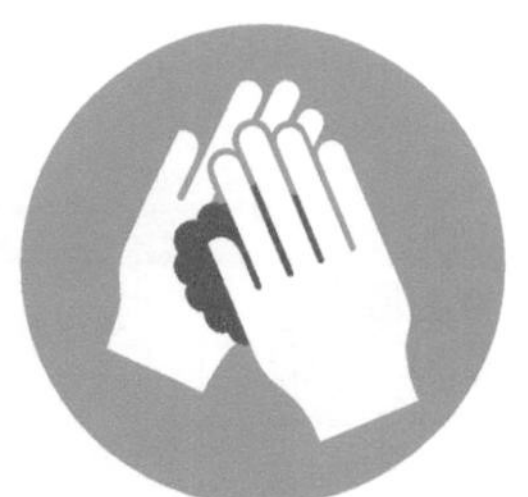

AUTHORS' ACKNOWLEDGEMENTS

Heulwen and Sharon would both like to thank Swansea University for their support and in particular Dr John Gammon.

Thanks also go to the authors who have contributed to this book:

- Chantal Patel – Legal Aspects of Nursing chapter
- Keith Bradley-Adams – Mental Health chapter
- Jill John, Sally Williams & Alyson Davies – Child Health chapter
- Emrys Jenkins – Learning Disability chapter
- Jonathan Hinkin – Infection Control chapter
- Christopher Goffin – Lecturer, Swansea University
- Professor Steve Edwards – Swansea University
- Lisa-Jayne Barson – Student Nurse
- Melanie-rae Conroy – Student Nurse
- Jason Hiorns – Student Nurse
- Cerys Jones – Student Nurse
- Ryan Lane – Student Nurse
- Kim Stockwell – Student Nurse

Without their hard work and expertise we would not have been able to produce such a comprehensive publication. We would also like to thank our families and friends for their support, patience and encouragement during the long process of developing this book.

Finally, we would like to thank the publishing team and review panel who helped us with the development of ideas in individual chapters. In particular we would like to thank:

- David Harrison
- Dawn Phillips
- Kelly Miller
- Rachael Muirhead
- Mel Beard
- Linda Dhondy
- Helen MacFadyen
- Sue Gard
- Sarah Beanland
- Paul Nash
- Alison Prior
- Lynette Miller

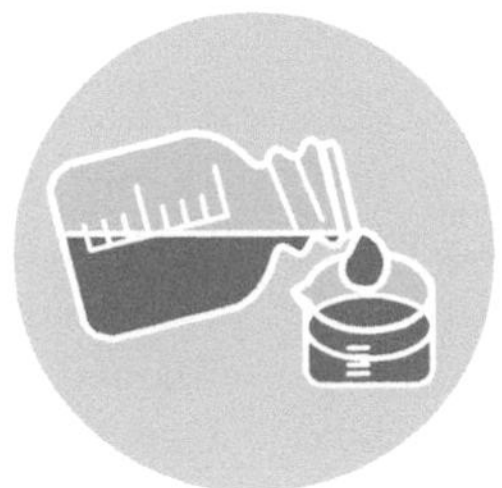
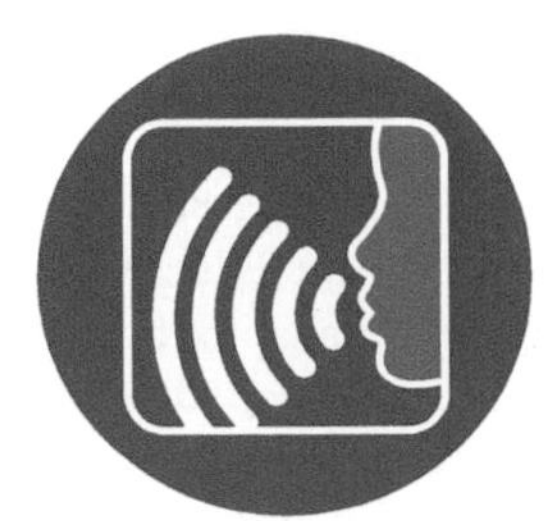
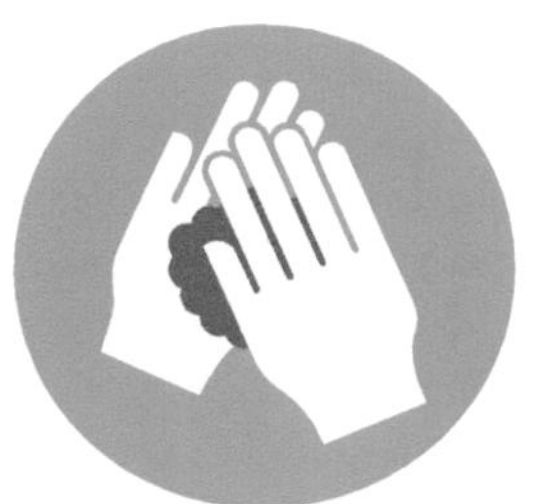

PUBLISHER'S ACKNOWLEDGEMENTS

We are grateful to the following for permission to reproduce copyright material:

Figures

Figures on page 32, page 33 adapted from *The ACP Guide to the Structure of the NHS in the UK*, Association of Clinical Pathologists (Galloway, M. 2009); Figure 2.1 from *Wellness: Concepts and Applications*, 6th ed., McGraw-Hill (Anspaugh, D.J., Hamrick, M.H. and Rosato, F.D. 2003) p. 4, reproduced by permission of The McGraw-Hill Companies, Inc; Figure 2.2 from Selected psychosocial models and correlates of individual health-related behaviours, *Medical Care*, 15 (5 Suppl.), pp. 24–46 (Becker, M.H. *et al.* 1977), Copyright © 1977, © Lippincott-Raven Publishers, with permission from Wolters Kluwer Health; Figure 2.3 adapted from *Community as Partner: Theory and Practice in Nursing*, 3rd ed., Lippincott, Williams and Wilkins (Anderson, E.T. and McFarlane, J. 2000) p. 166; Figure 3.1 from *Health Promotion: Models and Values*, 2nd ed. (Downie, R.S., Tannahill, C. and Tannahill, A. 1996) 'Tannahill's model of health promotion', Figure 4.1, p. 59, by permission of Oxford University Press; Figure 3.2 from Knowledge and control in health promotion: a test case for social policy and social theory, *The Sociology of Health Service*, edited by J. Gabe, M. Calnan and M. Bury (Beattie, A. 1994), pub. Routledge, with permission from Taylor & Francis Books (UK); Figure 3.3 from *Healthstyle: A Self-Test*, University of Florida, Institute of Food and Agricultural Science (UF/IFAS) (Bobroff, L.B. 1999) Retrieved 23 March 2003, from http://edis.ifas.ufl.edu/BODY_HE778. Copyright 1999 by UF/IFAS, reprinted with permission; Figure 3.4 adapted from A stage planning programme model for health education/health promotion practice, *Journal of Advanced Nursing*, 36(2), pp. 311–320 (Whitehead, D. 2001), with permission from John Wiley and Sons; Figures 7.3, 7.5 from NIH/Warren Grant Magnusen Clinical Center, National Institutes of Health; Figures 7.4, 24.6 Wong-Baker FACES Pain Rating Scale, from Hockenberry, M.J., Wilson, D., *Wong's essentials of pediatric nursing*, ed. 8, St. Louis, 2009, Mosby, Used with permission. Copyright Mosby; Figure 7.7 from Alison Twycross, Kingston University – St George's University of London; Figure 8.1 adapted from *Learning Disabilities* 3rd ed., Churchill Livingstone (Gates, B. 1997), Copyright Elsevier 1997; Figure 8.2 from *The Same as You? A review of services for people with learning disabilities* (Scottish Executive 2000) p. 9, http://www.scotland.gov.uk/Resource/Doc/1095/0078271.pdf, public sector information licensed under the Open Government Licence v1.0, http://www.nationalarchives.gov.uk/doc/open-government-licence/; Figure 8.6 from *Health Action Planning and Health Facilitation for people with learning disabilities: good practice guidance*, HMSO (HM Government 2009) p. 65, Crown Copyright material is reproduced with permission under the terms of the Click-Use Licence; Figures 9.2, 9.3 from *A Theory for Nursing: Systems, Concepts, Process*, Delmar (King, I.M. 1981), with permission from the author; Figure 10.2 from *Care Planning – a guide for nurses*, Pearson Education Ltd (Barrett, D. Wilson, B. and Woolands, A. 2008); Figures 13.1, 13.3, 13.6, 13.8, 13.9, 13.10, 13.11, 13.12, 13.13, 13.16, 13.18, 13.19, 13.20, 13.21, 13.25, 13.27, 13.28, 13.29, 13.30, 13.31, 13.32 from Manual handling illustrations © Edge Services (2006) reproduced by kind permission of EDGE Services – The Manual Handling Training Co. Ltd (01904 677853) sourced from People Handling & Risk Assessment Key Trainer's Certificate course materials; Figure 13.4 from Manual handling illustrations © Edge Services (2008) reproduced by kind permission of EDGE Services – The Manual Handling Training Co. Ltd (01904 677853) sourced from People Handling & Risk Assessment Key Trainer's Certificate course materials; Figure 13.7 from Manual handling illustrations © Edge Services (2010) reproduced by kind permission of EDGE Services – The Manual Handling Training Co. Ltd (01904 677853) sourced from People Handling & Risk Assessment Key Trainer's Certificate course materials. The views expressed in this text book, generally and with specific reference to manual handling, do not necessarily reflect the views, approach, company policies or course content of training programmes of EDGE Services – The Manual Handling Training Co. Ltd; Figure 13.15 from Health and Safety Executive, Crown Copyright material is reproduced with permission under the terms of the Click-Use License; Figure 14.51a courtesy of the Krames StayWell Company; Figure 15.1 adapted from *Fever and the Regulation of Body Temperatures*, Charles C. Thomas Publisher Ltd (BuBois, E.F. 1948); Figure 15.2 adapted from Elaine N. Marieb and Katje

Hoehn, *Human Anatomy & Physiology*, 8th Edition © 2010. Reprinted by permission of Pearson Education, Inc., Upper Saddle River, New Jersey; Figure 15.4 adapted from *MRHA04144: Thermometer Review: UK Market Survey 2005*, MRHA Evaluation Report (Crawford, D., Greene, N. and Wentworth, S. 2005) Figure 1, p. 3, Crown Copyright material is reproduced with permission under the terms of the Click-Use Licence; Figure 16.3 adapted by Clement Clarke for use with EN13826/EU scale peak flow meters – date of preparation 7 October 2004, with permission from Clement Clarke International Ltd; Figure 16.4 adapted by Clement Clarke for use with EU/EN13826 scale PEF meters only – date of preparation 7 October 2004, with permission from Clement Clarke International Ltd; Figure 18.3 from The Knoll scale of liability to pressure sores, *Guide to the practice of nursing*, St Louis: Mosby, pp. 83–86 (McFarlane, S. and Castledine, G., 1977), Copyright Elsevier 1977; Figure 19.1 from The eatwell plate, Department of Health in association with the Welsh Government, the Scottish Government and Food Standards Agency in Northern Ireland, © Crown copyright material is reproduced with the permission of the Controller of HMSO and Queen's Printer for Scotland; Figure 19.2 from *The 'MUST' Report – nutritional screening of adults: a multidisciplinary responsibility. Development and use of the 'Malnutrition Universal Screening Tool' (MUST) for Adults*, edited by Professor Marinos Elia, The Malnutrition Universal Screening Tool (MUST) is reproduced here with the kind permission of BAPEN (British Association of Parental and Enteral Nutrition); Figure 20.8 from *Essential Nursing Skills*, Mosby (Nicol, M. *et al.* 2000), Copyright Elsevier 2000; Figure 23.4 from sample medication administration record, Copyright © Chief Pharmacists in Wales; Figure 23.61 property of Trudell Medical International (TMI), used under permission from TMI; Figure 24.7 from *Cancer Pain Relief*, 2nd ed., World Health Organization (WHO 1996); Figure 25.3 from Royal Alexandra Hospital for Children; Figures 25.4, 25.11, 25.17 from *2010 Resuscitation Guidelines* (Nolan, J.P. (ed.) 2010) Copyright © Resuscitation Council (UK), Reproduced with the kind permission of the Resuscitation Council (UK).

Tables

Table 7.2 from Bee, Helen, L.; Boyd, Denise, A., *Developing Child, The, 11th © 2007.* Printed and Electronically reproduced by permission of Pearson Education, Inc., Upper Saddle River, New Jersey; Table 10.6 from *Nursing Diagnoses – Definitions and Classification 2009–2011.* Copyright © 2009, 1994–2009 by NANDA International. Used by arrangement with Blackwell Publishing Limited, a company of John Wiley & Sons, Inc; Table 16.3 from *The Royal Marsden Hospital Manual of Clinical Nursing Procedures*, 7th ed., Wiley-Blackwell (Dougherty, L. and Lister, S. 2008), with permission from John Wiley & Sons Ltd; Table 18.2 from *An Investigation of Geriatric Nursing Problems in Hospital*, Churchill Livingstone (Norton, D., McLaren, R. and Exton-Smith, A.N. 1975), Copyright 1975; Table 19.1 from Global Database on Body Mass Index – Table 1: The International Classification of adult underweight, overweight and obesity according to BMI http://apps.who.int/bmi/index.jsp?introPage=intro_3.html, World Health Organization; Table 20.2 adapted from *Nelson Textbook of Pediatrics*, Saunders (Behrman, R.E. 1992) p. 107; Table 24.8 from *Pain: Clinical Manual*, 2nd ed., Mosby (McCaffery, M. and Pasero, C. 1999), Copyright Elsevier 1999.

Text

Extracts on page 10, page 60, page 77, page 78, page 79 from *The Code: Standards for Conduct, Performance and Ethics for Nurses and Midwives*, Nursing and Midwifery Council (NMC) (NMC 2008); Box 3.1 from The social readjustment rating scale, *Journal of Psychosomatic Research*, 11(2), pp. 213–218 (Holmes, T.H. and Rahe, R.H. 1967), Copyright 1967, with permission from Elsevier; Box 5.1 from *ICN Code of Ethics for Nurses*, International Council of Nurses, 2006 Copyright © 2006 by the ICN – International Council of Nurses; Box on page 130 from Ten steps to successful breastfeeding – The Baby-Friendly Hospital Initiative, http://www.unicef.org/programme/breastfeeding/baby.htm#10, with permission from UNICEF, http://www.unicef.org/; Box 7.2 from *What to do if you're worried a child is being abused*, 19 May 2003 (Department of Health 2003) pp. 3–4, Crown Copyright material is reproduced with permission under the terms of the Click-Use Licence; Extract on page 244 from *Record Keeping: Guidance for nurses and midwives*, Nursing and Midwifery Council (NMC) (NMC 2009); Box 10.2 adapted from *Interviewing: Principles and Practices*, 10th ed., McGraw-Hill (Stewart, C.J. and Cash, Jr., W.B. 2002) pp. 55–60, reproduced by permission of The McGraw-Hill Companies, Inc; Box on pages 377–78 adapted from *Global Recommendations on Physical Activity for Health* (WHO 2010) pp. 17, 23, 29, © World Health Organization 2010, World Health Organization; Box on page 528 from The dos and don'ts of contact lens wear http://www.bcla.org.uk/en/consumers/consumer-guide-to-contact-lenses/the-dos-and-donts-of-contact-lens-wear.cfm, The British Contact Lens Association; Extract on page 528 from Definitions – Types of Ocular Prostheses (artificial eye), National Artificial Eye Service; Box on page 598 from Richard Hogston and Barbara Marjoram, *Foundations of Nursing Practice*, published 1999, Palgrave Macmillan, reproduced with permission of Palgrave Macmillan; Extract on page 742 from Undertreated pain: Could it land you in court?, *Nursing*, 32, 9, p. 18 (LaDuke, S. 2002), Copyright © 2002 Lippincott Williams, with permission from Wolters Kluwer Health; Box on page 761 from *Decisions relating to cardiopulmonary resuscitation: A joint statement from the British Medical Association, the Resuscitation Council (UK) and the Royal College of Nursing*, October (BMA 2007) p. 3, http://www.resus.org.uk/pages/dnar.pdf, British Medical Association; Extracts on pages 806–807, page 810 from *The Royal Marsden Hospital Manual of Clinical Nursing Procedures*, 7th ed., Wiley-Blackwell (Dougherty, L. and Lister, S. 2008), with permission from John Wiley & Sons Ltd.

Photographs

(Key: b-bottom; c-centre; l-left; r-right; t-top)

Page 3 Granada International: (tc). Rex Features: Everett Collection (tl). Page 4 Corbis: Bettmann (bl). Rex Features:

Nils Jorgensen (tr). 7 Mediscan: (tc); Gregory Hale (c). Science Photo Library Ltd: John Cole (cl); James King-Holmes (cr). Wellcome Library, London: (tl). Page 9 Wellcome Library, London: Anne-Katrine Purkiss. Page 260 Pearson Education Ltd. Page 261 Pearson Education Ltd. Page 263 Marsden Weighing Machine Group Ltd: (b). SECA ltd. UK Medical Scales and Weighing Systems: (t). Page 265 American Academy of Dermatology. 292 Pearson Education Ltd. 293 Pearson Education Ltd. Page 301 Pearson Education Ltd. Page 303 Pearson Education Ltd. Page 305 Pearson Education Ltd. Page 330 Pearson Education Ltd. Page 331 Pearson Education Ltd. Page 333 Pearson Education Ltd. Page 353 MEDesign Ltd: (bl). Mediscan: Dumas (br). Phil-e-slide patient handling system, Ergo Ike Ltd. www.phil-e-slide-uk.com: (tr). Page 355 Mediscan: Dumas (br); Dumas (bl). Page 360 Mediscan: Dumas. Page 362 Phil-e-slide patient handling system, Ergo Ike Ltd. www.phil-e-slide-uk.com. Page 363 MEDesign Ltd. Mediscan: Dumas (br). Page 364 Mediscan: Dumas. Page 365 ARJO MED AB Ltd: (bl). Hoist and Shower Chair Company Ltd: (br). Page 395 ARJO MED AB Ltd. Page 397 Pearson Education Ltd. Page 398 Patterson Medical Ltd: (tc). Page 401 Heulwen Morgan-Samuel: (tl). Page 402 Heulwen Morgan-Samuel. Page 421 Alamy Images: D Hurst (tr). Pearson Education Ltd. Simon Evans/Photographers Direct: (bl). Page 422 Alamy Images: F1online digitale Bildagentur GmbH (tr). Art Directors and TRIP Photo Library: 10589175 (tl). Page 424 Corbis: Radius Images (tr). Elena Dorfmann: (bl). Jenny Thomas: (br). Science Photo Library Ltd: Godong (tl). Page 427 Pearson Education Ltd. Page 429 Pearson Education Ltd. Page 431 Elena Dorfmann. Barts and The London NHS Trust: (tr). Page 440 Pearson Education Ltd. Page 441 Pearson Education Ltd. Page 446 Pearson Education Ltd. Page 447 Jenny Thomas. Nonin Medical Inc: (tr). Page 463 Science Photo Library Ltd: Coneyl Jay. Page 467 Pearson Education Ltd. Page 469 Heulwen Morgan-Samuel. Pearson Education Ltd. Shutterstock.com: Rob Byron (tr). Page 470 Air Products and Chemicals 2007. Elena Dorfmann. Jenny Thomas. Page 471 Jenny Thomas. Page 473 Jenny Thomas. Page 474 Air Products and Chemicals 2007: (l). Page 476 Smiths Medical International: (tr). Page 479 Elena Dorfmann. Page 480 Elena Dorfmann. Jenny Thomas. Page 483 Jenny Thomas. Page 484 Jenny Thomas. Page 486 Jenny Thomas. Page 488 Wellcome Library, London. Page 498 Patterson Medical Ltd. Page 500 Pearson Education Ltd. Page 501 Pearson Education Ltd. Page 502 Pearson Education Ltd. Page 517 Pearson Education Ltd. Page 523 Jenny Thomas. Page 524 Jenny Thomas. Page 527 (l) Science Photo Library Ltd: David Parker (l). Fotolia.com/Corbis: (r). Page 533 Pearson Education Ltd. Page 534 Pearson Education Ltd. Page 535 Pearson Education Ltd. Page 536 Pearson Education Ltd. Page 537 Pearson Education Ltd. Page 539 Pearson Education Ltd. Page 549 EASE: (tr). Hill-Rom Services Inc: (cr). KCI Licensing Inc (Therapulse): (br). Page 554 Wolters Kluwer Health Medical Research. Page 563 Jenny Thomas. Page 566 Elena Dorfmann. Page 583 Pearson Education Ltd. Page 586 Pearson Education Ltd. Page 587 Pearson Education Ltd. Page 590 Pearson Education Ltd. Page 696 Science Photo Library Ltd: Saturn Stills. Page 698 Pearson Education Ltd. Page 699 Pearson Education Ltd. Page 701 Pearson Education Ltd. Page 702 Pearson Education Ltd. Page 705 Pearson Education Ltd. Page 710 Pearson Education Ltd. Page 717 Pearson Education Ltd. Page 718 Science Photo Library Ltd: Antonia Reeve. Page 722 Jenny Thomas. Page 723 Jenny Thomas. Page 724 Jenny Thomas. Page 725 Jenny Thomas. Page 726 Jenny Thomas. Page 731 Pearson Education Ltd. Science Photo Library Ltd: Mark Clarke (tl). Page 732 Pearson Education Ltd. Page 752 Pearson Education Ltd. Page 753 Jenny Thomas. Wellcome Library, London. Pages 763, 764, 765, 766 and 767 Reproduced with kind permission by Michael Scott and the Resuscitation Council (UK). Page 768 Science Photo Library Ltd: Adam Hart-Davis. Page 780 Homecraft Rolyan Ltd. Page 781 Elena Dorfmann. Page 782 Elena Dorfmann. Page 795 Jenny Thomas. Page 805 E M Clements Photography. Page 810 Science Photo Library Ltd: Faye Norman. Page 814 Science Photo Library Ltd: Peter Gardiner (t). Page 816 Science Photo Library Ltd: Scott Camazine (bl). Thinkstock: Hemera Technologies (br).

CHAPTER 1
HISTORICAL AND CURRENT NURSING PRACTICE

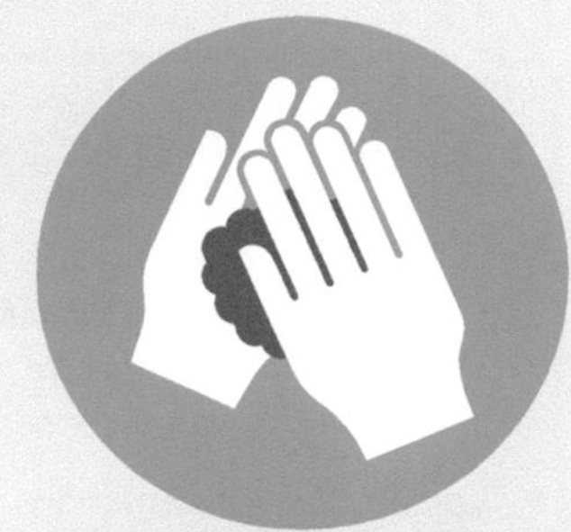

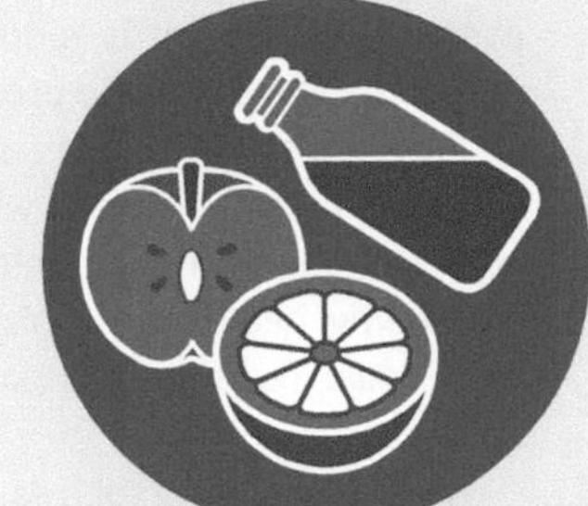

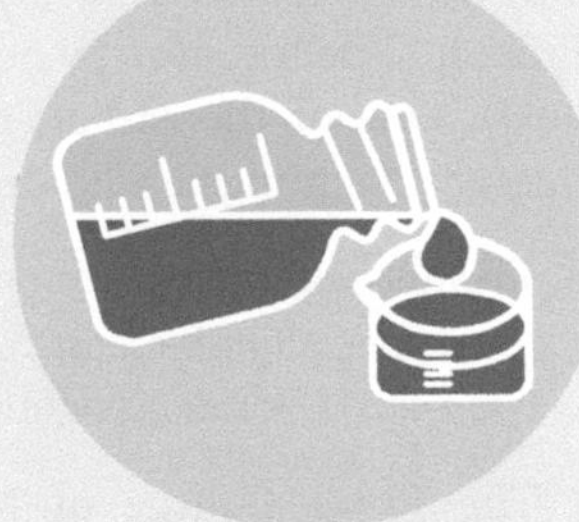

LEARNING OUTCOMES

After completing this chapter, you will be able to:

- Discuss historical and contemporary factors influencing the development of nursing.
- Identify the essential aspects of nursing.
- Identify the three main areas within the scope of nursing practice.
- Identify the potential settings for nursing practice.
- Discuss the organisation of nursing work.
- Describe the roles of nurses.
- Discuss the criteria of a profession.
- Describe factors that could influence current nursing practice.
- Discuss nurse education in the UK.
- Discuss the importance of research in nursing.

After reading this chapter you will be able to reflect on the nursing role in providing healthcare, the way care is organised and how nursing is classified as a profession. It relates to **Essential Skills Clusters (NMC, 2010) 1, 3, 4, 5, 7 and 12**, as appropriate for each progression point.

Ensure that you really understand this chapter by logging on to your complimentary **MyNursingKit** at **www.pearsoned.co.uk/kozier**. Complete the self-assessment tests to check your progress and utilise further activities to practise and confirm your understanding.

CASE STUDY

'After you clean up the patient in bed 4, would you mind giving Mr Rees his injection and make sure Mrs Watson has been prepped for theatre, and then go to pharmacy to pick up Mrs Smith's tablets for her to go home. Thanks.'

Typical? Well, instructions such as these echo through the corridors of hospitals. From bedpans to medicine rounds, one essential ingredient is required by the patient: care. But do nurses need a degree to provide care to patients?

A recent study by Allan and Smith (2009) found that there was a difference between what student nurses and registered nurses thought nursing entailed. Increasingly student nurses are seeing healthcare assistants (HCAs) delivering bedside care while registered nurses attend to the more technical tasks.

Media headlines such as nurses are 'too posh to wash' and 'too clever to care', compounded by the recent announcement that nursing is to become a graduate profession, led the Royal College of Nursing (RCN) Congress in 2004 to broach the idea that the caring component of nursing should be devolved to healthcare assistants so that nurses could concentrate on treatment and more technical tasks. However, an overwhelming 95% of nurses who voted in the Congress agreed that the caring role should not be delegated in this way.

Nursing does involve the 'basics' or 'fundamentals' of care but this should not be seen as a negative. Imagine caring for a person who is unable to care for their most basic human needs such as going to the toilet. Imagine the humiliation that person would feel having to rely on you to meet those needs. Some may say that this is unskilled work but nurses may miss important and subtle clues that can aid in the treatment and diagnosis of the patient if they fail to engage in fundamental nursing care. Indeed the Nursing and Midwifery Council (NMC, 2007) Essential Skills Clusters for Pre-registration Nursing Programme clearly states that nurses have a duty to provide care that is based on the highest standards, knowledge and competence. Nursing is more than the task itself, it is about holistically assessing and caring for the patient, which requires skill and professionalism.

INTRODUCTION

Nursing is said to 'touch' lives wherever they are lived (Mortimer and McGann, 2005). Despite this, nursing practice is difficult to define, even by nurses themselves (Finfgeld-Connett 2008). One of the earliest definitions of nursing came from Florence Nightingale who described nursing as:

> *Taking charge of the personal 'health' of individuals and to 'put' the individual in the best possible state and 'allow nature to act upon him'.* (Florence Nightingale (1859) cited in Meleis, 2006)

The Royal College of Nursing (RCN) (2003), however, defines the nurse as an 'enabler', bringing in the notion that patients have a role in caring for themselves.

> *Nursing is the use of clinical judgement in the provision of care to enable people to improve, maintain, or recover health, to cope with health problems, and to achieve the best possible quality of life, whatever their disease or disability, until death.* (RCN, 2003)

This chapter will explore historical and current nursing practice, considering the public's perception of nursing, nursing's professional status and the factors that influence nursing practice.

ACTIVITY 1-1

How would you define nursing? What are the characteristics of a good nurse?

PERCEPTION OF NURSING

Battleaxe, bimbo or angel, is this how the public perceives nurses? Well, according to a Mori Poll commissioned by the RCN in 1984, this was indeed how the public perceived nurses, with one in ten people (10%) seeing nurses as having sex appeal (Payne, 2000). However, a similar poll in 1999 showed that this perception of nurses has changed with only 6% of the public viewing nurses as having sex appeal (Payne, 2000). Despite this fact, the poll also showed that in the public's eyes the most famous nurses were Florence Nightingale, the Crimean war nurse, Hattie Jacques' 'matron' character and Barbara Windsor's 'saucy' character, both from the *Carry On* films (see Figure 1-1).

More recently there have been concerns about nurses' attitudes and professionalism (Maben and Griffiths, 2008). Holstrom (2008) makes an important observation, 'when things are going well' nurses are seen as angels, however 'when things aren't going well the image goes downhill'. These negative images of nurses not only affect patients but also impact upon the recruitment of young people into the profession with only 2% of nurses on the register under the age of 25 (Holstrom, 2008).

Since Florence Nightingale's era nursing has been inextricably linked with the female gender and although the perception that to be a good nurse you must be female has lessened in the public's eyes (Payne, 2000), it is a perception that is hard to shake off particularly when you consider the famous nurses highlighted by the public in the 1999 RCN poll (Payne, 2000).

In order to uncover the origins of some of these stereotypes of nurses, we must delve into the history of nursing.

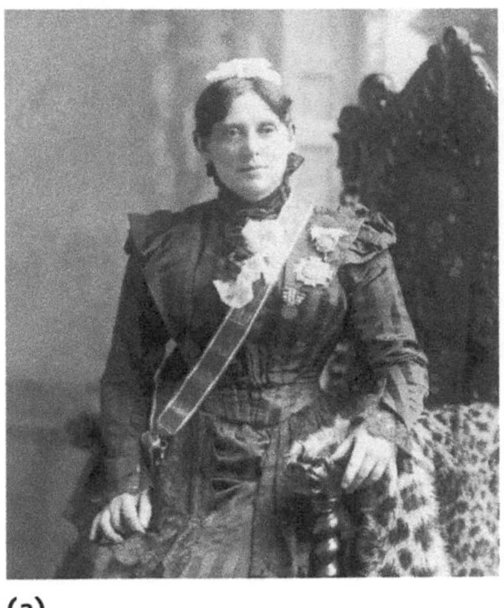
(a)

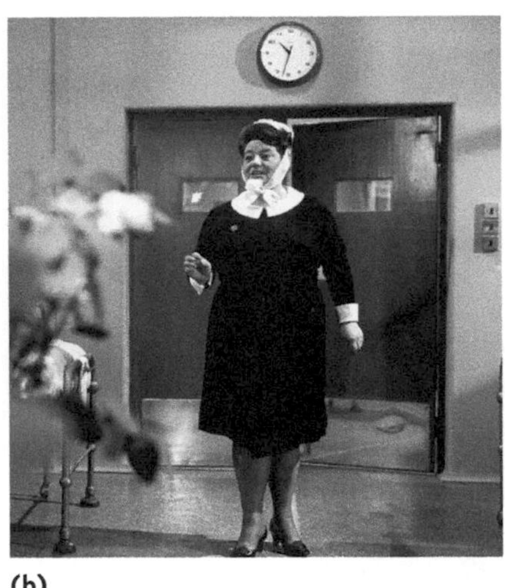
(b)

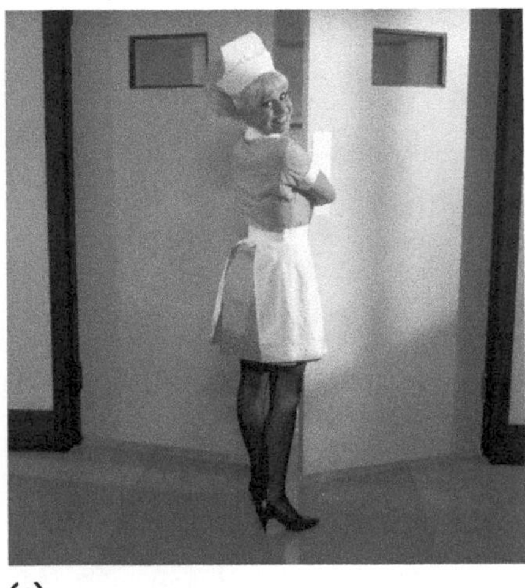
(c)

Figure 1-1 Public perception of nurses: (a) Florence Nightingale; (b) Hattie Jacques; (c) Barbara Windsor.
Source: (a) Rex Features; (b) and (c) Granada International.

ACTIVITY 1-2

What was your perception of nursing before entering the profession? What influenced this perception?

THE HISTORY OF NURSING

Until relatively recently, the history of nursing has had little attention from historians, despite its unique position in the history of healthcare and women (Mortimer and McGann, 2005). In fact, there is little written about nursing until the mid 19th century, when there was stark criticism of the nursing care provided to sick patients from physicians and philanthropists (Dingwall *et al.*, 1988).

The history of 'modern' nursing has been dominated by Florence Nightingale, although throughout history there is evidence of the existence of nursing. In fact the first written reference to nursing care can be found in the *Old Testament* where midwives cared for expectant mothers in their own homes. Other than this there are very few records of nursing pre-Christianity. However, it is interesting to note that medical history can be traced back over the past 6,000 years.

For centuries after the birth of Jesus Christ, the Roman Empire ruled most of Europe. During this time, physicians moved from being slaves to high-ranking Roman citizens, and nursing was finally considered as a vocation worthy of Roman ladies rather than female slaves.

It was also during this time that the first organised hospitals or *valetudinaria* were erected. These were built for Rome's most precious asset, its soldiers. Roman soldiers injured in battle needed to be placed somewhere where they could recover in readiness for their next battle as they were essential to the continuation of the Roman Empire.

In AD 335 Emperor Constantine ordered that Christianity be the official religion of the Roman Empire. It was during this time that some of the earliest nurses are recorded. Saint Helena, a British Princess and mother of Emperor Constantine, set up the first hospital in Jerusalem, while Fabiola, a high-ranking woman, gave up all her worldly goods in order to nurse. It seemed fashionable for high-ranking women within the Roman Empire to give up everything in order to nurse others. Indeed early religious values, such as self-denial, spiritual calling and devotion to duty and hard work, have dominated nursing throughout its history. Nurses' commitment to these values often resulted in exploitation and few monetary rewards. For some time, nurses themselves believed it was inappropriate to expect economic gain from their 'calling'.

It was probably during these early Roman times that nursing became a predominantly female vocation, possibly as a result of the nurturing and caring roles already undertaken by the women of the household. However, women were not always the sole providers of nursing care. For instance, during the Crusades several orders of knights were formed, including the Knights of Saint John of Jerusalem (also known as the Knights Hospitalers), the Teutonic Knights and the Knights of Saint Lazarus (see Figure 1-2), all of which provided nursing care to their sick and injured comrades. During these times, hospitals were built throughout Europe providing care to people with leprosy, syphilis and **chronic** skin conditions.

It appears that throughout history, war has played an important part in the development of the nurses' role. None more so than the Crimean War (1854–56), where British soldiers were dying from cholera and malaria soon after arriving in Turkey. The inadequacy of care given to soldiers led to a public outcry in Great Britain resulting in Florence Nightingale, a resident lady superintendent of a hospital for invalid women in London,

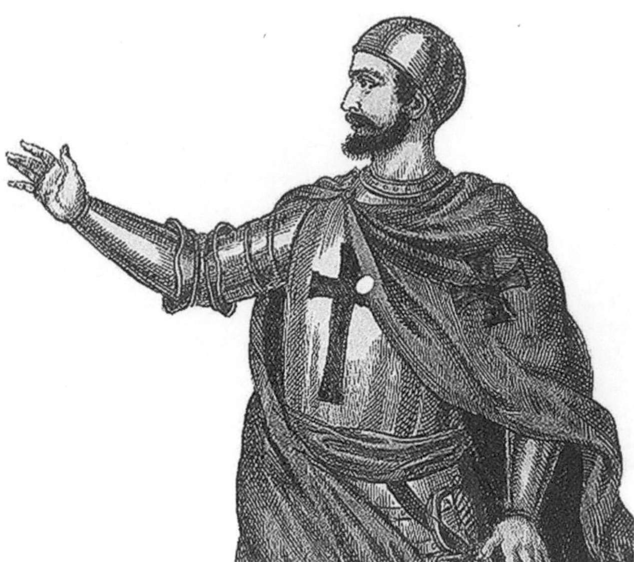

Figure 1-2 The Knights of Saint Lazarus.

volunteering her nursing services. The British government eventually gave permission for Florence Nightingale to take 38 nurses to Turkey in a bid to treat those soldiers suffering as a result of these two diseases (see Figure 1-3).

One other nurse, Jamaican-born Mary Seacole, also sought permission to care for the soldiers struck down by cholera and malaria in Turkey as she was incensed by the inadequacy of the care these soldiers were receiving (see Figure 1-4). However, she was refused permission on at least four occasions. Mary Seacole was shocked by this, believing that the decisions were based on racial discrimination. As a result she decided to travel to Turkey herself, and set up a British hotel at her own cost. Here she cared for and fed British soldiers often going into the battlefields to provide essential nursing care to those who needed it.

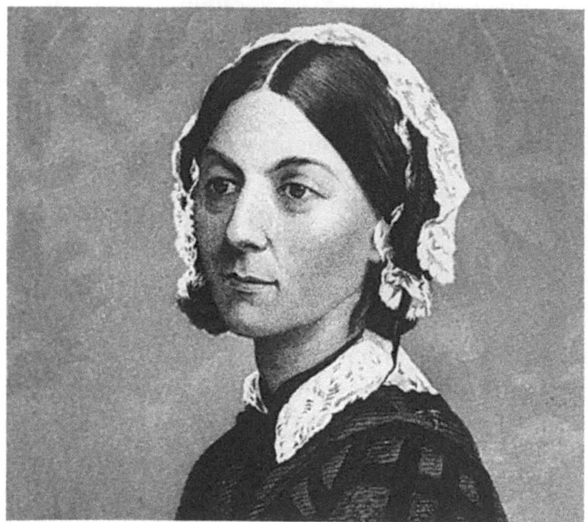

Figure 1-3 Florence Nightingale, founder of modern nursing
Source: Bettmann/CORBIS.

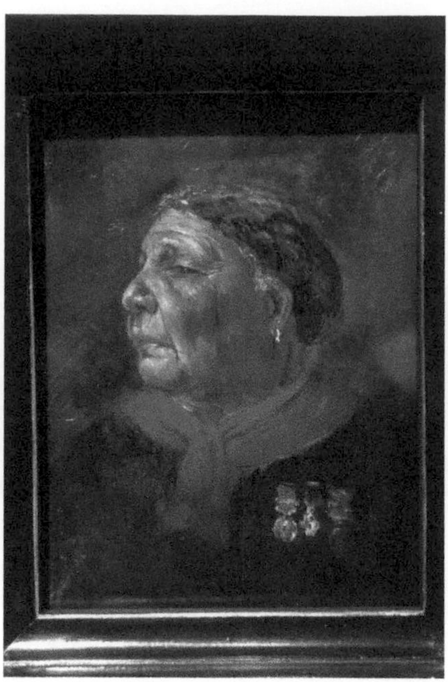

Figure 1-4 Mary Seacole.
Source: Rex Features.

After the Crimean War both Mary Seacole and Florence Nightingale arrived back in the UK as national heroines and were awarded several medals for their bravery during the war. Florence Nightingale's legacy led to a transformation in military hospitals by improving sanitation practices such as handwashing and also led to the establishment of the Nightingale Fund for the training of nurses, which continues today in the Florence Nightingale School of Nursing and Midwifery in King's College in London.

Florence was also instrumental in shaping the image of the nursing profession. Society now viewed nurses as *Guardian Angels* or *Angels of Mercy*. After Nightingale brought respectability to the nursing profession, nurses were viewed as noble, compassionate, moral, religious, dedicated and self-sacrificing; a view that encouraged middle-class women into the profession.

It is not only the Crimean War that led to the development of the nursing profession. During the First World War the Queen Alexandra's Imperial Military Nursing Services (QAIMNS) provided a 50,000-strong nursing workforce to the army. Many of these nurses worked near the front line in field hospitals' theatres. Again in the Second World War the QAIMNS were mobilised to provide nursing care at the front line under the charge of the Matron-in-Chief.

Following the Second World War the Army Medical Services, which included the QAIMNS, were reorganised and in 1949 the Queen Alexandra's Royal Army Nursing Corps was formed. Currently, military nurses from the Corps now serve on the front line across the world and also staff Ministry of Defence Hospital Units within the UK.

As a result of these wars the image of the nurse as heroine emerged. However, other perhaps more damaging perceptions of nurses have also emerged since the early 19th century. One such image is that of the *doctor's handmaiden*. This image evolved when women had yet to obtain the right to vote, when family structures were largely paternalistic and when the medical profession portrayed increasing use of scientific knowledge that, at that time, was viewed as a male domain.

Perceptions of nurses as 'angels' and 'handmaidens' linger to this day, however there is some evidence that society's views are changing. On the whole, the public see nurses as 'knowledgeable and skilled, yet . . . caring and compassionate' (Mullally, 2004: 17). However, Maben and Griffiths (2008) suggest that work is still needed to ensure nursing meets the challenges of the 21st century.

In order to continue improving the public's perception of nursing as a profession, the public needs to be made aware of nurses' current roles and responsibilities within healthcare. In order to do this we need to explore what current nursing practice involves.

CURRENT NURSING PRACTICE

'Nursing is not just one career; it is a set of careers linked by a belief in giving high quality care to patients' (Carter 2009). It is an ever-evolving profession offering new challenges to individuals embarking on this career pathway. There are many fields of practice within nursing covering a range of specialist care. However, four fields of nursing are offered to prospective students wanting to enter the profession: adult, mental health, child health and learning disability.

Adult Nursing

Adult nurses work with younger and older adults with both chronic and **acute** health conditions in a range of healthcare environments (see Chapter 2). Quality nursing care involves the use of a range of skills including caring, counselling, managing, teaching as well as practical and interpersonal skills. Adult nurses work at the centre of multidisciplinary teams alongside doctors, physiotherapists, dieticians, pharmacists and many others. Depending on the nurses' experience and education, adult nurses can hold positions at most levels of the NHS career framework.

Mental Health Nursing

It is thought that as many as one in three people suffer some form of mental health problem, most of which are cared for in the community. Mental health nursing is one of the most complex areas of nursing, as a key role and challenge is the formation of **therapeutic relationships** with the mentally ill patient and their family. Communication and interpersonal skills are key skills within mental health nursing. Like adult nurses, mental health nurses are at the centre of the multidisciplinary team working alongside general practitioners (GP), psychologists, social workers, psychiatrists and many others.

Child Health Nursing

Child health nurses care for children and young people in a range of healthcare settings (see Chapter 2). It involves not only caring for the child but also working in partnership with parents or guardians of that child. One of the challenges faced by children's nurses is communication. While adults are in the most part able to express what they feel and need, children may be unable to express in words what is needed. It is therefore up to the nurse to interpret behaviour intelligently. Like the other branches of nursing child health nurses are at the centre of the multidisciplinary team often working alongside doctors, hospital play staff, psychologists and social workers.

Learning Disability Nursing

Learning disability nurses care for individuals with a wide range of physical and mental health conditions. Learning disability nurses work in partnership with the individual with the learning disability, their family and carers. Learning disability nursing is usually provided in settings such as adult education, residential and community centres as well as patients' homes, workplaces and schools. Like the other branches of nursing, learning disability nurses work alongside a range of other professionals including psychologists, social workers, GPs and speech and language therapists.

THE CONCEPT OF CARING

At the core of each branch of nursing is the concept of care and caring (RCN, 2003; Barker and Buchanan-Barker, 2004). Care is a fundamental and important aspect of nursing, a point reiterated by the Nursing and Midwifery Council's essential skills clusters for student nurses (NMC, 2007). The RCN (2003) lists the defining characteristics of nursing as:

- caring
- an art
- a science
- patient centred
- holistic
- adaptive
- concerned with health education, health promotion and prevention of ill health
- evidence based.

Although it is claimed that nursing has lost its way in the 21st century with mixed views on the quality of nursing care, a report by Maben and Griffiths (2008) found that both patients and nurses considered quality nursing care to be at the centre of patient experience. Patients stated that they want to be valued and treated as human beings while nurses suggested that good nursing is 'how' not 'what'.

Quality nursing care is not only a priority for nurses and patients; it is at the core of the third and most ambitious phase of the government's 2001 NHS Plan. Lord Darzi (2008) set out his vision for this phase stating that the NHS should be clinically effective, personal and safe for all; a phase which focuses on quality at the heart of the NHS and gets 'the basics right every time'. According to Maben and Griffiths (2008) it is this phase that will pose nurses the biggest challenge, to re-affirm their role and aspire to be 'advocates, champions and guardians of quality' (2008: 11).

Although the challenges of the 21st century are clear for nursing practice, the focus of nursing care needs to remain on providing quality nursing care. In order to explore the concept of quality nursing care further it's vital to consider the recipients of nursing and the scope of nursing practice.

ACTIVITY 1-3

Reflect on what you consider to be quality nursing care.

Recipients of Nursing

The centrality of patient choice is a key concept within a modernised healthcare system (Barr *et al.*, 2008). Healthcare recipients are encouraged to become partners in their treatment and care. Patients now have 'choice'; choice of hospital at the point of GP referral (Barr *et al.*, 2008); choice of primary care services (DH, 2003); choice of where, when and how to get medicines (DH, 2003); and choice of care at the end of life, to name but a few.

Reforms to ensure patient choice is central to a modernised healthcare system have prompted a move to a consumerist view of healthcare (Newman and Vidler, 2006). This has led to 'patients' being referred to as 'customers', 'consumers' and 'service users'.

The terms consumer and service user are similar in that they refer to an individual, a group of people or a community that uses a healthcare service or commodity. Therefore a patient is said to be a consumer or service user. However the term patient can conjure visions of a passive recipient of healthcare. It implies an unequal relationship between them and the 'all knowing' healthcare professional (Neuberger, 1999). The word *patient* in fact comes from a Latin word meaning 'to suffer' or 'to bear'. Traditionally, the person receiving healthcare has been called a patient. Usually, people become patients when they seek assistance because of illness or for surgery. However, the term 'patient' is not suitable for all recipients of nursing care. With the emphasis on health promotion and prevention of illness, many recipients of nursing care are not ill. Nurses do not only provide support, information and care for individuals; they in fact also care for families and communities.

For these reasons, some nurses refer to recipients of healthcare as *clients*. A client is a person who engages the advice or services of another who is qualified to provide this service. The term *client* presents the receivers of healthcare as collaborators in the care, that is, as people who are also responsible for their own health. Thus, the health status of a client is the responsibility of the individual in collaboration with health professionals.

Scope of Nursing

Nurses provide care to a number of different parties, namely individual patients, families and communities as a whole. This nursing care usually involves a combination of the following areas: promoting health and preventing illness, restoring health and care of the dying.

Promoting Health and Preventing Illness

The World Health Organization's (1948) definition of health is 'a state of complete physical, mental and social well-being and not merely the absence of disease or infirmity', which implies engaging in attitudes and behaviour that enhance the quality of life and feelings of well-being. Nurses promote wellness in patients who are healthy or ill. This may involve individual and community activities to enhance healthy lifestyles, such as improving nutrition and physical fitness, immunisations, preventing drug and alcohol misuse, restricting smoking, and preventing accidents and injury in the home and workplace. See Chapter 3 for details.

Restoring Health

Restoring health focuses on the ill patient and it extends from early detection of disease through helping the patient during the recovery period. Nursing activities include the following:

- Providing direct care to the ill person, such as administering medications, baths and specific procedures and treatments.
- Performing diagnostic and assessment procedures, such as measuring blood pressure and examining **faeces** for **occult** blood.
- Consulting with other healthcare professionals about patient problems.
- Teaching patients techniques that aid recovery following illness, such as exercises that will accelerate recovery after a **stroke**.
- Rehabilitating patients to their optimal functional level following physical or mental illness, injury or drug **addiction**.

Care of the Dying

This area of nursing practice involves comforting and caring for people of all ages who are dying. It includes helping patients live as comfortably as possible until death and helping to support those coping with death. Nurses carrying out these activities work in homes, hospitals and extended care facilities such as *hospices*, which are specifically designed to care for dying patients and their families.

Settings of Nursing

There are many settings for nursing within the UK. Many nurses work in hospitals, but increasingly they work in patients' homes,

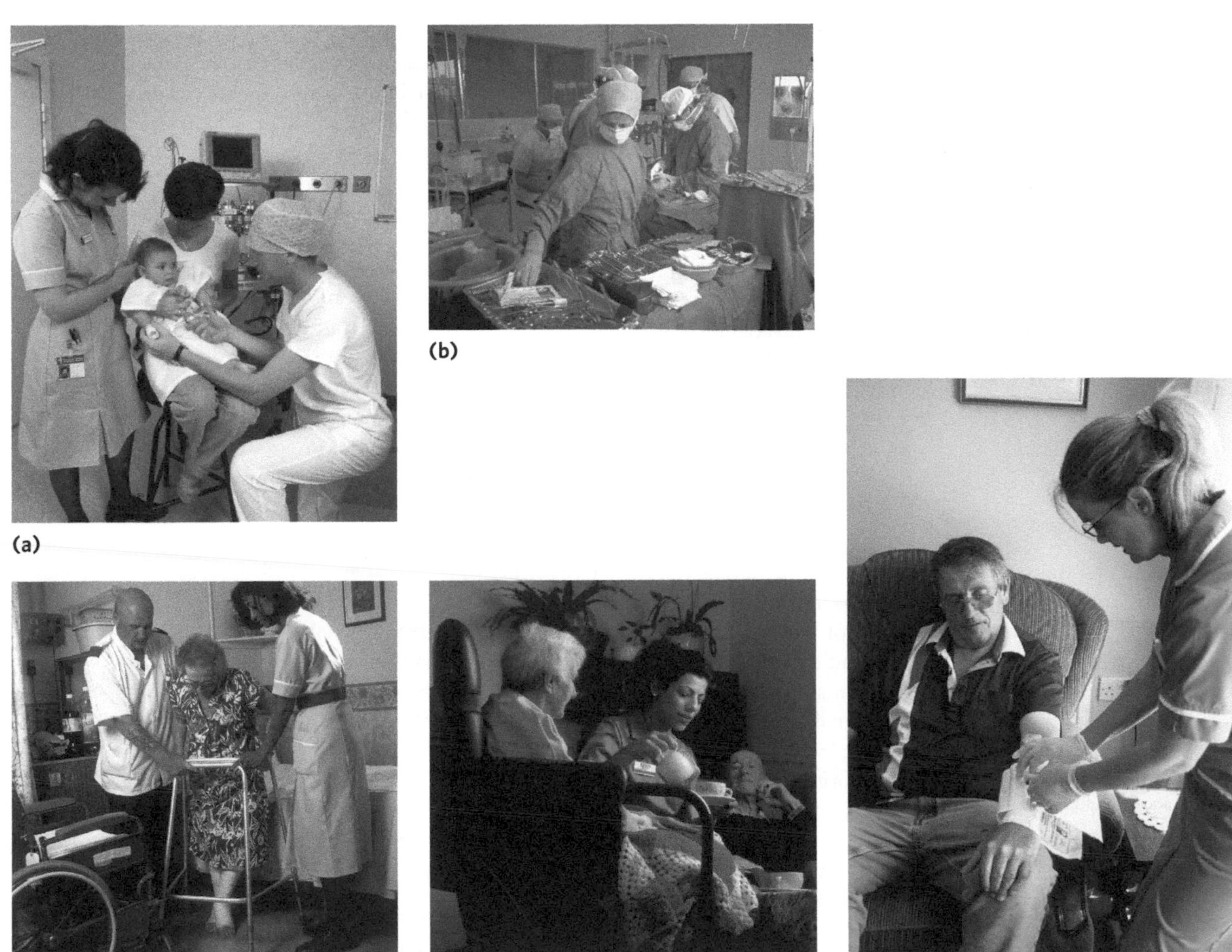

Figure 1-5 Nurses practise in a variety of settings: (a) hospital; (b) theatre; (c) nursing home; (d) residential care; (e) patient's home.
Source: (a) Creator/Wellcome Images; (b) and (c) Mediscan; (d) and (e) Science Photo Library Ltd.

long-term care, hospices, nursing homes, residential homes and general practitioner surgeries, among others (see Figure 1-5).

Nurses have different degrees of nursing **autonomy** and responsibility in these different settings but have many roles in common including providing care, education and support, acting as **advocates** and agents of change, and helping to determine health policies that affect their patients.

The Organisation of Nursing Work

Nursing care in the hospital setting has been traditionally organised into three broad models: **functional**, **team** and **primary nursing** (Thomas and Bond, 1990). More recently a fourth model was introduced; modular nursing (Anderson and Hughes, 1993). These organisation models serve to structure nursing care so as to maintain nursing values and ensure safe and coherent care delivery (Chan *et al.*, 2008).

Functional Nursing

This mode of organising nursing work is based purely on task allocation. The ward manager delegates tasks to individual nurses who have the skills to perform these tasks, but any decision making or responsibility lies with the ward manager. This is a fragmented method of organising nursing care. The focus is on the task rather than the patient.

Team Nursing

This mode of organising nursing work revolves around a team. The team leader coordinates the care provided and the responsibility and decision making lies with the team leader, resulting in the ward manager having less involvement and **accountability** for the care provided. Although the team leader is responsible for organising the patients' care, each individual nurse is accountable for his or her actions in accordance with the Code (NMC, 2008). Although widely used, this form of organisation has been criticised as just an extension of the task orientated and ritualised functional method of organising nursing care (Walsh and Ford, 1989).

Primary Nursing

Primary nursing is recognised as the gold standard method of organising nursing care. It involves the allocation of individual nurses to individual patients. The patient is the focus of the care rather than the task. It allows the nurse to assess, plan, implement and evaluate the care they provide to the patient and as a consequence the nurse has full responsibility and accountability for the care provided. This way of organising workload requires a team that can provide effective evidence-based care that is cost effective. The nurses need to have excellent clinical skills, communication skills and be experts in that particular field of nursing.

Modular Nursing

Modular nursing was proposed as a method of organising nursing care by Anderson and Hughes (1993). According to Chan *et al.* (2008) modular nursing is a mix of team and primary nursing. Nursing care is organised around small groupings of patients, called modules. Nurses are permanently assigned to that module and are responsible for the total care of that group of patients.

Community nursing, however, is organised differently. Nurses care either for patients in a particular geographical area or for patients on a general practitioner's list. Geographical nursing is the most common way of organising nursing care in the community according to the White Paper 'The New NHS' (DH, 1997). This White Paper proposed the development of Primary Care Groups in England and Local Care Groups in Wales that are geographically based. This means that community nurses are no longer linked to one general practitioner's practice but serve the community, which allows for sharing and pooling of resources and therefore is beneficial for patients.

ROLES AND FUNCTIONS OF THE NURSE

Nurses assume a number of roles when they provide care to patients, often carrying out these roles concurrently, not exclusively of one another. The roles required at a specific time depend on the needs of the patient and aspects of the particular environment.

Caregiver

The **caregiver** role has traditionally included those activities that assist the patient physically and psychologically while preserving the patient's dignity. The nurse may be required to provide a continuum of care from total nursing care for dependent patients to the supportive-educative care provided to patients who need assistance in attaining their highest possible level of health and wellness. Caregiving encompasses the physical, psychosocial, developmental, cultural and spiritual levels. The **nursing process** provides nurses with a framework for providing care (see Chapter 10) which they may provide themselves or delegate to others (e.g. healthcare assistants).

Communicator

Communication is integral to all nursing roles. Nurses communicate with a range of people; the patient, other healthcare professionals and support staff to name a few.

In the role of communicator, nurses identify patient problems and then communicate these verbally or in writing to other members of the multidisciplinary team. The quality of a nurse's communication is an important factor in nursing care. The nurse must be able to communicate effectively and accurately in order for a patient's healthcare needs to be met.

Teacher

As a teacher, the nurse helps patients learn about their health and the healthcare procedures they need to perform to restore or maintain their health. The nurse assesses the patient's learning needs and readiness to learn, sets specific learning goals in conjunction with the patient, enacts teaching strategies and measures learning. Nurses also teach other members of the multidisciplinary team, including support staff, in order to share expert knowledge.

Advocate

Advocacy is a key role for the nurse. The nurse has a duty to protect the patient and their human rights. The nurse may represent the patient's needs and wishes to other health professionals, such as relaying the patient's wish for information to medical staff. They also assist patients in exercising their rights and help them speak up for themselves (see Chapter 4).

Counsellor

Some nurses have the skills to counsel patients. Counselling is the process of helping a patient to recognise and cope with stressful psychological or social problems, to develop improved interpersonal relationships and to promote personal growth. It involves providing emotional, intellectual and psychological support to patients.

Leader

A leader influences others, to work together to accomplish a specific goal. The leader role can be employed at different levels: individual patient, family, groups of patients, colleagues or the community. Effective leadership is a learned process requiring an understanding of the needs and goals that motivate people, the knowledge to apply the leadership skills and the interpersonal skills to influence others.

Manager

The nurse manages the nursing care of individuals, families and communities. The nurse-manager also delegates nursing activities to support staff and other nurses, and supervises and evaluates their performance. Managing requires knowledge about organisational structure and dynamics, authority and accountability, leadership, change theory, advocacy, delegation, and supervision and evaluation.

Evidence-Based Practitioner

In order to provide individualised, holistic care that is based on the most recent evidence nurses need to refer to current research. However, in order to use research as a means of improving the care they provide they need to (a) understand the process and language of research, (b) have an awareness of issues relating to protecting the rights of human subjects (ethics), (c) recognise areas within care that need further investigation and research, and (d) be a discriminating user of research findings.

The Reflective Practitioner

Reflection within nursing is used as a means of articulating and developing knowledge embedded within practice (Benner *et al.*, 1996) and has been promoted as a way of enhancing learning since Dewey's (1933) writings. Boud *et al.* (1985) suggests that 'reflection in the context of learning is a generic term for those intellectual and affective activities in which individuals engage to explore their experiences in order to lead to new understanding and appreciations' (1985: 19). Schon (1983) agrees, stating that reflection is a means of uncovering the complex epistemology of practice. Atkins and Murphy (1993) suggest that reflection consists of three key stages, the first of which is the identification of uncomfortable feelings or thoughts, which is followed by a **critical analysis** of these feelings, leading to new perspectives being uncovered. However, this model can be criticised as focusing on negative experiences, indeed Belenky *et al.* (1986) suggest that positive thoughts and feelings can also lead to critical reflective evaluation and thereby promote self-awareness. In order to structure the reflective process nurses are encouraged to use reflective diaries or journals and also to implement a reflective framework.

Expanded Career Roles

Nurses are fulfilling expanded career roles in both the public and private sectors. Some of the expanded career roles are:

- **Nurse practitioner** – this is defined as 'a registered nurse who has undertaken a specific course of study of at least first degree (Honours)' (RCN, 2005) who sees patients with undiagnosed health problems; is autonomous; has decision-making and **problem-solving** skills; has advanced nursing skills which should include health education and counselling; has the authority to admit, discharge and refer patients; and is an effective leader and consultant (Figure 1-6).

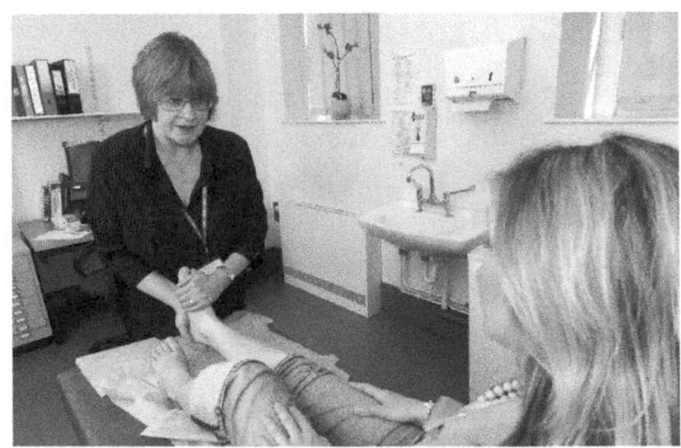

Figure 1-6 A nurse practitioner.
Source: Creator/Wellcome Images.

- **Clinical nurse specialist (CNS)** – is a nurse who has a relevant specialist qualification and is deemed by the employer to be competent to work in the speciality (UKCC, 1996). Miller (1995) states that a CNS has five main roles: clinical expert; researcher; consultant; teacher; and change agent.
- **Nurse researcher** – investigates nursing problems to improve nursing care and to refine and expand nursing knowledge. They are employed in academic institutions, teaching hospitals and research centres. Nurse researchers usually have advanced education at masters and doctoral level.
- **Nurse manager** – manages budgets, staffing and planning programmes. The educational preparation for nurse managers' positions is at least a degree in nursing and frequently a masters or doctoral degree.
- **Nurse educator** – is employed in higher education institutions to teach both pre- and post-registration nursing programmes. The nurse educator usually has a first degree, masters or doctoral degree and frequently has expertise in a particular area of practice.
- **Nurse consultant** – enhances the quality of healthcare provision and ensures that professional leadership is strengthened. A nurse consultant will usually have to perform skills that are complex and show a breadth of expertise over and above that of a clinical nurse specialist.
- **Nurse lead** – provides direction and leadership to all nurses and allied healthcare professionals involved in a particular speciality.

As nursing changes so do the roles and functions of the nurse. Indeed the above roles and functions aid the recognition of nursing as a profession.

NURSING AS A PROFESSION

Nursing is a profession. A profession is defined as an occupation that requires extensive education or a calling that requires special knowledge, skill and preparation, a profession is generally distinguished from other kinds of occupations by: (a) its requirement of prolonged, specialised training; (b) a body of knowledge based on research; (c) autonomy; and (d) a regulatory professional body.

Specialised Education

Specialised education is an important aspect of professional status. In modern times, the trend in education for the professions has shifted towards higher education. Within the UK there are three means of entry into registered nursing: the undergraduate diploma in nursing, the undergraduate degree in nursing and the postgraduate diploma in nursing, which are discussed in detail later in this chapter.

Body of Knowledge Based on Research

Nursing relies on a range of knowledge from different disciplines including biology, sociology and psychology. The creation of a body of knowledge that is distinct to nursing is vital to establish nursing as a profession. According to Aggleton and Chalmers (1986) for nursing to develop autonomous practices it must establish its own research base. From this research, nursing theories and **conceptual frameworks** are developed that contribute to nursing's knowledge base.

Autonomy

A profession is autonomous if it regulates itself and sets standards for its members. If nursing is to have professional status, it must function autonomously in the formation of policy and in the control of its activity. By defining its scope of practice, describing its particular functions and roles, and determining its goals and responsibilities in healthcare delivery, the **Nursing and Midwifery Council (NMC)** provides nurses with autonomy to practise within their particular expertise (see Chapter 5).

Regulating Professional Body

The Nursing and Midwifery Council is the nursing and midwifery professional regulating body that was created by an Act of Parliament in 2002 to protect the public by ensuring that high standards of care are provided to patients by nurses and midwives. It replaced the UK Central Council (UKCC). In order to achieve its aims the NMC maintains a register of all qualified nurses, midwives and specialist community public health nurses. It sets standards for practice, education and professional conduct and provides advice for nurses and midwives. It also considers allegations of misconduct or unfitness due to ill health.

The NMC is part of the **Council for Healthcare Regulatory Excellence (CHRE)**, which was set up in April 2003 by the National Health Service Reform and Health Care Professions Act 2002. The CHRE is funded by the Department of Health and must answer to the UK Parliament. It covers the nine regulators currently responsible for healthcare professions throughout the UK:

- General Chiropractic Council (GCC) regulates chiropractors.
- General Dental Council (GDC) regulates dentists, dental hygienists and dental therapists.
- General Medical Council (GMC) regulates doctors.
- General Optical Council (GOC) regulates dispensing opticians and optometrists.
- General Osteopathic Council (GOsC) regulates osteopaths.
- **Health Professions Council (HPC)** regulates 13 professions.
- Nursing and Midwifery Council (NMC) regulates nurses, midwives and specialist community public health nurses.
- Pharmaceutical Society of Northern Ireland (PSNI) regulates pharmacists.
- Royal Pharmaceutical Society of Great Britain (RPSGB) regulates pharmacists.

As a regulating body for the profession, the NMC sets out standards for nurses' conduct in and out of practice.

The Code: Standards for Conduct, Performance and Ethics for Nurses and Midwives

The purpose of this document is to clarify the expectation placed on nurses and midwives and also sets out the standard of care the public can expect to receive. The Code (NMC, 2008) clearly states that nurses and midwives are personally accountable for both their actions and omissions in practice and should be able to justify any decisions made. It goes on to say that the people who require care must be able to trust the nurse or midwife, stating that they should:

- Make the care of people their first concern, treating them as individuals and respecting their dignity.
- Work with others to protect and promote the health and well-being of those in a nurse's or midwife's care, their families and carers and the wider community.
- Provide a high standard of practice and care at all times.
- Be open and honest, act with integrity and uphold the reputation of the profession.

Although nursing is strictly controlled by its regulating body, the NMC, a number of factors influence current nursing practice.

ACTIVITY 1-4

Read 'The Code: Standards for Conduct, Performance and Ethics for Nurses and Midwives' (available from **www.nmc-uk.org**) and consider the standards that apply to your relationship with the patient.

FACTORS INFLUENCING CURRENT NURSING PRACTICE

To understand nursing as it is practised today and as it will be practised tomorrow requires an understanding of some of the social forces currently influencing this profession. These forces usually affect the entire healthcare system, and nursing, as a major component of that system, cannot avoid the effects.

Agenda for Change

In a bid to change the much disliked grading system for nurses, midwives and public health nurses, and as part of the modernisation of the National Health Service (NHS), the Agenda for Change pay strategy was implemented in December 2004 (RCN, 2009). This was the biggest change that the NHS had seen for 50 years (RCN, 2009a). Its aim was to ensure fair pay and a clearer system for career progression, paying NHS staff according to their skills and knowledge (Benton, 2003). However, there are claims that it has failed to deliver a fair deal for NHS staff (Mooney, 2009). A recent survey of nurses by the *Nursing Times* found that the main criticisms are inappropriate banding of staff, lack of career progression, and an unfair bias in favour of management (Staines, 2009).

Consumer Demands

Consumers of nursing services (the public) have become an increasingly effective force in changing nursing practice. On the whole, people are better educated and have more knowledge about health and illness than in the past. Consumers also have become more aware of others' needs for care. The ethical and moral issues raised by poverty and neglect have made people more vocal about the needs of minority groups and the poor.

The public's concepts of health and nursing have also changed. Most now believe that health is a right of all people, not just a privilege of the rich. Also, the patient has become an active participant in making decisions about the health and nursing care they receive. This is encouraged as the media emphasise that individuals must assume responsibility for their own health by obtaining a physical examination regularly, checking for the seven danger signals of cancer, and maintaining their mental well-being by balancing work and recreation. Interest in health and nursing services is therefore greater than ever. Furthermore, many people now want more than freedom from disease – they want energy, vitality and a feeling of wellness.

Family Structure

New family structures are influencing the need for and provision of nursing services. More people are living away from the **extended family** and the **nuclear family**, and the family breadwinner is no longer necessarily the man. Today, many single men and women bring up children, and in many two-parent families both parents work. It is also common for young parents to live at great distances from their own parents. These young families need support and frequently access social services and childcare centres.

Indeed, the image of the family is no longer two parents with children, particularly as the number of divorces granted in England and Wales reached 155,052 between 2004 and 2005 compared with 27,224 in 1961 (Office for National Statistics, 2005). One of the consequences of such a divorce rate is the increase in lone parents. Spencer (2005) suggests that lone parent families are much more likely to be hit by poverty and as a consequence more likely to have poorer health, which impacts on nursing services.

Information and Telecommunications

The Internet has already impacted on healthcare, with more and more patients becoming well informed about their health concerns. No longer the sole provider of health information, doctors and nurses may need to interpret Internet sources of information to patients and their families. Because not all Internet-based information is accurate, nurses need to become information brokers so they can help people to access high-quality, valid websites; interpret the information; and then help patients evaluate the information and determine if it is useful to them. Clark (2000) predicts that the difference between the future novice and expert nurse will be in knowing where to look for information and how to use it.

Over the past two decades there have been significant advances in the use of telecommunication in healthcare. It can be used to facilitate the delivery of nursing care to patients living in remote areas and also enable information exchange between healthcare professionals (Sarhan, 2009). NHS Direct, a national clinical service, utilises telecommunications to provide nurse-led help and advice for patients over the telephone and Internet. It is available to patients 24 hours a day seven days a week. Other forms of telecommunications used in practice include **telemedicine**, **telehealth** and **telecare**.

Legislation

Legislation about nursing practice and health matters affects both the public and nursing. Legislation related to nursing is discussed in Chapter 4. Changes in legislation relating to health also affect nursing. For example, the Hospital Complaints Procedure Act (1985) resulted in each health authority establishing a complaints procedure. This Act was reviewed by Professor Alan Wilson who found that the system for dealing with complaints relating to health services was confusing and bureaucratic. In 1996, a new complaints procedure was implemented nationwide. Since nurses are at the front line of healthcare, they need to be aware of the three stages of the new complaints procedure and its place within everyday nursing practice.

Ultimately, nurses should be aware of the limits that the law puts upon them as 'ignorance of the law is no defence' (Dimond, 2008: 4). See Chapter 4 for further discussion regarding the legal aspects of nursing.

Demography

Demography is the study of population, including statistics about distribution by age and place of residence, **mortality** (death) and **morbidity** (incidence of disease). From demographic data, the needs of the population for nursing services can be assessed. For example:

- The total population in the UK is increasing (Office for National Statistics, 2006). The proportion of elderly people has also increased, creating an increased need for nursing services for this group.
- The population is shifting from rural to urban settings. This shift signals an increased need for nursing relating to problems caused by pollution and by the effects on the environment of high concentrations of people. Thus, most nursing services are now provided in urban settings.
- Mortality and morbidity studies reveal the presence of risk factors. Many of these risk factors (e.g. smoking) are major causes of death and disease that can be prevented through changes in lifestyle. The nurse's role in assessing risk factors and helping patients make healthy lifestyle changes is discussed in Chapter 3.

Nursing Associations

Professional nursing associations have provided leadership that affects many areas of nursing. There are a number of different nursing associations that represent and support nurses within the UK. The International Council of Nurses (ICN) was established in 1899. Nurses from Great Britain, the USA and Canada were among the founding members.

The ICN provides an organisation through which member national associations can work together with the aim of representing nursing worldwide, advancing the profession and influencing health policy. The five core values of the ICN are visionary leadership, inclusiveness, flexibility, partnership and achievement (ICN, n.d.). The official journal of the ICN is the *International Nursing Review.*

The Royal College of Nurses (RCN) is a member of the International Council of Nurses and aims to promote excellence in practice and shape health policies in the UK. In 2003, the RCN published its first strategic plan that lays out its aims for the organisation as well as nursing as a whole. The strategic plan states that it aims to represent 'the interests of nurses and nursing and be their voice locally, nationally and internationally' (RCN, 2003: 3) and influence the government to implement policies that improve patient care and to build upon the value of nurses, healthcare assistants and nursing students (RCN, 2003).

Student nurses, along with registered nurses, can become members of the RCN and automatically become members of the Association of Nursing Students (ANS). Together with the universities' student union (the NUS) the ANS aims to ensure that the rights of the students are upheld and that they have a forum in which their voices can be heard.

Nurse Unions

The main nurse unions within the UK are the Royal College of Nursing (RCN) and Unison. As well as being a professional body for nursing, the RCN is also a trade union for nurses, midwives, healthcare support workers (nursing auxiliaries) and nursing students, and has over 370,000 members. Its members in general work within healthcare of some sort. However, Unison, the largest trade union in the UK with over 1.3 million members, deals with people working in any public service, such as the NHS, local authorities, schools and colleges, as well as utility providers such as electricity companies.

Nurses are advised to join a nurse union as membership generally includes indemnity insurance, an insurance that protects the member from personal claims against them by patients, colleagues or member of the public. Nurse unions also represent nurses locally, nationally and internationally, fighting for better pay and conditions and providing help and advice on a range of nursing issues including legal advice. The RCN also offers further education for nurses and is instrumental in the development of a number of clinical guidelines such as *The recognition and assessment of acute pain in children* (RCN, 2009b).

One of the most important criteria for a profession is a body of knowledge as stated earlier. Nurse education is key to the development of the individual nurse and to the development of the profession as a whole.

RESEARCH NOTE

The Facilitation of Self Management in Primary Care

Using a qualitative approach, Macdonald *et al.* (2008) explored practice nurse involvement in facilitation of self-management for patients with long-term conditions. Macdonald *et al.* (2008) used semi-structured interviews to elucidate key themes about self-management from 25 practice nurses in two primary care trusts (PCTs) in England. The analysis of the data focused on three stages of facilitation: early, intermediate and late stages.

In the early stages of facilitation most nurses felt that they were 'making sense of the patient' by categorising how the patient was going to cope and providing education about and ways of managing the condition. The intermediate stage of facilitation, on the other hand, explored the patients' beliefs and lifestyle behaviours, offering ways of coping with lifestyle changes. It also involved breaking information down into manageable portions for the patient. Some of the nurses felt that it was important to act as a role model; while others felt listening and encouragement were a vital part of facilitating self-management. Nurses recognised in the later stage that they were facing a long journey with some patients, and that it was up to them to maintain the momentum.

Implications for Practice

Since the advent of the general practice contract in the UK practice nurses' responsibilities for monitoring and recording patients' health status has significantly increased. Chronic and long-term conditions place a considerable burden on primary healthcare with practice nurses increasingly supporting patients with these conditions. The emphasis within current chronic condition management policy is that patients should be encouraged to manage their condition as far as possible: however, there has been little education offered for practice nurses in chronic condition management. Macdonald *et al.* (2008) adds that there needs to be clarification of the skills and competencies required by nurses to support patients with chronic conditions to help them to develop self-management skills.

Source: based on Macdonald, W., Rogers, A., Blakeman, T. and Bower, P. (2008) 'Practice nurses and the facilitation of self management in primary care', *Journal of Advanced Nursing*, 62(2): 191–199.

NURSE EDUCATION

Pre-registration Nurse Education

Pre-registration nurse education has adopted many guises over the past two decades. It is broadly described as post-compulsory education, which means that it takes place after compulsory education and has the purpose of providing a nursing workforce that is fit for practice and purpose (NMC, 2009).

Nurse education is a relative newcomer to higher education. Until the early 1990s the majority of student nurses undertook a hospital-based apprentice style course of nurse education. They were considered part of the workforce and were paid a salary. However, higher education institutions such as the University of Edinburgh have been offering pre-registration degree courses for nurses since 1960 (Weir, 1996). In the late 1980s nurse education was reformed and the Project 2000 (P2K) curriculum developed. This form of nurse education was university-based and students who embarked on this course were supernumerary. If successful, students would qualify with a university diploma or degree, as well as registration on to the appropriate part of the UK Central Council for Nursing, Midwifery and Health Visiting (UKCC) register. The course was made up of 18 months of a Common Foundation Programme followed by an 18-month Branch Programme, leading to registration as an adult nurse, child nurse, mental health nurse or learning disability nurse.

This form of nurse education reduced the amount of clinical experience student nurses were exposed to, but concentrated on the social sciences such as sociology and psychology. However, concerns were raised by clinical staff about the lack of clinical skills shown by students and newly qualified nurses. This resulted in the UKCC setting up a Commission for Nursing and Midwifery Education, which recommended in 1999 that there should be more emphasis on the development of competency in clinical skills within pre-registration nursing and midwifery programmes.

The recommendations set out by the UKCC (UKCC, 1999) were broadly accepted by the nursing profession and a new curriculum was developed, colloquially known as 'Fitness for Practice'. This course has a one-year Common Foundation Programme followed by a two-year Branch Programme with students receiving a bursary for the duration of the course. However, there is a shortened (two-year) pre-registration programme for graduates who have achieved an undergraduate degree in a health-related discipline.

In 2010, further changes have been made to pre-registration nurse education with new standards for pre-registration nursing being published and new programmes being introduced from September 2011 (NMC, 2010). These standards set out the knowledge, skills and attitudes student nurses must demonstrate in order to be fit for practice at the point of registration. The notion is that students will need to demonstrate generic competencies and field competencies. Field competencies relate to the four fields of nursing practice: adult, mental health, learning disabilities and child.

Entry onto Register

The NMC sets out clear criteria for entry onto its register, which includes evidence of course completion, a declaration of good health and good character along with a declaration of any police cautions or criminal convictions. The NMC currently recognises both the Diploma in Nursing and Degree in Nursing, which are both made up of 2,300 hours of practice and 2,300 hours of theory. The Higher Education Institution informs the NMC that the minimum hours have been met and that the applicant has indeed completed the course.

The Nursing and Midwifery Order states that the applicant has to declare that they are in good health and have good character in order to protect the public. The Order also states that the NMC requires evidence of good health and good character so that the NMC Registrar is satisfied that the applicant is capable of safe and effective practice. This has been included in the entry requirements following 'a number of high profile cases involving the health and character of doctors and nurses' (NMC, 2004).

Post-registration Nurse Education: Continuing Professional Development

Continuing professional development (CPD) refers to formalised education that is designed to enhance the knowledge and skills of practitioners. The NMC requires that each nurse must maintain their professional knowledge and competence (NMC, 2008) and as such continuing professional development plays a major role in maintaining this requirement. Also, nurses are required to show that they have met the Post-Registration Education and Practice (PREP) standards in order to maintain their registration. Currently, nurses have to undertake at least five days of learning activity relevant to their profession during a three-year period.

Continuing education and professional development is the responsibility of each practising nurse. Constant updating and growth are essential to keep abreast of scientific and technological change and changes within the nursing profession. A variety of educational and healthcare institutions conduct continuing education programmes. They are usually designed to meet one or more of the following needs: (a) to keep nurses abreast of new techniques and knowledge; (b) to help nurses attain expertise in a specialised area of practice, such as intensive care nursing; and (c) to provide nurses with information essential to nursing practice, for example, knowledge about the legal aspects of nursing. Post-registration nurse education currently comes in a number of formats, for example level 2 or 3 modules, first degrees, masters degrees and doctoral programmes.

Many post-registration nurse education programmes require the nurse to understand, apply, participate and initiate research as a means of improving and informing practice.

NURSING RESEARCH

Today, nurses are actively generating, publishing and applying research in practice to improve patient care and enhance the nursing scientific knowledge base. Although the focus for all nurses is use of research findings, in practice the degree of participation in research depends on the nurse's educational level, position, experience and practical environment.

As early as 1854, Florence Nightingale demonstrated the importance of research in the delivery of nursing care. When Nightingale arrived in the Crimea in November 1854, she found the military hospital barracks overcrowded, filthy, rat and flea infested, and lacking in food, drugs and essential medical supplies. As a result of these conditions, men died from starvation and diseases such as dysentery, cholera and typhus (Woodham-Smith, 1950: 151–167). By systematically collecting, organising and reporting data, Nightingale was able to institute sanitary reforms and significantly reduce mortality rates from contagious disease.

Clark and Hockey (1989) state that nurses have in the past depended upon other disciplines for the study of their own profession. However, the concept of research has been embraced within nursing curricula particularly since the integration of nurse education into higher education.

Nursing organisations such as the RCN have been crucial in supporting, promoting and developing nursing research within the UK (Parahoo, 2006). In 1995 the RCN and the London School of Hygiene and Tropical Medicine joined forces to form the Centre for Policy in Nursing Research and currently the RCN has an Institute of Research that aims to raise the profile of research in nursing by providing funding and resources.

Approaches to Nursing Research

There are two major approaches to investigating diverse phenomena in nursing research. These approaches originate from different philosophical perspectives and use different methods for the collection and analysis of data.

Quantitative Research

Quantitative research progresses through systematic, logical steps according to a specific plan to collect numerical information, often under conditions of considerable control, which is then analysed using statistical procedures. The quantitative approach is most frequently associated with positivism or logical positivism, a philosophical doctrine that emphasises the rational and the scientific (Polit and Beck, 2008). Quantitative research is often viewed as 'hard' science and uses **deductive reasoning** and the measurable attributes of human experience.

The following is an example of a research question that lends itself to a quantitative approach: what are the differential effects of continuous versus intermittent application of negative pressure on tracheal tissue during endotracheal suctioning?

Qualitative Research

The qualitative approach is often associated with naturalistic inquiry, which explores the subjective and complex experiences of human beings. Qualitative research investigates the human experience as it is lived through careful collection and analysis of narrative, subjective materials (Polit and Beck, 2008). Data collection and its analysis occur concurrently. Using the inductive method, data are analysed by identifying themes and patterns to develop a theory or framework that helps explain the processes under observation (Polit and Beck, 2008). The qualitative approach would be appropriate for the following types of research questions:

- What is the nature of the bereavement process in spouses of patients with terminal cancer?
- What is the nature of coping and adjustment after a radical prostatectomy?
- What is the process of family caregiving for elderly family relatives with Alzheimer's dementia as experienced by the caregiver?

Some examples of qualitative research studies are:

- Smith (2010): a study of how nurses at a national telephone triage centre made different use of the algorithms and organisational protocols to make decisions and give advice to parents with crying babies. Smith found that nurses used the 'crying baby' algorithm in various ways, depending on their experience and confidence with the algorithm.
- McLaughlin *et al.* (2010): this study investigated the motivation of nursing students, their reasons for entering nursing and the perceived influence of others in their decision making. They identified a number of motivators including self- and personal development, opportunities in nursing and the altruistic nature of caring for another person. They also found that family members offered a great deal of emotional and practical support to students.

CRITICAL REFLECTION

Let us revisit the case study on page 2. Now that you have read this chapter, think about the nurse's role in healthcare. Is nursing a profession that should devolve the caring element to healthcare assistants? Is it more important for the profession to move into more technical areas or is the current scope of nursing practice adequate?

CHAPTER HIGHLIGHTS

- Historical perspectives of nursing practice reveal recurring themes or influencing factors. For example, women have traditionally cared for others, but often in subservient roles. Religious orders left an imprint on nursing by instilling such values as compassion, devotion to duty and hard work. Wars created an increased need for nurses and medical specialties. Societal attitudes have influenced nursing's image. Visionary leaders have made notable contributions to improving the status of nursing.
- The scope of nursing practice includes promoting wellness, preventing illness, restoring health and care of the dying.
- Nurse practice is guided by legislation and it is the nurses' responsibility for knowing the law that governs their practice.
- Standards of clinical nursing practice provide criteria against which the effectiveness of nursing care and professional performance behaviours can be evaluated.
- Every nurse may function in a variety of roles that are not exclusive of one another; in reality, they often occur together and serve to clarify the nurse's activities. These roles include caregiver, communicator, teacher, advocate, counsellor, leader, manager and research consumer.
- With advanced education and experience, nurses can fulfil advanced practice roles such as clinical nurse specialist, nurse practitioner, educator, manager and researcher.
- A desired goal of nursing is professionalism, which needs specialised education; a unique body of knowledge based on research; autonomy; and a regulating professional body.
- Current nursing practice is influenced by the Agenda for Change, consumer demand, family structure, science and technology, information and telecommunications, legislation, demographic and social changes, nursing shortages and the work of nursing associations.
- Participation in the activities of nursing associations enhances the growth of involved individuals and helps nurses collectively influence policies that affect nursing practice.

ACTIVITY ANSWERS

ACTIVITY 1-1 Your definition of nursing may be very personal to you. Some of the attributes of a good nurse are:

- Highly qualified and trained
- Excellent communication skills
- Honest and trustworthy
- Sound character
- Empathetic and caring - sensitive to the needs of others
- Respect and value people as individuals
- A good listener
- A problem solver
- Professional.

Depending on your own experience you may have listed other attributes. It may be useful to consider why you have included other attributes.

ACTIVITY 1-2 Your personal perception of nursing before you entered into the profession could be based on:

- Personal experience of being a patient
- Personal experience of visiting a hospital or other healthcare environment
- Personal experience of someone you know who is a nurse
- The media
- Your personal expectations of the profession.

ACTIVITY 1-3 It is important not only to think about what you consider to be quality nursing care but also why you feel this way. Quality nursing care means a good experience for patients and is described by the National Nursing Research Unit (2008) as:

- A holistic approach to physical, mental and emotional needs, patient centred and continuous care
- Efficiency and effectiveness combined with humanity and compassion
- Professional, high-quality, evidence-based practice
- Safe, effective and prompt nursing interventions
- Patient empowerment, support and advocacy
- Seamless care through effective teamwork with other professions.

ACTIVITY 1-4 It would be reasonable to state that all the standards of the Code (NMC, 2008) apply to the relationship with the patient, however the following standards are of particular importance:

- Make the care of people your first concern, treating them as individuals and respecting their dignity
- Work with others to protect and promote the health and well-being of those in your care, their families and carers, and the wider community
- Provide a high standard of practice and care at all times
- Be open and honest, act with integrity and uphold the reputation of your profession.

REFERENCES

Aggleton, P. and Chalmers, H. (1986) 'Nursing research, nursing theory and the nursing process', *Journal of Advanced Nursing*, 11: 197–202.

Allan, H.T. and Smith, P.A. (2009) 'How student nurses' supernumerary status affects the way they think about nursing: a qualitative study', *Nursing Times*, 105: 43.

Anderson, C. and Hughes, E. (1993) 'Implementing modular nursing in a long-term care facility', *Journal of Nursing Administration*, 23: 29–35.

Atkins, S. and Murphy, K. (1993) 'Reflection: A review of the literature', *Journal of Advanced Nursing*, 18: 1188–1192.

Barker, P. and Buchanan-Barker, P. (2004) 'Caring as a craft', *Nursing Standard*, 19(9): 17–18.

Barr, D.A., Fenton, L. and Blane, D. (2008) 'The claim for patient choice and equity', *Journal of Medical Ethics*, 34: 271–274.

Belenky, M., Clinchy, B., Goldberger, N. and Tarule, J. (1986) *Women's ways of knowing: The development of self, voice and mind*, New York: Basic Books.

Benner, P., Tanner, C. and Chesla, C. (1996) *Expertise in nursing practice: Caring, clinical judgement and ethics*, New York: Springer.

Benton, D. (2003) 'Agenda for Change: Job evaluation', *Nursing Standard*, 17(36): 39–42.

Boud, D., Keogh, T. and Walker, D. (1985) *Reflection, turning experience into learning*, Worcester: Billing and Son.

Carter, P. (2009) 'Nursing is a set of careers linked by a belief in giving high quality care to patients', *The Independent*. Available from http://www.independent.co.uk/student/career-planning/getting-job/dr-peter-carter-nursing-is-a-set-of-careers-linked-by-a-belief-in-giving-high-quality-care-to-patients-167232 (Accessed 22/01/2010.)

Chan, E.A., Chung, J.W.Y. and Wong, T.K.S. (2008) 'Learning from the severe acute respiratory syndrome (SARS) epidemic', *Journal of Clinical Nursing*, 17(8): 1023–1034.

Clark, D.J. (2000) 'Old wine in new bottles: Delivering nursing in the 21st century', *Journal of Nursing Scholarship*, 32(1): 11–15.

Clark, J.M. and Hockey, L. (1989) *Further research for nursing*, London: Scutari.

Darzi, A. (2008) *High quality care of all: NHS next stage review final report*, London: DH.

Dewey, J. (1933) *How we think*, Boston: D.C. Heath.

DH (1997) *The new NHS: Modern, dependable*, London: The Stationery Office.

DH (2003) *Building on the best: Choice, responsiveness and equity in the NHS*, London: DH.

Dimond, B. (2008) *Legal aspects of nursing* (3rd edn), Harlow: Pearson Education.

Dingwall, R., Rafferty, A.M. and Webster, C. (1988) *An introduction to the social history of nursing*, London: Routledge.

Finfgeld-Connett, D. (2008) 'Concept synthesis of the art of nursing', *Journal of Advanced Nursing*, 62(3): 381–388.

Holstrom, R. (2008) *Recasting the nursing role*. Nursing Times. net. Available from http://www.nursingtimes.net/whats-new-in-nursing/acute-care/recasting-the-nursing-role/1907384.article (Accessed 22/01/2010.)

ICN – International Council of Nurses (n.d.) 'About the International Council of Nurses'. Available from http://www.icn.ch/abouticn.htm (Accessed 22/01/2010.)

Maben, J. and Griffiths, P. (2008) *Nurses in society: Starting the debate*, London: KCL.

Macdonald, W., Rogers, A., Blakeman, T. and Bower, P. (2008) 'Practice nurses and the facilitation of self management in primary care', *Journal of Advanced Nursing*, 62(2): 191–199.

McLaughlin, K., Moutray, M. and Moore, C. (2010) 'Career motivation in nursing students and the perceived influence of significant others', *Journal of Advanced Nursing*, 66(2): 404–412.

Meleis, A.I. (2006) *Theoretical nursing: Development and progress*, Philadelphia: Lippincott Williams and Wilkins.

Miller, L. (1995) 'The clinical nurse specialist: A way forward?', *Journal of Advanced Nursing*, 22: 494–501.

Mooney, H. (2009) *Half of nurses say agenda for change has failed.* Nursing Times.net. Available from http://www.nursingtimes.net/whats-new-in-nursing/management/half-of-nurses-say-agenda-for-change-has-failed/5004414.article?sm=5004414 (Accessed 22/01/2010.)

Mortimer, B. and McGann, S. (2005) *New directions in the history of nursing: International perspectives*, Oxon: Routledge.

Mullally, S. (2004) 'The shape of things to come', *Nursing Standard*, 18(17): 16–17.

National Nursing Research Unit (2008) 'High quality nursing care – what is it and how can we best ensure its delivery?', *Policy+*, 13: 1–2. Available from http://www.kcl.ac.uk/content/1/c6/04/37/71/PolicyIssue13.pdf (Accessed 15/12/2010.)

Neuberger, J. (1999) 'Let's do away with "patients"', *British Medical Journal*, 318(7200): 1756–1758.

Newman, J. and Vidler, E. (2006) 'Discriminating customers, responsible patients, empowered users: Consumerism and the modernisation of healthcare', *Journal of Social Policy*, 35(2): 193–209.

NMC – Nursing and Midwifery Council (2004) *NMC guidance: Requirements for evidence of good health and good character*, London: NMC.

NMC – Nursing and Midwifery Council (2007) *Essential skills clusters for pre-registration nursing programmes*, London: NMC.

NMC – Nursing and Midwifery Council (2008) *The Code: Standards for conduct, performance and ethics for nurses and midwives*, London: NMC.

NMC – Nursing and Midwifery Council (2009) *Review of pre-registration nursing education – phase 2*, London: NMC. Available from http://www.nmc-uk.org/Documents/Consultations/RPNE/9537%20NMC%20RPNE%2011%20Report.pdf

NMC – Nursing and Midwifery Council (2010) *Standards for pre-registration nursing education*, London: NMC.

Office for National Statistics (2005) *Divorces*, Newport: Office for National Statistics. Available from http://www.statistics.gov.uk/cci/nugget.asp?id=170 (Accessed 17/04/2007.)

Office for National Statistics (2006) *Population Estimates*, Newport: Office for National Statistics. Available from http://www.statistics.gov.uk/cci/nugget.asp?id=6 (Accessed 17/04/2007.)

Parahoo, K. (2006) *Nursing research: Principles, process and issues*, Basingstoke: Macmillan Press.

Payne, D. (2000) 'New year, new image', *Nursing Times*, 96(1): 14–15.

Polit, D.F. and Beck, C.T. (2008) *Nursing Research: generating and assessing evidence for nursing practice*, Philadelphia: Lippincott Williams and Wilkins.

RCN (2003) *Defining nursing*, London: RCN.

RCN (2005) *Nurse practitioner: A RCN guide to the nurse practitioner role, competencies and programme approval*, London: RCN.

RCN (2009a) *Agenda for change*. London: RCN. Available from http://www.rcn.org.uk/support/pay_and_conditions/agendaforchange (Accessed 22/01/2010.)

RCN (2009b) *The recognition and assessment of acute pain in children*, London: RCN.

Sarhan, F. (2009) *Telemedicine in healthcare 1: Exploring its uses, benefits and disadvantages*, Nursing Times.net. Available from http://www.nursingtimes.net/nursing-practice-clinical-research/telemedicine-in-healthcare-1-exploring-its-uses-benefits-and-disadvantages/5007796.article?sm=5007796

Schon, D. (1983) *The reflective practitioner*, London: Temple Smith.

Smith, S. (2010) 'Helping parents cope with crying babies: Decision making and interaction at NHS Direct', *Journal of Advanced Nursing*, 66(2): 381–391.

Spencer, N. (2005) 'Does material disadvantage explain the increased risk of adverse health, educational and behavioural outcomes among children in lone parent households in Britain? A cross-sectional study', *Journal of Epidemiological Community Health*, 59: 152–157.

Staines, R. (2009) *Agenda for change: Have hopes for fair pay faded?* Nursing Times.net. Available from http://www.nursingtimes.net/whats-new-in-nursing/management/agenda-for-change-have-hopes-for-fair-pay-faded/5004548.article (Accessed 22/01/2010.)

Thomas, L. and Bond, S. (1990) 'Towards defining the organisation of nursing care in hospital wards: An empirical study', *Journal of Advanced Nursing*, 15(9): 1106–1112.

UKCC (1996) *Registrar's Letter 7/1996 The Council's Standards for Education following PREP. Transitional arrangements – Specialist practitioner title/specialist qualification*, London: UKCC.

UKCC (1999) *Fitness for practice: The UKCC Commission for Nursing and Midwifery Education*, London: UKCC.

Walsh, M. and Ford, P. (1989) *Nursing rituals, research and rational actions*, Oxford: Heinemann Nursing.

Weir, R. (1996) *A leap in the dark: The origins and development of the Department of Nursing Studies at the University of Edinburgh*, London: Book Factory.

Woodham-Smith, C. (1950) *Florence Nightingale*, London: Constable and Co.

World Health Organization (1948) *Constitution of the World Health Organization Basic Documents*, Geneva: WHO.

CHAPTER 2
HEALTH, ILLNESS AND DISEASE

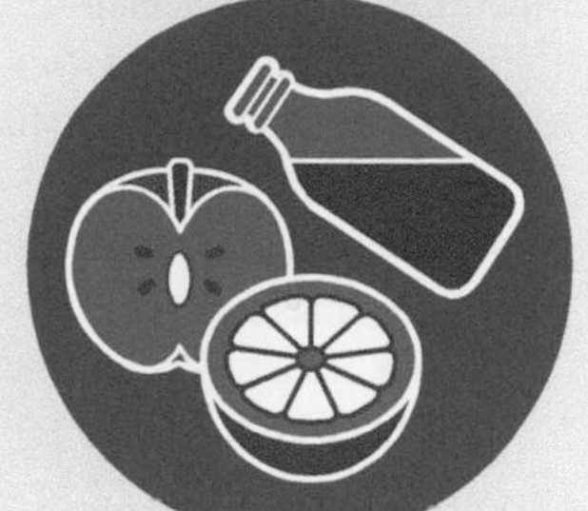

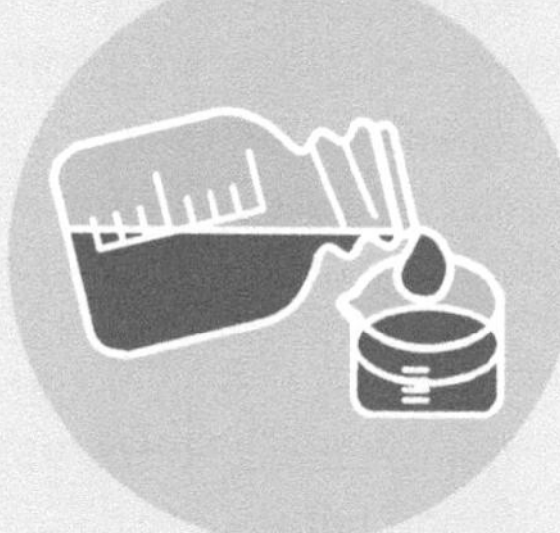

LEARNING OUTCOMES

After completing this chapter, you will be able to:

- Differentiate health, illness and disease.
- Identify factors affecting health status, beliefs and practices.
- Identify Parsons' four aspects of the sick role.
- Describe the effects of illness on individuals' and family members' roles and functions.
- Differentiate between the different dimensions of health.
- Identify common risk factors regarding family health.
- Identify various types of communities.
- Differentiate primary, secondary and tertiary healthcare services.
- Describe the functions and purposes of the healthcare services outlined in this chapter.
- Identify the roles of various healthcare professionals.
- Describe the factors that affect healthcare delivery.
- Discuss the different frameworks for the delivery of effective nursing care.

After reading this chapter you will be able to differentiate between health, illness and disease and be able to understand the impact chronic conditions such as anxiety can have on a person and their family's well-being. You will also be able to identify the type of care settings appropriate for an individual. This chapter relates to **all of the Essential Skills Clusters (NMC, 2010)**, as appropriate for each progression point.

Ensure that you really understand this chapter by logging on to your complimentary **MyNursingKit** at **www.pearsoned.co.uk/kozier**. Complete the self-assessment tests to check your progress and utilise further activities to practise and confirm your understanding.

CASE STUDY

George, a 49-year-old man, is admitted to a medical ward in a general hospital with chest pain and shortness of breath. He is accompanied by his daughter Susan. Susan informs the staff on the ward that she has seen her father have these 'attacks' on many occasions. George undergoes numerous diagnostic tests to establish the cause of the pain and breathlessness but all the results are normal. George's consultant decides that he can be discharged home as the chest pain and shortness of breath were probably as a result of anxiety. However, Susan is not particularly happy with this decision. She is afraid that George will suffer another 'attack' in the future.

You discuss the issues with Susan and George and find out that George has suffered for many years with anxiety and finds it difficult to interact with others. You also note from George's notes that he has had similar admissions into hospital in the past. Susan tells you that George has been having these 'attacks' since the death of his wife two years ago and has been drinking alcohol to alleviate the pain. As a result of his alcohol consumption, George has recently lost his job as a forklift driver.

INTRODUCTION

Nursing has a unique position within healthcare. The nurses' position provides them with the opportunity to influence people's lives and lifestyle choices. However, to help others nurses need to clarify their own understanding of health and wellness. Individuals have a unique view of the world of health, which is based on their life experiences and current healthcare. Patients' health beliefs also influence nurses' health practices. Some people think of health and wellness (or well-being) as the same thing or, at the very least, as accompanying one another. However, health may not always accompany well-being: a person who has a terminal illness may have a sense of well-being; conversely, another person may lack a sense of well-being yet be in a state of good health. For many years the concept of disease was the measure by which health was monitored. In the late 19th century the 'how' of disease (pathogenesis) was the major concern of health professionals. Currently, the emphasis on health and wellness is increasing. Indeed, the NMC (2007) Essential Skills Clusters state that nurses need to promote the health and well-being of their patients.

CONCEPTS OF HEALTH, ILLNESS AND DISEASE

Health, wellness and well-being have many definitions and interpretations. Familiarity with the most common aspects of these concepts is vital in interpreting how they may be perceived by individual patients.

A Positive View of Health

For some health means a state of well-being. Florence Nightingale saw health as a state of being well and using every power the individual possesses to the fullest extent (Nightingale, 1969). People with this view of health believe that remaining healthy requires continuous effort. Active steps are taken to maintain health, e.g. exercise and eating a healthy diet.

The World Health Organization (WHO) takes a more holistic view of health, defining health as 'a state of complete physical, mental, and social well-being, and not merely the absence of disease or infirmity' (WHO, 1948). This definition is concerned for the individual as a whole person functioning physically, psychologically and socially. It places health in the context of environment. People's lives, and therefore their health, are affected by everything they interact with – not only environmental influences such as climate and the availability of nutritious food, shelter, clean air to breathe and pure water to drink, but also other people, including family, friends, employers and other associates. It also equates health with a productive and creative life, focusing on the living state rather than on categories of disease that may cause illness or death.

A Negative View of Health

Traditionally health has been defined in terms of the absence of disease or illness. People with this belief see good health as normal and tend to take it for granted. Therefore they take few special actions to maintain their health. It is this view of health that underpins the western scientific medical model (see later in this chapter).

Dimensions of Health

Health is a holistic concept that has many dimensions. Anspaugh *et al.* (2008: 3–7) propose seven components of wellness (see Figure 2-1). To realise optimal health and wellness, people must deal with the factors within each component:

- **Physical.** The ability to carry out daily tasks, achieve fitness (e.g. pulmonary, cardiovascular, gastrointestinal), maintain adequate nutrition and proper body fat, avoid abusing drugs and alcohol or using tobacco products, and generally to practise positive lifestyle habits. Physical health is probably the easiest to recognise and measure. Consequently the focus for much of healthcare is on the physical well-being of the patient:

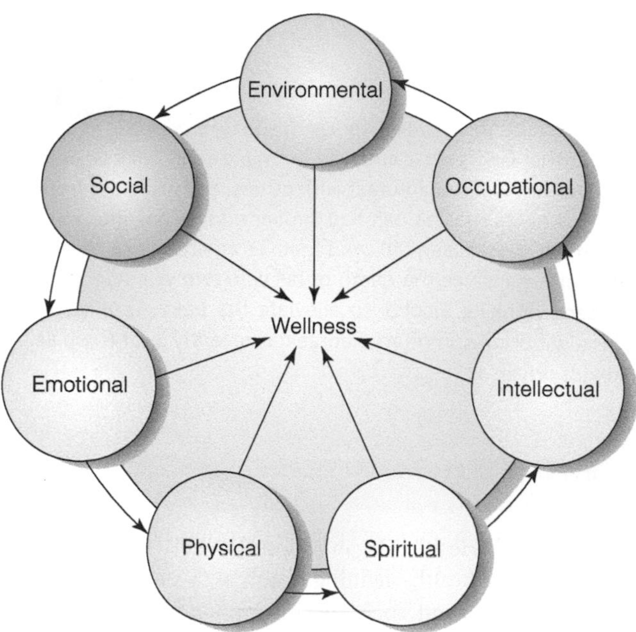

Figure 2-1 The seven components of wellness

Source: Wellness: Concepts and Applications, 6th ed., McGraw-Hill (Anspaugh, P.J., Hamrick, M.H. and Rosato, F.D. 2003) p. 4, reproduced by permission of the McGraw-Hill Companies, Inc.

- diagnostic investigations, e.g. blood tests and x-rays;
- health screening, e.g. mammograms for breast cancer;
- health prevention, e.g. immunisations.

Likewise many of the measures for improving health are aimed at the physical health of the person. Over recent years the Department of Health have implemented a range of health initiatives focusing on the physical element of health including:

- Healthy weight, Healthy lives (DH, 2008)
- Be Active, Be Healthy (DH, 2009a)
- Healthier Food Mark (rolled out in 2011 in England)
- Skilled for Health
- 5-A-Day.

- **Social.** The ability to interact successfully with people and within the environment of which each person is a part, to develop and maintain intimacy with significant others, and to develop respect and tolerance for those with different opinions and beliefs.
- **Emotional.** The ability to manage **stress** and to express emotions appropriately. Emotional wellness involves the ability to recognise, accept and express feelings, and to accept one's limitations.
- **Intellectual.** The ability to learn and use information effectively for personal, family and career development. Intellectual wellness involves striving for continued growth and learning to deal with new challenges effectively.
- **Spiritual.** The belief in some force (nature, science, religion or a higher power) that serves to unite human beings and provide meaning and purpose to life. It includes a person's own morals, values and ethics. Spiritual well-being can be described in terms of a number of characteristics (Carson, 1989):
  - sense of inner peace,
  - compassion for others,
  - reverence for life,
  - gratitude,
  - appreciation of both unity and diversity,
  - humour,
  - wisdom,
  - generosity,
  - ability to transcend the self,
  - capacity for unconditional love.
- **Occupational.** The ability to achieve a balance between work and leisure time. A person's beliefs about education, employment and home influence personal satisfaction and relationships with others.
- **Environmental.** The ability to promote health measures that improve the standard of living and quality of life in the community. This includes influences such as food, water and air.

The above seven components overlap to some extent, and factors in one component often directly affect factors in another. For example, a person who learns to control daily stress levels from a **physiological** perspective is also helping to maintain the emotional stamina needed to cope with a crisis.

Concepts of Ill Health

The terms illness and **disease** are often used interchangeably, but they have very different meanings. Illness indicates a condition that causes the individual a problem (Nordenfelt, 2007), causing them pain or harm (Naidoo and Wills, 2004). It is a highly personal state in which the person's physical, emotional, intellectual, social, developmental or spiritual functioning is thought to be diminished. It is not synonymous with disease and may or may not be related to disease. Illness is highly subjective; only the individual person can say he or she is ill, while disease can be described as a scientifically detectable alteration in body functions resulting in a reduction of capacities or a shortening of the normal life span.

The causation of a disease is called its **aetiology**. A description of the aetiology of a disease includes the identification of all causal factors that act together to bring about the particular disease. For example, the tubercle bacillus is designated as the biological agent of tuberculosis. However, other aetiological factors, such as age, nutritional status and even occupation, are involved in the development of tuberculosis and influence the course of infection. There are many diseases for which the cause is unknown (e.g. multiple sclerosis).

There are many ways to classify illness and disease; one of the most common is as acute or chronic. **Acute** illness is typically characterised by severe symptoms of relatively short duration. The symptoms often appear abruptly and subside quickly and, depending on the cause, may or may not require intervention by healthcare professionals. Some acute illnesses are serious (e.g. appendicitis may require surgical intervention), but many acute illnesses, such as colds, subside without medical intervention or with the help of over-the-counter medications.

Following an acute illness, most people return to their normal level of wellness.

A **chronic** illness is one that lasts for an extended period, usually six months or longer, and often for the person's life. Chronic illnesses usually have a slow onset and often have periods of remission, when the symptoms disappear, and exacerbation, when the symptoms reappear. Conditions such as arthritis, chronic obstructive pulmonary disease (COPD) and **diabetes** are considered as chronic illnesses.

ACTIVITY 2-1

When you discuss with George, if he feels healthy, he tells you that he eats well and does some exercise and feels 'healthy at the moment'. How may George define health?

MODELS OF HEALTH

A number of models have been developed to explain the complex concept of health:

- **Western scientific medical model** – health is identified by the absence of signs and symptoms of disease or injury.
- Role performance model – health is defined in terms of the individual's ability to fulfil societal roles, that is, to perform work.
- **Adaptive model** – health is a creative process; disease is a failure in adaptation or maladaption.
- **Eudemonistic model** – health is seen as a condition of actualisation or realisation of a person's psychological potential.
- **Agent-host-environment model** – health is an ever-changing state and involves interaction between the individual, the environment and the stressor that leads to illness or disease.
- **Health-illness continua** – health and illness are viewed as opposite ends of a health continuum. People move back and forth within this continuum day by day.

However, it is the medical model that dominates western society. This model is the narrowest interpretation of health. People are viewed as physiological systems with related functions, and health is identified by the absence of signs and symptoms of disease or injury. To laypeople it is considered the state of not being 'sick'. In this model the opposite of health is disease or injury.

FACTORS AFFECTING HEALTH AND WELL-BEING

There are many factors that affect the health of the individual. These factors may or may not be under conscious control. For example, people can choose healthy or unhealthy activities, however they have little or no choice over their genetic makeup, age, sex, culture and sometimes their geographical environments.

Internal Factors

Internal factors are generally described as non-modifiable factors affecting the biological, psychological and cognitive dimensions of the individual.

Biological Dimension

An individual's health can be influenced by hereditary factors, gender, age and developmental level. An individual's genetic makeup influences their biological characteristics, innate temperament, activity level and intellectual potential: it has been related to susceptibility to specific disease, such as diabetes and breast cancer. In some cases, genetic predisposition to health or illness is enhanced when parents are from the same ethnic origin. For example, people of African heritage have a higher incidence of sickle-cell **anaemia** and **hypertension** than the general population but may be less susceptible to malaria.

Gender influences the distribution of disease. Certain acquired and genetic diseases are more common in one gender than in the other. Disorders more common among females include osteoporosis and autoimmune disease such as rheumatoid arthritis. Those more common among males are stomach ulcers, abdominal hernias and respiratory diseases.

Age is also a significant factor. The distribution of disease varies with age. For example, arteriosclerotic heart disease is common in middle-aged males but occurs infrequently in younger people; such **communicable diseases** as whooping cough and measles are common in children but rare in older adults, who have acquired immunity to them.

Psychological developmental level has a major impact on health status. Consider these examples:

- Infants lack physiological and psychological maturity so their defences against disease are lower during the first years of life.
- Toddlers who are learning to walk are more prone to falls and injury.
- Adolescents who need to conform to peers are more prone to risk-taking behaviour and subsequent injury.
- Declining physical and sensory-perceptual abilities limit the ability of older adults to respond to environmental hazards and stressors.

Psychological Dimension

An individual's psychological state can significantly affect their health. The mind and body are inextricably linked and emotional responses to stressors can affect body function. For example, a student who is extremely anxious before an exam may experience urinary frequency and diarrhoea. A person worried about the outcome of surgery or about the behaviour of a teenager may chain-smoke. Prolonged emotional distress may increase susceptibility to organic disease or precipitate it. Emotional distress may influence the immune system through the central nervous system and endocrine alterations. Alterations in the immune system are related to the incidence of infections, cancer and autoimmune diseases.

Increasing attention is being given to the mind's ability to direct the body's functioning. Relaxation, meditation and biofeedback techniques are gaining wider recognition by individuals and healthcare professionals. For example, women often use relaxation techniques to decrease pain during childbirth. Other people may learn biofeedback skills to reduce hypertension.

Emotional reactions also occur in response to body conditions. For example, a person diagnosed with a terminal illness may experience fear and depression. *Self-concept* is how a person feels about self (self-esteem) and perceives the physical self (body image), needs, roles and abilities. Self-concept affects how people view and handle situations. Such attitudes can affect health practices, responses to stress and illness, and the times when treatment is sought. An example is the anorexic woman who deprives herself of needed nutrients because she believes she is too fat even though she is well below an acceptable weight level. Self-perceptions are also associated with a person's definition of health. For example, a 75-year-old man who can no longer move large objects as he was accustomed to do may need to examine and redefine his concept of health in view of his age and abilities, as he is no longer able to perform tasks in the same way.

Cognitive Dimension

Cognitive or intellectual factors can also influence health. An individual's lifestyle, including living conditions and patterns of behaviour, are influenced by sociocultural factors and personal characteristics. Lifestyle is considered a behaviour, a choice over which people have control and can have either positive or negative effects on health. The nurse is responsible for promoting healthy lifestyle choices including:

- regular exercise;
- weight control;
- reduced fat intake;
- reduced alcohol and tobacco intake;
- immunisation uptake;
- screening examinations and tests.

Practices that have potentially negative effects on health are often referred to as *risk factors*. For example, overeating, getting insufficient exercise and being overweight are closely related to the incidence of heart disease, **arteriosclerosis**, diabetes and hypertension. Tobacco use is clearly implicated in lung cancer, **emphysema** and cardiovascular diseases.

Spiritual and religious beliefs can significantly affect health behaviour. For example, Jehovah's Witnesses oppose blood transfusions. Likewise some fundamentalists believe that a serious illness is a punishment from God, for example if a child is born with a learning disability the parents may believe that they are being punished for a sin they have committed. Some religious groups are strict vegetarians; and Orthodox Jews perform circumcision on the eighth day of a male baby's life.

External Factors

External factors affecting health include the physical environment, standards of living, family and cultural beliefs, and social support networks.

Environment

Factors such as climate, pollution, radiation and chemicals can pose significant risk to individuals' health. Increasingly, people are becoming aware of their environment and how it affects their health.

Standards of Living

An individual's standard of living (reflecting occupation, income and education) is related to health, morbidity and mortality. Hygiene, food habits and the propensity to seek healthcare advice and follow health regimens vary among high-income and low-income groups.

Employment has been described as 'the glue that keeps our society together' (Smith, 1987). In fact, many people define themselves by way of their job or career, consequently employment has a significant effect on the health of the majority of individuals (Acheson, 1998). Employment is seen as inextricably linked to education, housing and general disadvantage, and as a result has acquired much attention from policy makers in the UK government. A recent document on tackling inequalities in health details some of the policies aimed at improving employment within the UK (DH, 2009b).

Family and Cultural Beliefs

The family passes on patterns of daily living and lifestyles to their children. For example the types and amount of food eaten, smoking, violence and abuse. These can have both a positive and negative effect on an individual's health.

Social Support Networks

Having a support network (family, friends or a confidant) and job satisfaction helps people avoid illness. People with inadequate support networks sometimes allow themselves to become increasingly ill before confirming the illness and seeking therapy. Support people can also provide the stimulus for an ill person to become well again (Hurdle, 2001).

ACTIVITY 2-2

What factors could be affecting George's health?

HEALTH AND ILLNESS BEHAVIOURS

Understanding human behaviour is central to improving health and wellness. In order to promote health and well-being nurses need to understand how and why individuals make decisions about their lives.

Behaviours are human actions or reactions to specified circumstances which Hubley and Copeman (2008) classify as:

- **Decision-based behaviour** – where a person makes a conscious decision to act in a particular way, e.g. a person's decision to eat healthily.

- **One-time behaviour** – an action that is carried out only a few times in their life, e.g. taking their child for immunisation.
- **Routine behaviour or habit** – regular action, e.g. washing hands after using the toilet.
- **Addictive behaviour** – dependency to a particular behaviour, e.g. drug abuse.
- **Custom or behavioural norm** – behaviour shared by a group of people, e.g. the diet of ethnic minorities.
- **Tradition** – behaviour that is passed down from generation to generation, e.g. avoidance of certain foods.
- **Lifestyle** – a collection of behaviours that make up a person's life, e.g. exercise and diet.

These behaviours are not always distinct from one another but overlap or may develop from one form of behaviour to another. For example, you may make a conscious decision to wear a seatbelt in a car which then becomes routine.

Illness Behaviour

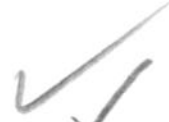

Illness behaviour is a coping mechanism which involves ways individuals describe, monitor and interpret their symptoms, take remedial actions and use the healthcare system. How people behave when they are ill is highly individualised and affected by many variables, such as age, sex, occupation, socio-economic status, religion, ethnic origin, psychological stability, personality, education and modes of coping.

The Sick Role

According to Parsons (1979), a sociologist, illness is socially deviant. He suggests that illness is not a biological or psychological condition but a social role and is characterised by the following rules:

1. Patients are not held responsible for their condition.
2. Patients are excused from certain social roles and tasks.
3. Patients are obliged to try to get well as quickly as possible.
4. Patients or their families are obliged to seek competent help.

Suchman (1979) expanded on this to describe five stages of illness: (1) symptoms, (2) sick role, (3) medical care contact, (4) dependent patient role and (5) recovery or **rehabilitation**. Not all patients progress through each stage. For example, the patient who experiences a sudden heart attack is taken to the emergency department and immediately enters stages 3 and 4, medical care contact and dependent patient role. Other patients may progress through only the first two stages and then recover.

Models of Behaviour

A number of models have been developed to describe human behaviour:

- **Biological model** – suggests that behaviour is influenced by biology and genetic makeup.
- **Motivational theory** – Maslow's theory (1943) suggests that people have a hierarchy of needs that affects their behaviour.
- **Cognitive dissonance theory** – suggests that uncomfortable information causes dissonance within the individual and changes behaviour.
- **Health belief model** – based on value expectancy theory, it suggests that a person will weigh up the 'pros' and 'cons' and change their behaviour accordingly (see Figure 2-2).
- **Stages of change model** – or transtheoretical model suggests that an individual will go through a number of stages: pre-contemplation, contemplation, trial, maintenance and **relapse**.
- **Social learning theory** – Bandura (1986) suggested that people learn through their own experiences.
- **Theory of reasoned action** – is based on value expectancy theory which suggests that a change in behaviour can be influenced by those around the individual.
- **Social network theory** – seeks to understand the behaviour of an individual in the social context in which it exists.
- **Social capital theory** – considers behaviour within the individual's social context and sees the cooperation of the community as beneficial in attaining change.
- **Innovations theory** – or diffusion theory suggests that information and ideas spread through communities.

Nurses play a major role in helping patients implement healthy behaviours. They help patients monitor health, they supply anticipatory guidance and they impart knowledge about health. Nurses can also reduce barriers to action (e.g. by minimising inconvenience or discomfort) and can support positive actions.

EFFECTS OF ILLNESS

Illness brings about changes in both the involved individual and in the family. The changes vary depending on the nature, severity and duration of the illness, attitudes associated with the illness by the patient and others, the financial demands, the lifestyle changes incurred, adjustments to usual roles, and so on.

Impact on the Patient

Ill patients may experience behavioural and emotional changes, changes in self-concept and body image, and lifestyle changes. Behavioural and emotional changes associated with short-term illness are generally mild and short lived. The individual, for example, may become irritable and lack the energy or desire to interact in the usual fashion with family members or friends. More acute responses are likely with severe, life-threatening, chronic or disabling illness. **Anxiety**, fear, anger, withdrawal, denial, a sense of hopelessness and feelings of powerlessness are all common responses to severe or disabling illness. For example, a patient experiencing a heart attack fears for his life and the financial burden it may place on his family.

Certain illnesses can also change the patient's body image or physical appearance, especially if there is severe scarring or loss of a limb or special sense organ. The patient's self-esteem and self-concept may also be affected. Many factors can play a part

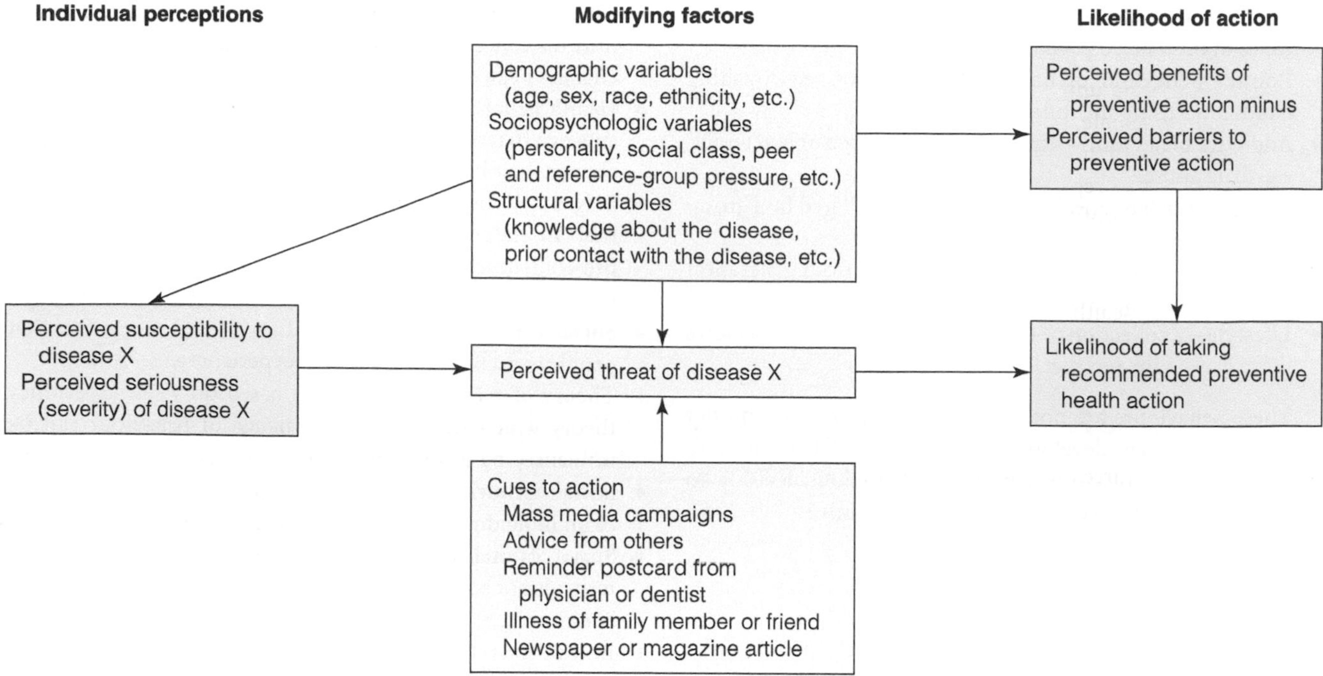

Figure 2-2 The health belief model

Source: 'Selected psychosocial models and correlates of individual health-related behaviors', by M.H. Becker *et al.*, 1977, *Medical Care*, *15*(5 Suppl.), pp. 27–46. Reprinted with permission from Wolters Kluwer Health.

in low self-esteem and a disturbance in self-concept: loss of body parts and function, pain, disfigurement, dependence on others, unemployment, financial problems, inability to participate in social functions, strained relationships with others and spiritual distress. Nurses need to help patients express their thoughts and feelings, and to provide care that helps the patient effectively cope with change.

Ill individuals are also vulnerable to loss of **autonomy**, the state of being independent and self-directed without outside control. Family interactions may change so that the patient may no longer be involved in making family decisions or even decisions about their own healthcare. Nurses need to support the patient's right to **self-determination** and autonomy as much as possible by providing them with sufficient information to participate in decision-making processes and to maintain a feeling of being in control.

Illness also often necessitates a change in lifestyle. In addition to participating in treatments and taking medications, the ill person may need to change diet, activity and exercise, and rest and sleep patterns.

Nurses can help patients adjust their lifestyles by these means:

- providing explanations about necessary adjustments;
- making arrangements wherever possible to accommodate the patient's lifestyle;
- encouraging other healthcare professionals to become aware of the person's lifestyle practices and to support healthy aspects of that lifestyle;
- reinforcing desirable changes in practices with a view to making them a permanent part of the patient's lifestyle.

Impact on the Family

A person's illness affects not only the person who is ill but also the family or significant others. The kind of effect and its extent depend chiefly on three factors: (a) the member of the family who is ill, (b) the seriousness and length of the illness, and (c) the cultural and social customs the family follows.

The changes that can occur in the family include the following:

- role changes;
- task reassignments and increased demands on time;
- increased stress due to anxiety about the outcome of the illness for the patient and conflict about unaccustomed responsibilities;
- financial problems;
- loneliness as a result of separation and pending loss;
- change in social customs.

ACTIVITY 2-3

Susan works full-time in a supermarket and is married with two children aged six years and four years. What affect could George's condition be having on Susan?

FAMILY HEALTH

The family is a basic unit of society. It consists of those individuals, male or female, youth or adult, legally or not legally related, genetically or not genetically related, who are considered by the others to represent the significant persons in their lives. In the nursing profession, interest in the family unit and its impact on the health, values and productivity of individual family members is expressed by family-centred nursing: nursing that considers the health of the family as a unit in addition to the health of individual family members.

Functions of the Family

The economic resources needed by the family are secured by adult members. The family protects the physical health of its members by providing adequate nutrition and healthcare services. Nutritional and lifestyle practices of the family also directly affect the developing health attitudes and lifestyle practices of the children.

In addition to providing an environment conducive to physical growth and health, the family creates an atmosphere that influences the cognitive and the psychosocial growth of its members. Children and adults in healthy, functional families receive support, understanding and encouragement as they progress through predictable developmental stages, as they move in or out of the family unit, and as they establish new family units. In families where members are physically and emotionally nurtured, individuals are challenged to achieve their potential in the family unit. As individual needs are met, family members are able to reach out to others in the family and the community, and to society.

Families from different cultures are an integral part of a country's rich heritage. Each family has values and beliefs that are unique to their culture of origin and that shape the family's structure, methods of interaction, healthcare practices and coping mechanisms. These factors interact to influence the health of families. Families of a particular culture may cluster to form mutual support systems and to preserve their heritage; however, this practice may isolate them from the larger society.

Families consist of persons (structure) and their responsibilities within the family (roles). A family structure of parents and their offspring is known as the **nuclear family**. The relatives of nuclear families, such as grandparents or aunts and uncles, compose the **extended family**. In some families, members of the extended family live with the nuclear family. Although members of the extended family may live in different areas, they may be a source of emotional or financial support for the family. A number of different types of family can be found in UK society:

- **Traditional** – both parents reside in the home with their children.
- **Two-career** – both partners are employed. They may or may not have children.
- **Single-parent** – one parent with children which may be caused by death of a spouse, separation, divorce, birth of a child to an unmarried woman or adoption of a child by a single man or woman.
- **Adolescent** – an adolescent parent with one or more children.
- **Foster** – children who can no longer live with their birth parents may require temporary placement with a family.
- **Blended** – existing family units who join together to form new families. Otherwise known as step or reconstituted families.
- **Intragenerational** – families where more than two generations live in the home.
- **Co-habiting** – consist of unrelated individuals or families who live under the same roof. Sometimes known as communal families.
- **Homosexual** – gay or lesbian families based on the same goals of caring and commitment seen in heterosexual relationships.
- **Single adults living alone** – individuals who live by themselves.

Communication within the Family

The effectiveness of family communication determines the family's ability to function as a cooperative, growth-producing unit. Messages are constantly being communicated among family members, both verbally and nonverbally.

Communication influences how family members work together, fulfil their assigned roles, incorporate family values and develop skills to function in society. Intrafamily communication plays a significant role in the development of self-esteem, which is necessary for the growth of personality and general well-being.

Families use both functional and dysfunctional methods of communication (Bomar, 2004). Open, honest, clear and direct communication improves family relations and allows individual growth and development. Bomar (2004) suggests that functional communication within the family should allow individuals to express their emotions. Functional families support one another and promote an environment which allows members to listen, empathise and reach out to one another during times of crisis.

When patterns of communication among family members are dysfunctional, messages are often communicated unclearly. Verbal communication may be incongruent with nonverbal messages. Power struggles may be evidenced by hostility, anger or silence. Members may be cautious in expressing their feelings because they cannot predict how others in the family will respond. When family communication is impaired, the growth of individual members is stunted. Members often turn to other systems to seek personal validation and gratification.

The nurse needs to observe intrafamily communication patterns closely. Nurses should pay special attention to who does the talking for the family, which members are silent, how disagreements are handled, and how well the members listen to one another and encourage the participation of others. Nonverbal communication is important because it gives valuable clues about what people are feeling.

Family Coping Mechanisms

Family coping mechanisms are the behaviours families use to deal with stress or changes imposed from either within or without. Coping mechanisms can be viewed as an active method of problem solving developed to meet life's challenges. Coping can be described as positive, negative, reactive or active (Shields, 2001) and has both positive and negative effects on the family. The coping mechanisms families and individuals develop reflect their individual resourcefulness. Families may use coping patterns rather consistently over time or may change their coping strategies when new demands are made on the family. The success of a family largely depends on how well it copes with the stresses it experiences.

Nurses working with families realise the importance of assessing coping mechanisms as a way of determining how families relate to stress. Also important are the resources available to the family. Internal resources, such as knowledge, skills, effective communication patterns and a sense of mutuality and purpose within the family, assist in the problem-solving process. In addition, external support systems promote coping and adaptation. These external systems may be extended family, friends, religious affiliations, healthcare professionals or social services. The development of social support systems is particularly valuable today because many families, due to stress, mobility or poverty, are isolated from the resources that would traditionally have helped them cope.

Risk for Health Problems

Risk assessment helps the nurse identify individuals and groups at higher risk than the general population of developing specific health problems, such as stroke, diabetes and lung cancer. The vulnerability of family units to health problems may be based on the maturity level of individual family members, heredity or genetic factors, sex or race, sociological factors and lifestyle practices.

Maturity Factors

Families with members at both ends of the age continuum are at risk of developing health problems. Families entering childbearing and child-rearing phases experience many changes in roles, responsibilities and expectations. The many, often conflicting, demands on the family cause stress and fatigue, which may impede growth of individual family members and the functioning of the group as a unit. Adolescent mothers, because of their developmental level and lack of knowledge about parenthood, and single-parent families, because of role overload experienced by the head of the household, are more likely to develop health problems. Many elderly persons feel a lack of purpose and decreased self-esteem. These feelings in turn reduce their motivation to engage in health-promoting behaviours, such as exercise or community and family involvement.

Hereditary Factors

Persons born into families with a history of certain diseases, such as diabetes or cardiovascular disease, are at greater risk of developing these conditions. A detailed family health history, including genetically transmitted disorders, is crucial to the identification of persons and families at risk. These data are used not only to monitor the health of individual family members but also to recommend modifications in health practices that potentially reduce the risk, minimise the consequences or postpone the development of genetically related conditions.

Gender or Race

Some family units or family members may be at risk of developing a disease by reason of sex or race. Males, for example, are at greater risk of having cardiovascular disease at an earlier age than females, and females are at greater risk of developing osteoporosis, particularly after menopause. Although it is sometimes difficult to separate genetic factors from cultural factors, certain risk factors seem to be related to race. Sickle-cell anaemia, for example, is a hereditary disease limited to people of African descent and Tay-Sachs is a neurodegenerative disease that occurs primarily in descendants of Eastern European Jews.

Sociological Factors

Poverty is a major problem that affects not only the family but also the community and society. Poverty is a real concern among the rising number of single-parent families, and as the number of these families increases, poverty will affect a large number of growing children.

When ill, the poor are likely to put off seeking services until the illness reaches an advanced state and requires longer or more complex treatment. Although the health of the people of industrialised nations has improved significantly during the past century, this progress has not benefited all segments of society, particularly the poor.

Lifestyle Factors

Many diseases are preventable, the effects of some diseases can be minimised or the onset of disease can be delayed through lifestyle modifications. Certain cancers, cardiovascular disease, adult-onset diabetes and tooth decay are among the lifestyle diseases. The incidence of lung cancer, for example, would be greatly reduced if people stopped smoking. Good nutrition, dental hygiene and use of fluoride – in the water supply, in toothpaste, as a **topical** application or as supplements – have been shown to reduce dental decay. Other important lifestyle considerations are exercise, stress management and rest. Today health professionals have the knowledge to prevent or minimise the effects of some of the main causes of disease, disability and death. The challenge is to disseminate information about prevention and to motivate families to make lifestyle changes prior to the onset of illness.

The Family Experiencing a Health Crisis

Illness of a family member is a crisis that affects the entire family system. The family is disrupted as members abandon their usual activities and focus their energy on restoring family equilibrium. Roles and responsibilities previously assumed by the ill person are delegated to other family members, or those functions may remain undone for the duration of the illness. The family experiences anxiety because members are concerned about the sick person and the resolution of the illness. This anxiety is compounded by additional responsibilities when there is less time or motivation to complete the normal tasks of daily living.

The family's ability to deal with the stress of illness depends on the members' coping skills. Families with good communication skills are better able to discuss how they feel about the illness and how it affects family functioning. They can plan for the future and adapt these plans as the situation changes. An established social support network provides strength, encouragement and services to the family during the illness. During health crises, families need to realise that it is a strength, not a sign of weakness, to turn to others for support. Nurses can be part of the support system for families, or they can identify other sources of support in the community.

During a crisis, families are often drawn together by a common purpose. In this time of closeness, family members have the opportunity to reaffirm personal and family values and their commitment to one another. Indeed, illness may provide a unique opportunity for family growth.

The Nurse's Role with Families Experiencing Illness

Nurses committed to family-centred care involve both the ailing individual and the family in the nursing process. Through their interaction with families, nurses can give support and information. Nurses make sure that not only the individual but also each family member understands the disease, its management and the effect of these two factors on family functioning. The nurse also assesses the family's readiness and ability to provide continued care and supervision at home when warranted. After carefully planned instruction and practice, families are given an opportunity to demonstrate their ability to provide care under the supportive guidance of the nurse. When the care indicated is beyond the capability of the family, nurses work with families to identify available resources that are socially and financially acceptable.

In helping families reintegrate the ill person into the home, nurses use data gathered during family assessment to identify family resources and deficits. By formulating mutually acceptable goals for reintegration, nurses help families cope with the realities of the illness and the changes it may have brought about, which may include new roles and functions of family members or the need to provide continued medical care to the ill or recovering person. Working together, nurses and families can create environments that restore or reorganise family functioning during illness and throughout the recovery process.

Death of a Family Member

The death of a family member often has a profound effect on the family. The structure of the family is altered, and this change may in turn affect how it functions as a unit. Individual members experience a sense of loss. They grieve for the lost person and for the family that once was. Family disorganisation may occur. However, as the family begins to recover, a new sense of normality develops, the family reintegrates its roles and functions, and it comes to grips with the reality of the situation. This painful blow takes time to heal.

After the death of a member, families may need counselling to deal with their feelings and to talk about the person who died. They may also want to talk about their fears and hopes for the future. At this time, families often derive comfort from their religious beliefs and their spiritual advisers. Support groups are also available for families experiencing the pain of death. It is often difficult for nurses to deal with grieving families because the nurses also feel the loss and feel inadequate in knowing what to say or do. By understanding the effect death has on families, nurses can help families resolve their grief and move ahead with life.

COMMUNITY HEALTH

Increasingly those requiring healthcare are being managed in the community. A community is a collection of people who share some attribute of their lives. It may be that they live in the same locality, attend a particular church or even share a particular interest such as gardening. Groups that constitute a community because of common member interests are often referred to as a *community of interest* (e.g. religious and cultural groups). A community can also be defined as a social system in which the members interact formally or informally and form networks that operate for the benefit of all people in the community. Five of the main functions of a community are:

- **Production, distribution and consumption of goods and services** – the community provides for the economic needs of its members.
- **Socialisation** – the transmission of values, knowledge, culture and skills to others in the community.
- **Social control** – the way in which the family and community maintain order within the community.
- **Social interparticipation** – community activities that are designed to meet people's needs for companionship.
- **Mutual support** – the community's ability to provide support to its members in times of need.

In community health, the community may be viewed as having a common health problem, such as a high incidence of infant mortality or of tuberculosis, HIV infection, or another communicable disease.

A healthy community:

- is one in which members have a high degree of awareness of being a community;
- uses its natural resources while taking steps to conserve them for future generations;
- openly recognises the existence of subgroups and welcomes their participation in community affairs;
- is prepared to meet crises;
- is a problem-solving community;
- possesses open channels of communication;
- seeks to make each of its systems' resources available to all members;
- has legitimate and effective ways to settle disputes that arise within the community;
- encourages maximum citizen participation in decision making;
- promotes a high level of wellness among all its members.

Community health nursing focuses on promoting and preserving the health of population groups.

Assessing the Community's Health

Several community assessment frameworks have been devised which can be utilised to identify community health needs and target health interventions where they are required. As an example, Anderson and McFarlane (2000) identify eight subsystems of the community for analysis. The subsystems are illustrated around a core, which consists of the people and their characteristics, values, history and beliefs. The first stage in assessment is to learn about the people in the community. Figure 2-3 shows some of the major components of the community core. Surrounding the core are the eight subsystems.

A community assessment needs to consider (Anderson and McFarlane, 2000):

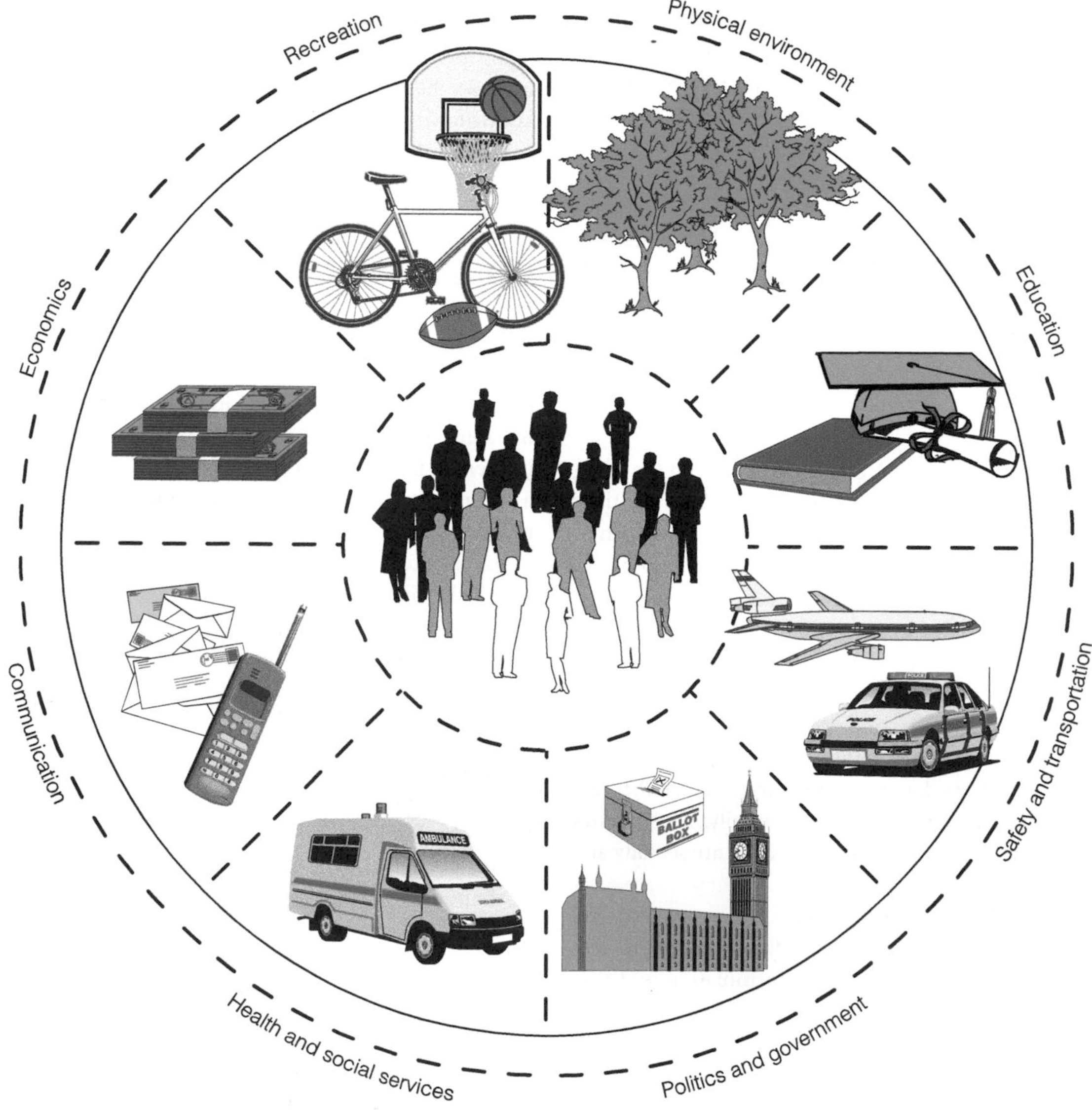

Figure 2-3 The community assessment wheel, the assessment segment of the community-as-partner model.
Source: *Community as partner: Theory and practice in nursing*, 3rd edn (p. 166), by E.T. Anderson and J. McFarlane, 2000, Philadelphia: Lippincott Williams and Wilkins.

- the physical environment
- education
- safety and transportation
- local and national politics and government
- health and social services
- communication
- economics
- recreation.

Community assessment data can be accessed from a number of sources including ordinance survey maps, local census data, employment statistics, health board statistics and health facilities, local telephone book, online services and libraries.

CULTURAL CARE

In order to provide quality care to individuals, families and the community as a whole, nurses must be informed about and sensitive to the cultural diversity of UK society. Cultural care is professional nursing care that is culturally sensitive, culturally appropriate and culturally competent respecting the patient's individuality. Cultural care is critical to meeting the complex nursing care needs of a given person, family and community. It is the provision of nursing care across cultural boundaries and takes into account the context in which the patient lives as well as the situations in which the patient's health problems arise.

- **Culturally sensitive** implies that the nurse possesses some basic knowledge of and constructive attitudes towards the health traditions observed among the diverse cultural groups found in the setting in which they are practising.
- **Culturally appropriate** implies that the nurse applies the underlying background knowledge that must be possessed to provide a given patient with the best possible healthcare.
- **Culturally competent** implies that within the delivered care the nurse understands and attends to the total context of the patient's situation and uses a complex combination of knowledge, attitudes and skills.

Culture can be defined as the nonphysical traits, such as values, beliefs, attitudes and customs, that are shared by a group of people and passed from one generation to the next (Tseng and Streltzer, 2008). Culture also defines how health is perceived; how healthcare information is received; how rights and protections are exercised; what is considered to be a health problem and how symptoms and concerns about the health problem are expressed; who should provide treatment and how; and what kind of treatment should be given.

Nurses must be aware that, although people from a given group share certain beliefs, values and experiences, often there is also widespread intra-group diversity. Major differences within groups may be due to such factors as age, gender, level of education, socioeconomic status and area of origin in the home country (rural or urban). Such factors influence the patient's beliefs about health and illness, practices, help-seeking behaviours and expectations of nurses. For these reasons, effort must be made and care taken to avoid the stereotyping of people from a specific group.

Countless conflicts in the healthcare setting can be predicted on cultural misunderstandings. Although many of these misunderstandings are related to universal situations, such as verbal and nonverbal language misunderstandings, the conventions of courtesy, sequencing of interactions, phasing of interactions, objectivity, and so forth, many cultural misunderstandings are unique to the delivery of nursing care. Cultural sensitivity is essential and it demands that nurses be able to assess and interpret a given patient's health beliefs and practices, and cultural needs.

Concepts Related to Cultural Care

All groups of people face issues in adapting to their environment: providing nutrition and shelter, caring for and educating children, dividing labour, developing social organisation, controlling disease and maintaining health. Humans adapt to varying environments by developing cultural solutions to meet these needs. Culture is a universal experience, but no two cultures are exactly alike. Cultural patterns are learned, and it is important for nurses to note that members of a particular group may not share identical cultural experiences. Thus, each member of a cultural group will be somewhat different from their own cultural counterparts.

Subculture

Large cultural groups often have cultural subgroups or subsystems. A subculture is usually composed of people who have a distinct identity and yet are related to a larger cultural group. A subcultural group generally shares ethnic origin, occupation or physical characteristics with the larger cultural group. Examples of cultural subgroups include occupational groups (e.g. nurses), societal groups (e.g. feminists) and ethnic groups.

Bicultural

Bicultural is used to describe a person who crosses two cultures, lifestyles and sets of values (Giger and Davidhizar, 1999). For example, a young man whose father is Asian and whose mother is British may honour his traditional heritage while also being influenced by his mother's cultural values.

Diversity

Diversity refers to the fact or state of being different. Many factors account for diversity: race, gender, sexual orientation, culture, ethnicity, socioeconomic status, educational attainment, religious affiliation, and so on. Diversity therefore occurs not only between cultural groups but also within a cultural group.

Assimilation

Assimilation is the process by which an individual develops a new cultural identity. Assimilation means becoming like the members of the dominant culture. The process of assimilation encompasses various aspects, such as behavioural, marital, identification and civic. The underlying assumption is that the person from a given cultural group loses their original cultural identity to acquire the new one. In fact, because this is a conscious effort, it is not always possible, and the process may cause severe stress and anxiety. Assimilation can also be described as a collection of subprocesses: a process of inclusion through which a person gradually ceases to conform to any standard of life that differs from the dominant group standards and, at the same time, a process through which the person learns to conform to all the dominant group standards. The process of assimilation is considered complete when the foreigner is fully merged into the dominant cultural group (McLemore *et al.*, 2001).

The concepts of assimilation and acculturation are complex and sensitive. The dominant society expects that all immigrants are in the process of acculturation and assimilation and that the world view that we share as nurses is commonly shared by our patients. Because we live in a society with many cultures, however, many variations of health beliefs and practices exist. Several other factors for cultural consideration include race, prejudice, stereotyping, discrimination and culture shock.

Race

Race is the classification of people according to shared biological characteristics, genetic markers or features. People of the same race have common characteristics such as skin colour, bone structure, facial features, hair texture and blood type. Different ethnic groups can belong to the same race and different cultures can be found within one ethnic group. It is important to understand that not all people of the same race have the same culture. Culture should not be confused with either race or ethnic group.

Prejudice

Prejudice is a negative belief or preference that is generalised about a group and that leads to 'prejudgement'. Prejudice occurs because either the person making the judgement does not understand the given person or his or her heritage, or the person making the judgement generalises an experience of one individual from a culture to all members of that group.

Stereotyping

Stereotyping is assuming that all members of a culture or ethnic group are alike. For example, a nurse may assume that all Italians verbally express pain loudly or that all Chinese people like rice. Stereotyping may be based on generalisations founded in research or it may be unrelated to reality. For example, research indicates that most Italians are likely to express pain verbally; however, a specific Italian patient may not do so. Stereotyping that is unrelated to reality is frequently an outcome of racism or discrimination. Nurses need to realise that not all people of a specific group have the same health beliefs, practices and values. It is therefore essential to identify a specific patient's beliefs, needs and values rather than assuming they are the same as those attributable to the larger group.

Discrimination

Discrimination, the differential treatment of individuals or groups based on categories such as race, ethnicity, gender, social class or exceptionality, occurs when a person acts on prejudice and denies another person one or more of the fundamental rights.

Culture Shock

Culture shock is a disorder that occurs in response to transition from one cultural setting to another. A person's former behaviour patterns are ineffective in such a setting, and basic cues for social behaviour are absent (Spectra, 2000). This phenomenon may occur when one moves from one geographic location to another or when a person immigrates to a new country. It may occur when a person is admitted into a hospital and has to adapt to a foreign situation. Expressions of culture shock may range from silence and immobility to agitation, rage or fury.

Ethnicity

Cultural background is a fundamental component of one's ethnic background or ethnicity, a group within the social system that claims to possess variable traits such as a common religion or language. The term *ethnic* has for some time aroused strongly negative feelings and often is rejected by the general population.

Religion

The third major component of a person's heritage is religion. Although the word has many definitions, religion may be considered a system of beliefs, practices and ethical values about divine or superhuman power or powers worshipped as the creator(s) and ruler(s) of the universe. The practice of religion is revealed in numerous cults, sects, denominations and churches. Ethnicity and religion are clearly related, and one's religion quite often is determined by one's ethnic group. Religion gives a person a frame of reference and a perspective with which to organise information. Religious teachings *vis-à-vis* health help to present a meaningful philosophy and system of practices within a system of social controls having specific values, norms and ethics. These are related to health in that compliance to a religious code is conducive to spiritual harmony. Illness is sometimes seen as the punishment for the violation of religious codes and morals. It is not possible to isolate the aspects of culture, religion and ethnicity that shape a person's world view. Each is part of the other and all three are united within the person.

Socialisation

Socialisation is the process of being raised within a culture and acquiring the characteristics of that group. Education – be it primary school, secondary school, college or nursing – is a form of socialisation. In addition, many people who have been socialised in cultures wherein traditional healthcare resources are used may prefer to use this type of care even when residing within a cultural setting with modern healthcare resources available.

HEALTHCARE DELIVERY: SETTINGS AND PROCESS

Healthcare in the UK has changed dramatically since the advent of the National Health Service in 1948. Healthcare in the 21st century is influenced by an ageing population and technological advances. However, the drive for a healthy society is an ever-increasing focus of the UK government with a range of initiatives aimed at improving the health of individuals, families and communities.

The population of the UK is ageing. In 2008, over 16% or 24 million people were aged 65 and over, while the percentage of the population aged 16 years and under dropped to 19% (Office of National Statistics (ONS), 2009). These statistics are compounded by a society that is becoming increasingly obese and physically inactive (The NHS Information Centre, Lifestyle Statistics, 2009).

Traditionally most healthcare needs have been met by the NHS. However, the strain on the NHS is overwhelming. In a bid to meet the ever-growing needs of the population and to modernise healthcare delivery in the UK, government ministers are planning a huge shake-up of current healthcare delivery systems. For example, the reform 'Commissioning a Patient Led NHS' aims to reorganise local healthcare bodies so that private firms can provide services such as district nursing and podiatry to patients in the community. Such reforms aim to improve patient care, save money and raise morale within the NHS, and are moving healthcare from the traditional hospital-based care to more diverse healthcare settings.

The National Health Service (NHS)

We tend to take the NHS for granted. But just think what healthcare was like before the NHS – a luxury that only a few could afford. Life in the 1930s and 1940s was tough especially during the Second World War. Infectious diseases such as tuberculosis, diphtheria and polio were rife and infant mortality was at an all-time high with one in 20 infants dying before they reached a year old.

Healthcare was generally free to workers who were on lower pay through National Health Insurance but this did not cover their wives or their children. Also, workers who earned a little more were unable to access free healthcare. This meant that many went without medical treatment or relied on dubious home remedies. Some doctors and hospitals, such as the Royal Free Hospital in London, however, did give their services for free to those poorer patients. Despite these efforts to provide medical care to patients it was recognised that there needed to be a fairer way of delivering healthcare in the UK.

The NHS was the result of decades of reports and campaigns to improve healthcare in the UK and began with the Dawson Report in 1920, which recommended a comprehensive healthcare system for the UK. In 1926 the Royal Commission on National Health Insurance was developed, which brought about the idea of publicly funded healthcare. Then during the Second World War the Emergency Medical Services sped up the process of a unified healthcare system. In 1941 the government commissioned an independent inquiry into healthcare across the UK and found that healthcare provision varied vastly. Then in 1942 the Beveridge report into social care identified a national health service as one of three essential elements for a viable social security system.

On 5 July 1948 the NHS was introduced and transformed the lives of millions of people almost instantly. However, its first few years were difficult. In post-war Britain, food was still being rationed; and building materials, fuel and housing were in short supply. This along with the fact that all those who were unable to afford healthcare in the past and now wanted access to its free medical care meant that the new NHS was put under extreme pressure.

It became apparent that the need far exceeded what was estimated, including the cost. The concept of the NHS was that medical care was free at the point of delivery but in 1952 a small charge for prescriptions was introduced as a means of recouping some of the costs. Despite these and other problems that have faced the NHS through the years it has been heralded as a success that has changed the lives of many within the UK.

The NHS today is somewhat different with more advanced medical procedures, coping with an increasing and ageing population and the advent of information technology. However, the concept of the NHS remains the same: to provide healthcare free at the point of delivery.

The primary purpose of the NHS is to provide care to the ill and injured and it is structured with this in mind. However, with increasing awareness of health promotion, illness prevention and levels of wellness, there is a drive for healthcare systems and the role of nurses to change.

Within the four countries of the UK – England, Wales, Scotland and Northern Ireland – there are significant differences in how the NHS is operated and structured (see *Boxes 2-1* and *2-2*, *Boxes 2-3* and *2-4*). However, the fundamental philosophy to provide essential services free at the point of delivery is the same throughout.

The NHS is the fourth largest employer in the world, currently employing 1.3 million, and is a key public service and the basis for the welfare state within the UK. It is an ever-evolving entity that is structured and managed by the UK government. Up until now the NHS has taken many guises, being structured by different reforms, White Papers and plans. A report by the Department of Health (DH, 2009c) outlines a five-year plan for the NHS, which aims to reshape the NHS to meet the challenge of delivering high quality care in a difficult financial climate. The vision of this report is that by 2015 the NHS should be preventative, people-centred and productive, giving patients greater choice and encouraging partnership.

BOX 2-1 Structure of the NHS in England (April 2009)

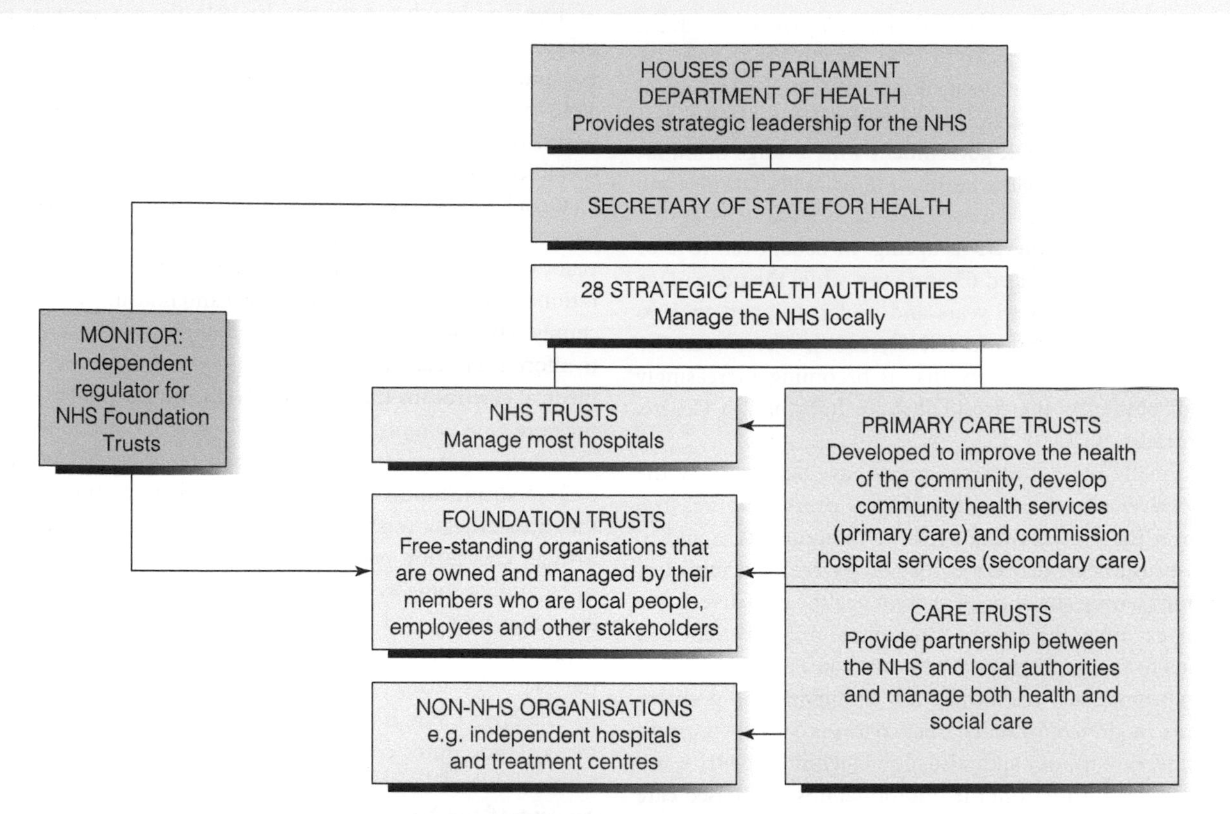

Source: Galloway, M. (2009) *The ACP guide to the structure of the NHS in the UK*. London: Association of Clinical Pathologists.

BOX 2-2 Structure of the NHS in Wales (April 2009)

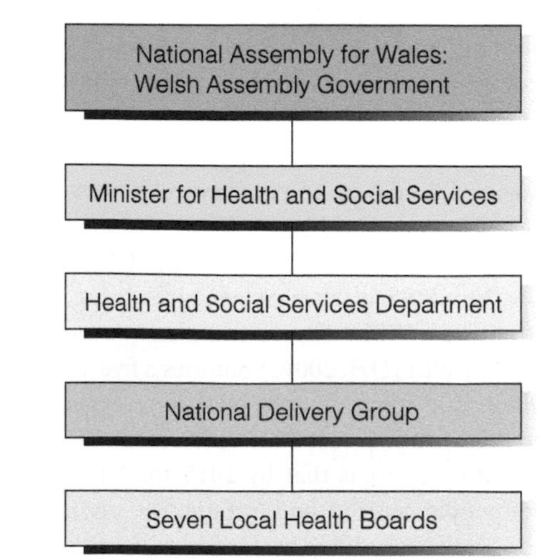

Source: adapted from Galloway, M. (2009) *The ACP guide to the structure of the NHS in the UK*. London: Association of Clinical Pathologists.

BOX 2-3 Structure of the NHS in Scotland (April 2009)

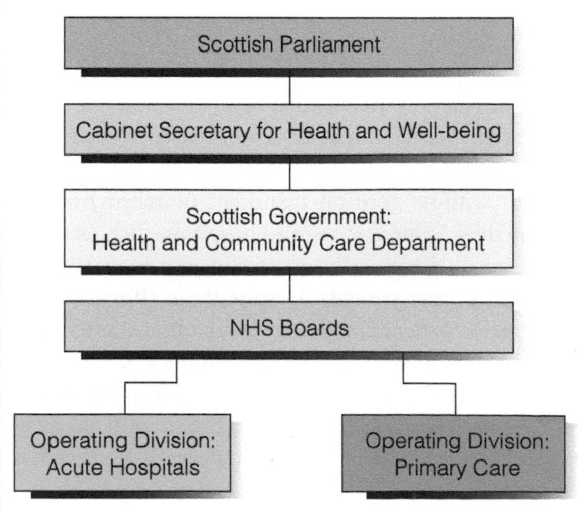

Source: adapted from Galloway, M. (2009) *The ACP guide to the structure of the NHS in the UK*. London: Association of Clinical Pathologists.

BOX 2-4 Structure of the NHS in Northern Ireland (April 2009)

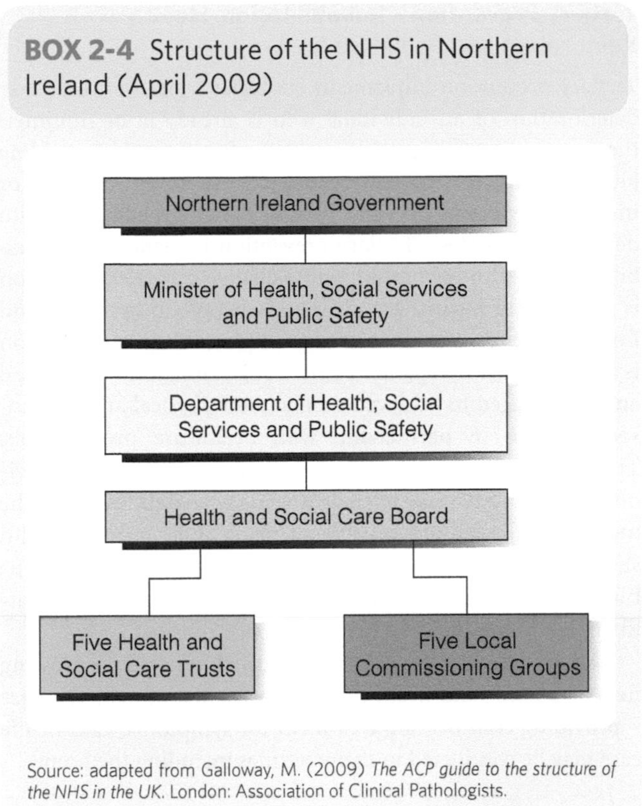

Source: adapted from Galloway, M. (2009) *The ACP guide to the structure of the NHS in the UK*. London: Association of Clinical Pathologists.

Types of Healthcare Agencies and Services

Both private and public sector providers deliver healthcare services within the UK. Some healthcare providers offer a number of different services to patients; for example, a hospital may provide acute inpatient services, outpatient clinics and accident and emergency services. Patients may be seen by any number and type of providers depending on their healthcare needs.

The NHS offers a range of services across primary and secondary care (see Figure 2-4). Primary care is usually the first point of contact for most people. It offers a range of services and provides access to a number of healthcare professionals, including general practitioners (GPs), nurses, dentists, pharmacists and opticians. The care provided usually deals with the treatment of minor injuries and illnesses as well as preventive care, such as services to help people stop smoking. Although primary care is concerned primarily with general healthcare needs there is a drive to provide more specialist services and treatments in the primary care setting.

Secondary care or acute care is the care provided in or by hospitals (NHS Trusts) and usually encompasses both elective care and emergency care. Elective care are those procedures that are seen as not urgent, not compulsory, routine or planned, while emergency care is care that is needed to maintain life or prevent further damage. Secondary care is offered by ambulance trusts, NHS Trusts, Local Health Boards (in Wales), Mental Health Trusts and Care Trusts.

Other healthcare services available include occupational health clinics, **physiotherapy** clinics, residential and nursing homes, rehabilitation centres and homecare agencies. These services can be offered by both the public and private sector.

Types of Healthcare Services

Three types of healthcare services are often described in correlation with levels of disease prevention: (a) primary prevention, which involves implementing strategies to improve health and prevent illness; (b) secondary prevention, which is concerned

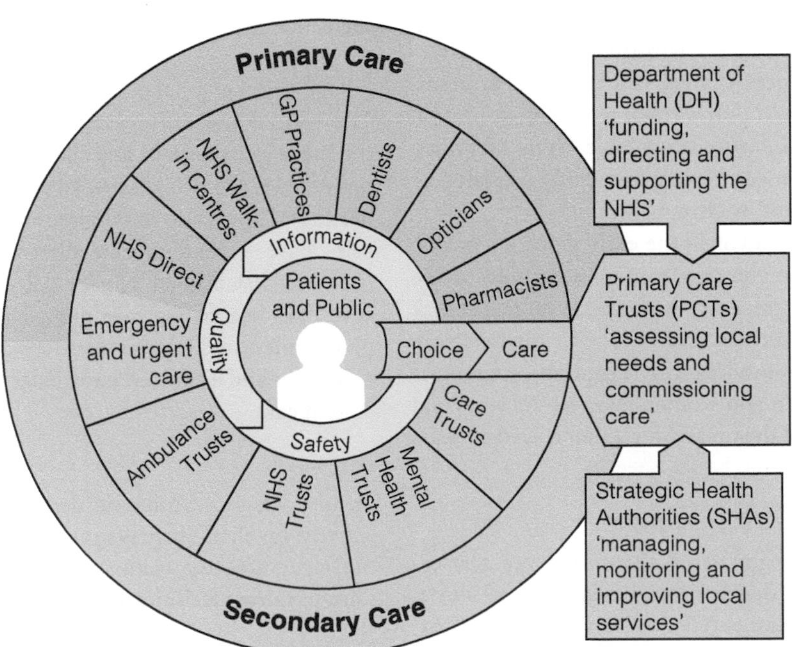

Figure 2-4 Types of healthcare services offered by the NHS.
Source: About the NHS, **http://www.nhs.uk/NHSEngland/thenhs/about/Pages/nhsstructure.aspx**

with the diagnosis and treatment of illness and disease; and (c) tertiary prevention, which involves rehabilitation and health restoration.

Primary Prevention – Health Improvement and Illness Prevention

When the NHS was established in 1948, one of its main principles was to improve health and prevent disease and not just treat those who are ill. However, much of the healthcare provided within the NHS is aimed at diagnosis and treatment of ill health.

Primary prevention is concerned with identifying factors that can affect health and educating people about these factors in order for those individuals to make lifestyle changes. In 2004, the Government issued a White Paper 'Choosing Health, Making Healthier Choices Easier' in a bid to improve the health of the nation. This report outlines the main health issues faced by the population and identifies strategies to tackle these. According to the report, the main priorities are to tackle health inequalities, reduction in the number of people who smoke, obesity, improving sexual health, improving mental health and encouraging sensible levels of alcohol consumption. The proposed strategy for tackling these problems involves raising awareness of health risks and implementing campaigns to educate people to make healthier lifestyle choices. The main principle of this document is emphasising the important role individuals play in maintaining their own health. Although this White Paper has not been superseded, a report in 2007 (DH, 2007) suggests that many of its recommendations have been achieved through government action, engaging communities and engaging people through information.

Illness prevention programmes may be directed at the patient or the community and involve such practices as providing immunisations, identifying risk factors for illnesses, and helping people take measures to prevent these illnesses from occurring. Illness prevention also includes environmental programmes that can reduce the incidence of illness or disability. For example, steps to decrease air pollution include requiring inspection of car exhaust systems to ensure acceptable levels of fumes. Environmental protective measures are frequently legislated by governments and lobbied for by citizens groups.

Primary prevention also involves the early detection of disease. This is accomplished through routine screening of the population and focused screening of those at increased risk of developing certain conditions. Examples of early detection services include the new bowel cancer screening programme introduced in 2006 for men and women aged 60–69 years and mammograms (an x-ray of the breast) for women aged 50 years and over.

Secondary Prevention – Diagnosis and Treatment

In the past, the largest segment of the healthcare services has been dedicated to the diagnosis and treatment of illness. Hospitals and general practitioner (GP) services have been instrumental in offering these complex services. Hospitals continue to focus significant resources on patients requiring emergency, intensive and round-the-clock acute care.

Tertiary Prevention – Rehabilitation, Health Restoration and Palliative Care

Tertiary prevention implements strategies to minimise further deterioration of an individual who is already ill or minimise the symptoms of that disease process, for example, providing kidney dialysis for a person whose kidneys do not function or insulin to a person who has Type 1 Diabetes mellitus (insulin dependent diabetes). Tertiary prevention is made up of rehabilitation, health restoration and palliative care. Rehabilitation is a process of restoring ill or injured people to optimum and functional levels of wellness, for example cardiac rehabilitation is a process by which patients with cardiac disease are supported and encouraged to achieve and maintain physical and psychosocial health in partnership with healthcare professionals. The goal of rehabilitation is to help people move to their previous level of health (i.e. to their previous capabilities) or to the highest level they are capable of given their current health status. Rehabilitation may begin in the hospital, but will eventually lead patients back into the community for further treatment and follow-up once health has been restored.

Sometimes, people cannot be returned to health. A growing field of nursing and healthcare services is that of palliative care – providing comfort and treatment for symptoms. End-of-life care may be conducted in many settings including the home.

Providers of Healthcare

The providers of healthcare, also referred to as the healthcare team or health professionals, are health personnel from different disciplines who coordinate their skills to assist patients and those who support them. Their mutual goal is to restore a patient's health and promote wellness. The choice of personnel for a particular patient depends on the needs of the patient. Health teams commonly include the nurse and some or all of the personnel that follow.

Nurse

The role of the nurse varies with the needs of the patient, the nurse's credentials, and the type of employment setting. A registered nurse (RN) assesses a patient's health status, identifies health problems and develops and coordinates care. As nursing roles have expanded, new dimensions for nursing practice have been established. Nurses can pursue a variety of practice specialties (e.g. critical care, mental health and oncology). Nurse practitioners and clinical nurse specialists have the appropriate education and advanced knowledge to provide direct specialist patient care.

Dentist

Dentists diagnose and treat dental problems. Dentists are also actively involved in preventive measures to maintain healthy oral structures (e.g. teeth and gums). Many hospitals, especially long-term care facilities, have dentists on their staff.

Dietician

When dietary and nutritional services are required, the dietician or nutritionist may be a member of a health team. A registered dietician has specialist knowledge about the diets required to maintain health and to treat disease. Dieticians in hospitals generally are concerned with therapeutic diets, may design special diets to meet the nutritional needs of individual patients, and supervise the preparation of meals to ensure that patients receive the proper diet.

Occupational Therapist

An occupational therapist (OT) assists patients with an impaired function to gain the skills to perform activities of daily living. For example, an occupational therapist might teach a man with severe arthritis in his arms and hands how to adjust his kitchen utensils so that he can continue to cook. The occupational therapist teaches skills that are therapeutic and at the same time provide some fulfilment. For example, weaving is a recreational activity but also exercises the arthritic man's arms and hands.

Technologists

Laboratory technologists, radiological technologists and pathologists are just three kinds of technologists in the expanding field of medical technology. *Pathologists* examine specimens such as urine, faeces, blood and discharges from wounds to provide exact information that facilitates the medical diagnosis and the prescription of a therapeutic regimen. The radiologist assists with a wide variety of x-ray film procedures, from simple chest radiography to more complex fluoroscopy. These technologists have highly specialised skills and knowledge important to patient care.

Pharmacist

A pharmacist prepares and dispenses pharmaceuticals in hospital and community settings. The role of the pharmacist in monitoring and evaluating the actions and effects of medications on patients is becoming increasingly prominent. A pharmacy assistant works in the pharmacy under the direction of the pharmacist.

Physiotherapist

Physiotherapists assist patients with musculoskeletal problems. Physiotherapists treat movement dysfunctions by means of heat, water, exercise, massage and electric current. Their functions include assessing patient mobility and strength, providing therapeutic measures (e.g. exercises and heat applications to improve mobility and strength) and teaching new skills (e.g. how to walk with an artificial leg). Some physiotherapists provide their services in hospitals; however, independent practitioners establish offices in communities and serve patients either at the office or in the home. Physiotherapy assistants also work with physiotherapists and patients.

Doctor

The doctor is responsible for medical diagnosis and for determining the treatment required by a person who has a disease or injury. Their role has traditionally been the treatment of disease and trauma (injury) but many doctors are now including health promotion and disease prevention in their practice. Some doctors are surgeons, oncologists, orthopaedists, paediatricians or psychiatrists.

Podiatrist

Podiatrists, previously known as chiropodists, diagnose and treat foot conditions. They may work within a hospital or privately.

Social Worker

A social worker counsels patients and support people to overcome their social problems, such as finances, marital difficulties and adoption of children. It is not unusual for health problems to produce problems in living and vice versa. For example, an elderly woman who lives alone and has a stroke resulting in impaired walking may find it impossible to continue to live in her third-floor apartment. Finding a more suitable living arrangement can be the responsibility of the social worker if the patient has no support network in place.

Spiritual Support Person

Chaplains, pastors, rabbis, priests and other religious or spiritual advisers serve as part of the healthcare team by attending to the spiritual needs of patients. In most facilities, local clergy volunteer their services on a regular or on-call basis. They usually offer regularly scheduled religious services. The nurse is often instrumental in identifying the patient's desire for spiritual support and notifying the appropriate person.

Healthcare Support Workers

Healthcare support workers are healthcare staff who assume delegated aspects of patient care. These tasks include bathing, assisting with feeding, and collecting specimens.

It is important to note that there can be significant overlaps among those providers who can perform certain healthcare activities. For example, a doctor, a nurse or a physiotherapist may be responsible for assisting a person with breathing problems.

Factors Affecting Healthcare Delivery

Today's healthcare users have greater knowledge about their health than in previous years and they are increasingly influencing healthcare delivery. Formerly, people expected a doctor to make decisions about their care but today patients are no longer passive recipients of healthcare but actively participate in their own healthcare, with many aware of how lifestyle affects health. However, it is not just the individual that affects the healthcare delivery system.

Increasing Number of Older Adults

By the year 2033 it is estimated that almost one quarter (23%) of the adult population in the UK will be over the age of 65 (Office for National Statistics, 2009). Chronic illnesses and disability are prevalent among this group who frequently require health and social care support.

The ageing population has changed the look of the NHS. Older adults are the main users of health and social care services. In 2003–04 43% of the NHS budget was spent on providing care for people aged 65 and over (Commission for Healthcare Audit and Inspection, 2006) but their needs have not always been met. However in 2001, the **National Service Framework** (DH, 2001) for older people was introduced in a bid to ensure that high-quality integrated health and social care is provided to older adults. It outlines a ten-year programme aimed at improving health and social care services for the older adult and considers the following (Baggot, 2004):

- age discrimination;
- person-centred care;
- intermediate care;
- general hospital care for older people;
- stroke prevention;
- falls;
- older people with mental health problems;
- the promotion of active, healthy life in older people.

Although the NSF has not been reviewed, there have been significant developments in government policy including *Opportunity age – meeting the challenges of ageing in the 21st Century* (Department of Work and Pensions, 2005) and *Independence, well-being and choice: our vision for the future of social care for adults in England* (DH, 2005), which set out plans for the future of health and social care for older adults.

Advances in Technology

Scientific knowledge and technology related to healthcare are rapidly increasing. Improved diagnostic procedures and sophisticated equipment permit early recognition of diseases that might otherwise have remained undetected. New antibiotics and medications are continually being manufactured to treat infections and multiple drug-resistant organisms. Surgical procedures involving the heart, lungs and liver that were nonexistent 20 years ago are common today. Laser and microscopic procedures streamline the treatment of diseases that required surgery in the past.

Computers, bedside charting and the ability to store and retrieve large volumes of information in databases are commonplace in healthcare organisations. In addition, as a result of the Internet and web, patients now have access to medical information similar to that of healthcare providers (although not all websites provide accurate information!).

These discoveries have changed the profile of the patient. Patients are now more likely to be treated in the community, utilising resources, technology and treatments outside the hospital. For example, years ago a person having cataract surgery had to remain in bed in the hospital for ten days; today, most cataract removals are performed on an outpatient basis in outpatient surgery centres. These technological advances and specialised treatments and procedures may come, unfortunately, with a high price tag.

Social and Economic Factors

Social and economic status has a profound impact on health. Social class particularly has an influence on the individual's health status. Life expectancy varies considerably between social classes (Office of National Statistics, 2007). People considered to be in the lower social classes (Social Class III–V, see Box 2-5) are at increased risk of dying from cardiovascular disease, including heart disease and stroke, than those who are in higher social classes (Social Class I–II) (DH, 2009b).

BOX 2-5 Registrar General's Classification of Social Class

SOCIAL CLASS I	Professional occupations
SOCIAL CLASS II	Managerial and technical occupations
SOCIAL CLASS III (N)	Skilled occupations, nonmanual
SOCIAL CLASS III (M)	Skilled occupation, manual
SOCIAL CLASS IV	Partly skilled occupations
SOCIAL CLASS V	Unskilled occupations

There are many theories why social class should influence health in this way. One such theory is that social class differences in health arise from social selection (Stern, 1983). This means that healthy people tend to move up the social classes whereas unhealthy people tend to stay in the lower social classes (IV and V). In other words the individual's health status produces social inequalities.

Access to Health Services

Access to healthcare services is essential to the maintenance of good health. However, it is not just access to any healthcare but to good quality healthcare that is essential. A number of factors impede such access, including financial barriers, geographic considerations and social class. For patients living in rural areas this may mean that they have to travel long distances for treatment. For example, coronary heart bypass surgery, a surgical treatment for coronary heart disease, is only offered in two hospitals in South Wales. This means that patients living in North Wales have to travel to Liverpool for this type of surgery.

There is also the issue that some treatments are available on the NHS in some parts of the country but not in others, otherwise known as the 'postcode lottery' of healthcare services. One such example is the 'Herceptin postcode lottery' where the drug was offered to breast cancer patients in some areas but not to those in other areas.

Demographic Changes

The characteristics of the UK population are ever evolving. There are certain points in an individual's life that makes him or her more prone to health problems. Accidents and injuries are the most likely cause of death in younger people, while cancers and circulatory diseases usually afflict the older age groups.

Despite people living longer, the prevalence of chronic illness and disability is still high. This means that although life expectancy has increased this is usually plagued by ill health or disability.

Health and healthcare delivery in the UK is dependent on a number of factors including its setting and factors such as population demographics. However, effective healthcare delivery is also dependent on appropriate frameworks for the delivery of that care. Frameworks of care are basically ways in which effective and efficient health and nursing care is delivered to patients.

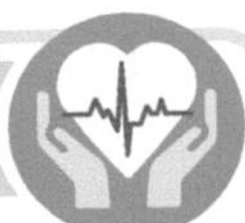

CRITICAL REFLECTION

Let us revisit the case study on page 19. Now that you have read this chapter what is the difference between an acute and chronic illness? Which health belief models could you use in your explanation? How may George define health? What factors could affect George and his health?

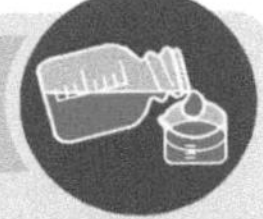

CHAPTER HIGHLIGHTS

- An individual's health beliefs influence their health practices.
- Most people describe health as freedom from symptoms of disease, the ability to be active and a state of being in good spirits.
- Internal variables include biological, psychological and cognitive dimensions. The biological dimension includes genetic makeup, sex, age and developmental level. The psychological dimension includes mind-body interactions and self-concept. The cognitive dimension includes lifestyle choices and spiritual and religious beliefs.
- External variables influencing health are physical environment, standards of living, family and cultural beliefs, and social support networks.
- Illness is usually associated with disease but may occur independently of it. Illness is a highly personal state in which the person feels unhealthy or ill. Disease alters body functions and results in a reduction of capacities or a shortened life span.
- Various theorists have described stages and aspects of illness. Parsons describes four aspects of the sick role. Suchman outlines five stages of illness: symptom experience, assumption of the sick role, medical care contact, dependent patient role, and recovery or rehabilitation.
- Nursing involves viewing the patient as an individual and in a holistic way.
- To ensure holistic healthcare, the nurse considers all components of health (health promotion, health maintenance, health education and illness prevention, and restorative-rehabilitative care) and recognises that disturbance in one part of a person affects the whole being.
- The family is the basic unit of society.
- The family plays an important role in forming the health beliefs and practices of its members.
- Family-centred nursing addresses the health of the family as a unit, as well as the health of family members.
- A community is a collection of people who share some attribute of their lives.
- For community assessment, eight subsystems proposed by Anderson and McFarlane can be used: physical environment, education, safety and transportation, politics and government, health and social services, communication, economics and recreation.
- Healthcare delivery services can be categorised as primary, secondary or tertiary and, generally, they can also be grouped by the type of service: (1) health promotion and illness prevention, (2) diagnosis and treatment and (3) rehabilitation.
- Hospitals provide a wide variety of services on an inpatient and outpatient basis.
- Various providers of healthcare coordinate their skills to assist a patient. Their mutual goal is to restore a patient's health and promote wellness.
- The many factors affecting healthcare delivery include the increasing number of older people, advances in knowledge and technology, socioeconomics, access to healthcare and demographic changes.

ACTIVITY ANSWERS

ACTIVITY 2-1 George appears to define health in physical terms linking health with a good diet and exercise and doesn't seem to recognise the psychological dimension of health.

ACTIVITY 2-2 Factors that may have influenced George's health include: loss of his wife, social isolation, alcohol consumption, and loss of his job.

ACTIVITY 2-3 Susan may now feel as if there is a change to her role within the family as she now has to care for her father. This places increased demands on her and her family which could lead to stress and anxiety.

REFERENCES

Acheson, D. (1998) Independent Inquiry into Inequalities in Health Report, London: The Stationary Office.

Anderson, E.T. and McFarlane, J. (2000) *Community as partner: Theory and practice in nursing* (3rd edn), Philadelphia: Lippincott Williams and Wilkins.

Anspaugh, D.J., Hamrick, M. and Rosata, F.D. (2008) *Wellness: Concepts and applications* (5th edn), New York: McGraw-Hill.

Baggott, R. (2004) *Health and healthcare in Britain*, Basingstoke: Palgrave Macmillan.

Bandura, A. (1986) *Social foundations of thought and action: A social cognitive theory*, New Jersey: Prentice-Hall.

Bomar, P.J. (2004) *Promoting health in families. Applying family research and theory to nursing practice*, Philadelphia: Saunders.

Carson, V.B. (1989) *Spiritual dimension of nursing practice*, Philadelphia: Saunders.

Commission for Healthcare Audit and Inspection (2006) *Living well in later life: A review of progress against the National Service Framework for Older People*, London: Commission for Healthcare Audit and Inspection.

DH (2001) *National Service Framework for Older People*, London: DH.

DH (2005) *Independence, well-being and choice: Our vision for the future of social care for adults in England*, London: DH.

DH (2007) *Choosing Health: Progress Report – April 2007*, London: DH.

DH (2008) *Healthy weight: Healthy lives*, London: DH.

DH (2009a) *Be active, be healthy: A plan for getting the nation moving*, London: DH.

DH (2009b) *Tackling health inequalities: 10 years on. A review of developments in tackling health inequalities in England over the last 10 years*, London: DH.

DH (2009c) *NHS 2010–2015: from good to great. Preventative, people-centred, productive*, London: DH.

Department of Work and Pensions (2005) *Opportunity age – meeting the challenges of the 21st century*, London: DWP.

Giger, J.N. and Davidhizar, R. (1999) *Transcultural nursing: Assessment and intervention* (3rd edn), St. Louis, MO: Mosby.

Hubley, J. and Copeman, J. (2008) *Practical health promotion*, Cambridge: Polity Press.

Hurdle, D.E. (2001) 'Social support: A critical factor in women's health and health promotion', *Health and Social Work*, 26(2): 72–79.

Maslow, A. (1943) 'A theory of human motivation', *Psychological Review*, 50: 370–396.

McLemore, S., Romo, H.D. and Baker, S.G. (2001) *Racial and ethnic relations in America* (6th edn), Needham Heights, MA: Allyn and Bacon.

Naidoo, J. and Wills, J. (2004) *Health promotion: Foundations for practice* (2nd edn), London: Bailliere Tindall.

Nightingale, F. (1969) *Notes on nursing: What it is, and what it is not*, New York: Dover Books. (Original work published in 1860.)

NMC – Nursing and Midwifery Council (2010) *Standards for pre-registration nursing education*, London: NMC.

Nordenfelt, L. (2007) 'The concepts of health and illness revisited', *Medicine, Healthcare and Philosophy*, 10: 5–10.

Office for National Statistics (2007) *Variations persist in life expectancy by social class.* Available from http://www.statistics.gov.uk/pdfdir/le1007.pdf (Accessed 5/3/2010.)

Office of National Statistics (2009) *Ageing.* Available from http://www.statistics.gov.uk/cci/nugget.asp?ID=949 (Accessed 5/3/2010.)

Parsons, T. (1979) 'Definitions of health and illness in the light of American values and social structure', in E.G. Jaco (ed.), *Patients, physicians, and illness* (3rd edn), New York: Free Press.

Shields, N. (2001) 'Stress, active coping and academic performance among persisting and nonpersisting students', *Journal of Applied Biobehavioural Research*, 6(2): 65–81.

Smith, R. (1987) *Unemployment and health: A disaster or a challenge?*, Oxford: Oxford University Press.

Spectra, R.E. (2000) *Cultural diversity in health and illness* (5th edn), Upper Saddle River, NJ: Prentice Hall.

Stern, J. (1983) 'Social mobility and the interpretation of social class mortality differentials', *Journal of Social Policy*, 12(1): 27–49.

Suchman, E.A. (1979) 'Stages of illness and medical care', in E.G. Jaco (ed.), *Patients, physicians, and illness* (3rd edn), New York: Free Press.

The NHS Information Centre, Lifestyle Statistics (2009) *Statistics on obesity, physical activity and diet: England*, London: The Health and Social Care Information Centre.

Tseng, W.S. and Streltzer, J. (2008) *Cultural competence in health care*, New York: Springer Science.

World Health Organization (1948) *Preamble to the constitution of the World Health Organization as adopted by the International Health Conference.* New York, 19–22 June 1946; signed on 22 July 1946 by the representatives of 61 States (Official Records of the World Health Organization, no. 2, p. 100) and entered into force on 7 April 1948.

CHAPTER 3
HEALTH PROMOTION

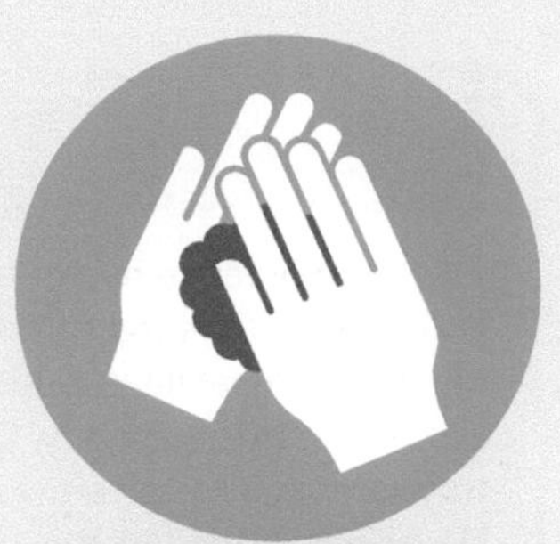

LEARNING OUTCOMES

After completing this chapter, you will be able to:

- Define health promotion.
- Identify various types and sites of health promotion programmes.
- Compare Tannahill models of health promotion with other available models.
- Explain the stages of health behaviour change.
- Discuss the nurse's role in health promotion.
- Discuss the importance of communication in health promotion.
- Assess the health of individuals.
- Develop, implement and evaluate plans for health promotion.

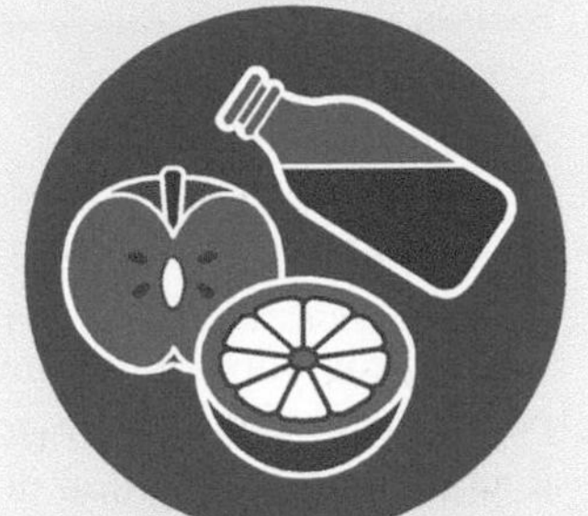

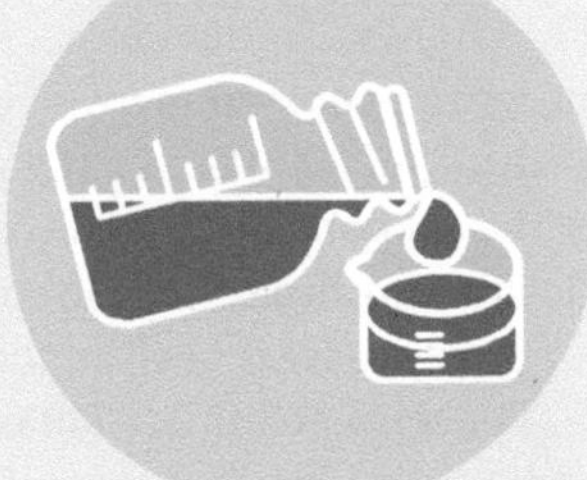

After reading this chapter you will be able to define and discuss the different types of health promotion. This chapter relates to **Essential Skills Clusters (NMC, 2010) 21 and 35**, as appropriate for each progression point.

Ensure that you really understand this chapter by logging on to your complimentary **MyNursingKit** at **www.pearsoned.co.uk/kozier**. Complete the self-assessment tests to check your progress and utilise further activities to practise and confirm your understanding.

CASE STUDY

You are a practice nurse running a cardiac rehabilitation programme in a GP surgery. You have a number of patients requiring cardiac rehabilitation after suffering **myocardial infarctions** and post-cardiac surgery. Fred Mainwaring, a 47-year-old factory worker, suffered a myocardial infarction two months ago. He briefly attended the hospital-run **cardiac rehabilitation programme** but decided that it wasn't doing him 'any good'. Although he gave up smoking for the first six weeks after the myocardial infarction, he has started back. He tells you that his father still smokes and it hasn't done him any harm.

INTRODUCTION

Health promotion is an important component of nursing (NMC, 2007) and is the responsibility of all healthcare professionals working in clinical practice and the government alike. The UK faces a number of health issues, some minor, some debilitating and some that carry high mortality rates such as coronary heart disease (CHD). Health promotion is the key to ensuring people are educated and encouraged to make healthy lifestyle choices.

This chapter will introduce you to the concept of health promotion and to the theories that underpin health promotion practice.

DEFINING HEALTH PROMOTION

The Ottawa Charter defines health promotion as 'the process of enabling people to increase control over, and to improve, their health' (WHO, 1986: 1). It goes on to say that health promotion is the responsibility of everyone, not just the health sector. Health and health promotion has therefore become the focus for policy makers in all sectors.

The term **health promotion** has been around since the 1970s and is used to encompass a plethora of strategies to improve the person's overall health including health education, illness prevention and health protection. Health promotion is not just focused on the prevention of disease but also on the person's social and mental health and revolves around a philosophy of wholeness, wellness and well-being.

According to the World Health Organization (WHO) health education comprises of 'consciously constructed opportunities for learning involving some form of communication designed to improve health literacy, including improving knowledge and developing life skills which are conducive to individual and community health' (1998: 4). Therefore health education is considered to be more wide-ranging than merely the communication of risk factors but also the development of skills such as self-awareness and decision making that will enable the individual to improve their health.

Alternatively, illness or disease prevention is seen as 'measures not only to prevent the occurrence of disease, such as risk factor reduction, but also to arrest its progress and reduce its consequences once established' (WHO, 1998: 4). According to Naidoo and Wills (2000) illness prevention can be divided into three categories:

- Primary prevention that seeks to avoid the onset of disease by detecting those groups that are at increased risk of developing disease and providing them with information, advice and counselling (e.g. immunisation).
- Secondary prevention that aims to shorten the episodes of illness and prevent progression of the disease (e.g. providing education healthy eating for diabetic patients).
- Tertiary prevention that aims to limit the effects and complications of the illness or disease process (e.g. rehabilitation for cardiac patients).

Health promotion is a priority for many healthcare professionals including nurses and is written into many of their job descriptions. In particular, community nurses, health visitors and community psychiatric nurses have a defined role in promoting the health of their patients and fostering effective working relationships with them while the patient is in their own home.

ACTIVITY 3-1

Consider what forms of health promotion you have received or been involved in.

HEALTH PROMOTION APPROACHES

According to Ewles and Simnett (2004) there are five approaches to health promotion:

- medical approach;
- behavioural change approach;
- educational approach;
- the client-centred approach;
- social change approach.

Although Ewles and Simnett (2004) present these approaches as distinct concepts, health promotion in practice can involve the use of a number of these approaches (Jones, 2000). In fact the approach used should suit the individual or community.

Medical Approach

The aim of this approach is to reduce **morbidity** and premature **mortality**. The driving force is to reduce disease and disability. It uses medical interventions such as immunisations and screening to prevent ill-health and premature death.

The medical approach is an expert led, top-down approach. It emphasises compliance rather than concordance or empowerment. It focuses on ill-health rather than the positive aspects of health and does not consider the social or environmental dimensions of health.

Behavioural Change Approach

The aim of the behavioural change approach is to encourage change in an individual's behaviour by changing their understanding of health and lifestyle choices. This approach assumes that human beings are rational decision makers who require information on which to base their health and lifestyle decisions.

This approach uses communication, education, persuasion and motivational techniques to encourage the individual to change their lifestyle behaviours. It tends to be expert-led and a top-down 'victim-blaming' approach.

Educational Approach

The educational approach to health promotion aims to provide knowledge and information for individuals to make an informed choice. This approach tends to focus on information-giving to individuals and groups through interpersonal channels, small groups and mass media. The main criticism of this approach is that it assumes that increasing knowledge will bring about behaviour and attitudinal change. It ignores the social, economic and social factors that affect health and lifestyle choices.

The Client-Centred Approach

Also known as the 'empowerment' approach, it aims to empower people to make healthy lifestyle choices. Self-empowerment, in health promotion terms, is defined as 'a process through which people gain greater control over decisions and actions affecting their health' (WHO, 1998: 6). In order to facilitate self-empowerment participatory learning techniques can be used to allow the individual to explore their values and beliefs as well as the environmental and social factors that influence their lifestyle choices (Homans and Aggleton, 1988). These participatory learning techniques can involve group work, problem solving and counselling.

Social Change Approach

The aim of this approach is to bring about changes in the physical, social and economic environment, thereby enabling people to enjoy better health. The focus is on changing society and not changing the behaviour of individuals. This involves the development of healthy public policies and legislation and creating supportive social and physical environments.

ACTIVITY 3-2

Consider what health promotion approaches are most commonly used in the hospital setting.

HEALTH PROMOTION MODELS

In order to provide structure for health promotion a number of health promotion models have been developed. These provide the underlying theoretical perspectives of health promotion and provide a framework for action.

One of the better known descriptive models of health promotion is Tannahill's model that describes health promotion as three interlinked circles that include health education, prevention and protection (see Figure 3-1). However, as the circles interlink there are overlaps between the following (Naidoo and Wills, 2001):

- preventive services, e.g. immunisation or cervical screening;
- preventive health education, e.g. smoking advice;
- preventive health protection, e.g. fluoridation of water;
- health education for preventive health protection, e.g. seat belt campaigns;
- health education, e.g. building life-skills with groups such as exercise programmes;
- health protection, e.g. implementing a workplace no-smoking policy;
- health education aimed at health protection, e.g. campaigning for protective legislation.

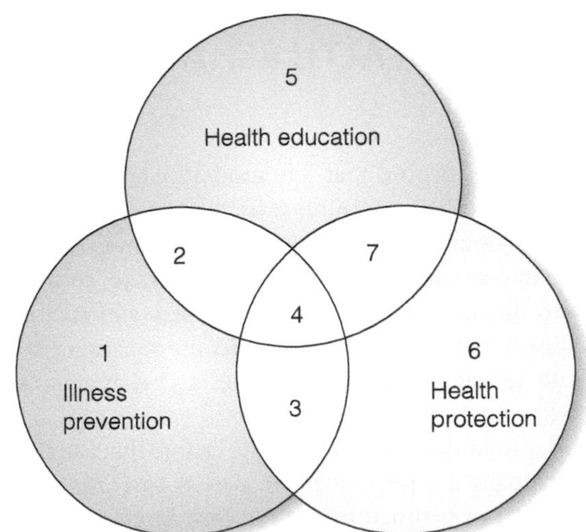

Figure 3-1 Tannahill's model of health promotion (1985).

Source: *Health Promotion: Models and Values*, 2nd ed. (Downie, R.S., Tannahill, C. and Tannahill, A. 1996) 'Tannahill's model of health promotion', Figure 4.1, p. 59, by permission of Oxford University Press.

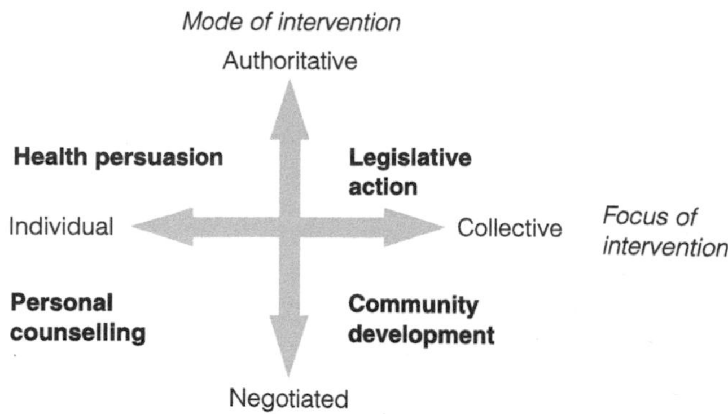

Figure 3-2 Beattie's model of health promotion (1991).
Source: Beattie, A. (1994).

Despite the simplicity of this model, it has many critics, some of which believe that it ignores the social and economic roots of ill health as it does not consider why the individual or community has behaviours that could lead to ill health. However, many argue that this model highlights the fact that it is difficult to change health behaviours using only one approach and that approaches need to complement one another. Indeed many aspects of health promotion practice overlap one another (Naidoo and Wills, 2001).

Beattie's model (see Figure 3-2), however, allows empowerment of the individual and the community and highlights the values and moral principles that underpin health promotion. This model allows the healthcare professional to consider the roots of ill health such as income, poverty, housing, etc. It shows the importance of partnership between the individual, the healthcare professional and the government.

The advantages of Beattie's model is that it allows the healthcare professional to question the actions used to deliver change and where a particular health promotion initiative fits into the overall strategy.

STAGES OF HEALTH BEHAVIOUR CHANGE

It is important to note that any model of health promotion activity needs to be underpinned by the patient's intention to change behaviour. For instance, in recent years there has been increased awareness of the links between diseases such as coronary heart disease (CHD) and particular lifestyle activities such as smoking and poor diet. However, people apparently still find it difficult to engage in health promoting behaviours such as eating a low fat diet.

In order to understand some of the factors that can influence the individual's decisions there is a need to consider Ajzen's (1991) model of planned behaviour. Icek Ajzen, a professor in psychology, developed this model in order to explain how behaviour can be changed in three steps:

- step 1 – the individual's attitude, determined by their beliefs about consequences;
- step 2 – the expectations of others;
- step 3 – the individual's perceived control and belief in their ability to change.

In order to change behaviour the individual must recognise the health benefit of making the change and also the consequence of not changing the behaviour (step 1). For example, an individual considering the incorporation of exercise into their life may think 'taking exercise will improve my health and being healthier would be good'.

However, some individuals may need outside influences in order to feel the need to change (step 2). For example, an individual considering incorporating exercise into their life may be more inclined to do so if they think 'my doctor thinks I should exercise more and what she thinks is important to me'.

Some individuals may feel that there are barriers to changing their behaviours and therefore may feel unable to change (step 3). For example, an individual considering incorporating exercise into their life may feel 'I don't have the facilities to exercise and this will make exercising difficult'.

In order to develop an effective health promotion programme it is vital that the healthcare professional establishes the individual's attitude and beliefs towards changing their behaviour and establishing their individual perceived obstruction to changing their behaviour (e.g. themselves, others or outside barriers or loci of control).

ACTIVITY 3-3

What factors may be influencing Fred's decision to continue smoking?

HEALTH PROMOTION ACTIVITIES

Health promotion programmes are found in many settings. Programmes and activities may be offered to individuals and families in the home or in the community setting and at schools, hospitals or in the workplace. Some health promotion programmes are aimed at the individual while others are aimed at groups, with the latter being more efficient but perhaps not the most effective as it can be difficult to ascertain if members of the group have understood what has been discussed. However, many people prefer the group approach, find it more motivating and enjoy the socialising and support.

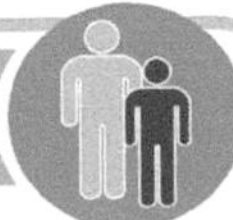

LIFESPAN CONSIDERATIONS

Health-Promotion Topics

Infants

Breastfeeding
Immunisations
Parenting skills for new parents

Children

Nutrition
Dental checkups
Immunisations
Safety promotion and injury control

Adolescents

Bullying - which can impact on psychological and physical health
Drugs
Peer group influences
Self-concept and body image
Nutrition and weight control
Alcohol abuse
Physical fitness
Personal safety
Smoking cessation
Sex education

Older adults

Dental/oral health
Exercise
Health screening recommendations
Hearing aid use
Immunisations
Medication instruction
Mental health
Malnutrition
Exercise
Preventive health services
Safety precautions
Smoking cessation
Weight control

Community-based programmes are frequently offered. The type of programme depends on the current health concerns and may include health promotion, specific protection and screening for early detection of disease (see the *Lifespan Considerations* box above for different health promotion topics). For example, there is a national policy set out by the Department of Health (DH) to offer influenza immunisation to specific at-risk groups within the community. Influenza, or 'flu', is a highly contagious acute viral infection that affects people of all ages. The signs and symptoms of the disease are fever, headache, aching muscles and a cough or other respiratory symptoms which most people recover from. However, for certain groups of people (see *Practice Guidelines*) it can cause serious illness and even death. Flu epidemics occur mainly in the winter months and can result in widespread disruption to healthcare and other services. As a result of the devastating effects both on the individual and healthcare services the DH health protection programme was developed.

School health-promotion programmes may serve as a foundation for children of all ages to gain basic knowledge about lifestyle and health issues. The school is the centre of the community; therefore by promoting health to school children it is thought that the health promotion message will reach the whole community. The school nurse may teach programmes about basic nutrition, dental care, drug and alcohol abuse, domestic violence and issues related to sexuality and pregnancy. Classroom teachers may include health-related topics in their lesson plans, for example, the way the normal heart functions or the need for clean air and water in the environment.

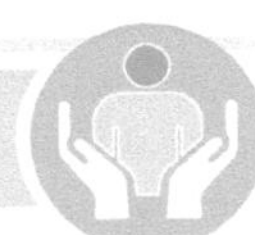

PRACTICE GUIDELINES

'At Risk' Groups Offered Influenza Immunisation

All those aged 65 years or over.

All those aged six months and over with the following health problems:

- chronic respiratory disease including asthma
- chronic heart disease
- chronic renal disease
- chronic liver disease
- diabetes
- **Immunosuppression** (e.g. splenic dysfunction and HIV infection).

Worksite programmes for health promotion have developed out of the need for businesses to control the rising cost of healthcare and employee absenteeism. Many industries feel that both employers and employees benefit from healthy lifestyles and behaviours. The convenience of the workplace setting makes these programmes particularly attractive to many adults who would otherwise not be aware of them or motivated to attend them. Health promotion programmes may be held in the company cafeteria so that employees can watch a film or attend a discussion group during their lunch break. Workplace programmes may be aimed at specific populations, such as accident prevention for the machine worker or back care programmes for individuals involved in heavy lifting; programmes to screen for high blood pressure; or health enhancement programmes, such as fitness information and relaxation techniques. Benefits to the worker may include an increased feeling of well-being, fitness, weight control and decreased stress. Benefits to the employer may include an increase in employee motivation and productivity, an increase in employee morale, a decrease in absenteeism and a lower rate of employee turnover, all of which may decrease business and healthcare costs (Mills, 2005).

Health promotion is the responsibility of the individual and society as a whole. However, health promotion is often associated with the healthcare sector and nurses in particular. Regardless of the setting, the nurse has a key role in health promotion.

The Nurse's Role in Health Promotion

Individuals and communities who seek to increase their responsibility for personal health and self-care require health education. The trend towards health promotion has created the opportunity for nurses to strengthen the profession's influence on health promotion, disseminate information that promotes an educated public, and assist individuals and communities to change long-standing health behaviours.

A variety of programmes can be used for the promotion of health, including (a) information dissemination, (b) health risk appraisal and wellness assessment, (c) lifestyle and behaviour change, and (d) environmental control programmes.

Information dissemination is the most basic type of health-promotion programme. This method makes use of a variety of media to offer information to the public about the risk of particular lifestyle choices and personal behaviour, as well as the benefits of changing that behaviour and improving the quality of life. Leaflets, posters, brochures, newspaper features, books and health fairs all offer opportunities for the dissemination of health-promotion information. Alcohol and drug abuse, driving under the influence of alcohol, hypertension and the need for immunisations are some of the topics frequently discussed. Information dissemination is a useful strategy for raising the level of knowledge and awareness of individuals and groups about health habits.

When planning information dissemination, it is important to consider factors such as cultural factors and different age groups. Knowing the best place and method to distribute information will increase the effectiveness. For example, some people who may be at risk from coronary heart disease may not go to their GP, therefore some GP practices have decided to do health assessments at shopping centres in a bid to identify and encourage people to adopt healthier lifestyles. This provides a stepping stone for providing information and suggesting resources for special needs – all done in a nonthreatening environment.

Lifestyle and behaviour change programmes require the participation of the individual and are geared towards enhancing the quality of life and extending the life span. Individuals generally consider lifestyle changes after they have been informed of the need to change their health behaviour and have become aware of the potential benefits of the change. Many programmes are available to the public, both on a group and individual basis, some of which address stress management, nutrition awareness, weight control, smoking cessation and exercise.

Health-promotion activities, such as the variety of programmes previously discussed, involve collaborative relationships with both patients and healthcare professionals. The role of the nurse is to work *with* people, not *for* them – that is, to act as a facilitator of the process of assessing, evaluating and understanding health. The nurse may act as advocate, consultant, teacher or coordinator of services. The nurse's role in health promotion can include:

- facilitating patient involvement in the assessment, implementation and evaluation of health goals;
- educating patients on ways of enhancing fitness, improving nutrition, managing stress and enhancing relationships;
- assisting individuals, families and communities to increase their levels of health;
- assisting patients, families and communities to develop and choose healthier options;
- reinforcing good health behaviours;
- acting as an advocate for community changes that promote a healthier environment.

These roles allow the nurse to work with individuals of all age groups and diverse family units or to concentrate on a specific population, such as new parents, school-age children or older adults. In any case, the nursing process is a basic tool for the nurse in a health-promotion role. Although the process is the same, the nurse emphasises teaching the patient (who can be either an individual or a family unit) self-care responsibilities.

RESEARCH NOTE

A Survey of Local Health Promotion Initiatives for Older People in Wales

Using a quantitative approach, Hendry *et al.* (2008) set out to describe the extent, content and regional variation of existing health promotion initiatives for older people in Wales. A questionnaire was sent to senior health promotion specialists across Wales. They found that in total there were 120 health promotion projects available in Wales. The largest promotion of health promotion initiatives focused on physical activity with three national and 42 local initiatives across Wales. Healthy eating, home safety and warmth, smoking, alcohol misuse and sexual health were poorly provided for.

Implications for practice

The provision of health promotion services for older people in Wales is patchy. There needs to be increased efforts to improve the number and effectiveness of health promotion interventions available to older people. It was noted that some ethnic groups and those in residential care homes had very little access to some of the initiatives.

Source: based on Hendry, M., Williams, N.H. and Wilkinson, C. (2008) 'A survey of local health promotion initiatives for older people in Wales', *BMC Public Health*, 8: 217. Available from **http://www.biomedcentral.com/content/pdf/1471-2458-8-217.pdf** (accessed on 15/12/10).

COMMUNICATION AND HEALTH PROMOTION

Communication is vital to the success of any health promotion programme or strategy. Communication between the nurse and patient allows opportunities to discover and uncover information, and develop client empowerment and participation. There are three forms of communication in humans: verbal, non-verbal and **metacommunication** (Edelman and Mandle, 2006).

Verbal Communication

When we think about communication, we automatically think 'verbal' communication. Verbal communication is the exchange of words, written and spoken, and is critical to the expression of oneself. Communication also involves listening to the words spoken or written. See the *Practice Guidelines* on how to actively listen.

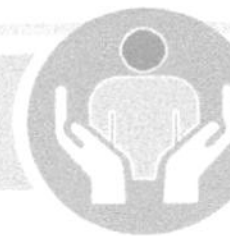

PRACTICE GUIDELINES

Active Listening

Active listening requires:

- Time - time to listen without interruptions.
- Encouragement - encouraging the individual to speak with nods, smiles and encouraging comments such as 'please go on'.
- Clarification - through questioning.
- Empathy - understanding how it feels for the individual.
- Interest - looking interested in what the individual has to say.
- Summarisation - summarising what the individual has said.

Verbal communication becomes even more difficult when an interaction involves people who speak different languages (see the *Practice Guidelines* below) or have hearing problems. Both patients and health professionals can experience frustration when they are unable to communicate verbally with each other.

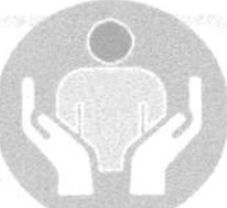

PRACTICE GUIDELINES

Verbal Communication with Patients Who Have Limited Knowledge of English

- Avoid slang words, medical terminology and abbreviations.
- Augment spoken conversation with gestures or pictures to increase the patient's understanding.
- Speak slowly, in a respectful manner, and at a normal volume. Speaking loudly does not help the patient understand and may be offensive.
- Frequently check the patient's understanding of what is being communicated. Be wary of interpreting a patient smiling and nodding to mean that they understand; the patient may only be trying to please the nurse and not understand what is being said.

For the patient whose language is not the same as that of the healthcare provider, an intermediary may be necessary. A translator converts written material (such as patient education pamphlets) from one language into another. An interpreter is an individual who mediates spoken communication between people speaking different languages without adding, omitting, distorting meaning or editorialising. A true interpreter has demonstrated ethical and interpreting skills and the knowledge and expertise required to function in a healthcare situation. In some hospitals a language line may be used, which is a 24-hour a day interpretation line. The nurse is able to have a three-way conference call with the patient and interpreter, in order to discuss clinical care. A language line aims to have an interpreter available on a phone within a few minutes of a request being made and covers all major international languages. Many hospitals that are located in culturally diverse communities have translators available on staff or maintain a list of employees who are fluent in other languages. Embassies, consulates, ethnic churches (e.g. Russian Orthodox, Greek Orthodox), and ethnic clubs may also be able to provide interpreters. However, asking a family member or other nonprofessional to interpret can create difficulties. Cultural rules often dictate who can discuss what with whom. Guidelines for using an interpreter are shown in the *Practice Guidelines* below.

PRACTICE GUIDELINES

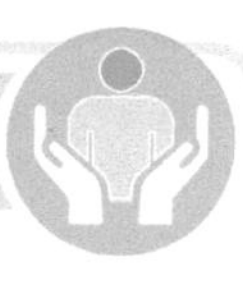

Using an Interpreter

- Avoid asking a member of the patient's family, especially a child or spouse, to act as interpreter. The patient, not wishing family members to know about his or her problem, may not provide complete or accurate information.
- Be aware of gender and age differences; it is preferable to use an interpreter of the same gender as the patient to avoid embarrassment and faulty translation of sexual matters.
- Avoid an interpreter who is politically or socially incompatible with the patient. For example, a Bosnian Serb may not be the best interpreter for a Muslim, even if he speaks the language, due to cultural differences.
- Address the questions to the patient, not to the interpreter.
- Ask the interpreter to translate as closely as possible the words used by the nurse.
- Speak slowly and distinctly. Do not use metaphors, for example, 'Does it swell like a grapefruit?' or 'Is the pain stabbing like a knife?'
- Observe the facial expressions and body language that the patient assumes when listening and talking to the interpreter.

Nonverbal Communication

Nonverbal communication can include the use of silence, touch, eye movement, facial expressions and body posture. The five senses form the basis for nonverbal communication (Edelman and Mandle, 2006). Nonverbal communication is particularly powerful. It can convey a person's inner feelings and thoughts and is not always congruent with what the person is verbally communicating.

The nurse needs to be aware of cultural differences with nonverbal communication. Some cultures are quite comfortable with long periods of silence, whereas others consider it appropriate to speak before the other person has finished talking. Many people value silence and view it as essential to understanding a person's needs or use silence to preserve privacy. Some cultures view silence as a sign of respect, whereas to other people silence may indicate agreement.

Touching involves learned behaviours that can have both positive and negative meanings. The nurse should be wary when using touch as some cultures believe that touch is considered magical and because of the belief that the soul can leave the body on physical contact, casual touching is forbidden. In some Asian cultures (e.g. people from India, Sri Lanka, Thailand and Laos), only certain older adults are permitted to touch the heads of others, and children are never patted on the head. Nurses should therefore touch a patient's head only with permission.

Metacommunication

According to Edelman and Mandle (2006) metacommunication refers to a message about a message. It is in fact impossible not to communicate. Metacommunication therefore is about reading between the lines, looking beyond what is verbally spoken.

Barriers to Effective Communication

Health promotion requires effective communication, in order to establish the factors that could lead to ill-health and to communicate the concepts of a healthy lifestyle. Some of the possible barriers to effective communication when promoting health include:

- unsuitable surroundings, e.g. no privacy;
- physical, mental or emotional state of the patient;
- the subject matter;
- the language used, e.g. jargon;
- health promoter's attitude/behaviour;
- fear.

ACTIVITY 3-4

How could you encourage a patient to change their unhealthy lifestyle choices?

THE NURSING PROCESS AND HEALTH PROMOTION

A key aspect of planning an effective health promotion strategy for an individual is a thorough assessment of the individual's health status. Identification of the individual health needs is the basis for the choice of interventions implemented.

ASSESSING HEALTH STATUS

Components of this assessment need to include information about the patient's past medical history, a physical examination, lifestyle assessment, social support review, health risk assessment, health beliefs review and life stress review.

Health History and Physical Examination

Information about the patient's past medical history along with a physical examination can detect any existing health problems. For example, patients may present with symptoms that may seem non-specific, such as tiredness and weight loss, however symptoms such as these may be indicative of an underlying disease such as type 2 diabetes. Physical examination, including blood tests and a detailed assessment of the patient's health history, can uncover diseases such as type 2 diabetes which, if undetected and untreated, could lead to the development of serious health problems such as a stroke or heart attack.

Type 2 diabetes is also known as maturity onset, or non-insulin dependent diabetes. It develops mainly in people older than 40 (but can occur in younger people). Currently in the UK about three in 100 people aged over 40, and about 10 in 100 people aged over 65, have type 2 diabetes. It is more common in people who are overweight or obese. It also tends to run in families.

Lifestyle Assessment

Lifestyle assessment focuses on the personal lifestyle and habits of the patient as they affect health. Categories of lifestyle generally assessed are physical activity, nutritional information, stress management and such habits as smoking, alcohol consumption and drug use. Other categories may be included. The goals of lifestyle **assessment tools** are to provide the following:

- an opportunity for patients to assess the impact of their present lifestyle on their health;
- a basis for decisions related to changing behaviours and lifestyle.

Several tools are available to assess lifestyle. A form for self-assessment of lifestyle is shown in Figure 3-3.

Social Support Review

Understanding the social context in which a person lives and works is important in health promotion. Individuals and groups can provide comfort, assistance, encouragement and information. Social support fosters successful coping and promotes satisfying and effective living (Pender *et al.*, 2010).

Social support contributes to health by creating an environment that encourages healthy behaviours, promotes self-esteem and wellness, and provides feedback that the person's actions will lead to desirable outcomes. Examples of social support include family, peer support groups, religious support systems (e.g. churches) and self-help groups (e.g. Weight Watchers).

According to Pender *et al.* (2010), authors of *Health Promotion in Nursing Practice*, the nurse begins a social support review by asking the patient to do a number of tasks:

- List individuals who provide personal support.
- Indicate the relationship of each person (e.g. family member, fellow worker or colleague, social acquaintance).
- Identify which individuals have been a source of support for five or more years.

This assessment allows the nurse and patient to discuss and evaluate the adequacy of their social support together and, if necessary, plan options for enhancing the support system.

Health Risk Assessment

A health risk assessment (HRA) is an assessment and educational tool that indicates an individual's risk for disease or injury. The individual's general health, lifestyle behaviours and demographic data are considered and compared to national data. The HRA includes a summary of the person's health risks and lifestyle behaviours with educational suggestions on how to reduce the risk. Specific HRAs exist such as the Framington Risk Equation (NICE, 2010), which aims to assess individual risk based on set factors known to be associated with cardiovascular disease such as hypertension and smoking.

Many HRA instruments are available today in paper-and-pencil as well as computerised forms. Recently, HRAs have begun to reflect a broader approach to health and health promotion. For instance, occupational health nurses can identify risk factors and subsequently plan interventions aimed at decreasing illness, absenteeism and disability.

Health Beliefs Review

Patients' health beliefs need to be clarified, particularly those beliefs that determine how they perceive control of their own health. Assessment of patients' health beliefs provides the nurse with an indication of how much the patient believes they can

Healthstyle: A Self-Test

Everyone wants good health. But many of us don't know how to be as healthy as possible. Health experts describe *lifestyle* as one of the most important factors affecting our health. In fact, it is estimated that 7 of the 10 leading causes of death could be reduced through common-sense changes in lifestyle. The first step in a healthier lifestyle is thinking about what we are doing now.

This brief self-test, developed by the Public Health Service, will let you know how well you are doing to stay healthy. The behaviors included in the test are recommended for most adult Americans. Some behaviors may not apply to persons with certain chronic diseases or handicaps, or to pregnant women. Such persons may need special advice from their doctor or other healthcare provider.

Cigarette Smoking

If you never smoke, enter a score of 10 for this section and go to the next section on *Alcohol and Drugs*.

	Almost Always	Sometimes	Almost Never
1. I avoid smoking cigarettes.	2	1	0
2. I smoke only low tar and nicotine cigarettes *OR* I smoke a pipe or cigars.	2	1	0
Smoking Score:			

Alcohol and Drugs

	Almost Always	Sometimes	Almost Never
1. I avoid drinking alcoholic beverages or I drink no more than 1 or 2 drinks a day.	4	1	0
2. I avoid using alcohol or other drugs (especially illegal drugs) as a way of handling stressful situations or the problems.	2	1	0
3. I am careful not to drink alcohol when taking certain medicines (for example, medicine for sleeping, pain, colds, and allergies) or when pregnant.	2	1	0
4. I read and follow the label directions when using prescribed and over-the-counter drugs.	2	1	0
Alcohol and Drugs Score:			

Eating Habits

	Almost Always	Sometimes	Almost Never
1. I eat a variety of foods each day, such as fruits and vegetables; whole grain breads and cereals; lean meats; dairy products; dry peas; beans; nuts and seeds.	4	1	0
2. I limit the amount of fat, saturated fat, and cholesterol I eat (including fat on meats, eggs, butter, cream, shortenings, and organ meats such as liver).	2	1	0
3. I limit the amount of salt I eat by cooking with only small amounts, not adding salt at the table, and avoiding salty snacks.	2	1	0
4. I avoid eating too much sugar (especially frequent snacks of sticky candy or soft drinks).	2	1	0
Eating Habits Score:			

Exercise/Fitness

	Almost Always	Sometimes	Almost Never
1. I do vigorous exercises for 20–30 minutes a day at least 3 times a week (examples include jogging, swimming, brisk walking, bicycling).	4	2	0
2. I do exercises that enhance my muscle tone for 15–30 minutes at least 3 times a week (examples include using weight machines or free weights, yoga and calisthenics).	3	1	0
3. I use part of my leisure time participating in individual, family, or team activities that increase my level of fitness (such as gardening, dancing, bowling, golf, baseball).	3	1	0
Exercise/Fitness Score:			

Stress Control

	Almost Always	Sometimes	Almost Never
1. I have a job or do other work that I enjoy.	2	1	0
2. I find it easy to relax and express my feelings freely.	2	1	0
3. I recognize early, and prepare for, events or situations likely to be stressful for me.	2	1	0
4. I have close friends, relatives, or others whom I can talk to about personal matters and call on for help when needed.	2	1	0
5. I participate in group activities (such as religious worship and community organizations) and/or have hobbies that I enjoy.	2	1	0
Stress Control Score:			

Safety

	Almost Always	Sometimes	Almost Never
1. I wear a seat belt while riding in a car.	2	1	0
2. I avoid driving while under the influence of alcohol and other drugs.	2	1	0
3. I obey traffic rules and the speed limit when driving.	2	1	0
4. I am careful when using potentially harmful products or substances (such as household cleaners, poisons, and electrical devices).	2	1	0
5. I avoid smoking in bed.	2	1	0
Safety Score:			

(continued)

Figure 3-3 Healthstyle: A Self-Test.

Source: 'Healthstyle: A Self-Test,' by L.B. Bobroff, 1999, University of Florida, Institute of Food and Agricultural Sciences (UF/IFAS). Retrieved 28 June 2011, from http://edis.ifas.ufl.edu/pdffiles/HE/HE77800.pdf.

Your Lifestyle Scores

After you have figured your scores for each of the six sections, circle the number in each column that matches your score for that section of the test. Remember: There is no total score for this self-test. Think about each section separately. You are identifying aspects of your lifestyle that you can improve in order to be healthier. So let's see what your scores reveal.

What Your Score Means to You (By Section)

Scores of 9 and 10

Excellent! Your answers show that you are aware of the importance of this area to your health. More important, you are putting your knowledge to work for you by practising good health habits. As long as you continue to do so, this area should not pose a serious health risk. It's likely that you are setting an example for the rest of your family and friends to follow. Since you got a very high test score on this part of the test, you may want to consider other areas where your scores indicate room for improvement.

Scores of 6 to 8

Your health practices in this area are good, but there is room for improvement. Look again at the items you answered with a 'Sometimes' or 'Almost Never.' What changes can you make to improve your score? Even a small change can help you achieve better health.

Scores of 3 to 5

Your health risks are showing. Would you like more information about the risks you are facing? Do you want to know why it is important for you to change these behaviours? Perhaps you need help in deciding how to make the changes you desire. In either case, help is available.

Scores of 0 to 2

Obviously, you were concerned enough about your health to take this test. But your answers show that you may be taking serious risks with your health. Perhaps you were not aware of the risks and what to do about them. You can easily get the information and help you need to reduce your health risks and have a healthier lifestyle if you wish. The next step is up to you.

YOU CAN START RIGHT NOW

The test you just completed included many suggestions to help you reduce your risk of disease and premature death. Here are some of the most significant:

Avoid cigarettes.

Cigarette smoking is the single most important preventable cause of illness and early death. It is especially risky for pregnant women and their unborn babies. Persons who stop smoking reduce their risk of getting heart disease and cancer. So if you're a cigarette smoker, think twice before lighting that next cigarette. If you choose to continue smoking, try decreasing the number of cigarettes you smoke and switching to a low tar and nicotine brand.

Follow sensible drinking habits.

Alcohol produces changes in mood and behaviour. Most people who drink are able to control their intake of alcohol and to avoid undesired, and often harmful, effects. Heavy, regular use of alcohol can lead to cirrhosis of the liver, a leading cause of death. Also, statistics clearly show that mixing drinking and driving is often the cause of fatal or crippling accidents. So, if you drink, do it wisely and in moderation.

Use care in taking drugs.

Today's greater use of drugs – both legal and illegal – is one of our most serious health risks. Even some drugs prescribed by your doctor can be dangerous if taken when drinking alcohol or before driving. Use prescription drugs as directed and discard out-dated medications. Excessive or continued use of tranquilizers (or 'pep pills') can cause physical and mental problems. Using or experimenting with illicit drugs such as marijuana, heroin, cocaine, and other street drugs may lead to a number of damaging effects or even death.

Eat sensibly.

Your eating habits are related to risk for high blood pressure, heart disease, and many forms of cancer. Good eating habits mean holding down the amount of fat (especially saturated fat), cholesterol, sugar, and salt in your diet. Include a wide variety of plant foods like whole grain foods, beans, nuts, fresh fruits, and vegetables in your daily diet. They contain nutrients as well as protective factors that may reduce your risk of chronic diseases. You'll feel better.

Exercise regularly.

Almost everyone can benefit from exercise – and there's some form of exercise almost everyone can do. (If you have any doubt, check first with your doctor). Usually as little as 20–30 minutes of vigorous exercise a day three times a week will help you have a healthier heart, tone up sagging muscles, and sleep better. Think about how these changes can improve the way you feel.

Learn how to handle stress.

Stress is a normal part of living. The causes of stress can be good (like a promotion on the job) or bad (loss of a spouse). Properly handled, stress does not need to be a problem. But unhealthy responses to stress – such as driving too fast, drinking too much, or prolonged anger or grief – can cause a variety of physical and mental problems. Even on a very busy day, find a few minutes to slow down and relax. Talking over a problem with someone you trust can often help you find a satisfactory solution. Learn to distinguish between things that are 'worth fighting about' and things that are less important.

Be safety conscious.

Think 'safety first' at home, at work, at school, at play, and on the highway. Buckle seat belts and place young children in child restraint seats. Children under 12 should sit in the back seat. Obey traffic rules. Keep poisons and weapons out of the reach of children, and follow label directions for care and use. Keep emergency numbers by your telephone – when the unexpected happens, you'll be prepared.

Figure 3-3 *(continued)*

influence or control health through personal behaviours. Several individuals have a strong belief in fate: 'Whatever will be, will be.' If people hold this belief, they do not feel that they can do anything to change the course of their disease. For example, educating diabetic patients about lifestyle changes such as diet and exercise would be made more problematic if the person believes they have no control over the outcome. In order to make changes in behaviour or lifestyle the individual needs to be motivated and ready to make those changes. Therefore a review of the individual's health beliefs is key to effective health promotion.

Life Stress Review

There is abundant literature about the impact of stress on mental and physical well-being. A variety of stress-related instruments have been found in the literature. For example, Holmes and Rahe (1967) developed a **Social Readjustment Rating Scale**, a tool that assigns numerical values to life events (see *Box 3-1*). Studies have shown that a high score is associated with the increased possibility of illness in an individual.

BOX 3-1 Social Readjustment Rating Scale

Life event	Impact score
Death of spouse	100
Divorce	60
Menopause	60
Separation from a living partner	60
Prison sentence	60
Death of close family member	60
Personal injury or illness	45
Marriage	45
Termination of employment or sacked	45
Marital reconciliation	40
Retirement	40
Change in health of family member	40
Work more than 40 hours per week	35
Pregnancy	35
Sex difficulties	35
Gain of a new family member	35
Business or work role change	35
Change in financial state	35
Death of a close friend	30
Change in number of arguments with spouse or partner	30
Mortgage or loan for a major purpose	25
Default in paying mortgage or loan	25
Sleep less than 8 hours per night	25
Change in responsibilities in work	25
Trouble with in-laws or children	25
Outstanding personal achievement	25
Spouse begins or stops work	20
Begin or end school	20
Change in living conditions	20
Change in personal habits	20
Trouble with boss	20
Change in work hours or conditions	15
Moving to new residence	15
Presently in pre-menstrual period	15
Change in schools	15
Change in religious activities	15
Change in social activities (more or less than before)	15
Minor financial loan	10
Change in number of family get-togethers	10
Holiday	10
Christmas approaching	10
Minor violation of the law	5

Life change units	Likelihood of illness in near future
300+	About 80%
150-299	About 50%
Less than 150	About 30%

The higher your life change score, the harder you have to work to get yourself back into a state of good health.

Source: Holmes and Rahe (1967).

PLANNING

Health-promotion plans are crucial to health improvement and need to be developed according to the needs, desires and priorities of the individual. The patient needs to be active in this process, deciding on health-promotion goals, the activities or interventions to achieve those goals, the frequency and duration of the activities, and the method of evaluation. During the planning process the nurse acts as a resource person rather than as an adviser or counsellor. The nurse provides information when asked, emphasises the importance of small steps to behavioural change, and reviews the patient's goals and plans to make sure they are realistic, measurable and acceptable to the patient.

Steps in Planning

According to Whitehead (2001), a senior lecturer at the University of Plymouth, in order for health promotion to be effective it needs to be systematically planned. As a result he developed a flowchart that maps the planning process (see Figure 3-4).

This model describes two approaches to health promotion: the empowerment approach, which usually focuses on the individual and their ability to take control in sometimes difficult situations in which the nurse acts as facilitator and advocate; while the preventive approach is generally derived from medical science and focuses on disease prevention.

1 *Identify the health promotion approach to be adopted.* The nurse will decide the approach that is most appropriate to the individual based on a number of factors including personality and resources. According to Whitehead (2001) the most common approach adopted is the preventive approach; however it is noted that many nurses are trying to break free from this framework to adopt more empowering approaches.

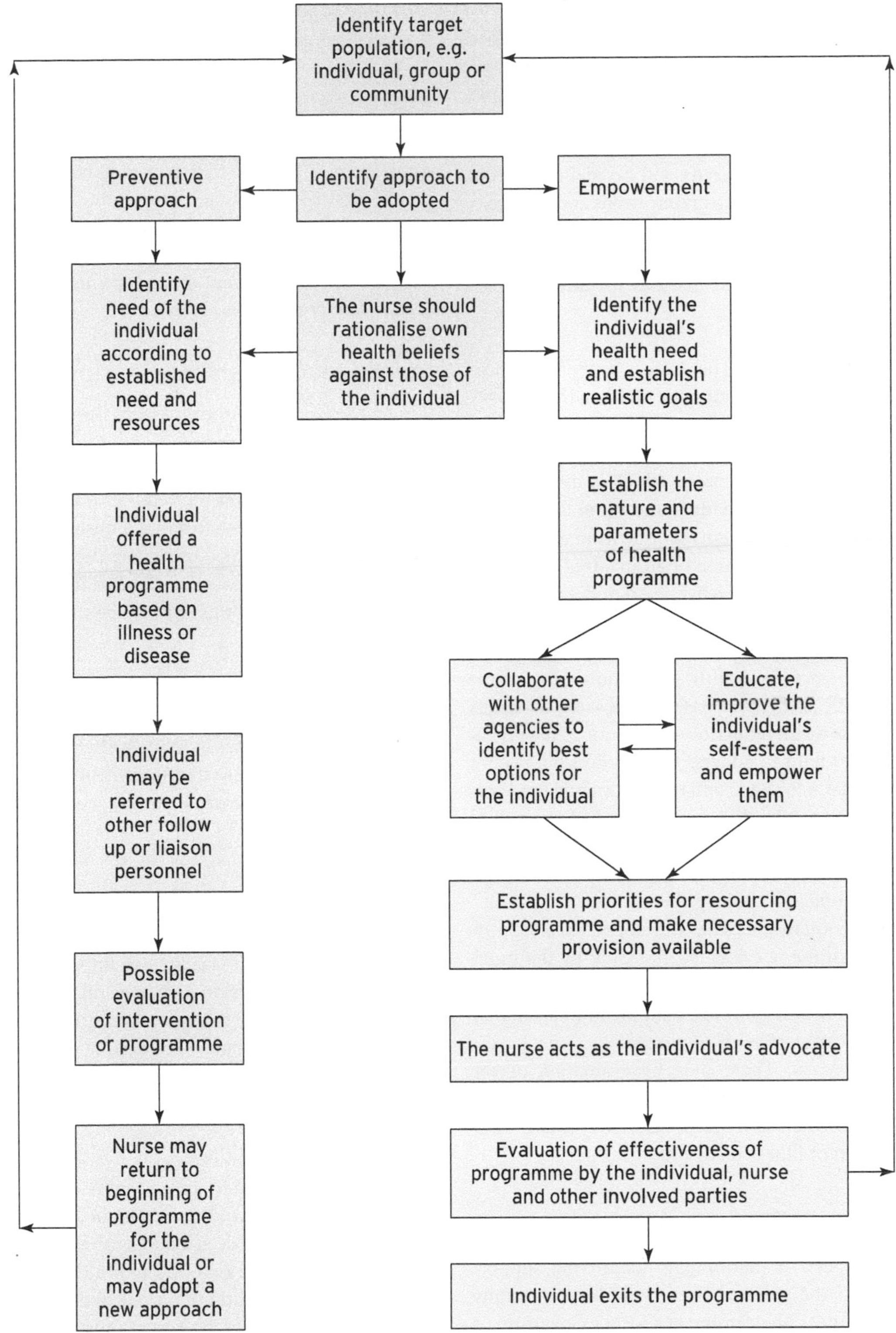

Figure 3-4 Planning health promotion.

Source: adapted from Whitehead, D. (2001b) 'A stage planning programme model for health education/health promotion practice', *Journal of Advanced Nursing*, 36(2): 311–320.

2 *Identify the individual's health needs*
   - *Empowerment approach:* These needs are established from the individual. This means that the individual will be assisted to decide their own health needs. For example, the individual may identify the need to stop smoking to improve their health.
   - *Preventive approach:* The needs will be identified from current established or 'expert-driven' needs and resources. For example, the individual may be entered onto a smoking cessation programme as smoking is known to be a risk factor for a number of diseases including cardiovascular diseases.

3 *Establish a health programme*
   - *Empowerment approach:* The health promotion programme is based on the nature of the health need, the individual's expressed wishes and is developed *with* the individual *not for* the individual. The individual is seen as an active part of this process, which is developed in collaboration with the individual and other appropriate agencies, for example dieticians for nutritional education for the obese. The programme often involves education, improving the individual's self-esteem and empowering the individual to make informed choices about their health.
   - *Preventive approach:* A health promotion programme is offered to the individual based on disease or illness management and risk reduction/prevention. These types of programmes tend to address the physical but do not consider societal, economic and environmental factors as they often focus on the disease or biological or medical problem rather than the socioeconomic or environmental dimensions of health.

4 *Evaluate the effectiveness of the programme*
   - *Empowerment approach:* The developed health promotion programme is evaluated not only by the nurse and other agencies but also by the individual. At this stage the nurse, in collaboration with the individual, may redefine or reset objectives if requested.
   - *Preventive approach:* There may be evaluation of the programme either by the nurse or by the individual. The evaluation is based on short-term behaviour change and/or modification of illness/disease status.

Exploring Available Resources

Another essential aspect of planning is identifying support resources available to the patient. These may be community resources, such as a fitness programme at a local gymnasium or educational programmes, such as stress management, breast self-examination, nutrition, smoking cessation and health lectures.

IMPLEMENTING

When developing a plan for promoting the health of an individual or group it is important to consider the types of nursing interventions needed to assist the individual. These may include providing support, counselling, facilitating, teaching, consulting and encouraging behaviour change.

Providing and Facilitating Support

A major nursing role is to support the individual. A vital component of lifestyle change is ongoing support that focuses on the desired behaviour change and is provided in a non-judgemental manner. Support can be offered by the nurse on an individual basis or in a group setting. The nurse can also facilitate the development of support networks for the patient, such as family members and friends.

Individual Counselling Sessions

If the nurse has the appropriate skills they may offer counselling sessions to individuals as part of the health promotion plan or if the individual has difficulties with the interventions or plan. The counselling relationship requires the nurse and individual to share ideas. In this sharing relationship, the nurse acts as a facilitator, promoting the individual's decision making in regard to the health promotion plan. Counselling may also be offered over the telephone but this may not be suitable for all patients.

Group Support

Group sessions provide an opportunity for participants to learn the experiences of others in changing behaviour. Group contact gives individuals a renewed commitment to their goals. Sessions are usually arranged according to the group needs and available resources.

Facilitating Social Support

Family and friends often play an important part in health promotion plans as they can facilitate or impede the efforts directed towards health promotion and prevention. The nurse's role is to assist the individual to assess, modify and develop the social support necessary to achieve the desired change.

Providing Health Education

Health education programmes on a variety of topics discussed earlier can be provided to groups, individuals or communities. Group programmes need to be planned carefully before they are implemented. The decision to establish a health promotion programme must be based on the health needs of the people; also, specific health promotion goals must be set. After the programme is implemented, outcomes must be evaluated.

Encouraging Behaviour Change

Whether people will make and maintain changes to improve health or prevent disease depends on many interrelated factors. To help patients succeed in implementing behaviour changes, the nurse needs to understand the stages of change and effective interventions that focus on progressing the individual through the stages of change.

CRITICAL REFLECTION

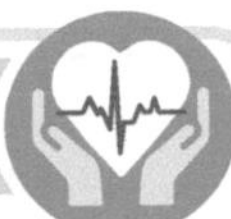

Let us revisit the case study on page 40. Now that you have read this chapter how would you encourage Fred to change his behaviours? What health promotion approach would you adopt? What support could be available for Fred?

CHAPTER HIGHLIGHTS

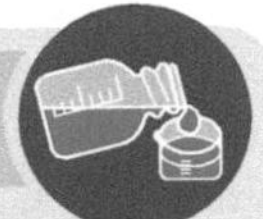

- Health promotion is not just focused on the prevention of disease but also the person's social and mental health and revolves around a philosophy of wholeness, wellness and well-being.
- Tannahill's model describes health promotion as three interlinked circles that include health education, prevention and protection.
- Beattie's analytical model of health promotion highlights the values and moral principles that underpin health promotion.
- The nurse's role in health promotion is to act as a facilitator of the process of assessing, evaluating and understanding health. It is the opportunity for nurses to strengthen the profession's influence on health promotion, disseminate information that promotes an educated public, and assist individuals and communities to change long-standing adverse health behaviours.
- A complete and accurate assessment of the individual's health status is basic to health promotion. Lifestyle assessment tools give patients the opportunity to assess the impact of their present lifestyle behaviours on their health and to make decisions about specific lifestyle changes.
- Health-promotion plans need to be developed according to the needs, desires and priorities of the patient.
- The nurse acts as a resource person, provides ongoing support, and supplies additional information and education in a nonjudgemental manner in order to help individuals change their lifestyles or health behaviours.
- During the evaluation phase of the health-promotion process, the nurse assists patients in determining whether they will continue with the plan, reorder priorities or revise the plan.

ACTIVITY ANSWERS

ACTIVITY 3-1 You may have been in receipt of or involved in a number of health promotion initiatives:

- health education, e.g. exercise programmes;
- illness prevention, e.g. immunisation programmes;
- health protection, e.g. implementing a workplace no-smoking policy.

ACTIVITY 3-2 The two health promotion approaches commonly used in the hospital setting are:

- the medical approach, e.g. screening;
- the educational approach, e.g. providing information leaflets or videos which aim to improve the individual's health.

ACTIVITY 3-3 Assess your own lifestyle choices. What factors influence your decision to continue with an unhealthy lifestyle choice?

ACTIVITY 3-4 You could encourage a patient to change their unhealthy lifestyle choices by:

- providing support, e.g. referral to support groups;
- dealing with the addiction/habit, e.g. referral to a GP for nicotine replacement;
- listening to the factors that influence his/her decisions;
- empowering the patient to make healthy choices, e.g. offering solutions/advice regarding the factors that are influencing his or her choices;
- providing written and verbal information.

REFERENCES

Ajzen, I. (1991) 'The theory of planned behaviour', *Organizational Behaviour and Human Decision Processes*, 50: 179–211.

Beattie, A. (1994) 'Knowledge and control in health promotion: a test case for social policy and social theory' in J. Gabe, M. Calnan and M. Bury (eds) *The Sociology of Health Service*, Routledge.

Downie, R.S., Tannahill, C. and Tannahill, A. (1996) *Health Promotion: Models and Values* (2nd edn), Oxford: Oxford University Press.

Edelman, C.L. and Mandle, C.L. (2006) *Health promotion throughout the lifespan*, St. Louis: Elsevier Mosby.

Ewles, L. and Simnett, I. (2004) *Promoting health: A practical guide*. Edinburgh: Bailliere Tindall.

Hendry, M., Williams, N.H. and Wilkinson, C. (2008) 'A survey of local health promotion initiatives for older people in Wales', *BMC Public Health*, 8: 217. Available from http://www.biomedcentral.com/content/pdf/1471-2458-8-217.pdf (Accessed 15/12/2010.)

Holmes, T.H. and Rahe, T.H. (1967) 'The social readjustment rating scale', *Journal of Psychosomatic Research*, 11(8): 213–218.

Homans, H. and Aggleton, P. (1988) *Social aspects of Aids*, Lewes: Falmer Press.

Jones, L. (2000) 'What is health?' in J. Katz, A. Peberdy and J. Douglas (eds) *Promoting health knowledge and practice*, London: Macmillan.

Mills, P.R. (2005) 'The development of a new corporate specific health risk measurement instrument, and its use in investigating the relationship between health and well-being and employee productivity', *Environmental Health: A Global Access Science Source* 4, 1. Available from http://www.ehjournal.net/content/pdf/1476-069X-4-1.pdf (Accessed 21/4/2007.)

Naidoo, J. and Wills, J. (2000) *Health promotion: Foundations for practice* (2nd edn), London: Bailliere Tindall.

Naidoo, J. and Wills, J. (2001) *Health studies: An introduction*, Basingstoke: Palgrave.

NICE (2010) *Lipid modification: Cardiovascular risk assessment and the modification of blood lipids for the primary and secondary prevention of cardiovascular disease*, London: NICE.

NMC – Nursing and Midwifery Council (2010) *Standards for pre-registration nursing education*, London: NMC.

Pender, N.J., Murdaugh, C.L. and Parsons, M.A. (2010) *Health promotion in nursing practice* (6th edn), Upper Saddle River, NJ: Prentice Hall.

Whitehead, D. (2001) 'A stage planning programme model for health education/health promotion practice', *Journal of Advanced Nursing*, 36(2): 311–320.

WHO (1986) *Ottawa Charter for Health Promotion*, Geneva: WHO. Available from http://www.who.int/hpr/NPH/docs/ottawa_charter_hp.pdf (Accessed 26/7/2010.)

WHO (1998) *Health for all for the 21st century*, Geneva: WHO.

CHAPTER 4
LEGAL ASPECTS OF NURSING

Chantal Patel

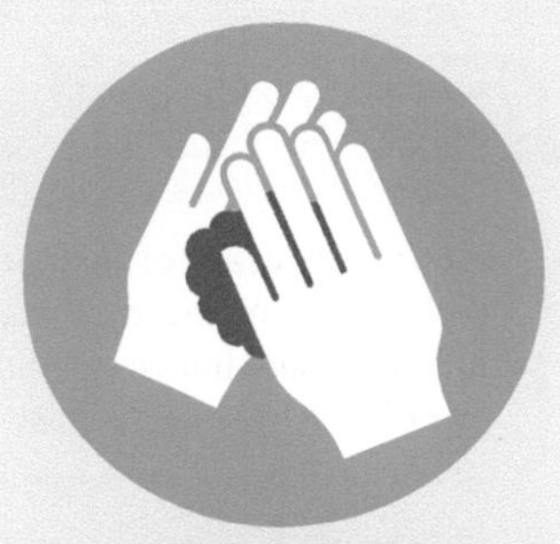

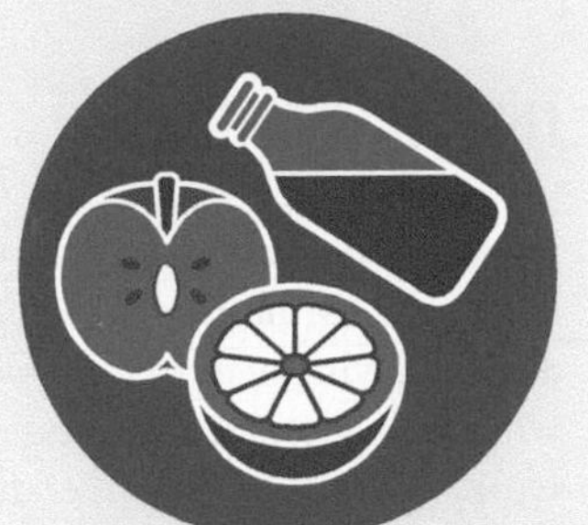

LEARNING OUTCOMES

After completing this chapter, you will be able to:

- Define the term 'law'.
- Outline the relevance of law to healthcare.
- Understand the importance of legal awareness in nursing practice.
- Understand the court system.
- Understand your obligations and duties to your employer and professional body.
- Understand and explain the basic principles in relation to consent.
- Understand the basic principles in relation to accountability.
- Understand the basic principles in relation to confidentiality.

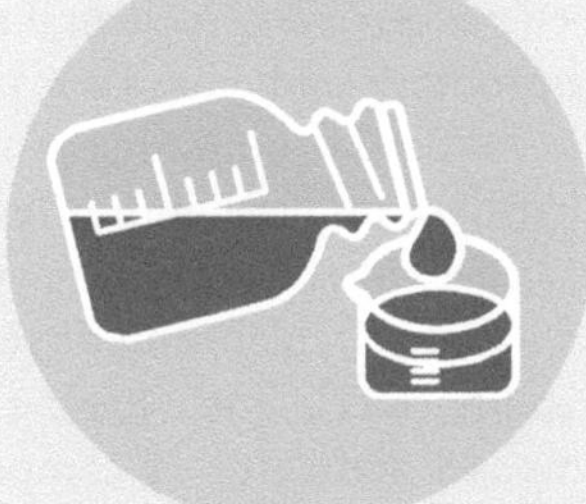

This chapter will help you consider the legal aspects of caring for patients and their families. It relates to **Essential Skills Clusters (NMC, 2010) 7, 8, 11, 12, 15, 20, 34 and 39**, as appropriate for each progression point.

Ensure that you really understand this chapter by logging on to your complimentary **MyNursingKit** at **www.pearsoned.co.uk/kozier**. Complete the self-assessment tests to check your progress and utilise further activities to practise and confirm your understanding.

CASE STUDY

Julie is 38 years of age. She is admitted to the ward in the early hours of the morning following a road traffic collision. Julie is stable but is awaiting surgery for a displaced fracture of her right femur. Whilst on the ward, her 'husband' calls. The nurse in charge doesn't want to wake Julie so decides to give full details of Julie's condition and progress to her 'husband'.

INTRODUCTION

Nursing practice involves the carrying out of a number of activities such as the provision of physical and psychological care and the giving of advice. However, such care should be delivered within an acceptable professional, legal and contractual framework. It is therefore imperative that nurses are aware of their obligations and liabilities as they are accountable for the care they provide. Knowledge of the law is important for two reasons:

- delivery of care is consistent with current legal principles;
- to protect the nurse from potential lawsuits.

GENERAL LEGAL CONCEPTS

There are a number of ways of defining 'law'. Law can be interpreted both as a set of prohibitive rules supported by court sanctions if the rules are breached and rules that govern behaviour. Under such an interpretation, law has a wider remit. It prohibits and guides our professional behaviour. In addition nurses need to be aware of rules that affect their clinical practice that have no legal authority but nevertheless are as important as legal rules, such as organisational policies and procedures as well as circulars and directives issued by the Department of Health (DH). The Nursing and Midwifery Council (NMC) imposes standards of competence and conduct that must be achieved by all nurses.

Functions of Law in Nursing

The law:

- provides a framework that informs the nurse which actions are legally permissible;
- helps in maintaining a standard of practice by making nurses accountable.

Sources of Law

The United Kingdom is not a single entity. It comprises of four countries: England, Wales, Scotland and Northern Ireland. This chapter deals with law as related to England and Wales. In so far as the health service is concerned, the law is as it applies to England and Wales. Scotland and Northern Ireland have different legal jurisdictions but the same principles would apply. Increasingly there are differences emerging as each devolved country adopts a rule that best suits its people.

Devolution in Wales, Scotland and Northern Ireland

Devolution arose as a result of the granting of powers from the central UK government to the governments of Scotland, Northern Ireland and Wales.

The Scottish Parliament is entitled to make primary legislation in relation to health law and policy. One such example is the passing of the Adults with Incapacity (Scotland) Act 2000.

The Northern Ireland Assembly has limited powers. The Welsh Assembly now has law making powers, following from a yes vote in the recently held referendum.

Before passing an Assembly Measure, the National Assembly for Wales must first have Legislative Competence for that particular issue. To get this competence, the Welsh Assembly must apply to the UK Government. Once received, a law can be passed at the National Assembly for Wales. From then on, the power to make any future laws on that issue remains with the National Assembly for Wales. This will not apply to Assembly Bills as, following on from a yes vote in the referendum on the law making powers of the National Assembly for Wales, the Assembly will have gained the powers to pass laws on all subjects in the devolved areas listed in Schedule 7 of the Government of Wales Act 2006.

Welsh laws apply only to Wales. However, the UK Parliament in Westminster retains the power to introduce laws which still affect Wales.

The National Assembly for Wales debates and passes these laws, which are often proposed by the Welsh Government. However, any Assembly Member, Assembly Committee or the Assembly Commission can propose one of these laws, and if the proposal receives a majority vote, through the various stages of scrutiny, then it becomes law.

As a result of these changes it is essential to ensure that the policies and laws you apply in your practice relate to the country you work in.

Nurses are not exempted from law and that means nurses need to obey the law just like any other citizen. They may be accountable both in the criminal as well as civil courts. The English legal system is governed by **common law** rules (derived from decisions made in Court), Parliament and The European Union. **Criminal law** is concerned about actions that affect society at large whilst **Civil law** deals with disputes between two parties. The sources of law are shown in Box 4-1.

BOX 4-1 Sources of Law

- Legislation: Acts of Parliament normally referred to as Statutes: e.g. the National Service Act 1977.
- Judicial decisions - decisions from court cases also known as Common law: e.g. *R* v *Weller* (2003) in criminal cases and *Paton* v *BPAS* (1978) in civil cases.
- European Community and Human Rights law: e.g. the Human Rights Act 1998 and the European Community Act 1972 permit the use of European decisions in domestic cases.
- Received wisdom - judges may consider both legal scholars as well as public opinion when deciding the outcome of novel and complex cases.
- Professional codes - the codes of conduct as issued by the NMC are not law in themselves but judges can use these in order to ascertain what would be considered good practice in a particular clinical field.
- Law from other countries - when judges are confronted with a novel issue or an issue that has not been considered previously by the courts, they may seek guidance from other jurisdictions: e.g. American Court decisions. These are merely persuasive and not binding.

Types of Laws

- **Public law**: refers to a body of law that deals with relationships between individuals and the government and its agencies. An important aspect of public law is criminal law which seeks to take actions via a criminal court against those who pose a threat to the safety and welfare of the public. Examples are murder, manslaughter, assault, theft and fraud.
- **Private law**: refers to a body of law that deals with relationships amongst private individuals usually pursued through a civil court. Examples are breach of contract, negligence and breach of privacy.

Kinds of Legal Actions

There are two kinds of legal actions:

1. **Civil actions**: a patient alleges that the nurse has been negligent in the care that has resulted in harm.
2. **Criminal actions**: an individual has committed an act that is not in the interests of society at large, for example, assaulting a patient.

Civil Liability

All nurses owe patients, colleagues and visitors a duty of care. This essentially means that the nurse should ensure that the welfare of the patient and others are not compromised by the nurse's actions. Where the patient is injured as a result of the nurse's actions, the patient may take action in the civil courts against the nurse if they are self-employed or against the employer if the nurse is an employee. The complainant will claim that the nurse has breached their duty of care by acting negligently which has resulted in the patient being harmed. For the patient to succeed, they need to establish, on a balance of probabilities, that the standard of care given fell below what would be considered reasonable. The purpose of the claim is to seek compensation for the injuries sustained as a result of the breach. There are a number of elements to establishing that medical treatment was negligent. Nursing and medical opinion often differ over treatment for a particular ailment and it is a valid defence if it can be shown that the treatment was in accordance with the views of 'a responsible body of medical opinion'. It is imperative that the nurse documents clearly the reasons for a particular treatment.

Further, even if the patient can show that the standard of care was negligent, the patient still has to prove that the negligence actually caused the injury. This is often the trickiest part of a claim. The medical/nursing practitioner may claim that the injury arose from the illness itself and not from the treatment; or that the injury would have come about in any event. Detailed medical/nursing evidence will be called with specialists arguing for each side.

The Meaning of the 'Duty of Care'

In most cases of negligence the key issue is whether the nurse is in breach of the standard of care. The test in English law is whether the nurse fell below 'the standard of the ordinary skilled man exercising and professing to have that skill' (The **Bolam Test**). The nurse need not possess the highest expert skill. It is sufficient for the nurse to demonstrate that their practice falls within what would be accepted by their peers or a particular clinical practice. A general nurse will therefore be assessed in terms of the relevant skills possessed by general nurses. A similar approach would be taken with midwives, specialist nurses and so on (*Bolam* v *Friern HMC* [1957]). This test essentially means that where the profession is divided as to what is the appropriate management, the nurse is unlikely to be found negligent provided that the reasons proferred have a logical basis. In *Bolitho* v *City and Hackney Health Authority* [1998], the House of Lords stated:

> *. . . the court has to be satisfied that the exponents of the body of opinion relied upon can demonstrate that such opinion has a logical basis.*

Nurses are under an obligation to take care to prevent harm to another when providing a service. Nurses do not owe a duty of care to complete strangers unless they decide to assist the person. The moment the nurse decides to help, they would be accepting responsibility for any actions taken for the person. Any action that causes further harm is likely to raise the issue as to whether the duty of care has been breached. This will be assessed as set out under the 'Bolam test'.

In order for a claim of negligence to be successful, the complainant or patient must prove on a balance of probabilities the harm resulted from the breach of the duty of care. In practice this is very difficult to show given the complexity of medical cases and the fact that patients may have underlying illnesses which make it difficult to say with any certainty that the harm was as a result of a breach of duty of care. In *Chester* v *Ashfar* [2002] the House of Lords held that the patient was entitled to damages as she had not been warned of the potential risks when undergoing spinal surgery. Though the surgeon had not been negligent in the way he operated, he was negligent for failing to inform her of the potential risks that in fact occurred. The patient was able to establish a link between the breach of duty of care and the injury she sustained.

BOX 4-2 Case Example

Failure to keep accurate medical checks by a midwife such as blood pressure monitoring led to brain damage. Laura gave birth to twins following a caesarian section. Ordinarily her blood pressure should have been monitored every 15 minutes. The midwife caring for her did not check her blood pressure for two and half hours and left her alone. By the time another midwife realised that Laura's blood pressure was too high, it was too late to provide her with the required treatment (Alleyne and Harding, 2002). The husband fought a three-year battle which culminated in an out-of-court settlement of £750,000.

Criminal Liability

In some cases nurses' actions may attract criminal liability, for example where a patient has been assaulted or abused or where a patient has died in suspect circumstances. A trial will take place in order to ascertain whether the nurse is guilty of the criminal act and the burden is on the prosecution to establish the guilt of the nurse beyond reasonable doubt. The purpose is to punish the nurse either by imprisonment, community order or fine.

BOX 4-3 Case Example

Edward Ruddick, 48, was convicted by a Teesside Crown Court jury of assaulting a pensioner in his care. Ruddick was accused of forcefully standing on Reg Hulse's foot after becoming annoyed with him. He was found guilty by a majority verdict of 10 to two of assault occasioning actual bodily harm against Reginald Hulse (Passant, 2010).

The Structure of the Courts

English law adopts a hierarchical system when dealing with legal claims (see Figure 4-1). The hierarchical system permits a series of appeals in the same case until it reaches the United Kingdom Supreme Court. Some cases may be referred to the European Court of Justice or to the European Court of Human Rights. It allows for a system of precedent which gives certainty to the law, prevents arbitrary decisions, treats like cases alike and provides a rational basis for decision making. Lower courts such as the magistrates' courts, county court or **High Court** are bound by decisions made by a higher court such as the **Supreme Court**. The nurse should be aware of where the cases have been heard in order to inform clinical practice. Decisions from the Supreme Court will be binding on lower courts unless there is some distinguishing feature that is materially different from a decided case.

HUMAN RIGHTS ACT 1998

The Human Rights Act (HRA) 1998 came into force in October 2000. The Act consists of rights and freedoms that are set out in the European Convention of Human Rights (ECHR). It is unlawful to act in a manner that is incompatible with a Convention right. In a healthcare environment, the nurse must be aware of the rights and freedoms of patients that are protected by the HRA. These rights do not have equal status. They are categorised as:

- **Absolute rights:** these cannot be withdrawn or made subject to conditions (Article 2).
- **Limited rights:** these apply in circumstances where the State needs to act to safeguard society at large. For example, the right to liberty under Article 5 can be limited by the legal requirement of imprisonment where a person has been found guilty of a criminal act such as murder.
- **Qualified rights:** these require a balance to be struck between the interests of the individual and that of other individuals, society and the public interest. It is legitimate to interfere if it is proportionate and in the interests of everyone such as the maintaining of public order and safety (Article 8).

These are the main rights incorporated into the Human Rights Act 1998:

- Article 2: Right to Life
- Article 3: Prohibition of Torture
- Article 4: Prohibition of Slavery and Forced Labour
- Article 5: Right to Liberty and Security
- Article 6: Right to a Fair Trial
- Article 7: No Punishment Without Law
- Article 8: Right to Respect for Private and Family Life
- Article 9: Freedom of Thought, Conscience and Religion
- Article 10: Freedom of Expression
- Article 11: Freedom of Assembly and Association
- Article 12: Right to Marry
- Article 14: Prohibition of Discrimination
- Article 16: Restrictions on Political Activity of Aliens
- Article 17: Prohibition of Abuse of Rights
- Article 18: Limitation on Use of Restrictions on Rights.

Structure of the Courts

United Kingdom Supreme Court
This is the most senior domestic court. It hears appeals from the Court of Appeal and in exceptional cases the High Court

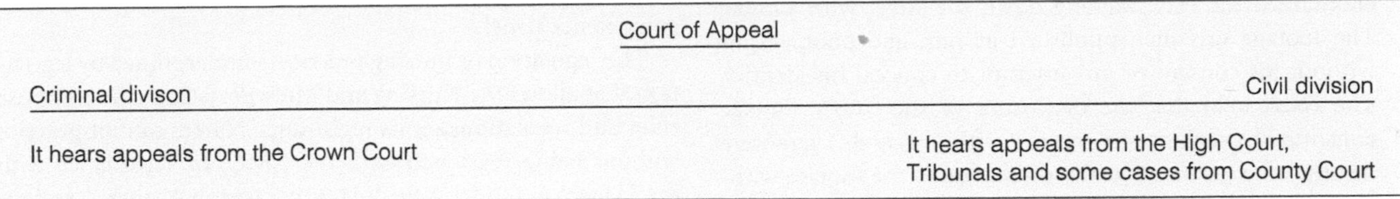

Court of Appeal
Criminal divison
It hears appeals from the Crown Court
Civil division
It hears appeals from the High Court, Tribunals and some cases from County Court

High Court

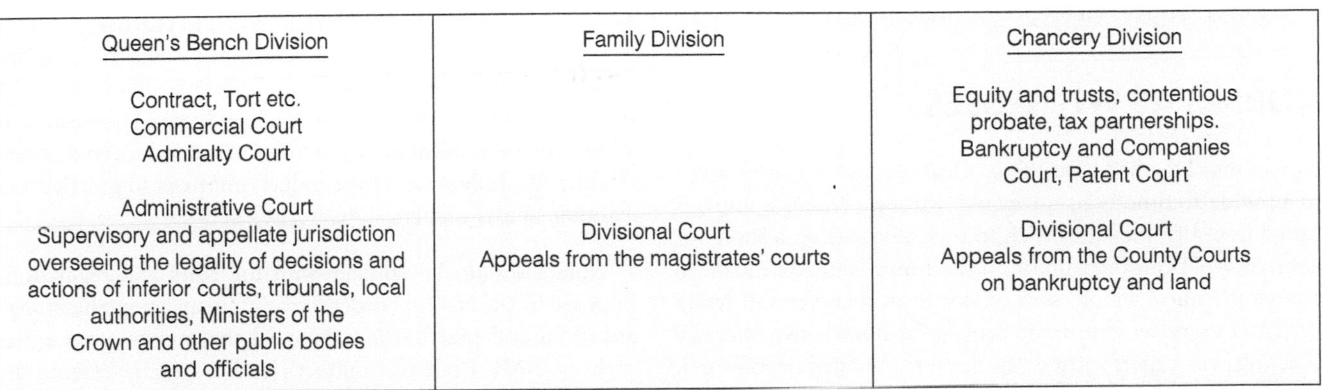

Crown Court	County Courts
Trials for indictable offences, appeals from magistrates courts, cases for sentence	Majority of civil litigation subject to nature of claim

Magistrates Courts	Tribunals
Trials of summary offences, committals to the Crown Court, family proceedings courts and youth courts	Hear appeals from decisions on immigration, social security, child support, pensions, tax and lands

Figure 4-1 Structure of the courts in UK.

The most relevant of these to nursing practice are:

- **Article 2: The right to life.** There is a positive obligation on the State to protect life. This obligation means that a patient or their representative may take legal action where denial of treatment may lead to the death of the patient. However, this positive obligation should not be interpreted as an obligation to continue to provide treatment if it is not clinically indicated. In *A NHS Trust* v *D and Others* (2000), the courts considered whether the clinical team looking after a 19-month-old child with severe medical problems could be allowed to cease treatment, including resuscitation, on the grounds that it would not be in the child's best interests. The parents strongly opposed the application considering it to be premature. In considering the conflicting views that could not be resolved by discussion or by seeking further medical opinions, Mr Justice Cazalet stated that the court's clear respect for the sanctity of human life imposed a strong obligation in favour of taking all steps capable of preserving life, save in the most exceptional circumstances. In this case, however, he held that there could be no Article 2 infringement because the treatment authorised (non-resuscitation) was made in the best interests of the child.
- **Article 3: The prohibition of torture.** This provides that 'no one shall be subjected to torture or to inhuman or degrading treatment or punishment'. In *Tanko* v *Finland* [1994], the European Commission on Human Rights refused to exclude the possibility that: '. . . a lack of proper medical care in a case where someone is suffering from a serious illness could in certain circumstances amount to treatment contrary to Article 3.'
- **Article 8: The right to respect for private and family life.** This concerns the right to respect for private and family life, home and correspondence. It is one of the most dynamically

interpreted provisions of the HRA. It can apply to personal care from same gender staff, the use of lifting devices and to complex end-of-life issues. This right is however a qualified right which means such a right can be interfered with if the circumstances are justified. In *Peck* v *UK* (2003) CCTV cameras filmed Mr Peck walking down the street with a knife. The footage was then published as film and photographs without his consent or any attempt to conceal his identity. The court held that the disclosure of the CCTV footage constituted a serious interference with Article 8. There were insufficient reasons to justify disclosure of the footage without the man's consent and without masking his identity. Accordingly the disclosure of material was a disproportionate interference with his private life.

NURSES AS WITNESSES

Nurses may be called to testify in a legal action or may be asked to provide testimony as an expert witness. Where a nurse is called to testify, they may wish to seek advice from a lawyer or alternatively from their union. If the nurse is the defendant in a case, the nurse should seek advice from a lawyer and retain the latter's services in order to protect the nurse's own interests. If acting as an expert witness, the nurse should demonstrate that they have special training, experience or skill in a particular area. The role of an expert witness is to provide assistance to the judge or jury to understand the evidence pertaining to a particular case.

REGULATION OF NURSING PRACTICE

Nurses face four fields of accountability: the civil and criminal courts, disciplinary proceedings of the employer and the Nursing and Midwifery Council Code of Conduct, and the competence panel.

The regulation of nursing practice is underpinned by legislation that allows the Nursing and Midwifery Council to impose rules and regulations on its registrants. Nurses cannot practice without being registered with the NMC. In accordance with the Health Act 1999, Schedule 3, paragraph 8, there are four fundamental functions of the regulatory body:

- to keep a register of members admitted to practice;
- to determine the standards of education and training for admission to practice;
- to give guidance about standards of conduct and performance;
- to provide a framework for administering procedures and rules for dealing with misconduct, unfitness to practice and other similar matters.

Nurses should be familiar with the rules and regulations imposed by the NMC in order to maintain an acceptable standard of clinical practice. It is essential that nurses are familiar with the NMC Code of Conduct (see *Box 4-4*). In essence the NMC makes it clear that the nurse will be accountable for any actions or decisions they make. The nurse should be prepared to justify any decisions taken.

BOX 4-4 The Code: Standards of conduct, performance and ethics for nurses and midwives

The people in your care must be able to trust you with their health and well-being.

To justify that trust, you must

- make the care of people your first concern, treating them as individuals and respecting their dignity
- work with others to protect and promote the health and well-being of those in your care, their families and carers, and the wider community
- provide a high standard of practice and care at all times
- be open and honest, act with integrity and uphold the reputation of your profession

Source: **www.nmc-uk.org**

BOX 4-5 Case Example

A nurse was found guilty of misconduct when she failed to administer prescribed medication to two patients A and B. In both cases the prescribed medication had been signed for and left in the room of both patients. Patient A was in the bathroom at the time and the medication for Patient B was found in a tablet crusher in his room. Though the patients did not come to any harm, the panel concluded that the nurse fell short of the standard of practice expected for someone in her position. It decided to suspend her for a period of six months.

Source: Conduct and competence panel held on the 2, 3 and 4 of August 2010 available at **www.nmc-uk.org**

LEGAL ROLES OF NURSES

Nurses have three separate interdependent legal roles, each with rights and associated responsibilities: as the provider of a service, an employee and a citizen. Nurses are expected to provide safe and competent care. Implicit within these roles are several legal concepts:

- Liability is about taking responsibility for the nursing activity even if ordered by the doctor. It is no defence to claim that you acted on orders. The nurse must ensure that they have the relevant skill and competence when treating patients.
- The standard of care is judged by the reasonableness of your actions in the circumstances. The nurses' actions are judged in relation to the 'Bolam test'.
- Nurses are bound by their contractual obligations to their employer. They are expected to deliver care in accordance with the express and implied terms of their contract of employment.

A contract of employment is essentially one of personal service which gives rise to duties and obligations on both sides. The contract of employment consists of a number of implied duties. These are:

- **Duty of faithful service.** Since the relationship between you and the employer is one of trust and confidence, you are expected to serve the employer faithfully. This is a fundamental obligation. A breach of this obligation may result in a breach of contract. In essence you are expected to perform your duties carefully and competently with due regard for the interests of the employer. A potential conflict may arise between your professional organisation and that of the employer but it is accepted that an employer will not require you to act in a manner that is inconsistent with your professional obligations. Examples of a breach of the duty of faithful service include: persistent lateness; incompetence; willful neglect; theft; strike; go-slow; work-to-rule; sit-ins; and competing with the employer whilst still employed.
- **Duty to obey lawful and reasonable orders.** You are expected to obey all lawful and reasonable orders. You can be dismissed by the employer for failing to obey. However, you are not expected to obey orders that are manifestly unlawful: for example, where you are instructed to administer medication in dosage not supported by the British National Formulary.
- **Duty to use skill and care.** You must perform your duties competently using reasonable skill and care as well as protecting the employer's property.
- **Duty not to accept bribes, gifts or commissions.** As an employee you undertake not to accept bribes, gifts and commissions. It is the case that patients often wish to reward the nurse for the care given. This can be in monetary form. Should this be the case you should inform your employer. Most NHS organisations keep a register of gifts.
- **Duty of confidentiality.** You are under a contractual duty not to disclose any confidential information to an unauthorised person. Maintaining confidentiality within the NHS can be difficult at times given the number of employees likely to be involved in the care management of the patient. It is accepted that information can be shared within the NHS family unless the patient expressly forbids it. It would not be acceptable for you to discuss the care of a patient with another nurse not involved in the management of the patient.
- **Duty of disclosure.** You are not expected to disclose facts that are adverse to your interests including misconduct except in response to a direct question. There is, however, a duty to disclose the misconduct of subordinates even if it incriminates you.

ACTIVITY 4-1

On your way to the canteen you find a woman on her own giving birth in the corridor. In such a case what care are you reasonably expected to give?

SELECTED LEGAL ASPECTS OF NURSING

Accountability

Nurses are familiar with the concept of **accountability** but it is frequently misunderstood. A research project carried out by the Royal College of Nursing found that nurses were frequently confused and uncertain of their accountability in practice, in particular when working in a multi-disciplinary context (Savage and Moore, 2004). The NMC (2002a) also highlighted the confusion surrounding the nature of accountability as a result of the number of queries they received from nurses, midwives and health visitors.

Accountability is defined by Lewis and Batey (1982) as:

The fulfilment of a formal obligation to disclose to referent others the purposes, principles, procedures, relationships, results, income and expenditures for which one has authority. This disclosure is systematic, periodic, and carried out in consistent form. Disclosure occurs so that decisions and evaluations can be made and reckoning carried out. As a formal obligation, accountability is an institutional requirement expected of one participating in an organisation. It is not based on the peculiar whims of individual personalities but instead on official mandates and positional requirements of the agency.

In a nutshell accountability means that you are answerable to others such as your employer, professional body and the law as to the actions you have taken which you must justify. In justifying your actions, you need to account for your conduct, competence and integrity. The NMC expects the nurse to account for their acts as well as their omissions. The NMC states (NMC, 2004b):

You are personally accountable for your practice. This means that you are answerable for your actions and omissions, regardless of advice or directions from another professional.

It is imperative that the nurse provides care in accordance with their competence. It is no defence to say that you were instructed to carry out a particular order or that you wanted to help the patient.

BOX 4-6 Case Example

Joanne Evans, a newly qualified community nurse, attended to an elderly lady as a favour to her colleagues. It was not until she arrived at the home was she aware that Mrs Thomas would require an insulin injection. Mrs Thomas who was partially blind normally injected herself with the use of a pen. However on that day the pen jammed. Joanne thought she had an insulin syringe in her car but had none. She decided to use a normal syringe and converted the dose. She miscalculated and administered 10 times the prescribed dose of 36 units. It was only later that night that she realised she had made a mistake but by then Mrs Thomas had already died. The coroner found that Mrs Thomas had been unlawfully killed. The NMC imposed an interim conditions of practice order for 18 months.

Source: NMC Conduct and Competence Panel, 10 August 2010; BBC News, 25 March 2009.

In clinical settings, the term accountability and responsibility are often used as interchangeable terms. Responsibility is, however, defined in the English dictionary as 'having control or authority over someone or something'. Hence responsibility means taking control over what you do for your patients and if the patient is harmed in the process you will need to account for how it happened.

The purpose of accountability is four-fold:

- to protect the patient from harm;
- to mete out appropriate sanctions to deter poor practice;
- to provide a regulatory system that ensures that nurses are answerable to a higher authority;
- to educate others in order to prevent future mistakes.

Accountable to whom?

The nurse is accountable to:

- Society through its public law regime: nurses are subject to the same legal constraints as any other citizen. There are, however, specific rules generally derived from various Acts of Parliament and Common law that guide nurses in their day-to-day clinical practice, for example the **Mental Capacity Act 2005**, Health and Safety Act 1974, Offences Against the Person Act 1861 as well as common law rules relating to confidentiality and consent in children. A breach may attract criminal liability, in particular if the patient sustains an injury.
- The profession through its regulatory body (the NMC): nurses are accountable to their regulatory body as a result of the Nurses, Midwives and Health Visitors Act 1997 and the Nursing and Midwifery Order 2001. Any breach in the standard of care is reported to the regulatory body who conduct an investigation. A range of actions can be taken to safeguard the public. These are: no further action need be taken; conditions imposing restrictions on what the nurse can do unsupervised; suspension for a period of time; and removal from the register.

  The standards by which the nurse will be held to account are set out in *The Code: Standards of conduct, performance and ethics for nurses and midwives* (NMC, 2008a). The nurse will be answerable to the 'fitness to practise' panel that judges the actions of the nurse in accordance with the average practitioner. The NMC uses a similar approach to the 'Bolam test'. One key difference to note is that in law harm to the patient must be shown whilst in professional standards no harm need be shown other than the breach of the code. The NMC has, for example, investigated and determined the suitability of the nurse to be on the register in the following:
  - physical, sexual or verbal abuse;
  - theft;
  - failure to provide adequate care in an appropriate environment;
  - poor documentation;
  - failure to administer medicines safely;
  - not disclosing unsafe practice deliberately;
  - committing criminal offences such as fraud;
  - lack of competence despite opportunities to improve.
- Patient: the patient is entitled to receive appropriate care and where the patient claims that the care provided was below what would be considered reasonable, the patient is entitled to sue the nurse or the employer of the nurse under the principle of vicarious liability through the civil courts.
- Employer through the contract of employment: the contract of employment sets out the general terms and conditions of employment and the appropriate standards of care. NHS employers are guided by the profession's code of conduct in determining the appropriate standard. In addition, the employer may issue policies, procedures and protocols to guide practice. Where there is a breach, the employer is entitled to take action against the nurse in line with its agreed disciplinary policy.

BOX 4-7 Questions to Consider

Can you be liable for failing to provide adequate care for the patient?

Yes, a nurse was found guilty of gross negligence when she failed to help a patient in a nursing care home suffering from an epileptic fit that lasted two hours (bbcnews.co.uk, 19 March 2008)

Can action be taken against you for suggesting that a patient can benefit from going to church?

Yes, both the employer and the NMC would agree that you would not be respecting the patient's dignity. It is important that when you advise patients that you remain neutral by providing a range of potential solutions to an issue. Your religious views are of no interest to the patient unless the patient seeks religious or spiritual guidance. In such cases the hospital chaplain should be called to provide such advice (nursingtimes.net, 26 May 2009)

In Summary

Nursing practice today is more complex as nurses are being called upon to take on roles previously carried out by junior doctors. It is therefore essential that nurses understand the obligations and duties owed not only to the patient but also to the employer and the general public at large. Understanding accountability is key to providing an acceptable standard of care. This requires the nurse to be familiar with the professional standards of conduct, the employers' organisational policies, procedures and protocols, and judicial decisions affecting clinical practice. Thus there is an implied duty that the nurse will ensure that they update their knowledge continuously.

Consent to Treatment

The law forbids any touching of another person without their implicit or explicit agreement. In the context of health, it would be unlawful to provide care for a patient without agreement. Consent to medical or nursing treatment is defined as an agreement between the patient and the provider of care that a number of interventions will be taken to enable the patient to recover from whatever illness/disease they suffer from. It is imperative that nurses know that the patient has consented to the treatment before proceeding with any interventions. However, the legal rules relating to consent are complex to the extent that you will need to apply general legal principles to practical situations that are often complicated. The law places an emphasis on the concept of **capacity**. In a nutshell the patient should demonstrate an understanding of the necessary intervention for their consent to be valid. There are three essential elements for consent to be valid:

1 The individual gives voluntary consent without coercion.
2 Capacity: in *Re T (Adult: Refusal of Treatment)* [1992], the Court of Appeal held that the right to decide presupposes an ability or a capacity to do so. Where the patient fully understands the nature of the treatment and its consequences, the patient is entitled to accept or refuse the treatment even if the refusal leads to death. Disregarding the patient's right of **self-determination** can amount to trespass to the person and is actionable in law. The test for determining whether the patient is capable of making the required decision is based on the ability of the patient to understand the nature of the treatment and the consequences of refusing the treatment. Nurses should ensure that they provide the relevant information in order to assist the patient in determining whether to accept or refuse treatment.
3 Reasonably informed: the law is clear that part of a nurse's duty is to give advice and information to patients so that they understand the nature of the treatment proposed and can make a choice (*Hills* v *Potter* [1983]). The duty to give information is drawn from two areas of law: the law of trespass and the law of negligence.
    - **Trespass to the person:** provided that the nurse has explained in broad terms the nature of the treatment and the patient has agreed, no cause of action will arise.
    - **Negligence:** the nurse must also inform the patient of the various risks associated with the treatment. Failure to disclose relevant risks will not vitiate the consent but a cause of action may arise in negligence.

Conclusion

It is important for the nurse to be familiar with the legal rules concerning consent to treatment as a failure to obtain appropriate consent can lead to action in trespass or negligence.

Incapacity

The law provides a framework for dealing with patients who lack capacity. The Mental Capacity Act 2005 (MCA) and its guiding principles ensure that their rights and interests are at the heart of the decision-making process. You can only act on behalf of the patient where the patient has been assessed as lacking capacity in accordance with the Act. Where you suspect that the patient may be unable to make a decision, you are expected to proceed by applying each of the five guiding principles (see *Box 4-8*). Documenting the assessment is essential

BOX 4-8 The Five Guiding Principles as Set Out Under the Mental Capacity Act 2005

1 A person must be assumed to have capacity unless it is established that he or she lacks capacity.
2 A person is not to be treated as unable to make a decision unless all practicable steps to help him or her to do so have been taken without success.
3 A person is not to be treated as unable to make a decision merely because he or she makes an unwise decision.
4 An act done, or decision made, under this Act for or on behalf of a person who lacks capacity must be done, or made, in his or her best interests.
5 Before the act is done, or the decision is made, regard must be had to whether the purpose for which it is needed can be as effectively achieved in a way that is less restrictive of the person's rights and freedom of action.

in order to establish authority for the proposed intervention. (It is also important to note that the MCA definition is 'decision specific', that is, a person could have the capacity to make a decision on a specific issue but not on another.)

Breach in the Standard of Care

Nurses owe a duty to take reasonable care not to cause harm to the patients they are attending. They are required to give advice and information to the standard of the ordinary nurse (*Bolam* v *Friern HMC* [1957]). The *Bolam* test is judged by reference to what information a respected body of nurses would have given in the same circumstances. However, in *Bolitho* v *City and Hackney HA* [1997], the courts have the right to reject a practice if it does not stand up to scrutiny.

- Free of undue influence: the law provides that an adult of sound mind is entitled to decide what happens to their body. Consequently, patients can refuse treatment even if it results in death. Nurses and family members are not entitled to coerce or unduly influence the patient when making a decision. They should have complete freedom to arrive at whatever decision they consider appropriate in terms of their own life plan.

BOX 4-9 Case Example

In *Re T (Adult: Refusal of Treatment)* [1992], a woman who initially consented to a caesarean section changed her mind following a visit from her mother, a person with strong views on the use of blood, and would only proceed without blood products. When *Miss T* later required a blood transfusion, the court held that her refusal of treatment had been negated by the undue influence of her mother, her refusal of treatment was not freely given and so the transfusion could proceed.

Where one of the elements for a valid consent, i.e. capacity, adequate information and free of undue influence is missing, then it will be doubtful as to whether the patient has consented to the treatment. One key element is capacity and the law recognises that some patients may not have the relevant capacity to make decisions for themselves.

The code of practice to the Mental Capacity Act 2005 (Department for Constitutional Affairs, 2007) suggests a series of steps before determining the patient's **incapacity**. In the first instance you are expected to explain to the patient the nature of the proposed treatment:

1 using simple language and, where appropriate, pictures and objects rather than words;
2 arranging for the person to have the information in their preferred language;
3 consulting whoever knows the person well on the best methods of communication.
4 choosing the best time and location where the person feels at ease;
5 waiting until the person's capacity improves before requiring a decision.

Where it is shown that the patient is unable to make the decision, you should assess the patient's capacity under the two tests provided for in the Mental Capacity Act 2005:

- Is there a permanent or temporary impairment or disturbance to the functioning of the mind or brain?
- If there is, how far is it affecting the person's ability to make a decision? Consider the factors that might impair decision making, for example, pain, under the influence of alcohol or drugs, head injury, stroke. These factors do not in themselves indicate incapacity.

In addition to the above, you then need to consider the functional part of the two tests approach. The law provides that a person is incapable if they are unable:

- to understand the nature of the treatment being proposed;
- to retain the information long enough to make a decision;
- to use the information as part of the decision-making process;
- to communicate that decision by any means.

Once the patient's incapacity has been determined, any treatment provided should be carried out in the best interests of the patient.

Best Interests

The Mental Capacity Act 2005 provides a checklist of factors that must be considered when determining whether care and treatment is in the best interests of a person who lacks capacity. This ensures that the wishes of the person and views of those caring for them are taken into account.

When determining whether care and treatment is in an incapable patient's best interests, you must:

- consider all the relevant circumstances;
- consider whether the decision can wait until the person regains capacity;
- as far as reasonably practicable, allow the person to participate in their care and treatment;
- not be motivated by a desire to bring about the death of the patient;
- consider, so far as is reasonably ascertainable:
  - the person's past and present wishes and feelings (and, in particular, any relevant written statement made when they had capacity);
  - the beliefs and values that would be likely to influence their decision if they had capacity;
  - other factors that they would be likely to consider if they were able to do so;
  - take into account, if it is practicable and appropriate to consult them, the views of: anyone named by the person

as someone to be consulted on the matter in question or on matters of that kind; anyone engaged in caring for the person or interested in their welfare.

In addition, before proceeding to any treatment in the patient's best interests, you need to consider whether there is an alternative way of dealing with the problem that would be less restrictive of the patient's rights and freedom of action.

The law provides that any provider of care regardless of qualifications should assess whether the patient has the relevant capacity. However, it is recognised that in complex cases other professionals may be called upon to assist in the determination of capacity.

Miscellaneous Matters

The Mental Capacity Act 2005 has two formal powers that allow a third party to make decisions on behalf of a person who lacks decision-making capacity. These powers can give the designated decision maker the right to consent to or refuse medical treatment. Where a designated decision maker with authority is in place, their consent must be obtained before care and treatment can lawfully be given.

Health and Welfare Lasting Powers of Attorney

A power allowing another to consent on behalf of a person who lacks capacity can be created through a health and welfare lasting power of attorney (LPA). The LPA must be created by the person (the donor) when they are capable and can only come into force when the person lacks capacity and the LPA has been registered with the Office of the Public Guardian.

Advanced Decisions

The law provides that a competent patient is entitled to set out their refusal of treatment in writing should they become incapacitated. Such a directive is binding on all healthcare professionals.

Independent Mental Capacity Advocate (IMCA)

There is a recognition that some patients may have no one to advocate on their behalf. In cases requiring serious treatment or decisions, an IMCA should be instructed who will make representations about the patient's wishes and feelings. The IMCA will be entitled to consult the notes and interview relevant people to assist in their task.

The Court of Protection

The Court of Protection deals with people who lack capacity. The Court can also appoint deputies and give them powers to make ongoing decisions for incapable adults.

Office of the Public Guardian

The Office of the Public Guardian is responsible for the supervision of deputies appointed by the Court of Protection and for supporting deputies in their role. It also has a role in protecting people subject to the Court's powers from abuse or exploitation by:

- keeping a register of LPAs;
- keeping a register of orders appointing deputies;
- supervising deputies appointed by the Court;
- receiving reports from attorneys;
- dealing with enquiries and complaints about deputies or attorneys.

Confidentiality

There is a public perception that nurses are well equipped to maintain confidences. Yet at the same time, nurses may turn to friends and family when facing difficult times. **Confidentiality** is a key aspect of trust that allows patients to divulge their most intimate psychological and physical problems, including submitting themselves to physical examinations. There is a legal as well as a professional and contractual duty for nurses to keep confidential what patients tell them. This duty is however not absolute. There are circumstances that impose an obligation on nurses to breach confidentiality and circumstances where the law allows the nurse to divulge information belonging to the patient. In both these situations the nurse should divulge the information to the relevant person or authority. This duty is a public interest rather than a private one as it is important for patients to trust the nurse. Therefore whether a breach is permissible or not would depend on balancing the public interests against the right of the patient to privacy.

ACTIVITY 4-2

Considering Julie in the opening case study.

1 Is the information about Julie's condition and progress subject to the rules of confidentiality?
2 Consider whether Julie's health information is of a private and intimate nature.
3 Has the nurse disclosed information without the consent of the patient?

The NHS Confidentiality Code of Practice for NHS staff (DOH, 2003) describes what a confidential service should look like as well as providing guidance to all healthcare professionals.

The duty of confidentiality is governed by common law in the main. There are, however, a number of statutory measures that are applicable in restricted circumstances (see *Box 4-10*).

BOX 4-10 Statutory Measure Applicable in Restricted Circumstances

Human Rights Act 1998	Article 8 of the Convention on Human Rights provides that 'everyone has the right to respect for his private, family life, home and correspondence'.
Public Health (Control of Diseases) Act 1984 (notifiable diseases)	Notifiable diseases or food poisoning must be reported to the relevant authority usually to a public health officer.
Abortion Act 1967	Abortions must be reported to the Chief Medical Officer.
Births and Death Registration Act 1953 (notification of births and deaths)	A midwife is under a duty to inform the district medical officer of the birth within six hours and parents are under a legal obligation to register the infant within 42 days. This also applies to stillbirths.
Road Traffic Act 1988 section 70 as amended by the Traffic Act 1991	Every citizen including nurses must provide the police on request with information that might identify a driver alleged to have committed a traffic offence.
Human Fertilisation and Embryology Act 1990 as amended by the Human Fertilization and Embryology (Disclosure of Information) Act 1992	The Human Fertilisation and Embryology Authority keeps a register of those who have undergone infertility treatment as well as children born as a result of such treatments. Therefore doctors providing such a service must provide the names of patients undergoing such treatment.
NHS Venereal Diseases Regulations 1974	There is a strict prohibition of sharing information related to sexually transmitted diseases, e.g. with an insurance company (even with the patient's consent) or with the GP, unless the patient requests so.
Prevention of Terrorism (temporary provisions) Act 2000	Nurses must report any suspicions that a person has been involved in terrorist activities.

Common Law Duty of Confidentiality

There is a general obligation on the part of nurses to keep patient information confidential (*Prince Albert* v *Strange* (1849)). However, it may be difficult for the nurse to know what information can be shared.

In order to establish a breach, three aspects must be present (*A-G* v *Guardian NewsPapers Ltd* (No. 2) (1990)):

- The information is not generally available or known. Intimate details of patient information would qualify.
- In a healthcare environment, patient information is likely to give rise to an obligation of confidence.
- That the information has been divulged without the permission of the patient and is detrimental to the person.

BOX 4-11 Case Example

In *X* v *Y and Others* [1988], a health authority employee passed on to a newspaper information obtained from the medical records of two doctors who were HIV positive. The doctors worked in the area and the newspaper wished to publish the details. The court granted the doctors an injunction preventing publication, holding that the public interest in preserving the confidentiality of hospital records outweighed any public interest in the freedom of the press, because victims of the disease ought not to be deterred by fear of discovery from going to hospital for treatment.

Exceptions to the duty of confidentiality are as follows:

- Disclosure with the consent of the patient subject to the nurse having provided relevant information and the ability of the patient to understand why the information needs to be disclosed.
- Disclosure for the purposes of care and treatment. It is inevitable within a health environment that information will be shared. This is permitted only where the information is being shared amongst those who are involved in the care of the patient.
- Disclosure at the specific request of the patient. In *C* v *C* [1946], the judge held that it was permissible to disclose strictly confidential matters when requested to do so even if there were stringent conditions on non-disclosure as in special clinics.
- Disclosure in the public interest. It is recognised that the courts need to strike a balance between the interests of individual and that of the public. This public interest duty is broad in nature and covers:
  - the protection of a third party: the law permits non-disclosure in some circumstances where a third party's interests outweigh those of the public;
  - prevention and detection of crimes: the nurse is entitled to divulge relevant information where they have knowledge that a patient is likely to commit or has committed a serious crime and this must be done to the relevant authority;

- interests of justice: the court has the power to order disclosure in the interests of justice and a refusal to do so will amount to contempt of court;
- the public good: in some circumstances the law permits disclosure if it is in the public interest to do so.

Data Protection Act 1998

The Data Protection Act 1998 provides additional safeguards regarding the protection of medical and nursing confidentiality. The key features of the Data Protection Act 1998 relate to the protection of personal data. Personal data are defined as 'any information relating to an identified or identifiable person; an identifiable person is one who can be identified directly or indirectly in reference to an identification number or to one or more factors specific to his physical, physiological, mental, economic, cultural or social identity' (Data Protection Directive, Article 2). The law regulates the processing of personal information under a set of eight principles (see *Box 4-12*).

BOX 4-12 Eight Principles for Processing Personal Information

Fairly and lawfully processed	Patient's information must be processed in accordance with the law. One of the following purposes must be met: consent of the patient, vital interests of the patient, legal and/or contractual obligation, public function or on a balance of interests. Essentially the nurse must make it clear to the patient the reasons for the gathering and recording of the information and who would have access to this material. In addition the patient is entitled to have access to this information unless they are likely to be harmed by the disclosure of the information.
Processed for limited purposes	Data must not be used for a new incompatible purpose without the subject's consent. For example, should you wish to use patient's data as part of your studies, you will need to ask for permission from the patient.
Adequate, relevant and not excessive	Data must not be amassed without a justifiable reason.
Accurate	An ongoing duty, thus data must be kept under constant review. For example, a review of 'specific warnings' on patient's notes should be undertaken at regular intervals.
Not kept for longer than is necessary	Information no longer necessary should be discarded or if such information is being kept, it should be done with the consent of the patient.
Processed in line with individual's rights	Patients have a right of access to their data, care should be taken as to what you record. Patients cannot be denied access unless there is a good reason for doing so.
Kept securely	Patient information should be guarded against accidental damage, loss or destruction as well as unauthorised data processing such as accessing medical notes of famous people when there is no personal involvement in the provision of care. In addition computerised records should be password protected and staff must ensure that they do not share passwords and they log out when away from the computer terminal.
Not transferred to countries without adequate protection	Information should not be transferred unless there is a contractual agreement between the countries.

Conclusion

Nurses should be aware of this key duty to maintain patient confidentiality as a breach may attract legal, professional and contractual sanctions that can lead to the nurse being barred from practising.

Documentation

Patients' nursing and medical notes are legal documents and can be produced in court as evidence. It is therefore important for the nurse to accurately document the care given. Many months or years may have elapsed before a case comes to court. The only way of ascertaining liability is by scrutinising the accuracy of the documentation. An incomplete or insufficient record can lead the court to determine that the care was not of a reasonable standard. The nurse is expected to document care in accordance with guidance provide by the NMC. It is not acceptable for the nurse to argue that there was insufficient time to accurately record the care of the patient. Indeed the law expects documentation to be done contemporaneously.

Reporting Unsafe Practices

Nurses are under a legal and professional duty to report unsafe practices that endanger the health and safety of patients. Examples include a colleague under the influence of alcohol or failure to adhere to accepted protocols when administering medication. However, it is not easy to report colleagues as the nurse may feel disloyal, may fear disapproval from others or fear that the reporting may scupper their chances of promotion. It is therefore important for the nurse to adopt the following approach:

- If concerned about the activity of another colleague, discuss it with someone trusted who will be supportive.
- Report it at the lowest possible level in the organisational hierarchy (e.g. student to nurse in charge, staff nurse to ward sister, etc.).
- Provide a clear and factual account of the incident.
- As you are a material witness, ensure you keep a copy of the account as you are likely to be questioned on its contents.

All NHS organisations have whistle-blowing policies that enable a nurse to be protected when disclosing malpractice. You should be familiar with the policies before deciding to report. If in doubt you may wish to seek advice from Public Concern at Work (www.pcaw.co.uk).

Legal Responsibilities of Student

Nursing students are legally responsible for their own actions and liable for their own negligent acts carried out during their clinical placements. It is imperative when they perform their duties that they do so within the scope of professional nursing. The provision of treatment, whether it is in the administration of an injection or oral medicines, should be done in accordance with accepted practice. The student nurse is judged to the same standard of skill and competence as qualified staff.

CRITICAL REFLECTION

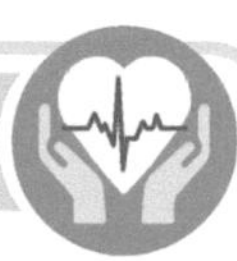

This chapter has explored the British legal system, the functions of the nurse, the nurse's legal obligations, duty and standards of care and the legal aspects of nursing in great depth. Reflect on the case study on page 56 and explore the issues related to Julie's care and the conversation the nurse had with Julie's 'husband' and its implications for the patient, the 'husband' and the nurse. Some points to consider are:

- the Human Right's Act
- the Mental Capacity Act
- the code
- standards of care
- best interest
- issues of confidentiality.

CHAPTER HIGHLIGHTS

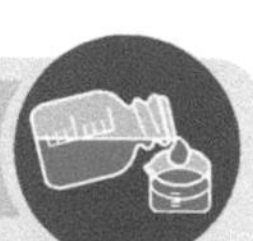

- Nursing care should be delivered within an acceptable professional, legal and contractual framework.
- Law can be interpreted both as a set of prohibitive rules supported by court sanctions if the rules are breached and rules that govern behaviour.
- The law provides a framework that informs the nurse which actions are legally permissible; and helps in maintaining a standard of practice by making nurses accountable.
- There are two types of law: public law and private law.
- There are two types of action: criminal action and civil action.
- All nurses owe patients, colleagues and visitors a duty of care. This essentially means that the nurse should ensure that the welfare of the patient and others is not compromised by the nurse's actions.
- The Human Rights Act 1998 consists of rights and freedoms that are set out in the European Convention of Human Rights (ECHR).
- Nurses may be called to testify in a legal action or may be asked to provide testimony as an expert witness.
- Nurses face four fields of accountability: the civil and criminal courts, disciplinary proceedings of the employer, the Nursing and Midwifery Council Code of Conduct, and the Competence Panel.
- Nurses have three separate interdependent legal roles, each with rights and associated responsibilities: as the provider of a service, an employee and citizen.
- Implicit within the nurse's role are three legal concepts: liability, standards of care and contractual obligations.
- Accountability means that you are answerable to others such as your employer, professional body and the law as to the actions you have taken which you must justify.
- The law forbids any touching of another person without their implicit or explicit agreement.
- There are three essential elements for consent to be valid: voluntary consent without coercion, the individual has capacity to give consent and that they have the necessary information to give informed consent.
- There are five guiding principles as set out under the Mental Capacity Act 2005.

- Confidentiality is a key aspect of trust that allows patients to divulge their most intimate psychological and physical problems.
- The Data Protection Act 1998 provides additional safeguards for regarding the protection of medical and nursing confidentiality.
- Patients' nursing and medical notes are legal documents and can be produced in court as evidence.
- Nurses are under a legal and professional duty to report unsafe practices that endanger the health and safety of patients.
- Nursing students are legally responsible for their own actions and liable for their own negligent acts carried out during their clinical placements.

ACTIVITY ANSWERS

ACTIVITY 4-1 You are only expected to provide her with reasonable care using your skills. You are not expected to provide her with the same level of care that a midwife could give. For example, you would be expected to phone for obstetric help.

ACTIVITY 4-2

1. There is a general obligation on the part of nurses to keep patient information confidential (*Prince Albert* v *Strange* (1849)). In Julie's case the information provided by the nurse to the 'husband' was subject to the rules of confidentiality.
2. Julie's health information is of a private and intimate nature. The information is not generally available or known.
3. The nurse has disclosed information without the consent of the patient, meaning that there has been a breach of confidentiality.

REFERENCES

Alleyne, R. and Harding, T. (2002) 'Hospital blamed for twin's mother's death' available at **www.telegraph.co.uk**, 19 January.

bbcnews.co.uk (2008) 'Nurse found guilty of gross negligence' available at **www.bbcnews.co.uk** (Accessed 19/03/2008)

bbcnews.co.uk (2009) 'Nurse's insulin overdose "horror"', 25 March.

Department for Constitutional Affairs (2007) *Mental Capacity Act 2005 code of practice*, London: The Stationery Office.

Department of Health (DH) (2003) *Confidentiality: NHS code of practice*, London: Department of Health.

Lewis, F. and Batey, M. (1982) 'Clarifying autonomy and accountability in nursing services', *Journal of Nursing Administration*, 12(9): 13–18.

Nursing and Midwifery Council (NMC) (2008a) *The Code: Standards of conduct, performance and ethics for nurses and midwives*, London: NMC.

NMC (2002a) 'Indemity insurance for nurses and midwives', *NMC Spring News* 1:5.

NMC (2004b) *Midwives' rules and standards*, London: NMC.

NMC (2010) *Standards for pre-registration nursing education*, London: NMC.

Passant, A. (2010) 'Nurse found guilty of attack on Stockton patient' at **www.gazettelive.co.uk**, 14 August.

Savage, J. and Moore, L. (2004) 'Interpreting accountability: An ethnographic study of practice nurses, accountability and multidisciplinary team decision-making in the context of clinical governance' available at **www.rcn.org.uk**.

Cases

A-G v *Guardian Newspapers Ltd No 2* (1990) 3 ALL ER 545

A NHS Trust v *D and Others* 2000 55 BMLR 19

Bolam v *Friern HMC* [1957] 1 WLR 582

Bolitho v *City and Hackney HA* [1998] AC 232

C v *C* [1946] 1 All ER 562

Chester v *Afshar* [2002] EWCA 724

Hills v *Potter* [1983] 3 All ER 716

Peck v *UK* 2003 36 EHRR 41

Prince Albert v *Strange* (1849) EWHC Ch J20

Re T (Adult: Refusal of Treatment) [1992] 3 WLR

Tanko v *Finland* [1994] 18 EHRR CD 179

X v *Y and Others* [1988] 2 All ER 648

FURTHER RESOURCES

Essential Reading

Dimond, B. (2008) *Legal aspects of nursing* (5th edn), Harlow: Pearson.

Griffith, R. and Tengnah, C. (2010) *Legal and professional issues in nursing* (2nd edn), Exeter: Learning Matters.

Further Reading and Websites

To keep up to date with changes in health law the following is recommended:

www.bailii.org.uk: British and Irish Legal Information Institute, which provides free access to law reports from the UK courts.

www.dh.org.uk: outlines government policy on health in England.

http://www.opsi.gov.uk/legislation/uk.htm: gives full text of legislation and statutory instruments.

And for Welsh and Scottish government health policy and publications: **http://wales.gov.uk/topics/health** and **www.scotland.gov.uk/Topics/Health.**

www.nmc-uk.org: for advice and guidance on nursing practice always refer to *The Code: Standards of conduct, performance and ethics for nurses and midwives.*

Nursing and Midwifery Council (NMC) (2004) *Complaints about unfitness to practice: A guide for members of the public*, London: NMC. This guide informs you how the NMC sets out to protect members of the public.

www.echr.coe.int/ECHR/EN/Header/case-law/HUDOC/HUDOC+database gives information on the most up-to-date cases in the European Courts.

www.opsi.gov.uk/ACTS/acts1998/ukpga_19980042_en_1: a copy of the Human Rights Act 1998 can be found here.

www.dh.gov.uk: the Department of Health has good information on consent including model consent forms.

www.justice.gov.uk: the Ministry of Justice site gives detailed legal guidance on the Mental Capacity Act 2005.

Health Act 1999 Schedule 3 paragragh 8 available at **www.statutelaw.gov.uk/content.aspx?...parentActiveTextDocId...activetextdocid**

Nurses Midwives and Health Visitors Act 1997 at **www.opsi.gov.uk/acts/acts1997/ukpga_19970024_en_1**

Nursing and Midwifery Order 2001 **www.opsi.gov.uk/si/si2002/20020253.htm**

Data Protection Act 1998 (commencement no 2) Order 2008 available at **www.legislation.gov.uk**

European Community Act 1972 at **www.opsi.gov.uk/acts/acts1972/ukpga_19720068_en-1**

Department of Health (DH) (2006) *Records Management: NHS code of practice*, London: The Stationery Office.

Nursing and Midwifery Council (NMC) (2009) *Record keeping: Guidance for nurses and midwives.* London: NMC.

www.pcaw.co.uk: provides guidance to employees if they have concerns about whistle blowing on potentially harmful practices that may affect the public.

Selected Bibliography

Montgomery, J. (2003) *Health care law* (2nd edn), Oxford: Oxford University Press.

Griffith, R. and Tengnah, C. (2010) *Legal and professional issues in nursing* (2nd edn), Exeter: Learning Matters

CHAPTER 5
PROFESSIONAL AND ETHICAL ASPECTS OF NURSING

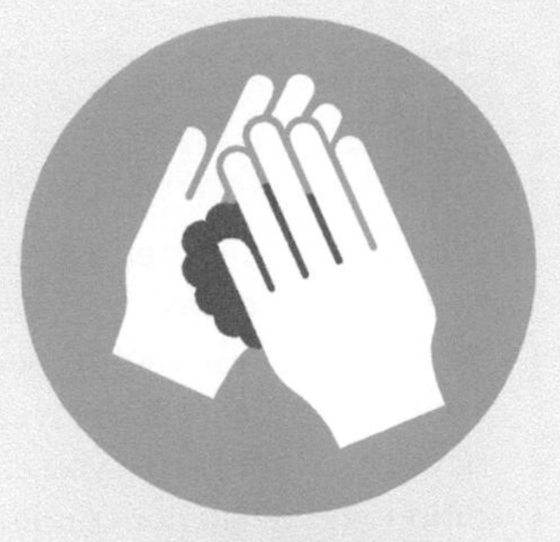

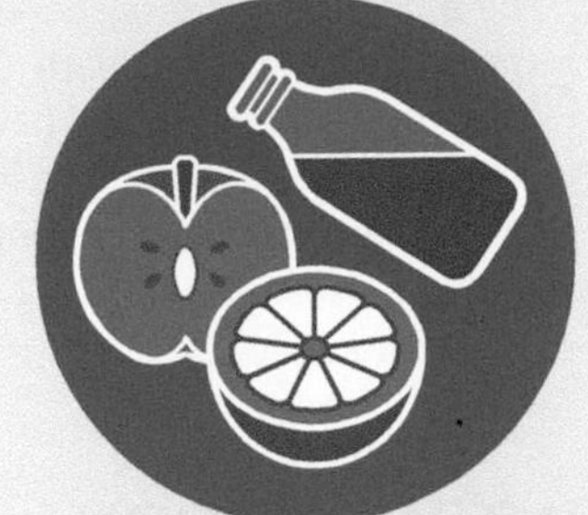

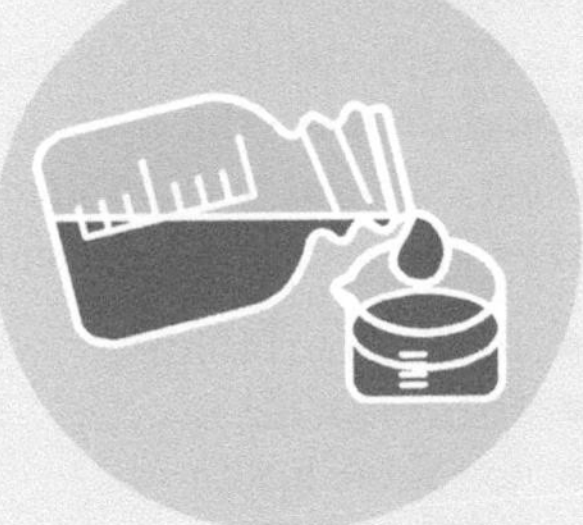

LEARNING OUTCOMES

After completing this chapter, you will be able to:

- Explain how cognitive development, values, moral frameworks and codes of ethics affect moral decisions.
- Explain how nurses use knowledge of values transmission and values clarification to make ethical decisions and facilitate ethical decision making by patients.
- When presented with an ethical situation, identify the moral issues and principles involved.
- Explain the uses and limitations of professional codes of ethics.
- Discuss common ethical issues currently facing healthcare professionals.
- Describe ways in which nurses can enhance their ethical decision making and practice.
- Discuss the advocacy role of the nurse.

After reading this chapter you will be able to reflect on the nursing role in providing healthcare, the way care is organised and the rationale for some of the decisions made. It relates to **Essential Skills Clusters (NMC, 2010) 1, 2, 3, 4, 6, 7, 11, 18, 34**, as appropriate for each progression point.

Ensure that you really understand this chapter by logging on to your complimentary **MyNursingKit** at **www.pearsoned.co.uk/kozier**. Complete the self-assessment tests to check your progress and utilise further activities to practise and confirm your understanding.

CASE STUDY

Euthanasia is currently against the law in Great Britain. You have over the past few weeks nursed a 46-year-old woman diagnosed with motor neurone disease. Claire is a softly spoken lady with a very caring and supportive family. They have often spoken to you about the difficulties of Claire's condition and when her condition deteriorates she would hate to be a burden to her husband and children and would 'hate to have an undignified death' (her words). They have taken you into their confidence and have told you that when Claire is discharged they are going to look at ways of helping her to die and in fact have been storing up medication so that when the time comes Claire, with her husband David's help, will choose when and where she will die. Both Claire and David have begged you not to tell anyone as they are now desperate for Claire to be discharged. Prior to Claire's imminent home discharge a multidisciplinary team meeting is held where you, as the nurse looking after Claire, are invited to give your opinion and advice based on evidence in relation to Claire's discharge. Both Claire and David will be present at the meeting.

Nurses face many moral and professional dilemmas in practice. This chapter will consider professional and ethical aspects of nursing.

INTRODUCTION

Ethics is derived from the Greek word *Ethos* which when you look at different dictionaries define it in numerous but not dissimilar ways. The literature (Thompson *et al.*, 2006; Tschudin, 2004) states that ethics is about values, beliefs, principles and moral judgements. Thompson *et al.* (2006) further explains that ethics is 'social custom' which relates to the right and wrong in the theory and practice of human behaviour. Thompson *et al.* (2006) go further and define ethics as being concerned with 'the study and practice of what is good and right for human beings' (2006: 5).

Within the unique nurse–patient relationship nurses face a multitude of ethical dilemmas. According to the *ICN code for nurses: Ethical concepts applied to nursing* (ICN, 2005), nurses have four areas of responsibilities:

- to promote health
- to prevent illness
- to restore health
- to alleviate illness.

Nurses deal with intimate and fundamental human events such as birth, death and suffering. They are the ones who are there to support and advocate for patients and families facing difficult choices. As a result, nurses should consider the morality of their own actions when they face the many ethical issues that surround such sensitive areas.

The present cost-driven environment of nursing care (e.g. inadequate staffing and inadequate provision of resources) creates new moral problems and intensify old ones, making it more critical than ever for nurses to make sound moral decisions. Therefore, nurses need to (a) develop sensitivity to the ethical dimensions of nursing practice, (b) examine their own and their patients' values, (c) understand how values influence their decisions, and (d) think ahead about the kinds of moral problems they are likely to face. This chapter explores the influences of values and moral frameworks on the ethical dimensions of nursing practice and on the nurse's role as a patient advocate.

VALUES

Values are our personal beliefs and attitudes about a person, object, idea or action. Values are important because they influence decisions and actions, including nurses' ethical decision making. Even though they may be unspoken and perhaps even unconsciously held, questions of value underlie all moral dilemmas. Of course, not all values are moral values. For example, people hold values about work, family, religion, politics, money and relationships, to name just a few. Values are often taken for granted. In the same way that people are not aware of their breathing, they usually do not think about their values; they simply accept them and act on them.

A value set is the small group of values held by an individual. People organise their set of values internally along a continuum from most important to least important, forming a value system. Value systems are basic to a way of life, give direction to life and form the basis of behaviour – especially behaviour that is based on decisions or choices.

Beliefs and attitudes are related to, but not identical to, values. People have many different beliefs and attitudes, but only a small number of values. Beliefs (or opinions) are personal interpretations that the individual accepts as being true. They are based more on faith than fact and may or may not be true. Beliefs do not necessarily involve values. For example, the statement 'I believe if I study hard I will get a good grade' expresses a belief that does not involve a value. While statements such as 'Good grades are really important to me. I believe I must study hard to obtain good grades' involves both a belief and a value.

Attitudes relate to the person behaving towards someone or something in an uncritical or conditioned way (Thompson *et al.*, 2006). While a stated belief is a person's interpretation and therefore changes easily, an attitude may be more long lasting. Attitudes are often judged as bad or good, positive or negative, whereas beliefs are judged as true or false. Attitudes have thinking and behavioural aspects, but feelings are an especially important component because they vary so greatly among individuals. For example, some patients may feel strongly about their need for privacy, whereas others may dismiss it as unimportant.

Values Transmission

Values are learned through observation and experience. As a result, they are heavily influenced by a person's sociocultural environment – that is, by traditions, cultural, ethnic and religious groups; and by family and peer groups. For example, if a parent consistently demonstrates honesty in dealing with others, the child will probably begin to value honesty.

Personal Values

Although people derive values from society and their individual subgroups, they internalise some or all of these values and perceive them as personal values. People need societal values to feel accepted, and they need personal values to have a sense of individuality.

Professional Values

Nurses' professional values are acquired during socialisation into nursing from codes of ethics, nursing experiences, teachers and peers. Waters (2005) states that the core fixed values of nursing are:

- compassion
- teamwork
- versatility
- making a difference.

Ritchie and Hall (2009) provide a further breakdown of these core values by stating that there are secondary characteristics which they acknowledge is diverse and interchangeable:

- Creative
- Innovative
- Surprise
- Constant challenge
- Intelligence
- Demanding
- Rewarding
- Sensitive
- Emotional Intelligence
- Listening skills
- Brave
- Life and death
- Intimacy
- Care
- Diversity
- Cope
- Always learning
- Enabler
- Mutual respect
- Give and take
- Communication
- Vital
- Practical
- Professional careers

Values, whether personal or professional, can be developed. Indeed there is an expectation that nurses as part of their personal and professional development identify and examine their own values in a process of values clarification. A principle of values clarification is that no one set of values is right for everyone. When people can identify their values, they can retain or change them and thus act on the basis of freely chosen, rather than unconscious, values. Values clarification promotes personal growth by fostering awareness, empathy and insight. Therefore, it is an important step for nurses to take in dealing with ethical problems.

Clarifying the Nurse's Values

Nurses and student nurses need to examine the values they hold about life, death, health and illness. One strategy for gaining awareness of personal values is to consider one's attitudes about specific issues such as designer babies or cloning, asking: 'Can I accept this, or live with this?', 'Why does this bother me?', 'What would I do or want done in this situation?'

Clarifying Patient Values

To plan effective care, nurses need to identify patients' values as they influence and relate to their particular health problem. For example, a patient with failing eyesight will probably place a high value on the ability to see or a patient with chronic pain will value comfort. Normally, people take such things for granted. When patients hold unclear or conflicting values that are detrimental to their health, it can sometimes be difficult for a nurse who values life to manage a patient that 'self harms' for example. In such cases, value clarification and identification can be used to help with the situation. Table 5-1 provides some examples of behaviours that may require the nurse to clarify the patient's personal values.

The following process may also help patients clarify their values:

1 **List alternatives.** Make sure that the patient is aware of all alternative actions. Ask 'Are you considering other courses of action? Tell me about them.'
2 **Examine possible consequences of choices.** Make sure the patient has thought about possible results of each action. Ask: 'What do you think you will gain from doing that?', 'What benefits do you foresee from doing that?'

Table 5-1 Behaviours that May Indicate Unclear Values

Behaviour	Example
Ignoring a health professional's advice	A patient with heart disease who continues to smoke against nursing and medical advice.
Inconsistent communication or behaviour	A diabetic who enjoys sweet food but denies eating them; yet blood results demonstrate otherwise.
Numerous admissions to a healthcare environment for the same problem	An alcoholic who has repeated admissions although he states that he only had one drink.
Confusion or uncertainty about which course of action to take	An 18-year-old boy who is a newly diagnosed epileptic has frequent weekend admissions as he cannot accept that he is an epileptic. This affects his ability to socialise with his friends.

3 **Choose freely.** To determine whether the patient chose freely, ask 'Did you have any say in that decision?'; 'Do you have a choice?'
4 **Feel good about the choice.** To determine how the patient feels, ask 'How do you feel about that decision (or action)?' Because some patients may not feel satisfied with their decision, a more sensitive question may be 'Some people feel good after a decision is made; others feel bad. How do you feel?'
5 **Affirm the choice.** Ask 'What will you say to others (family, friends) about this?'
6 **Act on the choice.** To determine whether the patient is prepared to act on the decisions, ask, for example, 'Will it be difficult to tell your wife about this?'
7 **Act with a pattern.** To determine whether the patient consistently behaves in a certain way, ask 'How many times have you done that before?' or 'Would you act that way again?'

When implementing these seven steps to clarify values, the nurse assists the patient to think each question through, but does not impose personal values. The nurse offers an opinion only when the patient asks for it – and then only with care.

MORALS AND ETHICS

The terms morals (Latin) and ethics (Greek) were derived from similar meanings: that regarding the rights and wrongs of 'social custom'. Morals are now linked with behaviour or standards of behaviour, while ethics is more about the science or study of morals (Beauchamp and Childress, 2001). Ethics are generally perceived as a set of standards that encompass the norms of a community. It can be defined as a set of values that define right and wrong or a guide to decisions relating to moral duty and obligations.

Bioethics is a branch of ethics concerned with the interdisciplinary field of medicine, and includes, for example, nursing, medical and paramedic ethics. Bioethics considers moral implications in relation to decisions within healthcare. The NMC *Code of professional conduct* (2008) and *The guidance on professional conduct for nursing and midwifery students* (2010) hold both qualified and student nurses accountable for their ethical conduct.

Morality (or morals) is similar to ethics and many use the terms interchangeably. Morality usually refers to private, personal standards of what is right and wrong in conduct, character and attitude. Sometimes the first clue to the moral nature of a situation is an aroused conscience or an awareness of feelings such as guilt, hope or shame. Another indicator is the tendency to respond to the situation with words such as *ought*, *should*, *right*, *wrong*, *good* and *bad*. Moral issues are concerned with important social values and norms; they are not about trivial things.

Nurses should distinguish between morality and law. Laws do reflect the moral values of a society, and they can offer guidance in determining what is moral. However, an action can be legal but not moral. For example, an order for full resuscitation of a dying patient is legal, but one could still question whether the act is moral. On the other hand, an action can be moral but illegal. For example, if a child at home stops breathing, it is moral but not legal to exceed the speed limit when driving to the hospital. Legal aspects of nursing practice are covered in Chapter 4.

Nurses should also distinguish between morality and religion, although the two concepts are related. For example, according to some religious beliefs, women should undergo procedures such as female circumcision that may cause physical mutilation. Other religions or groups may consider this practice to be a violation of human rights (Sala and Manara, 2001).

Moral Development

Ethical decisions require nurses to think and reason before making a decision. Reasoning is a cognitive function and is, therefore, developmental. Individual moral or ethical values develop over time. Moral development, the process of learning to tell the difference between right and wrong and of learning what ought and ought not to be done, is a complex process that begins in childhood and continues throughout life.

Theories of moral development attempt to answer questions such as:

- How does a person become moral?
- What factors influence the way a person behaves in a moral situation?

Two well-known theorists of moral development are Lawrence Kohlberg (1969) and Carol Gilligan (1982). Kohlberg's theory emphasises rights and formal reasoning; Gilligan's theory emphasises care and responsibility, although it points out that people use the concepts of both theorists in their moral reasoning.

Moral Frameworks

Moral frameworks are different frameworks that provide nurses with guidance when faced with difficult moral situations. Frameworks can help a nurse develop a strategy to investigate a situation further to help with the decision-making process. Nurses are often faced with difficult situations, for example on whether to withhold treatment or not; by examining the facts these decisions are more readily achieved. There are several moral theories that philosophers have developed, e.g. consequences (teleology), principles and duty (**deontology**).

Consequence-based (teleological) theories look to the consequences of an action in judging whether that action is right or wrong. Utilitarianism views a good act as one that brings the most good and the least harm for the greatest number of people. This approach is often used in making decisions about the funding and delivery of healthcare. Trusts or local health boards may have to decide whether they agree to fund treatment for a terminally ill patient or fund treatment for a group of people (for the greater good).

Duty-based (principles-based, deontological) theories are about promoting 'good outcomes'. Deontologists believe in telling the truth and not lying; fundamental principles should be followed whatever happens. Deontologists believe that a dying patient should be told that they are dying even though doctors and family have requested that the patient should not be told if at all possible.

A moral model or framework guides moral decisions, but does not determine the outcome. This can be illustrated by imagining a situation in which a frail, elderly patient has insisted that he does not want further surgery, but the family and surgeon insist otherwise. Two nurses have each decided that they will not help with preparations for surgery and that they will work through proper channels to try to prevent it. Using consequence-based reasoning, Nurse A thinks, 'Surgery will cause him more suffering; he probably will not survive it anyway; and the family may even feel guilty later.' While Nurse B, using principles-based reasoning, thinks, 'This violates the principle of autonomy. This man has a right to decide what happens to his body.'

Moral Principles

Moral principles are broad, general statements based on concepts such as autonomy justice, etc. Moral principles provide the foundation for moral rules, which are specific prescriptions for actions. Many authors suggest many concepts of moral principles (Kozier *et al.*, 2008; Beauchamp and Childress, 2001) but fundamentally the following are usually considered: autonomy, nonmalificence, beneficence, justice, fidelity, veracity and accountability.

Autonomy is to make one's own decisions. Nurses who follow this principle recognise that each patient is unique, has the right to be what that person is, and has the right to choose personal goals.

Honouring the principle of autonomy means that the nurse respects a patient's right to make decisions even when those choices seem to the nurse not to be in the patient's best interest. It also means treating others with consideration. In a healthcare setting this principle is violated, for example, when a nurse disregards patients' subjective accounts of their symptoms (e.g. pain). Finally, respect for autonomy means that people should not be treated as an impersonal source of knowledge or training. This principle comes into play, for example, in the requirement that patients provide **informed consent** before tests, procedures, research or being a teaching subject, can be carried out.

Nonmaleficence is to 'do no harm'. Although this would seem to be a simple principle to follow, in reality it is complex. Harm can mean intentionally causing harm, placing someone at risk of harm and unintentionally causing harm. In nursing, intentional harm is never acceptable. However, placing a person at risk of harm has many facets. A patient may be at risk of harm as a known consequence of a nursing intervention that is intended to be helpful. For example, a patient may react adversely to a medication. Unintentional harm occurs when the risk could not have been anticipated. For example, while trying to catch a patient who is falling, the nurse grips the patient tightly enough to cause bruises to the patient's arm.

Beneficence is 'doing good'. Nurses are obligated to do good, that is, to implement actions that benefit patients and their support persons. However, doing good can also pose a risk of doing harm. For example, a nurse may advise a patient about a strenuous exercise programme to improve general health, but should not do so if the patient is at risk of a heart attack.

Justice is often referred to as fairness. Nurses often face decisions in which a sense of justice should prevail. For example, a nurse making home visits finds one patient tearful and depressed, and knows she could help by staying for 30 more minutes to talk. However, that would take time from her next patient, who is a diabetic and needs a great deal of teaching and observation. The nurse will need to weigh the facts carefully in order to divide her time justly among her patients.

Fidelity means to be faithful to agreements and promises. By virtue of their standing, nurses have responsibilities to patients, employers, government and society, as well as to themselves. Nurses often make promises such as 'I'll be right back with your pain medication' or 'I'll find out for you.' Patients take such promises seriously, and so should nurses.

Veracity refers to telling the truth. Although this seems straightforward, in practice choices are not always clear. Should a nurse tell the truth when it is known that it will cause harm? Does a nurse tell a lie when it is known that the lie will relieve anxiety and fear? Lying to sick or dying people is rarely justified. The loss of trust in the nurse and the anxiety caused by not knowing the truth, for example, usually outweigh any benefits derived from lying.

Nurses must also have professional accountability and responsibility. According to *The code of professional conduct* (NMC, 2008), 'nurses are personally accountable for their practice, and must always be able to justify their decisions', which the NMC defines as being answerable for any actions or omissions that the nurse might make. Meanwhile, responsibility refers to the accountability or liability associated with the duties undertaken by the nurse. Thus, the ethical nurse is able to explain the rationale behind every action and recognises the standards to which they will be held accountable/liable.

NURSING ETHICS

No one profession is responsible for ethical decisions, nor does expertise in one discipline such as medicine or nursing necessarily make a person an expert in ethics. As situations become more complex, input from all caregivers becomes increasingly important.

It is nationally and internationally recognised that ethical issues are increasing due to the complexity of healthcare provision and advancing research and science. In 2000 there were 20 clinical ethics committees established in the UK. By 2010 there were 87 such committees with some hospitals employing ethicists. The aims of the committees are:

- to promote the development of ethics support in clinical practice in the UK;
- to promote a high level of ethical debate in clinical practice;

- to facilitate communication between all UK clinical ethics committees.

The ethics committees are multidisciplinary and while it is recognised that each committee has various functions a survey carried out in 2002 identified the following as core (UK Clinical Ethics Network, 2010):

- 54% frequently contribute to trust policies and guidelines;
- 20% frequently interpret national guidelines;
- 37% frequently provide ethical education within the trusts;
- 66% frequently provide ethical support to clinicians.

The UKCC Clinical Network committee examines and comments on issues such as withholding and withdrawing treatment, do not resuscitate orders, advance directives, consent, capacity, refusal of treatment and confidentiality.

Codes of Ethics in Nursing

A code of ethics is a formal statement of a group's ideals and values. It is a set of ethical principles that (a) is shared by members of the group, (b) reflects their moral judgements over time, and (c) serves as a standard for their professional actions. Codes of ethics usually have higher requirements than legal standards, and they are never lower than the legal standards of the profession. Nurses are responsible for being familiar with the code that governs their practice.

Nursing codes of ethics have the following purposes:

- Inform the public about the minimum standards of the profession and help them understand professional nursing conduct.
- Provide a sign of the profession's commitment to the public it serves.
- Outline the major ethical considerations of the profession.
- Provide ethical standards for professional behaviour.
- Guide the profession in self-regulation.
- Remind nurses of the special responsibility they assume when caring for the sick.

International and national nursing associations have established codes of ethics. The International Council of Nurses (ICN) first adopted a code of ethics in 1953 and the most recent revisions (2005) states that nurses have four fundamental responsibilities:

- to promote health
- to prevent illness
- to restore health and
- to alleviate suffering.

The need for nursing is universal. Inherent in nursing is respect for human rights, including cultural rights, the right to life and choice, to dignity and to be treated with respect. Nursing care is respectful of and unrestricted by considerations of age, colour, creed, culture, disability or illness, gender, sexual orientation, nationality, politics, race or social status.

Nurses render health services to the individual, the family and the community and co-ordinate their services with those of related groups.

BOX 5-1 The Code

The *ICN code of ethics for nurses* (2006) has four principal elements that outline the standards of ethical conduct.

1 Nurses and People

The nurse's primary professional responsibility is to people requiring nursing care.

In providing care, the nurse promotes an environment in which the human rights, values, customs and spiritual beliefs of the individual, family and community are respected.

The nurse ensures that the individual receives sufficient information on which to base consent for care and related treatment.

The nurse holds in confidence personal information and uses judgement in sharing this information.

The nurse shares with society the responsibility for initiating and supporting action to meet the health and social needs of the public, in particular those of vulnerable populations.

The nurse also shares responsibility to sustain and protect the natural environment from depletion, pollution, degradation and destruction.

2 Nurses and Practice

The nurse carries personal responsibility and accountability for nursing practice, and for maintaining competence by continual learning.

The nurse maintains a standard of personal health such that the ability to provide care is not compromised.

The nurse uses judgement regarding individual competence when accepting and delegating responsibility.

The nurse at all times maintains standards of personal conduct which reflect well on the profession and enhance public confidence.

The nurse, in providing care, ensures that use of technology and scientific advances are compatible with the safety, dignity and rights of people.

3 Nurses and the Profession

The nurse assumes the major role in determining and implementing acceptable standards of clinical nursing practice, management, research and education.

The nurse is active in developing a core of research-based professional knowledge.

The nurse, acting through the professional organisation, participates in creating and maintaining safe, equitable social and economic working conditions in nursing.

4 Nurses and Co-workers

The nurse sustains a co-operative relationship with co-workers in nursing and other fields.

The nurse takes appropriate action to safeguard individuals, families and communities when their health is endangered by a co-worker or any other person.

Source: *ICN code of ethics for nurses*, International Council of Nurses, 2006, Geneva: Imprimeries Populaires. Reprinted with permission.

The Nursing and Midwifery Council has recently updated *The code: Standards of conduct, performance and ethics for nurses and midwives* (NMC, 2008) to encompass not only professional conduct and performance but also ethics. The code states that:

- The people in your care must be able to trust you with their health and well-being.
- To justify that trust, you must make the care of people your first concern, treating them as individuals and respecting their dignity.
- Work with others to protect and promote the health and well-being of those in your care, their families and carers, and the wider community.
- Provide a high standard of practice and care at all times.
- Be open and honest, act with integrity and uphold the reputation of your profession.
- As a professional, you are personally accountable for actions and omissions in your practice and must always be able to justify your decisions.
- You must always act lawfully, whether those laws relate to your professional practice or personal life.
- Failure to comply with this code may bring your fitness to practice into question and endanger your registration.

Making Ethical Decisions

Ethical dilemmas differ from problems. Problems can be solved whereas ethical dilemmas require a choice to be made. Responsible ethical reasoning is rational and systematic and should be based on ethical principles and codes rather than on emotions, intuition, fixed policies or precedent (that is, an earlier similar occurrence).

BOX 5-2 Examples of Nurses' Obligations in Ethical Decisions

- Maximise the patient's well-being.
- Balance the patient's need for autonomy with family members' responsibilities for the patient's well-being.
- Support each family member and enhance the family support system.
- Carry out hospital policies.
- Protect other patients' well-being.
- Protect the nurse's own standards of care.

A good decision is one that is in the patient's best interest and at the same time preserves the integrity of all involved. Nurses have ethical obligations to their patients, to their employers and to other healthcare professionals. Therefore, nurses must weigh competing factors when making ethical decisions. Although ethical reasoning is principle-based and has the patient's well-being at heart, being involved in ethical problems and dilemmas is stressful for the nurse. The nurse may feel torn between obligations to the patient, the family and the employer. What is in the patient's best interest may be contrary to the nurse's personal belief system. In settings in which ethical issues arise frequently, nurses should establish support systems such as clinical supervision, counselling and debriefing sessions to allow expression of their feelings.

Many nursing problems are not moral problems at all, but simply questions of good nursing practice. An important first step in ethical decision making is to determine whether a moral situation exists. The following criteria may be used:

- A difficult choice exists between actions that conflict with the needs of one or more persons.
- Moral principles or frameworks exist that can be used to provide some justification for the action.
- The choice is guided by a process of weighing reasons.
- The decision must be freely and consciously chosen.
- The choice is affected by personal feelings and by the particular context of the situation.

Although the nurse's input is important, in reality several people are usually involved in making an ethical decision. Therefore, collaboration, communication and compromise are important skills for health professionals.

CLINICAL ALERT

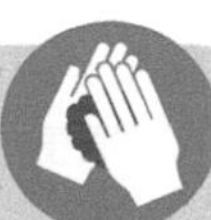

Ethical behaviour is contextual - what is an ethical action or decision in one situation may not be ethical in a different situation.

Strategies to Enhance Ethical Decisions and Practice

Several strategies help nurses overcome possible organisational and social constraints that may hinder the ethical practice of nursing and create moral distress for nurses. You as a nurse should do the following:

- Become aware of your own values and the ethical aspects of nursing.
- Be familiar with nursing codes of ethics.
- Respect the values, opinions and responsibilities of other healthcare professionals that may be different from your own.
- Strive for collaborative practice in which nurses' function effectively in cooperation with other healthcare professionals.

SPECIFIC ETHICAL ISSUES

Some of the ethical problems the nurse encounters most frequently are issues relating to patients who want a baby that increase the survival of a child (designer babies), euthunasia, organ transplantation, end-of-life decisions, withdrawing food and fluids, and breaches of patient confidentiality.

'Designer Babies'

Advanced scientific technology enables doctors to screen embryos. 'Designer babies' is a colloquial term applied to babies who are screened to determine sex and genes and for genetic disorders. There is much controversy and debate around this subject area, i.e. is it morally right?

Organ Transplantation

Organs for transplantation may come from living donors or from donors who have just died. Ethical issues related to organ transplantation include allocation of organs, selling of body parts, involvement of children as potential donors, consent, clear definition of death, and conflicts of interest between potential donors and recipients. In some situations, a person's religious belief may also present conflict. For example, certain religions forbid the mutilation of the body, even for the benefit of another person.

End-of-Life Issues

The increase in technological advances and the growing number of older adults have expanded the ethical dilemmas faced by healthcare professionals. Providing patients, who are at the end of life, with information and professional assistance, as well as the highest quality of care and caring, is of the utmost importance. Some of the most frequent disturbing ethical problems for nurses involve issues that arise around death and dying. These include euthanasia, assisted suicide, termination of life-sustaining treatment, and withdrawing or withholding of food and fluids.

Euthanasia

Euthanasia, a Greek word meaning 'good death', is popularly known as 'mercy killing'. Active euthanasia involves actions to directly bring about the patient's death, with or without patient consent. An example of this would be the administration of a lethal medication to end the patient's suffering. Regardless of the caregiver's intent, active euthanasia is forbidden by law and can result in criminal charges of murder.

Active euthanasia is giving patients the means to kill themselves if they request it (e.g. providing pills or a weapon). Some countries have laws permitting assisted euthanasia for patients who are severely ill, near death and who wish to kill themselves. In any case, the nurse should recall that legality and morality are not one and the same. Determining whether an action is legal is only one aspect of deciding whether it is ethical. The question of euthanasia is still controversial in the UK today with individuals still facing imprisonment if they assist in a 'mercy killing'.

Passive euthanasia involves the withdrawal of extraordinary means of life support, such as removing a ventilator or withholding special attempts to resuscitate a patient (e.g. do not resuscitate orders).

Withdrawing or Withholding Food and Fluids

It is generally accepted that providing food and fluids is part of ordinary nursing practice and, therefore, may be a moral duty. However, when food and fluids are administered by tube to a dying patient, or are given over a long period of time to an unconscious patient who is not expected to improve, then some consider it to be an extraordinary, or heroic, measure. A nurse is morally obligated to withhold food and fluids (or any treatment) if it is determined to be more harmful to administer them than to withhold them. The nurse must also honour competent patients' refusal of food and fluids.

ACTIVITY 5-1

Discuss how you would manage the care of a patient following an attempt to self-abort, if the nurse looking after her disagreed with abortion and the patient had been admitted to your ward under your colleague's care following the attempt.

Confidentiality

In keeping with the principle of autonomy, nurses are obligated to respect patients' privacy and confidentiality. Sharing of patient information should almost always be undertaken with the patient's consent, and this information should be related to their healthcare. Patients should be able to trust nurses to divulge only the appropriate information at all times, as outlined by the Caldicott principles (2008), the Data Protection Act (1998) and the Department of Health (DH, 2010).

The NMC (2008) code of conduct states that nurses must:

- respect people's right to confidentiality;
- ensure people are informed about how and why information is shared by those who will be providing their care;
- disclose information if they believe someone may be at risk of harm, in line with the law of the country in which they are practising.

Patients must be able to trust that nurses will reveal details of their situations only as appropriate and will communicate only the information necessary to provide for their healthcare. Computerised patient records make sensitive data accessible to more people and emphasise issues of confidentiality. Nurses should help develop and follow security measures and policies to ensure appropriate use of patient data. For example, nurses should not give their system security codes to unauthorised persons to allow access to computer files.

ADVOCACY

Advocacy in nursing is an essential component of nursing practice (Hanks, 2008). When people are ill, they are frequently unable to assert their rights as they would if they were healthy. Nurses are very often the advocate for a patient in their care and either inform the patient or speak up on behalf of the patient by presenting the patient's views and acting in the patient's best interests. Advocacy is about providing choices and informed choice.

If a patient lacks decision-making capacity, is legally incompetent or is a minor, these rights can be exercised on the patient's behalf by a designated individual. It is important, however, for the nurse to remember that patient control over health decisions is a western view. In other countries and societies, such decisions may normally be made by the head of the family or another member of the community. The nurse must ascertain the patient's and family's views and honour their traditions regarding the locus of decision making.

The Advocate's Role

The overall goal of the patient advocate is to protect patients' rights. An advocate informs patients about their rights and provides them with the information they need to make informed decisions. The code states that the nurse must act as an advocate for those in their care, helping them to access relevant health and social care, information and support.

An advocate supports patients in their decisions, giving them full or at least mutual responsibility in decision making when they are capable of it. The advocate must be careful to remain objective and not convey approval or disapproval of the patient's choices. Advocacy requires accepting and respecting the patient's right to decide, even if the nurse believes the decision to be wrong.

In mediating, the advocate directly intervenes on the patient's behalf, often by influencing others. An example of acting on behalf of a patient is asking a doctor to review with the patient the reasons for and the expected duration of therapy because the patient says he always forgets to ask the doctor.

BOX 5-3 Values Basic to Patient Advocacy

- The patient is an autonomous being who has the right to make choices and decisions.
- Patients have the right to expect a nurse-patient relationship that is based on shared respect, trust, collaboration in solving problems related to health and healthcare needs, and consideration of their thoughts and feelings.
- It is the nurse's responsibility to ensure the patient has access to healthcare services that meet health needs.
- It is the nurse's responsibility that the patient has access to all the information that they need to make informed decisions.

Advocacy in the Community Setting

Although the goals of advocacy remain the same, caring for a person at home poses unique concerns for the nurse advocate. For example, while in the hospital, people may operate from the values of the hospital and the healthcare professionals. When they are at home they tend to operate from their own personal values, and may revert to old habits and ways of doing things that may not be beneficial to their health. The nurse may see this as noncompliance; nevertheless, patient autonomy must be respected provided the patient has been presented with informed choices.

Professional and Public Advocacy

Nurses who function responsibly as professional and public advocates are in a position to effect change. To act as an advocate in this arena, the nurse needs an understanding of the ethical issues in nursing and healthcare, as well as knowledge of the laws and regulations that affect nursing practice and the health of society (see Chapter 4).

Being an effective patient advocate involves the following:

- being assertive;
- recognising that the rights and values of patients and families must take precedence when they conflict with those of healthcare providers;
- being aware that conflicts may arise over issues that require consultation, confrontation or negotiation between the nurse and administrative personnel, or between the nurse and doctor; or nurse, patient, family members and members of the multidisciplinary team;
- working with community agencies and lay practitioners;
- knowing that advocacy may require political action – communicating a patient's healthcare needs to government and other officials who have the authority to do something about these needs.

Dignity and Respect

An individual has an ethical and moral right to dignity and respect. Dignity and respect should underpin all nursing care (WAG, 2003). According to Article 8 of the Human Right Act 1998 each individual has a right to respect for his or her private and family life and there should be no interference by a public authority except in certain circumstances for the protection of health or morals.

Individuals also have a right for others to respect these basic human rights especially when vulnerable (e.g. in a caring environment). According to the RCN (2008: 8):

> *Dignity is concerned with how people feel, think and behave in relation to the worth or value of themselves and others. To treat someone with dignity is to treat them as being of worth, in a way that is respectful of them as valued individuals.*

In care situations, dignity may be promoted or diminished by: the physical environment; organisational culture; the attitudes and behaviour of the nursing team and others; and the way in which care activities are carried out. When dignity is present people feel in control, valued, confident, comfortable and able to make decisions for themselves. When dignity is absent people feel devalued, lacking in control and comfort. They may lack confidence and be unable to make decisions for themselves or feel humiliated, embarrassed or ashamed.

Dignity applies equally to those who have capacity and to those who lack it. Everyone has equal worth as human beings and must be treated as if they are able to feel, think and behave in relation to their own worth or value.

The nursing team should, therefore, treat all people in all settings and of any health status with dignity, and dignified care should continue after death.

Maintaining the dignity of patients in practice is about treating each individual with respect, talking and listening to patients, and not undermining their requests, concerns or problems. Valuing their choices, offering support and providing privacy (e.g. drawing the curtains around the bedside when taking the patient to the bathroom) are all essential. If the patient wishes to discuss personal issues then you must provide enough personal space where you are not overlooked or overheard. Ensure that there are adequate supplies of sheets and blankets and provide efficient non-judgemental support to the patient with their activities of daily living (e.g. incontinence, helping with eating and drinking, managing an odorous wound, covering the patient when helping them to wash). While these apply to both a hospital and home environment it is important that when visiting a patient at home, for example, that the nurse is non-judgemental regarding the home environment, maintains confidentiality and discretion when visitors are in the home, and provides reassurance to allay any fears that the patient may have. Remember to treat patients as you would like yourself or a member of your family to be treated, i.e. with dignity and respect.

EQUALITY AND DIVERSITY

Equality is about promoting a fairer society – where all can participate and have the opportunity to reach their potential. It is supported by legislation designed to address unfair discrimination which may be based on membership of a particular group.

Diversity is about recognising and valuing difference in its broadest sense: for example, creating a working culture and practices that recognise, respect, value and harness difference for the benefit of the organisation and the individual. There can be no equality of opportunity if difference is not recognised and valued. The areas covered are:

- age
- faith
- race
- disability
- gender
- sexual orientation.

Disability Discrimination

The Disability Discrimination Act 1995 as amended by the Special Educational Needs and Disability Act 2001 gives disabled students rights (and of course responsibilities). Disabilities include:

- specific learning difficulty (e.g. dyslexia),
- hearing loss,
- medical conditions.

It is the organisation's responsibility to disclose and make reasonable adjustments, when equality and diversity is compromised. Placements have a joint responsibility along with HEIs not to discriminate against students. Of course if a student does not disclose a disability then reasonable adjustments cannot be made.

The Equality Commission for Northern Ireland, in partnership with the Department of Health, Social Services and Public Safety, have developed the document 'Racial Equality Good Practice Guide', with the aim of meeting the needs of the community including individuals from black, minority ethnic and traveller backgrounds. The document highlights nine key issues: resources and staffing issues, staffing, ethnic monitoring of patients, communication, diet, religion, patient choice, patient complaints and user perspectives.

CRITICAL REFLECTION

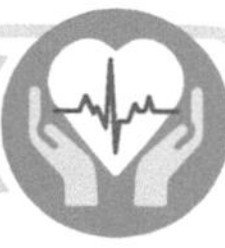

Revisit the case study on page 72. Now that you have read this chapter, discuss and consider what you think are the key issues that you need to consider both from a professional and personal aspect. Do you think that what Claire and David are considering is the right option, taking into account both your and their values? What is your role as Claire's advocate, regarding patient confidentiality and the moral principles in relation to Claire, David and their family?

The following points may be considered when exploring the case study and your own values and judgements:

- ethics
- morality
- beneficence
- values both professional and personal
- beliefs and attitudes
- dignity
- autonomy
- empathy
- communication
- advocacy
- collaboration
- teamwork
- the law.

CHAPTER HIGHLIGHTS

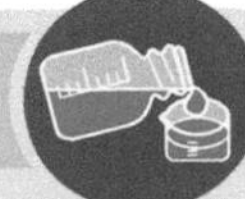

- Values give direction and meaning to life and guide a person's behaviour.
- Values are freely chosen, prized and cherished, affirmed to others, and consistently incorporated into one's behaviour.
- Values clarification is a process in which people identify, examine and develop their own values.
- Nursing ethics refers to the moral problems that arise in nursing practice and to ethical decisions that nurses make.
- Morality refers to what is right and wrong in conduct, character or attitude.
- Moral issues are those that arouse conscience, are concerned with important values and norms, and evoke words such as *good*, *bad*, *right*, *wrong*, *should* and *ought*.
- Three common moral frameworks (approaches) are consequence-based (teleologic), principles-based (deontologic) and relationships-based (caring-based) theories.
- Moral principles (e.g. autonomy, beneficence, nonmaleficence, justice, fidelity and veracity) are broad, general philosophical concepts that can be used to make and explain moral choices.
- A professional code of ethics is a formal statement of a group's ideals and values that serves as a standard and guideline for the group's professional actions and informs the public of its commitment.
- Nurses' ethical decisions are influenced by their moral theories and principles, levels of cognitive development, personal and professional values, and nursing codes of ethics.
- The goal of ethical reasoning, in the context of nursing, is to reach a mutual, peaceful agreement that is in the best interests of the patient; reaching the agreement may require compromise.
- Nurses can enhance their ethical practice and patient advocacy by clarifying their own values, understanding the values of other healthcare professionals, and becoming familiar with nursing codes of ethics.
- Patient advocacy involves concern for and actions on behalf of another person or organisation in order to bring about change.
- The functions of the advocacy role are to inform, support and mediate.
- Dignity and respect are essential when caring for a patient in your care.
- Treat all individuals equally and without discrimination regardless of age, faith, race, disability, gender and/or sexual orientation.

ACTIVITY ANSWERS

ACTIVITY 5-1 An abortion or miscarriage is a traumatic experience for the individual, family and nurses and it may often be against the individual's, family's or nurse's culture. There are professional issues to be considered and the following are some of the points you may wish to consider in your answer:

- effective communication
- confidentiality
- duty of care
- ethics
- morality
- collaboration
- teamwork
- law
- advocacy.

REFERENCES

Beauchamp, T. and Childress, J. (2001) *Principles of biomedical ethics* (5th edn), Oxford: Oxford University Press.

Caldicott (2008) *Principles into practice* (2008), Cardiff: Welsh Assembly Government.

Data Protection Act (1998) **http://www.legislation.gov.uk/ukpga/1998/29/contents** (Accessed 27/06/2011).

DH (2010) *Confidentiality: the NHS Code of Practice. Supplementary guidance: public interest disclosure*, Leeds: Department of Health.

Gilligan, C. (1982) *In a different voice*, Cambridge, MA: Harvard University Press.

Hanks, R. (2008) 'The lived experience of nursing advocacy', *Nursing Ethics*, 15(4).

ICN (2006) *ICN code for nurses: Ethical concepts applied to nursing*, Geneva: Imprimeries Populaires.

Kohlberg, L. (1969) 'Stage and sequence: The cognitive-developmental approach to socialisation', in D.A. Goslin (ed.), *Handbook of socialisation theory and research* (pp. 347–480), Chicago: Rand McNally.

Kozier, B., Erb, G., Berman, A., Snyder, S., Lake, R. and Harvey, S. (2008) *The fundamentals of nursing: Concepts, process and practice*, Harlow: Pearson Education.

NMC (2008) *The code of professional conduct – standards for conduct, performance and ethics*, London: NMC.

NMC (2010) *Standards for pre-registration nursing education, Annexe 3*, London: NMC.

NMC (2010) *The guidance on professional conduct for nursing and midwifery students*, London: NMC.

Ritchie, D. and Hall, C. (2009) *What is nursing? Theory and practice*, Exeter: Learning Matters.

RCN (2008) *Dignity at the heart of everything we do*, London: RCN.

Sala, R. and Manara, D. (2001) 'Nurses and requests for female genital mutilation: Cultural rights versus human rights', *Nursing Ethics*, 8: 247–258.

Thompson, I., Melia, K., Boyd, K. and Horsburgh, D. (2006) *Nursing Ethics* (5th edn), Edinburgh: Churchill Livingstone.

Tschudin, V. (2004) *Ethics in nursing*, China: Elsevier Ltd.

UK Clinical Ethics Network (2010) available from www.ethics-network.org.uk/

WAG – Welsh Assembly Government (2003) *Fundamentals of care*, Cardiff: Welsh Assembly Government.

Waters, A. (2005) 'Nursing is the most emotionally rewarding career', *Nursing Standard*, 19(30): 22–28.

FURTHER RESOURCES

Fundamentals of Nursing Dignity http://www.rcn.org.uk/__data/assets/pdf_file/0010/191737/003_292.pdf

International Code for Nurses: Code of Ethics for Nurses http://www.icn.ch/icncode.pdf

Summary of the Human Rights Act 1998 http://www.direct.gov.uk/en/Governmentcitizensandrights/Yourrightsandresponsibilities/DG_4002951?cids=Google_PPC&cre=Government_Citizens_Rights

The code: Standards of conduct, performance and ethics for nurses and midwives http://www.nmc-uk.org/

The Human Rights Act 1998 http://www.opsi.gov.uk/acts/acts1998/ukpga_19980042_en_4

Equity and Diversity http://www.dhsspsni.gov.uk/eq-raceeqhealth

CHAPTER 6
MENTAL HEALTH

Keith Bradley-Adams

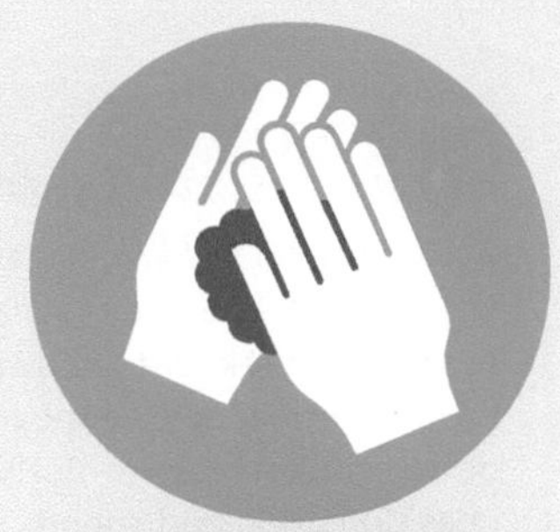

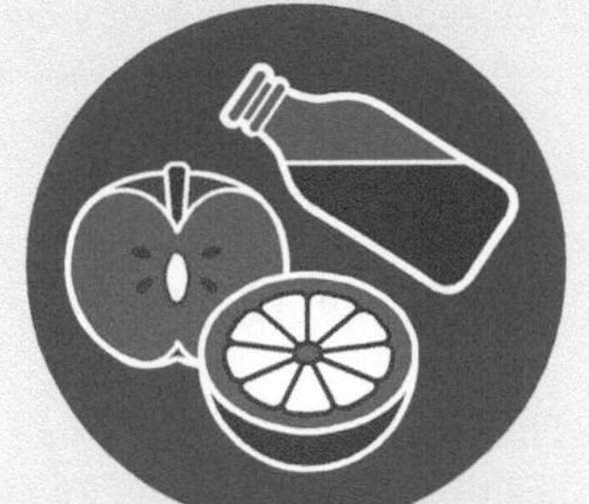

LEARNING OUTCOMES

After completing this chapter, you will be able to:

- Differentiate between the terms mental health and mental illness/disorder.
- Demonstrate an awareness of a range of disorders including: anxiety; post-traumatic stress disorder; depression; mania; bipolar disorder; schizophrenia; dissociative disorder; self-harm and suicide; dementia; and personality disorder.
- Describe appropriate interventions to be employed when nursing elderly confused patients.

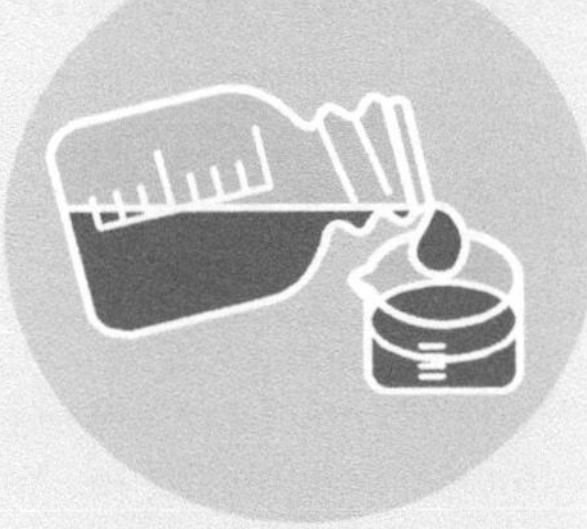

After reading this chapter you will be able to differentiate between the terms mental health and mental illness/disorder; demonstrate awareness of disorders and describe appropriate interventions. This chapter relates to **Essential Skills Clusters (NMC, 2010) 1–13 and 16**, as appropriate for each progression point.

Ensure that you really understand this chapter by logging on to your complimentary **MyNursingKit** at **www.pearsoned.co.uk/kozier**. Complete the self-assessment tests to check your progress and utilise further activities to practise and confirm your understanding.

CASE STUDY

Betty is an 83-year-old woman being nursed on a medical ward. She lives alone in what was the family home before her husband, Derek, passed away four years ago. Betty's children have all grown up and moved away and she rarely sees them or her grandchildren. Betty was admitted suffering from a chest infection and spends most of her day in bed apparently sleeping. Betty is a very quiet lady and never initiates conversations with staff, visitors or other patients. When Betty does respond to others she appears rather confused and disorientated. What do you think is Betty's most likely diagnosis? What could you do to help Betty if she was under your care? After reading this chapter you will be able to identify nursing strategies to support Betty.

INTRODUCTION

This chapter discusses some of the major themes in mental health nursing. Its principle focus is the aetiology and care of the more commonly diagnosed psychotic and neurotic disorders. Students should take note that the main role of the psychiatric nurse is to develop a **therapeutic relationship** with their clients and to work with them towards solutions of their problems as they perceive them. This is underpinned by the **humanistic** approach to person-centred care, valuing each client as idiopathic, i.e. an individual with needs which, even when they may be similar to those of others, are always unique to that person.

DEFINING MENTAL HEALTH

ACTIVITY 6-1

Before reading the definition below what do you think the term 'mental health' means? What sort of people may have 'mental health'? Do you know anyone with mental health?

When discussing our general (physical) health most 'lay' people seldom confuse the terms '*health*' and '*illness*'. However there is widespread confusion and misuse of these terms when discussing mental health. Many lay people assume that when discussing mental health we are actually discussing illness, this is simply not true. Health and illness are different concepts whether we are discussing our physical well-being or our psychological well-being.

Try asking a group of your peers 'Does anyone have mental health?' and see what responses you get. Most people will automatically equate this question with illness and accuse you of calling them 'mad'. Each and every one of us will almost certainly experience mental health; many of us will probably experience mental ill-health too.

The World Health Organization (WHO) (2005) assert that 'There is no health without mental health' and define health as 'a state of complete physical, mental and social well-being and not merely the absence of disease or infirmity'. The WHO goes on to say 'Mental health is clearly an integral part of this definition. The goals and traditions of public health and health promotion can be applied just as usefully in the field of mental health as they have been in heart health, infectious diseases and tobacco control'.

Mental health therefore is not simply the absence or avoidance of **mental disorder**. Rather it is as a state of wellness or well-being in which persons are able to function to the optimum level of their own innate ability, achieving their own life goals and thus realising their full potential. This would include all aspects of potential including relationships, work, education, etc.

As most people are able to achieve this and continue to lead lives where they are able to realise their potential (provided of course that they have a realistic view of what their true potential is and that if any barriers to achievement exist then they are not health barriers) then it is true to say that most therefore experience 'mental health'. Indeed even those who do suffer periods of ill-health will almost certainly also experience periods of health.

It is estimated that as many as one in four adults will be affected by mental illness at some point in their lives. This could be a brief, acute episode or an **enduring**, chronic condition. It could be a one-off experience or an illness that returns on two or more occasions. Often such 'breakdowns', as most lay people refer to these episodes, are linked to stressful life events such as bereavement, loss of a job, etc.

Individuals' experiences of mental disorder may be brief or **transient** or long-lasting and enduring. Some individuals will experience long periods of 'wellness' interspersed with short periods of disorder, for others their experience may be long periods of disorder with short periods of wellness. We refer to these periods of disorder as **relapse** and much of the focus of contemporary mental healthcare is on relapse prevention.

Mental health is a vital component of our overall health status. As the WHO states: 'There is no health without mental health', a declaration that serves to remind us of the need to consider the whole person. All aspects of our well-being are intrinsically linked and care must be based on an integrated biological, psychological and sociological assessment. This **paradigm** is properly referred to as a **bio-psycho-social model**, a **whole-person approach** or (more commonly) a **holistic approach**.

The alternative term **complex needs** is sometimes applied to this association of conditions.

Herberts and Eriksson (1995) hold a holistic view of health which they describe as being 'multi-dimensional' and say that all aspects of our health reflect three different dimensions: (a) health as behaviour, (b) health as being, (c) health as becoming. These dimensions describe our efforts to avoid illness, to cope with illness should it occur, and to move on and adopt future health behaviours. 'Health as being' demonstrates a truly holistic state the authors describe as 'characterised by a striving for a kind of balance or harmony in one's inner state. One understands the connection between physical and mental elements, between body and soul, between internal and external elements' (Herberts and Eriksson, 1995).

Mental ill-health is often referred to as 'mental illness' although it is more appropriate to refer to it as **mental disorder**. Both the *International Classification of Diseases* 10th edition (ICD-10) (WHO, 2007) and the *US Diagnostic and Statistical Manual of Mental Disorders* 4th edition (DSM-iv) (American Psychiatric Association, 2000) adopt this term. The term 'illness' appeared in the 1983 Mental Health Act but was replaced with the term 'disorder' in the 2007 Mental Health Act. Section 1(2) of the 2007 Act states: 'In this Act "*mental disorder*" means any disorder or disability of the mind; and "*mentally disordered*" shall be construed accordingly.'

The redrafting of the Act in 2007 amended the 1983 Act and abolished the four categories of mental disorders, introducing instead the simplified term of disorder. (Note that the Mental Health Act (2007) applies to England and Wales only. For Scotland please refer to the Mental Health (Care and Treatment) (Scotland) Act 2003, for Northern Ireland the Mental Health (Northern Ireland) Order 1986 applies.)

'Disorder' is a wide-ranging term which includes a series of neurotic and psychotic disorders such as depression, schizophrenia, bi-polar disorder, etc. Under the terms of the 2007 Act mental disorders do not include addiction to alcohol or drugs and therefore persons can neither be compulsorily detained nor treated for these behaviours alone. They may be detained if they are found to be experiencing a concurrent disorder however. Many patients present with both substance misuse and mental disorder and are said to have a dual diagnosis.

ACTIVITY 6-2

Jeff is a 59-year-old man with a diagnosis of chronic alcohol abuse. His GP wishes to have him admitted to hospital but Jeff is refusing to go. Can he be treated against his wishes under a compulsory treatment order? If he entered care on a voluntary basis and was experiencing auditory hallucinations (hearing voices) could he be detained if he wished to leave?

It is important to understand the difference between the **Mental Health Act (1983)** (as amended by the MHA 2007) and the **Mental Capacity Act (2005)**. (Note that the Mental Capacity Act (2005) only applies to England and Wales. For Scotland the Adults with Incapacity (Scotland) Act (2000) applies whilst for Northern Ireland there is no equivalent Act at the time of writing. However, the Bamford Review (DHSSPS 2007) has recommended that NI adopts similar legislation to the rest of the UK.)

The Mental Capacity Act (2005) provides a statutory framework to empower and protect vulnerable people who are not able to make their own decisions. The Act requires care staff and others to no longer assume that individuals may permanently lack capacity due to disorder or disability. Instead decisions should be made for patients on the basis that the person is unable to make that particular decision at that time. The whole Act is underpinned by a set of five key principles:

- a presumption of capacity – every adult has the right to make his or her own decisions and must be assumed to have capacity to do so unless it is proved otherwise;
- the right for individuals to be supported to make their own decisions – people must be given all appropriate help before anyone concludes that they cannot make their own decisions;
- that individuals must retain the right to make what might be seen by others as eccentric or unwise decisions;
- that anything done for, or on behalf of, people without capacity must be in their best interests; and
- that anything done for, or on behalf of, people without capacity should be the least restrictive of their basic rights and freedoms.

The Act applies to any adult who lacks decision-making capacity and may include those suffering from **dementia**, learning disability (especially severe learning disability), brain injury, severe mental disorder, etc. It also applies to those with temporary incapacity due, for example, to alcohol or drugs, unconsciousness, severe pain, trauma, etc. It is important to bear in mind that the Mental Capacity Act (2005) applies to all individuals, even those who are detained under the Mental Health Act (1983).

Detention under the Mental Health Act (1983) cannot be over-ruled by the Mental Capacity Act (2005). Whilst a patient may insist, for example, that they believe it is in their best interests to leave a care setting if they are lawfully detained then they would not be able to do so. The Mental Health Act always 'trumps' the Mental Capacity Act therefore. However, where an incapable patient requires electro-convulsive therapy (ECT) a second opinion doctor (SOAD) is not entitled to authorise such treatment where:

- there is a valid and applicable advance decision refusing ECT;
- an attorney with authority under a lasting power of attorney (LPA) refuses consent;
- a deputy with authority refuses consent.

The Mental Capacity Act (2005) also introduced the **Deprivation of Liberty Safeguards (DoLS)**. These came into effect in April 2009 and brought new responsibilities and legal duties on registered care homes and hospital in-patient services. The Deprivation of Liberty Safeguards represent an important new protection for people in hospitals and care homes who may need to be deprived of their liberty in order to protect them from serious harm. DOLS do not apply if a person is detained in hospital under the Mental Health Act (1983). However, they do apply if a person is under **guardianship**. The purpose of guardianship is to enable patients to receive care in the community where it cannot be provided without the use of compulsory powers. Section 7 of the Mental Health Act (2007) allows for guardianship under the auspices of a council on the recommendation of two doctors and an application by an approved social worker or nearest relative.

DOLS apply to anyone who:

- is aged 18 or older;
- is suffering a disorder or disability of the mind;
- lacks the capacity to give consent to their care/treatment;
- is receiving care or treatment that might amount to a deprivation of liberty under Article 5 of the European Convention of Human Rights.

If there is no alternative but to deprive such a person of their liberty, the safeguards say that a hospital or care home must apply to the council (for care homes) or to the primary care trust (for hospitals) for authorisation. The council or primary care trust is known as the supervisory body.

The supervisory body must assess the person concerned to see whether they:

- are deprived of their liberty;
- come under the new law;
- are being deprived of their liberty in their best interests.

Sometimes there is no alternative other than to deprive a person of their liberty, provided of course that this action is in their best interests. Some examples are:

- someone resists being admitted to a place of safety and they are restrained and/or sedated so that they can be admitted;
- staff have complete control over the care and movement of someone for a considerable time;
- the institution has decided that someone cannot be released into the care of others, or allowed to live somewhere else;
- carers ask for someone to be discharged to their care and this is refused;
- someone is not able to maintain social contacts because of restrictions placed on their seeing others.

A key principle of the Mental Health Act (2007) is that compulsory detention and treatment orders should only be applied to those individuals for whom 'appropriate medical treatment is available'. This change means that those persons who in the past may have been detained under a treatment order either for a condition that is untreatable or where the specialist care required is not available may no longer be detained.

This could mean, for example, that if a person suffering from **anorexia nervosa** and lives in an area where no specialist treatment centres are located then they should not be detained unless they are also suffering from another condition/disorder for which treatment is available and that they are also refusing that treatment.

This amendment is a fundamental change to the 1983 Act and reflects society's changing approach to the care of the mentally ill. It means that where compulsory detention occurs it is with an intention to treat the individual, and not simply as an excuse to exclude them from society.

The introduction of the **Care Programme Approach** (1991) was an attempt to deliver integrated and coordinated services which placed the needs of the individual patient at its heart. Its four main intended outcomes were:

- systematic arrangements for assessing the health and social needs of people accepted into specialist mental health services;
- the formation of a care plan which identifies the health and social care required from a variety of providers;
- the appointment of a key worker to keep in close touch with the service user and to monitor and coordinate care; and
- regular review and, where necessary, agreed changes to the care plan.

The policy has been revised on two occasions since (1999 and 2006) but the commitment to delivering individual care designed to support and maintain persons in the community through a named care coordinator remains the principle focus.

Although stigma still exists there is a wider acceptance and tolerance of mental disorder. Many celebrities now openly discuss their experiences of bi-polar disorder, depression, schizophrenia and other disorders. There are even hospitals and clinics which appear almost exclusively to treat celebrities, or anyone else with the means to fund their own care. However, when we think of these clinics we are most likely to think of treatments for misuse of alcohol or drugs.

The term **rehabilitation** or rehab is often applied to this care although strictly speaking rehabilitation refers to any therapeutic process intended to assist a person to return to their own habitat or home. This would include therapies such as physiotherapy as well as the psychological therapies to which this term is usually applied. In reality of course holistic care would involve a range of therapies to assist the service user to return to good health and promote future health. Rehabilitation therefore must focus on all needs, whether they are psychological, physiological or social needs. Generally the term is taken as meaning a return to the life or lifestyle the individual enjoyed before the disorder, i.e. their **premorbid** state. The process of managing a condition without curing it is termed **palliative care**: for many disorders this is the best we can offer our service users yet this term is seldom applied to mental disorder.

CLASSIFICATION OF MENTAL ILLNESS

Traditionally and historically in all care settings there is a requirement to divide illnesses or diseases into categories. There are practical reasons for this of course. It is logical, for example, to care for patients in a specialised care setting with dedicated staff expert in the required care, i.e. orthopaedic care, gynaecological care, etc. This division of services is based on the

medical model of care, a model that emphasises the need to identify and treat (i.e. manage or prevent) illness. This model is contrasted by the **social model** of care which offers an alternative approach, the emphasis on changing or adapting the individual lifestyle of the service user or of society at large to reduce 'problems' or their impact on society.

Recognising Mental Disorders

The signs and symptoms of mental disorder will vary greatly from individual to individual. When caring for those experiencing mental disorder it is crucial that nurses focus on the symptoms or experience of the individual and not overly concern themselves with a diagnosis. The nomenclature may be argued as being of little worth anyway when you consider the huge variety of dementias or indeed consider the equally diverse range of symptoms associated with schizophrenia. It is true to say that with all mental disorders the severity and longevity of an episode of ill health may vary greatly from individual to individual, and for individuals experiencing one or more episodes these episodes may differ from one another in the same regard. However, whilst disorders continue to be named, and sufferers consequentially labelled, it is necessary to have an understanding of what the terms mean. The more common disorders are described below.

The Person with Anxiety

Anxiety may be described as a normal physical and psychological reaction to stress. For example, a fear of heights or of dogs could be seen as nature's way of ensuring that we remove ourselves from harm and preserve ourselves at all costs. It is the psychological element of the stress response, and is in reality the body preparing for 'fight or flight' (Cannon, 1929). For some individuals low levels of anxiety may produce a beneficial effect. This paradoxical response to stress is common amongst athletes who perform better when the demand (whether external or internal) for them to do so is at its highest. This belief that certain types of stress may in fact be good for you originates from the work of Selye (1975) who coined the term **eustress** (literally good stress) to describe it.

ACTIVITY 6-3

Try asking your colleagues how far in advance they start their assignments. Is it the day they are handed out in class or the day before they are due to be submitted? Many students report that they function best when the stress of meeting a looming deadline is suddenly thrust upon them. Others will of course report a contrary view. We are all individuals after all!

Anxiety disorders are the most common of all mental disorders, affecting as many as 6% of the population. They are more common in women than in men. Although there are no absolute predictors of the likelihood to develop panic attacks many individuals who have a history of **phobias** will go on to develop panic disorders. There are a number of psychological theories which attempt to explain why some individuals experience anxiety disorders whilst others do not, for example:

- Freudian psychology explains anxiety as a product of stressful birth and early separation.
- Behaviouralist psychology describes it as a learned maladaptive response.
- Humanistic psychology asserts that anxiety is a result of denial of the true self.

It is unlikely that any one of these, or other approaches, alone can adequately account for anxiety, although for some individuals they may be strong predictors. For example, many clients who have experienced a traumatic birth may well go on to develop anxiety, those brought up by a phobic parent may well learn to develop the same responses, those struggling to come to terms with their sexuality may experience anxiety, etc. However, for many other individuals there will be no identifiable precursor, whilst others will experience stressful events without ever developing a disorder.

For some individuals anxiety may occur with very little stress and in a variety of settings. The term general anxiety disorder (GAD) has been applied to the suffering of anxiety concerning a range of issues. ICD-10 describes GAD as 'anxiety that is generalised and persistent but not restricted to, or even strongly predominating in, any particular environmental circumstances'. Rather more succinctly it describes GAD as being 'free-floating'.

ACTIVITY 6-4

Think of an occasion when you have felt anxious - attending an interview, sitting an exam, sitting your driving test, etc. How did you feel? What physical and psychological symptoms were present?

The signs and symptoms of anxiety are identical to those associated with stress. They are caused by an arousal of the body's natural defences and involve the release of hormones (adrenalin, noradrenalin, etc.) and it is the effects of these chemicals that we associate with stress and anxiety. The idiosyncratic response of each individual will differ, but some or all of the signs and symptoms shown in *Box 6-1* are likely to be present.

BOX 6-1 Psychological and Physical Symptoms

Psychological Symptoms

- Altered mood
- Avoidance
- Anger
- Depression
- Altered behaviours
- Increased or decreased appetite
- Tearfulness
- Sleep disturbance
- Hyper arousal/ alertness
- Reduced libido

Physical Symptoms

- Shortness of breath
- Tightness of chest
- Chest pain
- Increased heart rate
- Palpitations
- Dizziness
- Fainting
- Dry mouth
- Constipation or diarrhoea
- Muscle cramps or spasms
- Twitching
- Pins and needles
- Restlessness
- Sweating
- Sexual dysfunction
- Aches and pains
- Sleep disturbance

It is clear that the effects of anxiety may be extremely debilitating. The person suffering from anxiety disorder will find it impinges on their **global functioning**, affecting all aspects of their day-to-day living. Anxiety may affect the ability to form successful relationships, to seek education or employment, or to enjoy life's simple pleasures. This can become a self-perpetuating cycle, where the anxious person struggles to find work and happiness which in turn may increase anxiety. There are strong links between anxiety and poor physical health and also between anxiety and addictions.

Assessment and Interventions

When diagnosing general anxiety disorder it is necessary to first exclude other disorders. The disorder most commonly misdiagnosed as anxiety disorder is depression. Many screening tools have been developed over the years to assist clinicians in reaching a diagnosis (Becks Anxiety Inventory, Hamilton Anxiety Scale, Hospital Anxiety and Depression Scale, etc.) and although these tools are widely applied there is little evidence to suggest that any one tool is more accurate than others and clinicians must not rely on the screening tool alone. The **National Institute for Clinical Excellence** (**NICE**, 2004a) states: 'There is insufficient evidence on which to recommend a well-validated, self-reporting screening instrument to use in the diagnostic process, and so consultation skills should be relied upon to elicit all necessary information.'

NICE suggests that the clinician should first establish if the individual has experienced the signs and symptoms described previously and if no relevant **somatic** cause can be established then a diagnosis of anxiety may be made.

There are two main treatments available, **pharmacological interventions** or **psychosocial interventions**. Most individuals will receive a combination of both these approaches. It is important to discuss treatment options with the client and to coordinate a plan of care that meets the idiosyncratic wishes of the service user, not the clinician. This paradigm is of course supported in both person-centred-care and also the care programme approach.

Pharmacological Interventions

The long-term prescribing of **benzodiazepines** is no longer recommended. Whilst this was once the treatment of choice for many practitioners, particularly in the primary care setting, the potential for developing dependence on such drugs is well documented. Where pharmacological interventions are used today they should be for short-term (12–18 month) treatments only.

Some clients will remain on such treatments for longer periods, where this is the case their continued effectiveness should be considered and other treatment options discussed. Most clients will be prescribed anti-depressants rather than anxiolitics, the treatment of choice being **selective serotonin reuptake inhibitors (SSRIs)**. Some clients will receive **tricyclic antidepressants** rather than SSRIs, either because the SSRIs have not been effective or because the patient is able to tolerate one form of medication and not the other. When receiving SSRIs clients should receive sufficient support to help them manage their condition, particularly when withdrawing medication.

Psychological Interventions

Psychological interventions are believed to produce the longest-lasting beneficial effects for clients. They are the recommended treatment as they are both clinically effective and cost effective. The most common psychological interventions used in the treatment of anxiety are **cognitive behavioural therapy (CBT)** and **psycho-education**.

These therapies help clients identify a 'problem' or 'issue' and to seek a resolution. CBT encourages helping clients to identify what they think (**cognition**) and how they act (behaviour). The therapy involves proposing healthier alternatives and discussing these in order for the client to consider change.

For example, if a client reports feeling anxious in a certain situation they would be asked to discuss that specific situation in terms of thoughts, feelings (both physical and emotional) and actions taken or avoided. Each of these features will be analysed and discussed over a course of treatments, with the intention of helping the client to become more able to manage future events. Treatment may last from six weeks to six months, but is reported as being the most effective long-term solution to anxiety.

Other Interventions

Other interventions may include **relaxation therapy**. This involves educating the client to be able to relax, usually by undertaking a series of exercises designed to control breathing and heart rate. Audio tapes featuring a calming voice repeating the instructions whilst some gentle music plays in the background are a common tool to facilitate this. This technique may be applied individually or in groups.

The Person Experiencing Phobias

A **phobia** is an anxiety disorder which differs from general anxiety disorder in that it is focused on a specific issue rather than being global in nature. A phobia may be described as an irrational fear. The symptoms therefore would include a fear or loathing of a clearly defined situation or occurrence, e.g. an event or object (either animate or inanimate), without a rational cause and an extreme reaction when confronted with such stimuli. This would contrast with what may be considered rational fears, i.e. it may be considered rational to fear spiders in a country where deadly spiders are common but it would be irrational to fear the harmless spiders native to the UK and hence 'arachnophobia'.

When deciding if a fear is rational or not one must consider how the fear sits within the accepted 'norms' of society, taking account of the persons age, education, religion, cultural identity, etc. For example, Eurocentric views on witchcraft may differ from the African belief system so whilst a fear of witches (wicciphobia) may be considered irrational in a person of western European descent it may have a rational basis for someone from African descent.

One of the most common phobias in the UK is agoraphobia. Literally meaning 'fear of the marketplace' the term is applied to the irrational fear of going outdoors. Sufferers of phobias may vary greatly in their reaction to a stimulus. Mild symptoms may include increased heart rate or **respirations** whilst a severe reaction may comprise a panic attack.

Assessment and Interventions

All signs and symptoms for a phobia will be broadly identical to those of an anxiety disorder. Diagnosis would be made on history of predisposing factors, i.e. is it a general anxiety or an anxiety linked to a single identifiable cause. As with general anxiety disorder treatment options are psychological and pharmacological. The success rate of psychological interventions, particularly CBT, is very good and this remains the treatment of choice for sufferers of most phobias.

The Person Experiencing Stress and the Person Experiencing Post-Traumatic Stress Disorder (PTSD)

Stress is a normal physical and psychological response of the body to demands placed upon it. The signs and symptoms are as described under anxiety above. Abrupt or intermittent exposure to stress would generally result in short-term changes, whilst long-term exposure may result in stress-related illness. Chronic stress may effect almost every system in the body. Stress is associated with a whole raft of physical conditions such as raised blood pressure, increased risk of heart disease or stroke, sleep disturbance, infertility, etc. Psychological effects include increased susceptibility to anxiety disorder and depression.

Research suggests that men are more likely to experience stress-related illness than women. One of the factors believed to influence this is the relative reluctance of men to 'offload' stress. Whilst (generally) women are able to share emotional baggage with their peers men are more likely to find this uncomfortable and keep their feelings 'bottled up'. For some men, showing emotion may be perceived as a sign of weakness. This 'big boys don't cry' mentality is referred to as **limited self-disclosure**.

For many years it was believed that gastric ulcers were caused by stress. Recent research (Levy, 1989) has disproved this, it is now known that ulcers are caused by the presence of campylobacter organisms in the gut. However, stress may present itself in a number of other physical illnesses. There is a weight of evidence to support the belief that the body's immune system may be suppressed by exposure to stress. This occurs through a reduction in natural killer cell activity (Delahanty, 1997; Evans, 1995; Levy, 1987).

There are established links between stress and ill health (both physical and psychological) nevertheless. Holmes and Rahe (1967) undertook a review of 5,000 patients in a medical unit and discovered that almost all had been exposed to a stressful life event in the weeks or months prior to admission. From their study they developed a list of 43 stressful events that typically would precede the advent of illness. Their **social readjustment rating scale** ranks these events in order, those at the top being those most likely to initiate stress and subsequently ill health. The top 10 on their list are (Holmes and Rahe, 1967):

1. death of a spouse or child
2. divorce
3. marital separation
4. imprisonment
5. death of a close family member
6. personal illness or injury
7. marriage
8. dismissal from work
9. marital reconciliation
10. retirement.

Each of the categories on the scale carries a numerical value, with those at the top being the highest. The total of these points is used to determine the likelihood of ill health. Whilst significant events may be sufficient on their own to produce ill health a combination of lesser events may produce the same effect therefore. The effects of stress may not be immediately evident. After acute intense exposure to stressors individuals may suffer psychological illness at a later date.

This is generally referred to as **post-traumatic stress disorder (PTSD)** because of its strong association with traumatic events. A diagnosis of this disorder would require the individual to present with a stress disorder as a **sequelae** to a prior trauma. Whilst many believe that this is a relatively recent illness the first recording of an individual experiencing PTSD occurs in reports by Herodotus (490BC) of the Battle of Marathon.

PTSD has strong links to warfare, major catastrophes, road traffic accidents and even childbirth but it is impossible to predict its occurrence in any individual, or after any event, as such predictions will be confounded by the recognition that there appears to be no reliable means of predicting PTSD. A factor believed to influence individual susceptibility to developing

PTSD is the **locus of control** (Rotter, 1966). Whilst some individuals believe that they are able to influence or control events, and that they have control over their actions and responses (high internal locus), others feel that they have little control and that their destiny is controlled by others, or even by 'powers' outside their control (high external locus).

It is believed that individuals who feel they are in control of a situation to some degree are therefore less likely to experience it as traumatic, whilst those who perceive events as out of their control are more likely to view them as being traumatic. It is the absence of self-determination in these individuals at that time that produces the anxiety rather than the events themselves. This absence may be momentary (**transient**/acute) or long-lasting (permanent/chronic).

There is also a belief that individuals with existing neurotic traits are more at risk of developing PTSD, although again it seems impossible to proactively predict PTSD, only to be able to identify predisposing factors subsequently. Individuals with existing depressive disorders, anxiety disorders, compulsive behaviours, etc. are believed to be more at risk.

Assessment and Interventions

The signs and symptoms for PTSD will be similar to those of stress but will typically include an element of **pervasive thought**, i.e. memories forcing themselves into consciousness against your will. This may happen during waking hours (**flashbacks**) or when sleeping (**night terrors**). These pervasive thoughts or images are not to be confused with **hallucinations**. Pervasive or intrusive thoughts are the individual reliving a real experience, i.e. responding to real stimuli, rather than hallucinating which involves responding to or experiencing 'imagined' stimuli. (A more in-depth analysis of these phenomena is given later in this chapter.)

History of exposure to trauma is a key identifying factor. Generally PTSD will develop in the first six months after (post) the trauma. As this is a disorder caused by, or influenced by, the initial stress reaction at the time of the traumatic event the subsequent episodes (or symptoms) are referred to as **sequelae**. PTSD will also be differentiated from other neurotic disorders by its characteristic avoidance behaviours, hyper-arousal to stimuli and most importantly by the presence of intrusive thoughts.

Outbursts of aggression or terror may accompany these symptoms, particularly following sudden exposure to stimuli that remind the individual of the traumatic event, e.g. noises, flashes of light, etc. Avoidance of situations where exposure to such stimuli is likely (e.g. a firework display) is a common feature of individuals suffering PTSD.

Treatment will include psychosocial interventions (PSI) and pharmacological interventions. PSI will typically be CBT within a group of sufferers with similar disorders. Individual one-to-one CBT may also be offered. Often support networks exist for 'survivors' of traumatic events, and referral and engagement with such organisations may be of benefit for some sufferers.

Although sometimes referred to as 'shell shock' and believed by most lay persons to be a symptom of war PTSD appears to be more prevalent in non-military personnel exposed to catastrophic events. Survivors of natural disasters and of terrorist outrages are as likely, if not more likely, to develop symptoms. Fear *et al.* (2010) report that levels of PTSD amongst UK service personnel is 'relatively low' and that the most common mental health problem facing UK armed forces is alcoholism.

An anxiety disorder which is closely linked to PTSD is Da Costa's syndrome. This somatoform disorder (the physical manifestation of a psychological condition) is found almost exclusively in servicemen exposed to battle and has been referred to as 'Soldier's Heart' in some texts. Da Costa's syndrome produces chest pain, palpitations, exhaustion and other symptoms associated with **cardiac arrest** or myocardial infarction but with no real physical cause.

The Person Experiencing Obsessive-Compulsive Disorder

The occurrence of **intrusive thoughts** is not unique to PTSD. This phenomenon is also a feature of obsessive-compulsive disorder (OCD). Individuals experiencing OCD are often 'plagued' by persistent obsessive thoughts and by a compulsion to undertake tasks. The term obsessive is applied to these behaviours as the compulsion to undertake tasks, or rituals, may become all consuming. The intrusive thoughts are often distressing, and for some the ritualistic behaviours may be a means of trying to purge the thoughts, or at the very least provide distraction from them.

The pervasive thoughts are the thoughts of the person living the experience. There is no element of thought insertion or 'hearing voices'. The individual experiencing OCD is acting under their own **volition** or **impulse** and will not report being controlled by another. However, whilst the behaviours may be self-directed the individual will have little or no control over them, even when they recognise them as being unnecessary.

The compulsion to check that doors are locked, lights turned off, articles replaced in their correct location, etc. is an occurrence that many people will experience to some degree from time to time. These 'checking' behaviours are not to be confused with OCD. Whilst the activities may be broadly similar there are key differences between OCD and 'acceptable' behaviours.

To confirm a diagnosis of OCD there would be evidence that:

- The compulsion, driven by pervasive thoughts, to undertake rituals is so strong that it cannot be resisted. This is true even if the ritual has already been performed recently and/or repeatedly.
- The behaviours may have an underlying valid basis but because of their repetition or frequency they are broadly speaking senseless.
- Undertaking these routines interferes with the individual's ability to perform other activities of daily living and to continue to live their life in a manner of their choosing.
- The individual experiences acute anxiety.

Behaviours or rituals undertaken by individuals experiencing OCD tend to be very stereotypical. By this we do not mean that everyone experiencing OCD will perform the same practices, although certain behaviours are more common, but rather that for the individual patient their idiosyncratic behaviours will be the same, or similar, on each episode.

The intrusive thoughts provide the obsessional element of the disorder whilst the ritualistic behaviours are the compulsive element. Generally the behaviour is an attempt to reduce or remove the obsession. This is known as an **anankastic** behaviour. Experiencing intrusive thoughts may be extremely distressing. Such thoughts are often derogatory in nature, telling the individual they are unworthy or dirty, for example. The anankastic behaviours therefore try to resolve the thought by identifying what is at fault and attempting to put it right.

Common obsessions include:

- worrying about cleanliness of objects;
- worrying about personal health and hygiene;
- worrying about 'germs' or contamination;
- worrying about safety/security;
- fears about disposing of objects/property that 'may be needed';
- keeping everything in order or in its place;
- worrying about race, gender, religion, sexuality, etc.

Associated compulsive behaviours include:

- cleaning objects repeatedly;
- hand washing or bathing;
- using bleach or disinfectant excessively;
- checking doors, windows, appliances, etc.;
- hoarding or collecting things;
- arranging things in a precise order or position;
- repeating acts in a ritualistic way;
- repeating words, phrases, chants or prayers.

The compulsive behaviours are generally directly linked to the obsessive thoughts, i.e. anankastic. For example, if experiencing obsessive thoughts about dirt or contamination the individual is likely to exhibit compulsive washing and cleaning. Failing to act upon the obsessive thoughts will induce anxiety in the individual and performing the ritual is intended as a means of reducing this anxiety. Paradoxically for many the belief that this activity has not been performed to the necessary standard drives the person to repeat the activity over and over. Any reduction in anxiety is short term therefore, being replaced with an anxiety that the performance was inadequate, and the compulsion to perform rituals increases exponentially.

Insight into the disorder and its debilitating effects often leads to depression. Unfortunately, a depressive episode in an individual suffering from OCD may increase and magnify the obsessive thoughts resulting in a subsequent increase in the compulsive behaviours. This in turn may deepen the depression. This can become a self perpetuating cycle of a seemingly intransigent nature for an individual not receiving support and intervention.

Assessment and Interventions

Generally a diagnosis is made on the basis of self reporting and of observation. Individuals experiencing OCD will be encouraged to maintain a diary recording their thoughts and their behaviours. With the sufferers permission others (family or friends) may be involved in the monitoring of these behaviours.

A likely diagnosis would be made where it became clear that:

- all thoughts and **impulses** are recognised as being those of the sufferer;
- the thoughts or impulses are unpleasantly repetitive;
- evidence of unsuccessfully resisting all or some of these acts exists;
- the acts are in themselves not perceived as pleasurable (n.b. the absence of anxiety is not considered as pleasurable).

As with other **neuroses** the treatments are either pharmacological, psychological or a combination of the two. Choice of treatment will depend on the severity of the disorder and the presence/absence of depression or anxiety disorder.

The diagnosis of mild, moderate or severe OCD will be made on the individual's experience of his or her symptoms. Generally the following diagnostic criteria apply:

- *mild*: intrusive thoughts are not too distressing, the individual is able to resist some compulsions, anxiety low or absent, no depression present;
- *moderate*: intrusive thoughts are sometimes distressing, compulsions are not inhibiting ability to function, moderate anxiety, mood lowered;
- *severe*: intrusive thoughts are persistent and/or very distressing, unable to resist most compulsions, high anxiety, chronic depression.

It is important that diagnosis and treatment is based on the individual's perception of their symptomology and their report of how their day-to-day functioning is impaired. Severe impairment of their ability to undertake activities of daily living would therefore be a severe OCD even if the individual reports that compulsions and behaviours are minimal.

Where the individual is experiencing mild symptoms with no other disorders then the treatment of choice is likely to be CBT. For moderate disorders a more intensive programme of CBT and possibly a course of anti-depressants such as selective serotonin reuptake inhibitors (SSRIs) is probable, whilst for severe OCD combined therapy comprising SSRIs and intensive CBT is essential.

A model of CBT that has proved successful in treating OCD is exposure and response prevention (ERP). This therapy involves exposing the individual to stimuli that are producing fear and anxiety. Exposure would be managed carefully in a 'safe' environment to ensure the service user's personal safety (emotional and physical) is not compromised. Exposure may be physical (real or actual) or psychological (imagined or mental).

- physical, handling dirty objects;
- psychological, picturing yourself in a situation.

Following exposure most individuals with OCD will feel the compulsion to engage in ritualistic behaviour in order to resolve the anxiety. The therapist will engage with the client and attempt to delay or even prevent the compulsive reaction. As time progresses the individual will be able to exert more and more control over their compulsion and the need to react will lessen.

Progress is incremental and praise for success at each stage is vital to provide reassurance and affirmation of progress. If the individual has more than one stimulus, or more than one compulsive behaviour, it is common to begin with the more easily achievable goals. The duration of each session should not exceed one hour and, depending on the severity of the disorder, will normally comprise of about ten hours of therapy.

The Person Experiencing Depression

Depression is the fourth most common cause of disability and illness in the world. Two out of every three (about 67%) of adults will experience an episode of depression so severe that it will interfere with their ability to undertake their normal routines (activities of daily living) at some point in their lives. It is the third most common reason for consultation in general practice in the UK and is the most common psychiatric disorder.

In depression the individual will hold fixed and unshakeable negative thoughts. These beliefs that nothing is worthwhile and that everything is hopeless are referred to as nihilistic thoughts or **nihilism**. The collective term for a group, or family, of related thoughts or beliefs is a **schema** so we sometimes refer to individuals harbouring nihilistic thoughts as having 'negative schema' or 'negative schemata': schemata is the plural of schema and suggests that more than one group of thoughts is involved.

The incidence of depression appears to be more common in women than in men. In the UK it is estimated that 25% of adult women will seek help for depression at some time in their lives compared to just 10% of men. This may be in part due to the well documented reluctance of men to visit their GP and talk about their emotions. It is believed that men will attend their GP to report **somatic** symptoms of depression (see below) but not their actual mood.

Depression, and other **affective disorders**, often occur during the perinatal period, i.e. the period immediately before or after childbirth. It is reported that as many as 17% of all mothers will experience clinical depression within the first 90 days following childbirth. Some mothers may also experience psychotic disorders during the perinatal period. Approximately six out of every thousand women will develop symptoms of **mania**, symptoms of **schizophrenia** or **puerperal psychosis**.

Walsh (2009: 63) reports that 'Men are more likely to try to deal with their depression themselves, and often take drugs and alcohol'. This is true not only of depression but also of all other mental disorder in males. However, this may be considered of greater concern in depression as the potential to self-harm, including catastrophic self-harm, is greater in men than in women. This is not because the disorder is, strictly speaking, different from one gender to another. The signs and symptoms of depression are common to all persons of all ages and from all backgrounds. Nevertheless there is a greater prevalence of certain signs and symptoms in males, (Royal College of Psychiatrists, 2006). These symptoms are:

- irritability
- sudden anger
- increased loss of control
- greater risk-taking
- aggression.

Men are also more likely to commit suicide. This is not because the symptoms are more severe in males but because men are more likely to engage in acts of violence, including self-directed violence, than women.

Everybody experiences a low mood from time to time and it is important to be able to differentiate between 'sadness' and depression. Depression may be described as being mild, moderate or severe. Mood is always low and the individual is likely to lack energy and motivation. This will be characterised by marked lethargy, fatigue, isolation and a lack of interest in socialisation and particularly an inability to enjoy anything, known as **anhedonia**.

Other commonly identified symptoms include:

- sleep disturbance
- low appetite
- poor concentration and attention
- low self-esteem
- low self-confidence
- feelings of guilt and unworthiness
- gloomy or pessimistic outlook
- thoughts of suicide or self-harm.

Because we can all experience periods of feeling low a diagnosis of depression would normally only be made if the symptoms persist for a period of two weeks or more. However, if the onset of the symptoms is unusually rapid and/or if the symptoms are particularly severe a diagnosis may be made earlier. Differentiating between mild, moderate and severe depression involves a careful screening of the individual to assess which symptoms are present. 'Grades' of depression would normally only be used on the first presentation. These 'labels' are for diagnosis only and do not necessarily inform the treatment. Any subsequent episodes are generally referred to as **recurrent depression** and the severity seldom included.

Symptoms of depression are generally listed as two separate categories, those that are almost always present and those that are often also present (probables and possibles). The WHO (1994) presents those symptoms as two tables in the *International Classification of Diseases vol. 10* (ICD-10). For ease of use these tables are sometimes referred to as Category A symptoms and Category B symptoms (see *Box 6-2*).

BOX 6-2 ICD-10 Categories

Category A symptoms

- depressed mood;
- loss of interest and enjoyment;
- increased fatiguability (becoming tired easily).

Category B symptoms

- reduced concentration and attention;
- reduced self-esteem and self-confidence;
- ideas of guilt and unworthiness (even in a mild type of episode);
- bleak and pessimistic views of the future;
- ideas or acts of self-harm or suicide;
- disturbed sleep;
- diminished appetite.

In mild depression sufferers would be expected to exhibit any two category 'A' symptoms plus at least two category 'B' symptoms. Moderate depression would feature at least two category 'A' features plus three–four category 'B' symptoms. Severe depression would involve all three category 'A' features plus four or more category 'B' symptoms. This may be presented as shown in Table 6-1.

In mild depression the symptoms will be less intense and would not normally last for a period greater than about two weeks. The individual will be able to continue to undertake most activities of daily living, albeit with difficulty on occasion. The term 'mild' should not trivialise the problems, the symptoms will be distressing for the individual and will have an impact on their ability to work, socialise, etc.

In moderate depression the symptoms will be more manifest, either because there will be a greater number/variety of symptoms presented or because the symptoms presented are of increased intensity. Episodes would last for at least two weeks and ability to undertake normal activities would be compromised to a greater degree.

In severe depression the symptoms will be deeper and wider, i.e. more of them and to a greater intensity. They will severely restrict the ability to undertake other activities. Feelings of guilt, worthlessness and hopelessness are so intense and these feelings will persist for weeks or even months.

Individuals experiencing depression will often show little variation in their mood from day to day. It is common to show a decrease in mood as the day goes on though as what little optimism the individual may have woken with has been eroded minute by minute. This alteration in mood during the day is referred to as **diurnal variation** of mood and is a key symptom in diagnosing depression.

Table 6-1 Categorising Depression

Severity/Symptoms	Category A	Category B
Mild	2	2
Moderate	2	3-4
Severe	3	4+

Historically depression was, until the late 20th century, described as being either endogenous (from within) or exogenous (from without). Exogenous depression is also called **reactive depression** or **adjustment disorder**. This was because it was believed that whilst some were born with an innate predisposition to depression others had it thrust upon them by their experiences, i.e. that it was either biological or reactive in origin. These terms are no longer used in contemporary psychiatry as there is no genetic cause or link to depression and that, even if a predisposing factor did exist, for most sufferers a depressive episode will follow a stressful event or stimulus.

Somatic causes are also ruled out as there are no biological tests that can conclusively indicate that a person is depressed. However, most individuals who are depressed will show evidence of changes to the **neurotransmitters** (chemical messengers) in the brain. It is unclear if these changes are a cause of the depression or an effect of the depression. The neurotransmitter associated with mood is **serotonin**.

Serotonin is found in the brain and central nervous system where it has various functions, including the regulation of mood, appetite, sleep, muscle contraction, and some cognitive functions including memory and learning. Compounds that can stimulate or suppress production and absorption of serotonin can therefore moderate mood. This action is the key to the antidepressants known as **selective serotonin reuptake inhibitors (SSRIs)**.

The stress-vulnerability model (Zubin and Spring, 1977), suggests that we each have the potential to develop mental disorder and that all we need is the right (or wrong) environment for a disorder to develop. This model has been further divided into individual factors:

- biological explanation
- psychodynamic explanation
- interpersonal explanation
- cognitive explanation
- social explanation.

These theories briefly can be described as suggesting:

- **biological theory** – a chemical imbalance of serotonin and norepinephrine;
- **psychodynamic explanation** – current **affect** is result of past-lived experiences and memories of childhood;
- **interpersonal explanation** – depression is a result of negative personal relationships and the lack of positive reinforcement in one's life;
- **cognitive explanation** – negative responses, feelings and thoughts are a result of the individual's interpretation or perception of their life events;
- **social explanation** – depression is a result of social vulnerability, such as poor housing, unemployment, etc.

Whatever the cause of depression when caring for an individual suffering from depression, whether mild, moderate or severe, nurses must be aware that the potential for the individual to self-harm and/or to attempt suicide are a real danger. Careful observation and monitoring are necessary to reduce this risk. It is important to remember that, paradoxically, depressed patients are more likely to attempt suicide when emerging from a severe depression. This is because when deeply depressed people lack the volition to undertake such acts.

Assessment and Interventions

Assessment of individuals with depression is usually undertaken through one to one interviews and history taking. Individuals are asked to describe their recent symptoms and to express their mood. This is not the rather clichéd 'patient on a couch being assessed by psychiatrist' as portrayed on TV or in movies. **Psychoanalysis** of this sort is extremely rare in contemporary psychiatry; it is a crude and subjective assessment that focuses on the analyst's interpretation of the client's thoughts and emotions rather than the client's own interpretation. An assessment that allows the client to discuss and describe their thoughts in an objective and person-centred manner is far more likely to be adopted.

An **assessment tool** is usually used to provide a structure to the interview and also to produce a score which helps to establish if depression is present and if so whether it is a mild, moderate or severe depression. Tools employed by professionals assessing clients include:

- Beck Depression Inventory
- Geriatric Depression Scale
- Hamilton Rating Scale
- Montgomery/Asberg Scale
- Zung Self-rating Scale.

Interventions will be single or combined use of pharmacological, psychological or possibly physical approaches. Pharmacological interventions will usually involve prescription of either tricyclic antidepressants or selective SSRIs. Psychological interventions will involve **talking therapies** such as CBT whilst physical interventions are limited to **electro-convulsive therapy (ECT).**

The efficacy of both SSRIs and tricyclic antidepressants appear to be broadly similar. For both groups of drugs roughly 65% of individuals experiencing depression will show some improvement within a few weeks of starting treatment. It is believed that up to 35% of individuals experiencing depression improve if prescribed placebos for the same period however, as some people will improve of their own accord. Whilst this may not sound the most convincing argument in favour of pharmacological interventions it does suggest that you are roughly twice as likely to improve if prescribed antidepressants compared to not being prescribed them.

LIFESPAN CONSIDERATIONS

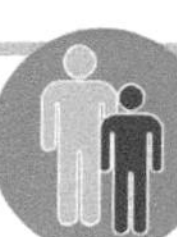

Causes of Depression

Children and Young People

- Older children may suffer depression due to hormonal influences due to puberty.
- Gender can be an influencing factor. Hankin and Abramson (2001) found that up to the age of 12 years both boys and girls experience depression equally. However, there is a higher incidence of depression in girls over the age of 12 years compared with boys of the same age.
- Loss of a parent.
- Bullying.
- As a result of changes in brain chemistry.

Adults

- Bullying in the workplace.
- Hormonal changes in females at puberty, during pregnancy, following childbirth and during menopause.
- Work related stress, e.g. those who work in high-stress jobs.
- Due to chronic disease such as coronary heart disease or cancer.

Older Adults

- Physical illness and pain.
- Isolation.
- Bereavement.
- Poverty.

Antidepressants do not work for every person or on every occasion. Sometimes they will work for one person during one depressive episode but not on subsequent episodes. Neither do they work instantly. Generally antidepressants will take between two and three weeks to build up their optimum concentration and for their effect to peak. For most individuals experiencing their first episode of depression a course of antidepressants will continue for up to six months or more after they stop exhibiting symptoms. Subsequent or recurrent depression may require longer courses of treatment.

This delayed effect, and the need to be weaned off the medication gradually, are key factors in caring for the person with depression. It is not uncommon for individuals to become frustrated with the apparent non-success of the drugs in the first couple of weeks after first taking them and therefore to cease treatment as they perceive it as ineffectual. It is best to wait for approximately one month before deciding if treatment is beneficial or not, if so then treatment should continue. If abruptly withdrawn then symptoms may rapidly return.

Individuals experiencing depression will exhibit nihilistic thoughts. In order to treat the depression it is necessary to change these negative thoughts and feelings into positive thoughts and emotions. CBT is a means of changing the way someone thinks and behaves and is proven to be an effective treatment in depression. Whilst pharmacological treatments are able to treat the symptoms of depression they cannot treat the causes: CBT is able to do this. Whilst CBT on its own may be of benefit for some individuals, particularly those experiencing mild depression, it is usually given in combination with pharmacological interventions.

CBT provides a means of changing thought processes and of turning negatives into positives. **Cognition** is the process of thinking, so changing how somebody thinks is the cognitive element of CBT. The process of transforming unhelpful thoughts into more positive thoughts requires a skilled therapist developing a trusting relationship with the client. This **therapeutic relationship** (also known as a therapeutic alliance) may take time to develop and once a bond develops it will take yet more time to achieve any real success. However, where client and therapist bond (**engagement**) then results may follow swiftly on. The process can quickly develop momentum and small changes can quickly become a succession of small, or even big, changes.

When treating depression a typical course of CBT would involve 6–8 sessions of an hour duration over a series of weeks. The client will usually be asked to complete a diary, detailing thoughts and actions, and may also given 'homework' to complete in between sessions. The homework would involve practising the techniques discussed in therapy. This is the 'behaviour' element.

Depression is one of the few disorders where a physical intervention may be considered. **Electro-convulsive therapy (ECT)** is an effective emergency treatment for resolving an acute severe depression. There is dispute over when, or if, ECT should be given. It is generally viewed as a treatment of last resort and will usually only be prescribed if other interventions are not working. The National Institute for Clinical Excellence (NICE, 2003) state that: 'ECT should be used to gain fast and short-term improvement of severe symptoms after all other treatment options have failed, or when the situation is thought to be life-threatening.'

ECT is a controversial treatment option. Some view it as a barbaric act. It works by inducing a grand mal epileptic-form fit. Despite countless investigations over many years nobody can actually demonstrate why this should have any therapeutic effect. However the evidence to show it does work is strong.

It is because of the doubt over why it works that many oppose the use of ECT, arguing it is not a proven cure. ECT is also controversial because of the risks involved. These include:

- The 'patient' will receive a general anaesthetic, with the risks that involves.
- Despite the use of muscle relaxants there is a possibility of injury during the induced seizure.
- It is unclear what the long-term effects of passing a current through somebody's brain may be. Evidence suggests that a person's memory may be damaged.

ECT would therefore only be given after a risk assessment has been undertaken. This would include demonstrating that ECT is the treatment of choice and that the benefits will outweigh the risks. Usually the patients consent would be sought, although it is possible to administer ECT against a person's wishes under both the Mental Health Act (1983) and Mental Capacity Act (2005). This only occurs in a relatively small but significant number of cases, about one in 10.

A course of treatment would normally consist of between 6 and 10 sessions, usually twice weekly. Most individuals who receive ECT are female, although this is probably in proportion to the incidence of depression in both genders. The course is usually completed within about a month so it is seen as a quick and relatively cost-effective treatment, despite its controversial status.

CLINICAL ALERT

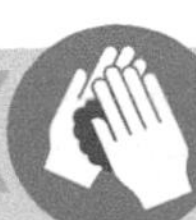

When nursing an individual experiencing depression it is vitally important to maintain close observations and to be vigilant to the risk of self harm and suicide. This is particularly so when their mood begins to elevate following a course of treatment (whether physical, psychological, pharmacological or combined therapies). Whilst severely depressed most individuals will lack the drive or volition to attempt suicide. However, as the symptoms begin to resolve they may regain this self-determination whilst still low enough to think that life is not worth living. The incidence of catastrophic violence towards oneself is at its peak during this phase of treatment.

Deliberate Self-Harm (DSH) and Suicide

Self-directed violence is the tenth largest cause of death in the UK and twelfth worldwide. Almost six times as many people die at their own hands than in wars each year. In Europe almost a third of all injury related deaths involve persons who inflicted the fatal injuries on themselves (WHO, 2005).

Suicide and self-harm are not only found in mental disorder, there may be cultural, religious or societal beliefs underpinning these behaviours. Depending where and how you live an individual may therefore view suicide as an affront to God or as an honourable act. In some cultures it is believed that suicides are condemned to eternal damnation, whilst for others it is a passport to Paradise. However, even within faith groups there is debate over this. Whilst some radical Islamists may believe that suicide bombing is a form of martyrdom (*Shahada*) and is acceptable in a holy war (*Jihad*) others dispute this, pointing out that suicide is expressly forbidden in the Qur'an.

This stance is taken by many faiths. Suicide is seen as a sin in Roman Catholicism, Islam, Judaism, Hinduism, etc. Despite the Catholic churches opposition to suicide it is acceptable in some other Christian faiths: both Methodism and Quakerism allow suicide under certain circumstances. Religions that do permit suicide include Shintoism, where Hari Kiri is an act of honour, and Jainism, where starving oneself to death is acceptable as an act of protest.

From a philosophical standpoint suicide may be seen as an expression of self-determination. It is the ultimate choice, whether to live or die. One could even argue that anyone who engages in any 'unhealthy' activity (smoking, drinking, over eating, etc.) is in fact killing themselves, albeit incrementally. Even those who support the right to suicide would accept, however, that generally the desire to ends one's life stems from feelings of severe distress, either physical, psychological or both. Many individuals can therefore imagine circumstances where they may consider suicide. For some individuals suicide can be considered a rational choice therefore.

This would only be true if that choice is based on the individual's ability to weigh the information and come to a logical conclusion. This would require holding the capacity to make such a choice. Where an individual's capacity to reach a decision of such magnitude is absent or impaired then nurses have a duty of care to prevent them from harming themselves.

There is no single reason why an individual may commit suicide, although those experiencing mental disorder are more likely to attempt suicide than individuals without a disorder. Whether the individual has a disorder or not the likelihood is that this will be an act committed in desperation when no other viable solution is evident. Individuals who cannot perceive any hope would be considered to be at risk of attempting suicide, which is why suicidal thoughts (suicidal ideation) are a feature of severe depression. These thoughts fall into two categories:

- Active suicidal ideation – the individual is engaged in planning their suicide, e.g. choosing times or locations, buying rope, hoarding drugs, etc.
- Passive suicidal ideation – the individual has nihilistic thoughts, or wishes to die, but is not actively undertaking steps towards this goal.

This is not to say that all suicides and attempted suicides are premeditated however. For some this will be a spontaneous act performed on impulse. There is a dilemma for nurses in that some service users will often talk about suicide yet never harm themselves, whilst others will commit suicide without ever disclosing their ideation in advance.

Assessment and Interventions

The safety and well-being of the individual service user must be at the heart of any assessment and intervention. Whilst as nurses we should always respect the client's right to self-determination we also have a duty of care to protect individuals. This duty would over-ride the client's autonomy if there is any suspicion that the person is unable at that time to make a rational decision due to the absence of capacity. Where capacity is absent interventions must be the least restrictive in terms of the individual's basic human rights.

Persons expressing suicidal ideation will generally be responding to a **motive** or **drive**. This may simply be a desire to die, but is likely to have deeper resonance for the individual. Typically, but not exclusively, motives will include:

- a longing to die;
- the need to change or resolve an intolerable situation;
- a need to influence others;
- to escape;
- anger;
- as punishment;
- to test 'God's will';
- in response to **hallucinations** or **delusions**.

Assessment will involve use of an assessment tool to identify risk. Assessment tools are generally structured interviews designed to establish how likely it is that an individual will attempt suicide. Some of the more common assessment tools include:

- Beck's scale for suicide ideation;
- positive and negative suicide ideation inventory;
- reasons for living scale;
- suicidal behaviours questionnaire;
- KGV Psychiatric Assessment Scale.

These scales will ask the individual to answer questions such as:

- In the last month, have there been times when you felt that life wasn't worth living?
- Have you thought that you might be better off dead?
- Have you had any thoughts about taking your own life?
- Have you made any plans/preparations for taking your life?
- Have you actually tried to take your life recently?

Whilst these scales are well researched and proven to be reliable nurses should not become over dependent on them. They rely on the nurse receiving an honest response from the client, this cannot be guaranteed in practice. Developing a strong therapeutic relationship with an individual will help to facilitate enhanced honesty and openness and will engender an atmosphere of **reciprocity** and information sharing. If a person chooses not to disclose information a nurse who has developed a level of familiarity with the person may sometimes recognise changes in their behaviour that suggest that something is wrong. This involves the nurse's ability to interpret the subconscious.

In such cases it may be possible to almost intuitively suspect that a person is suicidal despite the evidence they are trying to present. Nurses must observe their service users closely and look for other clues that may suggest a person is preparing for suicide. Behaviours such as stockpiling medications, purchasing rope or hosepipe etc may indicate a serious intention to commit suicide. Similarly, behaviours linked to 'completing all unfinished business' such as preparing a will, apologising for misdemeanours, telling family and friends that 'whatever happens, I will always love you', etc. may suggest an intent to end one's life.

Knowing the history of the individual may be a key factor in recognising change. An awareness of what the person has done in the past may be a good indicator of things they may do in the future. Predisposing factors which may suggest that a person is likely to attempt suicide include:

- history of previous attempts
- history of deliberate self harm (DSH)
- depression
- substance misuse/dependence
- personality disorder
- social isolation
- unemployment or recent loss of work
- loss of loved one (e.g. death, divorce, etc.).

Whilst individuals of either gender and of any age may commit suicide it is more common in men than in women, and is more likely to involve a person of 45 or more.

The primary focus of interventions must be to prevent injury or death. **Enhanced observations** are a means of reducing the risk of self harm. One-to-one observations can also allow a therapeutic relationship to develop between the individual and the nurse. This relationship may help to dissuade a person from attempting to harm themselves. Because of this factor observation at this level is often referred to as 'supportive observation'.

Suicidal ideation is generally a symptom of mental disorder and as such the behaviour may only be resolved if the disorder is resolved. Depression and anxiety disorder are linked to suicidal ideation and the pharmacological interventions and psychological interventions previously described are likely to be employed as part of a treatment plan. For suicidal thoughts linked to substance misuse or psychotic disorders the interventions described below would be applied.

Deliberate Self-Harm

Self-harm is the term used to describe acts or omissions committed by an individual against themselves which result in harm or injury. The term is usually applied to conscious (i.e. deliberate) acts but may also refer to acts of negligence. Some critics argue that the term 'deliberate' is misleading as many individuals cannot control the impulses to self harm and do not consider their actions deliberate. Self-harming behaviours include:

- overdoses
- cutting yourself
- stabbing yourself
- sticking things in your body (pins, pencils, etc.)
- burning yourself
- colliding with heavy or immovable objects (e.g. banging your arm against a table or your head against the wall)
- scramming yourself
- pinching yourself
- biting yourself
- punching yourself
- swallowing inappropriate objects (stones, glass, etc.)
- pulling out hair.

Whilst the individual self-harming may often appear emotionally detached from the act usually self-harm occurs during an aroused emotional state, i.e. whilst experiencing distress. Acts may occur spontaneously or may be planned. They may be one-off events or part of a long-term pattern. For some individuals the acts can become **appetitive**.

DSH may also include acts of recklessness, where an individual engages in high risk behaviours knowing that they are harming themselves or endangering their lives in so doing. This blasé attitude is summed up by expressions such as 'I don't care if I live or die', etc. Behaviours associated with such beliefs may include:

- substance abuse
- sexual promiscuity
- reckless driving
- binge eating
- excessive exercise
- excessive dieting.

Although some refer to more serious episodes as **parasuicide** or a **suicidal gesture**, these terms are misleading. It suggests that the individual was attempting to kill themselves and failed, evidence suggests that most people who self-harm do not want to kill themselves so the link to suicide is not necessary. However whilst most individuals who self-harm will probably never commit suicide most suicides will have self-harmed previously so a correlation between the two behaviours is evident.

DSH is a relatively common occurrence. As many as 10% of young people will self-harm at least once in their life. The behaviour may occur at any age however. Increased incidence of DSH is associated with:

- teenagers
- gay, lesbian and bisexual individuals
- victims of abuse or bullying
- sub-cultures such as 'Goths' or 'Emos'
- females
- peer pressure
- alcohol and/or substance use.

It is impossible to estimate how common such behaviours are as it is likely that most persons who self-harm do so in secret. Behaviours are usually hidden from family, friends and healthcare professionals for as long as possible and are therefore under-reported. Victims of DSH are said to suffer in silence.

The **motives** or **drives** to self-harm may be complex and would vary from individual to individual. Victims often report feeling hopeless or lacking control over their lives. DSH may become a means of exerting control over an aspect of their life therefore. Keeping the behaviour secret may not be just to avoid punishment but to maintain this control and to take ownership of the behaviour. Others will describe the behaviours, particularly cutting, as a means of achieving 'release' and of resolving tension or inner turmoil.

DSH should not be thought of as a 'phase' or as an inconsequential act. The risks are serious and injuries may cause complications, permanent injury, disability or even death. Anyone who self-harms should be taken seriously and offered help.

Assessment and Interventions

Victims of DSH will often come to the attention of healthcare professionals following an injury being reported. The behaviour is often discovered rather than disclosed therefore. Some individuals will reveal the behaviour during assessment of other disorders such as depression, anxiety, personality disorder, etc. Screening tools for these disorders will usually form the basis for an initial assessment. Where it is known that an individual is engaged in DSH further assessment would be undertaken to identify the type of behaviour, the frequency and the severity of incidents.

The individual may also be asked to maintain a diary. This would help to not only record the occurrences but also to discuss the events that led to the behaviour. This may be the key to preventing or reducing future DSH.

Psychosocial interventions are the treatment of choice. The behaviour is associated with inappropriate coping mechanisms or **dyscopia** so a programme of care that helps an individual to develop new coping skills is the most likely treatment option. Cognitive behavioural therapy (CBT) offers a means of developing more appropriate thoughts and responses to situations and would therefore be a suitable treatment for DSH.

Giving voice to an emotion can be a means of coming to terms with it and ultimately resolving it. Group therapy sessions can offer an opportunity to share thoughts with other individuals who have similar experiences. This can help to lessen feelings of loneliness and to resolve negative feelings such as guilt or worthlessness.

For some individuals where the instability centres on conflict within their immediate family then family therapy may be offered. The family are able to work with a therapist to help resolve conflict and to move forward in unity.

Individual coping techniques may also be taught. **Psychoeducation** is a means of helping a person to learn about and to develop new skills or new behaviours to allow them to manage their own care. Distraction techniques or relaxation techniques may be taught, for example. These techniques allow the individual to focus on a behaviour that can alleviate distress without causing harm, e.g. exercise, music, art.

Injury aversion is a means of developing less harmful behaviours or techniques which replace the need to injure oneself. For example, using red felt-tip pens or ice cubes stained with red food die to mimic injuries. For some the need to see 'blood' could be met by these methods. Others will snap an elastic band against their skin as a less harmful alternative to cutting.

Diary keeping helps the individual identify why they wanted to harm themselves and how they felt after adopting the alternative behaviour. This can help to reinforce the change.

Diary keeping should take the form of an 'ABC' analysis:

- antecedents
- behaviour
- consequences.

This is a means of examining the events that led up to the behaviour, a description of the behaviour itself, and what the results of engaging in this behaviour were. By identifying these discrete stages it is possible to discover at which point a change may have prevented the behaviour continuing and also to suggest what intervention may have helped.

The Person Experiencing Mania

Mania may be described as an exaggerated sense of well-being, energy and optimism. Individuals experiencing this euphoric state may have difficulties with their ability to think logically and to make judgements. This may be evidenced by making rash decisions, behaving outrageously, engaging in harmful activities or holding 'strange' beliefs. The ability to work or to maintain relationships will be severely affected.

Individuals experiencing mania are unlikely to realise that there is anything wrong. They will feel 'on top of the world' and will have no insight into their condition. Paradoxically they are likely to suspect that there is something wrong with everyone else, for not feeling like they do. The ability to maintain a sense of realism may be absent and individuals experiencing mania are likely to become increasingly detached from mundane, day-to-day events.

The disorder is characterised by an abnormally elevated (high) mood which is likely to present as:

- increased activity
- increased irritability
- hyper-arousal
- garrulousness
- 'frenzied' behaviour.

Mania will be experienced in an idiosyncratic way by each individual and the severity of the symptoms will vary accordingly. At its lowest level mania is referred to as **hypomania**. Whilst still a serious mental disorder, hypomania may be described as a lowered state of mania. Persons experiencing hypomania may have little impairment to their ability to function 'normally' and may be able to enjoy a quality of life similar to their pre-morbid existence.

Whilst many of the signs and symptoms of mania will be present it would be to a degree where the increased activity levels would result in few changes. Individuals experiencing hypomania are at an increased risk of suicide. This is particularly true if the individual has any insight into their disorder. The increase in volition or drives may provide an impulse to commit suicide that would be absent in their pre-morbid state.

A more severe mania is referred to as **hypermania** and will involve an individual who is highly disordered. Individuals experiencing hypermania are likely to be grossly impaired and unable to attend to their day-to-day functions. The inability to sit still may even mean that they are unable to sit down long enough to eat a meal and, together with the increased activity and increased **metabolism**, means a risk of **malnutrition** may arise even in young, physically robust individuals. Such individuals will require food supplements and will probably rely on a diet of 'finger foods', i.e. those foods that can be eaten on the move such as sandwiches.

A rare but serious form of hypermania is the condition known as Bell's mania. This is the most severe form of the disorder and will involve an extremely exaggerated form of mania. Individuals experiencing Bell's mania will almost certainly require rapid tranquilisation to reduce the risk of harm. Individuals may otherwise suffer dehydration, malnutrition or exhaustion. There is a risk of cardiac arrest associated with this increased level of activity so sedation is in the individual's best interests.

Signs and symptoms of mania include emotional disturbances, altered thinking, increased activity and changed behaviour. These changes may include:

- emotional disturbances such as excitability, irritability and feelings of grandeur;
- altered thinking such as rapid flow of new ideas, leaping from one idea to another,* delusions, and hallucinations; (*Persons experiencing mania may display flight of ideas, a condition in which ideas flow rapidly and without interruption or knight's move thinking, a term which suggests that thoughts may leap around in an apparently haphazard fashion, constantly changing, moving first in one direction then another as a knight on a chess board may.)
- increased activity such as bursting with energy, inability to rest or sleep, increased libido;
- changed behaviour such as acting impulsively, expressing unrealistic goals or ambitions, grandiose behaviours, spending money excessively, taking risks, rapid movements, talking quickly, initiating or ending relationships, increased disinhibition.

It is important to consider that some of these symptoms occur in other psychological or mental disorders and may also be linked to somatic causes. They may also be single spontaneous acts, individuals will sometimes perform behaviours that others consider 'out of character'.

Assessment and Interventions

As with depression the main means of diagnosing depression is the use of rating scales:

- mood disorder questionnaire;
- mania rating scale;
- affective disorder evaluation;
- Beigel scale;
- Petterson scale.

Diagnosis is usually reached through a combination of observation and assessment using such scales. The scales are designed to enable individuals to identify and list their symptoms asking questions linked to changes in emotions, thoughts, activity levels, etc.

It is important to eliminate other possible causes of these behaviours. Somatic or physical disorders (such as hyperthyroidism) may present as an elevated mood so blood tests, etc. would be an important part of the screening process. Hypomania and mania may also be drug-induced states, so testing for the presence of stimulants such as cocaine, ecstasy, amphetamines, etc. or for steroids will also be required to eliminate these as causes of the hyper-arousal or hyper-alertness.

Limiting harm or accidental injury are important considerations and will be the central aim of interventions. A plan of care that involves reducing undertaking high-risk activities must be negotiated. This would include maintaining an adequate diet and sleep or rest. Participating in therapeutic activities may help to distract the individual from harmful activities. It is important to develop an atmosphere free from over-stimulation, such as noise. The care plan should include high levels of support and a negotiated set of realistic goals.

It may be necessary to set limits to reduce behaviours that are distressing to others, particularly if the individual is being cared for on an in-patient area. The need to collaborate together within a therapeutic relationship to develop a care plan which is individually tailored to meet the needs of the person experiencing mania is vital.

Psychological interventions will include:

- **psycho education** – designed to inform the individual about their condition and its management;
- **mood monitoring** – to identify when mood is becoming elevated;
- **developing coping skills** – to identify distraction techniques, less harmful behaviours, etc.;
- **CBT** may be of use to come to terms with the negative aspects of diagnosis.

Persons experiencing mania will almost certainly be offered pharmacological interventions. Major tranquillisers are the treatment of choice in reducing overt behaviours. It is believed that at least two-thirds of individuals experiencing mania will present with **delusions**, i.e. fixed false beliefs, usually related to feelings of grandeur or omnipotence. Because of this it is common to prescribe antipsychotic medication. These medications will not only reduce the psychotic symptoms but also reduce agitation, impulsivity and levels of physical activity. Less commonly individuals may be prescribed benzodiazepines, anxiolitic medications which will do little to reduce **psychoses** but may reduce other symptoms and promote sleep.

The drugs that are likely to be prescribed are shown in *Box 6-3*.

BOX 6-3 Likely Prescribed Drugs

'Typical' Antipsychotic drugs (early drugs, associated with severe side-effects) such as:

- Chlorpromazine
- Haloperidol
- Trifluoperazine
- Zuclopenthixol
- Flupenthixol
- Pericyazine.

'Atypical' antipsychotic drugs (more modern drugs, less likely to produce side-effects) such as:

- Amisulpride
- Ariprazole
- Clozapine
- Olanzapine
- Risperidone

Benzodiazepines such as:

- Temazepam
- Diazepam
- Nitrazepam
- Triazolam.

Antipsychotics work by exciting (increasing) or suppressing (reducing) the levels of neurotransmitters such as dopamine, serotonin, noradrenaline, etc. The action of these neurotransmitters is to regulate mood and behaviour so altering their levels produces corresponding changes in these areas. Unfortunately they will often produce side-effects which can be severe in some cases. The earlier typical antipsychotics in particular are seen to produce **extra-pyramidal side-effects** which can be similar to the effects of Parkinson's disease. The more modern atypical antipsychotics are less likely to produce these side-effects and are therefore the treatment of choice.

Both classes of antipsychotic drugs are also associated with anticholinergic side-effects such as dry mouth, blurred vision, etc. A mnemonic for remembering these side-effects is the 'ABCD'S of anticholinergic side-effects':

- Anorexia
- Blurry vision
- Constipation/Confusion
- Dry Mouth
- Sedation/Stasis of urine (inability to micturate).

Weight gain is commonly reported by persons prescribed these drugs and is generally seen as an undesirable side-effect. The side-effects associated with antipsychotics are a major concern in maintaining **concordance** with drug regimes, with many individuals not taking their medication as the side-effects can be so limiting. 'Self-medicating' with drugs such as cannabis is not uncommon, and may lead to further complications.

Benzodiazepines are sedating drugs which reduce anxiety and promote sleep. They may have a rapid effect on symptoms of mania. Whilst these drugs have few serious side-effects when compared to antipsychotics (although weight gain is still an issue) they are associated with dependence. They are therefore recommended for use in the short-term only.

The Person Experiencing Bipolar Disorder

Bipolar disorder was formerly called 'manic depression'. As both names suggest, the disorder features severe mood swings ranging from depression to mania, disorders which are poles apart. Individuals may exhibit either mania or depression or a mixed presentation featuring elements of both depression and restlessness concurrently. The symptoms of bipolar disorder are severe. The mood swings are grossly exaggerated and are significantly different from the normal highs and lows that most people experience in everyday life. Bipolar disorder can limit the quality of life of an individual, impairing relationships, work, etc.

Typically the disorder will develop between the ages of 17–25, with almost half of all sufferers experiencing their first episode between these ages. However, it is not uncommon at an earlier age and similarly may develop later in life, although it rarely commences after 40. Bipolar disorder has strong familial links, i.e. it 'runs' in families, although no genetic link has been identified. Although for a diagnosis of bipolar disorder to be made the individual should exhibit mood swings it is not uncommon for a presentation featuring moderate highs and severe lows, severe depression with hypomania, only slight variation from 'normal' (premorbid) behaviour in either state, massive swings, or any combination of highs and lows.

It is because for many individuals there is an absence of hypermania and/or severe depression that the term manic-depression is now not considered to be an accurate description. In psychological medicine the correct term for mood is 'affect' so disorders which produce changes in mood are referred to as 'affective disorders'. Bipolar disorder is sometimes (properly) referred to as bipolar affective disorder therefore.

The experience of depression or of mania will be as previously described, the differential feature of bipolar disorder is the swing from one disorder to the other. Diagnosis of bipolar disorder is notoriously difficult during the first episode. The individual may present with either depression or mania and be treated as though they are suffering from a single disorder.

Treatments for depression may elicit mania and treatments for mania may elicit depression, so treating either may potentially exacerbate the bipolar disorder. Treatments for the disorder walk a tightrope between relieving one set of symptoms without aggravating the other.

Assessment and Interventions

Assessment involves a combination of self reporting of symptoms and of observations/reports from family, friends or healthcare professionals. The assessment tools used for either mania or depression will be employed along with a global assessment tool, which asks questions linked to both high and low mood as well as psychotic symptoms.

Diagnosis of bipolar disorder would be made if it is possible to establish a pattern of mood changes which features one of the following characteristics:

- The individual presents with mania *and* has had at least one previous episode of mania, *or* one previous episode of depression, *or* one previous episode of mixed presentation.
- The individual presents with depression *and* has had at least one previous episode of depression, or one previous episode of mania, *or* one previous episode of mixed presentation.
- The individual presents with a mixed disorder.
- N.B. for each of these criteria affective symptoms will be present whilst psychotic symptoms may (or conversely may not) be present.
- An alternative diagnosis of **cyclothymia** may be made if the individual presents with mood swings which are not as severe as those in full bipolar disorder but (typically) are of longer duration. Some individuals will experience cyclothymia without developing bipolar disorder.

Interventions are likely to include both pharmacological and psychological approaches. Pharmacological treatments will be to either treat symptoms of depression, treat symptoms of mania or to stabilise mood. Keeping mood stable is referred to as **prophylaxis**. Drugs to treat affective elements of the disorder are as described for mania or depression previously as are those to treat psychotic symptoms if present.

Mood stabilisers are mainly drugs used to treat **epilepsy**. It is unclear why these drugs have an effect on mood, although they have been proven to be successful in stabilising mood swings in bipolar disorder for many years. Drugs used to stabilise mood include:

- lithium
- carbamazepine
- sodium valproate
- gabbapentin.

Of these drugs lithium is believed to be the most effective. However, it is also probably the least likely to be prescribed as the side-effects associated with the drug, and the complex monitoring required for individuals prescribed lithium, mean it becomes more difficult to secure concordance. Although theoretically cheaper it may prove to be more expensive in the long term due to the additional costs of monitoring. It may also be more problematic to get the dose right with lithium as too low a dose would not deliver a therapeutic effect whilst too high a dose may prove toxic. Generally individuals would be prescribed a low 'starter' dose initially and this would be increased incrementally. This can of course delay its effectiveness.

The monitoring, i.e. blood tests, involved usually mean that individuals would usually be prescribed lithium whilst a hospital in-patient or attending daily for out-patient care. Even if the dose is correct fluctuations in metabolism may effect its absorption, making it ineffective or even toxic. Dehydration is a common cause of this, so ensuring individuals drink plenty of fluids whilst on lithium is part of the nursing care involved in its use.

Monitoring side-effects will also be crucial in order to maintain concordance and, more importantly, to ensure that the individual does not suffer negative experiences. Side-effects associated with lithium include:

- polydipsia (drinking excessively)
- polyurea (passing urine excessively)
- weight gain
- blurred vision
- gastro-intestinal disturbances
- dry mouth.

Usually the extent of these effects are linked exponentially to the dose prescribed, i.e. the higher the dose the higher the incidence. Early warning signs of toxicity include:

- vomiting
- diarrhoea
- tremors
- unsteady gait
- slurred speech
- polydipsia.

(N.B. if you suspect that a person prescribed lithium is experiencing suspected toxicity you must seek medical help urgently. Failure to resolve toxicity rapidly can result in serious harm or even death.)

For some individuals atypical antipsychotics may also provide a stabilising effect. This seems to happen more commonly with olanzapine so this drug is frequently prescribed to individuals experiencing bipolar disorder as it may reduce major symptoms and provide long-term stability. Individuals experiencing a depressive phase will usually benefit from antidepressants or anxiolitics. These may also help to promote sleep in manic phases although they are used with caution at this stage as elevating mood would be an undesirable effect during mania. This is more likely to occur if tricyclic medications are prescribed, and less likely if prescribed SSRIs. Most individuals will be prescribed a combination of drugs however.

Psychological interventions may also prove to be effective in the treatment and management of bipolar disorder. Psychoeducation is a particularly important aspect of long-term care. Individuals need to be able to develop skills and knowledge to monitor their condition and, particularly if taking lithium, to be able to safely adhere to drug regimes.

Mood monitoring is a means of recording feelings and emotions to determine if a swing is occurring. They may also help to identify potential exacerbating factors to mood swings, i.e. those experiences which may cause an elevation or depression in affect. Many individuals will be encouraged to keep a mood diary to record these changes and precipitating factors.

Mood diaries allow individuals to identify those things that are helpful and also those things that are not, enabling them to participate in healthy activities and to forgo activities which appear detrimental. This empowering of individuals allows them to take control of the management of their own symptoms and is an important aspect of individual, person-centred care. They are particularly useful when used to identify those early warning signs of an imminent 'breakdown'. They allow the individual to seek help and support before the symptoms of their disorder become more severe or unmanageable.

Learning coping skills can help individuals come to terms with their disorder and to manage symptoms more effectively. They allow the individual to develop a greater understanding of the disorder and of how to adapt behaviours to alleviate individual symptoms. They also help to maintain a positive outlook and to recognise that whilst an individual may never be quite the same person as they were before their disorder they can still have a productive and enjoyable life.

Cognitive behavioural therapy may also be of use, particularly in managing depression during low moods or to treat anxiety about the disorder at other times. CBT can also help individuals cope with the stresses and strains of everyday life. Unresolved stress can exacerbate a dramatic mood swing, particularly if it produces anxiety and ultimately depression.

Family therapy may also be of benefit in helping the individual to maintain relationships. Bipolar disorder can place significant strain on relationships with friends and family. The individual displaying disinhibited behaviours or expressing disinhibited thoughts may say or do things which are likely to cause offence to those around them.

Working with families to ensure that an environment of care, support and trust can be maintained is vital to ensure that individuals can return to their previous lifestyle. Educating families is also important as their experience of the individual with bipolar disorder may be frightening or distressing. They may need to learn that positive outcomes are possible which will be of comfort to them and also help them to support their loved one. Family and friends can also be educated to recognise early warning signs of impending mania or depression and to identify symptoms of lithium toxicity (if appropriate).

Children may need reassurance and support too. Older children, particularly young adults, may worry that they will develop the disorder. Younger children may believe that they are somehow the cause of the problem. Educating the whole family is vital therefore. For many individuals with bipolar disorder and/or their families joining a self-help group may be of benefit.

This may be of particular benefit to carers who need support from others to maintain their own health and well-being. Carer fatigue or breakdown in relationships is often a factor in relapse of bipolar disorder so supporting the family supports the individual.

The Person Experiencing Schizophrenia

Schizophrenia is a severe mental disorder which affects thoughts, emotions and behaviours. Approximately 1% of the adult population will experience schizophrenia and are most likely to have their first episode between the ages of 15 and 35. Although for some their experience will have a significant effect on their ability to form relationships, find employment, etc. for others their experience of schizophrenia will not prevent their ability to lead a 'normal' life.

There is no known cause of schizophrenia although evidence suggests that a **familial tendency** exists. Whilst schizophrenia occurs in 1% of the population 15% of those who have a close family member who has schizophrenia are likely to develop the disorder. This familial link suggests that persons related to those with schizophrenia are fifteen times more likely to have schizophrenia than those who do not have a relative with the disorder. Whilst nature appears to play a part therefore nurture has an impact too.

Some studies suggest that exposure to viral infections at an early age, or even in-utero, may predispose an individual to schizophrenia. Exposure to stress, particularly within relationships or family, may exacerbate the condition. Use of street drugs, particularly cannabis, may also trigger episodes.

The common perception of an individual experiencing schizophrenia, led by irresponsible reporting in the media and over-dramatisation of the disorder in fiction, is of a violent person with multiple personalities. This is far removed from the truth. Very few persons experiencing schizophrenia commit violent crime; only 2% of all murders in the UK are committed by individuals with a mental disorder.

It is also common to hear the disorder referred to as 'split personality'. This term is derived from the name schizophrenia which literally means 'divisions (or splits) of the mind'. Blueler (1911) chose this term for the disorder as he believed it implied divisions or **schisms** between thoughts, emotions and actions, rather than multiple personalities. The disorder was first described by Kraeplin (1896) who termed it **dementia praecox** or dementia of the young as he believed the presence of bizarre behaviours, increasing social isolation, self neglect, and confused thoughts were evidence of dementia in persons of a young age.

The symptoms of schizophrenia are generally described as being **positive** or **negative** in nature (Bleuler, 1911). Some critics argue that these terms are slightly misleading as they may be interpreted as suggesting that there are benefits to experiencing those symptoms described as positive. However, if the simple mathematical meaning of these terms is applied then it can be argued that what Bleuler actually meant is that the disorder adds one set of behaviours and takes away another. What the terms really imply therefore is that whilst one set of symptoms may provide motivation to undertake actions, the others reduce all drives and have a regressive impact on activity.

Positive symptoms of the disorder involve altered perception and thoughts and are characterised by:

- hallucinations
- delusions
- thought insertion, withdrawal, and broadcasting
- **somatic passivity phenomena**.

(Further description of what these terms mean is presented later in this chapter.)

The presence or absence of these symptoms, usually referred to as 'first rank symptoms' (Schneider, 1959), is not a sufficient cause to rule out, or indeed rule in, a diagnosis of schizophrenia. Whilst they were believed to be a robust diagnostic tool half a century ago it is now clear that roughly one in 10 (10%) of those who exhibit these symptoms are not experiencing schizophrenia, whilst conversely almost two in 10 (20%) of those with schizophrenia will not present with these symptoms. Schneider also overlooked impaired cognition, or **thought disorder**, which is present in many persons experiencing schizophrenia.

Hallucinations may involve any or all of the five senses (sensory modalities). They are essentially an erroneous perception, believing that something is there that in reality is not. The terms used to identify these hallucinations are

- **auditory hallucinations** – hearing voices or other sounds;
- **visual hallucinations** – seeing things;
- **tactile hallucinations** – feeling sensations or objects either touching the individual or that the individual can touch or feel;
- **olfactory hallucinations** – smelling things;
- **gustatory hallucinations** – tasting things.

A hallucination essentially is hearing, seeing, feeling, smelling or tasting, something that in reality is not actually there.

These experiences whilst generally considered always to be unpleasant by those who have never experienced them may in fact sometimes be interpreted as pleasant by the person experiencing them. Some individuals compare them to dreams which may be pleasant or unpleasant depending on the subject matter. Unfortunately for the majority of persons the experience is mostly an unpleasant one. Even if the subject matter is pleasant the feeling of having something outside your body exerting influence or control would be distressing for most individuals.

Hallucinations are not the same as illusions. An illusion is the misperception of an actual external stimuli, i.e. seeing, hearing, tasting, feeling, or smelling something that really is present, but perceiving it as being different to what it actually is. For example, if a person believes that there are rats running across the floor without any apparent external stimulus to produce this perception it would be a hallucination. However, if they mistakenly believed that an item on the floor, a shoe for example, was a rat this would be an illusion.

It is not uncommon for people without any disorders to misperceive perceptions on occasion. This is particularly evident in persons just entering or emerging from sleep who mistake persons or places that are familiar to them. These phenomena are not considered evidence of disorder and are referred to as a **hypnagogic** state if occurring while falling asleep or a **hypnopompic** state when awaking. Hallucinations are also different from imagined, almost real, sensations which may be experienced when awake such as daydreams.

The most common hallucinations experienced by persons with schizophrenia are auditory hallucinations, hearing voices. These voices may appear to come from inside the individuals own head or from outside their body. Although it varies from individual to individual external voices are usually considered to be the most unpleasant. Often there will be two voices undertaking a conversation with one another but discussing the person 'hearing' these voices, usually in the third person: 'look at her, ugly bitch' etc.

The content is generally negative or spiteful and is therefore distressing. The voices can appear even more real if they give a running commentary on the individual's behaviour as it occurs 'She's eating toast again', etc. Voices will sometimes give the person instructions or orders to undertake an activity or task. These **command hallucinations** often involve unpleasant tasks or activities and may be perceived as a punishment by the individual.

Visual hallucinations can take a variety of forms, lights, shapes, moving images, etc. Most commonly they are of animal-like or human-like beings. They may be a reassuring presence or a frightening presence and may vary in intensity and meaning. As with auditory hallucinations however they are more likely to be unpleasant.

Gustatory hallucinations are also usually unpleasant and may involve being able to 'taste' faeces or rotting flesh, etc. Olfactory hallucinations are similar in that generally they are of unpleasant smells; they may affect behaviour as often the individual will perceive the smell as emanating from themselves. Both olfactory and gustatory hallucinations are relatively uncommon in mental disorders, but more typical of medical disorders such as **organic brain disease** than mental disorders.

Tactile hallucinations are often unpleasant too. A common example is 'formication' (a feeling of ants or similar insects crawling over one's body) or being touched (especially sexually) by someone who is not there.

The perception of whether the experiences are pleasant or unpleasant may be based on if the individual has **insight** into their condition. For some knowing that these sensations are not real provides reassurance, conversely for others this can make them all the more distressing. Hallucinations cannot be explained by, or grounded in, the person's age, religion, culture, etc. and the perception of the significance of the event may be based upon a delusional interpretation of the hallucination.

Delusions are false fixed beliefs based on a misinterpretation of reality. So whilst an hallucination may be a false perception (or a perception of something not actually present) a delusion has a basis in reality but is not an accurate perception of that reality. For a belief to be described as a delusion it must meet three diagnostic criteria:

- **certainty** – the individual is absolutely convinced it is true;
- **incorrigibility** – the belief is fixed and unshakeable, even if presented with contradictory evidence;
- **falsity** – it must be untrue.

It is important to consider factors such as age, education, ethnicity, religion, culture, etc. when deciding if a belief is a delusion. It is possible for an individual to hold a belief that is common to their society or upbringing, but which would appear at odds to the beliefs held in others from a different background. It is only when the belief is contrary to those held by one's peers that they would be seen to be delusional therefore. For example it would not be unusual for a child to believe in the Easter Bunny, it would be unusual for an adult to do so however.

Delusions are regarded as being **congruent** (in keeping) with the individual's mood or **incongruent** (not in keeping) with the individual's mood. They are also placed in the categories of being either bizarre or non-bizarre. Congruent or incongruent delusions would involve those that appear to reflect the affect or mood of the individual. For example, if a person felt elated and believed that they possessed super-powers this may be considered congruent, whilst a person who is low in mood would have congruent delusions if they believed they were dying. Conversely a person may exhibit incongruent delusions if they were to appear elated at the perceived thought of their death or low at their perceived ability to be all conquering. It could be argued of course if a person saw their 'powers' as a burden such thoughts may be congruent. Applying the terms congruent or incongruent would depend on the individual's value judgement therefore.

Bizarre delusions are those that cannot be explained in terms of the person's background or experiences, whilst a non-bizarre delusion could be a mistaken interpretation of events that could potentially occur. For example if an individual being detained as an in-patient believes the government are keeping him locked up so he can't tell everyone his story then this may be a non-bizarre deluded misinterpretation of real events. However, if he believed that the clinical staff were aliens who intended to take him away in their spacecraft it may be considered bizarre, as such beliefs are not generally explainable within the real world.

Non-bizarre delusions may be unlikely or implausible to others but are at least potentially possible. Bizarre delusions are equally unlikely and implausible but crucially would not be considered as being remotely possible by most others.

Whilst delusions can be many and varied there are some themes which appear to be more common. Examples of common delusions include:

- **grandiose delusions** – believing you possess power or status;
- **persecutory delusions** – believing you are being spied upon or followed;
- **control delusions** – believing that another person, persons or force controls you;
- **nihilistic delusions** – beliefs focusing on death and disaster;
- **delusional jealousy** – belief that your partner is being unfaithful;
- **delusion of guilt or sin** – a belief that you have committed a crime;
- **delusion of reference** – a belief that insignificant remarks have personal meaning;
- **erotomania** – a belief that another person, often a celebrity, is in love with you;
- **somatic delusion** – a belief that your body is changed or abnormal.

Most grandiose, persecutory, somatic, guilt, jealousy and reference delusions would be considered non-bizarre. Delusions of control and nihilistic delusions are usually considered bizarre.

Another positive symptom of schizophrenia is thought disorder. Thoughts become disorganised and concentration may be significantly impaired. For some it is as though thoughts are being shared, that they can read the minds of others and/or that others can read their thoughts. These symptoms are referred to as thought insertion, thought withdrawal, thought broadcasting, thought blocking, and thought echo.

- **Thought insertion** – a belief or sensation that your thoughts are not really your own but have been placed in your mind by an external source.
- **Thought withdrawal** – a belief or sensation that your thoughts are somehow being extracted from your mind by an external source.
- **Thought broadcasting** – a belief or sensation that your thoughts can be heard or read by others.
- **Thought blocking** – a belief or sensation that your thought processes can be switched off, or your memory deleted, leaving you with a blank mind.
- **Thought echo** – a belief or sensation that you hear your thoughts spoken aloud, either simultaneously or within moments of you thinking them.

These symptoms can be very distressing for the individual and will almost certainly effect their ability to function 'normally'. They will make it difficult to maintain stable relationships, work, or engage in other activities of daily living.

The final positive feature of schizophrenia is **somatic passivity phenomena (SPP)**. This is the belief that you are a passive recipient of physical sensations from an external source. It can be described as a disorder of **volition**, i.e. that individuals are unable to prevent themselves doing things. Individuals who have SPP and have awareness of the sensation of being controlled often refer to themselves as being 'possessed'.

Individuals experiencing SPP may be at an increased risk of self-harm. Either because they are 'compelled' to harm themselves or, more commonly, in an attempt to remove a foreign body, such as a micro-chip or camera for example, they believe to be inside them.

'Negative symptoms' are those things that schizophrenia takes away from the individual. They refer to loss of interest, loss of energy, blunting of emotions and blunting of affect. In the long term these negative symptoms may prove to be more life-limiting than the positive symptoms.

Bleuler (1911) was the first person to identify these negative symptoms, sometimes described as the 'Four As':

- **Avolition**; lack of motivation.
- Anhedonia; inability to experience pleasure.
- **Asociality** or **Autism**; lack of ability to form social relationships.
- **Alogia**; poverty of speech.

These symptoms are often misunderstood by individuals experiencing schizophrenia and by their significant others. Whilst it is easy to recognise the positive symptoms as evidence of schizophrenia it is more difficult to recognise the negative symptoms as being caused by the disorder. For some carers the behaviours are not seen as genuine, and it is not uncommon for them to think negative symptoms are little more than the individual 'feeling sorry for themselves' or 'being lazy'. It is more common for individuals experiencing negative features, or their families/friends, to attribute them to 'over-medication' and to believe that they are being 'drugged'. Unfortunately this can cause problems with concordance.

This belief that negative symptoms are a side-effect of antipsychotic medication persists despite evidence to the contrary, i.e. that some individuals who experience negative symptoms will continue do so even if they are not currently taking antipsychotics and that some individuals taking antipsychotics will not demonstrate negative symptoms. The most telling evidence though is the rather simple fact that Bleuler first described negative symptoms in 1911, whilst the first antipsychotic medication (chlorpromazine) was not invented until 1950, some 39 years later.

Assessment and Interventions

There is no single diagnostic measure to establish if an individual has schizophrenia. Diagnosis is usually made on the basis of self reporting, feedback from others and from observation. Assessment must include details of personal history and current social circumstances.

There are several tools available to aid assessment, although none have been proved to be sufficient on their own to form a diagnosis. Tests include:

- Brief Psychiatric Rating Scale (BPRS);
- Camberwell Family interview;
- Clinical Global Impression (CGI);
- Krawiecka, Goldberg and Vaughan (KGV) Psychiatric Assessment Scale (Kraweicka *et al.*, 1977);
- Mental State Examination (MSE);
- Positive and Negative Syndrome Scale (PANSS);
- Scale for the Assessment of Negative Symptoms (SANS);
- Wisconsin Test.

The International Classification of Diseases (ICD-10) recommends that a diagnosis of schizophrenia should only be made if the individual has at least one of the following symptoms:

- thought echo, thought insertion or withdrawal, and thought broadcasting;
- delusions of control, influence, or passivity, clearly referred to body or limb movements or specific thoughts, actions, or sensations; delusional perception;
- hallucinatory voices giving a running commentary on the patient's behaviour, or discussing the patient among themselves, or other types of hallucinatory voices coming from some part of the body;
- persistent delusions of other kinds that are culturally inappropriate and completely impossible, such as religious or political identity, or superhuman powers and abilities (e.g. being able to control the weather, or being in communication with aliens from another world).

Diagnosis may be made in the absence of one of these symptoms if at least two of the following symptoms are present:

- persistent hallucinations in any modality, when accompanied either by fleeting or half-formed delusions without clear affective content, or by persistent over-valued ideas, or when occurring every day for weeks or months on end;
- breaks or interpolations in the train of thought, resulting in incoherence or irrelevant speech, or neologisms;
- catatonic behaviour, such as excitement, posturing, or waxy flexibility, negativism, mutism, and stupor;
- 'negative' symptoms such as marked apathy, paucity of speech, and blunting or incongruity of emotional responses, usually resulting in social withdrawal and lowering of social performance; it must be clear that these are not due to depression or to neuroleptic medication;
- a significant and consistent change in the overall quality of some aspects of personal behaviour, manifest as loss of interest, aimlessness, idleness, a self-absorbed attitude, and social withdrawal.

A diagnosis of schizophrenia should only be made when these symptoms have been clearly present for most of the time during a minimum period of one month or more. A diagnosis should not be made, however, without first excluding any relevant somatic causes such as organic brain disorder or during states of drug intoxication or withdrawal.

Hallucinations in particular are associated with drug use. Examples of substances which may induce hallucinations include:

- lysergic acid diethylamide (LSD or acid)
- skunk (a stronger version of cannabis or marijuana)
- cocaine
- heroin
- phenylcyclohexylpiperidine (PCP or angel dust)
- psilocin (magic mushrooms)
- alcohol.

It is necessary therefore to undertake blood tests, and of course to ask individuals about their lifestyles, to exclude drug use as a cause of hallucinations. It is possible for hallucinations induced by substances to persist for some time after ceasing using the product. It is even possible for the symptoms to worsen during withdrawal; this paradoxical effect is commonly observed when withdrawing from either alcohol or heroin.

Some individuals will experience schizophrenia as a one-off episode of psychoses, the positive symptoms of which never return. However, for many the disorder will be characterised by a series of 'breakdowns', i.e. several episodes of positive symptoms, generally separated by prolonged periods of negative symptoms.

The management of the disorder involves interventions to manage the positive symptoms, the negative symptoms and relapse prevention. For individuals with a known history of schizophrenia it is sometimes possible to identify subtle changes in mood or behaviour which may precipitate a breakdown. These changes are known as **prodromes** or **prodromal changes** or occasionally **pre-psychotic changes**.

Such signs, symptoms, emotions, etc. will be unique to each individual, although they may be broadly similar to the experiences of others. However, the unique, or idiosyncratic, nature of these changes allows us to refer to them as a **relapse signature**. This term reflects the fact that, just like a signature, the symptoms are unique to the individual yet easily recognisable to them and often to others too. This ability to identify these behaviours allows the individual to recognise relapse at an early stage.

Birchwood *et al.* (2000) describes a relapse signature as 'A pattern of psychological changes taken together and often occurring in a predictable sequence, indicating a potential further psychotic episode'. It is the fact that these behaviours almost always occur in such a recognisable pattern that allow the service user to recognise them as prodromal change. They are often referred to as **early warning signs (EWS)** as they are such a reliable predictor of forthcoming relapse.

The term schizophrenia applies to a wide range of disorders or conditions with contrasting presentations on occasion. The diagnosis of schizophrenia will usually be accompanied by a sub-type dependant on the symptoms displayed. Examples of schizophrenia include:

- Paranoid schizophrenia: the most commonly occurring of all schizophrenias. Symptoms include intrusive thoughts (hallucinations and delusions) of a persecutory nature. These thoughts may be episodic or continual.
- Disorganised schizophrenia: previously referred to as 'hebephrenia' or 'hebephrenic schizophrenia' symptoms include incoherence of speech and exhibiting strange or bizarre behaviours. Persons suffering from disorganised schizophrenia may experience few, or no, hallucinations or delusions. Behaviours may include inappropriate emotional responses.
- Catatonic schizophrenia: the rarest of schizophrenias true catatonia involves torpor and mutism, where individuals do not respond to any stimuli. **Cerea flexibilitas** or **waxy flexibility** may also be present, where individuals can be manipulated into shapes or positions which they will hold for hours. Paradoxically individuals may exhibit catatonic excitement where they become increasingly overactive and animated.
- Schizoaffective disorder: individuals exhibit symptoms of schizophrenia along with an affective disorder, i.e. a disorder of mood such as depression or mania.
- Undifferentiated disorder: individuals exhibit many or all of the classic symptoms of schizophrenia, without quite meeting a specific category.
- Residual schizophrenia: this term refers to the chronic long-lasting symptoms of schizophrenia exhibited by some individuals for months or years after the acute phase of the disorder. There is usually an absence of positive features and the disorder is characterised by negative symptoms. The term 'burnt-out' schizophrenic was inappropriately applied to this disorder for many years.

Residual schizophrenia can only be diagnosed in an individual who has a previous diagnosis (i.e. a history) of a schizophrenic disorder and has exhibited one or more acute episodes featuring positive symptoms. Residual schizophrenia is a later stage of the disorder characterised by persistent, long-term negative symptoms.

Whilst these negative symptoms may be **enduring** they should not be considered irreversible. Psychosocial interventions such as cognitive behavioural therapy are proven to be very successful in helping to lessen, or even eradicate, these symptoms. It is for this reason that the description 'burnt-out' is so inappropriate. It suggests that there is no hope for these individuals and that active interventions would be of no use. This could not be further from the truth. Individuals with residual schizophrenia are able to enjoy happy and productive lives with support from their family and friends and of course mental health services.

Interventions involve both psychological and pharmacological interventions. The management of positive symptoms is likely to be primarily through pharmacological interventions, typically through antipsychotic medication. These drugs are able to control most of the positive symptoms in approximately 80% of those prescribed them. They are not a cure however; they simply reduce the level of symptoms to a level which makes it possible for the individual to cope more readily. The way in which they do this varies depending on the nature of the drug.

Chlorpromazine was the seminal antipsychotic drug, produced originally in the 1950s. It was the first of a group of drugs (the phenothiazines) that became known as 'major tranquillisers'. This first wave of antipsychotics, usually referred to as 'typical antipsychotics', include:

- chlorpromazine
- droperidol
- haloperidol
- perphenazine
- prochlorperazine
- thioridazine
- trifluoperazine
- zuclopenthixol.

These drugs were very sedating and would reduce physical activity almost to the same extent as they reduced mental activity. Although more humane, or at any rate less barbaric, than many other early treatments phenothiazines were still quite a crude tool. Amongst its many nicknames chlorpromazine became known as the 'chemical cosh' as those who received high doses found the effect of taking the drug similar to being bludgeoned into unconsciousness.

Phenothiazines work by interfering with neurotransmitters in the brain. They slow the uptake of **dopamine**, a neurotransmitter associated with the positive symptoms of schizophrenia and also with 'excitable' and 'pleasurable' behaviours. Phenothiazines are highly sedating, an effect that may have been welcomed by some of those caring for disordered individuals though perhaps not by the individuals prescribed them. This class of drugs are associated with a range of undesirable side-effects including disturbances to almost every system, automatic nervous system, cardiovascular system, central nervous system, etc.

However, the effects which many will experience are within two broad groups:

- anticholinergic effects
- extrapyramidal effects.

Anticholinergic substances are those that block or otherwise inhibit the secretion or uptake of **acetylcholine**, a neurotransmitter that is required to manage certain motor movements as well as being involved in memory and sleep. If unable to uptake acetylcholine appropriately the effects are primarily linked therefore to interference with sleep pattern, impaired memory and, more noticeably, disturbances in involuntary fine motor movements. Persons experiencing anticholinergic side-effects to medication are also likely to complain of dry mouth, blocked nasal passages, blurred vision, constipation, sensitivity to sunlight (photophobia), etc.

The extrapyramidal system is the area of the brain concerned with the coordination of complex and fine movements as well as maintaining posture. The term 'extrapyramidal' simply means 'outside the pyramid' and refers to the fact that this network of nerves is outside the pyramid-shaped area of the medulla where most of the autonomic nervous system is located.

Interruption to transmission of signals in the extrapyramidal system produces symptoms akin to those experienced in Parkinson's disease. Symptoms include rigidity, 'mask like' face, pill rolling and other tremors, drooling, festinant gait, etc.

One of the more distressing symptoms is tardive dyskinesia, a condition characterised by repetitive, involuntary, aimless movements of the lower face (mouth, tongue, lips, cheeks and jaw) and also occasionally in the limbs, particularly the extremities. Persons experiencing tardive dyskinesia exhibit facial grimacing, rhythmical movements of mouth, tongue and jaw, tongue protrusion, lip smacking and licking, puckering and pursing of the lips, and rapid eye blinking. 'Fidgety' movements of the fingers and hands may also occur.

Other common side-effects include sexual dysfunction, weight gain, galactorrhea and gynecomastia. A rare disorder which has been identified in some individuals prescribed phenothiazines is neuroleptic malignant syndrome (NMS), a complex disorder characterised by fever, muscle clonicity, altered mental status (ranging from irritability and restlessness to unconsciousness) and autonomic instability (**arrhythmia**, hyper and hypo tension). NMS is an uncommon effect but is potentially fatal and therefore requires immediate support and intervention.

Because of the range and severity of these symptoms a second generation of antipsychotics was developed. These 'atypical' antipsychotics are less likely to produce side-effects, although some are still reported. As with the first generation, typical antipsychotics their action is not fully understood. Examples of atypical antipsychotics include:

- amisulpride
- ariprazole
- clozapine
- olanzapine
- quetiapine
- risperidone
- sulpiride.

Atypical antipsychotics also work on neurotransmitters in the brain. Whilst they may still produce extrapyramidal side-effects they are significantly less likely to do so. Incidence of Tardive dyskinesia is also greatly reduced in comparison to typical antipsychotics. However, the prevalence of weight gain, diabetes mellitus, sexual dysfunction and fatigue remain high.

The significant side-effects are a factor to overcome in maintaining concordance. Individuals may require high levels of **engagement** and support to ensure that treatment continues. It may be that pharmacological interventions are not the treatment of choice for some individuals if the side-effects outweigh any perceived improvement.

Whilst pharmacological interventions are effective in the treatment of the positive symptoms of schizophrenia the negative symptoms respond better to psychological interventions. CBT is seen as an effective measure to help individuals come to terms with their experiences. Along with psychoeducation CBT can provide a means of maintaining individuals in the community and reducing the risk of relapse.

CBT may be offered by any member of the multidisciplinary team, but is most commonly applied by nurses or psychologists. CBT is applied in combating negative symptoms by enabling and empowering individuals to:

- identify how their problems impact on their life;
- separate helpful behaviours from unhelpful behaviours;
- think about how their life could be different;
- learn new ways to think about their behaviours;
- learn new behaviours or habits;
- feel positive about themselves;
- set and achieve realistic goals.

Because the negative symptoms of schizophrenia can have such an impact on relationships family therapy may be an intervention worth considering. Family therapy can teach families to learn more about the disorder and about coping strategies to support individuals in the community. An individual experiencing schizophrenia may be more sensitive to stress, so educating families to reduce pressurising individuals and to avoid conflict and arguments is a key intervention.

Social support is a vital component of relapse prevention. It is usual to establish a holistic multi-agency approach to address some of the practical problems of day-to-day life. Whilst some individuals will live independent lives, for others the support of agencies such as day hospitals, drop-in centres, community nurses, sheltered housing, work experience, etc. will be necessary.

Psychoeducation is a key part of relapse prevention, with the primary aim of ensuring individuals are able to recognise and respond appropriately to prodromal symptoms or EWS. However, such education can also target healthy eating and exercise regimes to help combat the almost inevitable weight gain associated with antipsychotic medication. This is important as it not only offers a holistic health intervention but also increases the likelihood of concordance, thus reducing incidence of relapse.

Other interventions linked to maintenance of good physical health and good psychological health include avoidance of alcohol and illicit drugs, particularly those linked to inducing psychosis. Incidence of relapse in individuals who engage in such activities is high. It is unclear why this may occur. It may be because of the psychoactive effects of some of these drugs or it may simply be because individuals who self-medicate are often those who demonstrate poor concordance with prescribed medications. Smoking cessation is a desirable, though often unrealistic, goal too. The negative symptoms of the disorder make it very difficult to engage with individuals in health promotion.

The Person Experiencing Dissociative Disorders

Dissociative disorders – a range of disorders characterised by an interruption to the usual assimilation of perception, cognition, and physical responses. As individuals we each base our unique sense of personal identity, perception of reality and understanding of continuity on our interpretation and understanding of the world as we understand it. This belief is built on the interconnection between one's thoughts, emotions, feelings, perceptions, memories, etc. These factors are therefore said to share an association with one another. Disruption to this continuum results in an absence of this association, i.e. a dissociation.

Individuals experiencing dissociation may report feeling disconnected or removed from reality, as though viewing themself through a camera. Dissociation may be described as an absence of the 'united self' and individuals may see their experiences dispassionately or disinterestedly as though they were occurring to somebody else. A common feature of the disorder is the individual transforming emotional experiences into physical symptoms, for example emotional distress is converted into palpitations or in extreme cases paralysis. For this reason the disorder is sometimes referred to as conversion disorder. Dissociative disorders were formerly known as hysteria although this term is now considered inappropriate.

It can be argued that to a certain extent we each convert emotions into physical responses, e.g. stress reactions, etc. Dissociation may also be a form of coping with stressful emotions and could be described as a defence mechanism or coping mechanism therefore. This is a subconscious activity however, we have no conscious control over this reaction. Dissociative disorders differ from a 'normal' response in terms of their intensity and frequency therefore.

The individual experiencing dissociative disorder is likely to present with persistent and repeated episodes of dissociation. These episodes will result in an interruption to their ability to undertake activities of daily living. The disorder has links to other disorders, occurring as a symptom of, or co-morbidly alongside, disorders such as anxiety disorder, depression, PTSD, phobias, etc.

The ICD-10 (WHO, 1994) identifies five different types of dissociative disorder:

- dissociative amnesia
- depersonalisation disorder
- dissociative fugue
- dissociative identity disorder
- dissociative disorder not otherwise specified.

Dissociative amnesia – characterised by blocking out memories of events or occurrences too traumatic or emotionally overwhelming to think about. Typically the individual will forget basic personal details, such as their name, and other autobiographical detail such as recent events, etc. Dissociative amnesia may be divided into several subtypes:

- **Localised amnesia** – no memory of specific events (usually traumatic) that took place within an identifiable timescale (e.g. a survivor of a terrorist attack who has no memory of the incident).
- **Selective amnesia** – only small parts of events that took place within a specified time-frame can be recalled (e.g. a victim of an assault who recalls only some parts of the episode).
- **Generalised amnesia** – prolonged loss of memory which may encompass the individuals entire life – sometimes called retrograde amnesia.
- **Continuous amnesia** – memory loss occurs in a specified timescale usually encompassing the period from the time of the event to the present – sometimes called anterograde amnesia.
- **Systematised amnesia** – a loss of memory for a specific category of information (e.g. an individual may appear to wipe all memories about one specific person).

Depersonalisation disorder – characterised by an enduring and persistent feeling of detachment. The feeling that one is unable to influence events but only to observe them. Individuals experiencing depersonalisation disorder will perceive themselves as passive observers to their own life.

Dissociative fugue – characterised by sudden and unexpected travel away from the individuals usual surroundings. Such journeys can be short (in terms of both time and distance) or long (in both terms). Dissociative fugue is an uncommon disorder, the individual in a fugue state is unaware of their identity and other autobiographical details. This is also a feature of epilepsy, which would need to be excluded as a possible cause.

Dissociative identity disorder – characterised by the presence of two or more distinct personalities or alter-egos. These personalities seem to co-habit the individual and can lead separate lives, having their own personalities, experiences and memories. These alternate personalities force themselves in to consciousness periodically and the presenting personality will generally have no awareness of the existence of the others. This is seen as the most serious of all dissociative disorders.

Dissociative disorder not otherwise specified – this is something of an all-encompassing term which refers to all dissociative disorders that do not sit within the former definitions.

The individual would experience symptoms such as a marked dysfunction in memory, identity and consciousness.

Assessment and Interventions

The origins or causes of the disorder would usually involve a recent traumatic experience. Dissociation is a response to uncomfortable emotions and is a coping mechanism or defence mechanism intended to repress these emotions. Separating thoughts from reality can create an escape for such individuals by allowing them to experience an alternative reality where trauma is absent or if present appears to be happening to somebody else.

There is an argument proposing that dissociation is a learned technique and occurs as a deliberate response to trauma or anxiety. This is supported by reports of individuals who have experienced abuse or bullying who sometimes describe entering a trance-like state to get through it. Whilst this may occur in some individuals generally dissociation is a subconscious act.

Assessment would involve physical and psychological assessments. Dissociation may be linked to somatic causes such as substance use and organic brain disorders so physical assessments (bloods, EEG, etc.) are necessary to exclude these causes. Psychological assessments will involve use of diagnostic tools such as:

- Dissociative Disorders Interview Schedule (DDIS);
- Structured Clinical Interview for Dissociative Disorders (SCIDD).

Interventions are likely to be primarily psychological, although pharmacological interventions such as anxiolitics may be of benefit for some individuals. Psychosocial interventions such as CBT and counselling are the recommended interventions in dissociative disorders. This is likely to take place over a long time. The individual is likely to have deep-seated anxieties and to have experienced a significant traumatic event. The establishment of a therapeutic relationship is vital if recovery is to occur. Psychoeducation of family and friends may also be considered to help them come to terms with the disorder and also to ensure that they are able to support their loved one in the community over a long term.

The Person Experiencing Personality Disorder

Personality disorders are a range of individual behaviours or patterns of behaviour which become a major characteristic of the individual's lifestyle. These behaviours are persistent and enduring and will determine how an individual interacts with others. Behaviours tend to be fixed and inflexible and will differ significantly from societal norms. They are often described as 'antisocial' or 'negative' behaviours. Individuals with personality disorders are likely to display a disregard for the feelings of others and to display no guilt or remorse.

Contemporary psychiatry views the disorders formerly known as **psychopathy** and **sociopathy** as personality disorders. Individuals who may previously be described as a 'psychopath' or a 'sociopath' should now be referred to as having a 'personality disorder' therefore.

Behaviours may develop early during an individual's personal development or later in adult life. They will have an impact on the individual's ability to develop significant relationships and ability to function; many individuals experiencing a personality disorder will be unable to meet these basic personal goals. The behaviours are identifiable by their deviation from those deemed acceptable in the individual's society and the individual will seem to think and behave 'differently'.

Where individuals with personality disorders are involved in relationships they often have an ulterior motive at heart. They may actually value relationships, but only where this relationship is able to provide a 'reward'. Individuals with personality disorders are usually manipulative and can be superficially charming. Some disordered individuals may be able to inspire warmth or affection in others, but will not reciprocate this. Individuals with a personality disorder may view other human beings as a 'tool' to be used to achieve a specific purpose or to fill a need.

Insight into this condition may cause distress in the individual, however insight is uncommon. Most individuals experiencing personality disorder will exhibit **egocentric** behaviours, i.e. behaviours associated with self need or self-gratification. Such selfish behaviours may occur in individuals without this disorder of course, although individuals with personality disorder are likely to exhibit egocentric behaviours which are underpinned by **egosyntonic** cognition. This means that the individual does not perceive their behaviours to be 'abnormal' but instead perceives themselves as being 'normal' and others who do not share their beliefs as 'abnormal'.

Personality disorders usually emerge during childhood or adolescence and will persist into later life. It is unclear why some individuals develop these behaviours, although some studies suggest that they are more common in individuals who have suffered abuse, either physical, emotional or sexual, during childhood.

Personality disorders are far more common than many people realise. It is reported that between 40–70% of individuals in a typical psychiatric ward will have an element of personality disorder in their make-up and roughly half this number (30–40%) of individuals being treated in the community by psychiatric services will be similarly affected.

Personality disorders are notoriously difficult and controversial to diagnose. Some critics remain sceptical about whether the disorder even exists, and a 'Mad or Bad' debate has persisted since the disorder was first described by Cleckley (1941). The wide-ranging nature of the presenting characteristics make diagnosis difficult, so for that reason both ICD-10 and DSM-iv offer a range of sub-types of personality disorder. People may display the signs of more than one personality disorder.

Disorders are divided into clusters of similar types and may be presented as shown in *Box 6-4*.

BOX 6-4 Disorder Clusters

- Cluster A: 'Suspicious'
- Cluster B: 'Emotional and impulsive'
- Cluster C: 'Anxious'

Specific disorders identified within each cluster are as follows.

Cluster A: Suspicious

- Paranoid personality disorder
- Schizoid personality disorder
- Schizotypal personality disorder

Cluster B: Emotional and impulsive

- Antisocial, or dissocial personality disorder
- Borderline, or emotionally unstable personality disorder
- Histrionic personality disorder
- Narcissistic personality disorder

Cluster C: Anxious

- Obsessive-compulsive (aka anankastic) personality disorder
- Avoidant (aka anxious/avoidant) personality disorder
- Dependent personality disorder

Each of these disorders is characterised by an inability to form relationships of any real meaning and will have a serious impact on the capacity to lead a rewarding and fulfilling life.

Assessment and Interventions

Personality disordered individuals may present with a variety of symptoms or problems. Accurately diagnosing the nature and extent of these, and importantly, eliminating other disorders may be an onerous task. Observation of behaviours and interpretation of reported behaviours may require significant input. This task should be made easier, although some would argue that this is not always the case, by grouping sets of similar behaviours into the clusters described above.

These clusters are formed on the basis of them sharing common themes or threads that are projected or manifested as behaviours by the individual. Diagnosis therefore can be made on the evidence of reported thoughts and observed and reported behaviours. It is important to consider that behaviours should be measured against the cultural and ethnic background of the individual and not those of the nurse/clinician.

Assessment will normally involve completion of a schedule, table or questionnaire such as the Hare Psychopathy Checklist-Revised (PCL-R). This is a diagnostic tool used to rate the predisposition to psychopathic or antisocial traits in an individual. The tool helps identify those behaviours associated with the disorders such as lack of a conscience or sense of guilt, lack of empathy, egocentricity, pathological lying, repeated violations of social norms, disregard for the law, shallow emotions, and a history of bullying/victimising others.

By assessing individuals' behaviours via a twenty item symptom rating scale healthcare professionals are able to measure the degree of psychopathy in the individual and compare this to that of a psychopath. Although not without fault, not least as it is a subjective measure being applied to someone who may well be a pathological liar, the PCL-R is seen as one of the best means of assessing individuals believed to be experiencing personality disorders.

Although specific tests or criteria may be applied to each cluster, in general individuals experiencing personality disorder are likely to exhibit:

- contradictory, divergent and discordant beliefs, influencing mood, cognition and behaviours;
- behaviour patterns are persistent and enduring;
- abnormal behaviours are insidious and all encompassing and are markedly different to 'normal' responses;
- symptoms emerge during childhood or adolescence and continue into adulthood;
- sufferers exhibit high levels of anxiety and agitation, particularly late in its course;
- individual's generally have significant problems in work and personal relationships.

Individuals with personality disorders will show fixed patterns of behaviour which will differ (deviate) from social and cultural 'norms'. There will be no relevant organic (somatic) disorder or other functional mental disorder which could account for these behaviours.

Interventions for individuals experiencing personality disorders include both pharmacological interventions and psychological interventions. Although pharmacological interventions are not appropriate or recommended for all personality disorders it is likely that for most individuals with such disorders pharmacological interventions will form an element of their care. Medications commonly prescribed for the treatment of personality disorders are similar to those prescribed in the treatment of other psychosis, such as schizophrenia or bi-polar disorder. These drugs include:

- antipsychotic drugs
- antidepressants
- mood stabilisers.

Antipsychotic drugs may be of benefit for individuals exhibiting the disorders in cluster 'A' above. They can reduce symptoms of paranoia and, if also present, any delusions or hallucinations. Antidepressants can help with the affective elements (disturbance to mood or emotions) in the cluster 'B' disorders. Evidence suggests that selective serotonin reuptake inhibitors (SSRIs) can reduce impulsivity and aggression in cluster 'B' behaviours too. All antidepressants may also reduce anxiety in cluster 'C' disorders. Mood stabilisers may also be prescribed to combat features such as impulsivity and aggression in cluster 'B' disorders.

Pharmacological interventions are also recommended where individuals with a personality disorder also develop depression or schizophrenia. The evidence supporting the effectiveness of psychological interventions in treating personality disorders is not very strong. Bateman and Tyrer (2004) describe the limited evidence as being 'encouraging', most other reports suggest that not enough evidence exists at present to form an opinion.

Therapies that are used in working with individuals with personality disorders include:

- counselling
- dynamic psychotherapy
- cognitive therapy
- cognitive analytical therapy
- cognitive behavioural therapy
- dialectical behaviour therapy.

The purpose of each of these therapies (briefly) is to help individual's to think about their present thoughts or behaviours, their previous thoughts or behaviours, or their previous experiences and to identify how these may influence current thoughts and behaviours. The purpose of this is to help them recognise unhelpful or malignant thoughts, emotions or acts and to develop healthier patterns of behaviour.

The chosen treatment may be undertaken either individually or in a group. Often this will be as part of an in-patient treatment package, although some community provision exists. The choice will also be based on the preference of the therapist, the nature of the disorder, and the treatment available in the locality. Less commonly treatment choice may also be based on the choice of the individual experiencing the disorder. Despite best practice suggesting that individuals should be able to participate in planning their care, under CPA for example, the provision of services in the locality will determine what can be offered.

The Person Experiencing Dementia

All mental disorders are classified as either being **functional** or **organic** in origin. Functional disorders are those conditions where impairment is present but no identifiable somatic (physical) cause can be identified. Organic disorders, or syndromes, include those conditions where the physical structure of the brain (i.e. the organ) is the cause of the illness. This includes conditions where the brain becomes altered due to illness or injury. In medical terms we would say the brain has suffered an **insult**. The World Health Organization define organic brain disorders as: 'A range of mental disorders grouped together on the basis of their having in common a demonstrable aetiology in cerebral disease, brain injury or other insult leading to cerebral dysfunction' (WHO, ICD-10, 1994).

Organic brain disorders may be **transient** (acute) or **enduring** (chronic). Many adults have experienced transient organic brain disorders, without ever realising that was the correct diagnosis for their ailment. The chances are that you are one of them.

ACTIVITY 6-5

Imagine that you had consumed a poisonous substance which had entered your blood stream and travelled to your brain. This poison results in a disturbance in the multiple higher cortical functions including memory, thinking, orientation, comprehension, calculation, learning capacity, language and judgement.

Acute organic brain disorders are temporary cerebral conditions, from which most individuals are expected to recover; acute disorders are therefore usually reversible. Examples of the most common causes of acute organic brain disorders include:

- infections
- head injury
- chemical
- cerebral **anoxia**
- metabolic and endocrine
- epilepsy.

If treated promptly and appropriately it is expected that recovery rates for individuals experiencing acute organic brain disorders are:

- 75% are expected to recover within the first three weeks;
- 20% will recover within three months;
- 5% will become chronic or die.

For those who do not respond to treatment and whose symptoms persist for a period of three months or longer the disorder is considered to be chronic. Chronic organic brain disorders are usually caused by damage to the organic structure of the brain by accident or illness. The permanent or enduring nature of these insults means that the duration of the disorder will be permanent or enduring too. In many instances the condition, whilst not improving, will remain stable (**plateaued**) over many years.

Whilst it is not uncommon for many individuals to experience chronic disorders of this nature the more common experience will be of a disorder which becomes more widespread or severe over time. This pattern of insidious deterioration characterised by progressive, irreversible damage is termed **dementia**. The term dementia (which literally means 'deprived of mind') should only be applied to those chronic states where irreversibility exists and where the illness persists for a minimum period of six months.

The most common causes of dementia are:

- **Alzheimer's disease**
- vascular dementia
- Lewy body type dementia.

We often hear these diseases referred to as a dementia. Strictly speaking this is not correct as although these diseases are the cause of the dementia they are not a dementia themselves.

Generally in the early stages of the disease no dementia may be evident. In Alzheimer's disease, for example, individuals can be diagnosed with the disease but not develop a dementia for a number of years. The disease only becomes a dementia when the individual with a diagnosis of Alzheimer's disease begins to exhibit the signs and symptoms of dementia.

Alzheimer's disease is the most common cause of dementia in the UK with almost 750,000 individuals currently experiencing this disorder. Although the causes of Alzheimer's disease are unknown, research suggests that it begins in specific areas of the brain, principally in the **cortex**. The regions affected are those primarily concerned with memory, language, reasoning and judgement. This is why typical early symptoms of the disease are short-term memory loss followed by language dysfunction, behavioural changes, etc.

The disease process involves causing **neurons** to degenerate and lose their ability to function. Degeneration is characterised by deposits of the protein **beta amyloid**, which typically occur outside and around neurons, and by the depletion of the protein tau, which results in the formation of twists and tangles in the tiny fibres, or tubules, which connect them. These changes are referred to as the formation of **neuritic plaques** and **neurofibrillary tangles**.

Some studies suggest that it is the formation of these plaques and tangles that cause Alzheimer's disease by changing the ability of the neurones to process and transmit information. Others suggest that they lead to a reduction in blood supply to the cortical region, causing the death of brain cells. Evidence suggest there is also a reduction in the neurotransmitter **acetylcholine**, which is associated with attention and *may* (evidence is conflicting on this feature) also affect memory. Alzheimer's is an insidious, progressive disease. Over time more damage occurs within the brain and symptoms become more severe.

There are no identifiable predictive factors to determine the likelihood of an individual developing Alzheimer's disease. It is probable that the disease is linked to a combination of factors rather than one single factor. Suggested predisposing factors include:

- age
- genetics
- environment and lifestyle
- general health.

Age is the most significant predictor of Alzheimer's disease. The risk increases exponentially with age (see Table 6-2).

Table 6-2 Prevalence of Alzheimer's Disease by Age

Age	Incidence
40-65	1/1,000
66-70	1/50
71-80	1/20
81+	1/5

There is a common belief that Alzheimer's disease 'runs in families'. To a certain extent this may be true. Longevity of life does run in families; if your grandparents and parents lived to a ripe old age the likelihood is that you will to. As is demonstrated above the older one is the more likely they are to develop Alzheimer's so sharing a gene pool that predisposes you to a long life also predisposes you to Alzheimer's disease.

Evidence to demonstrate direct genetic inheritance is limited. Any link is likely to be because of the predisposition to longevity of life rather than an 'Alzheimer's gene'. However, inheritance is more common in individuals where early onset occurs so a genetic link should not be ruled out. This is particularly true in individuals who have defects on certain **chromosomes**, particularly chromosomes 14 and 21, and incidence of Alzheimer's is more common in these individuals.

In some individuals instead of having a pair of chromosomes as normal they have an additional third chromosome, this is known as a **trisomy**. Individuals with **Down's syndrome** have an additional chromosome present in the 21st pair. This condition is known as **trisomy 21**. Incidence of early onset Alzheimer's disease is more common in individuals with Down's syndrome. **Trisomy 14 (mosaicism)** is a very rare disorder, which also has links to early onset dementia. Generally, however, the incidence of Alzheimer's disease in families with no previous history of Alzheimer's is only slightly lower than in families with a history of the disease.

There are no demonstrable links to any environmental factors, although many have been suggested. Earlier links to aluminium, which resulted in many individuals throwing out their saucepans, have subsequently been disproved. However, evidence does suggest that individuals who smoke, have high blood pressure or high **cholesterol** levels also are more likely to develop Alzheimer's disease.

There is also evidence to suggest that individuals who have had severe head injuries or whiplash injuries also appear to be at increased risk of developing dementia. Also individuals who have suffered frequent low-impact blows to the head, such as boxers or footballers who often 'headed' a heavy leather ball are at an increased risk.

Links have been suggested between incidence of Alzheimer's disease and other diseases, although generally these are poorly evidenced. Diseases such as periodontal gum disease, cardiovascular disease, vitamin 'C' deficiency, vitamin 'E' deficiency, etc. have all been reported to have possible links. Paradoxically the major life limiting diseases (cancer, coronary heart disease, etc.) are less common in individuals with Alzheimer's disease.

Vascular Dementia

Vascular dementia occurs when the blood supply to the brain becomes interrupted, either due to a blockage or rupture in one of the many arteries or through disease in the blood vessels. When the damage occurs due to blocked or ruptured arteries it is known as a **cerebro-vascular accident (CVA)** or in layman's terms a 'stroke'. The area of the brain starved of blood, and more importantly oxygen, will quickly die. A collection of dead cells or dead tissue due to oxygen depletion is referred to as an **infarct** and the interruption to the blood supply causing an infarct as an **infarction.**

The effects of an infarction will depend on which area of the brain the infarct occurs in. The individual may experience physical problems such as impairment to speech, fine and gross motor skills, continence, etc. They may also experience psychological disturbances such as memory loss, poor concentration, altered affect, etc. Occasionally the individual may develop hallucinations in any or all modalities. Olfactory (smell) hallucinations are often found in individuals post CVA. The condition may remain stable for many years, or may worsen rapidly, depending on the nature of the infarction and if other infarctions occur.

Vascular dementia may result from a single infarct or multiple infarctions. It can also be caused by disease processes, particularly by hardening or thickening of the arteries, limiting the blood supply. This process is known as **atherosclerosis**.

In some individual's vascular dementia results due to a combination of these factors. It is possible to experience brief temporary changes to blood supply that may produce effects similar to a CVA, such as temporary weakness, slurred speech, or blurred vision. These episodes are known as **transient ischaemic attacks** and although not necessarily a precursor to more serious episodes should be investigated as a matter of priority.

Although infarctions generally occur in the arteries on the surface (**cerebral cortex**) of the brain they may occur deeper within the organ. The smallest arterial branches are called perforators and these penetrate the deeper layers of the brain, the white matter or '**sub-cortex**', to supply it with blood. A specific disease where interruption is due to atherosclerosis of these blood vessels is Binswanger's disease, or sub-cortical vascular dementia.

Many individuals who have multi-infarct dementia will have infarctions in both the surface region and inner layers of the brain. These individual's may present with a range of physical and psychological impairments which can severely impact on their abilities to care for themselves. Changes in behaviour or ability can change rapidly, some relatives of those affected in this way describe vascular incidents as resembling having something switched off or unplugged.

Vascular dementias are more common in individuals who would normally be considered to be in the high-risk groups for other CVAs, i.e. those individuals who have:

- a history of strokes (personal history and family history)
- high blood pressure
- high cholesterol
- diabetes
- a cardiovascular disease
- obesity
- a sedentary lifestyle
- a high alcohol intake.

For some individuals a diagnosis of mixed dementia may be reached. This refers to a disorder where both Alzheimer's disease and vascular dementia occur together.

The third most common cause of dementia is Lewy body disease, also known as Alzheimer's with Lewy bodies. This disease is similar to Alzheimer's and also features abnormal structures developing in the brain and the depletion of acetylcholine. Lewy bodies are different from plaques and tangles, although similar, and may occur together. Individuals with Lewy body disease may also display symptoms similar to Parkinson's disease as they will also have disruption to the **dopamine** levels in the brain.

Lewy body dementia is difficult to diagnose as its presentation is so similar to Alzheimer's. The onset tends to be more rapid, which may aid diagnosis although this often suggests a vascular dementia as these feature rapid onset too. Individuals with Lewy body dementia will present with a range of symptoms which could be confused for Alzheimer's disease, Parkinson's disease or a combination of both. The only way to accurately diagnose the disorder is through post-mortem examination of the brain.

Although Alzheimer's disease is the most common cause of dementia there are in fact at least 80 different dementias, some texts argue the exact figure to be in excess of 100, probably by classifying sub-divisions of identified disorders as disorders in their own right. Other less common causes of dementias are shown in *Box 6-5*.

BOX 6-5 Less Common Causes of Dementias

- Binswanger's disease
- Creutzfeldt-Jacob disease (CJD)
- Down's syndrome
- HIV and AIDS
- Huntington's disease
- **Korsakoff's psychosis**
- Kuru
- Normal pressure hydrocephalus
- Parkinson's disease
- Pick's disease
- Tertiary syphilis
- **Wernicke's encephalitis.**

If using the region of the brain affected by the disorder as a criteria for classification then two broad categories may be demonstrated, those occurring in the cortex (cortical dementias) and those occurring deeper within the brain (subcortical dementias):

- Cortical dementias occur where disease or disorder effects the cerebral cortex. This region of the brain is concerned with cognition, memory and language – the higher cortical functions. Individuals experiencing cortical dementia would typically exhibit symptoms such as memory impairment and aphasia – the inability to recall words or understand language. Alzheimer's and Creutzfeldt-Jakob disease are examples of cortical dementia.

- Subcortical dementias occur where disease or disorder effects the subcortex (the brainstem/hindbrain, the medulla and the reticular formation). Individuals experiencing subcortical dementia would typically exhibit symptoms such as changes in emotion, attention and motivation. Parkinson's disease, Huntington's disease, and HIV dementia are examples of subcortical dementia.

These terms are slightly misleading as both categories of illness can cause damage to both cortical and subcortical areas. As the disease progresses it is likely that individual's will experience a deficit in **global functioning**, evidence that all regions are affected. There are dementias where both parts of the brain tend to be affected quite early on in the course of the disorder, such as multi-infarct dementia.

All organic brain disorders, and hence all dementias, share a common set of signs and symptoms. Each individual will experience dementia in their own unique, idiopathic way and may therefore not exhibit all of these. Where symptoms are evident they may exist to a greater or lesser degree in every individual. The progressive nature of dementias means that in most cases the individual will show a greater range, and more pronounced, set of symptoms as the disease advances.

Typical signs and symptoms include:

- poor short-term memory;
- poor concentration;
- 'concrete' thought;
- disorientation in time, place and person;
- failure to understand simple instructions;
- unable to perform simple calculations;
- reduced or absent capability to retain fresh information;
- inability to correctly adopt terminology and names (dysphasia);
- impaired ability to perform simple tasks safely, loss of ability to perform the activities of daily living;
- impulsive behaviour, emotional instability, disinhibited behaviour, etc.;
- mood disturbances;
- hallucinations, delusions and confabulation;
- progressive physical deterioration;
- incontinence.

Disorientation in time, place and person involves features such as:

- day/night inversion;
- unaware of day, date, month, season, year;
- unable to recognise familiar persons or places (the inability to recognise familiar persons, objects, places, etc., is sometimes referred to as *'jamais vu'*, the opposite of *'déjà's vous'* where a person believes that new experiences are familiar).

While these are the most commonly occurring symptoms of dementia, it is important to remember that everyone is unique. No two individuals are likely to experience dementia in exactly the same way. Over time levels of support and intervention will need to increase as the person becomes less able to safely manage their daily activities.

Note that individuals with Lewy body dementia may have broadly similar symptoms but may also exhibit fluctuations in their levels of confusion, show symptoms similar to Parkinson's disease and experience hallucinations, commonly visual hallucinations featuring people or animals.

Where an individual presents with the symptoms tabled above, particularly those concerned with memory, language and concentration, then a diagnosis of organic brain disorder is likely. If these symptoms persist then this would equate to a dementia, although further tests will be necessary to confirm this.

Assessment and Interventions

Initial assessment is likely to follow either self-referral or referral from a relative or friend/carer, to primary care. Often this will be as a result of the individual experiencing lapses of memory, i.e. periods of forgetfulness or confusion, problems recalling words or names, etc. Primary care teams will usually refer the individual to specialist services, e.g. memory clinic, specialist nurse, psychiatrist, etc. depending on local arrangements and service provision.

At the first meeting it is probable that the individual will receive a range of physical and psychological assessments, or have arrangements made for follow up screening. Physical assessments are likely to include:

- blood tests to rule out hyperthyroidism, vitamin deficiency, etc.;
- brain scans – electro encephalographs (EEG) or magnetic resonance imaging (MRI) to eliminate an intercranial neoplasm, etc.;
- cardiovascular tests – electro cardiograms (ECG) to ensure symptoms are not due to anoxia through poor **cardiac output**, etc.
- urinalysis; to rule out infections, drugs, etc.

The purpose of these tests is to rule out other possible somatic causes for the symptoms presented. Some individuals who experience changes in affect, behaviour, cognition, etc. do so as a result of somatic disorders rather than as a result of a dementia. Another means of eliminating such causes is to only make a diagnosis of dementia if these changes persist for a period of six months or more.

Psychological assessments will include two main tests:

- Mini Mental State Examination (MMSE)
- Beck Depression Inventory (BDI) or Geriatric Depression Scale (GDS).

This is in order to establish if the individual has dementia whilst at the same time ruling out an alternative diagnosis of depression. The clinical impression of both disorders, particularly in the early stages, is easily confused. Other tests that may be employed include the Bristol Activities of Daily Living Scale (BADLS) which Bucks *et al.* (1996) report as correlating well with the MMSE and having the advantages of being user friendly.

The National Institute for Health and Clinical Excellence (NICE, CG 42, 2006) recommend that a standardised tool (or test) be applied to determine if an individual is suffering from dementia. This allows clinicians to undertake an evaluation of individuals which assesses the higher cortical functions; memory, attention, concentration, language, etc. Tests which facilitate this assessment include:

- the Mini Mental State Examination (MMSE);
- 6-item Cognitive Impairment Test (6-CIT);
- Cambridge Cognitive Examination (Cam Cog);
- Addenbrooke's Cognitive Examination – Revised (ACER);
- General Practitioner Assessment of Cognition (GPCOG);
- Clock-drawing Test.

The Mini Mental State Examination (MMSE) was originally produced by Folstein *et al.* (1975), published in journals and available for free use. However, it has since become copyrighted and its use now incurs a cost. Despite this potential barrier it remains the most widely used assessment tool in dementia care. It is a necessary component of the assessment process required before anti-dementia medication can be prescribed (NICE, CG 42, 2006).

The purpose of such tests is to examine functioning within the eight major subscales:

- orientation
- language
- memory
- attention
- praxis
- calculation
- abstract thinking
- perception.

Whilst the MMSE is able to demonstrate a global assessment of these abilities other tests are able to assess each area individually. Tests such as the Cambridge Cognitive Examination (Cam Cog), for example, are seen by some clinicians to have advantages over the MMSE as it is better able to do this. The MMSE features a series of questions which, if all answered correctly, would produce a score of 30 points. Whilst consideration must be given for education, reading ability and physical health needs generally scores are interpreted thus:

- 0–9 severe dementia
- 10–20 moderate dementia
- 21–24 mild dementia
- 25–30 no dementia (sometimes referred to as 'intact' or 'normal').

There is a need to ensure that due regard is given to levels of education and also to social class with the MMSE, Cam Cog and other tests as evidence suggests that these variables can influence results significantly (Huppert *et al.*, 1995).

Whilst usually a low score will indicate the presence of dementia it is still necessary to exclude other psychological or physical causes. Scores of 25–30 are considered by some clinicians as evidence of the presence of a mild cognitive impairment (MCI) a condition characterised by impairment to memory and cognition but not of sufficient severity to warrant the diagnosis of Alzheimer's disease. A diagnosis of MCI does not indicate an early dementia, evidence suggest that between 85–90% of individuals diagnosed with MCI do NOT go on to develop dementia.

Early diagnosis is vital in ensuring that individuals are able to gain the maximum benefit from interventions. In most areas specialist practitioners such as 'Admiral nurses' or 'Anti-dementia nurses' are responsible for managing services. Individuals with a diagnosis, or suspected diagnosis, of dementia should always be referred to these services in order to access the necessary pharmacological and psychological interventions. Correct diagnosis is particularly important for individuals with Lewy Body dementia as there is evidence to suggest that these individuals are at increased risk of experiencing adverse reactions to certain pharmacological interventions.

Interventions

Dementias are incurable. All interventions are concerned with arresting or decelerating the onset or progress of the disorder and with managing the symptoms. Alleviating the carer's burden is a vital component of comprehensive dementia care. Holistic assessment of the individual should include assessment of the relationship(s) with significant others and where necessary ensure that support and education for them is available. Recognising and celebrating the role of the carer can decrease incidence of carer distress and depression and delay or even prevent admission to hospital or care homes.

There is a widely held belief, increasingly gaining greater recognition, that pharmacological treatments for dementia should not be considered as the first-line treatment for dementia but should only be considered as a second-line approach. Best practice therefore involves placing non-pharmacological options as the treatment of first choice (Douglas *et al.*, 2004). Psychosocial interventions are primarily aimed at maintaining individuals in the community with their family and friends for as long as possible.

Psychoeducation, teaching individuals and their carers about the condition and of coping strategies to avoid conflict, is a useful means of promoting independence. Learning how to live with the condition and to maintain control over it for as long as possible is central to this. The concept of 'personhood' is important in dementia care, i.e. that the individual is a person with dementia, not a demented person. So promoting independence, choice, the right to self-determination, etc. are important concepts.

Psychosocial interventions may be of limited use in dementia. The declining cognition and memory of the individual will reduce the effectiveness of such techniques. However, therapies that may be of some benefit are **reality orientation, validation therapy** and **reminiscence therapy**. These are well-established interventions and are commonly applied, although the evidence supporting their use is mixed.

Woods *et al.* (2009) adopt the term **cognitive stimulation** to describe a range of therapeutic interventions whose intended purpose is to enhance cognitive functioning and social functioning in older adults with dementia. Their systematic review of the available evidence supports the belief that there is little cognitive benefit for the individual with dementia, but that there may be social benefits from increased engagement.

The benefits of engagement are not only limited to improved social skills. Even simple 'befriending', i.e. getting to know the individual as a person and becoming a friend, can have this effect. Involving persons with dementia in structured purposeful activities can:

- enhance physical, psychological, emotional and social (i.e. holistic) health;
- promote self-esteem and self-worth;
- provide opportunities for social interaction and emotional release;
- allow individuals to experience pleasure, and enhance the quality of life;
- allow the individual with dementia to realise their fullest potential;
- help them to rediscover themselves;
- enhance independence;
- emphasise positive features of ageing, not negative features of ageing.

Psychological therapies will not add years to the life of a person with dementia, but can add life to their years. They can make the difference between living and existing.

Reminiscence is an exercise which involves recollections of memories from the past. Applied as a therapy the technique involves discussion of past memories either in a group or one-to-one setting. The focus is on stimulating the memories of previous events in the long-term memory in the belief that the current short-term memory may be maintained or improved. Whilst there is some evidence that this technique may help individuals experiencing retrograde amnesia there is little evidence to demonstrate that it is of use with sufferers of dementia. Primarily because these individuals will lack cognitive abilities.

However, the therapy is still a useful process in caring for individuals with dementia as applying this technique is a means of maintaining social skills and promoting feelings of self-worth. Reminiscence is a familiar and enjoyable experience for most individuals. The notion of 'chatting about the good old days' with a group of friends is something that many people, young and old alike, indulge in from time to time. It is not uncommon to overhear a group of mature nurses reminiscing about their student days for example. This is basic social interaction and is a vital part of what makes life enjoyable for most people.

Individuals with dementia are often not afforded this luxury, particularly in some care settings. Encouraging engagement can be rewarding and beneficial. It allows social skills to remain intact and reduces the occurrence of challenging behaviours. It is about giving the individual with dementia a sense of worth, belonging and importance, recognising they are still able to participate in and enjoy social activities. It is an approach that remembers that individuals with dementia are people first and 'patients' second.

A range of materials can be employed to stimulate reminiscing, which can involve all modalities, e.g.:

- visual: photographs, slides, books or magazines, etc.;
- audio: radio, CDs, playing instruments, etc.;
- smell; carbolic soap, etc.;
- taste: 'old fashioned' sweets, etc.;
- tactile: fabrics, textures, etc.

Engaging in reminiscence appears to reduce **challenging behaviours** such as wandering, aggression, etc. and helps to maintain social skills. However, perhaps the real value of reminiscence is that it allows carers to feel as though they are actively participating in the care of their loved one. Carers can find 'not being able to do anything' particularly frustrating so reminiscence allows them to engage in an activity that is rewarding for both them and their loved one. Great care must be taken to ensure that memorabilia used in reminiscence does not induce distress. For example, baby's toys, clothing, etc. may remind a person of a lost child. Getting to know the individual will help reduce the risk of this potential harmful effect.

Reality orientation (RO) involves carers assisting the individuals orientation in terms of time, place and person. This can be achieved by providing stimulus via verbal or visual cues. As with reminiscence there is limited evidence to suggest that this therapy has any long-lasting influence on cognition but does help to promote and maintain social skills and engagement. This therapy can be in one-to-one or group settings.

Individuals with dementia will become increasingly disorientated or confused and may shun social interaction. These symptoms and behaviours may become worse in an environment that lacks stimulating activities. RO attempts to provide stimulation, social interaction and improve cognition.

The purpose of RO is to enable carers and professionals to provide structured interventions in the home. It is centred on a belief that individuals with mild to moderate dementia may improve their orientation through continually and repeatedly being told facts or given reminders. In RO individuals with dementia are surrounded by familiar objects (photographs, videos, scrap books, maps, flashcards, etc.) that can be used to stimulate their memory. The carer will engage the individual in conversations about these items and try to stimulate memory, whist at the same time trying to link this to the 'here and now'.

Many care homes, hospital wards and even private homes will feature a reality-orientation board, usually a magnetic white board on which information can be changed easily. The board would incorporate such information as current season, month, date, year and day of the week. It may also include comments about general news and weather. Ideally it would be located near a window to facilitate orientation to time of day, season, weather, etc.

RO can also be adapted for individuals experiencing more severe or advanced dementia. However, when used with this group of dementia sufferers it may be necessary to provide the stimulus in a way that makes it easier to understand, perhaps just using visual images or simple questioning. Subject matter may need to be more basic and could be limited to talks about the weather or seasons or even about the individual themselves. It is important to remember that the individual is an adult and must be treated with dignity and respect. Individuals must also be free to express their individuality by refusing to participate if they so wish.

Validation therapy is a technique that involves confirmation and affirmation rather than confrontation. Many individuals with dementia will experience dysphasia and not remember words or expressions. This can make communication extremely challenging. However, it is possible on occasions to interpret the emotion being expressed even if the words cannot be interpreted. Validation therapy involves 'validating' the individual's conversation by acknowledging the underlying meaning.

The therapy is based on the general principle of validation, the acceptance of both the reality and the personal truth of the experience of another. It has a basis in behavioural and cognitive techniques and originated in care of older persons without dementia, where it is believed to be of benefit. Its benefit in older persons with dementia is questionable, however. Just as with RO the main benefit of this approach in dementia care appears to be the befriending that occurs.

Psychosocial interventions may have the potential to prolong independence, promote safety and reduce the incidence of 'challenging behaviours'. In individuals with mild to moderate dementia they may help maintain daily living skills. Their greatest benefit is almost certainly their influence on the dynamics in the care environment and relationship. They empower individuals and their families and encourage socialisation and interaction. Supporting carers is as important as supporting the individual with dementia and a truly holistic approach to dementia care must involve caring for carers.

Pharmacological interventions have two primary aims: to treat behavioural symptoms of dementia and to arrest or decelerate the rate of decline. Pharmacological interventions concerned with symptom maintenance are generally those drugs used in mainstream adult psychiatry to alleviate symptoms such as agitation, poor sleep pattern, hallucinations etc. Interventions to halt the rate of decline are usually referred to as **anti-dementia medication** or as **drugs for dementia**.

Symptom maintenance, if considered necessary, will normally involve treating the main presenting feature where an individual exhibits either with challenging behaviours, low affect, or disturbed sleep. Challenging behaviours are likely to be treated with either anxiolitics or antipsychotic medication depending on the nature of the behaviour. Antidepressants may be prescribed to alleviate depression or to increase appetite. The drugs used are as described earlier in this chapter, but would normally be lower dosages.

Anti-Depressants

Anti-depressants may be prescribed where the individual experiences a significant degree of depression in addition to dementia. Care must be taken to monitor side-effects such as sedation and unsteady gait. Paradoxical effects such as irritability or agitation may also arise in some individuals. A particular concern when prescribing tricyclic antidepressants is the possible side-effects (constipation, reduced micturation, confusion, etc.) which are a particular concern in the elderly. In contemporary psychiatry therefore it is more likely that an individual will be prescribed **Selective Serotonin Reuptake Inhibitors (SSRIs)**. Side-effects are less common and less severe generally with SSRIs.

Some individuals with vascular dementia will display frequent and excessive mood swings, known as emotional lability. SSRIs appear to act as a preventative measure in managing this symptom so are commonly prescribed to individuals with a diagnosis of vascular dementia.

Anxiolytics

Anxiolytics, such as benzodiazepines, may be prescribed for short-term use in the management of anxiety and agitation. They may prove to be of use in treating the very anxious individual whose anxiety is interfering with his/her ability to undertake day-to-day tasks, the activities of daily living. Anxiolitics are also classed as 'minor tranquillisers' and may be used to treat agitation in individuals who are too sensitive to major tranquillisers to be considered for treatment with them. This may include many individuals with Lewy body dementia who appear sensitive to major tranquillisers. Anxiolitics may also be used to treat hallucinations in this group of individuals.

Anti-Psychotics

Anti-psychotics may be prescribed to manage behavioural problems in dementia such as aggression, restlessness, irritability, etc. This class of drugs can be particularly sedating and should be considered as the treatment of last resort. Other common side-effects include extrapyramidal symptoms and paradoxical excitement. However, after sedation the greatest concern is the risk of **hypotension**, or low blood pressure, a common cause of falls in the elderly. Individuals prescribed anti-psychotic medication must be monitored closely to reduce the risks of possible harmful side-effects.

It is more common for individuals who are prescribed anti-psychotics to receive the newer atypical drugs. These have fewer reported side-effects than the older drugs but are still linked to side-effects such as sedation and unsteadiness. Whilst these drugs are successful in the management of the positive symptoms of schizophrenia they are not suitable for the individuals with dementia who are most likely to experience hallucinations and delusions, those with Lewy body dementia. Individuals with Lewy body dementia appear to be particularly sensitive to antipsychotic drugs and experience marked, possibly fatal, increase in the severity of side-effects. Their use in these individuals therefore must be undertaken with extreme caution.

Hypnotics

Many individuals with dementia will experience day/night inversion, this is a form of disorientation to time where individuals appear to prefer to remain awake at night and to sleep in the day. This disruption to the normal **circadian rhythm** may be linked to physical (somatic) causes such as certain kidney disorders so these must be excluded. Treatment of sleep disorders is likely to involve hypnotic medication, such as benzodiazepines.

Hypnotics or sleeping tablets should only be prescribed as a short-term treatment. They are not recommended for long-term use. If taken for long periods hypnotics may lose their effect. There is also a risk of dependency on benzodiazepines. Withdrawal from a hypnotic after more than a few weeks use can be difficult and can even cause rebound insomnia.

Poor sleep may also be a symptom of depression, and some doctors prefer to use anti-depressants to treat both symptoms simultaneously, generally giving the maximum recommended daily dose in one dose taken at night. Individuals with Lewy body dementia sometimes have particularly poor sleep pattern, and the drug clonazepam (Rivotril) may be especially helpful.

Anti-Dementia Medication

Dementia may be treated with anti-dementia medication (ADM). This is a group of drugs called acetylcholinesterase inhibitors or ACE inhibitors. In the UK three ACE inhibitors, donepezil (Aricept), galantamine (Reminyl) and rivastigmine (Exelon) are licensed for prescribing to individuals with a diagnosis of Alzheimer's disease. Under NICE guidelines these drugs are only deemed suitable for individuals with Alzheimer's disease and not other dementias. They are only recommended for individuals with dementia of moderate severity, i.e. those with a MMSE score of between 10 and 20 points.

A 'conditional' licence has been issued for the use of memantine hydrochloride (Ebixa) for individuals with *moderate to advanced* Alzheimer's disease, i.e. an MMSE score of 21–30. There is little evidence at present to allow NICE to recommend use of this medication in all individuals with moderate to advanced dementia so prescription is currently limited to use in trials.

Aricept, Exelon and Reminyl work in Alzheimer's disease but not in other dementias because of the chemical changes associated with this disorder. Research has shown that there is a reduction in the quantity or potency of, or ability to absorb, the neurotransmitter **acetylcholine** in individuals with Alzheimer's disease. This neurotransmitter is broken down by the enzyme acetylcholinesterase so drugs which can inhibit the action of this enzyme will increase acetylcholine levels.

Ebixa has a different action. Ebixa acts on the neurotransmitter **glutamate**, which is secreted in excessive amounts when brain cells are damaged by Alzheimer's disease. Calcium is attracted to glutamate and high levels of glutamate result therefore in high calcium levels, and this causes the brain cells to be damaged further. Ebixa can protect brain cells by adhering to excess glutamate preventing calcium from so doing.

At present, there is no cure for dementia. Drugs for dementia are effective in arresting the progress of Alzheimer's disease and may also be of benefit in dementia with Lewy bodies, although not licensed in the UK for this group of individuals. There are no effective treatments for multi-infarct dementia, or for any other dementia.

CRITICAL REFLECTION

Let us revisit the case study on page 84. Now that you have read the chapter, is Betty experiencing depression, dementia, mild cognitive impairment or delirium? What tests (physical and psychological) would be considered? How can you befriend Betty and develop a therapeutic relationship with her? What biological, psychological and social interventions may be of benefit to Betty? Do these address her holistic needs? How best can we support Betty to return to the community and to live the life of her choice?

CHAPTER HIGHLIGHTS

- Mental health is not simply the absence or avoidance of mental disorder, it is as a state of wellness or well-being in which persons are able to function to the optimum level of their own innate ability, achieving their own life goals and thus realising their full potential.
- It is estimated that as many as one in four adults will be affected by mental illness at some point in their lives.
- The Mental Capacity Act (2005) provides a statutory framework to empower and protect vulnerable people who are not able to make their own decisions.
- The signs and symptoms of mental disorder will vary greatly from individual to individual. When caring for those experiencing mental disorder it is crucial that nurses focus on the symptoms or experience of the individual and not overly concern themselves with a diagnosis.
- Anxiety may be described as a normal physical and psychological reaction to stress.
- For some individuals low levels of anxiety may produce a beneficial effect. This belief that certain types of stress may in fact be good for you originates from the work of

Selye (1975) who coined the term **eustress** (literally good stress) to describe it.

- Anxiety disorders are the most common of all mental disorders, affecting as many as 6% of the population.
- A **phobia** is an anxiety disorder which differs from general anxiety disorder in that it is focused on a specific issue rather than being global in nature.
- **Stress** is a normal physical and psychological response of the body to demands placed upon it.
- Individuals experiencing OCD are often 'plagued' by persistent obsessive thoughts and by a compulsion to undertake tasks.
- Depression is the fourth most common cause of disability and illness in the world. Two out of every three adults will experience an episode of depression so severe that it will interfere with their ability to undertake their normal routines at some point in their lives.
- **Electro-convulsive therapy (ECT)** is an effective emergency treatment for resolving an acute severe depression. ECT is a controversial treatment option and some view it as a barbaric act. It works by inducing a *grand mal* epileptic-form fit. Despite countless investigations over many years nobody can actually demonstrate why this should have any therapeutic effect. However, the evidence to show it does work is strong.
- Suicide and self-harm are not only found in mental disorder, there may be cultural, religious or societal beliefs underpinning these behaviours.
- Self-harm is the term used to describe acts or omissions committed by an individual against themselves which result in harm or injury. The term is usually applied to conscious (i.e. deliberate) acts but may also refer to acts of negligence.
- Mania may be described as an exaggerated sense of well-being, energy and optimism. Individuals experiencing this euphoric state may have difficulties with their ability to think logically and to make judgements. Individuals experiencing mania are unlikely to realise that there is anything wrong.
- Bipolar disorder was formerly called 'manic depression' and features severe mood swings ranging from depression to mania, disorders which are poles apart.
- Schizophrenia is a severe mental disorder which affects thoughts, emotions and behaviours.
- **Hallucinations** may involve any or all of the five senses (sensory modalities); auditory, visual, tactile, olfactory and gustatory.
- Dissociative disorders are a range of disorders characterised by an interruption to the usual assimilation of perception, cognition, and physical responses.
- Personality disorders are a range of individual behaviours or patterns of behaviour which become a major characteristic of the individual's lifestyle.
- The most common causes of dementia are Alzheimer's disease, vascular dementia and Lewy body type dementia.

ACTIVITY ANSWERS

ACTIVITY 6-1 You should now know what mental health is and why it is very different to illness/disorder. Mental health may be maintained through health promotion; mental disorder is likely to require intervention.

ACTIVITY 6-2 Jeff would not normally be detained under the MHA (1983) for treatment for an addiction. His hallucinations may be a symptom of his alcohol use or could be linked to another disorder such as schizophrenia. He could potentially be detained for this, particularly if the voices are commanding him to undertake acts that may represent a risk to himself or others.

ACTIVITY 6-3 Stress can indeed be good for you as it can provide the motivation to perform at the optimal level. People often refer to this as 'focus' or being 'in the zone'. We seldom refer to this as stress however and usually associate the term with the more negative emotions.

ACTIVITY 6-4 The physical and psychological symptoms described above will be similar to those most of us will experience when sitting exams, etc. but hopefully they did not prevent us from continuing. Some people are almost literally paralysed by these fears and experience severe anxiety.

ACTIVITY 6-5 If you have ever been drunk then you have done just that. Thankfully these symptoms will have resolved as the poison (alcohol) is eliminated. The effects of the poison are temporary therefore but still equate to an acute organic brain disorder.

REFERENCES

American Psychiatric Association (2000) *Diagnostic and statistical manual of mental disorders* (4th edn), Washington: American Psychiatric Association.

Bateman, A.W. and Tyrer, P. (2004) 'Psychological treatment for personality disorders', *Advances in Psychiatric Treatment*, 10: 378–388.

Birchwood, M. Spencer, E. and McGovern, D. (2000) 'Schizophrenia; early warning signs', *Advances in Psychiatric Treatment*, 6: 93–101.

Bleuler, E. (1911, 1950) *Dementia praecox or the group of schizophrenias*, translated by Zinkin, J., New York: International Universities Press (out of print).

Bucks, R.S., Ashworth, D.L., Wilcock, G.K. and Siegfried, K. (1996) 'Assessment of activities of daily living in dementia: Development of the Bristol Activities of Daily Living Scale', *Age and Ageing*, 25: 113–120.

Cannon, W. (1929) *Bodily changes in pain, hunger, fear and rage*, New York: Appleton.

Cleckley, H.M. (1941) *The mask of sanity*, St Louis: Mosby

Delahanty, D. *et al.* (1997) 'Chronic stress and natural killer cell activity after exposure to traumatic death', *Psychosomatic Medicine*, 59(5): 467–476.

Department of Health (1983) *The Mental Health Act*, London: The Stationery Office.

Department of Health (2007) *The Mental Health Act*, London: The Stationery Office.

Department of Health, Social Services and Public Safety (2007) *The Bamford Review of mental health and learning disability (Northern Ireland)*. Belfast: DHSSPS.

Douglas, S., James, I. and Ballard, C. (2004) 'Non-pharmacological interventions in dementia', *Advances in Psychiatric Treatment*, 10: 171–177.

Evans, D. *et al.* (1995) 'Stress-associated reductions of cytotoxic T lymphocytes and natural killer cells in asymptomatic HIV infection', *The American Journal of Psychiatry*, 152: 543–550.

Fear *et al.* (2010) 'The mental health of UK military personnel revisited', *The Lancet*, 375 (9727): 1666.

Folstein, M.F., Folstein, S.E. and McHugh, P.R. (1975) '"Mini-mental state". A practical method for grading the cognitive state of patients for the clinician', *Journal of Psychiatric Research*, 12(3): 189–198.

Hankin, B.L. and Abramson, L. (2001) 'Development of gender differences in depression: An elaborated cognitive vulnerability-transactional stress theory', *Psychology Bulletin* 127: 1–40.

Herberts, S. and Eriksson, K. (1995) 'Nursing leaders and nurses' view of health', *Journal of Advanced Nursing*, 22: 868–878.

Holmes, T.H. and Rahe, R.H. (1967) 'The Social Readjustment Rating Scale', *Journal of Psychosomatic Research*, 11(2): 213–218.

Huppert, F.A., Brayne, C., Gill, C., Paykell, E.S. and Beardsall, L. (1995) 'CAMCOG – a concise neuropsychological test to assist dementia diagnosis: Socio-demographic determinants in an elderly population sample', *Journal of Clinical Psychology*, 34(Pt 4): 529–541.

Kraeplin, E. (1896) *Psychiatrie 5*. Leipzig: Barth.

Krawiecka, M., Goldberg, D. and Vaughan, M. (1977) 'A standardised psychiatric assessment scale for rating chronic psychotic patients', *Acta Psychiatrica Scandinavica*, 55: 299–308.

Levi, S. (1989) 'Campylobacter pylori and duodenal ulcers: The gastrin link', *The Lancet*, 333(8648): 1167–1168.

Levy, S. (1987) 'Correlation of stress factors with sustained depression of natural killer cell activity and predicted prognosis in patients with breast cancer', *Journal of Clinical Oncology*, 5: 348–353.

National Institute for Clinical Excellence (2003) *Technology Appraisal Guidance 59; Guidance on the use of electroconvulsive therapy*, London: NICE.

National Institute for Clinical Excellence (2004a) *Clinical Guideline 22 Anxiety: Management of anxiety (panic disorder, with or without agoraphobia, and generalised anxiety disorder) in adults in primary, secondary and community care*, London: NICE.

National Institute for Clinical Excellence (2004b) *Clinical Guideline 9 Eating disorders: Core interventions in the treatment and management of anorexia nervosa, bulimia nervosa and related eating disorders*, London: NICE.

National Institute for Clinical Excellence (2006) *Clinical Guideline 42 Dementia: Supporting people with dementia and their carers in health and social care*, London: NICE.

National Institute for Clinical Excellence (2007) *National Clinical Practice Guideline 51. Drug Misuse; Psychosocial interventions*, London: NICE.

NMC (2010) *Standards for pre-registration nursing education*, London: NMC.

Rotter, J. (1966) 'Generalized expectancies for internal versus external control of reinforcements', *Psychological Monographs*, 80, Whole No. 609.

Royal College of Psychiatrists (2006) *Men and depression*. Available at **http://www.rcpsych.ac.uk/mentalhealthinformation/mentalhealthproblems/depression/mendepression.aspx** (Accessed 17/5/2010.)

Schneider, K. (1959) *Clinical psychopathology*, New York: Grune and Stratton.

Selye, H. (1975) 'Confusion and controversy in the stress field', *Journal of Human Stress*, 1: 37–44.

Walsh, L. (2009) *Depression care across the lifespan*, Chichester: Wiley-Blackwell.

Woods, B., Spector, A.E., Prendergast, L. and Orrell, M. (2010) 'Cognitive stimulation to improve cognitive functioning in people with dementia (Protocol) 2', available at Aguirre *et al. Trials* 2010, 11: 46 **http://www.trialsjournal.com/content/11/1/46.** (Accessed 21/5/2010.)

World Health Organization (1994) *ICD-10, Classification of mental and behavioural disorders*, Geneva: WHO.

World Health Organization (2007) *International statistical classifications of diseases and related health problems* (10th revision, Geneva: WHO. Available from **http://apps.who.int/classifications/apps/icd/icd10online/** (Accessed 5/7/2011.)

World Health Organization (2005) *Promoting mental health*, Geneva: WHO.

World Health Organization (2005) *The solid facts on unintentional injuries and violence*, Geneva: WHO.

Zubin, J. and Spring, B. (1977) 'Vulnerability – a new view of schizophrenia', *Journal of Abnormal Psychology*, 86(2): 103–124.

CHAPTER 7
CHILD HEALTH

Jill John, Sally Williams and Alyson Davies

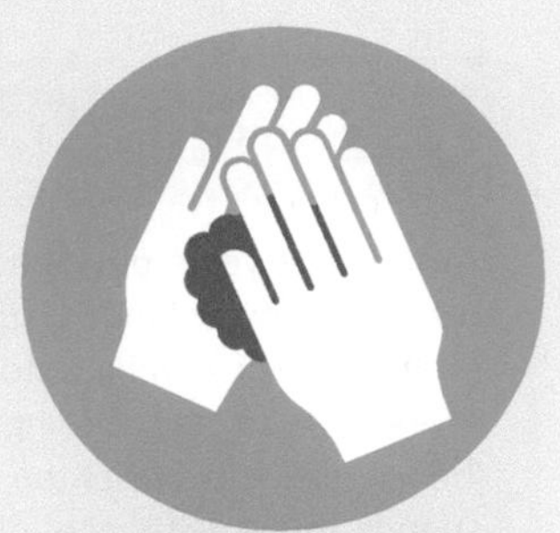

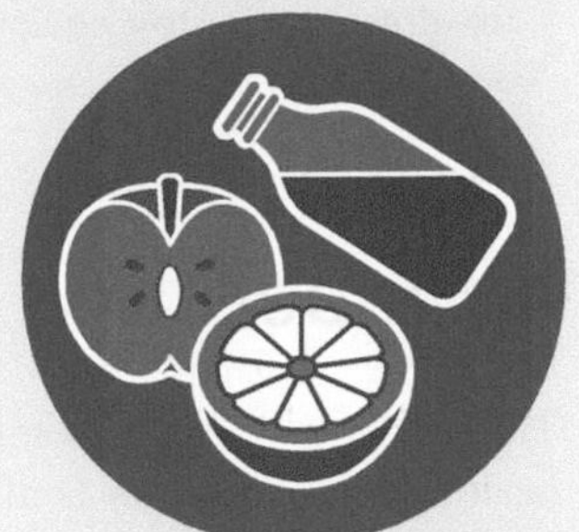

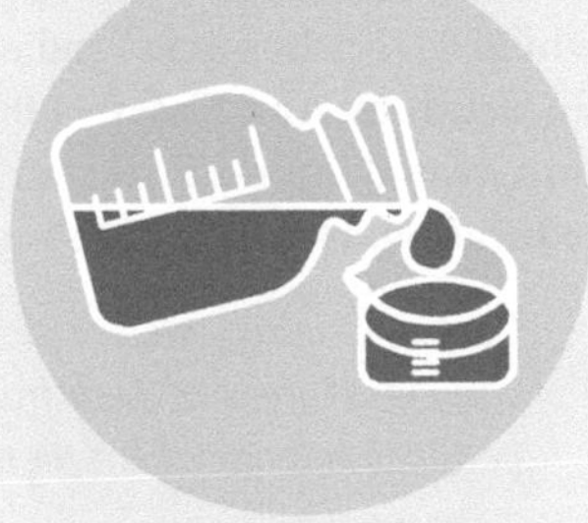

LEARNING OUTCOMES

After completing this chapter you will be able to:

- Define family centred care and understand how this is facilitated in practice.
- Understand the importance of assessment, planning, care delivery and evaluation of children and young people.
- Understand the physical and psychological needs of infants and children.
- Understand the importance of pain assessment tools in the management of children's pain.
- Develop an awareness of the issues influencing children and young people's mental health.
- Understand the rights of the child and safeguarding issues.

After reading this chapter you will be able to focus on the care, compassion and communication aspects required to safely and effectively manage the care of a child and their family. It relates to **Essential Skills Clusters (NMC, 2010) 1-8**, as appropriate for each progression point.

Ensure that you really understand this chapter by logging on to your complimentary **MyNursingKit** at **www.pearsoned.co.uk/kozier**. Complete the self-assessment tests to check your progress and utilise further activities to practise and confirm your understanding.

CASE STUDY

Amy is five years old. She is to be admitted to hospital for a tonsillectomy (planned surgery). Amy is apprehensive and excited about coming into hospital. She is invited to attend a preparation day. During the day Amy and her dad meet 'her nurse', Amy visits the ward and sees 'her bed'. Amy also spends time with the play specialist who has uniforms to dress up in, toy equipment and a book of photographs showing what will happen on the day that Amy goes to theatre. Amy thinks it is great fun and is looking forward to coming in and seeing everyone again. She is admitted and her stay is uneventful. She recovers quickly and does not appear stressed or unhappy during her stay. Amy leaves and her dad comments that the preparation day had really helped her.

INTRODUCTION

This chapter discusses some of the major themes in child health. It will focus on family centred care and how this can be facilitated by the nurse in practice. It will also consider the importance of applying the nursing process when managing children and young people and will explore both the physical and psychological needs of infants and children.

WHAT IS FAMILY CENTRED CARE?

The concept of family centred care (FCC) is multi-faceted, has evolved over the past 50 years and will continue in its importance and significance well into the 21st century. It was initially developed as a functional approach within acute care settings for children (e.g. hospitals) and was first examined and written about in depth by Ann Casey (1988), a children's nurse who worked in Great Ormond Street for many years before entering nurse education. Her definition is poignant and still relevant today:

> *Care of children, well or sick, is best carried out by families with varying degrees of help from suitably qualified members of the healthcare team whenever necessary* (1988: 8).

Family centred care embraces the caring of a child or young person within the context of their **family** with the nurse recognising the importance of this in their everyday delivery of care. It is a socially constructed concept so that the definitions are often dependent on the society from which they emerge, the evolution of nursing theory and a nurse's response to these (Coleman, 2002, cited in Smith *et al.*, 2002). It cannot be discussed today without including the rights of the child or young person in relation to the provision, protection and participation of their healthcare (see later in the chapter).

Family centred care is therefore broadly about working in partnership with parents and other family members. Several frameworks have been developed in different countries to guide nurses in the facilitation of family centred care but, as is often the case, at times some of these models remain difficult to implement. One of many frameworks that aids the transition of this concept into nursing practice is Hutchfield's (1999) (see Figure 7-1).

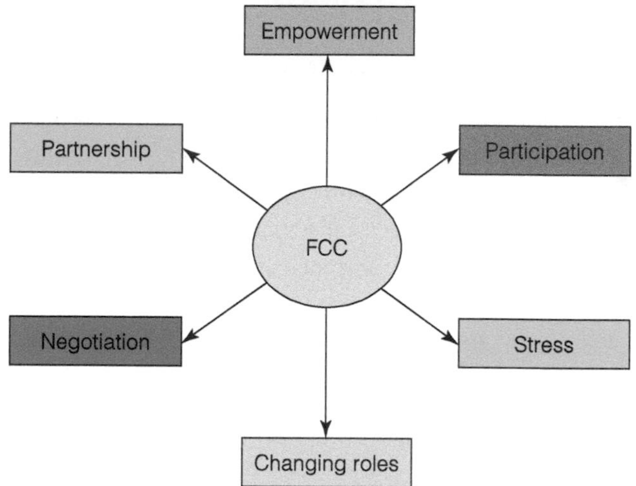

Figure 7-1 Concepts of family centred care.
Source: based on Hutchfield, 1999.

Hutchfield (1999), however, found that the key elements of FCC were seen to be:

- respect for parents,
- a concern for the family well-being,
- collaborative working (in the form of partnership),
- shared decision making,
- effective communication,
- involving the parents in the care of their child.

A more contemporary definition of family centred care is:

> *The professional support of the child and family through a process of involvement, participation and partnership underpinned by empowerment and negotiation* (Smith et al., 2002: 22).

These important concepts and practice examples are discussed below.

Negotiation

One definition of negotiation is 'producing an agreement on a course of action' (Oxford Dictionary, 2010) which when applied to the care of children and young people indicates the need for good communication, collaboration and openness whereby caring roles are established.

Undoubtedly a key fundamental concept in family centred care is that it is essential that health professionals have the skills to negotiate with the child and family. Simplistically put it identifies the need for discussion of who is doing what, when and how in relation to the care of the child. An agreement must be reached without any expectations or impositions being placed on any party (Newton, 2000). However, this may change on a daily or even hourly basis according to the family's needs both socially, personally and financially. Additionally there is also a need to understand the context in which negotiation takes place as there is no generic approach and every child and family will differ in their difficulties and issues.

The Evidence Base - Negotiation Failure

Unfortunately, research indicates that negotiation fails quite frequently and nurses often only pay lip service to applying the concept to nursing practice. Neill (1996) examined the experiences of participation in the care of children which revealed that there was an expectation of parents to automatically look after their children when they were in hospital and they were present. They demonstrated feelings of being left to 'get on with it' whilst they wanted to negotiate with staff to establish their role and that of the nurses. Dearmun's (1992) previous study, which included students, also identified similarities in that it was taken for granted that parents would be involved in their child's care and would take over if they were present.

The Evidence Base - Positive Negotiation

However, in contrast Taylor (2000), when comparing partnerships in the community and hospital, felt the difference in experience was due to the power of nurses being reversed when the nurse is seen as a visitor in the home. There are undoubtedly other factors that affect the different experiences, one of which is that there is more of a one-to-one relationship with a familiar, trusted and respected health professional.

Most of the research conducted in this area has been within secondary care (hospitals) and it is important to gain a balanced view clearly to identify the problems that occur when children and young people are in hospital.

But if negotiation is not happening with parents how can this be facilitated and how can nurses develop these skills? If there is a good role model they can be shadowed as a strategy to strengthen the nurses' negotiation style but if not then the cycle will be repeated. Indications for nurse education are the need to prepare students suitably with negotiating skills if they are to work effectively with parents and children (Smith *et al.*, 2002).

Empowerment

This is the process of either enabling or transferring power from one individual to another, and within family centred care has usually involved first a process and then an outcome.

This is a complex and multidimensional concept so for the purpose of this chapter it is important to clearly define and simplify its meaning. Information giving is often seen as the main tool for empowerment. Informed families are able to perform nursing care (including technical skills) and this helps them to develop coping strategies to allow them to have some control over the situation they might find themselves in with a sick child. Informed families, for example, are in a better position to give **informed consent** for an intervention that might be planned for their child. Some families will be keen to learn technical skills whilst others will want more time to exchange information with professionals and observe others performing skills. Teaching is integral to family centred care and hence empowerment and information giving.

Children's nurses possess the necessary theoretical knowledge to empower children and their families. However, Kawik (2006) found that although parents were willing to participate in their child's care, some nurses were reluctant to relinquish their control of the care. Other research studies have shown that nurses frequently assume that every parent will be involved actively in their child's care and leave them to do the care, when the reality is that they frequently don't know what they can or are able to do and lack information on how their roles interact with the nurses' (Coyne, 2003; Shields and Nixon, 2004). An important part of the nursing assessment is to determine the information needs of a family and information should be given systematically if empowerment is going to occur.

Changing Roles

It is difficult in the present day to define a 'family' as it can mean different things to different people and over the past 20 years or so there have been enormous changes to the structure of families. The idealised picture of two parents and 2.4 children has long gone. A family has been frequently defined as immediate relatives of an individual but more appropriately it should incorporate anyone, related or not, who is significant to both the child and their parents.

It is important that nurses respect and cooperate with the family. The nurse will therefore act as an equal partner and facilitator of care. The changing of roles indicates that nurses need to shift from a professionally centred view of healthcare to a more collaborative one that recognises that the families are viewed not only as a constant in the child's life but their values and priorities are central to the care that is planned for the child. It is important in the current healthcare climate that healthcare professionals working with children, young people and their families recognise diverse families and cultural and religious influences without compromising the safety and welfare of the child. Regardless of their capabilities it is important to recognise a family's strengths and coping methods and to emphasise their importance (including siblings) and essential role in the care of their child whether in hospital or at home. Ultimately, however, it must be in the child's best interests to have their family involved in their care.

Partnership

Partnership generally implies that there is an equal relationship between two entities (or in this case people).

The importance of parental participation and partnership approaches are now clearly identified as being paramount in both the delivery of health and social care (DH, 1989). It is important therefore that professionals working with children and their families have knowledge and understanding of parenting. Understanding the relative 'normal' but often diverse nature of parenting practitioners should be able to communicate and collaborate with parents in a more open and facilitative manner.

However, realistically working in partnership with families is not always easy and includes facilitating and enabling the child and parents to make a key contribution to the care and management of their child. In order to do this the practitioner will have to apply their knowledge of the individual child and family through observation, discussion and mutual trust and respect of each other's roles so that a true partnership approach can be facilitated in an appropriate, meaningful and culturally sensitive manner (Smith *et al.*, 2002). It means therefore that parents and nurses can work together in the delivery of care and not that parents will substitute for nurses providing nursing care.

ACTIVITY 7-1

Gemma is a nine-year-old known epileptic who has been admitted to accident and emergency after having a fit whilst out shopping with her mother. Gemma is normally very well controlled on her medication. How might the staff work in partnership with them both in regard to Gemma's immediate care?

Stress

The delivery of family centred care can be unquestionably stressful for both the families and the professional, and the practice continuum tool at the end of this section indicates how family and professional stress might be reduced by the flexibility of this tool. However the philosophy of family centred care must be upheld in that parents/carers should be allowed to be present to love and emotionally support their children and therefore reduce separation anxiety and stress for children, a factor that has been well documented since the 1950s. Nurses are in a prime position to help alleviate parents' potential distress and anxieties by maintaining constant contact with them and negotiating on a regular basis. For example, parental participation can be stressful not only regarding the teaching of technically difficult procedures but financially, socially and personally for families, and nurses need to be sensitive to this and the differences in childcare rearing in the 21st century including cultural issues.

Families from different cultures will frequently lack knowledge of what is considered to be appropriate behaviour for themselves and their children in hospital and they need help and advice about these issues. Therefore if there is a language/cultural barrier it should be addressed sooner rather than later otherwise it can be increasingly stressful for the child, their family and the health professionals dealing with them. It is inappropriate at times to use the child as an interpreter as their perceptions and understanding will be very different from that of their parents and they may give a very different message when translating information from the health professional to their parents. It is safer to use identified persons, either other health professionals and/or the hospital translation service. This is just as important for families who are caring for their children at home if they have to give care after discharge. It is well documented that children with common conditions such as **asthma** and eczema may have frequent readmissions due to non-compliance with treatments. However, non-compliance (that is not giving or giving the wrong treatment or medication) is often associated with cultural and language difficulties which have not been adequately addressed by the health professional.

Participation

Participation is defined as 'having a share or taking part' and cannot occur in relation to the care of children and young people either in hospital or at home without partnership, empowerment and negotiation, all equally important concepts of family centred care.

Thirty years ago the notion of working with children and their families in both the decision making and involvement of care would have seemed wholly inappropriate; parents were seen as amateurs who frequently got in the way of professionals trying to do their jobs. Unfortunately, research indicates that this can still be the case today. While Simons *et al.* (2001) identified that staff believed that they involved and allowed participation of parents in the care and treatment of their children, Hallstrom *et al.* (2002) highlighted that many nurses suggested that parents were only partly involved in decisions concerning their child's care. However, the role of the parents in caring for their child is nowadays fully acknowledged (if not always accepted) by most health professionals and is expected or even taken for granted.

Today parents are present (if not all) a considerable amount of time at their hospitalised child's bedside. They may witness countless examinations, tests and interventions by several members of the multi-disciplinary team who although they almost always explain and obtain verbal consent may still leave parents feeling at a loss as how they could be more involved. Parents do not usually want to make a final decision but do want to participate in both decision making and the actual care of their child. Parental involvement and subsequent participation is frequently nurse led where as partnership infers equality between all parties. For children admitted to hospital as either a planned or emergency case, participation can start as early on

No involvement	Involvement	Participation	Partnership	Parent-led
Nurse-led	Nurse-led	Nurse-led	Equal status	Parent-led

Figure 7-2 The practice continuum tool.
Source: based on Smith *et al.*, 2002.

as in the ambulance. Paramedics now also recognise the importance of family centred care.

The importance of family centred care cannot be overstated and although a very familiar concept in children's nursing for many years we still have a long way to go to improve the care of children and young people in both hospital and the community. Appropriately trained children's nurses need to be working in all areas where children and young people receive healthcare and these nurses need to be professionally updated. This was recommended way back in 1959 in the Platt Report and currently in the Department of Health 2004 *National Service Framework* (NSF) for Children, Young People and Maternity, and many local and national policies and guidelines. Yet we still fail to fully acknowledge this today in areas such as accident and emergency units and community health. However, with nursing fast becoming a graduate profession all nurses working with children and their families, if educated effectively, can implement family centred care successfully.

The Practice Continuum Tool

The Practice Continuum Tool (see Figure 7-2) had been developed in recent years specifically for use in clinical practice and it acknowledges some of the key elements of family centred care. It indicates and simply demonstrates the flexibility required to deliver family centred care and is timeless in regard to this evolving concept. More importantly it clearly indicates that families can be facilitated to move in either direction at any time according to the child's and family's needs. This tool can be used and adapted for the care of children, young people and their families in any setting. It was developed using a combination of research and practice experience and provides practitioners with a dialogue they can use with children and their families to articulate family centred care in meaningful and hopefully achievable ways.

CARING FOR SICK CHILDREN

Care Delivery – Assessment, Planning, Delivery and Evaluation

Child-rearing ideologies have changed significantly over the past century. These ideologies have a significant impact on the way society perceives the family unit, children and the way services surrounding children and young people are planned and delivered. In the 1920s and 1930s theorists such as Truby King advocated methods that specifically emphasised regularity of feeding, sleeping and bowel movements. Parents were led to believe that the adherence to a generally strict regimen was supposed to build character by avoiding cuddling and other attention. Another theorist at this time, John B. Watson, believed that children should be treated as young adults. He warned against the inevitable dangers of a mother providing too much love and affection. Watson also recommended the avoidance of children sitting on a parent's lap!

Today parenting styles continue to evolve. There has been a shift away from routines and emotional detachment. Parents will develop their own parenting style according to their experiences and beliefs, social influences and culture. The nurse's role is therefore to ensure that the child's and family's routine is promoted within the constraints of the hospital environment and that parents feel supported during this stressful experience.

The role of the parent of a hospitalised child has also undergone a dramatic transformation over the past 50 years. Research carried out in the 1950s by Spence, Bowlby and Robertson (Alsop-Shields and Mohay, 2001) highlighted some of the detrimental effects of hospitalisation on the child's emotional and physical well-being. This included the psychological damage caused by maternal deprivation and separation anxiety (the psychological and physical effects on children when they were separated from their mothers for short periods of less than two weeks, for example). Spence *et al.* studied the child's behaviour and described the process in a series of different stages (Bowlby, 1960b):

- **Protest:** in this phase a child cries, screams, is inconsolable, is uncooperative, shuns strangers, and tries to get attention.
- **Despair:** in the next phase the child does not cry, is quiet, withdrawn, lethargic, looks sad and pathetic, is classed as good, and does not join in play.
- **Detachment:** is the last phase where the child shows normal behaviour, is active, adapts well, shows resignation not contentment, turns away from the mother, and will go to anyone.

The publication and media coverage of the research, such as the emotionally provocative film 'A two-year-old goes to hospital' by Bowlby and Robertson (1952), not only heightened professional interest in the well-being of children in hospital but also increased public awareness surrounding the emotional effects of hospitalisation and provided a catalyst for change in the care of children and young people in hospital.

Even in the 1970s parents brought their sick children into hospital and had to leave the child in the hospital in the care of the nurses and doctors. There was little encouragement for parents to stay with the child and no facilities or provisions for them. Instead they were encouraged to only visit daily for an hour or two.

A Department of Health Report in 1991, the 'Welfare of Children and Young People in Hospital' (DH, 1991), and a 1993 report by the Audit Commission 'Children First' (Audit commission, 1993), both recognised the importance of adopting a 'family centred care' approach to the care of sick children and their families to promote and enhance the psychological well-being of hospitalised children.

Assessment of the sick child will aid the practitioner in determining care priorities. The child who presents with a general history of being unwell will be assessed using a recognised framework. This framework should provide information relating to the child's clinical and physical status, but also needs to consider social, psychological and emotional needs.

Trigg and Mohammed (2006: 84) suggest that the assessment process aims:

> *To obtain information via observation, history taking and physical examination, which will form a baseline for immediate action and ongoing assessment, and assist in developing your plan of action.*

Initial assessment of responsiveness, **vital signs** and immediate history taking from the parents will determine the need for immediate intervention following the **advanced paediatric life support** algorithms (**www.resus.org.uk**). If the child appears stable and not at immediate risk of deterioration then a more thorough assessment can be undertaken before intervention is required.

One of the commonly used models for the assessment, planning, delivery and evaluation of children in hospital is based on the Roper, Logan and Tierney's **activities of daily living (ADL) model** as described in Chapter 9. This model is used with the family centred philosophy of care embedded within each aspect. Care also has to be considered within a developmental framework which recognises the child's physical, psychological, social and moral stage of development. The framework in the *Practice Guidelines* (below) demonstrates some of the considerations necessary when utilising the ADL framework with children and young people.

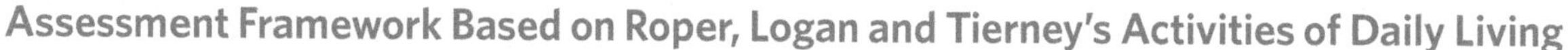

PRACTICE GUIDELINES

Assessment Framework Based on Roper, Logan and Tierney's Activities of Daily Living

1. ***Maintaining a safe environment*** - Is the child usually cared for in a cot or a bed? Height of the bed? Are cot sides appropriately maintained and designed for young children? Are plug sockets covered? Is all necessary medical equipment out of the child's reach? Is the ward area designed for children? Are all rooms which contain dangerous equipment or medication kept locked? Where are hazardous cleaning materials kept on the ward?
2. ***Communicating*** - What is the child's age and cognitive ability? Is the nurse using appropriate language and nonverbal cues to maximise the child's understanding? Is the nurse using appropriate body language to encourage the child to communicate? Does the child have any special words to describe needs that only the parents may be aware of, for example a special comforting toy or blanket may be given a special name only the family will be familiar with? What is the child's reading age? Are the child's nonverbal communication behaviours indicating pain?
3. ***Breathing*** - Infants under the age of six months are obligatory nose breathers, has the nasal airway been compromised by secretions? Respiratory rates in children differ according to their age and activity level - is the rate appropriate for the child's age? Children are most at risk of respiratory arrest, therefore appropriate assessment, planning and prompt intervention may be necessary if the child's respiratory rate and depth are abnormal. Is the ward area adequately prepared should a paediatric arrest occur?
4. ***Eating and drinking*** - Is the child's fluid intake compromised? Has input and output been recorded? Are all breastfeeds recorded in terms of duration? Is the food available on the ward appropriate for the child? What milk does the baby usually have and does the ward have a supply? What are the child's likes and dislikes? Can the child feed themselves? Accurate recording of the timing and quantity of feeds can be delegated to the parents; however they will need support and encouragement to maintain the records accurately.
5. ***Elimination*** - Is the infant/toddler in nappies? If so all of the time or just at night time? Have nappies been weighed to ensure an accurate output is recorded for infants? Can the child use an adult toilet or do they require a special seat or step? Are they self-caring or will they need assistance? Does the child have any special language or signs that might indicate they need the toilet? What is the nature and consistency of the child's stool?
6. ***Personal cleansing and dressing*** - Does the child get bathed in the morning or evening? Do they bath or shower? Do the parents use any particular soap, creams or lotions and if so these may need to be prescribed if the child is an inpatient? Can the child brush their own teeth or do they need assistance?
7. ***Controlling body temperature*** - Normative temperatures differ according to age therefore the temperature has to be recorded and considered in relation to the child's age. Infants and children under the age of five are more at risk of suffering from febrile convulsions if they become pyrexial. Has the child ever suffered from febrile convulsions, if so how did they react/behave? Is the child dressed appropriately in relation to their temperature? Is the room temperature appropriate for the child/infant?

8 ***Mobilising*** - Developmentally is the child's movement appropriate for their age? Are they at risk of falling, climbing and rolling? Have the risks to the child's safety been considered and minimised? Are all movements appropriate for the child's age? Have the child's needs been compromised by illness? Are all manual handling regulations being complied with?

9 ***Working and playing*** - What does the child like to play with and is there provision on the ward? Is the child's behaviour normal, are they interested in playing? Is there an onsite teacher or play specialist that can be available to visit the child and provide play equipment? Are the child's wider educational needs being met? Is the child's development normal for the age of the child?

10 ***Expressing sexuality*** - What is the age of the child and is their behaviour normal? Does the older child or adolescent have a partner? Is the older adolescent sexually active? Is the adolescent in need of further sexual health advice or health promotion?

11 ***Sleeping*** - How and when does the infant or child sleep? What is their normal pattern which encourages sleep; do they have a particular routine? Is the sleep pattern normal; are they sleeping more/less as a result of illness?

Some children however will be assessed as having an acute, potentially life-threatening illness and care priorities will differ accordingly. The accurate assessment and identification of an acutely ill child can affect the long-term outcomes for the child. Action needs to be taken immediately and necessary interventions should be commenced in accordance with APLS guidelines. Hockenbury *et al.* (2003) defines acute illness as symptoms severe enough to limit activity and require medical attention. When children first develop symptoms, however, it is often difficult to distinguish between a mild, self-limiting condition and the early stages of a severe, potentially life-threatening, acute illness.

This places greater emphasis on the initial assessment process, but also highlights the need for ongoing assessment and evaluation of care and interventions. There is also a greater responsibility placed on the role of the practitioner when dealing with young children who are developmentally unable to verbally communicate and cognitively unable to explain symptoms.

The practitioner needs to know the normal clinical vital signs for the age group they are caring for to be able to identify the abnormal and act accordingly. Table 7-1 identifies the normal heart rates, respiratory rates and blood pressures for children of different ages.

Rapid neurological assessment may also be necessary to identify the seriously ill child. Adult orientated neurological assessment tools are inappropriate for use in preverbal and young children. AVPU is a widely used paediatric neurological assessment tool which is specifically designed for this age group:

A = ALERT
V = Respond to VOICE
P = Respond to PAIN
U = UNRESPONSIVE.

Table 7-1 Normal Vital Signs for Children of Different Ages

Age of the child	Heart rate	Respiratory rate	Blood pressure
1 month	100-180	30-80	85/50
6 months	120-160	30-60	90/53
1 year	90-140	20-40	91/54
2 years	80-140	20-30	91/56
6 years	75-100	20-25	96/57
10 years	60-90	17-22	102/62
12 years	55-90	17-22	107/67
16 years	50-90	15-20	117/67

Source: adapted from Williams and Asquith (2000).

Another aspect of assessment involves taking a detailed history. In paediatric nursing the role of the parents in providing a detailed history of the events surrounding a child's illness or accident is vital. Parents will be able to identify the illness pattern or recount the events of an accident. They will be able to identify normal behaviour patterns and responses from both a physical and psychological perspective.

Communication skills with parents and children will also have to be adapted according to the child's age and understanding. The parents may well provide most of the history and information, but it is important to remember the child's need to be involved and have a voice whenever possible. Play can be considered a universal language for communicating with children and where necessary the skills of a specially qualified play therapist should be utilised to communicate with children. This can be particularly valuable in preparing a child for a clinical intervention such as cannulation. Through the use of toys and play equipment the intervention can be explained to the young child and the child can be appropriately psychologically prepared.

Other useful techniques for communicating with children are Story Telling, I Messages, Third Person Techniques, Facilitative Responding, Dreams, What If Questions, Three Wishes, Rating Game, Word Association Game and Sentence Completion (Hockenbury *et al.*, 2003).

Once the child and family have been assessed then care priorities can be identified and a plan of care can be followed. At all times this care plan should be discussed with the child and family and the evidence-based rationale should be explained. This supports the ethos of family centred care and can help empower the parents to increase their knowledge and parenting skills. It has been demonstrated that collaborative care planning and delivery with parents decreases their future dependence on health services (Hockenbury *et al.*, 2003).

ACTIVITY 7-2

Aaron is an 11-year-old boy admitted following a fall from his bike whilst out with his friends. He briefly lost consciousness.

What should you consider in your assessment of Aaron following his admission?

Care Needs

Care delivery will usually be negotiated with the parents and roles should be discussed to identify what the parents will continue to provide for the child during hospitalisation and what the nurse's role will be. Most parents of hospitalised children stay with the child, where possible, most of the time the child is on the ward and provide basic physical and psychological care needs such as feeding, hygiene, oral care, toileting and positioning, comfort, play, love and attention.

When the child requires more clinical interventions the parent can support the nurse in providing psychological support for the child; for example, comfort and holding during cannulation and blood taking. When more complex interventions are required parents usually prefer the nurse to retain the responsibility and undertake the necessary intervention: for example the recording of fluids given via an intravenous line and pump. It is important for the roles and responsibilities to be clearly discussed and negotiated to ensure all involved have identified the role boundaries, thus ensuring continuity of care for the child and family. Where possible this should be clearly documented within the patient's care plan. The NMC reminds practitioners that any care devolved to parents remains the responsibility of the qualified nurse (NMC, 2008). Before delegating any nursing care to parents nurses need to consider carefully the skills, abilities and demands placed on the parents, and the potential liability which surrounds care delegation, teaching and assessing.

However, some parents of chronically ill children will have more specialist nursing skills and be able to continue delivering these skills within the hospital setting. Some parents will be used to managing **enteral** feeding via nasogastric or gastrostomy tubes, others may have responsibility for giving intravenous antibiotics and physiotherapy, some may care for fully ventilated complex care children at home and may want to continue to have the **locus of control** whilst their child is in a hospital setting.

Other parents of chronically ill children, however, may view a period of hospitalisation as a chance to take a step back from being both the nurse and the parent and may ask the nursing staff to deliver the child's personal and nursing care needs whilst they are hospitalised. Utilising a family centred approach, the needs of the parents and child should be considered and all parents have the right to negotiate a level of involvement that is appropriate for their needs.

PHYSICAL DEVELOPMENT OF THE CHILD

The physical development of a child begins with prenatal development. The 'Germinal Stage' begins on day one where conception takes place – the female ovum and male sperm unite. Once fertilised the female egg or ovum forms a zygote and implants in the wall of the uterus. The next stage, the 'Embryonic Stage', involves rapid cell division which creates the embryo. The outer layer of cells, the chorion, contains the cells which form the placenta and umbilical cord. The inner membrane becomes a sac known as the amnion; this becomes filled with amniotic fluid in which the developing embryo floats. The mass of cells then differentiate to become several types of cells that will go on to become skin, sense receptors, nerve cells, muscles, circulatory system and the internal organs – liver, kidneys, pancreas, etc. This process is called organogenesis. Once the process of organogenesis is complete the developing organism is then called a foetus. This occurs around eight weeks after conception (Bee and Boyd, 2010).

The 'Foetal Stage' involves rapid growth and organ refinement. By about 12 weeks the sex organs can be seen on ultrasound. By week 24 the foetus can survive outside the uterus with intensive care nursing in a neonatal intensive care unit. After 30 weeks the developing foetus can hear, smell, is sensitive to touch and light (Bee and Boyd, 2010). Normal term delivery occurs from 38 weeks.

Labour is divided into three stages. Stage 1 involves dilatation and effacement of the cervix. The cervix will open to about 10cm. Stage 2 involves the delivery of the baby; Stage 3 is delivery of the placenta. Once delivered the baby has to rapidly adjust to being outside the uterus.

Physical development continues from birth to adulthood and beyond. The physical development of children cannot be viewed in isolation, however, and it is important to consider the multifaceted nature of a child's development – physical, psychological, social, moral and cultural. The child's development will be influenced by external factors such as their environment, experience and socialisation, and internal factors such as genetics, personality traits and characteristics.

Physical development begins with a set of primitive reflexes which are present at birth. Table 7-2 identifies some of the primitive reflexes which are present in newborn babies and the age at which these reflexes should disappear. A newborn developmental assessment would involve the healthcare professional assessing the presence of these reflexes as well as the baby's responsiveness, feeding and general behaviour.

A newborn baby has colour vision although they are short sighted, with an optimal visual range of 20–25cm; they begin to discriminate between voices and are able to taste flavours. Although a foetus can mimic a sucking action as young as 15–18 weeks gestation, mature coordination of sucking, swallowing and breathing is not present until 35 to 36 weeks gestation (Hockenberry *et al.*, 2003).

Physical development proceeds with a rapid rate of development in the first two years of life. There are two main patterns

Table 7-2 Reflexes Present in Newborn Babies

Reflex	Stimulation	Response	Age
Grasp reflex	Stimulate the palm of the baby's hand with your finger	Baby will grab your finger tightly	Disappears around 4 months
Moro reflex	Expose baby to a sudden loud noise	Extension of arms and legs with arching of back	Disappears around 3-4 months
Walking reflex	Hold baby up and touch soles of feet on a flat surface	Baby will mimic a walking action of legs	Disappears around 8 weeks
Rooting reflex	Stimulate baby's cheek	Baby turns head and opens mouth looking for nipple to attach to for feeding	Eventually develops voluntary control over head and neck around 3 weeks

Source: Bee, Helen L., Boyd, Denise A., *Developing Child, The, 11th © 2007.* Printed and electronically reproduced by permission of Pearson Education, Inc., Upper Saddle Eiver, New Jersey.

of physical development – cephalocaudal which essentially describes a child physically developing from the head downwards and proximodistal where development occurs from the centre outwards to the limbs.

The newborn infant's gross motor skills develop gradually during the first few months of life. The baby will develop increasing control over head and neck, torso, then arms, eventually gaining mastery of hand control, and then more defined fine motor skills such as finger movements. The same applies to the legs – gross mass muscle movement is gradually replaced by more refined control over individual limbs and eventually the feet. Thus the infant will replace gross mass muscle movement with more refined, controlled, calculated movement of extremities. This follows the patterns described above – cephalocaudal and proximodistal. The infant will learn to control the head and neck, before the arms, hands then fingers. Likewise, they learn to control legs before feet and then toes.

Put more simply, the infant will learn to control the head, and then learn to roll over, and then sit before crawling, standing, walking and running, skipping and riding a bicycle. By around five months the infant will learn to roll and has a whole hand or palm grasp, they begin sitting unsupported by around 7–9 months and learn to transfer objects between hands before mastering a 'pincer grasp', eventually walking by 10–12 months. The child develops more controlled hand coordination allowing basic grasping of a crayon by the age of two years (Bee and Boyd, 2010). An infant is expected to double their birth weight by the age of 5–6 months and treble it by the end of their first year. A two-year-old toddler is approximately half their full adult height.

The rate of physical growth and development in the school years tends to be at a slower pace until another rapid growth spurt during adolescence. During puberty hormones secreted by the thyroid, adrenal glands, leydig cells of testes (males)/ ovaries (females) and in the pituitary influence the development of the adolescent brain, bones, muscle and primary and secondary sexual characteristics. The average age of menarche in females of industrialised countries is 12½ to 13½ (Bee and Boyd, 2010), and occurs after the female experiences a significant growth spurt. For males the growth spurt starts later but is usually more significant and can continue longer.

Feeding and Nutrition

Adequate nutrition is fundamental to a child's growth and development. The World Health Organization (WHO) plays a pivotal role in giving health professionals and policy maker's guidance to ensure nutritional advice given to parents worldwide is up to date and evidence based.

In 2003, the WHO and the United Nations International Emergency Fund (UNICEF) published a joint global strategy for the feeding of infant and young children. This strategy aimed to revitalise the world's attention on the impact that feeding practices have on the nutritional status, growth and development, health and survival of infants and young people (WHO, 2003). This recommends that all infants are exclusively breastfed for the first six months of life. The policy also highlights the importance of nutritionally adequate, safe complementary feeding (weaning) starting at six months with breastfeeding continuing for the first two years:

> *Breast milk contains all the nutrients that an infant needs in the first 6 months of life, including fat, carbohydrates, proteins, vitamins, minerals and water* (WHO, 2009: 19).

The value and potential benefits of breastfeeding for the baby include less infections and decreased risk of some chronic conditions (see the *Practice Guidelines*). The benefits for mothers include increased rate of weight loss, and decreases in the risk of some types of cancer.

PRACTICE GUIDELINES

Benefits of Breastfeeding

Benefits for the infant include:

- decreased incidence of diarrhoea
- decreased incidence of otitis media
- decreased risk of *Haemophilus influenza* meningitis
- decreased risk of urinary tract infections
- decreased risk of obesity in later life.

Benefits for the mother include:

- decreased risk of postpartum haemorrhage
- decreased risk of breast cancer
- decreased risk of ovarian cancer
- increased rate of weight loss.

Source: *Infant and young child feeding - model chapter for textbooks for medical students and allied health professionals* (WHO, 2009).

Breast milk is easily digested by the infant and has bioactive factors which increase the infant's immature immune system. This provides extra protection for the infant in the first few months of life before the maturation of their own immune system. This is particularly important in the first few days of breastfeeding where the infant receives 'colostrum' from the mother which has essential immunoglobulins.

Breast milk contains 88% water (see Table 7-3), and even in hot climates the WHO (2009) suggests there is no need to supplement feeding with water or juice. This could in fact be detrimental to the production of milk in the baby as this relies on a balance defined by infant demand which then regulates the supply, or production.

There are two main hormones which regulate milk production in the breastfeeding mother. These are prolactin and oxytocin. As the baby suckles sensory impulses sent to the brain stimulate production of these hormones in the pituitary gland of the brain. Prolactin stimulates production of milk in the alveoli tissues of the breast. Oxytocin stimulates the cells around the alveoli to contract and thus encourage the flow of milk from the alveoli to the milk ducts in the nipple. This is commonly referred to as the 'let down reflex' and when initiated can cause the mother to ooze milk from both breasts whether the baby is attached and feeding or not!

Table 7-3 Composition of Breast Milk

Composition of breast milk	Per 100mls
Water	88%
Fat	3.5g
Lactulose	7g
Protein	0.9g

Source: based on WHO (2009).

To encourage breastfeeding rates health professionals in many trusts are specially trained to give advice, support and physical guidance to ensure the baby is attaching to the breast appropriately and feeding sufficiently. The 'Baby Friendly Hospital Initiative' (BFHI) (see the *Practice Guidelines*), was launched in 1992 by the WHO and identifies ways in which hospitals can actively promote breastfeeding and increase rates among the local population. This includes a reflection of the commitment to the promotion of breastfeeding through trust policy and providing specialist training for health professionals to enable them to support women wishing to breastfeed their babies.

PRACTICE GUIDELINES

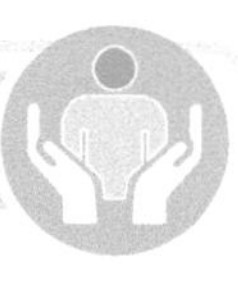

Ten Steps to Successful Breastfeeding

1. Have a written breastfeeding policy that is routinely communicated to all healthcare staff.
2. Train all healthcare staff in skills necessary to implement this policy.
3. Inform all pregnant women about the benefits and management of breastfeeding.
4. Help mothers initiate breastfeeding within a half hour of birth.
5. Show mothers how to breastfeed and how to maintain lactation even if they should be separated from their infants.
6. Give newborn infants no food or drink other than breast milk, unless medically indicated.
7. Practice rooming-in - allow mothers and infants to remain together - 24 hours a day.
8. Encourage breastfeeding on demand.
9. Give no artificial teats or pacifiers (also called dummies or soothers) to breastfeeding infants.
10. Foster the establishment of breastfeeding support groups and refer mothers to them on discharge from the hospital or clinic.

Source: Ten steps to successful breastfeeding - The Baby-Friendly Hospital Initiative, **http://www.unicef.org**

Breastfeeding mothers should be comfortable and relaxed; this will promote optimal conditions for infant feeding. Mothers should be encouraged to feed on demand and allow the infant to feed from the first breast until they are satisfied and spontaneously release the breast. If the infant still appears unsettled and hungry then the other breast should be offered. It is important that the baby empties the first breast completely because the composition of the first milk the baby suckles – the fore milk – differs to that of the hind milk which comes later in the feed. The hind milk is richer in fat and is therefore necessary for optimum growth and development.

It is important in all areas of the hospital to promote an environment which helps mothers feel comfortable, relaxed and able to breastfeed if they are attending any clinic environment. Promotion of dignity and providing comfortable appropriate facilities is of paramount importance.

Should a mother choose to give artificial formula the manufacturer's guidance should be followed to ensure the formula is reconstituted (if in powder format), stored and handled appropriately. Advice may need to be given to ensure the risk of infection associated is minimised, such as careful washing of hands, sterilisation of equipment and safe storage of reconstituted feed and safe feeding practices.

Supplementary feeding or weaning should start at six months, starting with small amounts of pureed, very well mashed, semi-solid foods offered twice, then three times a day. Baby rice or porridge are usually the first foods to be introduced, followed by fruit and vegetable purees.

At around eight months of age soft finger foods can be introduced and the consistency of the purees can become thicker with some small soft lumps. By this age the infant needs 3–4 meals a day. The infant should be introduced to a wide variety of flavours, ensuring a healthy balanced diet. The British Dietetic Association (BDA) suggests a diet which is low in salt, sugar and saturated fats (BDA, 2007). Care must also be taken when preparing foods to ensure the consistency is appropriate for the age group to prevent the risk of choking. For this reason whole nuts are inappropriate for young children. The WHO (2009), stresses, however, that there is insufficient evidence relating to the avoidance of certain foods, such as nuts, shellfish, cow's milk and eggs to reduce the risk of allergy. The BDA (2007) recommends introduction of these foods in children's diets unless there is a family member with a food allergy. In such cases the specific food should not be introduced until the child is over three years old.

By the age of one year the child should be eating the same types of foods as the rest of the family, and encouraged to experience a wide variety of flavours and textures. Where possible the mother should continue to offer breastfeeds until the child is two years old.

PSYCHOLOGICAL DEVELOPMENT OF CHILDREN AND YOUNG PEOPLE

Children and young people's psychological development is very different to that of adults; they view the world very differently resulting in a significantly altered perspective for many reasons. Children and young people (CYP) are physically smaller, their intellectual, social, emotional, reasoning and problem solving abilities are still in development and undergoing a process of maturation, all of which become refined and shaped by the child/young person's experience.

A number of theories are found within the literature which attempt to explain children and young people's psychological development. The theories attempt to provide an explanation of the psychological and intellectual development of the child and young person as they mature thus providing insight into their world view. No one theory can adequately explain the child and young persons' development and it may be useful to take an eclectic approach in using these theories when caring for and understanding children and young people.

Knowledge for Practice

Despite initiatives to ensure children and young people (CYP) are cared for in specific care settings by appropriately qualified and experienced nurses (RN Child) it is common for non-children's nurses to encounter CYP in a variety of care situations from community-based care settings (e.g. GP surgeries, home, clinics) through to more complex settings (e.g. A&E, ICU). Thus it is essential for all practitioners to have a clear understanding of children and young people's psychological development.

Perspective

The child or young person's perspective is influenced by their psychological development – cognitive, psychosocial – which influences their interpretation of events. The child/young person may express themselves in 'unusual' language (which is appropriate for their developmental age) or may feel threatened and vulnerable by what the nurse perceives to be a simple care event (e.g. temperature taking, blood pressure). The practitioner must develop insight into the CYP perspective, so that they can tailor their care, language and responses to the CYP needs.

Development

As practitioners it is vital to have insight into what is considered to be normal development so that any changes, delays in meeting milestones or inappropriate development can be detected and appropriate referrals or interventions can take place. Parents may also seek advice on their child's development and will want to discuss any issues to reassure themselves their child is progressing normally or to allay any anxieties they may have. Advice can then be given on how to maintain and promote the child's psychological development, especially during sickness or admission into hospital.

Communication

It is vital that nurses communicate with CYP clearly, concisely and in an understandable manner using the appropriate language tailored to the CYP appropriate developmental level. This should enable children and young people to be aware of the care which is being delivered and enable them to make informed decisions about what is to happen to them. Also an understanding of development gives the practitioner insight into the rich and varied language that may be used by CYP to express themselves, to describe events or interact with healthcare professionals.

Environment

The environment needs to be tailored to the child and young person's needs to enable them to feel psychologically comfortable, build trust and feel less fearful of what may happen. Bright colours, cartoon characters, toys, age appropriate decor can all be used. A cold, non-child oriented environment can make the child feel isolated, frightened and fearful.

Coping Mechanisms

Children and young people cope in very different ways compared to adults. Some children will play out events with toys, drawing or become aggressive or hiding away due to fear. Regression may occur; this is where the child returns to a previous developmental stage where they feel psychologically safe and less threatened by the need to cope with their own development and the demands of being in a care setting.

Therefore the healthcare professional needs to gain insight into the psychological development of the child and young person in order to fully understand the ways in which they interpret events and communicate their feelings about the healthcare situation.

Piaget's Theory of Cognitive Development

Piaget's theory of cognitive development is the most frequently cited theory used to underpin explanations and research into children and young people's experiences and conceptualisation of health and healthcare.

Piaget's theory suggests that each person has a **schema** or pattern about particular events or situations. These schemas or patterns are the building blocks of intelligence. Learning occurs through assimilation and accommodation. Assimilation occurs when new knowledge is incorporated into the schema and accommodation means that existing knowledge is changed to meet existing demands and challenges (Harris and Butterworth, 2002).

Piaget's theory of cognitive development is a classical stage theory. This means that certain developmental events 'belong' to different ages; for ease the child's development is divided into age groups. However, this is not to say that the child's development for that stage is completed by the prescribed age, rather the child or young person moves into the next stage in a way that is appropriate for that individual. The theory deals with four main stages.

Sensorimotor Stage: 0–2 Years

This stage is characterised by learning through the senses where the infant learns through the stimulation of their sight, touch, hearing, smell and taste. Infants enjoy the textures of new objects by touching them and sucking them. Bright colours can provide strong contrast which attract the infant's gaze and stimulate visual development. The infant acquires a basic understanding of cause and effect learning: that crying brings comfort and that smiling provokes a reciprocal interaction. This is the beginning of the child's ability to control the environment around them. During this stage the child acquires object permanence. This is where the child realises that an object or person still exists despite not being visible or present. It is suggested that this begins at around 6–8 months of age and is achieved at around 18 months (Harris and Butterworth, 2002). During this time stranger and separation anxiety develop. Egocentricity begins in this stage, where the infant views and responds to the world solely from their own viewpoint and needs. The infant in the early months of this stage is profoundly egocentric, where they have little sense of self and all needs are instantly met by the parent(s)/carers. This progresses so that by 4–6 months the infant begins to realise they are separate from their parents and are beginning to learn and recognise that they can shape events around them according to their needs and desires. At this stage communication skills are developing rapidly with symbols being used to communicate. The child has the ability to understand language and infer what they want but the actual verbal skills are maturing hence the use of symbols; this is known as general symbolic functioning (Gross, 2005). The child enjoys manipulating the environment, learning about which activities, behaviours and interactions influence events and people around them. The learning in this stage progresses from reflexive through to repetitive and finally imitative learning.

Implications for Practice

Object Permanence

Stranger anxiety and separation anxiety (protest, despair, and denial) can develop where the infant realises that even though their parents/carers may not be in sight they still exist. The infant resists separation and being cared for by strangers. Maintaining the attachment with parents is vital to avoid these anxieties developing, thus ensure that parents remain with their child throughout the care process or if not possible then minimise the separation time.

The older infant/child will realise that medicines can be hidden in drinks, etc. and so avoid hiding them. Through gentle explanation and allowing the child to see what will happen the child is able to adjust and prepare for the event. There will not be any nasty surprises. This will ensure that trust can be built up between the nurse and child who should not feel they have been tricked.

Imitation

Demonstrate procedures to children using toys (teddy/doll) in order to allay fears and explain what is to happen.

General symbolic function

Use symbols (pictures, hand gestures, toys) and simple language to explain and demonstrate procedures.

Sense, pleasure, play

Mobiles, bright toys, music all stimulate the infant and help to maintain development.

Preoperational Stage: 2–7 Years

This stage is characterised by magical thinking which is used to interpret and make sense of often confusing events and the adult world they encounter. Magical thinking occurs due to the child's lack of experience and understanding of the social rules and complexity of language and behaviour around them.

Egocentricity is a feature of this stage and it advances from the sensorimotor stage. The world is viewed and interpreted solely from the child's perspective; they do not understand that events can be interpreted differently by others or appreciate that there are other perspectives. The child is also unable to differentiate between what is subjective (personal and private) and what is objective (public knowledge and what is true) (Harris and Butterworth, 2002). A sense of personal power develops as they learn to understand and control events from their own perspective.

The child's thinking is concrete and so they think in absolutes. Expressions will be taken literally as the child does not have the ability to infer (e.g. there are eyes in the back of my head – the child will look for the eyes). The world is a very black and white place so that thoughts are polarised (e.g. people are very nice or very horrible). The child lacks the ability to think in relative terms and realise that there are shades of grey. They can only deal with one idea at a time so instructions and requests need to be made in stages to ensure the child understands what is required of them. Time is poorly understood as it is an abstract concept, thus 10 minutes can seem a very long time and is often underestimated. As a result the child needs to understand time in concrete terms in relation to events such as sleeps or TV programmes. The child has a sense of animism and will imbue non-human or inanimate articles with living or moving properties (e.g. cardboard box = boat or horse). It is often difficult for them to distinguish cause and effect. The body is seen as a global entity at this stage so pain sticks into the body as a whole rather than occurring in a specific part.

Children are influenced by surface features of objects. Thus they have difficulty understanding that if a liquid, weight or shape changes its appearance the mass remains the same in terms of its volume or weight of shape (e.g. a triangle inverted is still a triangle but the child will perceive it as a different shape; a tall beaker and a short tumbler contain the same volume of water yet the child perceives the tall beaker as holding more water). The child does not have the concept of reversibility until about seven years of age. As a result they do not grasp that there are opposite reactions and events can be reversed.

Transductive reasoning occurs. This is where the child recognises that objects or people have particular characteristics. Having learnt the rule the child then applies the rule indiscriminately until they learn to discriminate the differences. For example, a cat has four legs, fur, a tail, whiskers and a wet nose. A dog has four legs, fur, a tail, whiskers and a wet nose. Therefore a cat and a dog are the same. Or two doctors wear white coats. Nurses wear white tops. Therefore nurses and doctors are the same.

Syncretic thought means the child can only classify objects or people by one aspect at a time.

Implications for Practice

Concrete Thinking

Explanations need to be unambiguous and facts presented in a black and white way (e.g. this will hurt or hurt a lot). The child will struggle with the terms 'it will hurt a little bit more than last time'. Be careful of using analogies as the child's absolute thinking will mean they will take the analogy literally (e.g. lungs are like balloons – the child may become fearful as balloons burst and they will think their lungs will burst and not work anymore).

Magical Thinking

The child expects the nurse or doctor to be all powerful and to cure them of their illness or pain. They expect it to be magicked away. Use storytelling to work with the child and explain events and interventions (e.g. magic cream). The child may have imaginary friends who will need to be included and 'treated' too. If this is done it will help to calm and reassure the child and will save time in treatment as a result.

Events may be seen as reversible (e.g. death). Children will ask when the deceased person will return.

Egocentricity

The child has a sense of personal power so if they have been horrible to a sibling who is then hospitalised the child can feel guilty and responsible. They will feel they have influenced events. However, with careful and considerate explanation the child is able to decentre and understand some basic ideas with a different perspective.

The child will tie together two unconnected events because they have loomed large within their lives in a short space of time and they feel they are the focus for those events. Thus if a child has done something naughty and subsequently finds themselves in hospital they are likely to feel they have been punished for the transgression.

Conservation

This will influence the giving of medicines orally. 5mls of liquid presented in an oral syringe looks more than 5mls of liquid presented on a spoon. With regard to pain relief the child will expect analgesia to be given at the site of the pain and may struggle to grasp that oral analgesia will palliate the pain in their leg. Also, health promotion concepts can be difficult to grasp. If a child is encouraged to drink milk to give them healthy teeth and bones they will take this literally to mean their teeth and bones are made of milk. The child fails to understand that the nutritional content is extracted and absorbed.

Reversibility

The child will need explanations of events to ensure they understand what is happening and are not left to 'fill in the gaps' with magical thinking. Thus if the child is going to theatre and is having a 'magic sleep' (anaesthetic) they need to be told they will wake up.

Concepts of Illness

Phenomenism

The child will attribute the cause of their illness to a magical cause or a temporally or spatially remote cause (e.g. the wind gave me a cold because I wasn't wearing my coat) (Swanick, 1990).

Contagion

The child has some idea that illness can be 'caught' but the ideas are rudimentary and the child does not understand that proximity or contact with the illness is a feature of contagion. Also, the child may think that all illnesses are contagious, even chronic non-infectious illnesses (e.g. diabetes).

Body parts

The child will focus on what they can see or have had experiences of. They are aware of their bones; they can feel their heart beating; they are conscious of their brain as it helps them think. They can name 3–7 body parts.

Concrete Operational Stage: 7–11 Years

The child becomes increasingly logical at this stage and is able to classify and organise concepts. Judgements are now based on reasoning rather than emotion or magical thinking. The child attains conservation and reversibility as well as achieving the use of relativity. Cause and effect is now understood. A clearer understanding of the body is apparent.

Implications of Practice

Problem solving

The skills are now good, thus explanations can be factual, although models, drawings and diagrams are useful as the child's thinking is not totally on an abstract level. Diagrams, etc. reinforce the thinking and ideas to be absorbed.

Health promotion

It is now easier to discuss the issues around health promotion as the child can infer and has the ability to understand simple analogies as well as conserve.

Reversibility

This is attained so the child understands the concepts of healing and restoration of function to an injured limb.

Pain

This is still viewed as punishment; however the concept is more sophisticated. The child feels punished by the parents/guardians/carers who are meant to protect them. As a result the child may vent their anger on those caring for them, blaming them for their predicament.

Concepts of illness

Contamination

The child now has an understanding of cause and effect and will understand that contact with a causative factor is what causes illness (e.g. bad food = tummy ache) (Swanick, 1990).

Internalisation

Illness is located within the body but has an external cause (e.g. you breathe in cold air and get a cough) (Swanick, 1990).

Body parts

The child is able to understand the actions and workings of the body (e.g. the heart is a pump pushing blood around the body through small pipes called blood vessels) (McEwing, 1996).

Formal Operational Stage: 12+ Years

This stage is characterised by the development of abstract thinking and logical thought. The young person is able to problem solve using several strategies albeit they are still limited by experience and development. They are able to formulate hypotheses about the world around them which gives them the opportunity to experiment and test them out. The egocentricity appears to return as the young person focuses on their own perspectives and thoughts. This enables them to disengage from their parents/carers and develop their thinking, ideas, values and beliefs based on their own aspirations, knowledge and ideology. They become philosophical and idealistic in their pursuit of understanding the complexities of the adult world. The sense of self is developed via peer groups who facilitate the development of self-esteem and self-awareness. However, the young person is psychologically vulnerable leading to over intellectualisation and dramatisation of events.

Other writers (e.g. Erikson) discuss the psychosocial development of the young person. The period of adolescence is hallmarked by a search for identity where the young person seeks to develop a sense of self and identity whilst developing their values and beliefs. Self-esteem and body image are developed through contact with the peer group and the achievement of social competence (Gross, 2005; Bee, 2006).

Implications for Practice

Explanations

These can become more adult in nature – factual and discussing concepts.

Philosophical/idealistic

The young person can think about long-term outcomes in relation to their health although the reality of the health behaviours can remain an abstract issue due to the developmental need to risk take and the idealistic nature of their thinking. For example, with alcohol intake they are aware of the dangers but feel they are immune to them as they are 'invincible'. Health breakdown and ageing are not a reality at this age for a healthy young person. This is the personal fable which they carry. The failure to achieve personal goals is particularly devastating as it confounds hopes and aspirations regardless of the magnitude of the illness or injury.

Self-Esteem

This is fragile and can be easily dented. Belonging to the peer group is vital in establishing and confirming a sense of self. The peer group is a place to experiment, discuss ideas and formulate personal values and beliefs. Rejection is perceived acutely. This is also true of being within a relationship and any subsequent breakdown.

Risk-Taking Behaviour

This is a normal part of adolescent behaviour which links into the development of their thinking, values and social competence within the peer group. Risk-taking behaviour allows the young person to test out hypotheses and understand the consequences of that behaviour. Risk-taking behaviour also enables a sense of mastery to develop.

Concepts of Illness

Psychological

Psychological and emotional pain is perceived acutely.

Physiological

The young person understands the mechanisms of trauma, illness and the accompanying explanations. Be aware of using confusing jargon and use understandable lay terms.

PLAY

Play is the fundamental way in which children enjoy their childhood and is essential to their quality of life (Play England, 2009; McArdle, 2001). Through play the child is able to act on the world around it, make sense of it and attempt to understand their place within society (Welsh Assembly Government, 2001; Sturgess, 2003). Play is not a unitary concept but a complex, highly intense and highly individualised concept and behaviour comprising many different aspects; it is found across all societies and age spans (Fisher *et al.*, 2008). The right for the child to play is endorsed by the United Nations Convention on the Rights of the Child and the Welsh Assembly Government (2001) who state that it is an essential part of the child's life which encompasses their cultural heritage and facilitates self-esteem, confidence and positive mental health (Milligan and Bingley, 2007; McArdle, 2001).

Play is defined as:

> *. . . freely chosen; personally directed, intrinsically motivated behaviour that actively engages the child . . . Play can be fun or serious. Through play children explore social, material and imaginary worlds and their relationship with them, elaborating all the while a flexible range of responses to the challenges they encounter.* (Children's Play Council, 2000)

Play is about engaging in activities which are removed from the 'real' world but mimic it. Play should provide not only physical enjoyment but mental effort and emotional satisfaction (Garvey, 1977; Sheridan, 1999). Play has several characteristics:

- It is enjoyable.
- There is no extrinsic goal, it is intrinsically motivated.
- It is spontaneous and voluntary.
- It is chosen freely.
- It is about active enjoyment.
- It is related to what is not play.
- It is linked with creativity, problem solving, language, social roles and cognitive development.

Play encourages the development and refinement of skills which will be needed in adulthood, it allows children to explore the possibility of the world around them and develop a sense of mastery over themselves and what is going on around them (Harris and Butterworth, 2002; Gross, 2005).

Social Character of Play

Play interactions in infancy are mainly between a child and adult. Infants and children enjoy the company of an adult but do become increasingly able to play alone. As they become older so playmates assume greater importance and are an essential part of the socialisation process.

Solitary Play

The infant/child plays independently and alone. They may enjoy the presence of other children but make no effort to be involved with them or speak to them. The child's interest is centred solely on their own activity.

Onlooker

The child watches other children playing but does not enter the play activity. There is an active interest in observing the interaction of others but no move to participate.

Parallel

The child plays independently among others. They may play with similar toys to other children. Each child plays as they see fit neither influencing nor being influenced by those around them. They play alongside but not with other children.

Associative Play

The children play together engaged in a similar activity, however there is no organisation or division of 'work', leadership or goals. Each child plays according their own wishes, although similar play behaviours can be found amongst the children through copying.

Cooperative Play

This play is organised; the children play in a group with other children. The children discuss and plan activities for the purpose of accomplishing an end goal (e.g. drama, game, role playing). The group is loosely formed but there is a sense of belonging. There is an end goal and its attainment is achieved through the organisation of activities, 'work', roles and leadership which is closely controlled (McArdle, 2001).

Table 7-4 Types of Play

Types of play	Play activity	Application in practice
Free play	Child is allowed 'free rein' to choose all activities	Provide range of toys to choose from if child immobile - teddy, books, pen and paper
		Access to play area or play room
Organised play	Structured into activities	Painting (use aprons and absorbent sheet to mop up water)
		Colouring
		Story telling - child makes up story or nurse does as they care for child Singing as you care for child
Messy play	Finger painting, clay modelling	Modelling clay
		Finger paints in bed
		Water play with bowl and jug (if child in bed) or cup and water if in small area (e.g. A&E)
Creative play	Junk modelling, painting	Colouring
		Paper to make aeroplanes or shapes (useful if child is waiting or confined to bed)
		Growing cress on blotting paper if child in for long stay
		Keep puppet in your pocket or small toy to amuse child
Dramatic play	Role play, e.g. house	Child can be the hero of a story fighting the 'monster' of pain
		You can be the rescuer rescuing the child and making the child better
Formal games	Board games, card games	Useful if teaching child/young person about their condition, and management of the condition

Source: McArdle (2001).

Types of Play

There are various types of play that a child may engage in (see Table 7-4). The purposes of play include (Sturgess, 2003):

- sensori-motor development;
- intellectual development;
- socialisation;
- creativity;
- developing self-awareness;
- developing a sense of self and self-control;
- language development;
- development of problem-solving skill;
- therapeutic value: release from tension and stress; emotional expression;
- moral value: develops moral values and beliefs; codes of behaviour.

Play normally occurs in a child-oriented environment which provides stimulation for the child to explore, investigate and develop enjoyment. The presence of a permission-giving adult is required and they may be called upon to become involved in the play (Jun-Tai, 2008). This is particularly pertinent in settings which are not familiar to the child (e.g. hospital).

Play and the Sick Child

Coming into contact with the healthcare system and a number of unknown healthcare professionals is a particularly daunting and anxious experience for the majority of children. They are admitted or seen within an alien environment and are expected to comply with procedures and adapt relatively quickly to what is happening. This induces fear and anxiety and can make the child feel as if they are being punished in some way. Play has an immensely significant role in ensuring that the whole process of care is as comfortable and as least traumatic as possible. The Department of Health (DH, 2004) stated that play was a vital component of the child's care when in hospital and that it should be organised and delivered by qualified hospital play specialists. It is essential that all nurses coming into contact with children and young people have knowledge of play which should be an integral part of their role. Play enables the nurse to work comfortably with the child, building confidence, trust and a relationship which facilitates the delivery of care, treatment and procedures. Play is the key means by which nurses can communicate with the children in their care but also they in turn can understand and gain insight into the child's experiences and needs through play (Jun-Tai, 2008).

PRACTICE GUIDELINES

Why Do Nurses Need to Know About Play?

- Gives insight into the child and young person's development.
- Detection of emotional and behavioural issues.
- Allows child to communicate in a manner which they find safe.
- Enables adults to communicate ideas, information, allay fears.
- Used as distraction during painful and distressing procedures.
- Gives insight into how children can come to harm (e.g. accidents, places to play).
- Enables parents to take a role in the child's care.
- Health professional can use play to teach about their roles and work.
- Educate parents about safety in play.

Play in hospital has many functions which are invaluable. From a nursing perspective play enables the building of a relationship and trust before procedures are carried out. Children are often fearful and apprehensive of what will happen and their expectations are heightened. Play provides a means to relax the patient and acts as a distracter from pain and procedures as well as a means of the nurse and child to get to know each other and develop a positive rapport which will underpin their relationship during the stay.

ACTIVITY 7-3

Jamie is three years and has been admitted to the unit for investigations for failure to thrive. He is anxious and holds tight to his mother. Jamie needs a blood test and is prepared using anaesthetic cream to the backs of his hands.

What sort of activities might the nurse consider to distract Jamie from the impending blood test?

Play introduces normality into the environment at a time when the child is vulnerable, fearful and in need of distraction and comfort. A familiar activity is introduced which engages the child and develops their interest away from the immediate potential 'threat' of being dislocated from home, family and friends. Through playing the child can express themselves and understand the need to be in hospital. Play enables the child to work through their feelings, fears and anxieties so that hospital can become a positive experience. This may reassure parents about their child who may have had limited contact with healthcare. Play can be used to maintain normal family interactions which reassures the child and parents that their relationship can continue. Parents may be uncertain about what they can and can't do within hospital, feeling there are unspoken rules. They may have had little experience of seeing their child in pain, ill or fearful. With support and encouragement parents are able to maintain their role as play mate, comforter and engage in normal parenting activities through play. Parents are an invaluable resource as they can play with and distract the child or young person whilst the nurse delivers care and treatment. This also holds true for the siblings who may have felt excluded and uninformed during the stay. Play helps them to be involved and informed and ensures they can continue their playful relationship with each other as well as enabling them to understand the situation and express their own concerns.

Through play the impact of pain is lessened, and function is restored, as are skills lost through injury or illness. Play can provide an opportunity to assess the child for the type of injury, levels of pain they are experiencing, etc. enabling the healthcare professional to develop a plan of care which is individualised and can meet the child's needs. It can be used to engage children in treatments, making them fun whilst achieving the goals of care (Jun-Tai, 2008). Thus play aids recovery by making it faster and reducing the length of stay in hospital (McArdle, 2001; McArdle and Huff, 2001).

Play is an invaluable method for giving information in a meaningful way and enables the nurse to deliver the information at the appropriate developmental level using the appropriate language to meet the child's needs. Again parents can be involved in this process and find this valuable as information is given to their child. They also learn strategies for coping with their child's distress if care is to be delivered following discharge. Thus play is used not only to inform but to facilitate the child's coping abilities with a familiar activity.

Teddy Bear Clinics

These clinics have proved popular with children and have been successful in reducing the fear associated with hospital admission. The children attend a clinic where through role play their bears are examined, treated and made better. They also are given stickers and certificates. As the bears are treated so the children visit the different areas of the hospital they might attend and observe the treatment they may receive if they were a patient. The clinic gives the children the opportunity to ask questions and familiarise themselves with the hospital and staff, demystifying the experience and allaying any concerns they may have. In turn this develops the staff's skills in communication and therapeutic play (Zimmerman and Santen, 1997; Campbell and Brown, 2008; Terry and Davies, 2011).

Pre-Admission Programmes

These programmes are aimed primarily at children and families who are booked for a planned admission into hospital. The children attend the programme at the hospital where, through a morning of playful activity, they are able to understand what is to happen. The children have the opportunity to dress up in small nurses'/doctors' uniforms, play with toy equipment, see and feel the 'real' equipment, visit the bed area and ward and meet the staff. The children are given the opportunity to ask questions and explore the physical environment. The staff meet children in a relaxed atmosphere and the therapeutic relationship begins which will underpin a successful admission (Jun-Tai, 2008; McArdle and Huff, 2001; Muller *et al.*, 1992).

Children require an atmosphere that will foster and promote their ability to play and this includes appropriate toys and the presence of a permission-giving and trusted adult. Also the play may need to be initiated and organised in the first instance by the CYP nurse or play specialist in order to support the child, to feel they can play. Play enables the child to discover ways of coping as well as involving parents and siblings in the healthcare encounter.

Play is not a luxury or optional extra when delivering care; it is an essential and integral part of every nurse's role when caring for children and young people.

Children and Young People's Experience of Pain

Infants, children and young people can and do experience and perceive pain in a number of ways. Pain is the most distressing aspect of a disease, injury or hospitalisation (RCN, 2009b). Physical pain, both acute and chronic, arise as a result of trauma, infection or surgery, whereas psychological pain is experienced in response to psychosocial influences at home or in the community, the effects of hospitalisation, fears of pain, injury or change in body image (Kortesluoma and Nikkonen, 2004, 2006; Davies, 2009; RCN, 2009b). CYP understanding and interpretation of pain and the pain experience is shaped by a child's level of cognitive development as well as previous experiences. Indeed it has been found that children with cognitive impairment suffer significantly higher levels of pain more regularly than unimpaired children (RCN, 2009b; Carter *et al.*, 2002). Pain in infants and CYP requires effective assessment and management. Unrelieved pain can be severe and can have a number of physical and psychological consequences, which include extended stay, loss of function and mobility, loss of skills, lower self-esteem and self-efficacy, regression, withdrawal, depression and isolation (Davies, 2009; RCN, 2009b; Kortesluoma and Nikkonen, 2004, 2006).

Effective pain management is fundamentally linked to the effective assessment of pain and without such an assessment the subsequent pain management strategies are flawed as they will not be underpinned by good quality information to inform the care delivered. Assessing pain in an infant, child or young person is a challenging experience due to their cognitive level of development, the specific pain vocabulary used to express themselves and the fact that pain is a dynamic and complex experience which requires a multidimensional approach to assess it effectively. Thus the nurse needs to be able to interpret the information given to them as well as providing an accurate and effective pain assessment which is a critical step in the process of ensuring pain is managed successfully. This is an essential part of the nurse's role and care delivery.

It is essential that pain is assessed appropriately using a reliable, valid and measurable assessment on a regular basis. Indeed legally, ethically and morally healthcare practitioners have a duty of care to ensure that the children receive the highest standard of care so that their pain is relieved (DH, 2004; Simons and McDonald, 2006; NMC, 2008).

Patient-Centred Care

The following should be taken into account (RCN, 2009b):

- Children are listened to and believed.
- Parents/carers are listened to and their views respected ('Respecting the role of the parent is a significant part of providing services to children and young people' (National Service Framework Standards for Hospital Services, 2.17).
- At first contact, services should identify children and families who require extra support; for example, those who need interpreters or advocates and children in need including disabled children (National Service Framework Standards for Hospital Services, 3.2).
- Children and their families/carers are viewed as partners in care.
- Children and their families/carers are involved in shared decision making about individualised pain assessment and have the opportunity to ask questions.
- Children and their families/carers are informed of any potential risks and/or complications associated with pain assessment.
- Training is provided in the use of tools for parents/carers.

Myths and Misconceptions

Despite the body of policy and research on infant, children and young people's pain, providing robust evidence to underpin the practice of pain assessment and management, a number of pain myths and misconceptions still persist in practice (see Table 7-5). Such myths and misconceptions significantly undermine quality care and management as they negatively skew the practitioner's ability to listen to and understand the information imparted by the parent, child or young person. Thus the effectiveness of the assessment and subsequent management is flawed, leading to prolonged or even unrelieved pain (RCN, 2009b; Twycross, 2007, 2008).

Children and Young People's Understanding of Pain

Children and young people's interpretation and understanding of their pain is influenced by a number of factors – home background, previous experiences, family functioning, social

Table 7-5 Myths and Misconceptions about Children and Pain

Myth	Fact
Infants cannot feel pain.	Pain pathways (although immature) are present at birth and pain impulses are able to travel to and from the pain centres in the brain. Neonates exhibit behavioural, physiological and hormonal responses to pain.
Active children cannot be in pain.	Playing and being active or being distracted is one of the most effective ways in which infants, children and young people cope with pain. Some children and young people spontaneously use this method to focus away from their pain.
Children will always tell you when they are in pain.	Children may not report pain due to fear or a desire to please those around them. A child who conceals pain may do so in an attempt to avoid a further painful experience, such as a needle. Older children may not wish to appear weak by showing their pain, especially in front of their peers.
Children feel less pain than adults.	Younger children experience higher levels of pain than do older ones. For some, pain sensitivity seems to decrease with age. This may be due to cognitive development and the increasing ability to use coping strategies and to rationalise the pain.
Children forget pain quicker than adults.	Children can be traumatised by the pain episode and become fearful of further procedures or admissions. Children and young people's coping skills are not as well honed as an adult's and so they may be unable to rationalise what is happening.
It is unsafe to administer narcotics to children because they become addicted.	Addiction is rare. When used over a short period for pain narcotics are beneficial in resolving pain.
Narcotics always cause respiratory depression in children.	This is very rare. Children tolerate narcotic analgesia well. As long as it is given at the correct dosage and via the correct route it is safe.
Children cannot accurately tell you where it hurts.	Children can describe the intensity, location and meaning of their pain very clearly.
The best way to administer analgesia is by injection.	This method is unacceptable to children and young people. It is often the thing they fear most about hospital and pain relief.
Parents always know the best way to manage their children's pain.	Parents may not have seen their child in pain and can feel lost and vulnerable. They will need advice and support to care for their child in this situation.
Generally there is a usual amount of pain associated with any given procedure.	This is untrue and unacceptable as it can lead to children and young people not receiving adequate medication.
The less analgesia administered to children the better it is for them.	Unresolved pain leads to increased stress, delayed wound healing and a child who is fearful.
It is often being restrained during procedures rather than pain that children find distressing.	Restraint can be frightening but should not be assumed to be the cause of the child's distress as pain is heightened during fear-inducing procedures.

Sources: Collier, 1997; Twycross, 1998; Hospital for Sick Children, 2008; RCN, 2009b; Twycross (2011).

expectation, culture, religion/faith and their cognitive development (see Table 7-6). The nurse needs to have an understanding of the child's cognitive level and their interpretation of the pain experience not only for evaluating and understanding the pain experience but also for designing interventions to reduce the pain (Davies, 2009; RCN, 2009b; Twycross, 1998; McGrath, 1990).

Children and Young People's Pain Vocabulary

The expression of pain is also cognitively determined and it has been found that children have a rich and varied vocabulary to express their pain. Pain is an abstract concept and as such the word is not used until the child reaches the formal operation stage of their development (Hester *et al.*, 1992; Twycross, 1998; LaFleur and Raway, 1999). It has been found that definitions range from concrete to abstract. Children of 5–7 years define the pain by its locations and its physical properties (e.g. hurt); 8–10-year-olds discuss pain in relation to their feelings whilst young people discuss it in relation to how they feel psychologically (Gaffney and Dunne, 1986; Hester *et al.*, 1992; La Fleur and Raway, 1999). Children are socialised into the use of pain words by eight years of age.

Table 7-6 Children and Young People's Understanding of Pain

Sensorimotor stage 0–2 years	Preoperational stage 2–7 years	Concrete operational stage 7–11 years	Formal operational stage 12+ years
Preverbal concepts unknown	Pain is perceived as a physical and emotional punishment	Perceives pain physically and emotionally	Gives reason for pain
Interpret behavioural signs	The child wishes for the magical disappearance of pain	Increased awareness of body/organs	Perceives psychological pain
Realises it causes effect if cries	Nurse is all powerful and is perceived as someone who can magic away the pain	Fear of bodily harm and assault	Fears loss of control due to pain
Connects staff with pain/distaste of medicine	Cannot distinguish between cause and effect of pain and medication	Pain is viewed as a punishment	Lacks ability to cope using mature strategies and needs support
Realises if medicine hidden	Pain sticks into body where it occurs	Understands analgesia and pain relief - time	Pain damages self-esteem and self-efficacy
Distrusts unknown staff	Concerned with surface features of the pain and treatment	Understands the 'action' of analgesia and pain and method of administration	Expects nurse to know if they are in pain as it is a loss of face
Pain expressed in behaviour	Needs to complain of pain	Can locate pain accurately	Pain makes the young person vulnerable emotionally
Can point to pain	Can name and locate pain	Names pain	Pain erodes independence
			Thinks deeply about the meaning of the pain and its consequences
			Fear of disfigurement
			Fear of technology altering body image

Sources: McGrath, 1990; Woodgate and Kristjanson, 1995; Twycross, 1998; Kortesluoma and Nikkonen, 2004, 2006.

The language used to describe pain is varied, rich and colourful as well as being highly individual. Children and young people are able to provide excellent descriptors of their pain and it is essential that the healthcare practitioner gain insight into what is being communicated (Kortesluoma and Nikkonen, 2006). Jerret and Evans (1986) in a classic study found that children used a wide variety of words which ranged from concrete words through to more abstract expressions.

Specific pain descriptors used by children aged 5–9 years 6 months are shown in Table 7-7. The article by Kortesluoma and Nikkonnen (2006) should also be read to illustrate this issue further.

Table 7-7 Pain Descriptors Used by Children

Sensory	Affective	Evaluative
Lots of banging	Sad	Bad
Get it mostly	Unhappy	Ugly
Comes and goes	Drive you nuts	Awful
Buzzing	Bugged you	No good
Painful	Attacking	Different
Grabbing	Mean	Funny
Fall off	No strength	Terrible
Hitting	Scared	Not nice
Snow	Upset	Yucky
Ouch	Disappointed	Nagging
Sausages	Not well	Weird
Once and a while	Crying	Not good
Needle through	Hard	Like headache
Warm	Dizzy	A lot
Knife hit	Banging	Worst
Cymbals clapping	Falling	Really bad
Bullet	Chilling	Mild
Tickled	Sounds funny	Very sore
Off and on	Mosquitoes buzzing	Little bad
	Was bit	Feel worse
	Sometimes	

Pain Assessment: When?

Pain assessment should be an integral part of the care delivered and be an ongoing process whereby the infant, child or young person is observed, questioned and assessed. This is pertinent if analgesia is prescribed as there is a need to assess its efficacy. Routines of care should not interfere with this process or dictate when it occurs, the infant/child/young person is central to the care and it is their needs which should dictate when the assessment occurs and analgesia is required (Twycross, 2007).

Assessment points

- On admission – pain issues (vocabulary, behaviours, coping) can be discussed with the child and family.
- At regular intervals if the infant/child/young person is known to have pain.

Table 7-8 Framework for Assessing a Child's Pain

Child form	Parent form
Tell me what pain is.	What word(s) does your child use in regard to pain?
Tell me about the hurt you have had before.	Describe the pain experiences your child has had before.
Do you tell others when you hurt? If yes, who?	Does your child tell you or others when he or she is hurting?
What do you do for yourself when you are hurting?	How do you know when your child is in pain?
What do you want others to do for you when you hurt?	How does your child usually react to pain?
What don't you want others to do for you when you hurt?	What do you do for your child when he or she is hurting?
What helps the most to take your hurt away?	What does your child do for him- or herself when he or she is hurting?
Is there anything special that you want me to know about you when you hurt? (If yes, have child describe.)	What works best to decrease or take away your child's pain?
	Is there anything special that you would like me to know about your child and pain? (If yes, describe.)

Source: Adapted from Hester and Barcus (1986).

- When carrying out routine care if the child is experiencing pain.
- When unexpected or intense pain occurs as indicated by altered vital signs, behaviour changes or communication (Davies, 2009).

How to assess?

Due to its complexity and the individual needs of the child, children and young people's pain requires a multidimensional assessment – behaviour, physiological indicators and cognitive appraisal – which can be carried out in a number of ways. The key to assessment is to obtain a clear history regarding the infant, child's, young person's and family's experience of pain. It must be remembered that for some families this may be the first time they have seen their child in pain and will be uncertain of what to do or how to react. Therefore it is essential that a tactful and sensitive approach to care is taken using family centred care where roles and involvement are discussed and negotiated.

Family centred care: parents want and need to care for their child when they are in pain; they know their child best and are the experts on their child. It is essential that healthcare practitioners work with parents as their knowledge of their child is invaluable, especially if their child is preverbal, has a cognitive impairment or experiences chronic pain which underlies an episode of acute pain (RCN, 2009b; Carter, 2002; Simons *et al.*, 2001). Whilst nurses have judged parents to be involved in the process, parents have stated the opposite is true. They feel excluded, frustrated at not being involved and undervalued as a resource (Simons *et al.*, 2001). The parents must be involved as they can be active participants in the initial and ongoing assessment of their child's pain. The nurse is ideally located to support the family in learning about how to assess and manage their child's pain especially as the tools are easy to understand and use.

Pain history: the first step to gaining insight into the infant, child or young person's pain is to obtain a pain history. This should be done when the child is pain free or as comfortable as possible. The pain history provides insight into previous and present pain experiences, words used and coping strategies. A framework such as that formulated by Hester and Barcus is useful in providing a framework for assessment as it is child focused and provides both a child oriented and adult version of the same questions (see Table 7-8).

Behavioural assessment: this focuses on observing the behaviour of the infant, child or young person who is in pain. The nurse should observe any behaviours which are unusual or not part of the patient's repertoire when pain free. Such behaviours include: crying, screaming, shouting, pulling knees up to the chest, hitting out, refusing to accept comfort, rigid body/limbs, withdrawn and unusually quiet.

Physiological indicators: the vital signs taken by the nurse will indicate if the patient is stressed. The nurse should observe for sweating or clamminess of the child. Common signs of being in pain include **tachycardia**, **tachypnoea**, raised blood pressure, **pallor**. However, after a prolonged period of time these indicators may return to within normal parameters as the autonomic nervous system will act to stabilise the physiological status of the child.

Cognitive appraisal: this is a subjective assessment by the child who is able to communicate the intensity, location and degree of pain they are experiencing as well as the emotional 'hurt'. It is also an objective assessment for the nurse who is able to measure to some degree the intensity of the pain experience thus gaining clear insight into the infant/child/young person's perspective. Self-report is thought to be the gold standard for these reasons. However, if the child is preverbal or has cognitive impairment then an observer-rated tool may need to be used in order to assess the pain experience (RCN, 2009a).

Pain Assessment Tools

A number of validated pain assessment tools (PATs) are available to ensure assessment can be carried out in a child-centred manner. PATs are available for different groups of children and include (Davies, 2009; RCN, 2009b):

- Neonates and infants – CRIES (Krechel and Bildner, 1995) and NIPS.
- Non-verbal, cognitively impaired and anxious children – FLACC scale (Merkel *et al.*, 1997).
- Children over the age of four years – faces scales.
- Older children – visual analogue scales.
- Body outlines can help establish the location of the child's pain.
- Behavioural observational scales are the main method of assessment used in infants and children under three years. They can also be used in children who are cognitively impaired.

CRIES

This is an observer-related tool which assesses crying, requirements for oxygen, increase in vital signs, expression and sleeplessness. A score is provided for each parameter (see Figure 7-3).

Wong Baker Scale (1988)

This is an easily used and understood tool for children aged three years and upwards. The scale requires children to point to a face which feels like they do rather than requiring an understanding of numbers (see Figure 7-4).

DATE/TIME						
Crying – Characteristic cry of pain is high pitched. 0 – No cry or cry that is not high-pitched 1 – Cry high pitched but baby is easily consolable 2 – Cry high pitched but baby is inconsolable						
Requires O_2 for SaO_2 < 95% – Babies experiencing pain manifest decreased oxygenation. Consider other causes of hypoxemia, e.g., oversedation, atelectasis, pneumothorax 0 – No oxygen required 1 – < 30% oxygen required 2 – > 30% oxygen required						
Increased vital signs (BP* and HR*) – Take BP last as this may awaken child making other assessments difficult 0 – Both HR and BP unchanged or less than baseline 1 – HR or BP increased but increase in < 20% of baseline 2 – HR or BP is increased > 20% over baseline.						
Expression – The facial expression most often associated with pain is a grimace. A grimace may be characterised by brow lowering, eyes squeezed shut, deepening naso-labial furrow, or open tips and mouth. 0 – No grimace present 1 – Grimace alone is present 2 – Grimace and non-cry vocalisation grunt is present						
Sleepless – Scored based upon the infant's state during the hour preceding this recorded score. 0 – Child has been continuously asleep 1 – Child has awakened at frequent intervals 2 – Child has been awake constantly						
TOTAL SCORE						

Figure 7-3 CRIES Pain Assessment Tool.
Source: National Institutes of Health.

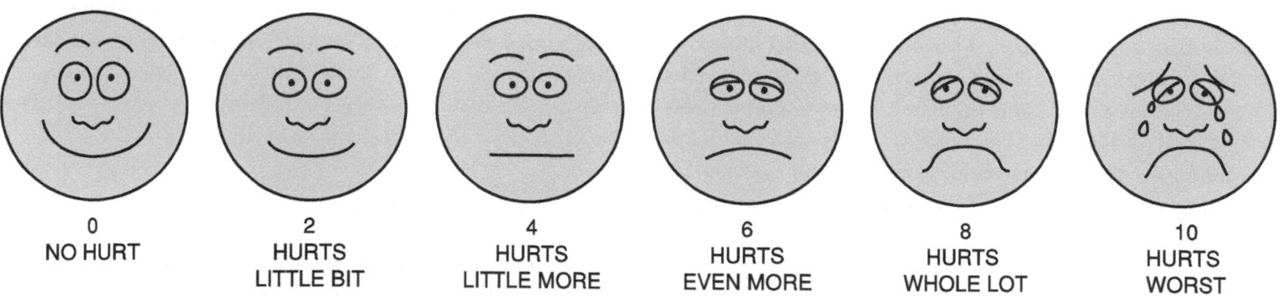

Figure 7-4 Wong-Baker FACES Pain Rating Scale
Source: from Hockenberry, M.J., Wilson, D.: *Wong's essentials of pediatric nursing*, ed. 8, St.Louis, 2009, Mosby. Used with permission. Copyright Mosby.

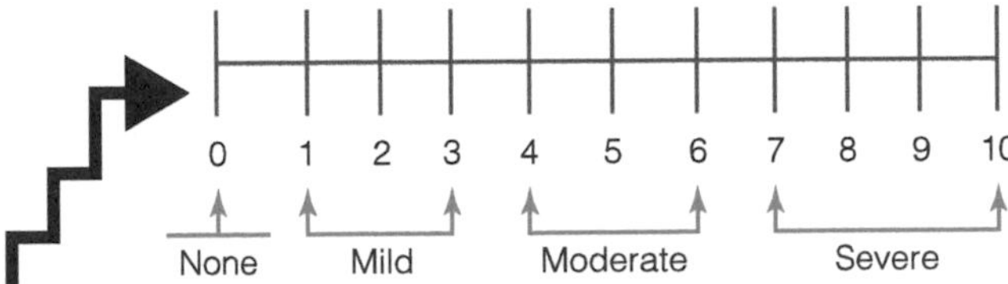

Figure 7-5 Numerical Pain Rating Scale.
Source: National Institutes of Health.

Numeric scales

These can be used with older children (9+ years) who have some understanding of numbers (see Figure 7-5).

A wealth of tools exists which are easily available for the practitioner to access both for the child who is able to communicate and for children with cognitive impairment (RCN, 2009b).

Management of Pain

Effective pain management begins with a belief that the infant/child/young person is in pain. Such a belief confirms to the child and family that their experience is valued and the care will be delivered empathetically. Also, both the nurse's personal practice and ward culture should be committed to providing effective, efficient evidence-based care in a timely manner; managing children's pain is a priority (Twycross, 2007, 2008).

Non-Pharmacological Method

Infants/children/young people are able to cope with quite significant levels of pain by using specific coping strategies. Practitioners need to have a knowledge of these so that coping can be facilitated whilst medication is organised or is being reassessed. Also, the patient could be taught to use these methods to enable coping until they are able to seek help (Kankkunen *et al.*, 2003).

PRACTICE GUIDELINES

Coping Strategies

Cognitive

- Distraction: singing, playing, games
- Relaxation: singing, daydreaming
- Guided imagery
- Positive self-talk: self-praise for coping
- Thought stopping: 'pain go'; 'pain stop'

Behavioural

- Hiding away: physical or psychological withdrawal, e.g. 'hiding' under bedclothes; daydreaming
- Fighting it: crying; shouting; pulling away
- Making it good: rocking; rubbing; patting; moving around.

Source: Kankkunen *et al.* (2003); Polkki *et al.* (2002); Woodgate and Kristjanson (1995).

The cognitive strategies distract the child's thought processes away from the pain acting as a psychological 'gate' which prevents the interpretation of pain impulses to be fully appreciated at the cortical level of the brain. Behavioural strategies act in such a way as to block the impulses reaching the brain and being interpreted and appreciated fully as pain.

Pharmacological Methods

This will centre on the assessment and prescription of medication to alleviate pain. Analgesia will be prescribed and must be administered according to the prescription and local drug administration policies used in conjunction with the NMC (2008) code of conduct. Analgesia will be given according to the severity of pain experienced by the child and reassessed to ascertain how well the pain has responded to the medication. The analgesic pain ladder provides guidance on the most appropriate analgesia to be given which is dependent on the child/young person's report of their pain (see Figure 7-6).

Thus once pain has been assessed, pain relieving interventions can be planned. For example, non-pharmacological strategies could be used whilst the analgesia is prepared and then administered. The next step is essential; the nurse must return to the patient and reassess their pain levels in order to assess the effectiveness of the analgesia. Without this process of assessment and reassessment the pain management will be flawed (see Figure 7-7).

In summary, pain assessment should be part of the care routine and integral part of the care which is delivered to the child and family. The PAT must be explained and used by all the family as they can be involved in the management of their child's pain so that effective management can be implemented to ensure the infant/child/young person is as comfortable as possible.

MENTAL HEALTH ISSUES IN CHILDREN AND YOUNG PEOPLE

It is widely recognised that good mental health is vital as it underpins the quality of children and young people's lives whose early childhood life experiences may influence the quality of their mental health. The ability to lead a positive, fulfilling

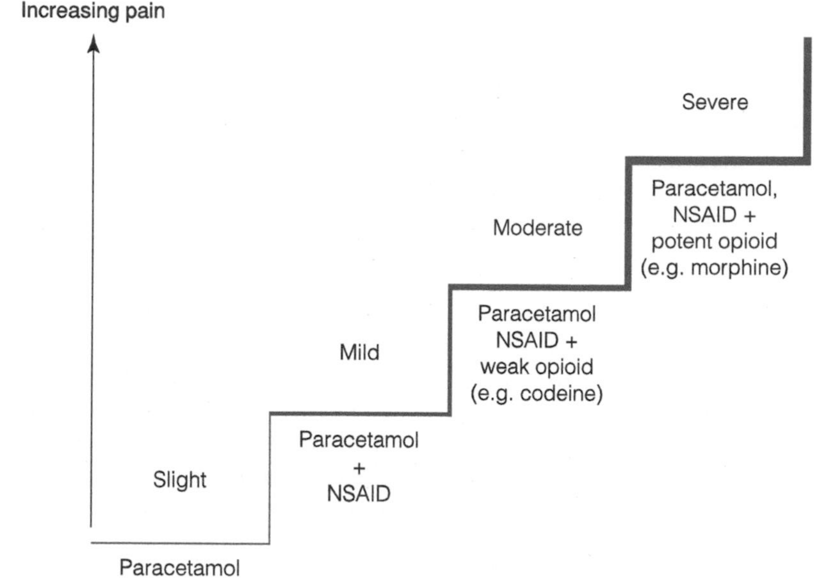

Figure 7-6 Analgesic Pain Ladder.
Source: http://www.gosh.nhs.uk/clinical_information/clinical_guidelines/cmg-guideline-00005

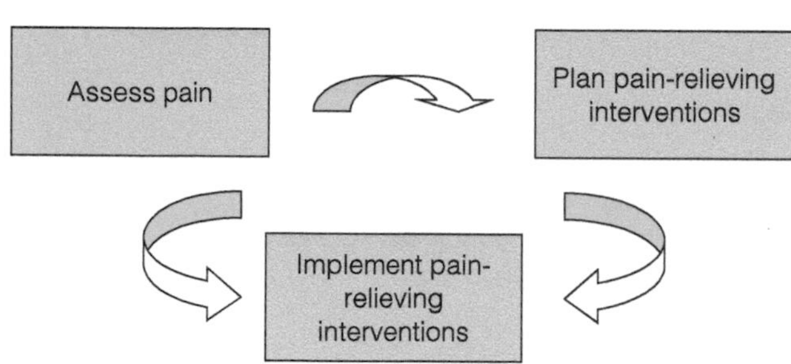

Figure 7-7 The pain management cycle.
Source: Alison Twycross, 2011.

life, cope with frustration, disappointment and stressful life events is laid down in those early family and social experiences of childhood where a functional family, support, confidantes and help should be available to enable the child to develop the skills to cope and be resilient when faced with adversity. Should this not occur, then the risks of developing a mental health problem increase leading to a lack of mature coping skills, low self-esteem, poor body image, social isolation and exclusion and dysfunctional relationships. Thus positive mental health and well-being are fundamental to the broader health and well-being of the child/young person (DH, 2009; DSCF/DH, 2008, 2009; DSCF, 2010; Parry-Langdon, 2008).

It has been recognised that the incidence of mental health problems amongst young people, especially those who are looked after, is rising. The prevalent problems appear to be emotional and behavioural disorders with those who experience a serious or chronic illness being significantly more at risk, especially boys (Immelt, 2006; Parry-Langdon, 2008; Bone and Knight, 2009; DSCF/DH, 2009). The most recent survey of children and young people's mental health found that 1.1 million children and young people less than 18 years of age had a diagnosable mental health disorder which required help from specialist services, of these 45,000 young people had a severe mental health problem (DCSF/DH, 2009; Green *et al.*, 2005) and 40% of those with a mental health problem were not receiving any specialist help. Recent reports suggest that one in five young people suffer with clinical depression. Despite public health initiatives to address self-harm and suicide amongst young people the incidence remains alarmingly high (WHO, 2005; Green *et al.*, 2005).

No one factor can be isolated which would explain such an increase yet it could be suggested that children and young people live in a complex society which they often struggle to understand and be part of (DSCF/DH, 2009; Parry-Langdon, 2008). The personal and social costs are high as disorders of childhood and adolescence can persist into the adult years leading to a person whose ability to function socially on all levels is impaired. Thus children and young people need support to deal with such complexities, be it within their families or by seeking external support through health and social care settings (Terry and Davies, 2011).

Mental health is not just a concern of specialists working within that field but is now recognised as being an issue for all health professionals who come into contact with children and young people. Those with mental health problems/issues may be encountered in a variety of healthcare settings as the child/young person seeks help for a specific mental health issue or comes into contact with healthcare professionals via other routes, e.g. GP, school nurse, A&E, admission to a general ward for a physical health problem which overlies the mental health issues, e.g. chronic illness (DCSF/DH, 2009; DCSF/DH, 2008; RCN, 2004) (see Table 7-9). This may be the first time the mental issue is addressed. Thus children and young people are

Table 7-9 Mental Health Problems in Children and Young People

Emotional disorders	Conduct disorders	Complex mental health problem
Separation anxiety	Conduct disorder	Depression
Phobic anxiety	Unsocialised conduct disorder	Self-harm
Social anxiety	Socialised conduct disorder	Eating disorders
Sibling rivalry	Oppositional defiant disorder	Suicide
Other emotional disorders		Neurodevelopmental disorders - autism, ADHD
Social functioning		

Source: based on WHO (2007).

vulnerable and require help and support in dealing with these issues. The care must be delivered sensitively as mental health problems carry a stigma which can isolate the child/young person leading to exclusion from their peers, community and families.

Early diagnosis and intervention has been found to have a positive effect, more severe problems in later life are prevented from developing, and youth offending is reduced as is self-harming behaviour. Also, the risk to the young person of becoming socially excluded or isolated is reduced, thus enabling them to achieve their potential (Dogra *et al.*, 2002; Dogra and Leighton, 2009).

ACTIVITY 7-4

Liam is 14 years old. He lives with his mother who is a single parent and unemployed, and his five siblings. His mother suffers with depression and Liam takes care of his siblings periodically when she cannot cope. The family live in social housing, a flat, in a deprived area of the town. Liam attends school and wants to do well but he is being bullied and is beginning to play truant to avoid the bullies. He has been in trouble with the police. He has begun to feel isolated and alone as he feels he has no one to talk to.

Identify the risk factors for Liam developing a mental health problem. What can be done to support Liam?

Who is At Risk?

It has been found that those who are at risk have a number of factors to be considered. Again no one factor is responsible for the development of mental health problems; they are caused by a combination of life events, background and personal characteristics which can precipitate the development of a problem (Green *et al.*, 2005; Parry-Langdon, 2008).

Boys: are more vulnerable than girls and twice as likely to have a conduct disorder. Also, the suicide rate is five times that of girls.

Social class: nearly three times as many children in lower socioeconomic groups had a mental health (MH) problem compared with children in higher groups. This is possibly due to a poorer environment materially/educationally/socially, and high stress levels due to lack of resources.

Substance misuse, smoking and alcohol use/misuse: there is a strong link between these behaviours and the development of mental health problems. This could be due to the actions of the substances themselves on the developing brain but also they add to the dysfunctional nature of lives which may already be chaotic and difficult to cope with (Ilomaki *et al.*, 2007). Substance misuse may also be a means to palliate the psychological distress being experienced by the child/young person.

Co-morbidity: the risk increases of a mental health problem occurring where there is a physical problem or ongoing mental health problem. Those who misused substances were found to have mental health problems (more than 40%) (Green *et al.*, 2005). Conduct disorders and emotional disorders were also found to be associated with substance misuse.

Physical ill health or problem: for example, speech and language problems, emotional problems.

Not all children and young people who live in these circumstances will develop a mental health problem. It is a combination of issues and events which heightens the risk significantly. Many children and young people cope with difficult circumstances and lives, yet it is the access to support, the emotional climate within the family and their ability to cope that is important in determining their vulnerability.

Factors to Consider

There are other factors which are more difficult to measure but need to be considered as precipitators for developing a mental health problem (see Table 7-10). The additional burden of these issues drains the child/young person's ability to cope and seek help. Thus they can become depressed and oppressed by the challenges of living in this situation but they do not seek help because they are afraid and isolated, believing they are alone and the only person going through this situation, they lack access to help or lack the physical resource needed to seek support. The factors affecting a child's mental health are shown in Figure 7-8.

Child

These are genetic influences and temperament.

Table 7-10 Factors Affecting a Child's Mental Health

Child risk factors	Family risk factors
Poverty	Learning disability
Family breakdown	Abuse
Single parent family	Domestic violence
Parent mental ill health	Prematurity or low birth weight
Parent criminality, alcoholism or substance misuse	Difficult temperament
Overt parental conflict	Physical illness
Lack of boundaries	Lack of boundaries
Frequent family moves/being homeless	Looked after children
Over-protection	Lack of attachment to carer
Failure to adapt to the child's developmental needs	Academic failure
Death and loss, including loss of friendships	Low self-esteem
Caring for a disabled parent	Shy, anxious or difficult temperament
	Young offenders
	Chronic illness

Source: RCN (2009a) and DH (2004).

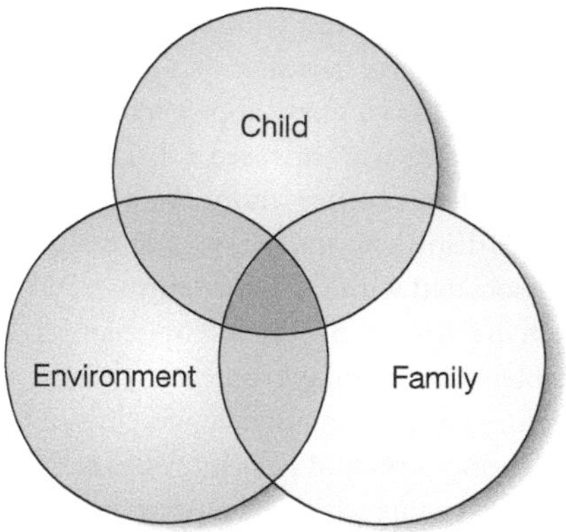

Child

Environment

Family

Figure 7-8 Factors affecting a child's mental health.

Family

Parental psychopathology: when the parents have MH problems they are no longer emotionally available to act as a confidante to their children. The emotional climate within the house also becomes heightened (Tulloch *et al.*, 1997; Evans *et al.*, 2005; Spender, 2007).

Parental education: where parents have no educational qualifications the incidence of mental health problems in children is four times higher than in households where the parents held a degree (Green *et al.*, 2005).

Harsh or inadequate parenting: parenting styles are important in developing warm, loving, trusting relationships with children. It is within the family that children learn social rules and norms, develop self-esteem and self-awareness. The best style is authoritative parenting which is warm and supportive but imposes boundaries appropriately. Authoritarian parenting is cold and harsh where discipline is imposed inappropriately. The child is made to feel they are a burden and lacks the warm environment to develop love, trust and confidants. *Laissez-faire* styles of parenting are characterised by a lack of disciplinary boundaries and the style can give rise to anxiety as the child wonders if they are cared for. The child becomes uncertain of what is appropriate. As a result it may be difficult to build self-esteem and a sense of self-efficacy without guidance and support.

Abuse/neglect: this is a significant risk factor as the child or young person feels trapped and oppressed by the behaviours and the emotional climate they are subjected to. Their self-esteem is eroded as is the sense of self-efficacy and coping. Depression occurs leading to an inability to seek help (Hawton, 2002; NICE, 2004; MHF, 2006).

Family discord: the emotional climate is important as it determines how psychologically safe the child/young person feels. In an environment where the family are functioning well the climate should be reassuring, mutually respectful and caring. This enables the child/young person to seek support and discuss issues with a confidante who is emotionally available. Where the family is dysfunctional and there is a lack of warmth, confidants and trust the child/young person can find themselves isolated, alone and oppressed by issues for which they need help.

Family type: the research has shown that mental health problems tend to be higher in families that have experienced breakdowns. As families change and reconstitute themselves so there is a loss of roles, confidants, support networks and friends (Ayyash-Abdo, 2002). Children and young people from non-intact families reported lower levels of self-esteem, increased anxiety, depression, suicidal ideation and attempts (Garnefski and Diekstra, 1997; Tulloch *et al.*, 1997). Boys tend to be more vulnerable to these changes as they lose roles they may have previously enjoyed. Girls fare better in step-parent families where new confidants can be found.

Environment

Income: the highest incidence of mental health problems occurs in households where the income is less than £100 per week.

Stressful life events: it was found that where children and young people had experienced a number of significant life events (e.g. bereavement, parents in jail, arrested by police, bullying, school refusal) their risk and incidence of mental health problems rose significantly.

Early separations from parents: lead to separation anxiety and loss of the primary attachment figure.

Adverse peer group influences: include substance misuse, vandalism and risk-taking behaviour.

Long-Term Outcomes

Early intervention and support is essential in order to prevent deteriorating mental health and provide the child/young person with access to helping services. If no help is provided the child/

young person's sense of hopelessness and helplessness increases leading to depression. This in turn erodes their coping skills and isolates them at a time when they need a confidant and support. If left unsupported the risk of poor long-term outcomes rises significantly as does the risk of self-harm and suicide.

These can include:

- Conduct and hyperkinetic disorders persist – 70%
- Antisocial behaviour
- Substance misuse
- Suicide
- Adult psychiatric disorders
- Depressive disorders
- Poor educational attainment
- Poor work histories
- Pregnancy or father children earlier
- Poor general health in early adult lives (ONS, 2005)

Protective Factors

There are a number of factors which would appear to provide psychological protection to the child/young person (RNC, 2009a):

- intelligence;
- living in a stable home environment;
- parental employment;
- good parenting;
- good parental mental health;
- activities and interests;
- positive peer relationships;
- emotional resilience and positive thinking;
- sense of humour.

They provide the warm, nurturing, positive atmosphere required in order to cope with the distress being experienced and give the child/young person a confidant who is easily accessed and who can provide access to help.

The mental health of the child/young person can be promoted by a number of approaches. Good strong family relationships, especially with the mother, who is still seen as the main confidant within the family, are vitally important. These nurture the individual emotionally and provide the arena in which to build confidence, social competence and self-esteem.

Schools are now involved in a broader educational role fostering healthy social and emotional development through circle time and development of emotional literacy. Child-friendly schools provide a good psychosocial environment which recognises the psychological needs of the child/young person. Schools are now providing access to counsellors, life skills teaching and community involvement (DH, 2004; WAG, 2001).

What To Do and Where To Go

A number of resources and helping services exist for CYP with mental health problems:

- primary care settings – GP, school nurse;
- voluntary sector – drop-in centres, support services targeted at young people;
- the Child and Adolescent Mental Health Services (CAMHS) team.

The practitioner must have a working knowledge of the help available to CYP whom they may encounter in the course of their work. The mental health issue may not be the presenting health problem but may be discovered during the healthcare encounter. Support can then be put in place and appropriate advice given to enable the young person to access help. This must be done by a practitioner who has knowledge, education and a focus for this area of CYP nursing.

ACTIVITY 7-5

Niamh is 15 years old and lives with her parents in a comfortable home in a good part of the town. The family is busy as both parents work long hours and when not in work spend time socialising with friends. Niamh attends the local school where she is achieving high grades. Her parents expect her to do well and go onto university. Niamh has little spare time as she studies and has several demanding hobbies. Her parents believe it is best she is kept busy to 'avoid hanging around street corners'. Niamh feels overwhelmed by her life and needs to confide in someone as she feels very tired and very down. She is unsure where to go or who to speak to.

Identify the risk factors for Niamh developing a mental health problem. What can be done to support Niamh?

CHILDREN'S RIGHTS IN HEALTHCARE

The ratification by the UK in December 1991 of the United Nations Convention on the Rights of the Child (UNCRC) (UN, 1989) has provided a framework that is widely respected for the development of national policies and laws to protect the rights of children throughout the world. It took decades of tireless work from non-government organisations (NGOs) such as Save the Children and UNICEF with all but two countries eventually ratifying the treaty. One of the main problems today is the lack of knowledge about the UNCRC amongst children and young people, and often professionals and others delivering services to them.

What is the UNCRC?

All 54 articles of the treaty apply to children and young people below the age of 18 and recognises not only their need for protection but acknowledge their rights regardless of race, gender, ethnic origin, religion, disability and age. However, one of the obligations of every country that ratifies the Convention is their requirement to indicate their progress made every five years (after the initial first two years) in implementing the Charter. The UN Committee will then respond to this after also comparing the report with those made by relevant organisations, voluntary and otherwise, such as NGOs. On receipt of the UN Committee's findings individual countries have to implement a plan to address any criticisms/observations within the following five years. This seems ironic considering the hazardous journey that some children still have towards adulthood including many atrocities that befall children and young people in both developing countries, countries at war and in many developed western countries. Below we discuss the necessity to apply a more rights-based approach to children and young people within healthcare, including examples of current good practice.

The ratification of the UNCRC has led to improved legislation and national policies in the UK with a rights-based agenda and approach, but it is important that these are implemented in all aspects of children's lives including socially, educationally and within their healthcare. Broadly speaking the Convention can be divided into three main parts – provision, protection and participation and these will be discussed briefly in relation to the delivery of healthcare to children and young people in the UK.

Provision of Healthcare

The provision of healthcare in the UK to children and young people has had a colourful history and only from the mid-20th century onwards has it been the 'norm' for children not only to survive but to also experience predominantly healthy lives. Hygiene, public health and the development of schooling has been a defining feature of 'modern childhood'. The impressive improvements in the UK and other developed countries in the areas of health and physical development of children are of course partly due to higher standards of living and advances in sanitation and nutrition.

Children's right to good healthcare is enshrined in various publications and policy documents including the UNCRC and the 1989 Children Act. In particular they are clearly indicated in Article 24 of the UNCRC which clearly states that they have:

> *the right to the highest attainable standard of health and health facilities of every type of healthcare that is available to them within their own culture/country.*

It is important to note that this clearly does not mean that children have the 'right to be healthy' but rather that they should have equal access to all health facilities available to children and young people in their own country. Equity was one of the founding principles of the NHS in 1946 and childhood poverty was going to be thing of the past. However it is well documented that inequalities in health provision still exist in the UK. The years following this new, free, health system did of course see a vast improvement of children's health although the topic was not given serious attention or adequately resourced as it was not very high on the political agenda at that time.

Health inequalities are linked to social inequalities and social exclusion with evidence indicating that poverty, homelessness, unemployment and various social breakdowns are significant factors to poor health and premature death (NAW, 2000a).

Health in childhood we now know is an important predictor for health in later life, and children who suffer the above mentioned are more likely to suffer ill health, behavioural disorders and under-achievement in school. Intergenerational cycles of health inequalities have persisted, with babies born to poorer families more likely to be born prematurely, being at greater risk of infant mortality and impaired development, having a greater likelihood of living in poverty themselves and developing chronic disease later in life (Hart, 1971; Acheson, 1998). Children's health and well-being are measured mainly in the form of children's ill health (morbidity) and the death rate (mortality).

Infant mortality figures, which are an acknowledged robust indicator of public health, are in most parts of Britain still falling steadily and are roughly half of what they were in the 1950s. The infant mortality rate below the age of one year and again below the age of five has been the major statistic for comparing 'child health' from one country to another and therefore measuring a country's progress. However, despite this, in 2009 at 4.8 per thousand live births (the lowest to date) infant mortality in the UK fell well behind the then 15 members of the European Union with Finland at 3.6 and Sweden at 3.2.

With a free at the point of delivery National Health Service and the monitoring and screening of pregnant mothers and young children this statistic is hard to explain but recent research by Mitchell *et al.* (2000) found that 1,400 lives could be saved a year if poverty were to be eradicated, taking into account some of the factors mentioned above. Measures of emotional health are sparce although there has been an increase in data collecting relating to children and young people's mental illnesses and behavioural problems in more recent years.

New Labour: The Changes that Affected Children and Young People

The new Labour government of 1993 came into power after 17 years of a Conservative government. It pledged to eliminate both poverty and social exclusion and did do more in this area than any preceding governments in recent political history. During their 13 years their National Childcare Strategy increased the workforce of childcare systems, after school activities were further extended, pre-school initiatives including breakfast clubs started as well as the Healthy Schools Initiative. At long last the availability of affordable childcare allowed many young mothers to get back to employment.

With regard to health Derrick Wanless was commissioned by the government (prior to the NHS spending review) to examine the potential future health trends and identify the factors determining the long-term finance and resource needs for the NHS. The findings indicated that the delivery of health services should not be postcode dependent and the principles of equity and evidence driven policy should continue to underpin the development of Child Health Programmes with the involvement of children and young people at all levels (Wanless, 2003).

BOX 7-1 Practice Example of Improving Health Provision - Sure Start

One of the most significant initiatives of recent years to address the inequalities in health has been a National Programme called Sure Start which started in England and Wales in 1999. Aimed at early intervention in families with pre-school children from predominantly disadvantaged areas the schemes have varied considerably from one locality to another. In some areas it is based on postcode lottery allocation, for example, improving community facilities/ support for mothers and young children or following an individual family's assessment of need, the subsequent support which may be in the form of one-to-one education/ provision.

The need to ensure children's survival has until recent years focused more on their physical health than their emotional or social well-being. The health and welfare services over time have reflected this by the development of comprehensive immunisation programmes, welfare foods and child health clinics. The move towards considering health rather than just sickness and disease means that we are now examining further ways of preventing ill health and promoting health rather than relying on a curative model (Underdown, 2007). The UN Convention states that all countries should assist one another in promoting children's health and well-being which means that children worldwide can benefit from healthcare knowledge and development, although the resourcing of this for developing countries is often not only difficult but at times impossible.

Protection

How have we addressed children's right to protection since ratifying the UNCRC? Article 19 of the UNCRC (UN, 1989) states that:

> *State parties shall take at all times the appropriate legislative, administrative, social and educational actions to protect children from all types of physical or mental violence, injury or abuse, neglect or neglective treatment, maltreatment or exploitation, including sexual abuse, which in the care of parents(s), legal guardians or any other person who has care of the child.*

Although ratified by the UK in 1991 international charters such as these are not enforceable by law. However, the Children Act 1989 had already taken into account the UNCRC charters after considerable debate, activity and discussions with various groups, although not children. The Convention put forward a new image of children; rather than just being objects of protection they are subjects of special rights and need to have a voice in everything that concerns them. Therefore developing and changing child protection systems over the years has been in relation to our views of children, child care and the abuse of children balanced against the parents/carers right to 'family life'. It has been a long and difficult journey and professionals working with children and their families have always had a difficult role in weighing up when to intervene in family life. The Children Act 1989 was therefore very welcomed to help provide everyone with a more structured approach by defining certain concepts in relation to family life.

The Children Act 1989 was not the first legislation in relation to the safeguarding of children and young people but it was the first to bring **public** and **private law** together and sought to establish a new basis for intervention in family life in cases of child abuse. This was done by placing the courts at the centre of the process. The Act opens with the 'welfare checklist' and continues by placing emphasis on to the 'ascertainable wishes and feelings of the child concerned'. Some very important concepts were also defined and identified:

- The 'welfare of the child' is of paramount importance in all decisions made.
- Wherever possible children should remain with their families.
- Children should be safe and protected by effective intervention if they are in danger.
- Children should always be kept informed and participate when decisions are made about them.
- Parents have responsibilities rather than rights and they only lose them when the child is adopted.
- Parents of children with special needs should be fully supported to bring the children up within the family.
- 'Significant harm' is defined.
- Children in 'need' are identified.

Child protection is a term that was used from 1989 by all agencies in the UK when there was a suspicion that a child (or children) was at risk of suffering from significant harm as defined within section 319 of the Children Act:

> *an effect on the physical, intellectual, emotional, social or behavioural development of the child and/or ill treatment which encompasses sexual abuse and other ill treatment, which are not physical.*

However, criticisms of this definition is that it is not detailed enough and making decisions about what is 'significant harm' are complex. They should be informed by a careful assessment of the child's circumstances plus discussion between the statutory agencies involved as well as the child and family. However, this definition did make social workers' and health professionals' jobs easier in that 'significant harm' has been the threshold that justifies intervention in family life in the best interest of the child/ren concerned and does therefore override the family's right to 'private life'.

Since the 1989 Children Act the emphasis has been to support and safeguard children within their own families. It importantly defined 'children in need' (in section 17) as those who require extra support and services to reach or maintain a satisfactory level of health and development. This includes children with physical disabilities and learning difficulties as well as chronically ill children and those living in poor socioeconomic circumstances. In recent times there has been greater investment in the provision of services for children in need including early years education and Sure Start programmes, as identified earlier.

It is important to include the definitions of child maltreatment in this chapter (see *Box 7-2*).

BOX 7-2 Definitions of Child Maltreatment

Physical abuse

This may involve hitting, shaking, throwing, poisoning, burning or scalding, and drowning, suffocating, or otherwise causing injury to a child which includes fabricating symptoms of or deliberately causing ill health to a child.

Emotional abuse

Is the persistent emotional ill-treatment of a child as to cause severe and persistent adverse effect on the child's emotional development? It may involve conveying to the child that they are worthless or unloved, inadequate, or valued only insofar as they meet the needs of another person, age or developmentally inappropriate expectations being imposed on children, causing children frequently to feel frightened, or the exploitation or corruption of children.

Sexual abuse

This involves the forcing or enticing a child or young person to take part in sexual activities, whether or not the child is aware of what is happening. The activities may include physical contact including penetration or non-penetrative acts. They may include involving children in looking at, or in the production of pornographic material, or encouraging children to behave in sexually inappropriate ways.

Neglect

Is the persistent failure to meet a child's basic physical and/or psychological needs, likely to result in the serious impairment of the child's health or development, such as failing to provide adequate food, shelter and clothing or neglect of or unresponsiveness to a child's basic needs emotional needs?

Source: 'What to do if you are worried a child is being abused', DH (2003: 3-4).

Unfortunately we know that many children suffer more than one type of abuse as listed above and these categories are how children are listed on the child protection register but only after there have been concerns raised and investigated (a section 47 inquiry) and the child/ren have been categorised as being 'at risk' of or suffering 'significant harm'.

Identification of child abuse is sometimes very difficult even for experienced practitioners but especially for nurses working in acute areas such as accident and emergency departments and children's wards, but there is more help and support available from specialist staff including liaison health visitors and named specialist nurses for safeguarding children.

The Evidence-Based Approach

Corby (2000) believes that the only safe definition is that of a judgement reached by a group of professionals involved on the examination of the circumstances of the child, normally at a child protection conference.

Child Protection Case Conference

The child protection case conference should be held within 15 working days of the initial strategy/discussion meeting when the Section 47 Inquiry was initiated. It brings together family members, the child where appropriate and those professionals most involved with them. As this is a legal process the family's solicitor is also present.

The appropriate social services manager and case worker will decide who to invite but a minimum of three agencies need to be present before the case conference can proceed and the child's voice should always be heard.

The purpose of the child protection conference is to share information, and detailed background reports and initial assessment about the child and their family are given. Multidisciplinary discussion follows about whether the child has been abused and whether the child or their siblings are at risk of future harm.

Members of the conference then decide if the child and their siblings are to be put on the child protection register and under which category. They then draw up an outline of the child protection plan and establish membership of the core group.

Child Protection Register

The child protection register is kept by local social services departments. This is a confidential list of children in that local authority area who are believed to be at risk of significant harm and who are currently the subject of an inter-agency child protection plan.

The child or children's names will stay on the register until it is believed that that they are no longer at risk of harm. On average this is for 1–2 years but is reviewed every six months. If a child on the register moves out of a local authority area information will be passed on to the new local authority.

All professionals working with children have access to the information in the database, on a need-to-know basis. The register contains details of the child's legal name, the name he/she is known by, date of birth, address, brothers and sisters and the category of abuse.

Safeguarding

This term is more increasingly used in relation to the protection of children and young people and it is a wider term than child protection. It importantly refers not only to minimising the danger of children's potential abuse but also promotes their health and welfare.

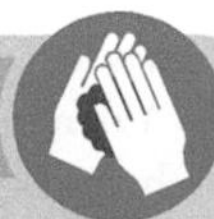

CLINICAL ALERT

Physical Abuse

Whereas physical abuse against children by their parents/carers has been outlawed by most of the EU countries, currently within the UK 'reasonable chastisement' remains legally acceptable despite professionals' and others' opinion. However, legislation has changed in relation to restricting other people such as teachers, nursery nurses and others working with children from meting out physical punishment.

Participation

Children and young people have been repeatedly overlooked in healthcare provision and services have been fragmented from one area to the next. However, in recent years there has been a growing acceptance that children and young people everywhere should participate more in making decisions about any issues that affect them including their healthcare. This has come from three main areas:

- the new sociology of childhood,
- the growing influence of the consumer,
- the children's rights agenda.

The UNCRC has undoubtedly had a large part to play in pushing the children's rights agenda to the forefront. The principle of children's right to participate in decision making is clearly indicated in Article 12.1 of the Convention and has been identified as a central underlying principle for children and young people in respect of all other rights:

> *States parties shall assure to the child who is capable of forming his or her own views the right to express those views freely in all matters affecting the child, the views of the child being given due weight in accordance with the age and maturity of the child.*

The Convention clearly sets out three levels that respect all children with regard to participation rights:

1. The right to be informed
2. The right to express views
3. The right to influence a decision.

The fourth level goes beyond the UNCRC and includes the sharing of power and responsibility for decision making although research has indicated that most children and adults prefer to stop at stage 3 and to share the decision making with people close to them.

Children's Participatory Rights is About Taking Part Not Taking Charge

However, until recent years it has been difficult to balance the differences between historical held beliefs about children, including that they should be 'seen and not heard', that they are the 'property of their parents' and that they have nothing valuable to contribute to adult life, with findings from research that contradicts such assumptions. Unfortunately this has also been the case in their healthcare decisions with an identified need for adult guidance, the need to reduce attempts to reason with them and in particular listen to their views and take them into consideration. Children, in particular those who are disabled, are frequently treated as an object of 'concern' or 'care' rather than as a citizen with rights.

RESEARCH NOTE

Non-Participation in Healthcare

Noyes' (2000) study of 18 young ventilator-dependent people interviewed them as well as their parents with regard to their health, social care and education. The findings included:

- a breach of the UNCRC in that they were not informed of their rights;
- those who were non-verbal did not have access to adequate communication systems and if they did people often did not understand them so their ability to freely express their views was restricted;
- an overwhelming finding was that they wanted to be placed at the centre of decision making with regard to their own lives.

The Need for Autonomy

Autonomy is defined as:

> *The capacity to think, decide and act freely and independently.* (Gillon, 1986; cited in de Cruz, 2004)

It is important that children have autonomy if they are going to be allowed to participate in their own healthcare but this is frequently constrained by well-meaning health professionals who believe that they know best. Allowing children and young people autonomy to express their views, for example on their proposed treatments, might not be in line with what is judged to be in their 'best interests'. This is a morally and ethically complex concept and cannot be discussed without examining the legislation around consent which goes beyond the remit of this book. However, examples below indicate changes in practice in relation to allowing children to participate in their own healthcare.

Consent Legislation with Regard to Children and Young People

Under section 3(1) of the Children Act 1989 the following can consent to their child's healthcare:

- parents with parental responsibility;
- married parents and mothers automatically;
- unmarried fathers if they are named on the birth certificate, or by agreement with the mother or application under section 4 of the Children Act;
- adoptive parents;
- 'de facto' carers have all the rights, duties, powers, responsibilities and authority which by law a parent has and include foster parents, teachers, baby sitters and other relatives.

Young people aged 16 or 17 can consent under the Family Law Reform Act 1969:

- to any surgical, medical and dental treatment;
- this does not cover the right to organ donation and blood;
- additional consent from the parent is not required, although can be given;
- parents need to consent for children with learning disabilities;
- this does not include consenting to taking part in research (clinical or other) this is covered by common law under the Gillick principle.

Children under 16 have no right in law to consent. Their right derives from common law or case precedent. A case that set a precedent was *Gillick* v *West Norfolk and Wisbech AHA* (1985), and led to what is known as the Gillick competency, when a child has reached a sufficient age, understanding and intelligence to make up their own mind about specific circumstances.

When do Children have the Capacity to Consent?

If they have:

- sufficient understanding and intelligence to understand what is fully proposed, and be
- capable of making a reasonable assessment of the advantages and disadvantages of the proposed treatment, and have
- sufficient discretion to make a wise choice in their own interests.

What Else Should be Considered?

The health professional needs to take into account:

- the child's age and intelligence – do they have 'sufficient understanding'? – Piaget believes this is directly related to age;
- that age alone is not a reliable indication of cognitive ability (Alderson, 1990);
- chronically ill children with 'lived experience' of illness (Fielding and Duff, 1999);
- that competency is more than a skill, it is a way of relating, and can be understood more clearly when each child's inner qualities are seen within a network of relationships and cultural influences (Alderson, 2002).

However, as discussed earlier, all health professionals understand the importance of working towards child and family friendly services as part of the philosophy of 'family-centred care'. This phrase has become well known within the UK children's nursing practice where the needs of the child should be considered within the context of the family unit and effective care depends on negotiation and partnership. Although family centred care is a welcome and evolving concept it has been slow in fully involving the child or young person in decision making. It is often chronologically age-related despite the fact that research indicates that children as young as five with a chronic illness can understand and comply with their treatments and medication (Alderson, 2002).

CLINICAL ALERT

Consent Forms for Invasive Medical Treatments and Surgery in NHS Hospitals

In recent years these have been changed to include the signature of a Gillick competent child or young person which they can sign (as well as or instead of) indicating informed consent that they as well as their parents have been involved in the process.

ACTIVITY 7-6

Hannah is 14 years old and was admitted to accident and emergency from school after falling and breaking her leg whilst playing netball.

Think about how you can ensure that Hannah is allowed to participate in her own care following her admission?

Policy and Law Changes to Adopt a more Rights-Based Approach

Children Act 2004

Recent government developments in acknowledging awareness of the importance of both the physical and mental health of children and young people was indicated in 2003 in the draft policy paper 'Every Child Matters' which followed the publication of the Laming Report, an enquiry into the death of Victoria

Climbie at the hands of her paternal aunt and her boyfriend. Presented in Parliament as the Children's Bill, then translated into the Children's Act 2004, it identified five main outcomes:

- being healthy
- staying safe
- enjoying and achieving
- making a positive contribution
- economic well-being.

These targets are linked to targets and health indicators for children and young people in the UK which include:

- further reducing the infant mortality rate, which has come down from 5.2 to 4.8 between 2005 and 2009;
- reducing the number of teenage pregnancies by 50% (TPU, 2006);
- improvements in access to child and mental health services;
- reducing the number of obese children in the under 11 age group.

Children's Commissioners were appointed in the four UK countries to act as independent champions for children, particularly those suffering disadvantage. They are high-profile independent bodies who have been established to monitor, promote and safeguard children's rights in the UK. The first appointment was in Wales in 2001 and their establishment is a recognition that children's needs and rights were not being recognised up until that point.

The **National Service Framework (NSF)** of 2004 was a blueprint to set health and social care standards for children, young people and maternity services. It focuses on child-centred interventions and has a remit to tackle both health inequalities and promote the health of children from conception to adulthood. The development of these standards involved service users and practitioners from many areas, but the evaluations of the standards are in their infancy. We can only hope that, combined with the above, we are now more fully addressing the rights of children and young people with regard to their health and well-being.

CRITICAL REFLECTION

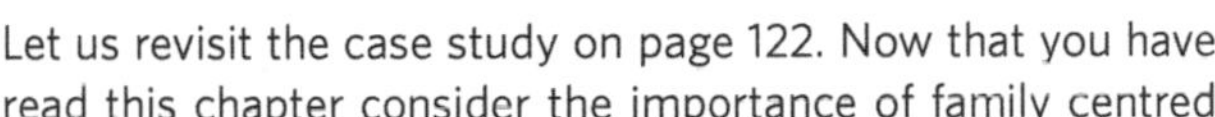

Let us revisit the case study on page 122. Now that you have read this chapter consider the importance of family centred care in Amy's case. Consider the importance of the use of play for children undergoing surgery.

CHAPTER HIGHLIGHTS

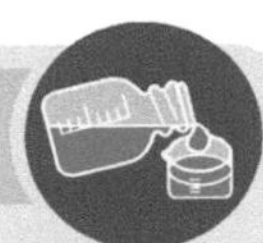

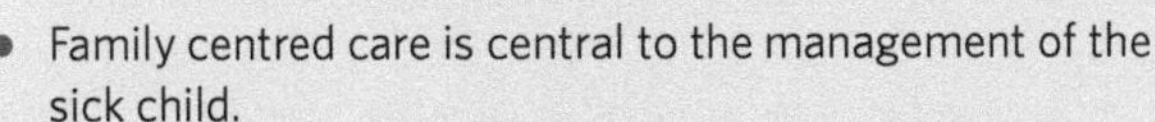

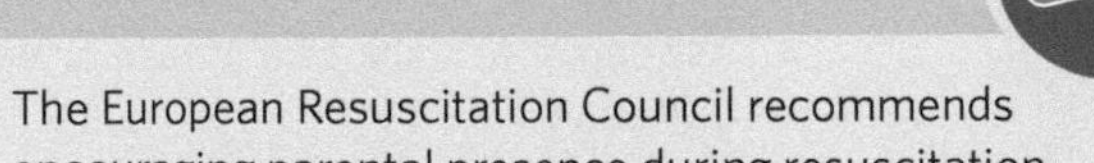

- Family centred care is central to the management of the sick child.
- Family centred care embraces the caring of a child or young person within the context of the family.
- Hutchfield (1999) stated that there are a number of key concepts of family centred care - negotiation, empowerment, changing roles, partnership, stress and participation.
- The nurses' role is to ensure that the child and family's routine is promoted within the constraints of the hospital environment.
- A child's separation from its mother can have a significant psychological and physical impact on the child.
- Assessment of the sick child will aid the practitioner in determining the care priorities.
- The assessment framework should provide information relating to the child's clinical and physical status, but also needs to consider social, psychological and emotional needs.
- Care delivery will usually be negotiated with the parents and roles should be discussed to identify what the parents will continue to provide for the child during hospitalisation and what the nurse's role will be.
- Paediatric basic life support is not a scaled-down version of that provided to adults. Specific techniques are required if optimum support is to be given.
- The European Resuscitation Council recommends encouraging parental presence during resuscitation.
- Physical development continues from birth to adulthood.
- The physical development of children cannot be viewed in isolation. It is important to consider the multifaceted nature of a child's development.
- Children and young people's psychological development is very different to that of adults: they view the world very differently resulting in a significantly altered perspective for many reasons.
- Play is a fundamental way in which children enjoy their childhood and is essential to their quality of life.
- Through play the child is able to act on the world around it, make sense of it and attempt to understand their place in society.
- Infants, children and young people can and do experience and perceive pain in a number of ways.
- Effective pain management is fundamentally linked to the effective assessment of pain.
- Children and young people face a range of mental health issues and problems.
- UNCRC recognises the child's need for protection regardless of race, gender, ethnic origin, religion, disability or age.

ACTIVITY ANSWERS

ACTIVITY 7-1

Some aspects you could have considered include:

- Recognise both Gemma's and her mother's knowledge and expertise in her condition.
- History of what happened leading up to the event including any recent illness, current medication, etc. Therefore exploring reasons why this may have happened.
- Assessment including vital signs and neurological observations if Gemma is not fully conscious, explaining to both why this is necessary.
- Discuss how Gemma's daily life activities are affected by her epilepsy.
- What support do they have? Consider and discuss if they need extra support (specialist nurse or other).

ACTIVITY 7-2

Some aspects you could have considered:

- Inform parents/carers of admission.
- Hourly vital signs including neurological observations and AVPU.
- History leading up to the event - if Aaron unable to remember then ask a friend who was with him.
- Reassurance and support.
- Care plan according to medical assessment and findings.
- Implement.
- Re-evaluate.

ACTIVITY 7-3

The nurse could:

- Use toys to 'play out' what is to happen to Jamie beforehand.
- Books and pictures to explain what will happen. Also story books can be read by you or parent/carer.
- Nursery rhymes: ask Jamie what his favourite rhyme is and ask him and his mum to sing it with you/or on their own during the blood test. You may set a number of times to sing it so that you could tell Jamie that it will all be over when you have sung it that number of times (show number on your fingers, e.g. three or four).
- Tell a story with Jamie as the hero because he is being brave.
- Ask parent/carer to tell Jamie's favourite story and ask Jamie to join in.
- Use toys to sing songs and tell stories. Hold them where Jamie is able to see and touch them.
- Finger puppets on your fingers to sing/tell stories, which will focus Jamie's attention.
- Bubbles: ask Jamie to count how many bubbles/watch the bubbles as you blow them.
- Ask Jamie to think of a phrase or words he can repeat whilst having his blood taken - this will act as a distracter.

ACTIVITY 7-4

The risk factors include:

- Parental mental health is poor so mother is not accessible as a confidante and support. Liam may in fact be providing support to his mother.
- Large family size means Liam takes on childcare activities and supports younger children physically and emotionally.
- Poor material environment - lack of opportunities.
- Lone parent family - stress is increased as the domestic burden falls on the lone parent and is disseminated to Liam.
- Unemployment, low income, poor social housing.
- Lack of opportunity to meet developmental needs and challenges.
- Lack of support or confidante outside family.
- Being bullied.
- Stigma of his background.
- Need to achieve is thwarted by bullying and truanting.
- Isolation and potential depression.
- Contact with police.
- Low parental expectation academically but high expectations domestically.

Support to include:

- Need for confidante and support.
- Relief of domestic load.
- Resolution of bullying following contact with school.

- School - contact with teachers to enable Liam to attend school regularly.
- Feeling he can be 'himself' and develop according to his needs.
- Help to improve levels of self-esteem and prevent worsening depression.
- Access to opportunities to develop (e.g. youth club).
- Services: school nurse, school counsellor, GP, HV (if visiting younger children the HV can act as a referral agent to other helping services), voluntary services, e.g. drop-in centres, Barnados (young carers schemes and other programmes), education welfare officer, youth offending team (if appropriate).

ACTIVITY 7-5 The risk factors include:

- High parental expectation.
- Apparent lack of parental interest - boundaries not clear.
- Lack of expressed affection and emotional nuturing.
- Lack of access to parents as confidants.
- Supportive environment is not apparent.
- Developmental needs not being met or allowed to develop due to very structured lifestyle.
- Life is very controlled and ordered leading to a lack of opportunity to develop a sense of autonomy and control.
- Beginning to feel out of control as others 'take over' and Niamh has to adapt to parents' expectations.
- Access to confidant.
- Early signs of depression.
- Loss of self-esteem.
- Isolation.

Support:

- Enabling Niamh to develop autonomy and control within her life.
- More opportunities to develop her choice of activities and structure her free time.
- Parenting style.
- Access to parents' time, attention, affection.
- Spending time together as a family.
- Decreasing isolation through family time and spending time with friends.
- Reducing parental expectation to realistic and supportive levels.
- Physical check up to ensure the tiredness is not due to a physiological problem.

Services:

- School nurse, school counsellor, teachers, GP, voluntary services (e.g. drop-in centres), primary mental health worker.

ACTIVITY 7-6 Give information pertinent to her age and understanding in a clear manner.

- If assessed as Gillick competent then verbal or written consent can be taken for treatment before her mother gets there, if it is necessary, but consent should always involve the child.
- Use a pain assessment tool that suits Hannah and she understands the process.
- Allow her choices of pain medication and how they are administered after explanation.

REFERENCES

Acheson, Sir D. (1998) *Inequalities in health: An independent inquiry*, London: The Stationery Office.

Alderson, P. (1990) *Choosing for children*, Oxford: Oxford University Press.

Alderson, P. (2002) 'Young children's healthcare rights and consent', in Franklin, B. (ed.) *The new handbook of children's rights*, London: Routledge.

Alsop-Shields, L. and Mohay, H. (2001) 'John Bowlby and James Robertson: Theorists, scientists and crusaders for improvement in the care of children in hospital', *Journal of Advanced Nursing*, 35(1): 50–58.

Audit Commission (1993) *Children first: A study of hospital services*, London: HMSO.

Ayyash-Abdo, H. (2002) 'Adolescent suicide: An ecological perspective', *Psychology in the Schools*, 39(4): 459–475.

Bee, H. (2006) *The developing child*, 11th edn, USA: Longman.

Bee, H. and Boyd, D.R. (2007) *The developing child* (12th edn), London: Pearson.

Bone, D. and Knight, D. (2009) 'The mental health of children and young people: The EMHA role', *Community Practitioner*, 82(1): 27–30.

Bowlby, J. and Robertson, J. (1952) 'A two-year-old goes to hospital' at: http://www.ncbi.nlm.nih.gov/pmc/articles/PMC1918555/pdf/procrsmed00418-0060.pdf

Bowlby, J. (1960) 'Separation anxiety', *International Journal of Psychoanalysis*, 41: 89–11.

British Dietetic Association (BDA) (2007) *Delivering nutritional care through food and beverage services: A toolkit for dieticians*, available at http://www.bda.uk.com

British Dietetic Association (2007) *Weaning infants onto solid foods*, Paediatric Group of the BDA. Available from http://www.child-nutrition.co.uk/weaning.pdf

Campbell, A. and Brown, S.T. (2008) 'The health teddy clinic: A innovative pediatric experience', *Teaching and Learning in Nursing*, 3: 72–75.

Carter, B., McArthur, E. and Cunliffe, M. (2002) 'Dealing with uncertainty: Parental assessment of pain in their children with profound special needs', *Journal of Advanced Nursing*, 38(5): 449–457.

Casey, A. (1988) 'A partnership model with child and family', *Senior Nurse*, 8(4): 8–9.

Children's Play Council. In *Play strategy for Harlow 2007–2012*, Harlow: Harlow Council www.harlow.gov.uk/pdf/1 (accessed 14 May 2010.)

Children's Play Council (2000) *Best play*, London: National Playing Fields Association.

Collier, J. (1997) 'Attitudes to children's pain: Exploding the pain myth', *Paediatric Nursing*, 9(10).

Corby, B. (2000) *Child abuse: Towards a knowledge base*, Buckingham: Open University.

Coyne, I. (2003) *A grounded theory of disrupted lives: Children, parents and nurses in the children's ward*, London: King's College University of London.

Davies, A. (2009) 'Pain assessment: Child', in Glasper, A., McEwing, G. and Richardson, J., *Foundation skills for caring*, London: Palgrave.

Dearmun, N. (1992) 'Perceptions of parental participation', *Paediatric Nursing*, 4(7): 6–9.

De Cruz, P. (2004) *Medical law*, London: Sweet and Maxwell.

Department for Children, Schools and Families (2010) *Keeping children and young people in mind – full government response to the CAMHS review*, London: DH.

Department for Children, Schools and Families/Department of Health (2008) *Children and young people in mind: the final report of the national CAMHS review*, London: DCSF/DH.

Department for Children, Schools and Families/Department of Health (2009) *Healthy lives, brighter futures: The strategy for children and young people's health*, London: DCFS.

Department of Health (DH) Home Office, Department of Education and Skills (Dfes) (2003) *What to do if you are worried a child is being abused*, DH, London.

Department of Health (1989) *Children Act*, London: HMSO.

Department of Health (1991) *Welfare of children and young people in hospital*, London: HMSO.

Department of Health (2004) *The National Service Framework for children, young people and maternity services*, London: DH.

Department of Health (2009) *New horizons: Towards a shared vision for mental health – consultation*, London: DCSF/DH.

Dogra, N. and Leighton, S. (2009) *Nursing in child and adolescent mental health*, Berkshire: Open University Press.

Dogra, N., Parkin, A., Gale, F. and Frake, C. (2002) *A multidisciplinary handbook of child and adolescent mental health for front-line professionals*, London: Jessica Kingsley.

Evans, E., Hawton, K. and Rodham, K. (2005) 'In what way are adolescents who engage in self harm or experience thoughts of self harm different in terms of help-seeking, communication and coping strategies?', *Journal of Adolescence*, 28: 573–587.

Fielding, D. and Duff, A. (1999) 'Compliance with treatment protocols: Interventions for children with chronic illness', *Archives of Disease in Children*, 80: 196–200.

Fisher, K.R., Hirsh-Pasek, K., Golinkohh, R.M. and Gryfe, S.G. (2008) 'Conceptual split? Parents and experts' perceptions of play in the 21st century', *Journal of Applied Developmental Psychology*, 29: 305–316.

Gaffney, A. and Dunne, E.A. (1986) 'Developmental aspects of children's definitions of pain', *Pain*, 26: 105–117.

Garnefski, N. and Diekstra, R.F. (1997) 'Adolescents from one parent, step-parent and intact families: Emotional problems and suicide attempts, *Journal of Adolescence*, 20(2): 201–208.

Garvey, C. (1977) *Play*, London: Fontana Books.

Green, H., McGinnity, A., Meltzer, H., Ford, T. and Goodman, R. (2005) *Mental health of children and young people in Great Britain 2004: A survey for the Office of National Statistics*, London: Palgrave Macmillan.

Gross, R.D. (2005) *Psychology: The science of mind and behaviour*, London: Hodder Arnold.

Hallstrom, I., Runeson, I. and Elander, G. (2002) 'An observation study of the level at which parents participate in decisions during their child's hospitalization', *Nursing Ethics*, 9: 202–214.

Harris, M. and Butterworth, G. (2002) *Developmental psychology: A student's handbook*, London: Taylor and Francis.

Hart, J. (1971) 'The inverse care law', *The Lancet*, 27 February: 405–412.

Hawton, K., Rodham, K., Evans, E. and Weatherall, R. (2002) 'Deliberate self-harm in adolescents: Self report survey in schools in England', *BMJ* 325: 1207–1211.

Hester, N.O. and Barcus, C.S. (1986) 'Assessment and management of pain in children', *Paediatrics: Nursing Upate*, 1(14): 2–6.

Hester, N.O., Foster, R.L. and Beyer, J.E. (1992) 'Clinical judgment in assessing children's pain', in Watt-Watson, J.H. and Donovan, M.I. (eds), *Pain management: Nursing perspective*, St. Louis: Mosby-Yearbook.

Hockenbury, M., Wilson, D., Kline, N. and Winklestein, M. (2003) *Nursing care of infants and children*, Missouri: Mosby.

Hospital for Sick Children (2008) http://www.gosh.nhs.uk/website/gosh/clinicalservices/Pain_control_service/Custom%20Menu_02?portal_status_message=&came_from=http%3A%2F%2Fcms.ich.ucl.ac.uk%2Fwebsite%2Fcms%2Fgosh%2Fclinicalservices%2FPain_control_service%2Fworkitems_view&message=&-C=

Hutchfield, K. (1999) 'Family centred care: A concept analysis', *Journal of Advanced Nursing*, 29(5): 1178–1187.

Ilomaki, E., Rasanen, P., Viilo, K. and Hakko, H. (2007) 'Suicidal behaviour among adolescents with conduct disorder – the role of alcohol dependence', *Psychiatry Research*, 150: 305–311.

Immelt, S. (2006) 'Psychological adjustment in young children with chronic medical conditions', *Journal of Pediatric Nursing*, 21(5): 362–377.

Jerrett, M. and Evans, K. (1986) 'Children's pain vocabulary', *Journal of Advanced Nursing*, 11: 403–408.

Jun-Tai, N. (2008) 'Play in hospital', *Paediatrics and Child Health*, 18(5): 233–237.

Kankkunen, P., Vehilainen-Julkunen, K., Pietial, A. and Halonen, P. (2003) 'Parents' use of non-pharmacological methods to alleviate children's postoperative pain at home', *Journal of Advanced Nursing*, 41(4): 367–375.

Kawik, L. (2006) 'Nurses attitudes and perceptions of parents' participation', *British Journal of Nursing*, 5(7): 430–434.

Kortesluoma, R.L. and Nikkonen, M. (2004) '"I had this horrible pain": The sources of and causes of pain experiences in 4–11-year-old hospitalised children', *Journal of Child Healthcare*, 8(3): 210–231.

Kortesluoma, R.L. and Nikkonen, M. (2006) '"The most disgusting ever": Children's pain descriptions and views of the properties of pain', *Journal of Child Healthcare*, 10(3): 213–227.

Krechel, S.W. and Bildner, J. (1995) 'CRIES: A new neonatal postoperative pain measurement score. Initial testing of validity and reliability', *Paediatric Anaesthesia*, 5(1): 53–61.

LaFleur, C.J. and Raway, B. (1999) 'School age child and adolescent perception of the pain intensity associated with three word descriptors', *Pediatric Nursing*, 25(1): 45–55.

McArdle, P. (2001) 'Children's play', *Child: Care, health and development*, 27(6): 509–514.

McArdle, P. and Huff, N. (2001) 'What is it?': Findings on preschoolers responses to play with medical equipment', *Child: Care, Health and Development*, 27(5): 451–462.

McEwing, G. (1996) 'Children's understanding of their internal body parts', *British Journal of Nursing*, 5(7): 423–429.

McGrath, P. (1990) *Pain in children*, London: Guilford Press.

Mental Health Foundation (2006) *Truth hurts*, London: MHF.

Merkel, S.I., Voepel-Lewis, T., Shayevitz, J.R. and Malviya, S. (1997) 'The FLACC: A behavioral scale for scoring postoperative pain in young children', *Pediatric Nursing*, 23(3): 293–297.

Milligan, C. and Bingley, A. (2007) 'Restorative places or scary places? The impact of woodland on the mental health and well-being of young adults', *Health and Places*, 13: 799–811.

Mitchell, R., Dorling, D. and Shaw, M. (2000) *Inequalities in life and death: What if Britain were more equal?* London: The Policy Press.

Muller, D.J., Harris, P.J., Wattley, L. and Taylor, J.D. (1992) *Nursing children: Psychology, research and practice*, London: Chapman and Hall.

National Assembly for Wales (2000a) *Better Health: BetterWales*, Cardiff: Health Promotion Division, NAW.

National Insititute for Clinical Excellence (2004a) *Self harm: The short-term physical and psychological management and secondary prevention of self harm in primary and secondary care. National Clinical Practice Guideline Number 16*, London: NICE. http://www.nice.org.uk/nicemedia/pdf/CG16FullGuidelione.pdf (Accessed 21/09/2010.)

National Institute for Clinical Excellence (2004b) *Eating disorders: National practice guidelines CG9*. London: NICE. Available from http://www.nice.org.uk/nicemedia/pdf/CG9FullGuideline.pdf.

National Statistics Online (2005) Social Trends 2005. London: NSO. Available from www.statistics.gov.uk/socialtrends35/

Neill, S. (1996) 'Parent's participation', *British Journal of Nursing*, 5(2): 110–117.

Newton, M.S. (2000) 'Family centred care: Current realities in parent participation', *Paediatric Nursing*, 26(2): 164–168.

Noyes, J. (2000) 'Enabling young "Ventilator-Dependent" people to express their views and experiences of their care in hospital', *Journal of Advanced Nursing*, 31(5): 1206–1215.

Nursing and Midwifery Council (2008) *The code of conduct: Standards of conduct, performance and ethics for nurses and midwives*, http://www.nmc-uk.org/Documents/Standards/nmcTheCodeStandardsofConductPerformanceAndEthicsForNursesAndMidwives_LargePrintVersion.PDF (Accessed 16/09/2010.)

Nursing and Midwifery Council (2010) *Standards for pre-registration nursing education*, London: NMC.

Parry-Langdon, N. (2008) *Three years on: Survey of the emotional development and well-being of children and young people*, Newport: ONS.

Play England (2009) *Charter for children's play*, National Children's Bureau London, http://www.playengland.org.uk/resources/charter-for-childrens-play.pdf (Accessed 14/05/2010.)

Polkki, T., Vehilainen-Julkunen, K. and Pietila, A. (2002) 'Parents' roles in using non pharmacological methods in their child's postoperative pain alleviation', *Journal of Clinical Nursing*, 11(4): 526–536.

Royal College of Nursing (2009a) *Mental health in children and young people: An RCN toolkit for nurses who are not mental health specialists*, London: RCN.

Royal College of Nursing (2009b) *The recognition and assessment of acute pain in children: Clinical practice guidelines*, London: RCN.

Royal College of Nursing Children and Young People's Mental Health (2004) *Every nurse's business*, London: RCN. Available at: http://tinyurl.com/d3xk3r (Accessed 21/09/2010.)

Sheridan, M. (1999) *Spontaneous play in early childhood from birth to six years*, Oxford: NFER, pp. 11–15, 69–73.

Shields, L. and Nixon, J. (2004) 'Hospital care of children in four countries', *Journal of Advanced Nursing*, 45: 475–486.

Simons, J., Franck, L.S. and Robertson, E. (2001) 'Parent involvement in children's pain care: Views of parents and nurses', *Journal of Advanced Nursing*, 36(4): 591–599.

Simons, J. and McDonald, L.M. (2006) 'Changing practice: Implementing validated paediatric pain assessment tools', *Journal of Child Health Care*, 10(2): 160–176.

Smith, L., Coleman, V. and Bradshaw, M. (eds) (2002) *Family centred care: Concept, theory and practice*, Hampshire: Palgrave.

Spender, Q. (2007) 'Assessment of adolescent self harm', *Pediatrics and Child Health*, 17(11): 448–453.

Sturgess, J. (2003) 'A model describing play as a child-chosen activity – is this still valid in contemporary Australia?', *Australian Occupational Therapy Journal*, 50: 104–108.

Swanick, M. (1990) 'Knowledge and control', *Paediatric Nursing*, 2(5): 18–20.

Taylor, J. (2000) 'Partnership in the community and hospital: A comparison', *Paediatric Nursing*, 12(5): 28–30.

Teenage Pregnancy Unit (TPU) (2006) Department of Health.

Terry, J. and Davies, A. (2011) 'Child and adolescent mental health'. In Davies, R. and Davies, A. *Children and young people's nursing: Principles for practice*, London: Hodder Education.

Trigg, E. and Mohammed, T. (eds) (2006) *Practices in children's nursing: Guidelines for hospital and community*, Edinburgh: Churchill Livingstone.

Tulloch, A.L., Blizzard, L. and Pinkus, Z. (1997) 'Adolescent-parent communication in self harm', *Journal of Adolescent Health*, 21: 267–275.

Twycross, A. (1998) 'Children's cognitive level and their perception of pain', *Paediatric Nursing*, 10(3): 24–27.

Twycross, A. (2007) 'Children's nurses' post operative pain management practices: An observational study', *International Journal of Nursing Studies*, 44: 869–881.

Twycross, A. (2008) 'Does the importance of a pain management task affect the quality of children's nurses post operative pain management practices?', *Journal of Clinical Nursing*, 17: 320–326.

Twycross, A. (2011) 'Principles of pain management and entitlement to pain relief'. In Davies, R. and Davies, A. *Children and young people's nursing: Principles for practice*, London: Hodder Education.

Underdown, A. (2007) *Young children's health and well-being*, Maidenhead: Open University.

United Nations (1989) *Convention on the rights of the child*, Geneva: UN.

Wanless, D. (2003) *The review of health and social care in Wales*, Cardiff: Welsh Assembly Government.

Welsh Assembly Government (WAG) (2001) *Children and young people: A framework for partnership*, Cardiff: WAG. Available from http://wales.gov.uk/docrepos/40382/40382313/childrenyoungpeople/403821/623995/q262a360_english1.pdf;jsessionid=fCXqMh9YhDLp8Qz2y02v7YxdXhG0FwLXQkhlPG8NjL1VsXtLPnWL!-42672990?lang=en

Welsh Assembly Government 2006 *Play in Wales: Play Policy Implementation Plan*, Cardiff: WAG, http://wales.gov.uk/dcells/publications/policy_strategy_and_planning/early-wales/playpolicy/implementationplane.pdf?lang=en (Accessed 6/5/2010.)

Williams, C. and Asquith, J. (2000) *Paediatric intensive case nursing*, London: Elsevier.

Woodgate, R. and Kristjanson, L.J. (1995) 'Young children's behavioural responses to acute pain: Strategies for getting better', *Journal of Advanced Nursing*, 22: 243–249.

World Health Organization (2003) *Global strategy for infant and young child fooding*, Geneva: WHO.

World Health Organization (2005) *World Health Organization: Child and adolescent injury prevention: A global call to action*, Geneva: World Health Organization.

World Health Organization (2007) *International statistical classification of diseases and related health problems* (10th edn), Geneva: WHO. Available from http://apps.who.int/classifications/apps/icd/icd10online/

World Health Organization (2009) *Infant and young children feeding – model chapter for textbooks for medical students and allied health professionals*, Geneva: World Health Organization.

Zimmerman, P.G. and Santen, L. (1997) 'Teddy says Hi!: Teddy bear clinics revisited', *Journal of Emergency Nursing*, 23(1): 42–44.

CHAPTER 8
LEARNING DISABILITY

Emrys Jenkins

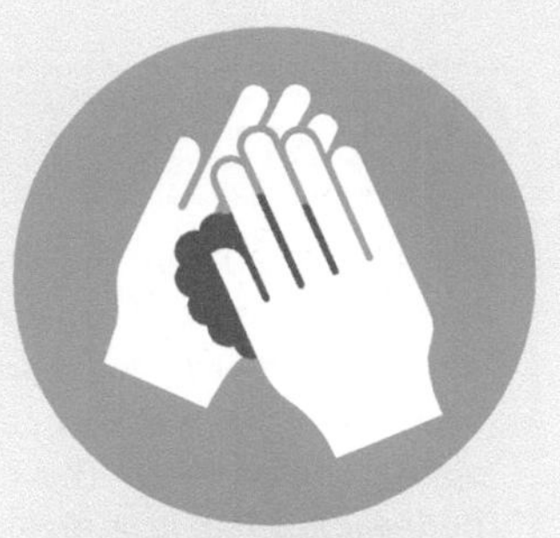

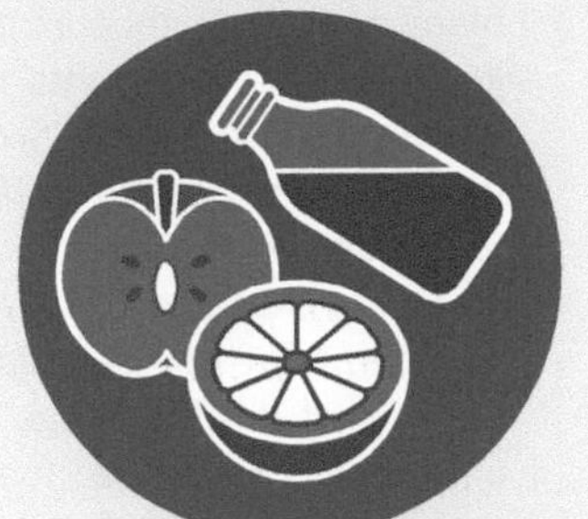

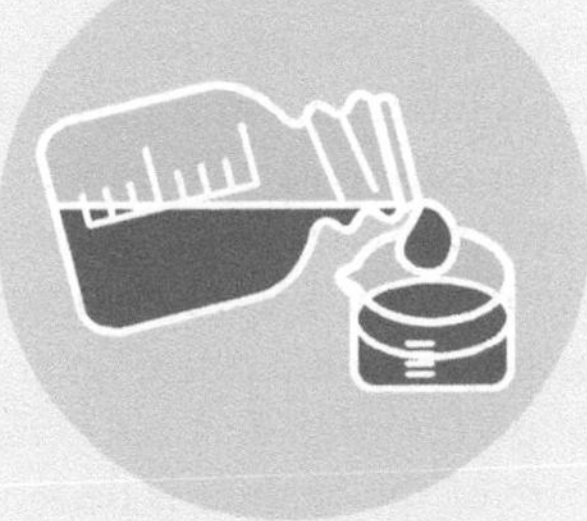

LEARNING OUTCOMES

After completing this chapter, you will be able to:

- Define learning disabilities with reference to biological, psychological and social factors and explain implications for prevention, recognition and intervention.
- Explain the relevance of the history of learning disabilities to current and anticipated policy and practice.
- Justify your own values position in respect of nursing people with a learning disability and helping their families and carers.
- Identify and differentiate the roles of all nurses in providing care to learning disabled people, families and carers.
- Explain and demonstrate relevant communication and nursing intervention skills with reference to evidence.

After reading this chapter you will be able to consider the care, compassion and communication aspects required to care for a learning disabled person and their families and carers. It relates to **Essential Skills Clusters (NMC, 2010) 1–8**, as appropriate for each progression point.

Ensure that you really understand this chapter by logging on to your complimentary **MyNursingKit** at **www.pearsoned.co.uk/kozier**. Complete the self-assessment tests to check your progress and utilise further activities to practise and confirm your understanding.

CASE STUDY

Aliya is a 20-year-old woman from Libya, who describes herself as 'reserved'. She moved to the UK five years ago and agreed to an arranged marriage with Qasim when she was 19. They have known each other since childhood and neither speak English well. The couple have lived in a small two-bedroomed flat in a highly populated area of Bristol where many of their neighbours belong to the same ethnic minority group. Both their parents and several aunts and uncles have homes very close by. Six weeks ago Aliya gave birth at the local hospital to a baby girl weighing just over 2kg. Communication problems arose during the antenatal period, and were exacerbated by Aliya's poor English and by lack of an interpreter being available. The labour was normal until the end of the first stage then the foetal heartbeat slowed and forceps were used to assist delivery. The umbilical cord was tightly wrapped round the baby's neck and she was asphyxiating, with a slow pulse, and little signs of life. Intubation seemed to prompt spontaneous breathing some eight and a half minutes after birth. The doctor noted a low Apgar score and flaccid paralysis. The baby was taken to the special care unit.

The next day approximately 24 hours after seeing her child taken away, Aliya saw a paediatrician and was told the baby had some level of cerebral palsy though it was unclear about how severe the condition would prove to be. The doctor explained she would like to keep the child in special care to monitor progress. Aliya did not appreciate or understand much of this, though she did realise that something was wrong with her child. She did not respond to the doctor, except to nod her head which was interpreted as apparent assent. The paediatrician then left. Nurses found her a few minutes later, very upset and tearful - she had thought her baby was dead. Staff contacted the family and Qasim came immediately, along with his brother and parents. His brother was able to act as an interpreter. Aliya and her baby left the hospital 10 days later to return home. The large family group of which she was part coped admirably with the emotional distress and immediate practical demands of caring for Aliya and the baby. They were reticent though polite about additional offers of help and the need for assessment and treatment for the baby. The health visitor, who has several years' experience of working in this community, is currently the main contact with the family.

INTRODUCTION

This chapter provides an introductory overview of learning disabilities and the particular contributions that health professionals, especially nurses, offer. It is not drafted as an absolutely comprehensive account of all that might apply to nursing people with a learning disability. Some specialist therapies, for example gentle teaching, are not referred to and some aspects of pertinent law are only referred to in general terms. The main core of the chapter is designed to help readers appreciate what learning disability means, what values apply, how knowledge from history and research can help us learn about it and how nurses can intervene (or not) in most helpful and effective ways. The first section addresses how we come to understand learning disabilities, its degrees, scope and forms set against a historical background and current policy and philosophy. Causes, recognition and prevention are outlined and a single illustrative example (Down's syndrome) provides a more detailed illustration. The second section encompasses key factors in assisting people so they can lead more fulfilling lives, characterised by respect, dignity, independence and choice. Risk and risk analysis inform this assistance as does effective communication and advocacy. Nurse contributions to working with families and health promotion, including sexual health, conclude this section. The final section explores contemporary issues, challenges and implications for learning disability nursing, including community and day care, responding to profound and multiple disabilities and challenging behaviour, and research issues.

UNDERSTANDING LEARNING DISABILITIES

The nature of learning disabilities

The UK government (DH, 2001e) defined learning disability as:

> *a significantly reduced ability to understand new or complex information, to learn new skills (impaired intelligence) along with a reduced ability to cope independently (impaired social functioning). The onset of disability is considered to have started before adulthood, with a lasting effect on development.*

Other definitions adopt medical and psychological language and criteria such as those found in classification systems, for example, *The ICD-10 classification of mental and behavioural disorders* (WHO, 1992) and the *Diagnostic and statistical manual of mental disorders* DSM-IV (APA, 1994). These tend to be applied when considering whether a person is entitled to specialist services. Significant limitations are recognised as applying to most definitions, not least because of anomalies in interpreting diagnostic information and test results. Legal definitions are similarly limited. The Mental Health Act 2007 amends some aspects of the 1983 Act (see for example, Part 1, Amendments to Mental Health Act 1983, Chapter 1, Changes to Key Provisions, Mental Disorder) where learning disability is defined as:

> *. . . learning disability means a state of arrested or incomplete development of the mind which includes significant impairment of intelligence and social functioning.*

Burton (1997) reviewed several definitions, identifying advantages and disadvantages of each. He proposed a composite definition that could apply in both health and social services as a practical way of identifying eligibility of those needing specialist help. This facilitates focusing resources on those with greatest need, without neglecting others falling beyond the remit of simpler definitions. Burton's work emphasises social impairment arising from primary intellectual disability (during childhood) and not from other causes, such as illness. People with a learning disability are likely to need help via appropriate, relatively specialist services/sources of expertise, in relation to:

- home making/independent living;
- occupation and employment;
- dealing with interpersonal situations.

This mirrors the Scottish government's approach insofar as implications for help are outlined (Scottish Executive, 2000):

> *People with learning disabilities have a significant, lifelong condition that started before adulthood, that affected their development and which means they need help to:*
>
> - *understand information;*
> - *learn skills; and*
> - *cope independently.*

Degrees and Scope of Learning Disability

It is difficult to identify precisely the number of people with a learning disability in the UK. Emerson and Hatton (2008) estimate that 1.5 million people in England have a learning disability with 13,500 people identified in Wales by means of local authority links (WAG, 2006). In Scotland, approximately 120,000 people have a learning disability (Scottish Executive, 2000). It is not uncommon to read (or hear) about degrees of learning disability from mild, moderate, to severe or profound, reflecting something of a traditional medical perspective on categorising disability. Policy makers, professionals and educators are tending to adopt an individual needs approach rather than categorising, though these terms and language remain common in practice (RCN, 2006b). Table 8-1 outlines a synopsis of these terms, based on more extensive details presented by Hardy *et al.* (2006) and the Royal College of Nursing (RCN, 2006b).

Learning disability has, unfortunately, a lengthy association with misconceptions and stereotypes that promote homogeneity of view, that people with learning disabilities are 'all the same', are 'unable to do anything for themselves' and 'cannot learn new skills' or how to be more independent. Students of nursing should appreciate the challenge they face in appreciating the person beneath or behind the language of labels and categories, to see them as individuals and not mere stereotypes linked to negative associations or 'labelling'. Learning disability is now generally thought of as mainly a social condition linked to people's social competence and skill. Most people with a learning disability live in their own homes with their families and do not require residential support services. They do need help from educational, social and community services including health services. Relevant professionals need to ensure effective links between the primary healthcare team, social services and voluntary and independent sectors. Most learning disabled people have similar health needs to anyone else and healthcare interventions will largely mirror those provided to anyone, via individualised means though with some adaptation that reflects particular needs, circumstances and abilities. Some people will have healthcare needs that transcend these general ones, perhaps including specific physical, behavioural, emotional or psychological needs that require some form of specialist nursing care within the multidisciplinary frame. People with challenging behaviours, for example kicking, biting or spitting, self-injurious behaviour, aggressive outbursts and swearing, require relatively intensive help and support.

A Brief History

Until recently, societal attitudes to learning disability have been characterised by intolerance, lack of understanding and

Table 8-1 Synopsis of Mild, Moderate, Severe and Profound Learning Disability

Mild	Moderate	Severe/profound
A clear majority, 75% or more, of people with learning disabilities are in this category. Most of these live independently, many with their own families and in employment without need for extra support from services, except in times of crisis.	Support needed for these individuals is higher with many needing some level of support with everyday tasks. People may have difficulty communicating their needs and are likely to live with parents, with day-to-day support, or in supported living schemes. These individuals are also likely to use a range of support services including day and outreach schemes.	People with severe and profound learning disability may have significant health problems and needs, perhaps higher rates of epilepsy, sensory problems and physical disabilities. Their needs are more complex including increased difficulty in communication. Sometimes as attempts to communicate are frustrated, individuals engage in behaviour that others consider challenging, Self-injury is particularly common in people with profound learning disability. In severe cases this can lead to additional disability, poor health and a significantly decreased quality of life. People with severe and profound learning disabilities can also be described as 'people with high support needs'. This more contemporary language is being used widely, and is included in government policies.

prejudice. We know very little about the lives of people with a learning disability before the 18th century, though Gates (1997: 40) provides an illustrative timeline beginning in the 1400s up until the 1990s.

Before the industrial revolution most people lived in rural, farming communities, and whilst some people were called, for example, 'village idiots', it is misleading to equate them with having a learning disability. Then, survival beyond infancy was unlikely if physical problems were present and mild learning disabilities would be difficult to recognise since fewer people were literate. Those people who did survive and had a learning disability would only have received help from their immediate families, if at all.

The Poor Laws of 1834 coincided with construction of asylums, institutions for people termed 'mad' or 'feeble minded'. Asylums, in keeping with the original meaning of the word, were a genuine attempt to provide safe sanctuary, commonly in picturesque locations. Unfortunately, these institutions developed strict uncompromising (and uncaring) milieu where 'inmates' were routinely denied choice and devalued. Segregation became the order of the day as admission to institutions (known as colonies) required certification as a 'mental defective' (Mental Deficiency Act 1913).

> *The self-sufficiency basis of these colonies depended on employing inmates as the main workforce. The Wood Committee (Wood Report, 1929) had envisaged that a range of abilities would be necessary to maintain the colonies. High-grade inmates (people with mild or borderline learning disabilities) would be required for jobs demanding skilled labour, medium-grade inmates for simple routine work and low grades for jobs that involved fetching and carrying. One significant feature of work related to the colony was that it was unpaid.* (Gates, 2007: 54)

Between 1918 and 1940 admissions to institutions rose as laws prompted further segregation of people regarded as 'defective', or 'feeble minded, insane, epileptics, drunks' and even 'musicians'. IQ (intelligence quotient) tests were introduced in the 1930s, with low scoring individuals classified as 'mentally defective' and ineducable. Figure 8-1 is based on Gates' work with some additional, recent (21st century) material.

After 1946, the new National Health Service (NHS) brought **medical model** approaches to **disability** and introduced the language of 'mental handicap'. Institutions became hospitals, inmates became patients and a new caring approach was advocated. Public perceptions of danger and degeneracy gradually shifted towards more sympathetic views of people in need of treatment and help, albeit with a continuing emphasis on segregation and isolation. The 1959 Mental Health Act distinguished between 'mental handicap' and 'mental illness' and began to explore notions of care outside hospitals. Standards of care remained generally poor, and 1967 saw the first of many scandals in service provision, including those at South Ockendon and Ely hospitals. *Better services for the mentally handicapped* was published by the DHSS in 1971 as a government response to these continuing scandals, laying the basis for community care provision.

> *Being in the institution was bad. I got tied up and locked up. I didn't have any clothes of my own, and no privacy. We got beat up at times but that wasn't the worst. The real pain came from being a group. I was never a person. I was part of a group to eat, sleep and everything . . . it was sad.* (MENCAP, 2010b [words of a former resident])

During the 1970s and 1980s hospitals were increasingly recognised as inadequate and community services provision began apace, supplemented by the developing concepts of 'Normalisation' and 'Social Role Valorisation' (Wolfensberger, 1972, 1980, 1983, 1984). These prompted a reappraisal of disability as different and distinct from a purely medical phenomenon, emphasising its social dimension, the normal facets of living, having a home, education, work and leisure. The normalisation ethos emphasises the unique value of the individual, rights to choice, opportunity and additional support needed for fulfilling potential. **Social role valorisation** (SRV) developed from normalisation (Wolfensberger, 1984) with an increased emphasis on providing valued roles for devalued people. Valued roles relate to receiving an education, developing and contributing to the community through participation, and with chances for independent and supported living, work and self-support. These lead to societal recognition of the individual as worthy, being treated respectfully, with dignity and given opportunities to contribute and be 'heard'. Brown and Benson (1992) outline John O'Brien's Five Essential Service Accomplishments that supplemented the SRV approach by providing care staff with direct means by which to promote valued activities by learning disabled people as participant members in communities. These are summarised as the right of learning disabled people to:

- take part in community life and to live and spend leisure time with other members of the community;
- experience valued relationships with non-disabled people;
- make choices, both large and small, in one's life: these include choices about where to live and with whom to live;
- learn new skill and participate in meaningful activities with whatever assistance is required;
- be valued and not treated as a second-class citizen.

The All Wales Strategy for the Development of Services for Mentally Handicapped People (AWS) was launched in 1983 and seen as something of a flagship.

> *If services are to fulfil their potential for creating positive outcomes in the lives of people with mental handicaps, they need to maintain a critical attitude which constantly examines their goals and activities in terms of the lives of the people they serve. . . . The All-Wales Strategy has a foundation of clear, specific and explicit values. This provides an opportunity to develop an evaluative approach that can be seen as useful to the development of services and relevant to the lives of those being served.* (Evans et al., 1988: 249-250)

By 1990, the NHS and Community Care Act placed the right of disabled people to be an equal part of society, with access to the necessary support in statute. By the early years of the 21st century, closing the old institutions (de-institutionalising) had

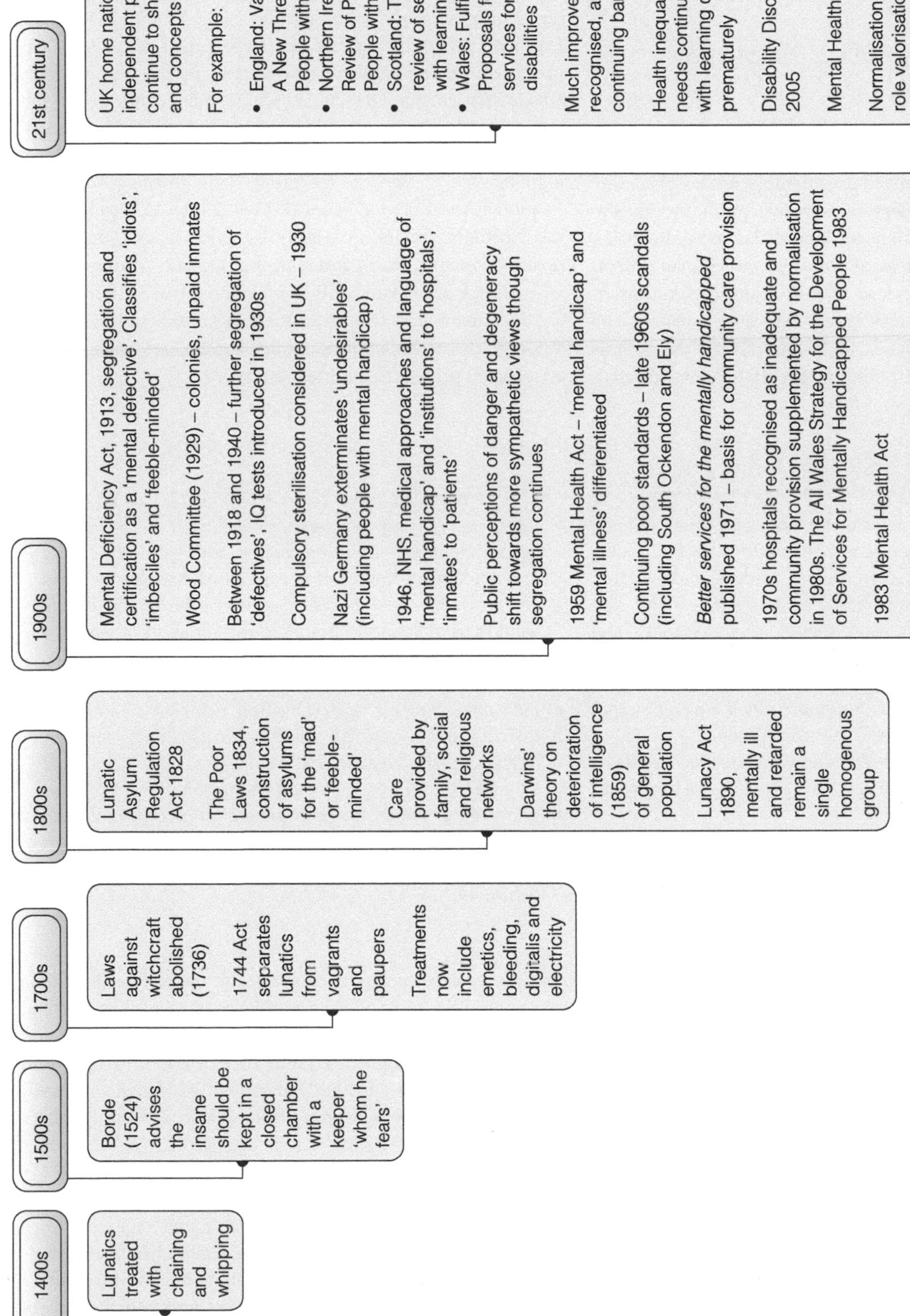

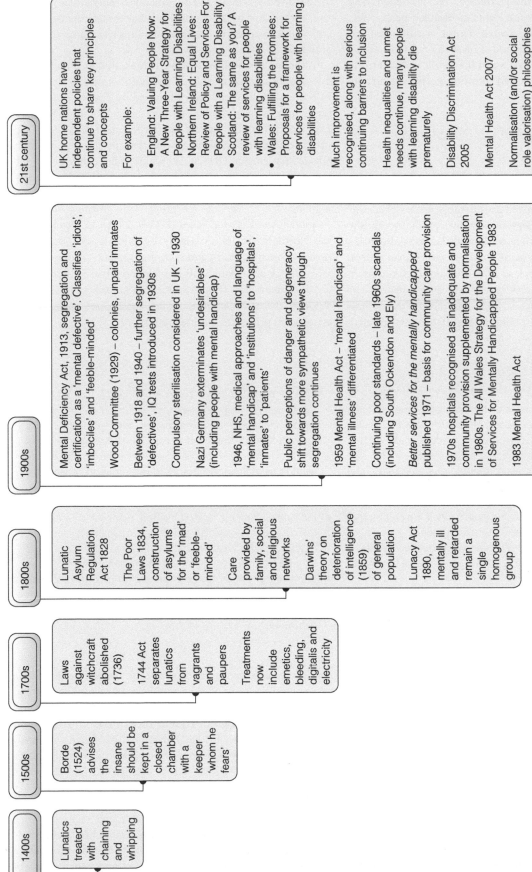

Figure 8-1 History, timeline.
Source: adapted from Gates, B. (1997: 40). Copyright Elsevier 1997.

largely been achieved and the Disability Discrimination Acts of 1995 and 2005 guarantee the rights of disabled people. Yet, many people continue to be denied decent accommodation, work and leisure opportunities and choices in education, effectively presenting service providers and the public with continuing challenges. These are reflected in more recent and current policy initiatives.

Twenty-first Century Policy, Philosophies and Evidence

The latter parts of the 20th century and beginnings of the 21st are generally regarded as times when the lives of people with a learning disability have improved considerably, not least because of more enlightened policy, service provision, public perception and involvement. Yet objectively, we should also recognise inadequacies and continuing areas of concern, rather than accept romanticised historical overviews of shifts from (institutional) misery to effective community based help and support (e.g. see Bredberg, 1999; Manthorpe, 2007). Race (2007) shows how some relevant examples of policy in the 1970s were created largely by professionals and bureaucrats, tending to be prescriptive, with a shift by 2001 towards broader statements of principle created via active consultation with a wide range of groups and disabled people themselves.

Although this shift is to be welcomed, doubts remain about how significantly people's lives have been improved. Since 2000, in Scotland, policy has been informed by *The same as you? A review of services for people with learning disabilities* (Scottish Executive, 2000). In England, the Department of Health (DH) produced *Valuing people: A new strategy for learning disability for the 21st century* (DH, 2001e) whilst Wales continued to follow policy development evolving from the 'All Wales Strategy' (Welsh Office, 1983) and *Fulfilling the promises: Proposals for a framework for services for people with learning disabilities* (National Assembly for Wales (NAW), 2001). In October 2002 the Northern Ireland Assembly established an independent review of mental health and learning disability. Although each UK country has created and implemented these different policy documents and strategies, there is considerable similarity amongst them. In synopsis, policy makers are pursuing the actions and principles outlined in *Box 8-1*.

BOX 8-1 Synopsis of UK Policy During 2000–2010

- Improved information provision for users and carers. People with learning disabilities need better information to make more informed choices. Government, professionals and the public need to better understand people with learning disabilities and their needs. More support is needed for carers including means of facilitating more flexible and fresh ideas for short breaks.
- Person-centred and needs-led approaches which put the individual at the heart of any decisions made.
- Joint working and improved teamwork between professionals, agencies and (crucially) including service users and carers as partners.
- Advocacy that realises more control for individuals over their lives and services.
- Community living that assists inclusion in education, leisure and recreation; in-day opportunities and particularly in employment. Improved access to mainstream services and less reliance on specialist services is promoted. People want to have their own homes in the community. Very few people should have hospital as their home, and other forms of shared living should reduce.
- Individual planning and transition planning to improve, reshape and reorganise services, employment opportunities, further education and day services that focus more on education, employment and personal fulfilment.
- Improved attention for both general and complex health needs.
- Improved responses to people who present challenging behaviour.

The Scottish Executive (2000) included a comparative review of financial resource utilisation in Scotland, England and Wales which illustrated health and local authorities in England (at that time) spending £59 each year on learning disability services for every person in the population. In Wales the figure was £63 whilst in Scotland, only £54 per person was spent (see Figure 8-2).

In Wales 74% of total spending went through local authority community care services, with only 58% in Scotland (Scottish Executive, 2000: 9), providing an obvious policy driver.

Clearly, all the UK home nations have pursued and updated/amended similar policies since the millennium (DH, 2009; Northern Ireland Assembly (NIA), 2005; Scottish Executive, 2008; Welsh Assembly Government (WAG), 2007) yet significant obstacles and problems remain. Learning disabled people continue to experience significant health inequalities including unmet needs in terms of, for example, **heart disease**, **stroke** and **diabetes** (DRC, 2006b). Snell (2009) outlines the urgency and implications of recognising premature deaths in people with learning disabilities and the Department of Health (England) confidential inquiry is running from March 2010 to February 2013. The **Disability Rights Commission (DRC)** (2006b) makes a raft of recommendations:

- Better primary care, ensuring people can register with a General Practitioner (GP) and have regular health checks.
- Improved staff training and prescribing including providing information and choice so that risks and benefits inform more balanced decision making.

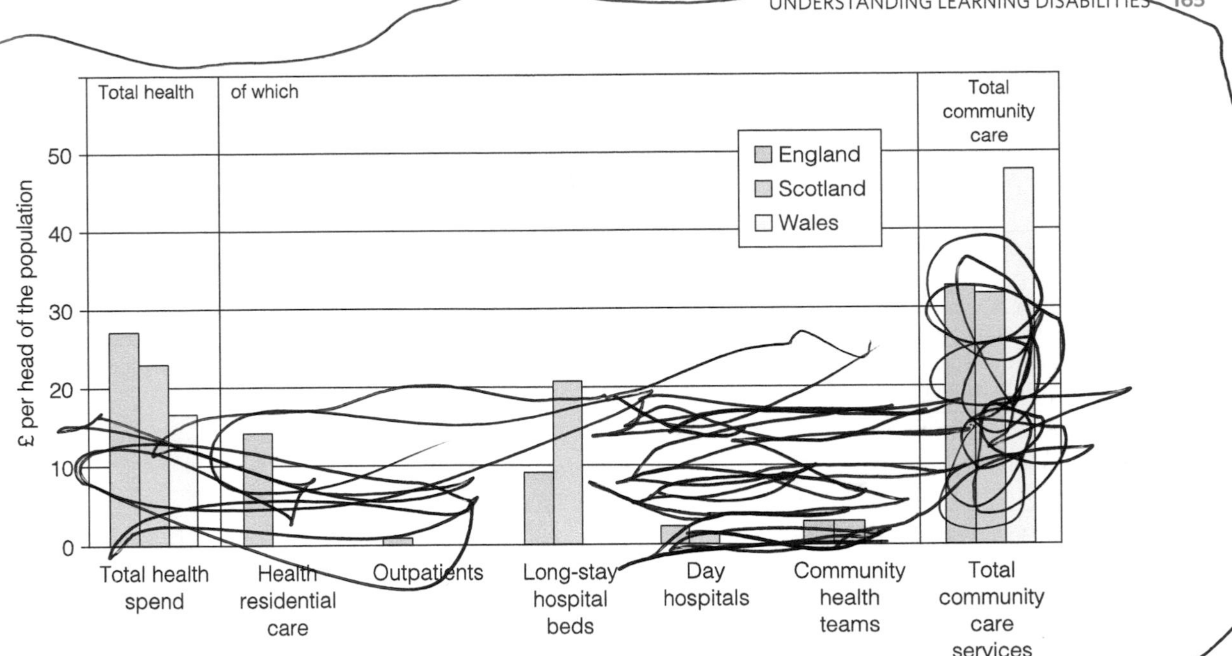

Figure 8-2 Where the money goes: England, Scotland and Wales compared.
Source: Scottish Executive (2000) *The Same as You? A review of services for people with learning disabilities*, p. 9.

- Effectively targeted health promotion (acknowledging challenging smoking and obesity rates and low staff expectations).
- More direct involvement of disabled people in influencing and leading service improvements.

There are particular implications for nurses in these health related domains. McCray (2003a) points to policy and economic incongruence that may lead to different agencies providing resource-led (not needs-led) services, and the key role of nurse as facilitator of interprofessional practice. Williamson and Johnson (2004) and Leyshon *et al.* (2004) present ways of ensuring health needs are met in mainstream primary care services with an emphasis on teamwork and inclusion. Researchers such as Brown (2005) and Gibbs *et al.* (2008) complement research into primary healthcare provision, illustrating that people with learning disabilities have increased and distinct health needs; are likely to require help from most healthcare systems, including general hospital and emergency services; and that these services can be much better delivered. Devine and Taggart (2008) and Harrison and Berry (2006) make similar points in respect of mental health and health visiting service provision respectively, that better meets the needs of people with learning disabilities.

Seemingly, despite enduring policy and general improvements in service provision, people with learning disabilities continue to experience marginalisation, social exclusion and lack of opportunities, educational, occupational and communal (Colley and Hodkinson, 2001; Gates, 1997; Hall, 2005; Manthorpe, 2007).

Richardson (2000) describes small scale research undertaken by a group of people with learning disabilities on themselves, showing how nursing staff supported 'ordinary living' and lifestyles that participants valued, yet concurrently also contributed to disempowerment, echoing the notion of inclusion being accompanied by some forms of exclusion (Colley and Hodkinson, 2001).

Adopting normalisation (and/or SRV) as the basis for service design and provision is being challenged (Manthorpe, 2007) with some authors advocating better means of promoting inclusion (Culham and Nind, 2003). Gates (2007) provides a detailed account that highlights serious questions (such as the possibility of service provider antipathy) and some pragmatic suggestions, for example that absolute answers will only be realised in a perfect society (with wholesome attitudes about difference and ability, etc.) and that this is utopian, inconceivable.

For decades, the institutional, hospital, medical models of care have been replaced by community-oriented services based on normalisation and SRV. Change seems inevitable, particularly since law and policy continue to promote rights for learning disabled people, along with evidence of continuing social exclusion. The implications for service development and service philosophies are broad, deep and challenging.

Causes, Presentations, Prevention and Counselling

Several distinct causes of learning disability are identified, affecting brain development before, during or soon after birth. Groups of specific features are indicative of particular syndromes or conditions. Causes include genetic factors, infection before birth, brain injury or damage at birth, brain infections or brain damage after birth. Whilst a large number of syndromes are known, including for example, **Down's syndrome, fragile X syndrome** and **cerebral palsy**, they apply to only a minority of people with learning disability. For the majority, a definitive cause remains unknown. Knowledge of causation is helpful in assisting understanding learning disability, not least in terms

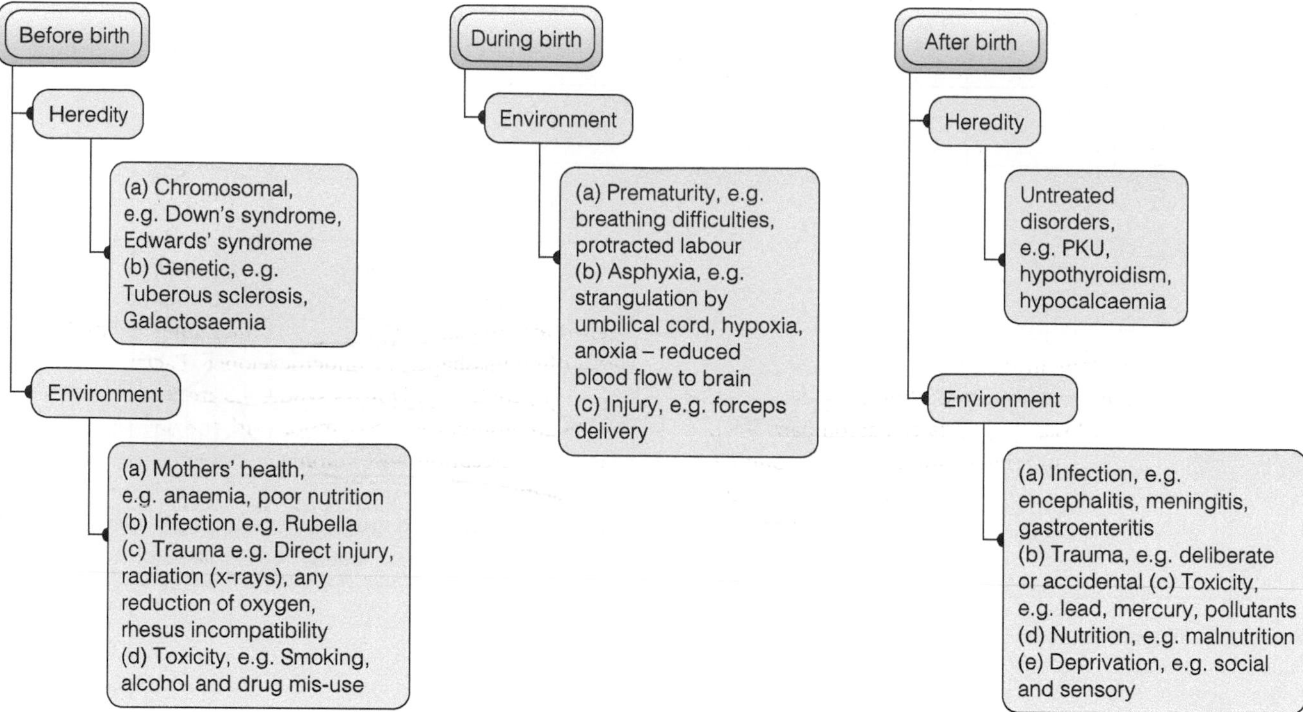

Figure 8-3 Causes of learning disability with selected examples.

of prevention and treatment, although for most people with a learning disability, knowing causation does not help significantly in meeting their needs. To ensure prompt recognition of problems, health visitors, doctors and educational psychologists undertake tests and developmental screening programmes, beginning soon after birth and continuing through childhood.

Every human cell contains 23 pairs of **chromosomes**, 1 from each parent with the exception of **gametes** (egg and sperm cells) which have only half the full complement. Pairs 1 to 22 are known as **autosomes** whist the 23rd pair are sex chromosomes. In women, this pair are the same, known as X chromosomes, in men they are different, known as X and Y. Each chromosome is made from a string of **genes** that individually, are responsible for specific characteristics such as height and eye, hair or skin colour. Generally, each gene is matched with a partner (similarly to pairs of chromosomes). Dominant genes are those which express their relevant characteristic, overriding their partners, whilst recessive genes produce characteristics only when both gene partners express the same characteristic. Figure 8-3 presents an overview of the causes of learning disability as they relate to progress of time and type of causative factor; heredity and environment.

Before Birth

An unborn baby who inherits particular genes or chromosomes that contribute to adverse effects on the central nervous system (brain and the spinal cord) will have a learning disability. One relatively common cause of inherited learning disability is Down's syndrome in which an additional chromosome exists (number 21) so that the person has a complete complement of 47 chromosomes in each cell (rather than 46, as 23 pairs). This is known as Trisomy 21. Alternatively, translocation of number 21 chromosome means that part of the chromosome attaches to another one either during formation of sperm/egg cells or very soon during foetal development. In its mosaic form, the person has some cells with the normal number and type of chromosomes and other cells with an additional chromosome. Further examples of chromosomal disorders include: **Edwards' syndrome** (Trisomy 18); **Cri-du-chat syndrome** (deletion of part of chromosome 5); and some that are specific to the sex chromosomes (X and Y), such as **Turner syndrome, Triple X syndrome** and **Klinefelter syndrome.**

Genetic disorders may be dominant or recessive, either linked with autosomes or the sex chromosomes. Autosomal dominat presentations include **tuberous sclerosis** (epiloia), **neurofibromatosis** and **Prader-Willi syndrome.** Autosomal recessive presentations include **phenylketonuria**, **maple-syrup disease**, **galactosaemia**, **Tay-Sachs disease** and **Hurler syndrome.** Sex-linked recessive presentations include X-linked **hydrocephalus**, **Hunter syndrome** and fragile X syndrome. Additional genetic presentations involve a number of different genes combining to produce complex features and effects. These include **Sturge-Weber syndrome**, hydrocephalus and **hypothyroidism**, as well as **congenital** conditions such as **spina bifida** and **cleft lip.** These chromosomal and genetic presentations each have similar and disparate features though the needs of people and the care they require are generally similar, albeit with unique (individualised) elements.

The developing brain and spinal cord may also be compromised if the mother has an accident or illness while she is pregnant. These include direct trauma to the foetus, any reduction of oxygen, infection such as **German measles (rubella)**, **cytomegalovirus** (herpes family) or **chickenpox**. Smoking, alcohol and drug misuse are all implicated in harmful effects on the developing foetus (Crome and Kumar, 2007; Manthorpe, 2007), as is poor nutrition, physical factors such as radiation (x-rays) which interfere especially harmfully with developing foetal cells, and **rhesus** incompatibility (rhesus negative mother carries a rhesus positive baby).

During Birth

Premature births often involve associated problems such as breathing difficulties and protracted labour, putting the vulnerable baby at increased risk. **Asphyxia** can accompany a lengthy second stage of labour, or strangulation by the umbilical cord. These invariably lead to either **hypoxia**, a reduced oxygenation of the blood or **anoxia**, an absence of oxygen. Both lead to reduced blood flow to the brain with a danger of brain tissue swelling and/or bleeding. Forceps delivery is implicated in direct trauma to the head with subsequent brain injury.

After Birth

Generally, inherited (for example, **PKU** and some metabolic conditions such as **hypocalcaemia** and **hypoglycaemia**) are only recognised in the post-natal period. This is why routine tests (for example, Guthrie Test and Tandem Mass Spectrometry) are undertaken during the days and weeks following birth.

Encephalitis is inflammation of the brain linked to viral infections such as rubella, whilst **meningitis**, inflammation of the membranes close to the brain and spinal cord, can both lead to learning disability. **Gastroenteritis** can lead to dehydration of sufficient severity that brain haemorrhage and damage result.

Trauma, either deliberate or accidental, can relatively easily damage the young person's brain with severe and permanent effects. Similarly, damage can result from the presence of toxins including mercury and atmospheric pollutants. Deprivation of food and fluids, especially if reaching the status of malnutrition, will impact negatively on the developing brain and general health of the child. Similarly, deprivation of sensory stimulation impedes physical and psychological development, as does social isolation.

ACTIVITY 8-1

Which factors can you identify that contributed to a newborn baby becoming brain injured?

One Example of Recognising and Acting on Presenting Features: Down's syndrome

It is clear that people present with a wide range of learning disabilities, and that each person will have their own unique characteristics. This section outlines typical features associated with Down's syndrome, as a single example for readers to begin to appreciate recognition, diagnosis, assessment, education and care provision principles. Detailed and extensive descriptions of particular syndromes can be found in Gates (1997) and Manthorpe (2007).

A person with Down's syndrome has a characteristic facial appearance and stature. This usually includes: an upward slant of the eyes associated with **epicanthic folds** of both eyelids and sockets sloping forward; flattening of nasal bridge and a rounded head and face with ears being low set; a small nose and high arched mouth palate. The tongue is often long and mobile and teeth often misshapen or underdeveloped. Facial resemblances between people with Down's syndrome are sufficiently characteristic to prompt easy recognition with the obvious dangers of mistaken perception and automatic stereotyping. A relatively short stature accompanies short and variable length fingers on angular, square-shaped hands, sometimes with degrees of **syndactyly** (webbing of digits). Cardiac problems are not uncommon as is poor peripheral circulation, sometimes leading to cyanosis of the face. Congenital heart problems may or may not present, though persistent cyanosis, poor feeding, breathlessness and **tachycardia** warrant attention and investigation, so that, for example, continuing problems do not lead to secondary pulmonary vascular disease or chronicity. A predisposition to infection results from poor immunological system responses, typically as frequent or more random respiratory infections. Significant numbers of people with Down's syndrome have hearing and/or sight problems. Diagnosis is usually possible quite soon after birth as physical features are identified and ultimately confirmed by chromosome test.

Degree of learning disability in people with Down's syndrome is very variable, so an individual approach is crucial. Help, support and treatment should be designed to meet the person's needs, physical, psychological and emotional, social and spiritual. This invariably requires appreciation of particular predispositions and interrelationships, that may on occasion, lead to increased risks to health and well-being, such as heart and respiratory problems, infections and obesity-linked problems. Care and interventions should mirror those provided for the public generally, with the additional or enhanced support that learning disability necessitates. Health providers are identified as needing to improve these aspects of their support and intervention strategies for learning disabled people (Gibbs *et al.*, 2008; Kerr *et al.*, 2005). Physical issues are likely to require appropriate intervention including, for example, **chemotherapy** (and possibly, surgery) for heart, circulatory and respiratory disorders, infections diabetes and sensory impairments.

Nursing care requires informed and sensitive communication with the person and their family/carers, underpinned by regard for independence. In most healthcare settings nurses will have many opportunities to support and encourage independence, not least in terms of everyday living activities such as dressing, feeding and maintaining personal hygiene. It should be noted that nurses require awareness of the effects and impact upon learning by the person, of their actions (behaviours). Inconsistency of approach will foster lack of clarity and ambiguity with negative consequences (see below). As well as this individual or micro-level approach, nurses, like all professionals, must recognise the importance of the social dimension including interpersonal relationships, cultural, organisational and systemic elements. These are intrinsic to normalisation and SRV that aim to improve individuals' lives through more socially and culturally oriented means. This represents a significant shift from the established, medically oriented (individual therapy approach) model of disability to more integral, social and community models (van der Gaag, 1998). Nurses then, must attend to the individual and his or her particular needs whilst recognising the crucial impact of the environment, particularly the social environment, upon the person with a learning disability. This demands from nurses, breadth and depth of knowledge (for example, about health, illness, development, learning disability, culture, and values) that they can use to best effect, to help and support the person with insight not just in the immediate term, during crises, but in more lifelong terms. Van de Gaag (1998) points out that everyone involved in the 'social care industry' has a responsibility to communicate in ways that break cycles of negativity that pervade interactions experienced by many people with learning disabilities. Nurses have significant contributions to make towards improving the lives of people with a learning disability, especially since health and social care policy is consistently aimed at more community and service user oriented provision. Nurses can assist in supporting ordinary patterns of life within the community; respect and treatment for individuals as individuals; and the additional professional help needed to achieve maximum potential.

Prevention and Counselling

Prevention in health and social care is described in three ways and each is applicable to learning disabilities nursing, including physical, emotional and social dimensions of development, health and well-being:

1. **Primary prevention** has two modes. First, actions designed to protect people from disease and disability by means such as immunisations, for example rubella immunisation. Second, education and health promotion, such as providing advice to expectant mothers in relation to nutrition, smoking, alcohol and drug use.
2. **Secondary prevention** aims to detect disease and difficulty as soon as possible so that treatment and remedial efforts can be swiftly instigated to best effect. Some disorders may be eradicated whilst others will have their progress slowed so that complications are reduced and disability limited, with beneficial impact upon lifestyle and independence. Examples include, routine testing for PKU and provision of low phenylalanine diets, and thyroid hormone treatment for those with hypothyroidism (virtually eradicated, largely due to secondary prevention).
3. **Tertiary prevention** is designed to improve the quality of life for those with longer-term conditions and problems so that complications and negative impact are reduced in severity. Learning disability nurses provide considerable tertiary prevention in the form of actions and activities, for example, working with individuals and families to promote development. This might include designing and running social or skill training programmes, and providing appropriate education and rehabilitation. Tertiary prevention is a key aspect of nurses' role and input, with proportionally greater emphasis and applicability than either primary or secondary prevention which tend to fall into the remit of other professionals and agencies. This tertiary, longer-term input by nurses requires appreciation that cause and effect relationships may be much more than simply linear. For example, irrespective of the cause of learning disability, people who have problems with mobility, movement, sight, hearing or communication are at increased risk of reduced learning opportunities as well as some form of social stigma, perhaps resulting in a lack of personal relationships with neighbours/others. Nurses need to appreciate and appraise those issues and factors that inhibit learning and functioning almost without reference to the primary cause of the learning disability. These issues and factors assume more importance than biological causes and nursing interventions should be designed to counter functional deficits.

These preventive approaches involve an integral communication and counselling dimension whereby professionals, including nurses, can explain and present information and evidence that assists people to make their own informed choices about actions, inaction and implications. For example, preconception and genetic counselling can explicate potential parents' biological status, clarifying the risk of having a child with inherited illnesses, such as cystic fibrosis or Down's syndrome, and the likelihood of passing them on to children, so that choices can be made in respect of avoiding or terminating pregnancy. Skilled and sensitive communication is also necessary when informing parents that child has a learning disability or is considered to be at risk of delayed development.

Medical treatment has a role to play, so that medical problems of hereditary, congenital or birth origins are treated promptly. Then, particular therapies may be used to ease symptoms, encourage learning and assist speech and language development. There is no medical treatment that raises intelligence quotients (IQ) but there are exercises and therapies which improve coordination, balance, memory and concentration skills. Treatment is designed to control more disabling symptoms and support independent living. Improving general health by ensuring a healthy balanced diet, exercise and rest are worthy contributions to overall development and complement specific therapies, such as speech, language and physiotherapy that improve communication skills, coordination and mobility.

Prevention (and education) also applies in community nursing and primary healthcare contexts, not least because people with a learning disability tend to be at more risk of health problems than others and have their problems overlooked (DH, 2001e; Lennox *et al.*, 2001; Minihan and Dean, 1990; Whittaker and McIntosh, 2000). It is imperative that health and social care agencies and practitioners work closely together and with people in receipt of services to adopt proactive and responsive healthcare.

FULFILLING LIVES: INDEPENDENCE AND WELL-BEING

Community Service Provision and Multidisciplinary Teamwork

In broad terms, recent and current UK policy and legislation have been designed to promote social inclusion. Learning disabled people are encouraged to access services, including social, educational, employment, accommodation and health services in the same ways as anyone else. The use of separate, specialised services for people with learning disabilities is being targeted towards those with the most complex needs, as a supplement to mainstream services. The independent and voluntary sectors also make significant contributions. The move away from institutionalised care to care in the community, along with improved integration, aims to reduce exclusion and marginalisation with a subsequent realisation of more independent living. This is easier stated than realised and there is widespread recognition that too few learning disabled people are benefiting from efforts to counter social exclusion.

Misconception and stereotyping by the public remain significant issues, including that learning disabled people cannot or do not wish to work, or are to be feared. In the learning disability nursing context, Sweeney and Mitchell (2009: 2761) explain how courses changed during the late 1980s into the 1990s and beyond to reflect 'a deeper knowledge and experience of community, public health and social work and care'. These changes were underpinned by the shift to community care with its family oriented and social care/inclusion ethos that has raised ongoing debate about the role of nurses, nursing and the health professions *vis-à-vis* social, welfare and education professions (see for example, Nehring, 2003; Northway *et al.*, 2005; Vere-Jones, 2007).

Early Years, Diagnosis, Intervention and Education

Diagnosis of learning disability may occur soon after birth in some cases, though the majority are likely to be made as a result of a recognition that the usual developmental milestones are not being met, for example through routine testing by health visitors. Sensitivity and high-quality communication skills are required to inform and support families during the period of testing and assessing, which may take a protracted period of time. The Children Act 1989 established local authorities as the lead agencies for ensuring the safety and well-being of children. Local councils are required to provide a range of services to 'children in need', for example those who are disabled, or unlikely to have a reasonable standard of health or development. Social workers conduct a multi-agency 'needs assessment', including health, social care and educational needs, and an appraisal of the needs of the child in tandem with the needs the family as a whole and carers. Typically, services include:

- short breaks
- holiday play schemes
- care at home
- some aids and adaptations
- relevant financial help and advice.

Placing the person/family at the centre of decision making is an oft quoted and visible value statement, yet particular professional cultures and customs tend to detract from collaboration, instead, driving the maintenance of existing power relations. McCray (2003b) identifies lack of understanding by nurses and social workers about interprofessional and service users relationships fuelled by conflicting values (e.g. department loyalty, bureaucracy).

As soon as a child is diagnosed, parents/families can access pre-school health services usually as input by the GP, health visitor or perhaps a specialist health visitor. Early support provision leads to improved attention to crucial developmental progress in respect of pre-linguistic skills, motor skills, and multi-sensory communication, for example through use of speech and language therapy, or physiotherapy. When full-time schooling nears, parents are faced with complex decisions about the type of schooling their child will benefit most from. In essence, the options fall into two categories:

- integration/mainstream (the child attends an ordinary primary school that is also able to provide additional support and help for them in the classroom);
- special education (special school, where more intensive and extensive help is available).

These decisions are informed by assessment for special educational needs (SEN) and the provision of a 'Statement of SEN' by the local educational authority. The legal rights of parents and guardians include the expression of their preferences for the child, in specialist or mainstream school, though these are not absolute.

Transitions, Continuing Education and Employment

When the child reaches 16 years of age, options are considered in respect of moving to a college place, a day centre or remaining in school until 19. The Valuing People Support Team and the Learning and Skills Council (LSC, 2005) detail help for individuals making these transitions so they can do courses that they want to; that help them get a job; which are enjoyable for their own sake and help people to learn new things, even if they are not looking for work; or join mainstream courses, and train while working.

After school, the social inclusion ethos aims to help people with learning disabilities engage with the world of work, wherever possible, as paid employment. Difficulties exist in the form of a general lack of understanding and appreciation by the community generally. Even in the 21st century there remain serious misconceptions, ignorance and prejudices about competence, and the 'dangers' in employing learning disabled people. The eventual outcome of this is that many people who could be almost self-sufficient are trapped into receiving financial support, effectively by a system of disincentives. Approximately 10% (or less) of people with learning disabilities are in employment, a situation compounded by low expectations and lack of training for employment (DH, 2003). To address these concerns, several initiatives are underway (DH, 2003):

- new government target for increasing numbers of people with learning disabilities in work;
- a new Workstep Programme will benefit people with learning disabilities;
- joint Department of Health/Department for Education and Employment scoping study into links between supported employment and day services;
- job brokers under the New Deal for Disabled People will have skills in working with people with learning disabilities;
- disabled people starting work will not lose Disability Living Allowance unfairly;
- learning Disability Partnership Boards to develop local employment strategies;
- better employment opportunities in public services for people with learning disabilities.

Housing and Accommodation

A place to live is regarded as a fundamental tenet of citizenship and the past three decades have witnessed many learning disabled people moving from large institutionally based living to community settings. For example, in houses and bungalows, housing networks, group homes, shared living/accommodation schemes, village schemes, rental and home ownership. Policy reflects a growing wish to help people with learning disabilities and their families to exercise more choice and preferences about their accommodation (DH, 2003). The evidence for benefits of particular types of housing on people's lives is mixed, with issues such as management style and staff training being equally as important (Felce and Emerson, 2001; Perry and Felce, 2005; Perry *et al.*, 2000).

> *. . . staffing levels within settings of a similar type were not a significant determinant of the level of interaction which residents received from staff. It is rather the way that staff work and the procedures they adopt for selecting and scheduling activities and arranging the support necessary to enable residents to participate fully (Emerson and Hatton, 1994) which are the key determinants of service quality. Jones et al. (1999) have demonstrated experimentally the beneficial impact of staff training. In their study, residents engaged in more activities at home as a result of staff being trained to give more assistance.* (Perry et al., 2000: 314)

The majority of people with learning disabilities reside with their families and only need to move should a crisis occur, such as ill health or death of a carer, a situation that demography suggests will increase as more people live with older relatives/carers in our ageing population. Planners and providers face several challenges. The Department of Health (DH, 2003) has identified that in some situations a culture exists whereby professionals adopt a 'take what you are given' stance, coupled with a less than enthusiastic approach to exploring living accommodation possibilities with people with learning disabilities.

Primary and Secondary Healthcare

In common with other marginalised groups, people with learning disabilities experience proportionally greater risks (than non-marginalised groups and individuals) associated with poverty (Palmer *et al.*, 2006), deprivation and poor health (Graham, 2004). The DRC (2006b) has identified that accessing primary care services is problematic and also, most worryingly, that some professionals' responses compound problems. Examples of people not being registered with a GP are explained by reference to them '. . . being difficult, overly demanding or aggressive' (Nocon and Sayce, 2008: 327) with questionable justification and little recourse once decisions are made. Practitioners sometimes explain access and registration problems by reference to people's impairments, effectively shifting responsibility to service users without recognition of service provider responsibility as legally defined in the Disability Discrimination Act 1995. Some staff continue to believe they are doing their best and that problems such as failures to attend appointments or follow advice are the result of users choices and actions. This is illustrative of diagnostic overshadowing (Jones *et al.*, 2008; Jopp and Keys, 2001), where physical health issues are perceived as part of the learning disability and not as valid concerns that warrant investigation. Identifying illness is made more difficult, for example, because of poor communication by staff and service users. Staff assume agreements offered by patients are indicative of informed understanding and inadequately check whether understanding of symptoms is accurate.

Of course, some staff are keen to improve practice, especially those with personal experience of disability and Nocon and Sayce (2008) present illustrative examples of good practice, including GPs offering recordings of consultations, allowing patients with a learning disability to listen again as a means of helping appreciation of diagnosis, treatment and advice. As one example of poor uptake of screening, Nocon and Sayce (2008: 328) identify that women with learning disabilities only have cervical screening at rates of 13% and 47%, whilst the general population have rates of 84% and 89%. In Wales, health checks for people with learning disabilities were introduced in 2006, England followed in 2008. People with a learning disability have an increased incidence of physical and mental health problems (Black and Hyde, 2004; Bollard, 1999; DH, 1998, 2001e, 2009; DRC, 2006b; Emerson and Hatton, 2008; Foundation for People with LD, 2001; Gates, 1997; Hardy *et al.*, 2006; Lindop and Read, 2000; Manthorpe, 2007; Marshall *et al.*, 2003; MENCAP, 2010a), including:

- visual impairment;
- hearing impairment;
- physical disability (for example, those seen in cerebral palsy);

- **epilepsy** (approximately 30%, increasing to 50% for those who have more severe learning disability;
- heart disease;
- respiratory problems;
- **Alzheimer's disease** (for example, people with Down's syndrome are living longer and seem to suffer higher rates of dementia than the general population);
- mental health problems;
- dental hygiene (unhealthy teeth and gums);
- body weight problems.

These problems and features are sustained for several reasons, including the effects of discrimination, disadvantage and social exclusion; inadequate knowledge of health needs, dependency, poor healthcare access often compounded by poor health service responses, poor literacy and communication problems.

The need for different agencies and professionals, including nurses and other providers, to work well together is paramount. The number, variety and characteristics of relevant organisations and individuals is extensive, including primary care providers, nurses, doctors, social workers, teachers, dentists, dieticians, chiropodists, therapists, commissioners of services, specialist teams, governance bodies (standard-setting and regulatory bodies) and government, local and national. The complexity of managing and monitoring these systems and individuals tends to diffuse responsibility so that accountability becomes ambiguous. Nocon and Sayce (2008: 330) outline some examples (Department of Health and national standard-setting and inspection bodies in particular) of 'buck-passing and a failure to ensure that physical health inequalities are adequately addressed'. Attempts to counter these barriers in England include the good practice guide on commissioning and providing health services for people with learning disabilities (DH, 1998) and the continuing emphasis on policy evolution and implementation in all the home countries. Despite the limitations of more macro, strategic and policy initiatives, there is evidence of good operational practice. Jackson and Read (2008) report a case study in Staffordshire, where health facilitators (for people with learning disabilities) based in primary care settings, work to improve access to primary care services through appraising and sustaining effective relationships at individual and organisational levels, achieving reduction and removal of barriers and impediments between services and professionals. (Other areas have included this role within existing positions such as community learning disability nurses.) Jackson and Read (2008) present a comprehensive account of how one person was helped and supported by a health facilitator and the team in the community and also prior, during and after hospital admission. This echoes Corbett's (2007) recognition of the necessity for people known to the patient with complex needs to provide additional support, for example during hospital admission, after surgery and perhaps during meals. Planning is crucial in this type of situation, involving open and frank dialogue between the patient, families/carers and community and hospital based professionals that has added benefits in terms of recognising and addressing myths, stereotypes and false apprehensions linked to hospital care. Similarly, in the city of Warrington, Harrison and Berry (2006) describe how health visitors provide an inclusive approach to healthcare for learning disabled people by engaging with them better and assisting their choice making, effectively demonstrating use of a public health model of healthcare that supports people through providing information that is both accessible and understood in respect of lifestyle and actions.

Whilst many learning disability nurses and policy makers have gradually shifted positions towards promotion of the autonomy of people with learning disabilities coupled with health promotion, some nurses seem not to appreciate this latter element of their work nor even that the language of healthcare (with its associations with predominantly physical issues and illness) is relevant (Turnbull, 2004). Obvious questions arise from these considerations: has the healthcare role been used to justify inclusion of learning disability nurses as members of the nursing profession generally? What relevance is the certainty that people with a learning disability have significant unmet healthcare needs? Although difference of view amongst professionals, academics and the public exists in tangible forms (literature) Turnbull seems to take a pragmatic route and suggests that whatever our views, the 'key issue for learning disability nurses would be to ensure that this role [health promotion] enhances their capacity to support the rights and independence of people with learning disabilities' (Turnbull, 2004: 63).

Normalisation, Independence, Rights and Risk-Taking

Normalisation

This, and its related concept of social role valorisation (Nirje, 1992; Race, 1999; Wolfensberger, 1972, 1984, 2000) is concerned with adopting valued means of providing services and help for people who are devalued. So, for example, normalisation (and SRV) promotes creating opportunities for learning disabled people to experience everyday activities and patterns of living that mirror those of mainstream society. In simple terms, it is about assisting people to live an ordinary life in an ordinary community and with the effect of building their esteem as a means to diminishing stigma associated with devalued status (for example as accompanying learning disability, mental illness or old age). Services adopting normalisation principles aim to enable living in 'normal' family situations, where relationships can develop and flourish, where schools educate all children together without segregation, where adult life incorporates close, including sexual, relationships and where learning disabled people can enjoy the opportunities, responsibilities, choices and decision making that most people value. In the 1970s and later, normalisation fuelled the development of community-based services with a concurrent reduction in hospital provision, in line with the drive to improve people's lives and choices. Normalisation has attracted strong advocates and protagonists with Culham and Nind (2003: 66) expressing examples of 'fierce debate' in Europe and the UK. At the positive end of the spectrum tangible benefits are ascribed (Culham and Nind, 2003: 69):

> *Normalisation-inspired activity has included de-institutionalisation, to be replaced by ever smaller group homes in ordinary houses in ordinary streets and the use of ordinary education, health and leisure facilities (KFC, 1980)* [King's Fund Centre, 1980].

More negatively, these authors comment that (Culham and Nind, 2003: 70):

> *The real legacy of the normalisation movement can be seen to be a status quo that has been largely unchallenged. The power dynamics in which professionals hold on to key decision-making is unthreatened (Aspis, 1997; Chappell, 1992). Schools, colleges and workplaces have been required to do little to respond to the needs and rights of people with an intellectual disability and nothing major in terms of their systems and structures. People with an intellectual disability are present in services for ordinary people, due mostly to their own attempts (or attempts by others 'on their behalf') to conform and be invisible* (Rapley, Kiernan and Antaki, 1998).

So, there are simultaneous yet contradictory perceptions of the utility of normalisation/SRV. First, that it has undoubtedly improved the lives of people with a learning disability, through impacts upon teaching skills required for development, achieving respect and dignity and creating opportunities and choices about living and working, and with whom (relationships). Second, that it represents a somewhat utopian model for service development and for removing prejudices. To assume that social prejudices, including those of devalued groups/people themselves, will be remedied by a relatively simple integration with 'normal' society seems naive and leans a little too heavily on the notion that mutual aid, support and beneficent attitudes and actions are more commonplace than they actually are. This is has especial resonance with societies where extended family networks are reducing and where increased numbers of people live on their own, where networks of families and friends are decreased or are temporary rather than enduring.

In the UK, present day services for people with learning disabilities are provided in keeping with an evolving appreciation of values, normalisation/SRV, social inclusion and person centred planning (DH, 2001e, 2009; Dowling *et al.*, 2007; Ritchie *et al.*, 2003; Thompson *et al.*, 2008). Person-centred planning is presented in more detail below.

Rights, Independence, Choice and Risk

UK policy has reflected the developing legal, civil and human rights of people with learning disabilities, their independence, choice, and social inclusion. Legal and civil rights are designed to remove discrimination, though almost invariably only partially effect their aims. Law does offer recourse for individuals to challenge decisions and actions, for example when they perceive being discriminated against because of disability (intellectual and/or physical) or their actions, behaviour and modes of expression, speech and talk. The Disability Discrimination Act 1995 stipulates rights of disabled people that support ending discrimination, for example in employment, buying/renting property or land. The Race Relations Acts 1976 and 2000 and the Sex Discrimination Act 1975 are other examples of attempts to promote fairness and equity throughout society. Civil rights (specific to a country or district) include eligibility to vote, to receive relevant benefits and have legal representation. Human rights (see the Human Rights Act, 1998 which became operational in the UK in 2000) include the right to life, freedom of speech, freedom from abuse and freedom to practice a religion of choice. Moral rights do not usually carry the power of other types, they originate from the general and gradual shifting of society's moral positions, depending on goodwill and intrinsic senses of 'right and wrong', for example that everyone has the right to be treated with dignity and respect.

People with learning disabilities are considered able to make their own decisions and exercise their autonomy, with appropriate support if needed. Herein lies something of a conundrum; what might count as a boundary for the learning disabled person's autonomy of decision making? What would count as a legitimate overriding of a person's decision, for example, acting against their wishes yet justifiably in their interests? For a more extensive account of this type of moral tension, see Holloway (2007). Redley and Weinberg (2007) support the shift from biomedical to social constructionist understandings of learning disability but examine the tensions and contradictions involved in exercising autonomy, particularly as self-determining, independent decision making by people deemed, by definition, to have compromised decision-making ability and who are likely to be life-long dependent on others, and who are always vulnerable. For most people, making choices and decisions is a welcome aspect of life that contributes to individuality and a sense of control, particularly in respect of major decisions, such as where to work, live, receive treatment or help and also who to confide in, trust, accept as a friend or intimate. For learning disabled people, appreciating and processing relevant information is often more difficult.

Adults, including those with learning disability, have a legal right to consent (Gillings-Taylor, 2004). In a minority of cases, incapacity may be appraised (DHSSPS, 2003; DH, 2001a, 2001b, 2001c; WAG, 2002) perhaps as required by a court, but most choices and decisions made by learning disabled adults can be honoured with the provision of adequate support that achieves verified understanding. This equates to valid consent and requires three criteria: (i) the person must be competent, able to decide; (ii) he or she must be acting freely without coercion; and (iii) sufficient and pertinent information must be provided in ways that ensure understanding (Gillings-Taylor, 2004).

Seeking informed consent means professionals have to appraise abilities and competence and then communicate effectively with the learning disabled person. As well as using aids and communication tools (Apraiz, 2001; Manthorpe, 2007; Sowney and Barr, 2007; van der Gaag, 1998) it is vital that professionals attend closely and purposively, listen actively, noticing non-verbal signs (eye contact, tone, body language, facial expression, gestures) and avoid making assumptions. Knowledge of the person will assist in appreciating subtle and complex expressions. Conclusions should be regarded as tentative and checked, perhaps through offering information in alternative ways, or in smaller volumes on multiple occasions. Where individuals are unable to decide independently, assistance should be provided after consideration of who is best placed to help and without self- or vested interest. Citizen Advocates (DH, 2001e) have an obvious role to play. Unfortunately, dealing adequately with communication issues is not always properly addressed (Cable *et al.*, 2003; DH, 2001a, 2001b, 2001e) with an association often made (erroneously) between decision making and learning disability that discounts the person's active involvement. In hospitals, disabled people are often not spoken with directly, nor are their decisions (about their health) sought and nor are they asked for consent to examination, treatment and care (Barr, 2004; Hutchinson, 2005; MENCAP, 2004b). These issues require attention to communication skills and also to attitudes so that practitioners are not only able to engage effectively with people and patients but also seek to do so rather than act (or decline to act) because of negative assumptions.

Promoting choice invariably includes some degree of risk for the individual and also, perhaps, for practitioners who may adopt defensive approaches as a means of dealing cautiously (too much so) with tensions between choice, empowerment, vulnerability and risk (Bertram and Stickley, 2005; Mullen *et al.*, 2008). This is especially relevant where a blame culture is perceived (Attree, 2007; Ehrich, 2006; Kerfoot, 2008) and can sometimes present as an illusory or 'Hobson's' choice, a 'take it or leave it' situation which does not constitute active choosing from valid options by the person.

Clear and relevant risk policies help to illuminate definitions of risk that take account of likelihood, implications and consequences and are an essential part of agencies and practitioners ensuring people with learning disabilities experience fulfilling lives. Risk and risk assessment are complex concepts and more comprehensive accounts can be seen in Sellars (2002) and Alaszweski and Alaszweski (2005). Illustrations of risk assessment and practice application can be found in Hogan *et al.* (2007), McNamara *et al.* (2008) and Stein (2005). These authors explore how serious, relevant perceived hazards or dangers are likely to occur, if at all, what should be provided, how and how often, and with which relevant safeguards. Legal requirements, the roles of emancipation, dignity and balance of actions and safeguards are all appraised against background issues such as negative aspects of bureaucracy (such as defensive practice) and the growth of litigation. Person-centred planning (PCP) lends itself to bridging the disparities and tensions involved, whilst actively valuing the disabled person's wishes and contributions as core in constructing and implementing life plans. In synopsis, key elements of risk assessment and management include:

- **Clarification of perceived risk** Collective dialogue and appraisal that adopts suitable language and expression will promote shared understanding of risk(s) and context(s).
- **Frequency** What do we know of, how often, or in what patterns the issue occurs? What, if any, precursors are identified?
- **Consequences** What are the implications and effects on the individual, families, carers, public and organisations? What implications and effects apply should the risk be avoided or action delayed?
- **Risk management** How can risks be managed and/or reduced? What safeguards and support are required? How should evaluation be planned and implemented?
- **Planning and collective agreement** Assessment should explicate the risk; how, when and why consequences are likely to happen; preferred ways of managing the risk and who has which responsibilities. Records of all meetings and contributions should be stored securely and highlight details of decisions agreed and their rationale.

ACTIVITY 8-2

Reflect on what you have just read and explore what risks might apply in a baby's childhood and what principles should guide how help is provided?

Communication

This section is designed to complement more detailed accounts of, and texts on, communication. After a very brief explanation of communication, the section addresses those issues, knowledge and skills that have particular relevance to learning disability nursing contexts.

Communication is fundamental to human life. It involves people sending and receiving messages that result in mutual understanding, a two-way process. It may take the form of words, spoken or written, and also other forms of presenting ideas and information, such as through art, imagery and music. Verbal communication refers to speech, and is intrinsically linked to tone of voice, volume, hesitancy and emphasis as well as to non-verbal or body language, facial expressions, eye contact, posture, gesture and spatial awareness (personal space). Combinations of all these produce complex messages that are interpreted in context, sometimes accurately, sometimes not. The complexity of communication, speech, language and perception is illustrated well through humour. Often, a joke can only be understood as funny because people appreciate relevant links and connections, the absurd often causes us to stop thinking for a moment and to see new connections and patterns that push our thinking in unanticipated directions (Greenwood and Levin, 1998: 107).

Most learning disabled people have some form of communication difficulty which may be caused or exacerbated by other sensory problems, such as visual or hearing loss. Total communication (MENCAP, 2010d) is way of thinking about how people communicate by constantly seeking and using best methods in context, at any given time including using:

- gestures, pointing, facial expressions;
- signing, for example, Makaton (2010), or Signalong (2010) or British Sign Language (2010);

PRACTICE GUIDELINES

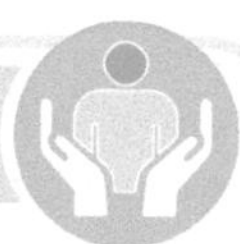

Communication Principles when Speaking with Learning Disabled People

- **Face-to-face communication** - each person with a learning disability, like all people, is an individual with specific communication needs and strengths. However, the principles below are useful for nurses to adopt when speaking with a person who is learning disabled.
- **Talk to the person** and attempt to clarify things that are unclear and check mutual understanding. If the person does not respond or if doubt persists, then they should be asked for permission to seek help/clarification from relevant carers.
- **Simple, commonplace language should be used**. Long sentences and elaborate language should be avoided. Instructions should be presented in small segments with each step clarified before proceeding sequentially, to guarantee mutual understanding.
- **Talk about things in the here and now**. Some people may find it difficult to understand the concept of time. Providing written information, for example, for appointment times, is better than merely telling the person to 'attend next Wednesday'. Visual materials including drawings, images, photos are useful in supporting and complimenting what is said.
- **Check that the person has understood**. Sometimes, a learning disabled person may seem to have understood, perhaps even repeating words expressed. This does not necessarily signify understanding. Nurses should seek responses in the persons' own words that paraphrase the nurses', indicating meaningful appreciation and understanding.
- **Literal uses of phrases, words and sentences**. Speaking figuratively or metaphorically, including colloquialisms such as 'Did you sleep a wink last night?' or 'I'm absolutely beat today' are unhelpful. Nurses should speak more literally, for example stating 'Did you sleep all night?' and 'I am very tired today'.

PRACTICE GUIDELINES

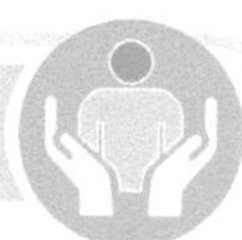

Principles When Using Written Communication with Learning Disabled People

When communicating in writing with people with a learning disability:

- Plan what and how you wish to present, taking care to adopt clear, easily recognised and plain text. Keep sentences short and minimise punctuation. Jargon, nomenclature and complex language are best avoided.
- If you must include difficult words or terms (health and social care are complex arenas) then only do so with accompanying simpler words and terms that explain the issue.
- Present materials in a logical sequence avoiding unnecessary detail.
- Bullet points and/or illustrative graphics can often assist clarification and emphasis of points that are made.
- Similarly, use of images, photos, sketches or symbols support understanding of text. Often, these may express key messages much more obviously than text alone. Note that abstract symbols are likely to detract from accurate perception - keep use of graphics to those that effectively convey messages.

- symbols, pictures representing words;
- objects, for example a cup could mean 'I am thirsty';
- photographs – used to show someone what a person wants, has been doing or wants to talk about;
- drawing;
- writing;
- speech, speaking whilst using other methods is recommended.

Box 8-1 and *Box 8-2* illustrate practice guidelines that should inform nurses' considerations and actions when communicating in person or in writing with people with a learning disability.

Nurses should not assume the person cannot speak and should use simple everyday language in short sentences. Any requests or instructions should be similarly phrased and conveyed in small sections that help checking of understanding before proceeding to the next part or section. If the person is not responsive or there is lack of clarity, only then should they be asked for permission to involve carers. Gestures and signing of key words, for example using Makaton, will help the person understand better than if only speech is used, as might aids like photos or symbols because visual information is often easier to interpret. Nurses must allow the person sufficient time to speak for themselves, perhaps allowing more time for more complicated issues, such as making appointments or negotiating medication or treatment choices. It is not uncommon for learning disabled people to find waiting, crowds or groups, or smaller spaces anxiety provoking, so nurses should minimise delays, for example, by offering the first appointment of the day to the person. During conversation, speak in the here and now. It may be that appreciating time is difficult for the person and so providing written details of appointments is better than simply asking them to 'return next Friday at 10am'. Again, using visual communication aids such as drawings, pictures or signs all assist in accurate perception and understanding, though checking thoroughly is essential. Even when the person repeats what has been said and agreed, it does not necessarily mean they have understood. Understanding is indicated if the person can recall agreements in paraphrased terms, that is, if they are able to use their own words and reflect accuracy of meaning, then understanding is evident. Words and sentences should be used in as literal a way as possible, because of added difficulty in understanding analogy or metaphor. So, for example, say 'it is hard to find your umbrella . . .' rather than 'it's like looking for a needle in a haystack'.

Using written communication demands clear and simple text (plain English), no jargon, short sentences and simple punctuation. Bullet points and story boxes help to highlight main points and can be easily supplemented by images, photos or symbols. Crucially, these images and symbols need to effectively supplement and convey messages and so using more abstract examples should be avoided, unless the person is known to be familiar with them. Often, placing images at one side with text adjacent makes for a clear and illustrative communicative message.

Unnecessary detail should be avoided and by using plain language details should be presented in a logical, one step at a time manner. Abbreviations are to be avoided. If difficult words are required they should be complemented by a list of descriptive terms in explanation. Short sentences that include a single idea or message are best as is minimal punctuation. Try not to include semicolons (;), colons (:), hyphens (-) or too many commas. Wherever possible, personalise the writing by using the individual's name and 'you', 'we' and 'I'. Consistency of word use should be adopted, for example, if the person understands the term 'treatment' do not substitute it later with 'therapy'.

Ferris-Taylor (2007) distinguishes between speech and language (language as a system of meaning) and notes that considerable discrepancies may exist between comprehension (what is perceived and understood) and expression (what is said) in people with learning disabilities. This, once again, highlights the crucial importance of nurses checking with the person about their shared understanding. Disability, discrimination and human rights legislation have placed more accessible forms of communication, including use of signs and pictorial symbol systems, in statute. Communication has shifted from 'person to person' contexts (focusing on the individual with learning disabilities as the 'problem') into more socially oriented models of disability with a concurrent recognition of a need for everyone to change the way we communicate with, and our attitudes towards, people with learning and communication difficulties. Interaction is everyone's responsibility and requires consideration of culture, race, environment and sensory perception. Effective communication requires active involvement with others and genuine opportunities for choosing, including choosing from relevant modes of technology, such as augmenting hearing, vision and communicative systems.

Van der Gaag (1998) also illuminates the social dimension to communication (as distinct from micro, person-to-person interaction) and uses the term 'professional myopia' to describe a professional tendency to focus on intrinsic aspects of communication difficulty, that is, difficulty arising within the person with a learning disability. The counter to this 'myopia' is to accept extrinsic sources of difficulty, those arising 'outside' of the individual. Examples of intrinsic difficulties include intelligibility, fluency and rate of speech, comprehension, recall, concentration skills and social skills.

These types of features are often linked with physical manifestations such as cleft palate, cerebral palsy, hearing and visual loss. All of these factors are interrelated to social and personal contexts, so that when learning disabled people live in places where they are not given chances to communicate they underutilise the communication skills they have. Invariably, this leads to reduction in self-esteem, social isolation, loneliness, acquiescence, frustration and anger. Van der Gaag (1998) suggests that challenging behaviour is often a means of communication that works for the learning disabled person, when other means have proved ineffective. So, once again, nurses need to learn about and appreciate micro and macro influences, personal, cultural and social dimensions to effective communication with people with a learning disability and their families and carers.

Research, like practice itself, is illustrative of the wide variety and complexity of both professional and personal issues experienced by individual learning disabilities' nurses and the profession as a whole. Specific examples of broad systemic and cultural influences include professional marginalisation (Talbot *et al.*, 2010: 173) and effects of language and discourse (for example, see Shaw, 2009). The Royal College of Nursing (RCN, 2011) has attempted to appraise relevant challenges and suggests actions required to assist future development. These include enhancing nurse education through promoting evidence-based approaches, helping the workforce to adopt inclusive and partnership approaches at local and national levels and to support and promote learning disability nursing leadership. These more systemic, organisational or macro elements should be viewed alongside the more micro, personal arenas that constitute nurses 'everyday' experiences.

Learning disabilities' nurses need to possess and demonstrate constructive levels of self-awareness in their interactions and relationships. Their personal values' systems and ethical standpoints impact significantly in what they do, how and to what effect, not least in respect of their research mindedness, reflective and critical thinking abilities. Relevant literature has echoed practical means of assisting nurses and organisations in understanding, appreciating and developing relevant knowledge skills and attributes. For example, clinical supervision (Lynch *et al.*, 2008; Sines and McNully, 2007) has provided time for nurses to reflect with competent colleagues to clarify, make sense and learn from practice experience in supportive, constructive ways. Similarly, emotional intelligence (Akerjordet and Severinsson, 2007; Goleman, 1996; McQueen, 2004; Stichler, 2006) is becoming better understood as a requirement for nurses and nursing practice. McCallin and Bamford (2007) illustrate links between emotional intelligence and interdisciplinary work, team effectiveness, quality of client care, staff retention and job satisfaction.

Person-Centred Planning and Working with Families

Person-centred planning (PCP) has some links with normalisation in that both are principled ways of influencing service development geared towards identifying what is needed to offer 'normal' opportunities for living, work, friendships and relationships for individuals with learning disabilities (DH, 2010: 3):

> *A number of reports and inquiries during the past three years have highlighted the continuing inequalities faced by many people with learning disabilities and the devastating effect this has had in some cases, including Death by Indifference (MENCAP, 2006), Healthcare for All (Department of Health 2008) and the Joint Ombudsman report Six Lives (The Stationery Office, 2009). In light of recommendations from these reports, it is particularly important that professionals ensure that they fully utilise the tools and support systems available through Health Action Planning (as part of person-centred planning) to recognise individuals' needs for 'reasonable adjustments' to enable vulnerable people to access healthcare and to get the care and treatment they need.*

Person-centred planning (PCP) (Alaszewski and Alaszewski, 2005; Carnaby and Cambridge, 2005; DH, 2001d; Ritchie *et al.*, 2003) represents a new way of working with people with disabilities. Rather than an agency or professional focus, PCP places the person at the heart of assessment and planning. Instead of professionals determining needs and aims for people, usually in multi-disciplinary team meetings, PCP requires a 'person-centred approach' that reflects precisely what the person with a learning disability sees as important to him or herself. Professionals' roles are to keep listening and learning what is important to the person and to take actions in tandem with the person, family and friends. This in turn requires an attitude illustrative of relationships characterised by 'power with' and not 'power over' (Sweeney and Sanderson, 2002: 1) effectively switching perception from disability first, person second to the opposite (person first, disability second).

Person-centred planning has a basis in principles associated with rights, freedom of choice and independence relevant to individuals making informed choices about how they live and what support is required. The person, family and friends are partners with professionals in understanding particular wishes and aspirations in ways that foster creative approaches to achievement and usually involve shared appraisal of conflict, safety and risk. PCP matches ability with aims as a step towards identifying necessary support systems that enable people to make valued contributions, a quite different ethos to the former service delivery mode that tended to fit people into categories. A collective, shared approach to taking agreed actions and building ongoing commitment is a dynamic feature of PCP that improves the life chances and opportunities of individuals and also broader service delivery and evaluative systems. PCP is useful for anyone, irrespective of their status or abilities, and differs from traditional assessment and care planning in that prescribed or pre-specified eligibility criteria are not used, so that excluding people is avoided. It does not replace all other forms of planning, instead it functions to ensure other planning systems complement PCP, making them effective for the person.

Different Approaches to PCP

PCP is designed to answer questions, 'Who are you and who are we in your life?' and 'What can we do together to achieve a better life for you now and in the future?' Different emphases apply in terms of ways that information is sought and detail about everyday life or development of plans for the longer-term future. All approaches use:

- questions – these help appreciation of the person and their life and situation;
- particular ways of engaging with people, working together and agreeing decisions.

Individuals may need to attend to different aspects of their lives at different times, using one planning style or another one at a different time, as needed. It might be a priority to learn about everyday matters first, and then move on to thinking about the future, or alternatively, people's dreams may figure first as the prominent element for consideration, with everyday issues following. Specific approaches include:

1. Essential lifestyle planning (Smull and Burke-Harrison, 1992) uses specific headings (for example, communication) to focus on a person's life in the present and represents a considerably detailed planning format suggesting how life may be improved. It facilitates people discovering and identifying what is important to them and the types/degrees of support needed.
2. Individual service design (Sanderson *et al.*, 1997) focuses on the past to help deepen the shared understanding about, and commitment to, the person, based on supporting people to become self-determining citizens.
3. Personal futures planning (Mount and Zwernik, 1988) involves a group of people committed to describing a person's current life and imagining what they would like in the future. It differs from PATH (see below) in that it assists learning about the person's life (PATH assumes this knowledge) and creates a vision for the future.
4. MAPs (Vandercook *et al.*, 1989) and PATH (Pearpoint *et al.*, 1993) focus predominantly on a desirable future or dream and what it would take to move closer to that. PATH places particular emphasis on direct and immediate planning linked with action.

Evidence that PCP is having positive effects on people's lives is provided by Robertson *et al.* (2005: 113):

> *. . . results . . . have indicated that PCP is both efficacious and effective in improving the life experiences of people with learning disabilities, benefits that come without significant additional service costs. It has also, however, indicated that some people are more likely than others to experience the benefits of PCP and that the benefits associated with PCP do not extend into certain areas of peoples' lives. The research has also identified some organisational factors that need to be attended to, for successful implementation.*

These authors stress the need for developing policy and practice so that as many people as possible are able to access benefits associated with PCP, and the need to confront inequalities in access and efficacy. O'Brien and Towell (2003) report positive changes in staff working to advance self-determination of people with learning disabilities. Robertson *et al.* (2005) illustrate the ongoing policy context and the need to clarify the impact of PCP, for example, on social exclusion, employment and health. Expectations are raised in terms of improved choice, control and individualisation of support (DH, 2005; Prime Minister's Strategy Unit, 2005; Routledge, 2006).

Working with Families

Families, like individuals, are unique and differences of need, resource availability and context will apply and be shaped by factors such as the age of the learning disabled person. Children with a learning disability present families and services with particular issues, which tend to shift as transitions to adulthood, maturity and older age occur. In the foreword of the report 'First Impressions' (Davies and Holstrom, 2005) Professor Barry Carpenter describes his own family experiences of having a child with Down's syndrome.

> *... my wife and I met professionals who were empathetic human beings and whose rich professional skills, combined with their humanity, had a powerful impact on our family life. But we met others who hid behind their professional labels, and whose intervention was a hindrance, and diminished our quality of life.*

Help from a variety of professionals including social, educational and health services, as well as voluntary and private organisations, raises the spectre of fragmented or disjointed provision with consequent frustrations and ineffectiveness. Person-centred planning is designed to assist professionals and families to work together better, to avoid, recognise and remedy negative attitudes, actions and effects. Relationships are the cornerstone of PCP and professionals, nurses included, need to explore, develop and enact a shared, agreed set of values that are demonstrative of mutual respect, trust and commitment to person-centred care. In our multicultural society, nurses need to appreciate the relevance of differing cultures, beliefs and values in relation to learning disabilities and recognise individuality, individual differences and implications for planning. This will avoid providing the same services to all, irrespective of background, and will require careful consideration about treatment modes, gender and dress codes, timing and providing information in appropriate languages. Power (2009) reviewed families' experiences (in Ireland) of accessing services, day care, special vocational training and respite places on behalf of their young adult children. This research presents evidence for concern that significant gaps exist between government rhetoric and service provision 'on the ground'. Most worryingly, Power shows that despite improved funding, the system often works for the system, not for the user, an antithesis for PCP.

Collaboration, by definition, includes sharing power, a challenge for more traditional professionals or those whose view it is that title and professional status equate (absolutely) to 'being right' all the time. The knowledge possessed by family members is often much more relevant and applicable to informed action and professionals must be open to acknowledging this. Additionally, involvement must apply to all family members who wish to be involved, and not limited, for example, only to those who the nurse meets regularly during visits. This may require managing timing of visits to ensure different family members are not excluded.

Providing information in ways that ensure families are effectively informed is a key role for nurses. Presenting information in ways that enhance understanding and routinely checking for feedback will enhance relationships, support and development. Davies and Holstrom (2005: 7) report half of parents interviewed saying 'they did not receive adequate information at the time of diagnosis, and were unsure where to go for information'. Of course, there is a balance to be struck between providing too little and too much information, and in ways that foster understanding. The same research cites other parents (Davies and Holstrom, 2005: 8):

> *... on the first visit they gave me too much information ... it's great there's so much out there but it can be too much to absorb. Even if your child doesn't have a disability you're adjusting to your life with a baby – you've just given birth, your lifestyle has changed, you're exhausted. On top of that you have to come to terms with something you hadn't anticipated; there is a danger of being bombarded.*

These authors outline six areas that parents of young children identify as warranting support:

- emotional support;
- information about their child's condition;
- information about services;
- accessing services;
- coordinating services;
- developing a 'whole picture' of the child.

The areas relating to services (information, access and coordination) have attracted continuing criticism from people with learning disabilities and their families, that they are complex and difficult to access (Manthorpe, 2007: 86). This is compounded by local variation, availability and differing lines of accountability. Manthorpe (2007) provides the examples of some areas having community learning disability teams whilst others do not, regular service reorganisations (with invariable upheavals) and frequent staff turnover. Also, as children grow and move through adolescence and adulthood to old age, the type and form of services required will similarly evolve.

Figure 8-4 is based on descriptions and illustrations presented by Barr (1996) and Gates (1997) and shows the types of services available, though readers should note that shape, structure and form of service provision is significantly 'localised' as described above. Nurses have parts to play in mainstream (generic) and specialist domains. They can work with families and individuals to help to improve or maintain physical and mental health. These are prerequisites for negotiating and

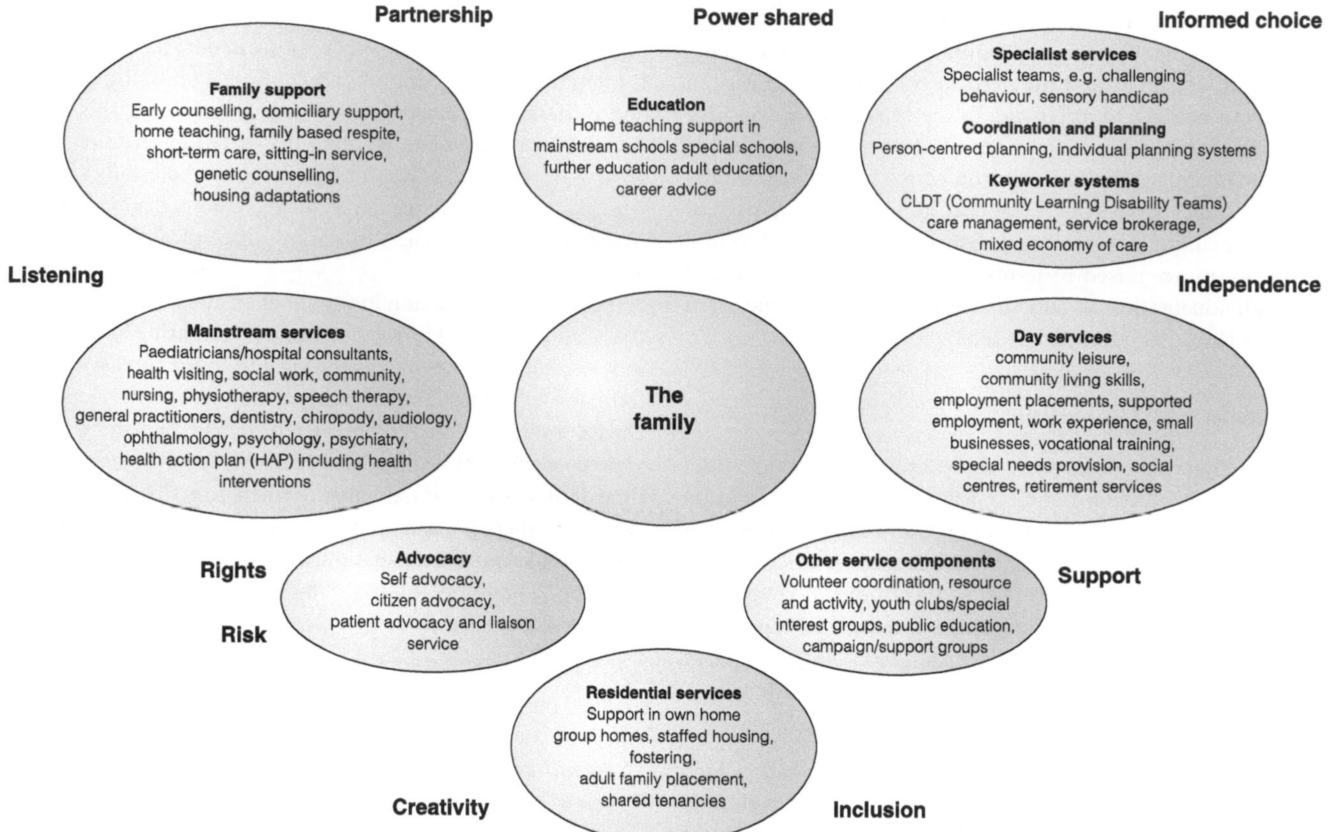

Figure 8-4 An illustration of service provision.
Source: based on Barr, O. (1996) and Gates, B. (ed.) (1997).

resolving barriers that impede goals and opportunities for learning disabled people. Health and avoiding or effectively treating illness, pave the way for optimal independence and ultimately, inclusion. Nurses contribute towards health promotion and education, preventive strategies and screening programmes, as well as training in life and social skills or employment prospects. Nurses need demonstrably good communication skills, including self-evaluative and intuitive dimensions.

Helping to Empower People and Advocacy

Advocacy and empowerment are inextricably related, since both involve contributing to the means that enable people to have increased control of their lives. Clement (2002) is critical of the lack of precision in definitions of these terms, and suggests that empowerment is a value insofar as it is a positive idea that applies to different situations whilst it also refers to how people should act, to 'empower' others. Advocacy means to speak up for someone (BILD, 2010) or:

> . . . *speaking or acting on behalf of oneself or another person or an issue with self-sacrificing vigour and vehemence* (Williams and Schoultz, 1979: 92)

Both can be understood in at least two dimensions: first, as people's subjective experience linked with their rights, choices and control that contribute to self-determining, autonomous living. Second, as a professional function concerned with anti-discriminatory practice, gauging rights and relevant responsibilities that inform safe and ethical practice (Gray and Jackson, 2002). Even cursory reflective attention reveals some dichotomy between advocacy and autonomy, in the sense that if I am autonomous then I (surely) have no need for someone else to speak up for me? Enter the notions of assertiveness and ethics as they relate to advocacy (see, for example, Bateman, 2000; Kubsch *et al.*, 2004; Porter and Yahne, 1995).

People with a learning disability, by definition, are relatively more vulnerable than others, and so part of supporting them has to be aimed towards minimising their dependency, ensuring they get and understand information that assists their self-advocacy and rights assertion. This micro-level dimension is supplemented by a wider role for advocacy as it impacts upon policy development and service development, where learning disabled people's and carers/families' views are instrumental in influencing design that meets need. Advocacy is now regarded as an essential policy and operational element in supporting people with learning disabilities with an increase in local advocacy groups being sustained (BILD, 2010). Many of these are based in the voluntary sector, often with some paid employees and with varying modes of operating. In most instances, advocacy training is provided to highlight main values, principles and responsibilities of the role and a system of ongoing monitoring and support for advocates. Gray and Jackson (2002) provide a detailed review and critique of a variety of forms of advocacy, whilst (in the same text) Walmsley (2002) compares and contrasts Self-Advocacy and Citizen Advocacy. Below, the three main types are explained.

Self-Advocacy

This is people being able to speak up for themselves, perhaps with support from friends, family, neighbours or professionals. Local self-advocacy groups provide a forum for people to offer mutual support, confidence building activities (such as role playing) and collective, more representative feedback about plans for organisation or service initiatives.

Citizen Advocacy

This involves establishing a friendship between a person with a learning disability and a local (usually lay) person. Because the relationship is based on friendship, trust and complete independence and separation from public bodies, expressing honest views is regarded as easier and more likely than if a professional sought feedback. If the learning disabled person needs support, then the friend is well placed to provide it so that views are communicated meaningfully. Citizen advocates are often volunteers who have been approved by a local group and are able to sustain advocate-partner relationships via friendship, trust and confidentiality. Advocates are linked with 'partners' by virtue of mutual interest and commitment. Usually, informal meetings and discussions are scheduled so that both parties can make informed decisions about acceptance. The person with a learning disability, of course, is the final arbiter of who should advocate for them. They are not relatives of the person and function always to help loyally represent their partner's own choices and decisions without adding any personal or biased influences. The relationship may endure for as long as either party wishes. Advocates are not substitutes for professionals, such as a nurse or social worker, or to cover holes and weaknesses in services which should otherwise be provided. Finally, citizen advocates are neither referees nor some form of arbitration in solving disagreements.

Instrumental or Issue-Based Advocacy

This refers to advocacy that addresses an outstanding issue that is likely to require particular knowledge, skill or expertise, for example, about housing, health, financial benefits or immigration. Usually, this form of advocacy involves remuneration and the duration of advocacy is linked with the outcome of the issue. Unlike citizen advocacy, concluding the arrangements is time oriented. Instrumental advocacy is not a discrete alternative to citizen or self-advocacy but complements them.

In all types and cases, advocacy relationships are confidential (to the learning disabled person and advocate partner). Where partnerships endure, it is not uncommon that they evolve toward longer-term friendships that add high-quality support and safeguards for people and their interests, particularly when people live in long-term, residential settings (BILD, 2010).

A Thought-Provoking Nursing Perspective

Advocacy and nursing share a lengthy history, perhaps unsurprisingly, since nurses spend considerable time with people who are in pain or anguish, or people who care for someone in pain or anguish, or who are dying and all of whom are especially vulnerable. Kubsch *et al.* (2004) present small scale, but extremely illustrative research that elaborates advocacy in nursing. The study differentiates nurses who act as simple 'go-betweens' (e.g. noticing a patient's need and calling for medical attention) and those who embrace advocacy as opportunities to responsibly (Kubsch *et al.*, 2004: 44):

> *. . . intercede as risk-takers and role-breakers when advocating for patient welfare within spiritual, moral-ethical, legal, political, and substitutive contexts.*

The study adopts Kohlberg's (1981) theory that outlines three levels of moral development. In level 1, the nurse acts as advocate as a means of avoiding punishment. The next level involves the nurse acting as advocate in line with policy, procedure or law and in doing so they gain affirmation from others. In level 3, the nurse acts as advocate because of the intrinsic qualities of doing good for and on behalf of, people, acting autonomously with self-determination, effectively being 'a risk-taker/role-breaker' in pursuing fairness. Figure 8-5 is a modified illustration of Kubsch's categories of nurse advocacy. The relevance and interrelationship of Kubsch's and Kohlberg's work for advocacy by nurses with learning disabled people and families are implicit. They are made explicit by reference (for example) to:

- **Legal advocate** – Disability Discrimination Acts 1995 and 2005, stipulation of rights in terms of employment, education, access to goods, facilities and services, including transport,

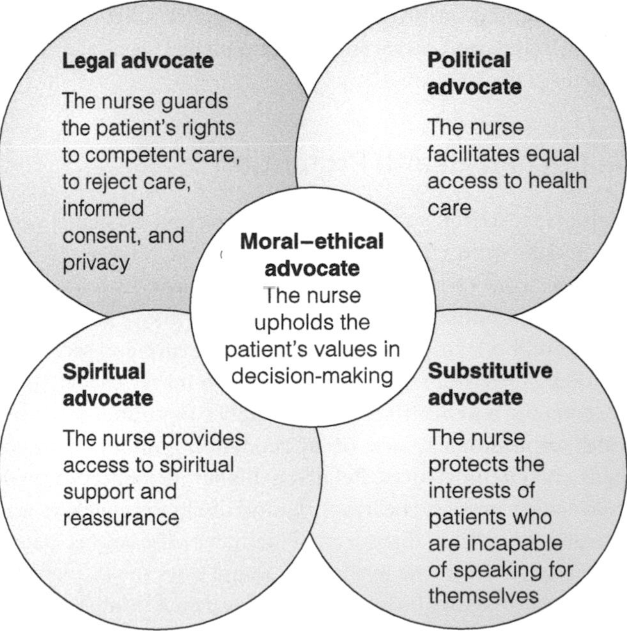

Figure 8-5 Nurse advocacy.
Source: based on Kubsch *et al.* (2004).

buying or renting land or property, and that public bodies promote equality of opportunity for disabled people.

- **Moral–ethical advocate** – PCP, policy and procedure that upholds the patient's values in decision and choice making as moral and ethical standards (not simply 'good practice' or kindness).
- **Political advocate** – Linking micro with more macro dimensions, such as the particular relevance of nursing in respect of equal access to, and provision of, healthcare.
- **Spiritual advocate** – spirituality in nursing is prompting increasing attention and research activity with a broad spectrum of views (Alaszewski and Alaszewski, 2005; Becker, 2009; Begley, 2009; Clarke, 2009; Duggleby *et al.*, 2009; Ellis and Narayanasamy, 2009; Leathard and Cook, 2009; Paley, 2009; Pesut, 2008). Narayanasamy *et al.* (2002) provide an account specifically in relation to learning disabilities.
- **Substitutive advocate** – learning disabled people are recognised as being generally more susceptible to exclusion and marginalisation. Even when some are capable of speaking for themselves, their voices are often unacknowledged. Nurses have a lengthy history as advocating for those unable to speak for themselves; in learning disability contexts they must move beyond being a 'go-between'.

Kubsch *et al.* (2004: 44) promote advocate for advocacy in nursing, characterising it as an independent complementary therapy, such are its claimed beneficial effects. The literature offers a more extensive and disparate set of claims and counter claims with authors like Willard (1996) suggesting advocacy is misplaced in nursing (due to its conceptual confusion with beneficence). More recent work tends to draw more positive connections between the role of the nurse and responsibilities for empowering, not as a single event, but a process of analysing, responding and whistle blowing, in practice allied to voicing responsiveness and active support of patients' needs and wishes (Vaartio *et al.*, 2006).

Health and Health Promotion

Health is inextricably related to well-being and social inclusion, and people with a learning disability are at greater risk of a wide spectrum of health problems. It is clear that people with learning disabilities experience relatively poor standards of healthcare, both in primary (community) care and secondary (hospital) provisions. We know they take up fewer invitations for screening and health checks, possibly compounded by some health professionals' lack of understanding about particular needs and circumstances. Relatively higher incidences of problems include: eyesight; hearing; physical disability; epilepsy; heart disorder; breathing disorder; Alzheimer's disease (as people with Down's syndrome live longer so too does the incidence of early onset of dementia); dental health; mental health and body weight (DH, 1998, 2001e, 2003; Emerson and Hatton, 2007; Jones *et al.*, 2008; Manthorpe, 2007; MENCAP, 2004a; NHSS, 2004; RCN, 2006a, 2006b; Scottish Executive, 2008; WAG, 2007). Reasons why people with a learning disability have a poorer health record are similarly wide ranging. Exclusion, marginalisation and discrimination contribute towards lack of education, knowledge and awareness and impaired access to healthcare. Poor levels of literacy impact negatively on information retention and use. Communication difficulties such as speech impediment and poor articulation tend to exacerbate stigma and negative attitudes that invariably lead to reduced concern by others. Prejudicial attitudes about sex education limit provision markedly. MENCAP (2004a) has identified that many general practitioners (GPs) have received little if any relevant training, and along with other health professionals (including nurses) exhibit 'diagnostic overshadowing' when they inaccurately attribute features to 'learning disability' per se, when the same features in other people would raise concerns.

Bollard (2002) and Harrison and Berry (2006) explain how nurses and health visitors can help counter these negative experiences, mainly through establishing and sustaining relationships with learning disabled individuals and their carers and adopting a health promotion approach. Ewles and Simnet (2003) explain that health promotion is concerned with improving health status of individuals and communities. Health is largely determined not by individuals, but by social, economic and environmental elements that are outwith individual control, so a central tenet of health promotion is to empower people to achieve better control over those parts of their lives that impact upon health (Ewles and Simnett, 2003: 23):

> *These twin elements - improving health and having more control over it - are fundamental to the aims and processes of health promotion.*

The World Health Organization's definition echoes the emphasis on people's control (WHO, 1986):

> *Health promotion is the process of enabling people to increase control over, and to improve, their health.*

Health is characterised not as a reason for living, but as a resource for everyday life linked with individual, social and environmental resources that enable needs to be met, or adaptation or coping with the environment. This represents a distinct shift from the more micro, individual, deficit focus (of traditional, illness model) towards approaches that involve empowerment, egalitarianism, partnership, collaboration, community partnership, self-determination, accessibility, mutual aid and shared responsibility (WHO, 1986). The congruence between these ideas and the principles and ethos driving 21st century learning disability services is demonstrable, reflecting Bollard's (2002) contentions that nurse–client relationships move to egalitarian forms, actively promoting autonomy and empowerment.

Health Action Plans (HAPs) for people with learning disabilities have been advocated in policy since 2001(DH, 2001e; HM Government, 2009) though they have existed in some form for much longer (Howatson, 2005). These plans specify what action is required, and by whom, to sustain and improve an individual's health, effectively acting as a system to connect disparate services and professionals (and relevant non-professionals) with the person. Normally, HAPs are constructed by and with service users, carers and professionals. Apart for the benefits for the individual, in functional terms (i.e. their use) HAPs enhance education and information availability for disabled people, carers and professionals, improve teamwork and service coordination and provide evaluative feedback on systems and outcomes.

The format of the HAP is not prescribed, though guidance is readily available (DH, 2002; HM Government, 2009). The plan must specify what needs to happen and who needs to be involved so that the person's health is maintained/improved mainly through connecting people with services and support. Health concerns and options for dealing with them are explicated, via co-ordination of different services and agencies. The written plan can be conceived as illustrating the extent to which service providers are meeting their legal obligations. Health facilitators function as the main co-ordinator, and Matthews (2003) and Howatson (2005) suggest that since carers are in a most advantageous position to notice changes, a key worker liaising with carers and a specialist learning disabilities nurse, would provide ideal health facilitator input. Health facilitators are well placed to provide continuing evaluation and amendment of HAPs, ensuring adherence to principles of choice, independence, rights and inclusion. Two types of health facilitation role are differentiated (DH, 2001e; HM Government, 2009) as:

- level one – service development work and informing planning and commissioning (strategic and organisational role); and
- level two – person-to-person work with people with learning disabilities (operational, practice role).

In practice settings, working with learning disabled people and carers, health facilitators must:

- identify and monitor/record health targets;
- support access to all health services including screening;
- ensure the HAP matches well person-centred and/or all other personal care plans;
- identify and monitor health education needs;
- monitor health outcomes via regular review and evaluation, making agreed changes where necessary.

Additionally, the following responsibilities apply:

- annual health checks for people living in residential care;
- single assessment process (National Service Framework for Older People) for older individuals with a learning disability;
- training for carers;
- quality appraisal and service evaluation;
- reporting discriminatory practice and any service deficits which limit health improvement.

Figure 8-6 is taken from the government guidance document 'Health Action Planning and Health Facilitation for people with learning disabilities: good practice guidance' and illustrates what learning disabled people, carers and professionals wanted in HAPs.

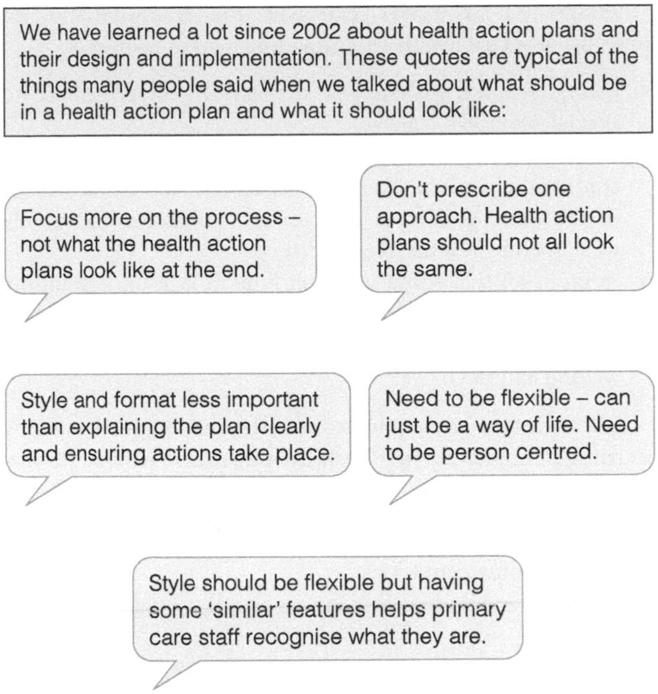

We have learned a lot since 2002 about health action plans and their design and implementation. These quotes are typical of the things many people said when we talked about what should be in a health action plan and what it should look like:

Focus more on the process – not what the health action plans look like at the end.

Don't prescribe one approach. Health action plans should not all look the same.

Style and format less important than explaining the plan clearly and ensuring actions take place.

Need to be flexible – can just be a way of life. Need to be person centred.

Style should be flexible but having some 'similar' features helps primary care staff recognise what they are.

Figure 8-6 A picture of a health action plan.
Source: HM Government, 2009: 65.

Sexual Health

Defining sexuality and sexual health is extremely difficult, with Wheeler (2001: 922) making reference to it as a complex area of life, an integral part of every person including issues of power, sensuality, integrity, decision making, identity, self-awareness, intimacy and relationships. This conceptual ambiguity presents added confusion when related to learning disability. Stereotypical views include people with learning disabilities being seen as potential sexual predators or childlike innocents requiring protection. Some parents of learning disabled children either deny, or prefer not to assist the transitions from child to adolescent to adult, denying opportunity for relationship formation (Aylott, 1999). The move to community care has led to some individuals living in accommodation that precludes adult relationship formation and/or privacy, with individuals having little control over who they live with, what work they do, and where and how they relax, including expression of sexuality (Wheeler, 2001: 924).

Fraser and Sim (2007) provide an extensive account of research and implications on sexual health needs of young learning disabled people in Scotland. This work identifies that learning disabled people have many similar experiences, needs, hopes and aspirations as other young people. Unfortunately, they also face particular barriers including problematic education and information access and provision. Discovering and elaborating the views of young people themselves about sexual health is also problematic. The evidence supports the claim that parents and carers have poor levels of awareness of available sexual health services, even those directed specifically at meeting the needs of young learning disabled people (Craik, 2002).

Fraser and Sim (2007) can assist nurses' appreciation of promoting sexual health and providing help in respect of:

- young people's wish to use mainstream, in preference to special, services;
- welcoming of services that are local, friendly, anonymous, confidential and that enable consultation with a practitioner of the same gender as themselves – all issues commonly welcomed by nondisabled peers;
- recognition that some staff continue to lack understanding about learning disability and some even continue to stigmatise them (examples include staff expecting literacy and writing abilities).

These factors are supported by relevant literature and the learning disability nursing/healthcare discourse with additional issues identified:

- flexible appointment systems;
- short appointment times;
- reactive systems, which require people to actively ask for help;
- physical access problems;
- poor inter-agency/services co-ordination;
- institutional discrimination (Powrie, 2002; Wood and Douglas, 2007).

As part of their health promotion role, nurses need to access resources and processes that help parents and carers discuss sexuality, health and well-being with their learning disabled children. When young people are not adequately supported or informed, significant risks apply, including unanticipated pregnancy or sexual abuse. Sant-Angelo (2000) illustrates the tensions between being so concerned about risk and preventing sexual abuse and exploitation that we are deterred from addressing people's sexual needs. Nurses need to carefully consider their own role, attitudes, values and expertise in respect of sexual health and well-being of people with learning disabilities.

LEARNING DISABILITY NURSING: CONTEMPORARY ISSUES, CHALLENGES AND IMPLICATIONS

Community and Day Care

The Nursing and Midwifery Council (NMC), the regulatory body for nurses, midwives and health visitors in the UK, has confirmed its review of pre-registration standards (NMC, 2010b). These standards will apply to all new pre-registration nursing education programmes that start from September 2011 and in all the rest by 2013. Learning disabilities nursing will become one of four fields of nursing, others being adult, mental health and children's nursing. Learning disabilities nurses care for individuals with a learning disability of any age, children included, aiming to maximise health and independence. Learning disabilities nurses will continue to work towards facilitating primary, secondary and tertiary care provision; and helping those with complex physical and mental health needs and problems. The emphasis on a values base that includes involvement from people with learning disabilities and carers will underpin the drive towards meeting the diverse needs of all individuals, of whatever background or ethnic origin, by nurses who have achieved prespecified practice competencies. Practice contexts will include primary, general, acute and prison settings. Mental healthcare will depend upon teamwork with both residential and community mental health teams working with learning disability nurses so that legislative requirements are met and, equally, if not more importantly, vulnerable people are safeguarded after effective risk appraisal and continuing evaluation.

Nurses need to navigate differing theoretical and practice domains, particularly in community settings and when in facilitation mode, appraising the relevance and applicability, for example, of either or both medical, social, and educational models of care and support. Whilst these models and approaches have tended to be characterised as different, discrete and conceptually distinct they each have strengths and weaknesses and need not absolutely be perceived as irreconcilable. Slevin and Sines (2005) outline how Baldwin and Birchenall (1993) adapt Beck *et al.*'s (1988) holistic model in ways that echo significant aspects of the learning disabilities nurses' role. These interrelated aspects are physical, emotional, intellectual, social and spiritual care with none taking precedence over any of the others. Collectively, they form a framework that is cogently applicable to the nurses' function in respect of therapist, educator, manager, advocate, counsellor and clinician. This holistic approach towards health and nursing encompasses physical, psychological and social aspects as well as primary, secondary and tertiary aspects (Sines *et al.*, 2009: 229). Holism demands holistic assessment, that includes identifying a person's needs, health status and social circumstances. For assessment to be comprehensive, and holistic, it requires collaboration by professionals, individuals and families/carers. Different professionals will contribute in particular ways, perhaps using standardised tools or mechanisms. Nursing assessment contributes significantly to the appreciation of health issues (especially relevant in view of the high level of unmet health needs among people with a learning disability) and Sines *et al.* (2009) stress the need for community nurses to carefully match assessment instruments and systems with the individual needs of the person with learning disabilities. The nursing assessment, based on a recognised model or theory base, can then supplement other assessment information to contribute, for example, to a PCP.

Assessment will inform health, education and other agencies of needs, actions and selected interventions and these are likely to comprise of active screening, health promotion and education along with mainstream service provision for identified health problems (DRC, 2006a; Harrison and Berry, 2006; Wood and Douglas, 2007). Community learning disabilities nurses will fulfil some of these assessment and service co-ordination/facilitation roles and are likely also to provide specialist input for people with more complex needs who are not able to benefit from mainstream services alone. Nurses should adopt care management roles only where needs are predominantly health oriented. Regular, continuing home visits and linking with additional support agencies and practitioners will include expertise in relation to, for example, behavioural and psychological techniques, epilepsy, mental health, primary care, acute hospitals and palliative care. Sines *et al.* (2009) advocate basing community nurses and learning disability teams in buildings and offices accommodating other members of the primary healthcare team and services, such as GPs, as a way of optimising communication and liaison (Sines *et al.*, 2009: 230):

> *. . . such links will assist in overcoming barriers to accessing primary and acute care services for the increasing number of people with learning disabilities who need to access such services. In contrast, the continued 'isolation' of community nurses within separate learning disability and social work networks will do little to inform other nursing colleagues of their role and possible contributions.*

Day care provision has proceeded apace with the ongoing reduction in older hospital accommodation and care in the community, initially mainly in the form of adult training centres (ATCs). Research into day care has provided a mix of positive and more unwelcome information. For example, the Scottish Executive (2000: 54) identified people were 'going to day centres for many years without a formal assessment' and that many described day care as boring and without direction. In Wales, *Fulfilling the promises* (WAG, 2001) revealed some variety in day provision with fewer larger day centres, though employment and benefits systems were problematic. *Valuing people* (DH, 2001e: 19) described day care as 'frequently failing to provide sufficiently flexible and individual support'. Cole *et al.* (2007) illustrate a shift during the past two decades, from people going to a day centre, to services supporting people in their workplaces, education classes and colleges, sports and leisure centres, community centres and around local villages and towns. Cole *et al.* (2007) present an extensive review of services and literature that they named 'Having a Good Day', because it reflected how services, opportunities and support could be provided and encouraged to assist people to take up ordinary opportunities and have ordinary lifestyles. The study explored and identified how services were working to help people 'have a good day' and also, what support is needed for services to address what they find difficult. Figure 8-7 is a synopsis of Cole *et al.*'s findings and conclusions.

Against this changing background of the shape and form of day care provision, the numbers of learning disabilities nurses had fallen (DH, 2007) by 37% between 1996 (12,105) and 2006 (7,583) with some nurses being seconded by the NHS to jointly managed community learning disability teams. The remainder work in community settings, including day care or residential, mental health or forensic services where they contribute to assessment and treatment provision. Because the learning disabilities nurses' role includes helping other professionals

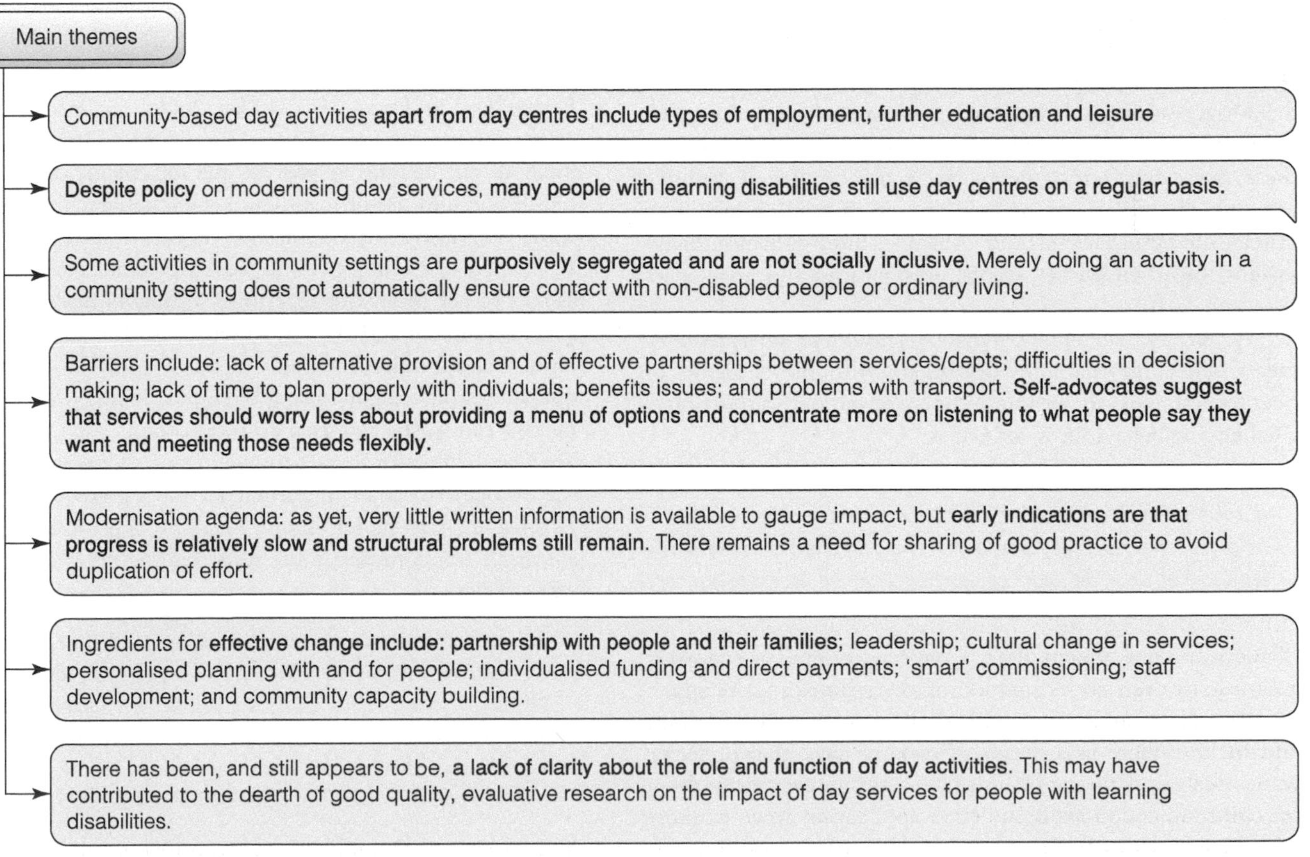

Figure 8-7 A synopsis of 'Having a good day'.
Source: based on Cole *et al.*, 2007 [emphasis added].

appreciate the value of health promotion, health facilitation (including liaising with primary care teams and hospitals) and service evaluation, development and planning (DH, 2007) their input to day service provision requires them to appreciate that working in a 'community setting does not equal social inclusion' (Cole *et al.*, 2007: xv). The learning disability nurse working in day care has significant opportunities to provide a health promotion and education emphasis to their work that sustains helpful networking and is genuinely socially inclusive (Bollard, 2002; Gates, 1997; Howatson, 2005; Sines *et al.*, 2009; Tilly, 2008) and avoids the traps of providing an illusion of inclusion and non-supportive interactions (Power, 2009).

Responding to Profound and Multiple Disabilities and Challenging Behaviour

It is difficult to estimate the numbers of people with these particular types of disabilities though the DH (2001e) cite estimates of approximately 210,000 in England alone and an expectation that proportionate numbers will increase in the future (Emerson, 2009). In Scotland, 4,000 to 5,000 people are thought to have complex needs (Scottish Executive, 2000). People with profound and multiple learning disabilities (PMLD) have an IQ below 20 with consequent limitation in understanding and communicating. The term 'multiple' is a literal reference to the presence of other additional impairments such as poor sight and/or hearing, epilepsy, swallowing problems, other chronic medical conditions, mental health problems and/or psychological problems and mobility problems. They need considerable help with most aspects of living including eating and drinking, washing and bathing, dressing and using the toilet. Some also exhibit challenging behaviour and self-injury. Despite these pervasive factors, people with profound and multiple learning disabilities can and do engage in relationships with others, and family, friends and loved ones often gain meaningful insight into their wishes, wants, personalities and preferences (Mansell, 2010).

The term 'challenging behaviour' should be interpreted to mean behaviour that provides others with the challenge of how to best assist the person to be involved and to contribute. Challenging behaviour is defined as:

> *culturally abnormal behaviour(s) of such an intensity, frequency or duration that the physical safety of the person or others is likely to be placed in serious jeopardy, or behaviour that is likely to seriously limit use of, or result in the person being denied access to ordinary community facilities.* (Emerson, 1995: 44)

Because a person with PMLD may have limited or no formal language or even no recognition of, or responses to, images, it presents carers and nurses with challenges on how to involve and include them as a means of seeking what they prefer or want. Healy and Noonan Walsh (2007) provide extensive detail on communication skills and their application when working with people with PMLD and MENCAP (2010c) provide guidance on consulting that illustrates how carers, nurses and others need to be creative in the ways they address seeking and establishing communication with a person with PMLD. The key elements are:

- finding out if the persons' (topic related) experiences have been positive or negative;
- establishing the degree of sensitivity used when communicating with the person;
- appraising body language, vocalisations and facial expressions to gauge some insight into what their 'signs' mean (how happy or unhappy do their expressions seem?);
- providing and presenting these appraisals and evidence to those able to make changes and relevant others, and recording experiences and decisions.

The DH (2007: 8) expresses how learning disabilities nurses working in inpatient care services should aim to provide excellent person-centred care, with the proviso that, ultimately, support is designed to return the person to life in their community. The Welsh Assembly Government (WAG, 2004) presents similar preferences that mean authorities are required to provide specialist arrangements for people with complex health needs in their communities, even in times of acute crisis. WAG recognises that there may be occasions when there is no alternative to residential support at least until a return home or to new, longer-term accommodation can be managed. In some instances, severity of behaviour can lead to people becoming virtually trapped in institutional care. Slevin and Sines (2005) present grounded theory research with 22 community learning disabilities nurses and outline interventions applicable in challenging behaviour contexts. These include the following:

- Behavioural interventions (McCue, 2000), qualified by the expression of need for additional specialist training. Specific methods include using positive reinforcement, diversion, redirection and use of tokens and chaining (teaching using small progressive steps). Stimulus transfer is illustrated via an example of a young girl who repeatedly drank cans of cola as part of her behaviour repertoire, leading to health problems. The nurse and the girl's mother worked to shift the rewarding stimulus (the cola) to water, with the eventual outcome of the daughter being as happy drinking water from the cola can, as she had been drinking cola.
- Therapeutic relationships, between nurses, clients and carers was recognised as an important factor, a prerequisite for establishing trust underpinning a holistic, and whole family approach. Some nurses in the study referred to a 'presence' with families.

  > *The support that you can give the family, I think that is a word that gets splattered about but the real support you can provide by visiting and making sure that you are available and that you do get back to them. You know that it is not just a paper exercise that you only say what you mean to people and then that you can carry that out.* (Slevin and Sines, 2005: 421)

- Multi-inclusive therapies that encompass several distinct role attributes or approaches. First as 'therapist', adopting interventions such as **relaxation therapy** and aromatherapy.

Second, as 'clinician', such as administering medication and injections. Third, eclectic approaches that combine other types of interventions and teamwork.

Slevin and Sines (2005) note the strength of view by those nurses interviewed that single, discrete methods/techniques are useful yet almost always insufficient. For example, even though behavioural interventions have a firm base in evidence, using them in a purely technical objectively oriented sense can be questioned in terms of creating distance between professionals and those receiving help. Nurses saw great appeal in combining behavioural with **humanist** (and caring) approaches. This caring element extended to their 'willingness to relinquish professional power and distance' to genuinely work 'with' people with learning disabilities and carers (Slevin and Sines, 2005: 421).

Perhaps unsurprisingly, Slevin and Sines link these mulit-inclusive and eclectic approaches with the learning disability nursing framework outlined by Baldwin and Birchenall (1993). This is an holistic framework based on Beck *et al.* (1988) which encompasses overlapping elements of physical, emotional, intellectual, social and spiritual care. Turnbull (2004) and Aldridge (2004) present similar sentiments, advocating breadth of approach through the use of the 'Ecology of Health Model' (Aldridge, 2004: 171). This differentiates learning disabilities nursing from other nurses', therapists' and social workers' practice and acknowledges the dynamism of working with individuals and their families, using a theoretical base that informs thinking and decision making. It brings together policy, values and practice to promote health, autonomy and social inclusion of people with learning disabilities.

In conclusion, people with PMLD and challenging behaviour present learning disability nurses (and others) with challenges, to apply their expertise in assessment, analysis and design of interventions that lead to optimum autonomy and independence for individuals in receipt of care and also to help carers develop relevant coping skills.

Research: Implications for Learning Disability Nursing

This section is not intended to introduce or replicate information and techniques in nursing research, how to refine suitable questions, review literature, identify and select relevant methods, sample, seek, gather and analyse data and disseminate conclusions. These fundamental issues in respect of research in nursing warrant reading and review/reflection of specialised texts such as Parahoo (2006) and/or Polit and Beck (2009). Additionally, skills associated with sharing, disseminating and publishing research are not addressed here. Readers interested in these issues should explore relevant texts/materials (for example, Albarran and Scholes, 2005; Appleton, 2008; Oermann and Hays, 2010). What follows is an outline of issues and questions about research that apply in learning disability nursing contexts.

In keeping with most aspects of modern life, health, social and welfare services have embraced the need for research to inform action and contribute to new insights, understanding and knowledge. This is clearly illustrated in policy, education and the evidenced-based practice discourses (DiCenso *et al.*, 2002; DH, 2007; NMC, 2004; Sackett *et al.*, 1997). The research discourse in nursing reflects a spectrum of views about the nature of evidence and research itself, summarised as the tensions between those who claim high-quality research must be objective, generalisable and valid, as seen in well designed randomised control trial (RCT) studies, to others who pay more credence to issues of practical application, contextualisation and meaningful interpretation. This spectrum is indicated in work by several nurse researchers and authors (Nolan and Bradley, 2008; Rolfe, 2002, 2005, 2006; Weaver and Olson, 2006). Against this ever-shifting background, recent evidence (specifically related to learning disability nursing) has concluded 'the current body of learning disability research is not fit for purpose in terms of its extent, quantity or quality' (Griffiths *et al.*, 2007: ii). The DH (2007: 47) has echoed this lack of quality and quantity of research in learning disability nursing and the consequent difficulties in provision of 'reliable, generalisable or verifiable insights'. Policy promotes that all learning disability nurses undergo postgraduate (research) education with a commitment to publish and for strategists to see merit in smaller scale research (such as individual projects) forming part of a more meaningful body of evidence, through consideration of (DH, 2007: 39):

> *. . . whether their future research strategies should incorporate opportunity to develop research that will inform future learning disability nursing practice and encourage small-scale projects to link in a coherent, thematic manner.*

Griffiths *et al.* (2007), and by association the DH endorsement of their 2007 review, is afforded critical attention by Caan and Toocaram (2008) who present a range of criticisms or charges. Examples with responses are in Table 8-2 below, as an illustration of the tortuous and interpretive nature of research, irrespective of its pedigree. (The hidden aim in including this is that readers take a more informed and critical view of research, in place of simply accepting what is included in textbooks, even this one, or journal articles or commissioned reports and policy.)

Differences of research philosophies and methodological premises can be found in a wealth of nursing literature. For example, Griffiths (2005) explains evidence-based practice in two broad ways, the traditional RCT that (sometimes) minimises the value of experience and subsequently fails to bond with the real nature of clinical practice, and the extreme alternative of an 'anything goes' mentality. The review concludes that whilst 'objectivity' can be challenged, evidence and claims still require standards and criteria for judging their worth and relevance. Luck *et al.* (2006) offer a 'bridge across the paradigms', using case study method to approach research in real-life nursing settings with a 'paradigmatic openness'. Nolan and Bradley (2008: 388) show how evidence-based practice has utility but that evidence per se is constituted of many kinds of information and that 'any single approach to determining care, no matter how popular, is likely to lead to a service that does not truly

Table 8-2 Criticisms and Charges

Criticism/charge	Comment*
The review is 'cursory and superficial'.	Perhaps, though the parameters of the work are openly stated and indicated in the title.
Relevant material is excluded. Muir-Gray's (1998) work in Anglia and Oxford is relevant, yet missing, as is work from grey literature (typically, unpublished theses and dissertations) including some seemingly relevant and potentially valuable work such as McVicar and Caan's (2005) overview of thesis work, studies involving partnerships with service users and advocacy and Broughton's (2002) feasibility study using attempts to use RCT as method in a community intervention context.	The crux of this criticism concerns the exclusion or loss of potentially valuable material with consequent effects on reduced numbers of studies included in the review. The report does outline search parameters though little attention is paid to making explicit the possibilities of existing and potentially useful work. An outsider view might pose questions about the 'added' quality of published *vis à vis* unpublished work with strictness of peer review systems (published work) generally held to add quality. Conversely, this does not necessarily mean unpublished work is of lower quality nor that it might not constitute a valuable source of valid evidence and information.
Approximately 15,000 items exist in Google Scholar between 1995 and 2006 under 'learning disabilities and nurs*', from which the most active researchers and sites could quickly have been identified. (Griffiths identified 175 relevant studies.)	Search parameters are different (the review outlines its own search boundaries). So (even though somewhat paradoxical) both viewpoints are valid. (Once more, the report has remained 'true' to its stated method - the key question is whether its boundaries were too narrow or limited, by choice of the reviewers?)
Muir-Gray's (1998) work included the learning disability specialist library (LDSL) for practitioners and it appears the review team did not include relevant evidence bulletins.	Another aspect that sits outside the reviews' boundaries, so technically the LDSL bulletins need not have been included. Yet, the charge that the boundaries are too limiting remains, with consequent questions about the reviews' comprehensiveness.
Web of Science, could find no personal contributions to this 'research base for learning disability nursing' by any of the review's three authors. This is an outsider's view of the field.	Technically accurate, yet even though some support is made for efficacy and quality being linked to 'insider' insight, the counter charge of some defensiveness is easily levied. (Non-learning disability nurses can surely learn from research into their practice by non-nurses?)
Review recommends nurses work more closely with other disciplines. Relevant evidence limited or missing - interprofessional studies research, e.g. Fran Stevens' family skills within Holland *et al.*, 1998; or Rachel Moxon's care planning skills within (Caan *et al.*, 2000). Re inclusion, the review seems to miss partnerships (Burls, 2007) and especially with children and school nurses, for example, for health facilitation (Caan *et al.*, 2005).	This criticism seems to most clearly illustrate the limitations re narrow boundaries of the review, yet even the most critical eye would (surely) acknowledge that not every single relevant study might be included in any review. (It remains an interpretive judgement whether the search and appraisal parameters were effective in identifying resources and materials sufficiently comprehensively to support the reviews conclusions.)
Several other issues raised and outlined, including involving service users as research partners, research fellowships and financial systems.	Probably legitimate challenges and concerns, though again in a purely technical sense these types of issue are outwith the review design. These broader, more systemic influences are surely relevant to any research design that is aimed to inform, critically?

* The comments aim to illustrate the spectrum of interpretations that often apply to published research - an attempt to push readers to think more divergently rather than accept unquestioningly.

meet the complex individual needs of patients'. Different types of evidence exist and require multiple ways of thinking and appraisal in respect of responding sensitively and appropriately to patients' preferences. Reed and Lawrence (2008: 422) explore relevant research trends, arguments and issues and advocate developing practice-based knowledge (as well as theory) that 'could give voice to the caregiver's knowledge and, in turn, enhance patient care and the satisfaction and retention of nurses'.

Despite the different (and also similar) perceptions, interpretations and passionate arguments amongst nurse researchers, authors and leaders, the intrinsic value of research remains undeniable. The NMC (2004: 13) endorses the crucial importance of research especially in complex and ever-changing healthcare environments that demand high standards of skill in relation to searching the evidence base, analysing, critiquing and using research in practice, including sharing and disseminating findings so practice can adapt and develop. Many practical examples exist of how research into learning disability nursing has contributed to improving the lives of learning disabled people as well as alerting us all to issues of concern. Some brief examples follow, not all are conducted exclusively by learning disability nurses.

Donovan (2002) and Kingston and Bailey (2009) address pain recognition and management with clients unable to communicate feelings verbally. Many types of non-verbal expression may be used to indicate pain and nurses need extensive knowledge of the person in avoiding making assumptions about causes. Diagnostic tests and pain assessment tools (individually designed as well as standardised) should be available and accessible in ways that help people with a learning disability to communicate their pain. Thomson *et al.* (2007) explain how a dedicated team of health facilitators contributed to innovative collaboration between practice, education and research personnel and the introduction of health action plans for learning disabled adults. Brown and Marshall (2006) present how cognitive behaviour therapy (CBT) is best used by properly trained learning disabilities nurses with people with a learning disability, taking account of particular cognitive and support needs.

Some research demonstrates an explicit congruence, or matching, with a learning disabilities nursing ethos that embraces inclusion, user involvement, participation and practice application. Many of these types of studies are described as 'inclusive' research. For example, Walmsley (2004) reviews research that includes people with learning difficulties as active participants, rather than passive subjects, and identifies areas of practice development that benefit from these collaborative approaches (Walmsley, 2004: 61–62):

> *I have sought to derive lessons from developments in inclusive research which might usefully be used in working with people with learning difficulties to promote health improvements. After more than a decade, it has begun to be possible to critique inclusive research, and build some pointers for professionals seeking to work inclusively. The naïve belief that if conditions are right somehow the effect of the impairment will disappear continues to be evident in some quarters. But a more detached perspective allows a recognition of the positive value of such approaches, and some of the limitations. Working alongside users and carers is just too important to improve practice, and improve lives. People with learning difficulties do have pressing health needs. It is important to draw out the best practice from research to support this, whilst not being distracted by overstated claims about what is both possible and achievable.*

These types of inclusive research demand careful consideration of relevant ethical issues. Smith (2008) considers exclusion from research as a means of avoiding difficult ethical concerns about autonomy and decision making by vulnerable people and marginalised groups. The main ethical tensions apply to sampling and recruitment, and assessing capacity of individuals re informed consent, thus avoiding coercion and exploitation. 'Responsible advocacy' (in keeping with principles of autonomy, beneficence, non-maleficence and justice) is recommended. Shields and Pearn (2007: 1196) conclude that inducements (rewards, including financial remuneration) are 'inappropriate when offered to those who are "ethically captive" in the sense that autonomy of choice may be compromised'.

Learning disability nursing presents a graphic history of the shift from custodial, depersonalised systems and institutions towards aspirations of person-centred, community oriented, holistic care. Learning disability nurses are continuing to strive to support learning disabled people so that they experience fulfilled lives, through inclusion and access to relevant health provision. They practice in complex professional milieu that present disparate principles, theoretical assumptions and even values, illustrated clearly by the tensions between medical, biopsychosocial or educational models. They require an extensive repertoire of skills and critically informed knowledge bases to fulfil their roles, including providing specialist healthcare as partners with learning disabled people, their families, carers and other professional and public groups in residential and community settings. These include primary, secondary and prison healthcare systems. They are faced by, and must seek to effectively counter exclusion, whether by ability, capacity, gender, race, religion, colour, age or health status acting both as advocate and as promoter of self-advocacy.

CRITICAL REFLECTION

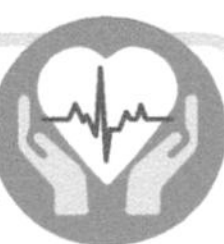

It is evident that there are several issues to consider when caring for Aliya before, during and after the birth of her baby. There are cultural and language barriers when providing care. There is also a need to consider the baby and family when nursing Aliya. Consideration should also be given to the ongoing care for all concerned. Reflecting on this case study should therefore include the above mentioned individuals, and from reading the chapter you should highlight the issues to be considered and provide a rationale for your decisions. Suggested points to consider are:

- language
- culture
- empowerment and advocacy
- causes of cerebral palsy
- primary, secondary, tertiary prevention
- counselling
- community care
- Mental Capacity Act
- independence and well-being
- primary and secondary health
- family support and guidance
- individual rights
- communication
- patient-centred planning (PCP)
- contemporary issues.

CHAPTER HIGHLIGHTS

- The issue of defining learning disability, problematic as it may be, has been illustrated as embracing IQ, behavioural and social dimensions.
- Learning disability can be the result of biological, psychological and social factors.
- Identifying the cause is crucial for preventive and appropriate interventions.
- The crucial impact of communication is writ large in one-to-one encounters between people, in teamwork and person-centred planning and in working effectively, and productively, with families.
- Understanding learning disability means nurses appreciate the relevance of helping with independence and living in a home of one's choice, engaging in meaningful employment and enjoying interpersonal and sexual relationships that most of us regard as fundamental elements of our productive lives.
- Nurses can facilitate or contribute to person-centred planning and needs-led approaches that include the individual in all decision making, illustrating the central roles of teamwork and communication.
- Nurses have particular and quite obvious roles in respect of improving the health status of people with a learning disability and contributing to assisting people with challenging behaviours.
- Primary and secondary healthcare are especially relevant in prevention and effective treatment for a raft of health problems, including impaired vision, hearing, physical disability, epilepsy, heart disease, respiratory problems, Alzheimer's disease (key for a population growing older), mental health issues, dental hygiene and weight problems.
- Supplementing the direct healthcare input role is advocacy, such as when the nurse ensures the learning disabled person is registered with a GP, has regular health checks and has a realistic health action plan.
- Nurses' extensive knowledge of aetiology and preventive strategies can enhance their counselling and health promotion roles including essentially sensitive health issues such as sexuality.
- Normalisation is undoubtedly linked to values orientation, service design and evaluation.
- Recent criticisms and alternatives have been explicated against a background (complex as it is) of promoting independence, asserting/supporting rights and comprehensive yet meaningful risk assessment and appropriate risk taking.
- Helping provide people with a learning disability, their loved ones and carers with assistance that reflects their legal, civil, human and moral rights is writ large at present and into the future.
- Challenges to nurses apply in terms of ageism, ethnicity and colour as well as labelling that adds weight to low expectations that are self-fulfilling.

ACTIVITY ANSWERS

ACTIVITY 8-1 Brain damage can be caused by many different factors, some of which have been discussed at the beginning of this chapter. On reflection (without revisiting the chapter) make a list of the ones you can remember and write at the side which are more likely to happen pre, during or post birth.

ACTIVITY 8-2 Individuals with learning disabilities have rights, choice and the need to be independent. Reflect back on the chapter and discuss these rights and include, e.g., the Disability Discrimination Act 1995, the Race Relations Acts 1976 and 2000, the Sex Discrimination Act and the Human Rights Act 1998. The 1975 civil rights (specific to a country or district) include eligibility to vote, to receive relevant benefits and have legal representation. All these should be considered in your reflection.

REFERENCES

Akerjordet, K., and Severinsson, E. (2007) 'Emotional intelligence: A review of the literature with specific focus on empirical and epistemological perspectives', *Journal of Clinical Nursing*, 16(8), 1405–1416.

Alaszewski, H.A. and Alaszewski, A.A. (2005) 'Person-centred planning and risk: Challenging the boundaries', in S. Carnaby and P. Cambridge (eds), *Intimate and personal care with people with learning disabilities* (pp. 183–197), London: Jessica Kingsley.

Albarran, J.W. and Scholes, J. (2005) 'How to get published: Seven easy steps', *Nursing in Critical Care*, 10(2): 72–77.

Aldridge, J. (2004) 'Learning disability nursing: A model for practice', in J. Turnbull (ed.), *Learning disability nursing* (pp. 169–187), Oxford: Blackwell Science.

APA (1994) *Diagnostic and statistical manual of mental disorders* (4th edn), Washington DC: American Psychiatric Association.

Appleton, J.V. (2008) 'Sharing evidence: Community practitioners writing for publication', *Community Practitioner*, 81(12): 22–25.

Apraiz, E. (2001) *Using pictures of paintings as aids to communication with people who have learning disabilities*, Reading: University of Reading.

Attree, M. (2007) 'Factors influencing nurses' decisions to raise concerns about care quality', *Journal of Nursing Management*, 15(4): 392–402.

Aylott, J. (1999) 'Is the sexuality of people with a learning disability being denied?' *British Journal of Nursing*, 8(7): 438–442.

Baldwin, S. and Birchenall, M. (1993) 'The nurse's role in caring for people with learning disabilities', *British Journal of Nursing*, 2(17): 850–854.

Barr, O. (1996) 'Developing services for people with learning disabilities which actively involve family members: a review of recent literature', *Health and Social Care in the Community*, 4(2): 103–101, 112.

Barr, O. (2004) *Promoting access. The experience of children and adults with learning disabilities and their families/carers who had contact with acute general hospitals in the WHSSB area and the views of nurses in these hospitals*, Londonderry: Western Health and Social Services Board.

Bateman, N. (2000) *Advocacy skills for health and social care professionals*, London: Jessica Kingsley.

Beck, C.M., Rawlings, R.P., and Williams, S.R. (1988) *Mental health psychiatric nursing* (2nd edn), St. Louis: Mosby.

Becker, A.L. (2009) 'Ethical considerations of teaching spirituality in the academy', *Nursing Ethics*, 16(6): 697–706.

Begley, A. (2009) 'Secular is good', *Nursing Standard*, 24(13): 26–27.

Bertram, G. and Stickley, T. (2005) 'Mental health nurses, promoters of inclusion or perpetuators of exclusion?' *Journal of Psychiatric and Mental Health Nursing*, 12(4): 387–395.

BILD (2010) Advocacy. Retrieved 20 July 2010, from http://www.bild.org.uk/04advocacy_about.htm

Black, P. and Hyde, C. (2004) 'Caring for people with a learning disability, colorectal cancer and stoma', *British Journal of Nursing*, 13(16): 970–975.

Bollard, M. (1999) 'Improving primary healthcare for people with learning disabilities', *British Journal of Nursing*, 8(18): 1216–1221.

Bollard, M. (2002) 'Health promotion and learning disability', *Nursing Standard*, 16(27): 47–53; quiz 54.

Bredberg, E. (1999) 'Writing disability history: Problems, perspectives and sources', *Disability and Society*, 14(2): 189–201.

British Sign Language (2010) *A guide to British sign language*. Retrieved 20 July 2010, from http://www.britishsignlanguage.com/

Broughton, S. (2002) 'Interventions to maximise capacity to consent and reduce anxiety in women with learning disabilities', unpublished MSc thesis, Hertfordshire: University of Hertfordshire.

Brown, H. and Benson, S. (eds) (1992) *A practical guide to working with people with learning disabilities*, London: Hawker.

Brown, M. (2005), 'Emergency care for people with learning disabilities: what all nurses and midwives need to know', *Accident and Emergency Nursing*, 13(4): 224–231.

Brown, M. and Marshall, K. (2006) 'Cognitive behaviour therapy, and people with learning disabilities: Implications for developing nursing practice', *Journal of Psychiatric and Mental Health Nursing*, 13(2): 234–241.

Burls, A. (2007) 'People and green spaces: Promoting public health and mental well-being through ecotherapy', *Journal of Public Mental Health*, 6(3): 24–39.

Burton, M. (1997) 'Intellectual disability: Developing a definition', *Journal of Intellectual Disabilities*, 1(1): 37–43.

Caan, W. and Toocaram, J. (2008) 'Learning disabilities is bigger than a cursory review', *British Journal of Nursing*, 17(2): 78–79.

Caan, W., Lutchmiah, J., Thomson, K. and Toocaram, J. (2005) 'Health facilitation in primary care', *Primary Health Care Research and Development*, 6: 348–6.

Caan, W., Streng, I., Moxon, R. and Machin, A. (2000) 'A joint health and social services initiative for children with disabilities', *British Journal of Community Nursing*, 5(2), 87–90.

Cable, S., Lumsdaine, J. and Semple, M. (2003) 'Informed consent', *Nursing Standard*, 18: 47–53.

Carnaby, S. and Cambridge, P. (2005) *Intimate and personal care with people with learning disabilities*, London: Jessica Kingsley.

Clarke, J. (2009) 'A critical view of how nursing has defined spirituality', *Journal of Clinical Nursing*, 18(12): 1666–1673.

Clement, T. (2002) 'Exploring the role of values in the management of advocacy schemes', in B. Gray and R. Jackson (eds), *Advocacy and learning disability* (pp. 50–71), London: Jessica Kingsley.

Cole, A., Williams, V., Lloyd, A., Major, V., Mattingly, M., McIntosh, B., *et al.* (2007). *Having a good day? A study of community-based day activities for people with learning disabilities*, London: Social Care Institute for Excellence.

Colley, H. and Hodkinson, P. (2001) 'Problems with "bridging the gap": the reversal of structure and agency in addressing social exclusion', *Critical Social Policy*, 21(3): 335–359.

Corbett, J. (2007) *Health care provision and people with intellectual disabilities: A guide for health professionals*, Chichester: Wiley and Sons.

Craik, J. (2002) *What you don't know won't harm you: A needs assessment about the relationships and sexual wellbeing of people with learning disabilities*, Glasgow: Greater Glasgow and Clyde NHS Health Board.

Crome, I.B. and Kumar, M.T. (2007) 'Epidemiology of drug and alcohol use in young women', *Seminars in Fetal and Neonatal Medicine*, 12(2): 98–105.

Culham, A. and Nind, M. (2003) 'Deconstructing normalisation: Clearing the way for inclusion', *Journal of Intellectual and Developmental Disability*, 28(1): 65–78.

Davies, J. and Holstrom, R. (2005) *First impressions: Emotional and practical support for families of a young child with a learning disability*, London: Foundation for People with Learning Disabilities.

Devine, M. and Taggart, L. (2008) 'Addressing the mental health needs of people with learning disabilities', *Nursing Standard*, 22(45): 40–48; quiz 50.

DH (1998) *The healthy way: How to stay healthy – a guide for people with learning disabilities*, London: HMSO.

DH (2001a) *Reference guide to consent to examination or treatment*, London: Department of Health Publications.

DH (2001b) *Seeking consent. Working with people with intellectual disabilities*, London: Department of Health Publications.

DH (2001c) *Valuing people: A new strategy for learning disability for 21st century*, Vol. 1, London: Department of Health.

DH (2001d) *Valuing people: A new strategy for learning disability for 21st century*, Vol. 2, London: HMSO.

DH (2001e) *Valuing people: A new strategy for learning disability for the 21st century*, Vol. 3, London: Department of Health.

DH (2002) *Action for health: Health action plans and health facilitation: Good practice on implementation for learning disability partnership boards*, London: HMSO.

DH (2003) *Valuing people, chapter 7 – Housing, fulfilling lives and employment*, London: HMSO.

DH (2005) *Independence, wellbeing and choice*, London: Department of Health.

DH (2007) *Good practice in learning disability nursing*, London: HMSO.

DH (2009) *Valuing people now: A new three-year strategy for people with learning disabilities. Executive Summary*, London: HMSO.

DH (2010) *Person-centred planning. Advice for professionals*, London: HMSO.

DHSS Department of Health and Social Security (1971) *Better services for the mentally handicapped*, London: HMSO.

DHSSPS (2003) *Consent – What you have a right to know: A guide for relatives and carers*, Belfast: DHSSPS.

DiCenso, A., Cullum, N. and Ciliska, D. (2002) 'Evidence-based nursing: 4 years down the road', *Evidenced Based Nursing*, 5(1): 4–5.

Donovan, J. (2002) 'Learning disability nurses' experiences of being with clients who may be in pain', *Journal of Advanced Nursing*, 38(5): 458–466.

Dowling, S., Manthorpe, J. and Cowley, S. (2007) 'Working on person-centred planning: From amber to green light?' *Journal of Intellectual Disability*, 11(1): 65–82.

DRC (2006a) *Equal treatment: Closing the gap*. Manchester: Disability Rights Commission.

DRC (2006b) *Equal treatment: Closing the gap*. Manchester: Disability Rights Commission.

Duggleby, W., Cooper, D. and Penz, K. (2009) 'Hope, self-efficacy, spiritual well-being and job satisfaction', *Journal of Advanced Nursing*, 65(11): 2376–2385.

Ehrich, K. (2006) 'Telling cultures: "cultural" issues for staff reporting concerns about colleagues in the UK National Health Service', *Sociology of Health and Illness*, 28(7): 903–926.

Ellis, H.K. and Narayanasamy, A. (2009) 'An investigation into the role of spirituality in nursing', *British Journal of Nursing*, 18(14): 886–890.

Emerson, E. (1995) *Challenging behaviour: Analysis and interventions in people with learning difficulties*, Cambridge: Cambridge University Press.

Emerson, E. (2009) *Estimating future numbers of adults with profound multiple learning disabilities in England*, Lancaster: CeDR, Lancaster University.

Emerson, E. and Hatton, C. (1994) *Moving out: The impact of relocation from hospital to community on the quality of life of people with learning disabilities*, London: HMSO.

Emerson, E. and Hatton, C. (2007) *The mental health of children and adolescents with learning disabilities in Britain*, Lancaster: Lancaster University.

Emerson, E. and Hatton, C. (2008) *People with learning disabilities in England*, Lancaster: Lancaster University.

Evans, G., Beyer, S. and Todd, S. (1988) 'Looking forward not looking back: The evaluation of community living', *Disability and Society*, 3(3): 239–252.

Ewles, L. and Simnett, I. (2003) *Promoting health. A practical guide* (5th edn), London: Bailliere Tindall.

Felce, D. and Emerson, E. (2001) 'Living with support in a home in the community: Predictors of behavioural development and household and community activity', *Mental Retardation and Developmental Disabilities Research Reviews*, 7(2): 75–83.

Ferris-Taylor (2007) 'Communication', in B. Gates (ed.), *Learning disabilities: Toward inclusion* (pp. 325–360), London: Elsevier.

Foundation for People with LD (2001) *Learning disabilities: The fundamental facts*, London: Foundation for People with Learning Disabilities.

Fraser, S. and Sim, J. (2007) *The sexual health needs of young people with learning disabilities*, Edinburgh: Health Scotland.

Gates, B. (ed.) (1997) *Learning disabilities* (3rd edn), London: Churchill Livingstone.

Gates, B. (ed.) (2007) *Learning disabilities: Towards inclusion*, London: Elsevier.

Gibbs, S.M., Brown, M.J. and Muir, W.J. (2008) 'The experiences of adults with intellectual disabilities and their carers in general hospitals: A focus group study', *Journal of Intellectual Disability Research*, 52(12): 1061–1077.

Gillings-Taylor, S. (2004) 'Why the difference? Advice to carers of women who have learning disability and women who do not', *Journal of Intellectual Disabilities*, 8: 176–189.

Goleman, D. (1996) *Emotional intelligence*. London: Bloomsbury.

Graham, H. (2004) *Socioeconomic inequalities in health in the UK: evidence on patterns and determinants*, London: Disability Rights Commission.

Gray, B. and Jackson, R. (eds) (2002) *Advocacy and learning disability*, London: Jessica Kingsley.

Greenwood, D.J. and Levin, M. (1998) *Introduction to action research*, London: Sage.

Griffiths, P. (2005) 'Evidence-based practice: A deconstruction and postmodern critique: book review article', *International Journal of Nursing Studies*, 42(3): 355–361.

Griffiths, P., Bennett, J. and Smith, E. (2007) *The research base for learning disability nursing: A rapid scoping review*, London: Nursing Research Unit, King's College London.

Hall, E. (2005) 'The entangled geographies of social exclusion/inclusion for people with learning disabilities', *Health and Place*, 11(2): 107–115.

Hardy, S., Woodward, P., Woolard, P. and Tait, T. (2006) *Meeting the health needs of people with learning disabilities*, London: Royal College of Nursing.

Haringey Council (2005) *Communication plan: Adults with learning disabilities guidelines*, from http://www.haringey.gov.uk/communication_plan_-_adults_with_learning_disabilities.pdf

Harrison, S. and Berry, L. (2006) 'Valuing people: Health visiting and people with learning disabilities', *Community Practitioner*, 79(2): 56–59.

Healy, D. and Noonan Walsh, P. (2007) 'Communication among nurses and adults with severe and profound intellectual disabilities: Predicted and observed strategies', *Journal of Intellectual Disabilities*, 11(2): 127–141.

HM Government (2009) *Health action planning and health facilitation for people with learning disabilities: Good practice guidance*, London: HMSO.

Hogan, D.P., Shandra, C.L. and Msall, M.E. (2007) 'Family developmental risk factors among adolescents with disabilities and children of parents with disabilities', *Journal of Adolescence*, 30(6): 1001–1019.

Holland, A.J., Hon, J., Huppert, F., Stevens, F. and Watson, P. (1998) 'Population-based study of the prevalence and presentation of dementia in adults with Down's syndrome', *British Journal of Psychiatry*, 172: 493–8.

Holloway, D. (2007) 'Ethical issues in learning disabilities', in B. Gates (ed.), *Learning disabilities: Toward inclusion* (pp. 67–81), London: Elsevier.

Howatson, J. (2005) 'Health action plans for people with learning disabilities', *Nursing Standard*, 19(43): 51–57.

Hutchinson, C. (2005) 'Addressing issues related to adult patients who lack the capacity to give consent', *Nursing Standard*, 9: 47–53.

Jackson, S. and Read, S. (2008) 'Providing appropriate healthcare to people with learning disabilities', *British Journal of Nursing*, 17(4): S6–10.

Jones, E., Perry, J., Lowe, K., Felce, D., Toogood, S., Dunstan, F., *et al.* (1999) 'Opportunity and the promotion of activity among adults with severe learning disabilities living in community housing: The impact of training in Active Support', *Journal of Intellectual Disability Research*, 43(3): 164–178.

Jones, S., Howard, L. and Thornicroft, G. (2008) '"Diagnostic overshadowing": Worse physical healthcare for people with mental illness', *Acta Psychiatrica Scandinavica*, 118(3): 169–171.

Jopp, D.A. and Keys, C.B. (2001) 'Diagnostic overshadowing reviewed and reconsidered', *American Journal of Mental Retardation*, 106(5): 416–433.

Kerfoot, K.M. (2008) 'From blaming to proactively changing the future: The leader's safety challenge', *Nursing Economics*, 26(4): 280–281.

Kerr, M., Felce, D. and Felce, J. (2005) *Equal treatment: Closing the gap. Final report from the Welsh Centre for Learning Disabilities*, Cardiff: Cardiff University.

KFC (1980) *An ordinary life: Comprehensive locally-based residential services for mentally handicapped people*, London: King's Fund Centre.

Kingston, K. and Bailey, C. (2009) 'Assessing the pain of people with a learning disability', *British Journal of Nursing*, 18(7): 420–423.

Kohlberg, L. (1981) *The philosophy of moral development: Moral stages and the idea of justice*, San Francisco: Harper Row.

Kubsch, S.M., Sternard, M.J., Hovarter, R. and Matzke, V. (2004) 'A holistic model of advocacy: Factors that influence its use', *Complementary Therapies in Nursing and Midwifery*, 10(1): 37–45.

Leathard, H.L. and Cook, M.J. (2009) 'Learning for holistic care: Addressing practical wisdom (phronesis) and the spiritual sphere', *Journal of Advanced Nursing*, 65(6): 1318–1327.

Lennox, N.G., Green, M., Diggens, J. and Ugoni, A. (2001) 'Audit and comprehensive health assessment programme in the primary healthcare of adults with intellectual disability: a pilot study', *Journal of Intellectual Disability Research*, 45: 226–232.

Leyshon, S., Clark, L.L., Epstein, L. and Higgins, S. (2004) 'Caring for people with learning disability using care management', *British Journal of Nursing*, 13(14): 845–847.

Lindop, E. and Read, S. (2000) 'District nurses' needs: Palliative care for people with learning disabilities', *International Journal of Palliative Nursing*, 6(3): 117–122.

LSC (2005) *Valuing people and post-16 education summary: Learning and Skills Council guidelines*, London: Learning and Skills Council.

Luck, L., Jackson, D. and Usher, K. (2006) 'Case study: A bridge across the paradigms', *Nursing Inquiry*, 13(2): 103–109.

Lynch, L., Hancox, K. and Happell, B. (2008) *Clinical supervision for nurses*. Chichester: Wiley-Blackwell.

Makaton (2010) *About Makaton*. Retrieved 20 July 2010, from http://www.makaton.org/about/about.htm

Mansell, J. (2010) *Raising our sights: Services for adults with profound intellectual and multiple disabilities*, London: Department of Health.

Manthorpe, J. (2007) 'Accessing services and support', in B. Gates (ed.), *Learning disabilities: Toward inclusion* (pp. 85–105), London: Elsevier.

Marshall, D., McConkey, R. and Moore, G. (2003) 'Obesity in people with intellectual disabilities: The impact of nurse-led health screenings and health promotion activities', *Journal of Advanced Nursing*, 41(2): 147–153.

Matthews, D. (2003) 'Action for health', *Learning Disability Practice*, 6(5): 16–19.

McCallin, A. and Bamford, A. (2007) 'Interdisciplinary teamwork: Is the influence of emotional intelligence fully appreciated?' *Journal of Nursing Management*, 15(4), 386–391.

McCray, J. (2003a) 'Interprofessional practice and learning disability nursing', *British Journal of Nursing*, 12(22): 1335–1344.

McCray, J. (2003b) 'Leading interprofessional practice: A conceptual framework to support practitioners in the field of learning disability', *Journal of Nursing Management*, 11(6): 387–395.

McCue, M. (2000) 'Behavioural interventions', in B. Gates, J. Gear and J. Wray (eds), *Behavioural distress: Concepts and strategies* (pp. 215–256), London: Harcourt.

McNamara, J., Vervaeke, S.L. and Willoughby, T. (2008) 'Learning disabilities and risk-taking behaviour in adolescents: A comparison of those with and without co morbid attention-deficit/hyperactivity disorder', *Journal of Learning Disability*, 41(6): 561–574.

McQueen, A.C.H. (2004) 'Emotional intelligence in nursing work', *Journal of Advanced Nursing*, 47(1), 101–108.

McVicar, A. and Caan, W. (2005) 'Research capability in doctoral training. Evidence for increased diversity of skills in nursing research', *Journal of Research in Nursing*, 10: 627–646.

MENCAP (2004a) *Treat me right! Better health care for people with intellectual disabilities*, London: MENCAP.

MENCAP (2004b) *Treat me right! Better health care for people with intellectual disabilities*, London: MENCAP.

MENCAP (2010a) *About learning disability*. Retrieved 29 June 2010, from http://www.mencap.org.uk/landing.asp?id=1683

MENCAP (2010b) *Changing attitudes*. Retrieved 1 July 2010, from http://www.mencap.org.uk/page.asp?id=1895

MENCAP (2010c) *Communicating with people with profound and multiple learning disabilities (PMLD)*, from http://www.mencap.org.uk/guides.asp?id=459

MENCAP (2010d) *What is communication*? Retrieved 20 July 2010, from http://www.mencap.org.uk/document.asp?id=14864

Minihan, P.M. and Dean, D.H. (1990) 'Meeting the needs of health services of persons with mental retardation living in the community', *American Journal of Public Health*, 80: 1043–1048.

Mount, B. and Zwernik, K. (1988) *It's never too early, it's never too late: A booklet about personal futures planning*, St. Paul, Minnesota: Governor's Planning Council on Developmental Disabilities.

Muir-Gray, J.A. and Northfield, J. (1998) *Research and development in learning disabilities*, Milton Keynes: NHS Executive Anglia and Oxford.

Mullen, R., Admiraal, A. and Trevena, J. (2008) 'Defensive practice in mental health', *New Zealand Medical Journal*, 121(1286): 85–91.

Narayanasamy, A., Gates, B. and Swinton, J. (2002) 'Spirituality and learning disabilities: A qualitative study', *British Journal of Nursing*, 11(14): 948–957.

National Assembly for Wales (2001) *Fulfilling the promises: Proposals for a framework for services for people with learning disabilities. Consultation Document*, Cardiff: National Assembly for Wales.

Nehring, W.M. (2003) 'History of the roles of nurses caring for persons with mental retardation', *Nursing Clinics of North America*, 38: 351–372.

NHSS (2004) *Health needs assessment report: People with learning disabilities in Scotland*, Edinburgh: National Health Service Scotland.

Northern Ireland Assembly (2005) *Equal lives: Review of policy and services for people with a learning disability in Northern Ireland*, Belfast: Northern Ireland Assembly.

Nirje, B. (1992) *The normalization principle papers*, Uppsala, Sweden: Centre for Handicap Research (Uppsala University).

NMC (2004) *Standards of proficiency for pre-registration nursing education*, London: Nursing and Midwifery Council.

NMC (2010a) *Standards for pre-registration nursing education*, London: NMC.

NMC (2010b) *Standards for pre-registration nursing education in the UK*, London: Nursing and Midwifery Council.

Nocon, A. and Sayce, L. (2008) 'Primary healthcare for people with mental health problems or learning disabilities', *Health Policy*, 86(2–3): 325–334.

Nolan, P. and Bradley, E. (2008) 'Evidence-based practice: Implications and concerns', *Journal of Nursing Management*, 16(4): 388–393.

Northway, R., Hutchinson, C. and Kingdon, A. (2005) *A vision for learning disability nursing: A discussion document*, The United Kingdom Learning Disability Consultant Nurse Network.

O'Brien, J. and Towell, D. (2003) *Person-centred planning in its strategic context – Towards a framework for reflection-in-action*, London: Centre for Inclusive Futures/Responsive Systems Associates.

Oermann, M. and Hays, J.C. (2010) *Writing for publication in nursing* (2nd edn), New York: Springer Publishing Company.

Paley, J. (2009) 'Keep the NHS secular', *Nursing Standard*, 23(43): 26–27.

Palmer, G., MacInnes, T. and Kenway, P. (2006) *Monitoring poverty and social exclusion*, York: Joseph Rowntree Foundation.

Parahoo, K. (2006) *Nursing research: Principles, process and issues*, Basingstoke: Palgrave Macmillan.

Pearpoint, J., O'Brien, J. and Forest, M. (1993) *PATH: A workbook for planning positive, possible futures and planning alternative tomorrows with hope for schools, organizations, businesses and families*, Toronto: Inclusion Press.

Perry, J. and Felce, D. (2005) 'Correlation between subjective and objective measures of outcome in staffed community housing', *Journal of Intellectual Disability Research*, 49(Pt 4): 278–287.

Perry, J., Lowe, K., Felce, D. and Jones, S. (2000) 'Characteristics of staffed community housing services for people with learning disabilities: A stratified random sample of statutory, voluntary and private agency provision', *Health and Social Care in the Community*, 8(5): 307–315.

Pesut, B. (2008) 'A reply to "Spirituality and nursing: A reductionist approach" by John Paley', *Nursing Philosophy*, 9(2): 131–137; discussion 138–140.

Polit, D.F. and Beck, C.T. (2009) *Essentials of nursing research: Appraising evidence for nursing practice*, London: Lippincott Williams and Wilkins.

Porter, N. and Yahne, C. (1995) 'Feminist ethics and advocacy in the training of family therapists', *Journal of Feminist Family Therapy*, 6(3): 29–47.

Power, A. (2008) '"It's the system working for the system": Carers' experiences of learning disability services in Ireland', *Health and Social Care in the Community*, 17(1): 92–98.

Power, A. (2009) '"It's the system working for the system": Carers' experiences of learning disability services in Ireland', *Health and Social Care in the Community*, 17(1): 92–98.

Powrie, E. (2002) 'Primary healthcare provision for adults with a learning disability', *Journal of Advanced Nursing*, 42: 413–423.

Prime Minister's Strategy Unit (2005) *Improving the life chances of disabled people*, London: Prime Minister's Strategy Unit.

Race, D.G. (1999) *Social role valorisation and the English experience*, London: Whiting and Birch.

Race, D.G. (2007) 'A tale of two White Papers: Policy documents as indicators of trends in UK services', *Journal of Intellectual Disabilities*, 11(1): 83–103.

RCN (2006a) *Meeting the health needs of people with learning disabilities*, London: Royal College of Nursing.

RCN (2006b) *Mental health nursing of adults with learning disabilities*, London: Royal College of Nursing.

RCN (2011) 'Learning from the past – setting out the future: Developing learning disability nursing in the United Kingdom. An RCN position statement on the role of the learning disability nurse', London: Royal College of Nursing.

Redley, M. and Weinberg, D. (2007) 'Learning disability and the limits of liberal citizenship: Interactional impediments to political empowerment', *Sociology of Health and Illness*, 29(5): 767–786.

Reed, P.G. and Lawrence, L.A. (2008) 'A paradigm for the production of practice-based knowledge', *Journal of Nursing Management*, 16(4): 422–432.

Richardson, M. (2000) 'How we live: Participatory research with six people with learning difficulties', *Journal of Advanced Nursing*, 32(6): 1383–1395.

Ritchie, P., Sanderson, H., Kilbane, J. and Routledge, M. (2003) *People, plans and practicalities: Achieving change through person-centred planning*, Edinburgh: SHS Trust.

Robertson, J., Emerson, E., Hatton, C., Elliott, J., McIntosh, B., Swift, P., *et al.* (2005) *The impact of person-centred planning*, Lancaster: Institute for Health Research, Lancaster University.

Rolfe, G. (2002) 'Faking a difference: Evidence-based nursing and the illusion of diversity', *Nurse Education Today*, 22(1): 3–12.

Rolfe, G. (2005) 'The deconstructing angel: Nursing, reflection and evidence-based practice', *Nursing Inquiry*, 12(2): 78–86.

Rolfe, G. (2006) 'Nursing praxis and the science of the unique', *Nursing Science Quarterly*, 19(1): 39–43.

Routledge, M. (2006) 'Person-centred planning and care management with people with learning disabilities', *Health and Social Care in the Community*, 14(4): 371–372.

Sackett, D.L., Richardson, W.S., Rosenberg, W. and Haynes, R.B. (1997) *Evidence-based medicine*, London: Churchill Livingstone.

Sanderson, H., Kennedy, J. and Ritchie, P. (1997) *People, plans and possibilities: Exploring person-centred planning*, Edinburgh: SHS Ltd.

Sant-Angelo, D. (2000) 'Learning disability community nursing: Addressing emotional and sexual health needs', in R. Astor and K. Jeffereys (eds), *Positive initiatives for people with learning difficulties: Promoting healthy lifestyles* (pp. 52–68), London: Macmillan.

Scottish Executive (2010) *The same as you? A review of services for people with learning disabilities*, Edinburgh: Scottish Executive.

Scottish Executive (2000) *The same as you? A review of services for people with learning disabilities*, Edinburgh: Scottish Executive.

Scottish Executive (2008) *Statistics release: Adults with learning disabilities implementation of 'Same as You?'*, Edinburgh: Scottish Executive.

Sellars, C. (2002) *Risk assessment in people with learning disabilities*, Oxford: Blackwell.

Shaw, S.A. (2009) 'Drawing on three discursive modes in learning disability nurse education', *Nurse Education Today*, 29, 188–195.

Shields, L. and Pearn, J. (2007) 'Inducements for medical and health research: Issues for the profession of nursing', *Journal of Clinical Nursing*, 16(7): 1196–1200.

Signalong Group (2010) *Signalong*. Retrieved 20 July 2010, from http://www.signalong.org.uk/publications/index.htm

Sines, D. and McNally, S. (2007) 'An investigation into the perceptions of clinical supervision experienced by learning disability nurses', *Journal of Intellectual Disabilities*, 11(4), 307–328.

Sines, D., Saunders, M. and Forbes-Burford, J. (eds) (2009) *Community health care nursing*, Chichester: Blackwell.

Slevin, E. and Sines, D. (2005) 'The role of community nurses for people with learning disabilities: Working with people who challenge', *International Journal of Nursing Studies*, 42: 415–427.

Smith, L.J. (2008) 'How ethical is ethical research? Recruiting marginalized, vulnerable groups into health services research', *Journal of Advanced Nursing*, 62(2): 248–257.

Smull, M.W. and Burke-Harrison, S. (1992) *Supporting people with severe reputations in the community*, Alexandria, VA: National Association of State Mental Retardation Program Directors.

Snell, J. (2009) 'UK government sets up inquiry into premature deaths in people with learning disabilities', *British Medical Journal*, 338: b227.

Sowney, M. and Barr, O. (2007) 'The challenges for nurses communicating with and gaining valid consent from adults with intellectual disabilities within the accident and emergency care service', *Journal of Clinical Nursing*, 16(9): 1678–1686.

Stein, W. (2005) 'Modified Sainsbury tool: An initial risk assessment tool for primary care mental health and learning disability services', *Journal of Psychiatric and Mental Health Nursing*, 12(5): 620–633.

Sweeney, C. and Sanderson, H. (2002) *Factsheet – person-centred planning*, Kidderminster: British Institute of Learning Disabilities.

Sweeney, J. and Mitchell, D. (2009) 'A challenge to nursing: An historical review of intellectual disability nursing in the UK and Ireland', *Journal of Clinical Nursing*, 18(19): 2754–2763.

Talbot, P., Astbury, G. and Mason, T. (2010) *Key concepts in learning disabilities*, London: Sage.

Thompson, J., Kilbane, J. and Sanderson, H. (eds) (2008) *Person-centred practice for professionals*, Maidenhead: McGraw Hill Open University Press.

Thomson, K., Gripton, J., Lutchmiah, J. and Caan, W. (2007) 'Health facilitation in primary care seen from practice and education', *British Journal of Nursing*, 16(18): 1156–1160.

Tilly, L. (2008) 'Enabling people with learning disabilities to manage their own health and well-being', *Medicine, Conflict and Survival, 24 Supplement 1*, S108–113.

Turnbull, J. (ed.) (2004) *Learning disability nursing*, Oxford: Blackwell Science Ltd.

Vaartio, H., Leino-Kilpi, H., Salanterä, S. and Suominen, T. (2006) 'Nursing advocacy: How is it defined by patients and nurses, what does it involve and how is it experienced?' *Scandinavian Journal of Caring Sciences*, 20(3): 282–292.

van der Gaag, A. (1998) 'Communication skills and adults with learning disabilities: Eliminating professional myopia', *British Journal of Learning Disabilities*, 26: 88–93.

Vandercook, T., York, J. and Forest, M. (1989) 'The McGill Action Planning System (MAPS): A strategy for building the vision', *Journal of the Association for Persons with Severe Handicaps*, 14: 205–215.

Vere-Jones, E. (2007) 'Does learning disability nursing have a future?' *Nursing Times*, 103(50): 11.

WAG (2001) *Fulfilling the promises*, Cardiff: Welsh Assembly Government.

WAG (2002) *Reference guide for consent to examination and treatment*, Cardiff: Welsh Assembly Government.

WAG (2004) *Learning disability strategy: Section 7 guidance on service principles and services responses*, Cardiff: WAG.

WAG (2006) *Personal social services statistics Wales 2005–06*, Cardiff: Welsh Assembly Government.

WAG (2007) *Statement on policy and practice for adults with a learning disability*, Cardiff: Welsh Assembly Government.

Walmsley, J. (2002) 'Principles and types of advocacy', in B. Gray and R. Jackson (eds), *Advocacy and learning disability* (pp. 24–37), London: Jessica Kingsley.

Walmsley, J. (2004) 'Involving users with learning difficulties in health improvement: Lessons from inclusive learning disability research', *Nursing Inquiry*, 11: 54–64.

Weaver, K. and Olson, J.K. (2006) 'Understanding paradigms used for nursing research', *Journal of Advanced Nursing*, 53(4): 459–469.

Welsh Office (1983) *All Wales strategy for the development of services for mentally handicapped people*, Cardiff: Welsh Office.

Wheeler, P. (2001) Sexuality: Meaning and relevance to learning disability nurses, *British Journal of Nursing*, 10(14): 920–927.

Whittaker, A. and McIntosh, B. (2000) 'Changing days', *British Journal of Learning Disabilities*, 28: 3–8.

WHO (1986) *Ottawa Charter for Health Promotion*, Geneva: World Health Organisation.

WHO (1992) *The ICD-10 classification of mental and behavioural disorders*, Geneva: Division of Mental Health, World Health Organization.

Willard, C. (1996) 'The nurse's role as patient advocate: Obligation or imposition?' *Journal of Advanced Nursing*, 24(1): 60–66.

Williams, P. and Schoultz, B. (1979) *We can speak for ourselves*, London: Souvenir.

Williamson, A. and Johnson, J. (2004) 'Improving services for people with learning disabilities', *Nursing Standard*, 18(24): 43–51; quiz 52–43.

Wolfensberger, W. (1972) *The principle of normalization in human services*, Toronto: National Institute on Mental Retardation.

Wolfensberger, W. (1980) 'The definition of normalisation: update, problems, disagreements and misunderstandings', in R.J. Flynn and K.E. Nitsch (eds), *Normalization, social integration and human services*, Baltimore: University Park Press.

Wolfensberger, W. (1983) 'Social role valorisation: A proposed new term for the principle of normalization', *Mental Retardation*, 21(6): 234–239.

Wolfensberger, W. (1984) 'A reconceptualisation of normalization as social role valorisation', *Mental Retardation (Canada)*, 34(7): 22–26.

Wolfensberger, W. (2000) 'A brief overview of social role valorisation', *Mental Retardation*, 38: 105–123.

Wood, R. (1929) *Report of the Mental Deficiency Committee*, London: HMSO.

Wood, R. and Douglas, M. (2007) 'Cervical screening for women with learning disability: current practice and attitudes within primary care in Edinburgh', *British Journal of Learning Disability*, 35: 84–92.

FURTHER RESOURCES

Weblinks

For the full text of Acts and Regulations mentioned in this chapter see **www.legislation.hmso.gov.uk**.

About Learning Disabilities
http://www.aboutlearningdisabilities.co.uk/how-define-categorise-learning-disabilities.html

Association of Chartered Physiotherapists for People with Learning Disabilities
http://www.acppld.org.uk/

British Institute of Learning Disabilities
http://www.bild.org.uk/

Department of Health – Learning Disabilities
http://webarchive.nationalarchives.gov.uk/+/www.dh.gov.uk/en/SocialCare/Deliveringadultsocialcare/Learningdisabilities/DH_4001805

Foundation for People with Learning Disabilities
http://www.learningdisabilities.org.uk

Hampshire County Council – Communicating with people with a learning disability
http://www3.hants.gov.uk/logos/cx-logos-corporatestandards/cx-logos-accessforall/cx-logos-accesslearning.htm

Health Encyclopedia – Diseases and Conditions
http://www.healthscout.com/ency/68/630/main.html

Helping parents with learning disabilities in their role as parents
http://www.scie.org.uk/publications/briefings/briefing14/index.asp

Just Advocacy (formerly known as Community Partners)
http://www.justadvocacy.org.uk/index.html

Learning Disability Wales
http://www.learningdisabilitywales.org.uk/llais.php

Meeting the health needs of people with learning disabilities
http://www.rcn.org.uk/__data/assets/pdf_file/0004/78691/003024.pdf

MENCAP
http://www.mencap.org.uk/page.asp?id=1684

Mental health nursing of adults with learning disabilities
http://www.rcn.org.uk/__data/assets/pdf_file/0006/78765/003184.pdf

MIND – Learning disabilities and mental health problems
http://www.mind.org.uk/help/people_groups_and_communities/learning_disabilities_and_mental_health_problems

National forum for people with learning disabilities
http://www.nationalforum.org.uk/view.asp?id=0

NHS Evidence – learning disabilities
http://www.library.nhs.uk/learningdisabilities/

PMLD network
http://www.pmldnetwork.org/resources/index.htm

Primary care service framework: management of health for people with learning disabilities in primary care
http://www.primarycarecontracting.nhs.uk/uploads/primary_care_service_frameworks

Psychiatric services for children and adolescents with learning disabilities
http://www.rcpsych.ac.uk/files/pdfversion/cr123.pdf

RCN Learning Disabilities page
http://www.rcn.org.uk/development/practice/social_inclusion/learning_disabilities

Speech and language therapy provision for adults with learning disabilities
http://www.rcslt.org/docs/free-pub/position_paper_ald.pdf

The Foundation for People with Learning Disabilities
http://www.learningdisabilities.org.uk/

This list is for UK learning disability nurses to share information, research and views, and is made available as one of the Yahoo! Health mailing list groups.
http://health.groups.yahoo.com/group/RNLDs/

Understanding individual needs
http://www.understandingindividualneeds.com

Welsh Centre for Learning Disabilities
http://medic.cardiff.ac.uk/archive_subsites/_/_/medic/subsites/learningdisabilities/index.html

CHAPTER 9
NURSING THEORIES, CONCEPTUAL FRAMEWORKS AND PATHWAYS

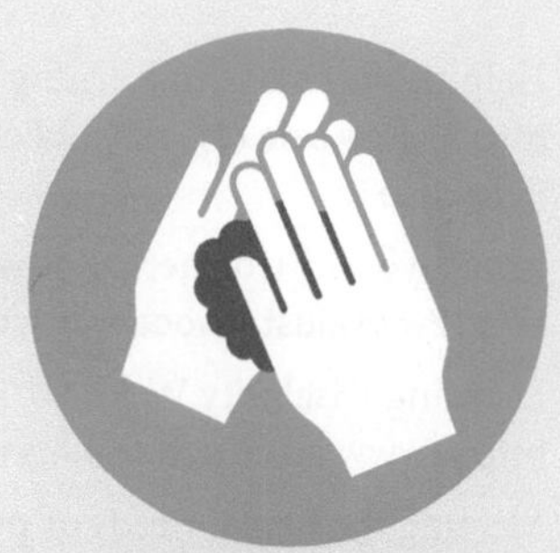

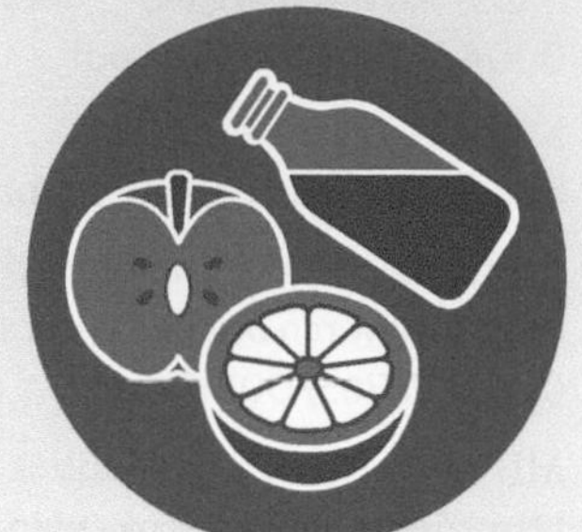

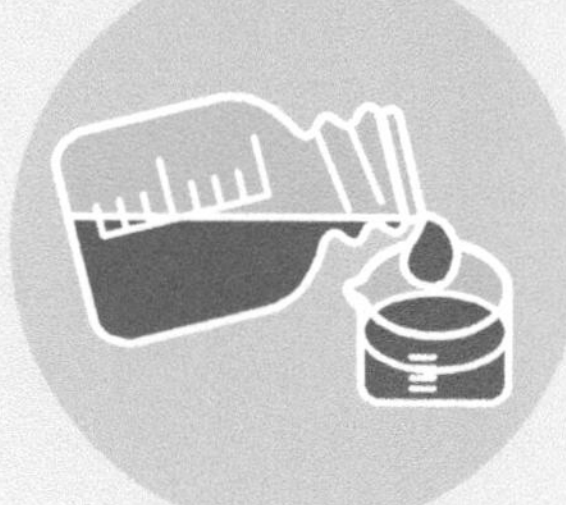

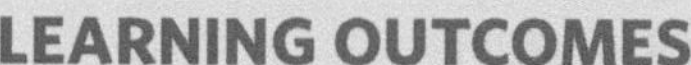

LEARNING OUTCOMES

After completing this chapter, you will be able to:

- Identify the purposes of nursing theory in nursing education, research and clinical practice.
- Identify the components of the metaparadigm for nursing.
- Describe the major purpose of theory in the social sciences and practice disciplines.
- Identify one positive and one negative effect of using theory to understand clinical practice.
- Discuss and identify an appropriate nursing model, conceptual framework and pathway for the individual in your care.

After reading this chapter you will be able to reflect on the nursing role in providing healthcare, the way care is organised and discuss the physical, social and psychological issues related to the care planning. It relates to **Essential Skills Clusters (NMC, 2010) 1, 2, 3, 4, 5, 6, 7, 9, 10, 11, 28**, as appropriate for each progression point.

Ensure that you really understand this chapter by logging on to your complimentary **MyNursingKit** at **www.pearsoned.co.uk/kozier**. Complete the self-assessment tests to check your progress and utilise further activities to practise and confirm your understanding.

CASE STUDY

Stephen is a 45-year-old businessman married with a five-year-old daughter. He has been admitted to your ward several times with an alcohol-related problem which has been managed effectively with medication. He has been advised during these previous admissions that unless he changes his lifestyle, permanent damage to his liver will occur, leading ultimately to an early death. He finds this very difficult as his business relies heavily on this social aspect to introduce new work for his company. On this admission his general condition has deteriorated and he presents to your care with **ascites**, **jaundice**, lack of coordination and cognitive instability. This admission is very challenging as there are physical, psychological and social aspects of care to be considered, both for the patient and the family. During the assessment it is important that you apply the appropriate nursing model and identify and initiate a **care pathway** to ensure best practice and individualised and holistic care for Stephen is assured.

Discuss and provide a rationale for your choice of appropriate model of nursing that will provide an effective framework to guide the care provided to Stephen.

INTRODUCTION

Nursing since its conception has had difficulty in distinguishing whether it is an art or a science. What is evident is that like all disciplines nursing has its own unique knowledge base. This knowledge base is developed through evidence-based practice. However, as with any knowledge a theory or framework guides the practitioner in utilising the knowledge effectively. These theories and/or frameworks are fundamental in ensuring or improving patient care.

THEORIES IN OTHER DISCIPLINES

A theory may be defined as a judgement, conception, proposition or formula relating to phenomena (Merriam-Webster, 1986). Theories projected in the 20th century, for example Freud's theory of the unconscious, Darwin's theory of evolution and Einstein's theory of relativity, influence nursing theory and practice. Inferences can be drawn, for example, from Marx's theory of alienation and student nurses can develop understanding and knowledge of behavioural issues relating to alienation and the social implications of this. Similarly, inferences can be drawn from Freud, Darwin and Einstein's theories which will enable students to apply these theories to enhance patient care.

The extent to which theories build on or modify previous theories varies with the discipline, as does the importance of theory in the discipline. Undergraduate music and art students often take some courses in theory, but these students generally focus on creating art or performing music. Management students study management theories, but the relationship between the theory of management and the practice of management is not quite as strong or evident as the relationship between the theory of physics and the practice of physics. This is because the practice of physics *is* theory and research, whereas the practice of management, teaching, nursing, art, music, law, clinical psychology and pastoral care is something else entirely. The term 'practice discipline' is used for fields of study in which the central focus is performance of a professional role (nursing, teaching, management, music). Practice disciplines are differentiated from the disciplines such as physics and chemistry, that have research and theory development as their central focus. In the practice disciplines, the main function of theory (and research) is to provide a basis and to aid in understanding the discipline's focus.

Context for Theory Development in Nursing

In the 19th century, Florence Nightingale thought that the people of Great Britain needed to know more about how to maintain healthy homes and to care for sick family members. Nightingale's *Notes on nursing: What it is, and what it is not* (1860/1969) was the first textbook on home care and community health. However, the audience for that text was the public at large, not a separate discipline or profession. To Nightingale, the knowledge required to provide good nursing was neither unique nor specialised. Rather, Nightingale viewed nursing as a central human activity grounded in observation, reason and commonsense health practices.

During the 1990s nursing within the UK and Europe followed that in the US by moving into institutions of higher education from the more traditional hospital placed schools of nursing, and indeed the 21st century has now moved to an all graduate profession. This 'new' way of learning developed something that Nightingale had not envisioned for nursing – a unique body of theoretical knowledge.

The more traditional sciences were often seen as role models for this purpose. Theories in the traditional sciences provided a foundation and direction for research. Research in these disciplines often produced tangible results: knowledge that could be used in efforts to control nature, disease and complex health issues due to worldwide travel.

The term 'practice discipline' was not in common use until the very end of the 20th century. Disciplines without a strong theory and research base were referred to as 'soft', a negative comparison with the 'hard' traditional sciences, which elicited scientific results. Many of the soft disciplines attempted to emulate the sciences, so theory and scientific research became a more important part of academic life, both in the practice disciplines and in the humanities.

Whereas theories in the traditional sciences provide a suitable framework for productive research, theories serve a different purpose in the social sciences and practice disciplines such as nursing. In these disciplines, theories work like lenses through which we may interpret things like market forces, industrial efficiency, the human mind, pain and suffering. Their usefulness comes from aiding interpretation of a phenomenon from unique perspectives, building new understandings, relationships and possibilities.

Defining Terms

Theoretical models and systems often use terms that can be difficult to understand but these terms are often used as part of the framework of the theory. Concepts are often called the building blocks of theories or the ideas on which it is based. Concepts are often hard to define because the definition has to include everything that the concept (idea) is made up of, and when the concept is applied or introduced, the outcome of its application. Concepts are easier to understand by example. For example, it is good practice to commence discharge planning for a patient on admission rather than leave it until discharge is imminent. However, theories are not always built like houses out of block-like concepts. Freud's theory of the unconscious not only required some new concepts it required a completely new model. Freud needed a model of the mind that could bring a host of human experiences (or concepts or phenomena) together under one mental roof: dreams, wishes, decisions, behaviours, feelings, anxieties, sexuality. Freud's theory of the mind included three new concepts: the ego, the id and the superego. It would not be right to say that Freud's theory of the unconscious evolved out of these concepts. Rather, these new concepts helped him create a model in which his larger idea, the unconscious, might be understood.

A **conceptual framework**, however, is a group of related ideas, statements or concepts. Freud's structure of the mind (id, ego, superego) could be considered a conceptual framework or model. The term conceptual model is often used interchangeably with conceptual framework, and sometimes with grand theories – those that consider a broad range of the significant relationships among the concepts of a discipline.

No scientific theory is purely objective, because each is developed in cultures and expressed in language. Theories offer ways of looking at or conceptualising the central interests of a discipline, and mathematical terms are often used to express both biological and chemical sciences. In the social and behavioural sciences such as sociology and psychology, theories attempt to explain relationships between concepts. Although it is helpful when these theories are presented in clear, specific, non-ambiguous language, they are most often presented in books that in turn generate other books of critique and explanation, which often complicates understanding of these concepts.

A **paradigm** is a term used broadly to describe both theory and practice; it refers to a pattern of shared understandings and assumptions about reality and the world. Paradigms include our notions of reality that are largely unconscious or taken for granted. For example it is common knowledge that jelly when set is fairly hard but if the jelly is not mixed properly or left out in the sunlight then it does not harden. This fact is based upon either experience or observation. Careful measurements and mixing of the jelly is always considered and the refrigeration of the jelly almost fundamental to its success (with decision making depending on external factors such as the weather).

THE METAPARADIGM FOR NURSING

In the late 20th century, much of the theoretical work in nursing focused on embracing relationships with four major concepts: person, environment, health and nursing. Because these four concepts can be superimposed on almost any work in nursing, they are sometimes collectively referred to as a metaparadigm for nursing, or key concepts of all theories. The term originates from two Greek words: *meta*, meaning 'with' and *paradigm*, meaning 'pattern'.

The following four concepts are considered to be central to nursing.

- **Patient** – the recipient of nursing care (includes individuals, families, groups and communities).
- **Environment** – the internal and external surroundings that affect the patient. This includes people in the physical environment, such as families, friends and significant others.
- **Health** – the degree of wellness or well-being that the patient experiences.
- **Nursing** – the attributes, characteristics and actions of the nurse providing care on behalf of, or in conjunction with, the patient.

Internationally, it can be argued that nurse theorists reflect a wide range of ideas about people, health, values and the world. Each nurse theorist's definitions of these four major concepts vary in accordance with scientific and philosophical orientation, experience in nursing and the effects of that experience on the theorist's view of nursing. A single metaparadigm or basis of nursing may be impossible given the variety of world views expressed in nursing models.

Nursing theories fall into one of two paradigms/concepts. One view reflects prevailing understandings in medicine and the healthcare system; the other view reflects emerging understandings in **transpersonal psychology**.

It is important to remember that any organised approach to understanding the world – including theories, social practices and people – can both illuminate and obscure what is of central importance to nurses.

PURPOSES OF NURSING THEORY

Direct links exist among theory, education, research and clinical practice.

In Education

Since the early 1970s and 1980s nursing theory was taught, delivered and became more firmly established in academia than in clinical practice. In the 1970s and 1980s, many nursing programmes identified the major concepts in one or two nursing models, organised these concepts into a conceptual framework and then attempted to organise the entire curriculum around that framework. However, in the 1990s and 2000 this was developed into more individualised holistic care of the patient and by 2012 the NMC will be working towards generic concepts which will ensure that the student nurse will be 'Fit for Purpose', 'Fit for Practice' in the continuously changing healthcare environment. Furthermore, the introduction of working towards an all graduate profession in Wales and Scotland in 2004 and 2005 respectively has developed further with Northern Ireland (2011) and England (2013) securing an all graduate profession, suggesting that nursing theory is fundamental to the nursing profession.

In Research

Nurse scholars have repeatedly insisted that nursing research identifies the philosophical assumptions or a theoretical framework on which it is founded on. That is because all thinking, writing and speaking is based on previous assumptions about people and the world. New theoretical perspectives provide an essential framework by identifying gaps in the way we approach specific fields of study such as symptom management or quality of life. Different theoretical perspectives can also help generate new ideas, research questions and interpretations.

Grand theories only occasionally direct nursing research. Nursing research is more often informed by mid-level theories that focus on the exploration of concepts such as pain, self-esteem and learning. Qualitative research in nursing and the social sciences can also be based on theories from philosophy or the social sciences (as previously noted). The term critical theory is used in academia to describe theories that help clarify how social structures affect a wide variety of human experiences from art to social practices. In nursing, critical theory helps explain how structures such as race, gender, sexual orientation and economic class affect patient experiences and health outcomes.

In Clinical Practice

Where nursing theory has been utilised in a clinical setting, its main contribution has been the facilitation of reflection, questioning and thinking about what nurses do. An increasing body of theoretical scholarship in nursing has been outside the framework of the formal theories. Benner (2000) and MacIntyre (2001) argue that formalistic theories are too often superimposed on the life-worlds of patients, overshadowing core values of the profession and our patients' humanity. Family theorists and critical theorists have encouraged the profession to move the focus from individuals to families and social structures. The focus is to bridge the gap between acute hospital and primary and community care settings. This will promote independence by providing enhanced services from the NHS in order to reduce, or prevent, unnecessary hospital admission (DH, 2007).

OVERVIEW OF SELECTED NURSING THEORIES/MODELS

The theories discussed in this chapter provide nurses with concepts of care provision holistically. Philosophies, conceptual frameworks/grand theories and mid-level theories are discussed. A philosophy is often an early effort to define nursing phenomena and serves as the basis for later theoretical formulations of theory. Examples of philosophies are those of Nightingale, Henderson and Watson. Conceptual models/grand theories include those of Orem, Roper, Logan and Tierney, Rogers, Roy, King and Casey; whereas mid-level theorists are Peplau, Leininger, Parse and Neuman. Only brief summaries of the author's philosophy, central theme and basic assumptions are included here.

Nightingale's Environmental Theory

Florence Nightingale, often considered the first nurse theorist, defined nursing more than 100 years ago as 'the act of utilising the environment of the patient to assist him in his recovery' (Nightingale, 1969). She linked health with five environmental factors: (1) pure or fresh air, (2) pure water, (3) efficient drainage, (4) cleanliness and (5) light, especially direct sunlight. Deficiencies in these five factors produced lack of health or illness.

These environmental factors attain significance when one considers that sanitation conditions in the hospitals of the mid-1800s were extremely poor and that women working in the hospitals were often unreliable, uneducated and incompetent to care for the ill. In addition to those factors, Nightingale also stressed the importance of keeping the patient warm, maintaining a noise-free environment, and attending to the patient's diet in terms of assessing intake, nutritional value, timeliness of the food and its effect on the person.

Nightingale set the stage for further work in the development of nursing theories. Her general concepts about ventilation, cleanliness, quiet, warmth and diet remain integral parts of nursing and healthcare today.

Peplau's Interpersonal Relations Model

Hildegard Peplau, a psychiatric nurse, introduced her interpersonal concepts in 1952 as one of the first models of psychiatric nursing care. Central to Peplau's theory is the use of a therapeutic relationship between the nurse and the patient.

Nurses enter into a personal relationship with an individual when a need is present. The nurse–patient relationship evolves in four phases:

1 **Orientation.** During this phase, the patient seeks help, and the nurse assists the patient to understand the problem and the extent of the need for help.

2 **Identification.** During this phase, the patient assumes a posture of dependence, interdependence or independence in relation to the nurse (relatedness). The nurse's focus is to assure the person that the nurse understands the interpersonal meaning of the patient's situation.
3 **Exploitation.** In this phase, the patient derives full value from what the nurse offers through the relationship. The patient uses available services based on self-interest and needs. Power shifts from the nurse to the patient.
4 **Resolution.** In this final phase, old needs and goals are put aside and new ones adopted. Once older needs are resolved, newer and more mature ones emerge.

To help patients fulfil their needs, nurses assume many roles: stranger, teacher, resource person, surrogate, leader and counsellor. Peplau's model continues to be used by clinicians when working with individuals who have psychological problems.

Henderson's Definition of Nursing

In 1966, Virginia Henderson's definition of the unique function of nursing was a major stepping stone in the emergence of nursing as a discipline separate from medicine. Virginia Henderson has been described as the *first lady of nursing*. An accomplished author, avid researcher and a visionary, she is considered by many to be the most important nursing figure in the 20th century. Like Nightingale, Henderson described nursing in relation to the patient and the patient's environment. Unlike Nightingale, Henderson saw the nurse as concerned with both healthy and ill individuals, acknowledged that nurses interact with patients even when recovery may not be feasible, and mentioned the teaching and advocacy roles of the nurse.

Henderson (1966) conceptualised the nurse's role as assisting sick or healthy individuals to gain independence in meeting 14 fundamental needs:

- breathing normally;
- eating and drinking adequately;
- eliminating body wastes;
- moving and maintaining a desirable position;
- sleeping and resting;
- selecting suitable clothes;
- maintaining body temperature within normal range by adjusting clothing and modifying the environment;
- keeping the body clean and well groomed to protect the integument;
- avoiding dangers in the environment and avoiding injuring others;
- communicating with others in expressing emotions, needs, fears or opinions;
- worshipping according to one's faith;
- working in such a way that one feels a sense of accomplishment;
- playing or participating in various forms of recreation;
- learning, discovering or satisfying the curiosity that leads to normal development and health, and using available health facilities.

Henderson has published many works and continues to be cited in current nursing literature. Her emphasis on the importance of nursing's independence from, and interdependence with, other healthcare disciplines is well recognised.

Rogers' Science of Unitary Human Beings

Professor Martha Rogers' (1914–1994) philosophy was that nursing was a learned profession that incorporated both science and art. She believed that an unitary human being is 'irreducible, indivisible, pan dimensional (four-dimensional) energy field identified by pattern and manifesting characteristics that are specific to the whole and which cannot be predicted from knowledge of the parts' and 'a unified whole having its own distinctive characteristics which cannot be perceived by looking at, describing, or summarising the parts'. This belief led her to develop the Science of Unitary Human Beings.

Rogers views the person as an irreducible whole, the whole being greater than the sum of its parts. *Whole* is differentiated from *holistic*, the latter often being used to mean only the sum of all parts. She states that humans are dynamic energy fields in continuous exchange with environmental fields, both of which are infinite. The 'human field image' perspective surpasses that of the physical body. Both human and environmental fields are characterised by pattern, a universe of open systems, and four dimensionality. According to Rogers (1970), unitary man:

- is an irreducible, four-dimensional energy field identified by pattern;
- manifests characteristics different from the sum of the parts;
- interacts continuously and creatively with the environment;
- behaves as a totality;
- as a sentient being, participates creatively in change.

Nurses applying Rogers' theory in practice (a) focus on the person's wholeness, (b) seek to promote symphonic interaction between the two energy fields (human and environment) to strengthen the coherence and integrity of the person, (c) coordinate the human field with the rhythmicities of the environmental field, and (d) direct and redirect patterns of interaction between the two energy fields to promote maximum health potential.

Nurses' use of noncontact therapeutic touch is based on the concept of human energy fields. The qualities of the field vary from person to person and are affected by pain and illness. Although the field is infinite, realistically it is most clearly 'felt' within several feet of the body. Nurses trained in noncontact therapeutic touch claim they can assess and feel the energy field and manipulate it to enhance the healing process of people who are ill or injured.

Orem's General Theory of Nursing

Dorothea Orem (1914–2007), founder of the Orem model of nursing, was a nurse academic. Orem's theory, first published in 1971, includes three related concepts: self-care, self-care deficit and nursing systems. Self-care theory is based on four concepts:

self-care, self-care agency, self-care requisites and therapeutic self-care demand. Self-care refers to those activities an individual performs independently throughout life to promote and maintain personal well-being. Self-care agency is the individual's ability to perform self-care activities. It consists of two agents: a self-care agent (an individual who performs self-care independently) and a dependent care agent (a person other than the individual who provides the care). Most adults care for themselves, whereas infants and people weakened by illness or disability require assistance with self-care activities.

Self-care requisites, also called self-care needs, are measures or actions taken to provide self-care. There are three categories of self-care requisites:

1 Universal requisites are common to all people. They include maintaining intake and elimination of air, water and food; balancing rest, solitude and social interaction; preventing hazards to life and well-being; and promoting normal human functioning.
2 Developmental requisites result from maturation or are associated with conditions or events, such as adjusting to a change in body image or to the loss of a spouse.
3 Health deviation requisites result from illness, injury or disease, or its treatment. They include actions such as seeking healthcare assistance, carrying out prescribed therapies, and learning to live with the effects of illness or treatment.

Therapeutic self-care demand refers to all self-care activities required to meet existing self-care requisites, or in other words, actions to maintain health and well-being (see Figure 9-1).

Self-care deficit results when self-care agency is not adequate to meet the known self-care demand. Orem's self-care deficit theory explains not only when nursing is needed but also how people can be assisted through five methods of helping: acting or doing for, guiding, teaching, supporting, and providing an environment that promotes the individual's abilities to meet current and future demands.

Orem identifies three types of nursing systems:

1 Wholly compensatory systems are required for individuals who are unable to control and monitor their environment and process information.
2 Partly compensatory systems are designed for individuals who are unable to perform some, but not all, self-care activities.
3 Supportive-educative (developmental) systems are designed for persons who need to learn to perform self-care measures and need assistance to do so.

The five methods of helping discussed for self-care deficit can be used in each nursing system.

Roper, Logan and Tierney's Activities of Living Model

Nancy Roper (1918–2004), Winifred W. Logan and Alison J. Tierney published in 1980 the first British model with adaptations in later years and most recently in 2000 (Roper *et al.*, 1980, 1981, 1983, 2000). The model was developed to support student nurses in their learning. Roper, Logan and Tierney (RLT) believe that nursing should embrace the living person as a whole entity and should be assessed as promoting holistic care (Roper *et al.*, 2000). The model was developed and influenced by Maslow (1954), a psychologist, and Virginia Henderson (1966). According to Barrett *et al.* (2009) there are five key issues that are intrinsic to the model:

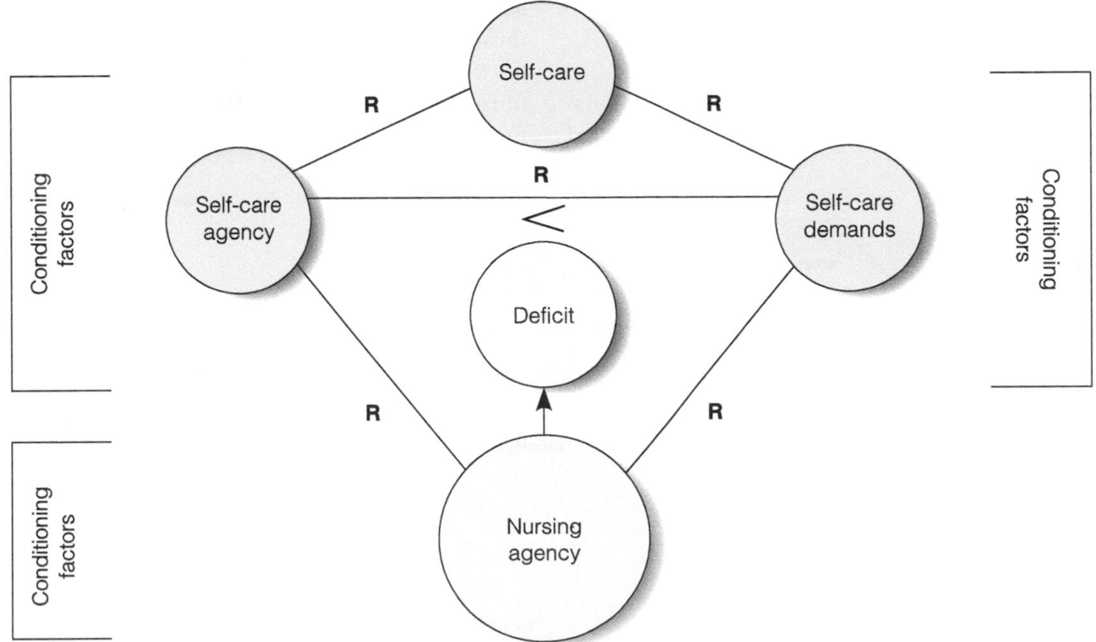

Figure 9-1 The major components of Orem's self-care deficit theory. R indicates a relationship between components; < indicates a current or potential deficit where nursing would be required.

Source: based on Orem, D.E. *et al.* (2001).

- individuality;
- the activities of living;
- a dependence–independence continuum;
- the progression of a person along a life-span continuum;
- influencing factors.

The RLT model (2000) is made up of 12 activities of daily living (see *Box 9-1*). These are activities that an individual will undertake during everyday living. Intrinsic to the 12 activities of living is the need to consider and assess biological, socio-cultural, psychological, environmental and politico-economic issues affecting health and well-being.

BOX 9-1 Activities of Living

1 Maintaining a safe environment
2 Communicating
3 Breathing
4 Eating and drinking
5 Eliminating
6 Personal cleansing and dressing
7 Controlling body temperature
8 Mobilising
9 Working and playing
10 Sleeping
11 Expressing sexuality
12 Dying

Once a comprehensive assessment of the patient has been undertaken then an identified healthcare need of the patient can be assigned to the appropriate activity of daily living, thus providing a framework for patient care.

King's Goal Attainment Theory

Imogene King (1923–2007) was recognised as a founder of nursing theory. Her theory of goal attainment (1981) was derived from her conceptual framework (see Figure 9-2). Her framework demonstrates the relationship of operational systems (individuals), interpersonal systems (groups such as nurse-patient), and social systems (such as educational system, healthcare system). She selected 15 concepts from the nursing literature (self, role, perception, communication, interaction, transaction, growth and development, stress, time, personal space, organisation, status, power, authority and decision making) as essential knowledge for use by nurses.

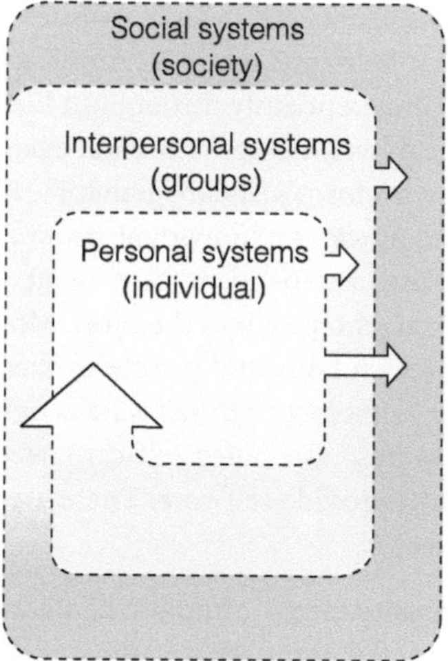

Figure 9-2 King's conceptual framework for nursing: dynamic interacting systems.

Source: *A Theory for Nursing: Systems, Concepts, Process* (p. 11), by I.M. King, 1981, Albany, NY: Delmar. Copyright Imogene M. King, with permission from the author.

Ten of the concepts in the framework were selected (self, role, perception, communication, interaction, transaction, growth and development, stress, time and personal space) as essential knowledge for use by nurses in concrete nursing situations. Within this theory, a transaction process model was designed (see Figure 9-3). This process describes the nature of and standard for nurse–patient interactions that leads to goal attainment – that nurses purposefully interact and mutually set, explore and agree

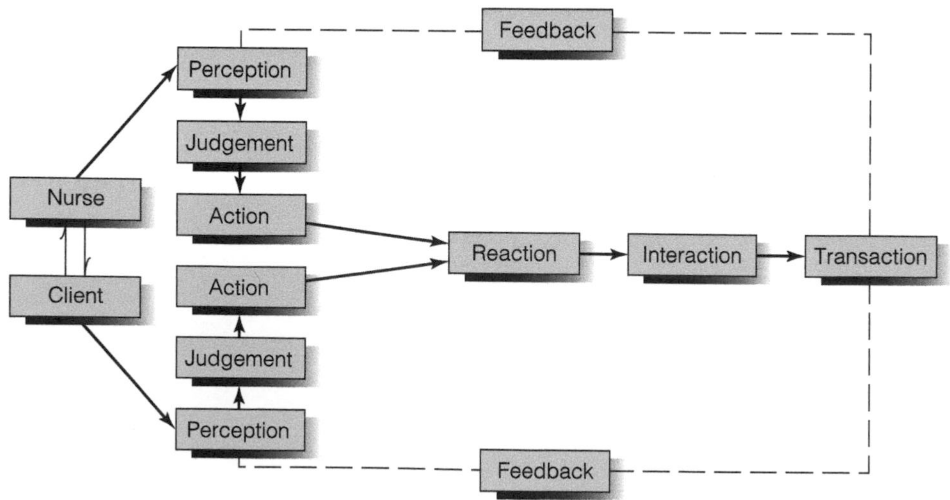

Figure 9-3 King's model of transactions.

Source: *A Theory for Nursing: Systems, Concepts, Process* (p. 145), by I.M. King, 1981, Albany, NY: Delmar. Copyright Imogene M. King, with permission from the author.

to the means to achieve goals. Goal attainment represents outcomes. When this information is recorded in the patient record, nurses have data that represent evidence-based nursing practice.

King's theory offers insight into nurses' interactions with individuals and groups within the environment. It highlights the importance of a patient's participation in decisions that influence care and focuses on both the process of the nurse–patient interaction and the outcomes of care.

Neuman's Systems Model

Betty Neuman (Neuman and Fawcett, 2002), a community health nurse and clinical psychologist, developed a model based on the individual's relationship to stress, the reaction to it, and reconstitution factors that are dynamic in nature. Reconstitution is the state of adaptation to stressors.

Neuman views the patient as an open system consisting of a basic structure or central core of energy resources (physiological, psychological, sociocultural, developmental and spiritual) surrounded by two concentric boundaries or rings referred to as lines of resistance (see Figure 9-4). The lines of resistance represent internal factors that help the patient defend against a stressor; one example is an increase in the body's leukocyte count to combat an infection. Outside the lines of resistance are two lines of defence. The inner or normal line of defence, depicted as a solid line, represents the person's state of equilibrium or the state of adaptation developed and maintained over time and considered normal for that person. The flexible line of defence, depicted as a broken line, is dynamic and can be rapidly altered over a short period of time. It is a protective buffer that prevents stressors from penetrating the normal line of defence. Certain variables (e.g. sleep deprivation) can create rapid changes in the flexible line of defence.

Neuman categorises stressors as intra-personal stressors, those that occur within the individual (e.g. an infection); interpersonal stressors, those that occur between individuals (e.g. unrealistic role expectations); and extrapersonal stressors, those that occur outside the person (e.g. financial concerns). The individual's reaction to stressors depends on the strength of the lines of defence. When the lines of defence fail, the resulting reaction depends on the strength of the lines of resistance. As part of the reaction, a person's system can adapt to a stressor, an effect known as reconstitution.

Nursing interventions focus on retaining or maintaining system stability. These interventions are carried out on three preventive levels: primary, secondary and tertiary.

- Primary prevention focuses on protecting the normal line of defence and strengthening the flexible line of defence.
- Secondary prevention focuses on strengthening internal lines of resistance, reducing the reaction and increasing resistance factors.
- Tertiary prevention focuses on readaptation and stability and protects reconstitution or return to wellness following treatment.

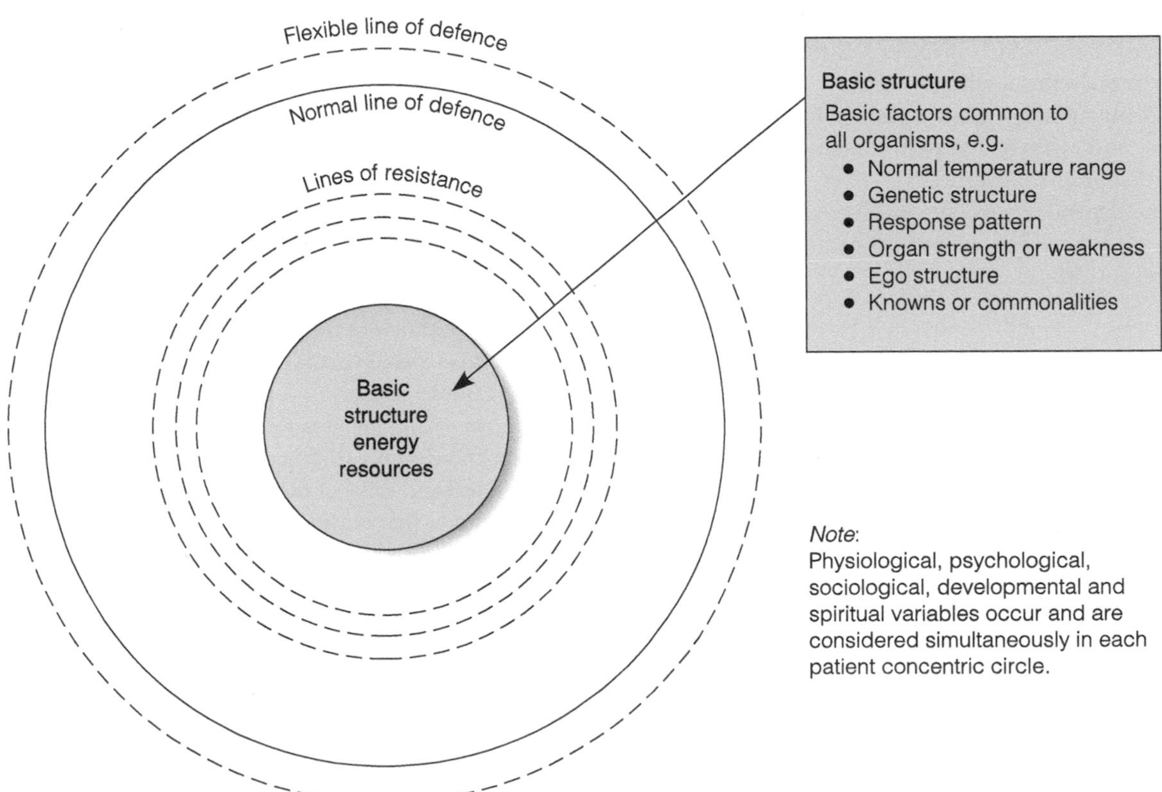

Figure 9-4 Neuman's patient system.

Source: Neuman, Betty; Fawcett, Jacqueline, *Neuman Systems Model, The*, 4th Edition, © 2002, pg 15. Reprinted by permission of Pearson Education Inc., Upper Saddle River, NJ.

Betty Neuman's model of nursing is applicable to a variety of nursing practice settings involving individuals, families, groups and communities.

Roy's Adaptation Model

Sister Callista Roy is a member of the Sisters of Saint Joseph of Carondelet. Roy is both a professor and nurse theorist, and defines adaptation as 'the process and outcome whereby the thinking and feeling person uses conscious awareness and choice to create human and environmental integration' (Roy, 1997: 44).

Roy developed the adaptation model in 1976 and focuses on the individual as a biopsychosocial adaptive system that employs a feedback cycle of input (stimuli), throughput (control processes) and output (behaviours or adaptive responses). Both the individual and the environment are sources of stimuli that require medication to promote adaptation, an ongoing purposive response. Adaptive responses contribute to health, which she defines as the process of being and becoming integrated; ineffective or maladaptive responses do not contribute to health. Each person's adaptation level is unique and constantly changing.

Individuals respond to needs (stimuli) in one of four modes (Roy, 1997):

1 The physiological mode involves the body's basic physiological needs and ways of adapting with regard to fluid and electrolytes, activity and rest, circulation and oxygen, nutrition and elimination, protection, the senses, and neurological and endocrine function.
2 The self-concept mode includes two components: the physical self, which involves sensation and body image, and the personal self, which involves self-ideal, self-consistency and the moral-ethical self.
3 The role function mode is determined by the need for social integrity and refers to the performance of duties based on given positions within society.
4 The interdependence mode involves one's relations with significant others and support systems that provide help, affection and attention.

The goal of Callista Roy's model is to enhance life processes through adaptation in the four adaptive modes.

Leininger's Cultural Care Diversity and Universality Theory

Madeleine Leininger, a well-known nurse anthropologist, put her views on transcultural nursing in print in the 1970s and 1990s and then in 2006 published her book *Culture care diversity and universality: A theory of nursing*.

Leininger states that care is the essence of nursing and the dominant, distinctive and unifying feature of nursing. She emphasises that human caring, although a universal phenomenon, varies among cultures in its expressions, processes and patterns; it is largely culturally derived. Leininger produced the Sunrise model to depict her theory of cultural care diversity and universality. This model emphasises that health and care are influenced by elements of the social structure, such as technology, religious and philosophical factors, kinship and social systems, cultural values, political and legal factors, economic factors and educational factors. These social factors are addressed within environmental contexts, language expressions and ethnohistory. Each of these systems is part of the social structure of any society; healthcare expressions, patterns and practices are also integral parts of these aspects of social structure (Leininger and McFarland, 2002). In order for nurses to assist people of diverse cultures, Leininger (2006) presents three intervention modes:

1 Culture care preservation and maintenance
2 Culture care accommodation, negotiation, or both
3 Culture care restructuring and repatterning.

Watson's Human Caring Theory

Dr. Jean Watson, a Professor of Nursing, a psychiatric and mental health nurse, believes the practice of caring is central to nursing; it is the unifying focus for practice. Her major assumptions about caring are that:

- Human caring in nursing is not just an emotion, concern, attitude or benevolent desire. Caring connotes a personal response.
- Caring is an intersubjective human process and is the moral ideal of nursing.
- Caring can be effectively demonstrated only interpersonally.
- Effective caring promotes health and individual or family growth.
- Caring promotes health more than does curing.
- Caring responses accept a person not only as they are now, but also for what the person may become.
- A caring environment offers the development of potential while allowing the person to choose the best action for these at a given point in time.
- Caring occasions involve action and choice by nurse and patient. If the caring occasion is transpersonal, the limits of openness expand, as do human capacities.
- The most abstract characteristic of a caring person is that the person is somehow responsive to another person as a unique individual, perceives the other's feelings and sets one person apart from another.
- Human caring involves values, a will and a commitment to care, knowledge, caring actions and consequences.
- The ideal and value of caring is a starting point, a stance and an attitude that has to become a will, an intention, a commitment and a conscious judgement that manifests itself in concrete acts.

(*Note*: From J. Watson, personal communication, 22 September 2002.)

Nursing interventions relating to human care are referred to as *carative factors*, a guide Watson refers to as the 'Core of Nursing'. Watson outlines the following 10 factors:

1 Forming a humanistic-altruistic system of values.
2 Instilling faith and hope.

3 Cultivating sensitivity to one's self and others.
4 Developing a helping-trust (human care) relationship.
5 Promoting and accepting the expression of positive and negative feelings.
6 Systematically using the scientific problem-solving method for decision making.
7 Promoting interpersonal teaching–learning.
8 Providing a supportive, protective or corrective mental, physical, sociocultural and spiritual environment.
9 Assisting with the gratification of human needs.
10 Allowing for existential-phenomenological forces (aspects from outside the individual or their area of control).

Watson's (1979) theory of human caring has received worldwide recognition as a major force in redefining nursing as a caring-healing health model.

Parse's Human Becoming Theory

Rosemarie Rizzo Parse's work is based on human becoming theory (1995) and is an alternative to the traditional nursing theory. The human becoming theory focuses on the lived experience and the interaction of individuals through their journey.

Parse's theory proposes three assumptions about *human becoming*:

1 Human becoming is freely choosing personal meaning in situations in the inter-subjective process of relating value priorities.
2 Human becoming is co-creating rhythmic patterns or relating in mutual process with the universe.
3 Human becoming is cotranscending multidimensionally (finding unique ways of living in many aspects of life), with the emerging possibles.

These three assumptions are based on finding different ways of living and focus on meaning, rhythmicity and cotranscendence.

- Meaning arises from a person's interrelationship with the world and refers to happenings to which the person attaches varying degrees of significance.
- Rhythmicity is the movement towards greater diversity.
- Cotranscendence is the process of reaching out beyond the self.

Parse's model of human becoming emphasises how individuals choose and bear responsibility for patterns of personal health. Parse contends that the patient, not the nurse, is the authority figure and decision maker. The nurse's role involves helping individuals and families in choosing the possibilities for changing the health process. Specifically, the nurse's role consists of illuminating meaning (uncovering what was and what will be), synchronising rhythms (leading through discussion to recognise harmony), and mobilising transcendence (dreaming of possibilities and planning to reach them).

The Parse nurse uses 'true presence' in the nurse–patient process. 'In true presence the nurse's whole being is immersed with the patient as the other illuminates the meanings of his or her situation and moves beyond the moment' (Parse, 1994: 18).

Casey's Partnership Model of Nursing

Until 2009, Anne Casey was editor of the *Paediatric Nursin[g]* journal which is published by the RCN. In 2002 she was made a fellow of the RCN for her services to paediatric nursing and nursing informatics. In 1988, while working in Great Ormond Street Hospital, London she developed a nursing model which focused on working in partnership with children and their families.

The model comprises of five concepts and the relationships between them (Casey, 1988):

- Child
- Family
- Health
- Environment
- Nurse.

This is broken down further as:

Child
Nurse
Ability of child/family to participate in care environment
Dependent – independent continuum
Functioning, growing and developing
Emotional
Social

Family
Partnership
Health
Conception–maturity continuum
Physical
Intellectual
Spiritual

The philosophy of the model, which is widely used by children's nurses in hospital and community settings across the UK, is that the families are the best people to care for the child with support from professionals when needed. Interesting to note is that according to Fawcett's analysis, the model is not a nursing model but a middle range theory (Fawcett, 1995).

CRITIQUE OF NURSING THEORY

Several nurse scholars have developed strong critiques of 20th century nursing theories, choosing to ground their work in philosophy or the social sciences (Benner, 2000; Munhall, 2007). The best theories in philosophy and the social sciences are often used in the humanities for the insights and perspectives that can be brought to literature and art. So far, other disciplines have not discovered a sufficiently unique or interesting perspective on the human condition in nursing theories.

Nursing scholars continue to debate whether grounding our research in the best theories from other disciplines is good or bad. Some think this detracts from the development of nursing as a separate discipline; others argue that nursing research becomes more relevant when informed by scholarship that addresses larger social concerns.

Theory can be used to broaden our perspectives in nursing and facilitate the altruistic (showing unselfish concern for the welfare of others) and humanistic values of the profession. At the same time, rational and predictive theory can produce language and social practices that are superimposed onto the

ents and do violence to the fragility of s in which to view the world through, nate or obscure; as a tool, theory can

ACTIVITY 9-1

Consider and reflect on what you have just read and highlight why a nursing theory/model is effective in patient care.

NURSING THEORY AND APPLICATION

The nursing process is a strategy by which nursing care is delivered. It was developed from a problem-solving approach as a means of delivering patient care incorporating philosophies, theories and models of nursing. While the nursing process originally was made up of four key stages:

- plan
- assess
- implement and
- evaluate

many would argue that a fifth component of the nursing process is nursing diagnosis (see Figure 9-5). The nursing process is cyclical and ongoing and can be revisited, reassessed, replanned, rediagnosed, reimplemented and re-evaluated at any point, which is fundamental to its effectiveness.

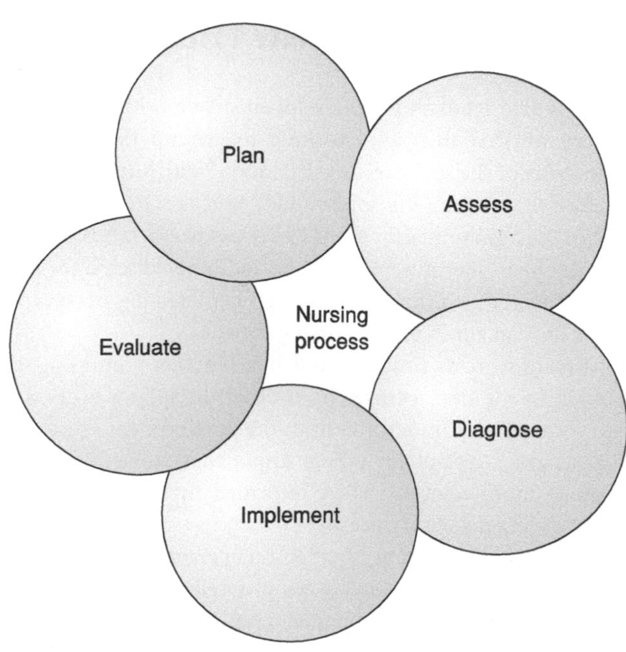

Figure 9-5 The nursing process.

Patient Pathway/Care Pathways/Integrated Care Pathways

According to the Department of Health (2007) a 'patient pathway' is 'the route that a patient will take from their first contact with a National Health Service member of staff (usually their GP through referral) to the completion of their treatment'.

A **care pathway** is a system that by mutual decision making, organisational policies, guidelines, etc. is incorporated into patient care to provide excellent, up-to-date care for a patient or group of patients over a clearly defined period.

Vanhaecht *et al.* (2007) define care pathways as:

(i) An explicit statement of the goals and key elements of care based on evidence, best practice and patients' expectations and their characteristics;
(ii) the facilitation of the communication among the team members and with patients and families;
(iii) the coordination of the care process by coordinating the roles and sequencing the activities of the multidisciplinary care team, patients and their relatives;
(iv) the documentation, monitoring, and evaluation of variances and outcomes; and
(v) the identification of the appropriate resources.

An integrated care pathway (ICP) is multidisciplinary and includes all aspects of patient care. According to WAG (2003) the Gold standard for development for ICPs are that they:

- are placed in an appropriate time frame;
- are written and agreed by a multidisciplinary team;
- are locally agreed standards based on evidence;
- form part of the clinical record/documentation;
- facilitate and demonstrate quality improvement;
- include patient milestones and clinical interventions.

The WAG (2003) also states that ICPs should work towards and/or include the following standards:

- Multidisciplinary
- Single documentation
- Use exception reporting
- Variance analysis
- Patient involvement
- Monitoring of the utilisation
- Cross boundaries
- Standard format
- Outcome orientated
- Built-in audit
- Evidence based.

National Service Frameworks

The Department of Health recognised the need to address the quality of care provided especially with specific patient groups, to ensure that the care provided was based on evidence and consistent wherever it was provided. The White Paper *Quality care and clinical excellence*, highlighted that National Service Frameworks (NSF) provide a systematic approach on which to tackle the agenda of improving standards and quality across healthcare sectors. NSFs are implemented in partnership with social care and other organisations.

National service frameworks:

- set national standards and define service models for a service or care group;
- put in place programmes to support implementation;
- establish performance measures against which progress within agreed timescales would be measured.

There are currently eight NSFs published with one other in publication:

- cancer;
- children, young people and maternity;
- coronary heart disease;
- diabetes;
- long-term conditions;
- mental health;
- older people;
- renal services;
- COPD (in production).

All of these can be accessed via the links at the end of the chapter.

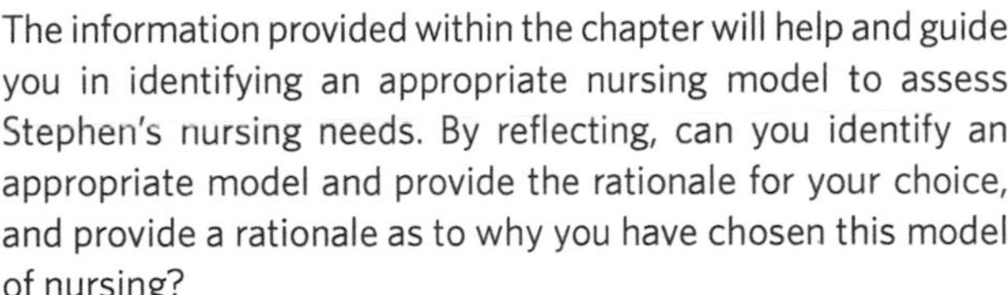
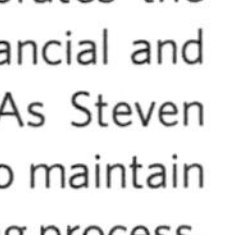

CRITICAL REFLECTION

The information provided within the chapter will help and guide you in identifying an appropriate nursing model to assess Stephen's nursing needs. By reflecting, can you identify an appropriate model and provide the rationale for your choice, and provide a rationale as to why you have chosen this model of nursing?

The Roper, Logan and Tierney (2000) model looks at the individual patient as a 'whole' and not from a disease-based approach (Barrett *et al.*, 2009). The model outlines both the 'normal' and the not so normal for each patient. Each of the 12 activities of daily life are placed on a continuum of dependence to independence. The model incorporates the physical, psychological, socio-cultural, politico-financial and environmental factors that influence healthcare. As Steven has been admitted he is dependent on the nurses to maintain his activities of daily living identified from the nursing process. The Roper, Logan and Tierney (2000) model could be considered as one of the most appropriate in this instance.

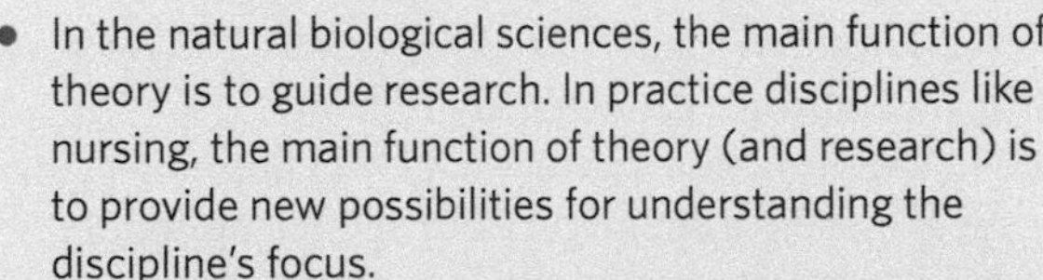
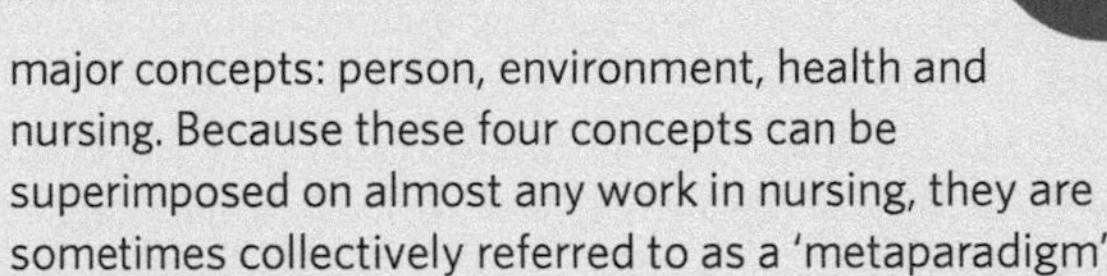
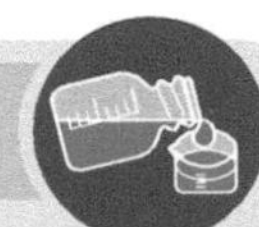

CHAPTER HIGHLIGHTS

- In the natural biological sciences, the main function of theory is to guide research. In practice disciplines like nursing, the main function of theory (and research) is to provide new possibilities for understanding the discipline's focus.
- To Nightingale, the knowledge required to provide good nursing was neither unique nor specialised. Rather, Nightingale viewed nursing as a central human activity grounded in observation, reason and commonsense health practices.
- During the latter half of the 20th century, disciplines seeking to establish themselves in universities had to demonstrate something that Nightingale had not envisioned for nursing - a unique body of theoretical knowledge.
- Theories articulate significant relationships between concepts in order to point to something larger, such as gravity, the unconscious or the experience of pain.
- Paradigms include our notions of reality that are largely unconscious or taken for granted. Most theories reflect the dominant paradigm of a culture, although some may grow out of a developing rival paradigm.
- In the late 20th century, much of the theoretical work in nursing focused on articulating relationships between four major concepts: person, environment, health and nursing. Because these four concepts can be superimposed on almost any work in nursing, they are sometimes collectively referred to as a 'metaparadigm' for nursing.
- It is important to remember that any organised approach to understanding the world - including theories, social practices and people - can both illuminate and obscure what is of central importance to nurses.
- Debates about the role of theory in nursing practice provide evidence that nursing is maturing, both as an academic discipline and a clinical profession.
- The application of a nursing model helps and guides a nurse when assessing, diagnosing, planning, implementing and evaluating patient care.
- Implementing an appropriate pathway provides clear guidelines, effective communication and effective ways of evaluating patient care.
- Quality is fundamental to the success of the National Health Service in order to provide excellent patient care. Successive governments have recognised this and developed National Frameworks based on evidence to support and guide practitioners in order to provide these standards nationally.

ACTIVITY ANSWERS

ACTIVITY 9-1 There is much discussion as to the purpose and effectiveness of a nursing model/theory. However, it is important to recognise that for optimum care provision an appropriate model or theory is followed when providing care. Demonstrating an understanding of each model provides the reader with the knowledge to utilise the most appropriate model for the optimum structure of their care delivery.

Thus a model/theory:

- provides structure;
- identifies the key points of patient care;
- links, theory, education, research and practice;
- provides individual, holistic nursing care.

REFERENCES

Barrett, D., Wilson, B., Woollands, A. (2009) *Care planning: A guide for nurses*, Harlow: Pearson Education.

Benner, P. (2000) 'The roles of embodiment, emotion and lifeworld for rationality and agency in nursing practice', *Nursing Philosophy*, 1(1): 5–19.

Casey, A. (1988) 'A partnership with child and family', *Senior Nurse*, 8(4): 8–9.

Department of Health (2007) *National Service Framework for Older People*, London: Department of Health.

Fawcett, J. (1995) *Analysis and evaluation of conceptual models of nursing* (3rd edn), Philadelphia: F.A. Davis.

Henderson, V.A. (1966) *The nature of nursing: A definition and its implications for practice, research, and education*, Riverside, NJ: Macmillan.

King, I.M. (1981) *A theory for nursing: Systems, concepts, process*, Albany, NY: Delmar.

Leininger, M.M. (2006) *Culture care diversity and universality: A theory of nursing* (2nd edn), New York: National League for Nursing Press.

Leininger, M.M. and McFarland, M.R. (2002) *Culture care diversity and universality: A theory of nursing* (3rd edn), New York: McGraw-Hill.

MacIntyre, R.C. (2001) 'Interpretive analysis', in P. Munhall (ed.), *Nursing research: A qualitative perspective* (3rd edn) (pp. 439–466), Boston: Jones and Bartlett.

Maslow, A. (1954) *Motivation and personality*, New York: Harper.

Merriam-Webster (1986) *Webster's Third New International Dictionary and Seven Language Dictionary*, Chicago: Merriman Webster.

Munhall, P.L. (ed.) (2007) *Nursing research: A qualitative perspective* (4th edn), Boston: Jones and Bartlett.

Neuman, B. and Fawcett, J. (2002) *The Neuman systems model* (4th edn), Upper Saddle River, NJ: Prentice Hall.

Nightingale, F. (1969) *Notes on nursing: What it is, and what it is not*, New York: Dover. (Original work published in 1860.)

NMC (2010) *Standards for pre-registration nursing education*, London: NMC.

Orem, D.E. (1971) *Nursing: Concepts of practice*, Hightstown, NJ: McGraw-Hill.

Orem, D.E., Taylor, S.G. and Renpenning, K.M. (2001) *Nursing: Concepts of practice* (6th edn), St. Louis, MO: Mosby.

Parse, R.R. (1994) 'Quality of life: Sciencing and living the art of human becoming', *Nursing Science Quarterly*, 7(1): 16–21.

Parse, R.R. (ed.) (1995) *Illuminations: The human becoming theory in practice and research*, New York: National League for Nursing Press.

Rogers, M.E. (1970) *An introduction to the theoretical basis of nursing*, Philadelphia: F.A. Davis.

Roper, N., Logan, W. and Tierney, A. (1980) *The elements of nursing*, Edinburgh: Churchill Livingstone.

Roper, N., Logan, W. and Tierney, A. (1981) *Learning to use the process of nursing*, Edinburgh: Churchill Livingstone.

Roper, N., Logan, W. and Tierney, A. (1983) *Using a model for nursing*, Edinburgh: Churchill Livingstone.

Roper, N., Logan, W. and Tierney, A. (2000) *The Roper, Logan and Tierney model of nursing*. Edinburgh: Churchill Livingstone.

Roy, C. (1997) 'Future of the Roy model: Challenge to redefine adaptation', *Nursing Science Quarterly*, 10(1): 42–48.

Vanhaecht, K., De Witte, K. and Sermeus, W. (2007) *The impact of clinical pathways on the organisation of care processes*. PhD dissertation Kuleuven, 154pp, Katholieke University Leuven.

Watson, J. (1979) *Nursing: The philosophy and science of caring*, Boston: Little, Brown.

Welsh Assembly Government (2003) *Innovations in care*. Wales: Welsh Assembly Government.

FURTHER RESOURCES

National Service Framework:
http://www.library.nhs.uk/
http://www.wales.nhs.uk/sites3/home.cfm?OrgID=334
http://www.nsfscot.org.uk/

CHAPTER 10
THE NURSING PROCESS

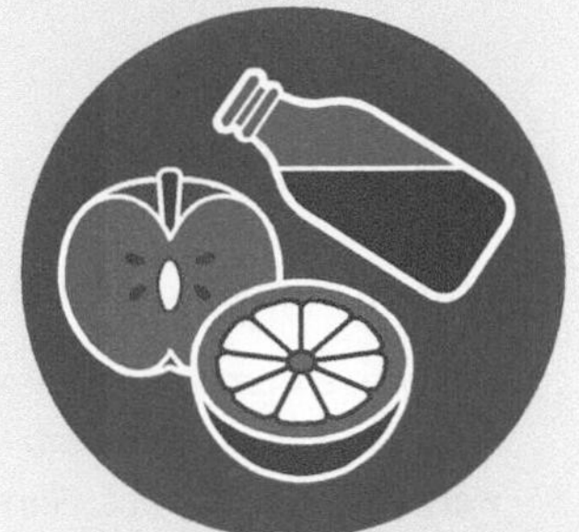

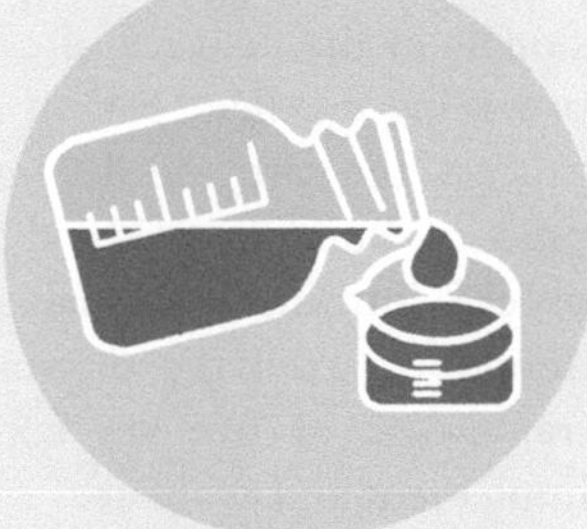

LEARNING OUTCOMES

After completing this chapter, you will be able to:

- Discuss the principles and the phases of the nursing process.
- Identify major characteristics of the nursing process.
- Identify the purpose of assessing.
- Discuss how communication is inherent in the nursing process.
- Discuss the importance of recognising when to use closed and open-ended questions.
- Compare the various frameworks and identify when, why and which one should be used when undertaking a nursing assessment.
- Discuss and debate the difference between a nursing diagnosis to that of a medical diagnosis.
- Discuss and evaluate the planning process and how it can impact on discharge planning.
- Compare and contrast the different types of care plans.
- Explain the key functions of writing goals/desired outcomes.
- List and explore the five activities of the implementing phase and discuss these in relation to patient care.
- Identify five components of the evaluation process.
- List the key skill required to utilise the nursing process effectively.
- Discuss the term 'critical thinking' and how this relates to nursing decision making and the nursing process.
- Recognise the components of quality assurance in healthcare.

After reading this chapter you will be able to devise a plan of care using the nursing process. You will also be able to reflect on the nursing role in providing healthcare, the way care is organised and the importance of recognising holistic individualised care to a confused patient. It relates to **Essential Skills Clusters (NMC, 2010) 1–10, 11, 14, 17, 19, 27, 28, 30**, as appropriate for each progression point.

Ensure that you really understand this chapter by logging on to your complimentary **MyNursingKit** at **www.pearsoned.co.uk/kozier**. Complete the self-assessment tests to check your progress and utilise further activities to practise and confirm your understanding.

CASE STUDY

Ethel is an 86-year-old widow, who lives with her daughter aged 53 years. Ethel was admitted to hospital following an episode of acute confusion. On admission to the ward Ethel's daughter, May, contributes to the assessment process and states that Ethel is normally a placid, kind lady and is grateful for any support that is offered to her. Leading up to this admission Ethel has refused to drink too much fluids, is frequently asking to go to the toilet to pass small amounts of concentrated urine and is a little bit aggressive.

INTRODUCTION

The International Council of Nurses, states that (ICN, 2010: 1):

> *Nursing encompasses autonomous and collaborative care of individuals of all ages, families, groups and communities, sick or well, and in all settings. Nursing includes the promotion of health, prevention of illness, and the care of ill, disabled and dying people. Advocacy, promotion of a safe environment, research, participation in shaping health policy and in patient and health systems management, and education are also key nursing roles.*

Nursing in the 21st century is a complex discipline, as it embraces multiple concepts, which have been noted above. In order to capture the multifaceted role of the nurse it is important that there is a structured, systematic patient-centred approach to the delivery of care.

It has been discussed in Chapter 9 how theories, models, care pathways and the nursing process guides healthcare professionals in the delivery of care. Fundamental to the success of providing excellent patient care is the theory, the science, the process, the care and the framework that guides and develops practice. Building on the theory and framework is the nursing process introduced by Hall as far back as 1955, which has been developed from the original four concepts into the current framework of five key concepts, i.e. assess, diagnose, plan, implement and evaluate.

The nursing process entails gathering (assessing) and analysing (diagnosing) information in order to identify patient strengths and potential or actual health problems (planning), developing (implementing) and continually reviewing (evaluating) a plan of nursing interventions to achieve mutually agreed outcomes. At every stage of the process, the nurse works closely with the patient to individualise care and build a relationship of mutual regard and trust.

ASSESSMENT AS PART OF THE NURSING PROCESS

While Hall originated the term 'nursing process' in 1955 in a lecture entitled 'The quality of nursing care', Johnson (1959), Orlando (1961) and Wiedenbach (1963) were among the first nurse theorists to use it to refer to a series of phases describing the process of nursing and Yura and Walsh were the first to introduce it into nursing in 1967. While there have been several adaptations and implementations of the nursing process, fundamentally it has remained unchanged in relation to the way the information is gathered and processed in relation to patient care.

The purpose of the nursing process (see Figure 10-1) is to identify patients' health status and actual or potential healthcare problems or needs, to establish plans to meet the identified needs, and to deliver specific nursing interventions to meet those needs. The patient may be an individual, a family or a group, commonly known in the clinical environment as APIE.

However, more recently Barrett *et al.* (2008) have added another phase to the nursing process which is the recheck phase (see Figure 10-2) (ASPIRE). Barrett *et al.* (2008) state that evaluation is different to rechecking and it is important to recheck the patient prior to making a valid evaluation. For example, you record a patient's blood pressure and note that it is high. You are aware that the doctor needs to be informed of the raised blood pressure, but prior to informing either the nurse in charge of the patient or the doctor you would recheck the blood pressure to make sure that you are evaluating the situation correctly.

Phases of the Nursing Process

Although nursing theorists may use different terms to describe the phases of the nursing process, the activities of the nurse using the process are similar. For example, diagnosing may also be called analysis, and implementing may be called intervention.

An overview of the five-phase nursing process is shown in Table 10-1. Each of the five phases is discussed in depth later throughout this chapter. The phases of the nursing process are not discrete entities but overlapping, continuing sub-processes (see Figure 10-3). For example, assessing, which may be considered the first phase of the nursing process, is also carried out during the implementing and evaluating phases and indeed is continuous throughout each phase. This occurs, for instance, while assisting a patient with personal hygiene the nurse continuously notes the patient's skin colour, any abnormal swelling, bruising or broken areas, and so on.

Each phase of the nursing process affects the others; they are closely interrelated. For example, if inadequate data is obtained during assessing, the nursing diagnoses will be incomplete or incorrect; inaccuracy will also be reflected in the planning, implementing and evaluating phases.

The nursing process is a systematic, rational method of planning and providing nursing care. Its goal is to identify a patient's healthcare status, and actual or potential health problems, to establish plans to meet the identified needs, and to deliver specific nursing interventions to address those needs.
The nursing process is cyclical; that is, its components follow a logical sequence, but more than one component may be involved at one time. At the end of the first cycle, care may be terminated if goals are achieved, the cycle may continue with reassessment or the plan of care may be modified.

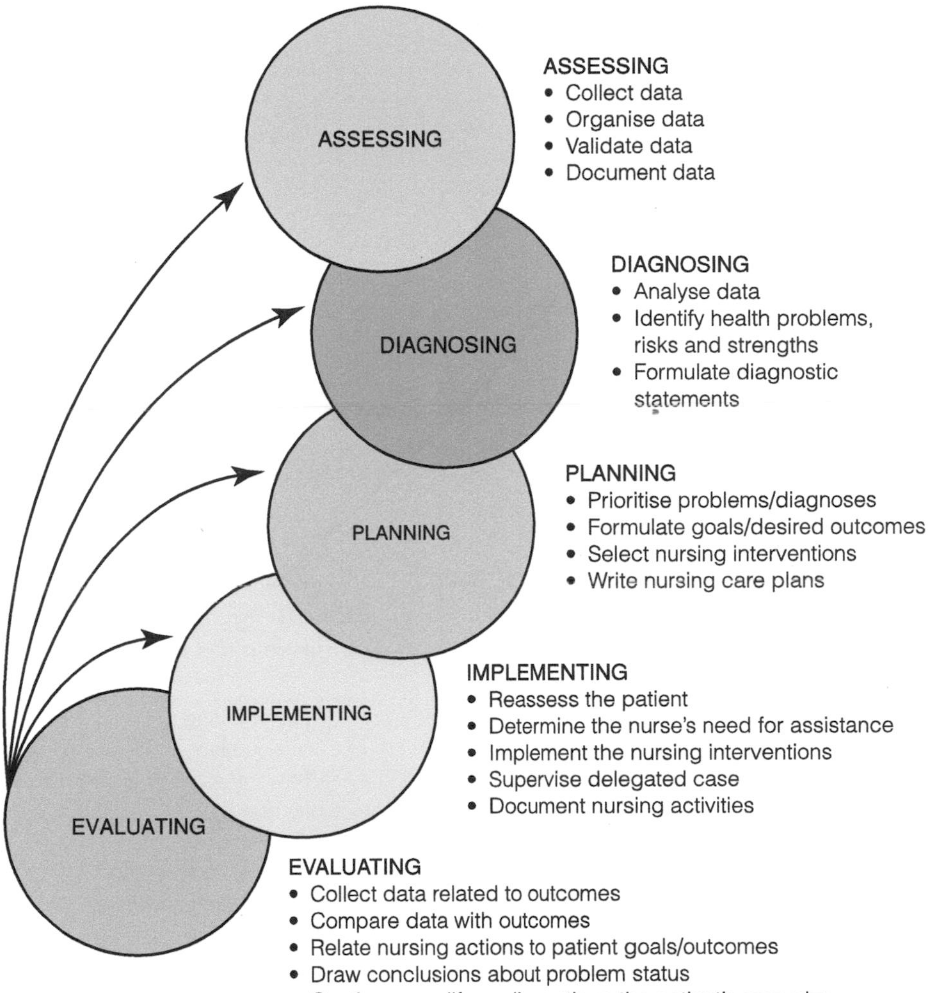
ASSESSING
DIAGNOSING
PLANNING
IMPLEMENTING
EVALUATING
ASSESSING
• Collect data
• Organise data
• Validate data
• Document data
DIAGNOSING
• Analyse data
• Identify health problems, risks and strengths
• Formulate diagnostic statements
PLANNING
• Prioritise problems/diagnoses
• Formulate goals/desired outcomes
• Select nursing interventions
• Write nursing care plans
IMPLEMENTING
• Reassess the patient
• Determine the nurse's need for assistance
• Implement the nursing interventions
• Supervise delegated case
• Document nursing activities
EVALUATING
• Collect data related to outcomes
• Compare data with outcomes
• Relate nursing actions to patient goals/outcomes
• Draw conclusions about problem status
• Continue, modify or discontinue the patient's care plan

Figure 10-1 The nursing process in action.

ACTIVITY 10-1

Explain and rationalise why and how you think the nursing process guides and directs patient care.

Characteristics of the Nursing Process

The nursing process has unique characteristics that enable responsiveness to the changing health status of the patient. These characteristics include its cyclic and dynamic nature, patient-centred ethos, focus on problem solving and decision making, interpersonal and collaborative style, universal applicability and use of **critical thinking**.

- The information gathered from each phase provides input into the next phase. Findings from evaluating are fed back into assessing. Hence, the nursing process is a regularly repeated event or sequence of events (a cycle) that is continuously changing (dynamic) rather than staying the same (static).
- The nursing process is patient centred, and focused on holistic care. The nurse organises the plan of care according to patient problems rather than nursing goals. In the assessment phase, the nurse collects data to determine the patient's habits, routines, needs, and the patient's normal practice/abilities enabling the nurse to incorporate patient routines into the care plan as much as possible.
- The nursing process is an adaptation of problem solving and systems theory. It can be viewed as parallel to but separate

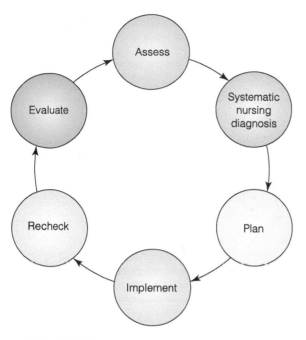

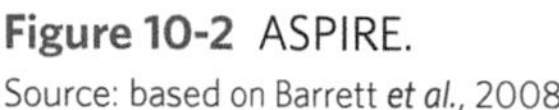

Figure 10-2 ASPIRE.
Source: based on Barrett *et al.*, 2008.

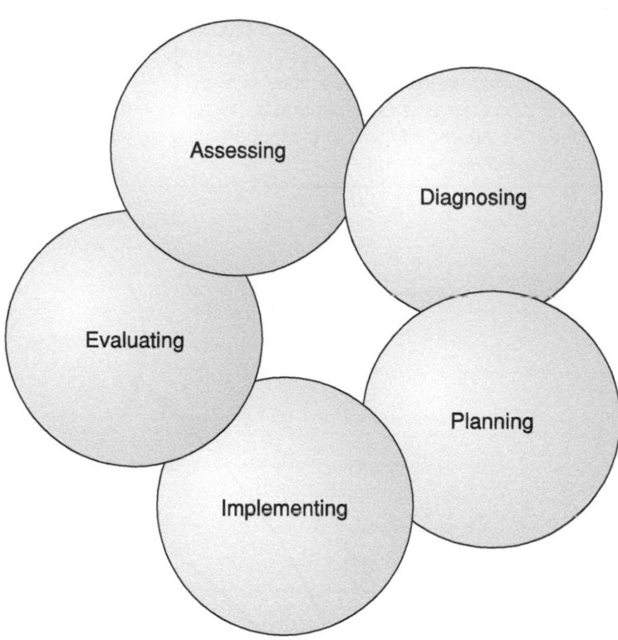

Figure 10-3 The phases of the nursing process.

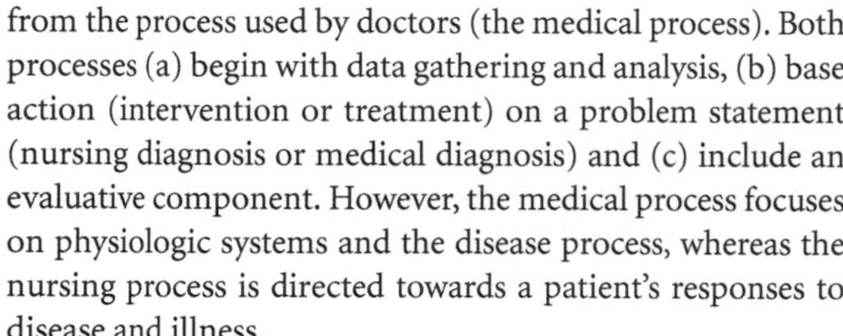

from the process used by doctors (the medical process). Both processes (a) begin with data gathering and analysis, (b) base action (intervention or treatment) on a problem statement (nursing diagnosis or medical diagnosis) and (c) include an evaluative component. However, the medical process focuses on physiologic systems and the disease process, whereas the nursing process is directed towards a patient's responses to disease and illness.

- Decision making is involved in every phase of the nursing process. Nurses can be highly creative in determining when and how to use data to make decisions. They are not bound by standard responses and may apply their repertoire of skills and knowledge to assist patients. This facilitates the individualisation of the nurse's plan of care.
- The nursing process is interpersonal and collaborative. It requires the nurse to communicate directly and consistently with patients and families to meet their needs. It also requires that nurses collaborate, as members of the healthcare team, in a joint effort to provide quality patient care.
- The universally applicable characteristic of the nursing process means that it is used as a framework for nursing care in all types of healthcare settings, with patients of all age groups.
- Nurses must use a variety of skills and attributes to carry out the nursing process. (See *Box 10-1*: references will be made to these skills throughout the chapter.)
- Fundamental to any skill or interaction is communication. Hayes and Llewellyn (2010) state that unless there is good communication how can we assess, diagnose, plan, implement, and evaluate patient care effectively. It is therefore imperative that the principle of communication is briefly discussed before exploring the nursing process further.

BOX 10-1 Examples of Fundamental Skills required in the Nursing Process

- Critical thinking
- Clinical judgement/decision making
- Self-awareness/self-assessment
- Reflection
- Interpersonal skills
- Collaboration/team working
- Intuition/tacit knowledge
- Record keeping

COMMUNICATION

Communication is fundamental to human life, and whether communication is voluntary or involuntary it exists within all human beings (McCabe and Timmins, 2006). It begins with the foetus in the womb, and at each stage of human life is intrinsic to development. Communication is a two-way process and is a complex interaction in which information passes between individuals. Communication is cyclical in nature, as it allows a message to be sent and received, and either confirmation of the receipt of the information or otherwise allows the sender to interpret the interaction as being successful or otherwise. Further communication may then develop.

Effective communication skills are essential within nursing and can be considered as one of the most important skills that are required for nurses to support patients and their families (Dougherty and Lister, 2011). Effective communication in

Table 10-1 Overview of the Nursing Process

Phase and description	Purpose	Activities
Assessing Collecting, organising, validating and documenting patient data	To establish a database including all relevant information about the patient response to health concerns or illness and the ability to manage healthcare needs	Establish a database: • Obtain a nursing health history. • Conduct a physical assessment. • Review patient records. • Review nursing literature. • Make appropriate referrals to members of the multidisciplinary team. • Update data as needed. • Organise data. • Validate data. • Communicate/document data.
Diagnosing Analysing and synthesising data	To identify patient strengths and health problems that can be prevented or resolved by collaborative and independent nursing interventions. To develop a list of nursing and collaborative problems	Interpret and analyse data: • Compare data against standards. • Group the information appropriately (generate tentative hypotheses). • Identify gaps and inconsistencies. • Identify and assess any risks that may be pertinent to the patient's safety and well-being. • Determine patient strengths, risks, diagnoses and problems. • Formulate nursing diagnoses and collaborative problem statements. • Document nursing diagnoses on the care plan.
Planning Determining how to provide patient care in order to prevent, reduce or resolve the identified patient problems; how to support patient strengths; and how to implement nursing interventions in an organised, individualised and goal-directed manner	To develop an individualised holistic care plan that specifies patient goals/desired outcomes, and related nursing interventions	Set priorities and goals/outcomes in collaboration with patient. Write goals/desired outcomes. Select nursing strategies/interventions. Consult other health professionals. Write nursing care plan/advanced care plan. Communicate care plan to relevant healthcare providers/ multidisciplinary team. Initiate early discharge plan from assessment.
Implementing Carrying out the planned nursing interventions	To assist the patient to meet desired goals/outcomes; promote wellness; prevent illness and disease; restore health; and facilitate coping with altered functioning	Reassess the patient and update the care plan, accordingly. Determine level/need of nursing assistance. Perform planned nursing interventions. Communicate what nursing actions were implemented. • Document care and patient responses to care. • Give verbal reports as necessary.
Evaluating Measuring the degree to which goals/outcomes have been achieved and identifying factors that positively or negatively influence goal achievement	To determine whether to continue, modify or discontinue the plan of care	Collaborate with patient and members of the multidisciplinary team and evaluate the data in relation to the desired outcomes. Measure (protocols, guidelines etc.) whether the goals/ outcomes have been achieved. Evaluate the nursing actions to patient outcomes. Make decisions on the effectiveness of the interaction/ intervention. Review and modify the care plan as indicated or discontinue the nursing care if the problem has been managed effectively and does no longer exist. Document achievement of outcomes and modification of the care plan.

nursing is pivotal in ensuring that holistic patient care is provided, patient autonomy and advocacy (NMC, 2008) is maintained, that the well-being of the patient is prominent and both the patient and family well informed. The unique relationship between a patient and the nurse encourages trust, honesty and intimacy. Nurses are at the forefront of care and therefore effective communication is essential when answering questions, advising and explaining (e.g. with regard to medication, conditions or procedures) to patients and their relatives. There are two types of communication – verbal and non-verbal – and it is important to recognise that verbal messages can be contradicted when non-verbal communication does not reflect what is being said.

Verbal communication

Verbal communication is the use of either the spoken or written word. The effectiveness of spoken words can depend on elements such as culture, language, tone of voice, speech rate, accents, jargon, type of questioning (open or closed) or a physical impairment of a patient (e.g. a patient who is hard of hearing). Written communication relies heavily on accuracy and comprehension of the individual who is communicating either by reading or writing. Language is very important in communication, as what is being said can be misinterpreted.

It is therefore important to speak clearly and concisely and make sure that what is being said is what is intended and that the receiver understands the message. Jargon such as medical terms should be avoided, in order to reduce anxiety. Language barriers such as accents, speed of delivery and tone should be considered and adaptations made as necessary. Humour is an important tool when caring for patients but care is needed so that it is used appropriately: for example, humour is not always appropriate when a patient or relative has received bad news.

Non-verbal Communication

Non-verbal communication does not rely on words but on other aspects of human behaviour, such as body language (e.g. personal appearance, eye contact, gestures, facial expressions, touch, or posture). It is one of the most powerful ways individuals communicate. For example, if you greet a patient in the morning with 'Good morning, how are you?' in an open and direct manner then it can be suggested that the receiver will be receptive of the greeting; conversely if the greeting is delivered in a closed manner, i.e. arms crossed in front of you, not directly looking at the individual, then this may be received in a negative manner. The way a person stands (gait) reflects attitudes, self-concept and physical wellness.

Personal appearances are important as they immediately give a first impression of whether the nurse is professional and takes their profession seriously: for example, wearing jewellery, a non-ironed uniform, etc. may suggest to the patient that the nurse is not very professional as if they are not bothered about the neatness of their uniform then it may suggest that they will have a similar attitude to nursing care. A well-groomed nurse suggests professionalism and adherance to local policies.

A gesture is simply a wave of a hand, or shifting of feet, and when accompanied with limited eye contact it can give an impression of disinterest or guilt, etc., whereas facial expression sets the tone of the interpersonal communication between the patient and the nurse. This is significant when, for example, a student nurse attends to a patient who has recently undergone surgery for a **stoma** formation following bowel cancer. The 'bag' needs changing and there is a strong putrid smell coming from the patient. Non-verbal communication, especially facial expressions, are fundamental to the well-being of the patient and how the patient perceives him or herself following such surgery.

Touch is highly significant when nursing a patient as it can offer empathy, sympathy, support, presence (of another) and caring. Touch is very important when caring for patients with a disability (e.g. blindness or deafness). However, care is needed as touch can sometimes be misconstrued and be perceived as a sexual gesture. Care is also needed with personal space, culture, etc.

Listening and silence are important aspects of non-verbal communication. They involve being fully attentive to the other party without being distracted. When actively listening to a patient it is important to demonstrate that they have been heard and understood. This can be achieved by paraphrasing, which involves repeating what has been heard using different words in order to confirm that the intended message has been both heard and understood. The inability of nurses to listen effectively can lead to patients feeling anxious. Another important aspect of communication is the hidden agenda when listening. For example, if a patient has been admitted with abdominal pain due to constipation, and during the assessment process you identify that the patient eats precooked meals, etc. with no vegetables or high fibre as he is unable to access the shops, then this contributes to your knowledge of his condition. Listening is used when the patient responds or discusses a situation and may through verbal communication inadvertently highlight an issue that they may not think is significant but has an adverse effect on the their overall condition. Silence allows the patient time to gather their thoughts and acceptance that they may need to speak about certain issues relating to their psychosocial or physiological condition.

In summary, communication is multifaceted and uses key skills such as clarification, reflection, probing, summarising and questioning during the assessment process and during any interaction with a patient and/or relative, and is essential in order to gather information to advise in the assessing and planning of patient care. According to the NMC (2008) every effort should be made to ensure that patient's language and communication needs are met.

Table 10-2 Types of Assessment

Type	Time performed	Purpose	Example
Initial assessment	Performed within specified time after admission to hospital, care home or at home	To establish a complete database for problem identification, reference and future comparison	Nursing admission assessment
Problem-focused assessment	Ongoing process integrated with nursing care	To determine the status of a specific problem identified in an earlier assessment	Hourly assessment of patient's liquid intake and urinary output in an intensive care unit or high-dependency area.
		To identify new or overlooked problems	Assessment of patient's ability to perform self-care while assisting with hygiene needs
Emergency assessment	During any physiological or psychological crisis of the patient	To identify life-threatening problems	Rapid assessment of a person's airway, breathing status and circulation during a cardiac arrest. Assessment of suicidal tendencies or potential for violence
Time-lapsed reassessment	Several months after initial assessment	To compare the patient's current status to baseline data previously obtained	Reassessment of a patient's functional health patterns in a home care or outpatient setting or, in a hospital, at shift change

THE NURSING PROCESS IN ACTION

Assessing

Assessing is the systematic and continuous collection, organisation, validation and documentation of data (information). Assessing is a continuous process carried out during all phases of the nursing process. For example, in the evaluation phase, assessment is undertaken to determine the outcomes of the nursing strategies and to evaluate goal achievement. All phases of the nursing process depend on the accurate and complete collection of data.

There are four different types of assessments: initial assessment, problem-focused assessment, emergency assessment and time-lapsed reassessment (see Table 10-2). Assessments vary according to their purpose, timing, time available and patient status.

Nursing assessments focus on a patient's responses to a health problem. A nursing assessment should include the patient's perceived needs, health problems, related experience, health practices, values and lifestyles. To be most useful, the data collected should be relevant to a particular health problem. Therefore, nurses should think critically about what to assess. The assessment process involves four closely related activities: collecting data, organising data, validating data and documenting data (see Figure 10-4).

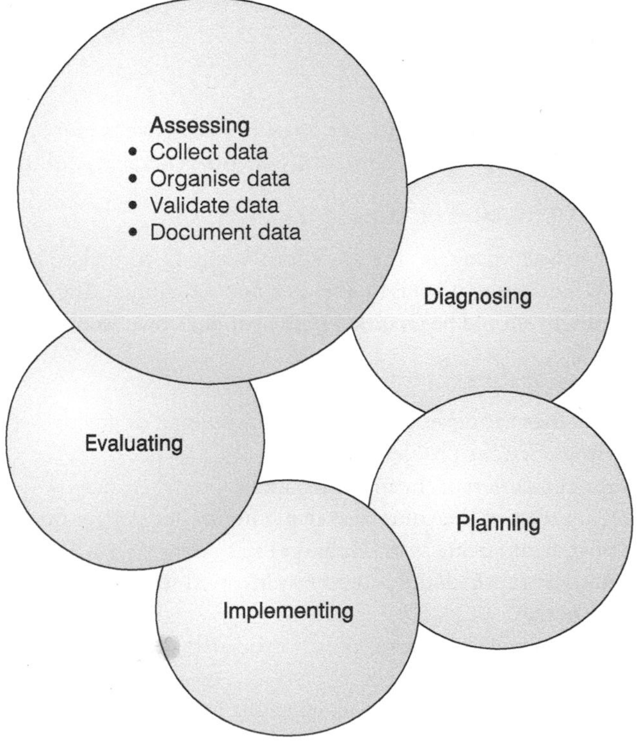

Figure 10-4 Assessing. The assessment process involves four closely related activities.

DATA/INFORMATION GATHERING

Collecting Data

Data collection is the process of gathering information about a patient's psychological, physical and social status which affects their health status. It must be both systematic and continuous to prevent the omission of significant data and reflect their changing health status.

A database is all the information about a patient; it includes the nursing health history (see below), physical assessment, the doctor's history notes and physical examination, results of laboratory and diagnostic tests, and material contributed by other health personnel. In order to collect and record this information accurately a nursing model or care pathway is used.

Patient data should include past history as well as current problems. For example, a history of recurrent or frequent falls, as well as an allergic reaction to penicillin is a vital piece of historical data. Past surgical procedures, complementary therapies and chronic diseases are also examples of historical data. Current data relate to present circumstances, such as pain, nausea, sleep patterns and religious practices. To collect data accurately, active participation must be engaged by both the patient and the nurse while contributions can be received from relevant relatives and carer.

Components of a Nursing Health History

In outline, these are as follows.

Biographic Data

Patient name, address, age, sex, marital status, occupation, religious preference, next of kin, family doctor/general practitioner.

Chief Complaint or Reason for Visit

The answer given to the question 'What is troubling you?' or 'What brought you to the hospital or clinic?' The chief complaint should be recorded in the patient's own words.

History of Present Illness

- Whether the onset of symptoms was sudden or gradual.
- How often the problem occurs.
- Exact location of the distress/pain.
- Character of the complaint (e.g. intensity of pain or quality of sputum, sickness or discharge).
- Activity in which the patient was involved when the problem occurred.
- Phenomena or symptoms associated with the chief complaint.
- Factors that aggravate or alleviate the problem.

Past History

- *Childhood illnesses*, such as chickenpox, mumps, measles, rubella (German measles), streptococcal infections, scarlet fever, rheumatic fever and other significant illness.
- *Childhood immunisations* and the date of the last tetanus immunisation.
- *Allergies* to drugs, animals, insects or other environmental agents, and the type of reaction that occurs.
- *Accidents and injuries*: how, when and where the incident occurred, type of injury, treatment received and any complications.
- *Hospitalisation for serious illnesses*: reasons for the hospitalisation, dates, surgery performed, course of recovery, and any complications.
- *Medications*: all currently used prescription and over-the-counter medications, such as aspirin, nasal spray, vitamins, herbal remedies or laxatives.

Family History of Illness

To ascertain risk factors for certain diseases, the ages of siblings, parents and grandparents, and their current state of health or, if they are deceased, the cause of death are obtained. Particular attention should be given to disorders such as heart disease, cancer, diabetes, hypertension, hyperlipidaemia (high cholesterol), obesity, allergies, arthritis, tuberculosis, bleeding, alcoholism and any mental health disorders.

Lifestyle

- *Personal habits*: the amount, frequency and duration of substance use (tobacco, alcohol, coffee, tea and illicit or recreational drugs).
- *Diet*: description of a typical diet on a normal day or any special diet, number of meals and snacks per day, who cooks and shops for food, ethnically distinct food patterns and allergies.
- *Sleep/rest patterns*: usual daily sleep/wake times, difficulties sleeping and remedies used for difficulties.
- *Activities of daily living (ADLs)*: any difficulties experienced in the basic activities of eating, grooming, dressing, elimination and locomotion.
- *Instrumental activities of daily living*: any difficulties experienced in food preparation, shopping, transportation, housekeeping, laundry, and ability to use the telephone, handle finances and manage medications.
- *Recreation/hobbies*: exercise activity and tolerance, hobbies and other interests and vacations.

Social Data

- *Family relationships/friendships*: The patient's support system in times of stress (who helps in time of need?), what effect the patient's illness has on the family and whether any family problems are affecting the patient.
- *Ethnic affiliation*: Health customs and beliefs; cultural practices that may affect healthcare and recovery. See also detailed ethnic/cultural assessment guide.
- *Educational history*: Data about the patient's highest level of education attained and any past difficulties with learning.
- *Occupational history*: Current employment status, the number of days missed from work because of illness, any history of accidents on the job, any occupational hazards with a potential for future disease or accident such as chemicals or industrial dust, the patient's need to change jobs because of past illness, the employment status of spouses or partners

and the way childcare is handled, and the patient's overall satisfaction with the work.

- *Economic status*: Information about how the patient is managing financially while in hospital and any consideration to effects to social benefits being received.
- *Home and neighbourhood conditions*: Home safety measures and adjustments in physical facilities that may be required to help the patient manage a physical disability, activity intolerance and activities of daily living; the availability of social and community services to meet the patient's needs.

Psychological Data

- *Major stressors* experienced and the patient's perception of them.
- *Usual coping pattern* with a serious problem or a high level of stress.
- *Communication style*: ability to verbalise appropriate emotion; nonverbal communication – such as eye movements, gestures, use of touch and posture; interactions with support persons; and the use of nonverbal behaviour and verbal expression.

Patterns of Healthcare

All healthcare resources the patient is currently using and has used in the past. These include the family doctor, specialists (e.g. ophthalmologist or gynaecologist), dentist, complementary practitioners (e.g. herbalist or reflexologist), health clinic or health centre; whether the patient considers the care being provided adequate; and whether access to healthcare is a problem.

Types of Data

Data can be subjective or objective. Subjective data, also referred to as symptoms data, are apparent only to the person affected and can be described or verified only by that person. Itching, pain and feelings of worry are examples of subjective data. Subjective data include the patient's sensations, feelings, values, beliefs, attitudes and perception of personal health status and life situation.

Objective data, also referred to as sign or presentations, are detectable by an observer or can be measured or tested against an accepted standard. They can be seen, heard, felt or smelled, and they are obtained by observation or physical examination. For example, a discoloration of the skin or a blood pressure reading is objective data. During the physical examination, the nurse obtains objective data to validate subjective data and to complete the assessment phase of the nursing process. Information supplied by family members, significant others or other healthcare professionals is considered subjective if it is not based on fact. If the patient's relative states, 'Dad is very confused today,' that is subjective data. However, if she were to state, 'Dad couldn't remember his address or phone number today,' that is objective data.

A complete database of both subjective and objective data provides a baseline for comparing the patient's responses to nursing and medical interventions. Examples of subjective and objective data are shown in Table 10-3.

Table 10-3 Examples of Subjective and Objective Data

Subjective	Objective
'I feel lightheaded when I get up to stand and walk.'	Blood pressure 85/45 Radial pulse 44 Skin pale and clammy
'I feel tired all the time and I do get short of breath when I walk short distances, and I used to be able to walk to the top of the mountain approximately 2.5 miles round trip'	Rapid or irregular heartbeat, pale gums and nail beds Patient always lethargic and tired Blood results confirm low haemoglobin Breathing difficulties, poor lung expansion
'No, I don't have post operative pain'	Blood pressure normal 120/80 Pulse regular 60 bpm Nonverbal communication demonstrates patient comfortable, i.e. body language

Sources of Data

Sources of data are primary or secondary. The patient is the primary source of data. Family members or other support persons, other health professionals, records and reports, laboratory and diagnostic tests, and relevant literature are secondary or indirect sources. In fact, all sources other than the patient are considered secondary sources.

The Patient

The best source of data is usually patients themselves, unless they are too ill, young or confused to communicate clearly. The patient can provide subjective data that no one else can offer.

Carers and Family Members

Family members, friends and caregivers who know the patient well often can supplement or verify information provided by the patient. They might convey information about the patient's response to illness, the stresses the patient was experiencing before the illness, family attitudes on illness and health, and the patient's home environment.

Carers and support workers are an especially important source of data for a patient who is very young, unconscious or confused. In some cases – a patient who is physically or emotionally abused, for example – the person giving information may wish to remain anonymous. Before gathering data/information from support people, the nurse should ensure that the patient, if mentally able, accepts such input. The nurse should also indicate on the nursing history/notes that the data/information was obtained from a support person/significant other.

Patient Records/Notes

According to the NMC (2008) it is the nurse's responsibility to keep 'clear and accurate records', which include collecting and entering data as well as any amendments made. Patient records include information documented by various healthcare professionals. Patient records also contain data regarding their occupation, religion and marital status. By reviewing such records before interviewing the patient, the nurse can avoid asking open-ended questions and can use closed questioning to confirm whether the information is still valid or has changed without unduly stressing the patient. Repeated questioning can be stressful and annoying to patients and cause concern about the lack of communication among health professionals. Types of patient records include medical records, records of treatment, laboratory results, x-rays, MRI and ultrasound. The reliance on such investigations is becoming increasingly more dependant and consultants look at this to support their initial diagnosis.

Medical records (e.g. medical history, physical examination, operative report, progress notes and consultations undertaken by doctors) are often a source of a patient's present and past health and illness patterns. These records can provide nurses with information about the patient's coping behaviours, health practices, previous illnesses and allergies.

Records of treatments provided by other health professionals, such as social workers, dieticians and all other members of the multidisciplinary team help the nurse obtain relevant data not expressed by the patient. For example, a dietician's/occupational therapist's report on a patient's diet and home conditions or ability to cope at home alone can also be helpful to the nurse conducting an assessment.

Laboratory records/results also provide pertinent health information. For example, the determination of thyroxine level allows health professionals to monitor the administration of levothyroxine treatment for the management of hypothyroidism. Any laboratory data about a patient must be compared to the laboratory's norms for that particular test and for the patient's age, sex, and so on.

The nurse must always consider the information in patient records in light of the present situation. For example, if the most recent medical record is 10 years old, the patient health practices and coping behaviours are likely to have changed. Older adults may have numerous previous records. These are very useful and contribute to a full understanding of the health history, especially if the patient's memory is impaired, but may take some time to examine thoroughly.

Healthcare Professionals

Because assessment is an ongoing process, verbal reports from other healthcare professionals serve as other potential sources of information about a patient's health. Nurses, social workers, physicians and physiotherapists, dieticians, speech therapists, for example, may have information from either previous or current contact with the patient. Sharing of information among professionals is especially important to ensure continuity of care when patients are transferred to and from home and healthcare agencies.

Data Collection Methods

The primary methods used to collect data are observing, interviewing and examining. Observation occurs whenever the nurse is in contact with the patient, family and/or carers. Interviewing is used mainly while taking the nursing health history. Examining is the major method used in the physical health assessment.

In reality, the nurse uses all four methods simultaneously when assessing patients. For example, during the patient interview the nurse observes, listens, asks questions and mentally retains information to explore in the physiological examination.

Observing

To *observe* is to gather data by using the senses. Observation is a conscious, deliberate skill that is developed through effort and with an organised approach. Although nurses observe mainly through sight, most of the senses are engaged during careful observations. Examples of patient data observed through the senses are shown in Table 10-4.

Observation has two aspects: (a) noticing the data and (b) selecting, organising and interpreting the data. A nurse who observes that a patient's face is flushed must relate that observation to, for example, body temperature, activity, environmental temperature and blood pressure. Errors can occur in selecting, organising and interpreting data. For example, a nurse might not notice certain signs, either because they are unexpected or because they do not conform to preconceptions about a patient's illness. Nurses often need to focus on specific data in order not to be overwhelmed by a multitude of data. Observing, therefore, involves discriminating among data that is distinguishing data in a meaningful manner. For example, nurses caring for newborns learn to ignore the usual sounds of machines in the clinical environment but respond quickly to an infant's cry or movement.

The experienced nurse is often able to attend to an intervention (e.g. give a bed bath or monitor an intravenous infusion) and at the same time make important observations (e.g. note a change in respiratory status or skin colour). The student nurse needs to learn to make observations and complete tasks simultaneously.

Table 10-4 Using the Senses to Observe Patient Data

Sense	Example of patient data
Vision	Overall appearance (e.g. body size, general weight, posture, grooming); signs of distress or discomfort; facial and body gestures; skin colour and lesions; abnormalities of movement; nonverbal communication (e.g. signs of anger or anxiety); religious or cultural artefacts (e.g. books, icons, candles, beads)
Smell	Body or breath odours
Hearing	Conscious or subconsciously observing the patient verbally or non-verbally communicating as appropriate considering the patient's ability (e.g. deafness, language barriers, speed of delivery and understanding)
Touch	Skin temperature and moisture; muscle strength (e.g. hand grip); pulse rate, rhythm and volume; palpatory lesions (e.g. lumps, masses, nodules)

Nursing observations must be organised so that nothing significant is missed. Most nurses develop a particular sequence for observing events, usually focusing on the patient first. For example, a nurse walks into a patient's room and observes, in the following order:

1 Clinical signs of patient distress (e.g. pallor or flushing, laboured breathing, and behaviour indicating pain or emotional distress).
2 Threats to the patient's safety, real or anticipated (e.g. whether the patient has or needs a bed side/cot rail).
3 The presence and functioning of associated equipment (e.g. intravenous equipment and oxygen).
4 The immediate environment, including the people in it.

INTERVIEWING

An interview is a planned communication or a conversation with a purpose, for example, to get or give information, identify problems of mutual concern, evaluate change, teach, provide support, or provide counselling or therapy. One example of the interview is the nursing health history, which is a part of the nursing admission assessment.

There are two approaches to interviewing: directive and nondirective. The directive interview is highly structured and elicits specific information. The nurse establishes the purpose of the interview and controls the interview, at least at the outset. The patient responds to questions but may have limited opportunity to ask questions or discuss concerns. Nurses frequently use directive interviews to gather and to give information when time is limited (e.g. in an emergency situation).

During a nondirective interview, or rapport-building interview, by contrast, the nurse allows the patient to control the purpose, subject matter and pacing. Rapport is an understanding between two or more people.

A combination of directive and nondirective approaches is usually appropriate during the information-gathering interview. The nurse begins by determining areas of concern for the patient. If, for example, a patient expresses worry about surgery, the nurse pauses to explore the patient's worry and to provide support. Simply noting the worry, without dealing with it, can leave the impression that the nurse does not care about the patient's concerns or dismisses them as unimportant.

Types of Interview Questions

Questions are often classified as closed or open-ended, and neutral or leading. Closed questions, used in the directive interview, are restrictive and generally require only 'yes' or 'no' or short factual answers giving specific information. Closed questions often begin with 'when', 'where', 'who', 'what', 'how', 'do (did, does)' or 'is (are, was)'. Examples of closed questions are: 'What medication did you take?', 'Are you having pain now? Show me where it is', 'How old are you?', 'When did you fall?' The highly stressed person and the person who has difficulty communicating will find closed questions easier to answer than open-ended questions.

Open-ended questions, associated with the nondirective interview, invite patients to discover and explore, elaborate, clarify or illustrate their thoughts or feelings. An open-ended question specifies only the broad topic to be discussed, and invites answers longer than one or two words. Such questions give patients the freedom to divulge only the information that they are ready to disclose. The open-ended question is useful at the beginning of an interview or to change topics and to elicit attitudes.

Open-ended questions may begin with 'what' or 'how'. Examples of open-ended questions are: 'How have you been feeling lately?', 'What brought you to the hospital?', 'How did you feel in that situation?', 'Would you describe more about how you relate to your child?', 'What would you like to talk about today?'

The type of question a nurse chooses depends on the needs of the patient at the time. Nurses often find it necessary to use a combination of closed and open-ended questions throughout an interview to accomplish the goals of the interview and obtain needed information.

BOX 10-2 Advantages and Disadvantages of Questioning Styles

Advantages of Open-Ended Questions

- They let the interviewee do the talking.
- The interviewer is able to listen and observe.
- They are easy to answer and non-threatening.
- They reveal what the interviewee thinks is important.
- They may reveal the interviewee's lack of information, misunderstanding of words, frame of reference, prejudices or stereotypes.
- They can provide information the interviewer may not ask for.
- They can reveal the interviewee's degree of feeling about an issue.

Disadvantages of Open-Ended Questions

- They take more time.
- Only brief answers may be given.
- Valuable information may be withheld.
- They often elicit more information than necessary.
- Responses are difficult to document and require skill in recording.
- The interviewer requires skill in controlling an open-ended interview.
- Responses require psychological insight and sensitivity from the interviewer.

Advantages of Closed Questions

- Questions and answers can be controlled more effectively.
- They require less effort from the interviewee.
- They may be less threatening, since they do not require explanations or justifications.

- They take less time.
- Information can be asked for sooner than it would be volunteered.
- Responses are easily documented.
- Questions are easy to use and can be handled by unskilled interviewers.

Disadvantages of Closed Questions

- They may provide too little information and require follow-up questions.
- They may not reveal how the interviewee feels.
- They do not allow the interviewee to volunteer possibly valuable information.
- They may inhibit communication and convey lack of interest by the interviewer.
- The interviewer may dominate the interview with questions.

Source: *Interviewing: Principles and Practices*, 10th edn (pp. 55–60), by C.J. Stewart and W.B. Cash, Jr, 2002, New York: McGraw-Hill. Adapted with permission.

A neutral question is a question the patient can answer without direction or pressure from the nurse, is open ended, and is used in nondirective interviews. Examples are: 'How do you feel about that?' or 'Why do you think you had the operation?' A leading question, by contrast, is usually closed, used in a directive interview, and thus directs the patient's answer. Examples are: 'You're stressed about surgery tomorrow, aren't you?' and 'You will take your medicine, won't you?' The leading question gives the patient less opportunity to decide whether the answer is true or not. Leading questions create problems if the patient, in an effort to please the nurse, gives inaccurate responses. This can result in inaccurate data.

Planning the Interview and Setting

Before beginning an interview, the nurse reviews available information, for example, previous nursing and medical notes, information about the current illness or literature about the patient's health problem. The nurse also reviews all available (previous and current) documentation that is relevant to the patient to identify what data must be collected and what data are within the nurse's discretion to collect based on the specific patient.

Each interview is influenced by the patient's condition and ability to contribute, time, place, seating arrangement or distance, and language.

Patient's Condition

Consideration should be given to the current health condition of the patient. For example, if the patient is very short of breath then it is inappropriate to ask extensive questions. In this case a minimal contribution from the patient is required and expected, in order to reduce anxiety, stress and exacerbation of the patient's condition.

Time

While nurses should plan interviews with all patients when they are physically comfortable and free of pain, and when interruptions by friends, family and other health professionals are minimal, this is not always avoidable especially in an acute setting. Nurses should schedule interviews with patients in their homes at a time selected by the patients wherever possible. The patient should be made to feel comfortable and unhurried.

Place

A well-lit, well-ventilated, moderate-sized room that is relatively free of noise, movements and interruptions encourages communication. In addition, a place where others cannot overhear or see the patient is desirable. It is important to recognise that some information the patient divulges is very personal as well as confidential and that moving to a more private area or room is necessary as an open ward is not private.

Seating Arrangement

A seating arrangement with the nurse behind a desk and the patient seated across creates a formal setting that suggests a business meeting between a superior and a subordinate. In contrast, a seating arrangement in which the parties sit on two chairs placed at right angles to a desk or table or a few feet apart, with no table between, creates a less formal atmosphere, and the nurse and patient tend to feel on equal terms. In groups, a horseshoe or circular chair arrangement can avoid a superior or head-of-the-table position and should be considered when patients are extremely vulnerable and of low self-esteem.

By standing and looking down at a patient who is in bed or in a chair, the nurse risks intimidating the patient, who may perceive the nurse as having greater status. When a patient is in bed, the nurse can sit at a 45-degree angle to the bed. This position is less formal than sitting behind a table or standing at the foot of the bed. During an initial admission interview, a patient may feel less confronted if there is a bedside table between the patient and the nurse. Sitting on a patient's bed hems the patient in and makes staring difficult to avoid.

Distance

The distance between the interviewer and interviewee should be neither too small nor too great, because people feel uncomfortable when talking to someone who is too close or too far away. The distance should be assessed individually and non-verbal communication, i.e. looking for body language signs, should dictate the appropriate distance. Some patients require more or less personal space, depending on their cultural and personal needs.

Language

Failure to communicate in language the patient can understand may be considered a form of discrimination. The nurse must convert complicated medical terminology into common English usage, and interpreters or translators are needed if the patient and the nurse do not speak the same language. Translating medical terminology is a specialised skill because not all persons fluent in the conversational form of the language are familiar with anatomic or other health terms. Interpreters, however, may make judgements about precise wording but also about subtle meanings that require additional explanation or clarification according to the specific language and ethnicity. They may edit the original source to make the meaning clearer or more culturally appropriate.

If giving written documents to patients, the nurse must determine that the patient can read in their native language. Live translation is preferred since the patient can then ask questions for clarification. Nurses must be cautious when asking family members, patient visitors or hospital nonprofessional staff to assist with translation. Services such as Language Line are available 24 hours a day in about 150 languages, for a fee paid by the local service provider. Many larger trusts and local health boards have established their own on-call translator services for the languages commonly spoken in their geographical areas.

Even among patients who speak English, there may be differences in understanding terminology. Patients from different parts of the country may have strong accents; less well-educated and teen patients may ascribe different meanings to words. For example, 'cool' may imply something 'good' to one patient and something 'not warm' to another. The nurse must always confirm accurate understandings.

Stages of an Interview

An interview has three major stages: the opening or introduction, the body or development, and the closing.

The Beginning of the Interview

The introduction can be the most important part of the interview because what is said and done at that time sets the tone for the remainder of the interview. The purpose of the introduction is to establish rapport and orient the interviewee.

Establishing rapport is a process of creating goodwill and trust. It can begin with a greeting ('Good morning, Mr. Thomas') or a self-introduction ('Good morning, I'm Samantha Peckering a student nurse') accompanied by nonverbal gestures such as a smile, a handshake and a friendly manner. The nurse must be careful not to overdo this stage; too much superficial talk can arouse anxiety about what is to follow and may appear insincere. In orientation, the nurse explains the purpose and nature of the interview, for example, what information is needed, how long it will take, and what is expected of the patient. It is important that the nurse also informs the patient that the information will be used to inform and instruct patient care working in collaboration with the patient.

PRACTICE GUIDELINES

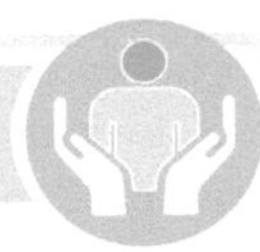

Communication During an Interview

- Listen attentively, using all your senses, and speak slowly and clearly.
- Use language the patient understands and clarify points that are not understood.
- Plan questions to follow a logical sequence.
- Ask only one question at a time. Double questions limit the patient to one choice and may confuse both the nurse and the patient.
- Allow the patient the opportunity to look at things the way they appear to him or her and not the way they appear to the nurse or someone else.
- Paraphrase to ensure that the patient has understood and that the nurse understands what the patient is conveying.
- Do not impose your own values on the patient.
- Avoid using personal examples, such as saying, 'If I were you . . .'
- Nonverbally convey respect, concern, interest and acceptance simply be self-aware.
- Use and accept silence to help the patient search for more thoughts or to organise them.
- Use eye contact and be calm, unhurried and sympathetic.

The Main Body of the Interview

In the body of the assessment interview, it is important the recognition is made to how the patient communicates to the nurse their thoughts, feelings, knowledge and perception of the responses made to questions from the nurse. Effective development of the interview demands that the nurse uses communication techniques that make both parties feel comfortable and serve the purpose of the interview.

Ending of Interview

The interview comes to an end when the nurse has obtained all the information that is needed, from both the patient and nurse's perspective in order to make an informed assessment. In some cases, however, a patient terminates it, for example, when deciding not to give any more information or when unable to offer more information for some other reason – fatigue, for example. The closing is important for maintaining rapport and trust and for facilitating future interactions. The following techniques are commonly used to close an interview:

- Offer to answer questions: 'Do you have any questions?', 'Is there anything you would like to know? I would be glad to answer any questions you have.' Be sure to allow time for the patient to answer or the offer will be regarded as insincere.
- Conclude by saying, 'Well, that's all I need to know for now' or 'Well, those are all the questions I have for now'. Preceding

a remark with the word 'well' generally signals that the end of the interaction is near.

- Thank the patient: 'Thank you for your time and help. The questions you have answered will be helpful in planning your nursing care.'
- Express concern for the person's welfare and future: 'Take care of yourself' or 'I hope all goes well for you.'
- Provide a summary to verify accuracy and agreement. Summarising serves several purposes: it helps to end the interview, it reassures the patient that the nurse has listened, it checks the accuracy of the nurse's perceptions, it clears the way for new ideas and it helps the patient to note progress and forward direction. 'Let's review what we covered in this interview.' Summaries are particularly helpful for patients who are anxious or who have difficulty staying with the topic. 'Well, it seems to me that you are especially worried about your hospitalisation and chest pain because your father died of heart attack five years ago. Is that correct? . . . I'll discuss this with you again tomorrow, and we'll decide what plans need to be made to help you.'
- If there is to be another planned meeting, include the day, time, place, topic and purpose: 'Let's get together again here on the 15th at 9:00 a.m. to see how you are managing then.' Or 'Mrs Smith, I will be responsible for visiting you three mornings a week to change your dressings. I will be in to see you each Monday, Wednesday and Friday between eight o'clock and noon. At those times, we can adjust your care if we need to.' Otherwise, state e.g. 'I shall be the nurse looking after you today, please ring the bell if you should need anything and I am not in the ward' or 'Staff Nurse x will be looking after you today, she is with another patient but I will bring her along to introduce you when she is free'.

EXAMINING

The physical examination/assessment is a systematic data-collection method that uses observation (i.e. the senses of sight, hearing, smell and touch) to detect health problems. The physical assessment is carried out systematically. It may be organised according to the examiner's preference, in a head-to-toe approach or a body systems approach. Usually, the nurse first records a general impression about the patient's overall appearance and health status, for example, age, body size, mental and nutritional status, speech, behaviour, mobility and risk assessments. Then the nurse takes measurements such as vital signs height, weight, visual acuity and skin integrity (see Chapter 18), and will also record baseline observations such as blood pressure, temperature, pulse and respirations.

DATA MANAGEMENT

Organising Data

The nurse uses a written (or computerised) format that organises the assessment data systematically. This is often referred to as a patient profile, nursing health history, nursing assessment or nursing database form. The format may be modified according to the patient's physical status such as one focused on musculoskeletal data for orthopaedic patients, the end of life pathways for terminally ill patients or the mental health computerised system: the Functional Analysis of Care Environments (FACE).

Nursing Conceptual Models

While the nursing process is a systematic, patient-centred method for structuring the delivery of nursing care, it is not enough on its own (Barrett *et al.*, 2008). Nursing models provide guidance and direction from the information gathered during the assessment process, to plan and deliver effective holistic nursing care. Most schools of nursing and healthcare settings have developed their own structured assessment format. Many of these are based on selected nursing theories (discussed earlier in Chapter 9). Four examples are Roper, Logan and Tierney's activities of living model, Gordon's functional health pattern framework, Orem's self-care model and Roy's adaptation model.

Body Systems Model

The body systems model focuses on abnormalities of the following anatomic systems:

- integumentary (skin) system
- respiratory system
- cardiovascular system
- nervous system
- musculoskeletal system
- gastrointestinal system
- genitourinary system
- reproductive system
- immune system.

Maslow's Hierarchy of Needs

Maslow's hierarchy of needs (see Chapter 2) clusters data pertaining to the following:

- physiological needs (survival needs)
- safety and security needs
- love and belonging needs
- self-esteem needs
- self-actualisation needs.

Validating Data

The information gathered during the assessment phase must be complete, factual and accurate because the nursing diagnoses and interventions are based on this information. Validation is the act of 'double-checking' or verifying data to confirm that it is accurate and factual. Validating data helps the nurse complete these tasks:

- Ensure that assessment information is complete.
- Ensure that objective and related subjective data agree.

- Obtain additional information that may have been overlooked.
- Differentiate between cues and inferences. Cues are subjective or objective data that can be directly observed by the nurse; that is, what the patient says or what the nurse can see, hear, feel, smell or measure. Inferences are the nurse's interpretation or conclusions made based on the cues (e.g. a nurse observes the cues that an incision is red, hot and swollen; the nurse makes the inference that the incision is infected).
- Avoid jumping to conclusions and focusing in the wrong direction to identify problems.

Not all data require validation. For example, data such as height, weight, birth date and most laboratory studies that can be measured with an accurate scale can be accepted as factual. As a rule, the nurse validates data when there are discrepancies between data obtained in the nursing interview (subjective data) and the physical assessment (objective data), or when the patient's statements differ at different times in the assessment. Guidelines for validating data are shown in Table 10-5.

To collect data accurately, nurses need to be aware of their own biases, values and beliefs, and to separate fact from inference, interpretation and assumption. For example, a nurse seeing a man holding his arm to his chest might assume that he is experiencing chest pain, when in fact he has a painful hand.

To build an accurate database, nurses must validate assumptions regarding the patient's physical or emotional behaviour. In the previous example, the nurse should ask the patient why he is holding his arm to his chest. The patient's response may validate the nurse's assumptions or prompt further questioning.

Documenting Data

To complete the assessment phase, the nurse records patient data. Accurate documentation is essential and should include all data collected about the patient's health status. Data are recorded in a factual manner and not interpreted by the nurse. For example, the nurse records the patient's breakfast intake (objective data) as 'coffee 200 ml, juice 100 ml, 1 egg and 1 slice of toast', rather than as 'appetite good' (a judgement). A judgement or conclusion such as 'appetite good' or 'normal appetite' may have different meanings for different people. To increase accuracy, the nurse records subjective data in the patient's own words. Restating in other words what someone says increases the chance of changing the original meaning.

DIAGNOSING

Diagnosing is the second phase of the nursing process, which is a system that is developing within nursing in the UK. Diagnosing is a pivotal step in the nursing process. All activities preceding this phase are directed towards formulating the nursing diagnoses; all the care-planning activities following this phase are based on the nursing diagnoses (see Figure 10-5). An important point to remember is that nursing diagnosis is not the same as a medical diagnosis, as a nursing diagnosis is formulated from the assessment of the patient.

Saint Louis University School of Nursing and Allied Health Professions sponsored the first national conference to identify nursing diagnosis in 1973. Subsequent national conferences occurred in 1975, 1980 and every two years thereafter.

Table 10-5 Validating Assessment Data

Guidelines	Example
Compare subjective and objective data to verify the patient's statements with your observations.	Patient's perceptions of 'feeling hot' need to be compared with measurement of the body temperature.
Clarify any ambiguous or vague statements.	*Patient*: 'I've felt sick on and off for 6 weeks.' *Nurse*: 'Describe what your sickness is like. Tell me what you mean by "on and off".'
Be sure your data consist of cues and not inferences.	*Observation*: Dry skin and reduced tissue elasticity. *Inference*: Dehydration. *Action*: Collect additional data that are needed to make the inference in the diagnosing phase. For example, determine the patient's fluid intake, amount and appearance of urine, and blood pressure.
Double-check data that are extremely abnormal.	*Observation*: A resting pulse of 30 beats per minute or a blood pressure of 210/95. *Action*: Repeat the measurement. Use another piece of equipment as needed to confirm abnormalities, or ask someone else to collect the same data.
Determine the presence of factors that may interfere with accurate measurement.	A crying infant will have an abnormal respiratory rate and will need quietening before accurate assessment can be made.
Use references (textbooks, journals, research reports) to explain phenomena.	A nurse considers tiny purple or bluish-black swollen areas under the tongue of an elderly patient to be abnormal until reading about physical changes of ageing. Such varicosities are common.

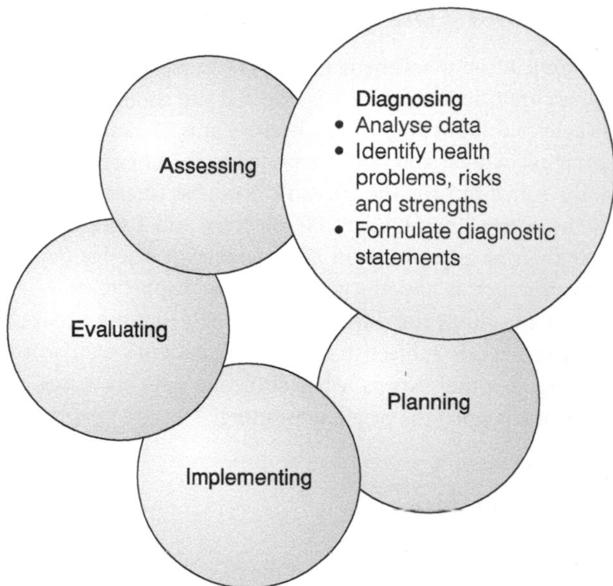

Figure 10-5 Diagnosing. The pivotal second phase of the nursing process, in which the nurse interprets assessment data, identifies patient strengths and health problems and formulates diagnostic statements.

International recognition came with the First Canadian Conference in Toronto in 1977 and the International Nursing Conference in May 1987 in Calgary, Alberta, Canada. In 1982, the conference group accepted the name North American Nursing Diagnosis Association (NANDA), recognising the participation and contributions of nurses in the USA and Canada. In response to their widening membership in 2002 NANDA relaunched itself as NANDA International (NANDA-I).

The continued development and use of nursing's standardised terminology by NANDA-I ensures patient safety through evidence-based care, thereby improving the healthcare of all people. NANDA-I develops nursing terminology reflecting nurses' clinical judgement in social psychological and spiritual dimensions of care (NANDA International, 2009). The members of NANDA International include staff nurses, clinical specialists, faculty, directors of nursing, deans, theorists and researchers.

In the UK, nursing practice currently adopts the NANDA system as there is no UK equivalent.

Nursing Diagnosis

To use the concept of nursing diagnosis effectively in generating and completing a nursing care plan, the nurse must be familiar with the definitions of terms used, the types and the components of nursing diagnosis. However, while nursing diagnosis is used in the UK, in many cases it is still used subconsciously.

Definitions

The term *diagnosing* refers to the reasoning process, whereas the term 'diagnosis' is a statement or conclusion regarding the nature of a phenomenon. The standardised NANDA names for the diagnoses are called diagnostic labels; and the patient's problem statement, consisting of the diagnostic label plus **aetiology** (causal relationship between a problem and its related or risk factors), is called a nursing diagnosis.

In 1990, NANDA adopted an official working definition of nursing diagnosis: '. . . a clinical judgement that nurses make about individual, family, to community responses to conditions/life processes. Based on that judgement, the nurse is responsible for monitoring of client responses, decision making culminating in a plan of care, and implementing interventions, including interdisciplinary collaboration and referral as required. The nurse is wholly or partly accountable for the desired outcome' (NANDA International, 2009).

This definition implies the following:

- Professional nurses (registered nurses) are responsible for making nursing diagnosis, even though other nursing personnel may contribute data to the process of diagnosing and may implement specified nursing care. The American Nurses Association *Standards of clinical nursing practice* (1998) (the US equivalent of the NMC), states that nurses are accountable for this phase of the nursing process. The Joint Commission on Accreditation of Healthcare Organizations (JCAHO) – the equivalent of the UK Department of Health – requires evidence of nursing diagnosis in patients' medical records as well (JCAHO, 2009).
- The domain of nursing diagnosis includes only those health states that nurses are educated and licensed to treat. For example, nurses are not educated to diagnose or treat diseases such as diabetes mellitus; this task is defined legally as within the practice of medicine. Yet nurses can diagnose and treat *deficient knowledge, ineffective coping* or *imbalanced nutrition*, all of which may accompany diabetes mellitus.
- A nursing diagnosis is a judgement made only after thorough, systematic data collection.
- Nursing diagnoses describe a continuum of health states: deviations from health, presence of risk factors and areas of enhanced personal growth.

Types of Nursing Diagnoses/Plan of Care

The five types of nursing diagnoses are actual, risk, wellness, possible and syndrome/chronic conditions.

- An actual plan/diagnosis is a patient problem that is present at the time of the nursing assessment. Examples are *ineffective breathing pattern* and *anxiety*. An actual nursing diagnosis is based on the presence of associated signs and symptoms.
- A **risk nursing plan/diagnosis** is a clinical judgement that a problem does not exist, but the presence of risk factors indicates that a problem is likely to develop unless nurses intervene. For example, all people admitted to a hospital have some possibility of acquiring an infection; however, a patient with diabetes or a compromised immune system is at higher risk than others. Therefore, the nurse would appropriately use the label *risk for infection* to describe the patient's health status. The National Patient Safety Agency has published a

document that makes risk assessment easy (see the website address at the end of the chapter).

- A wellness plan/diagnosis 'describes human responses to levels of wellness in an individual, family or community that have a readiness for enhancement' (NANDA International, 2009: 263). Examples of wellness diagnosis would be *readiness for enhanced spiritual well-being* or *readiness for enhanced family coping.*
- A **possible nursing diagnosis** is one in which evidence about a health problem is incomplete or unclear. A possible diagnosis requires more data either to support or to refute it. For example, an elderly widow who lives alone is admitted to the hospital. The nurse notices that she has no visitors and is pleased with attention and conversation from the nursing staff. Until more data are collected, the nurse may write a nursing diagnosis of possible delayed discharge due to social isolation related to unknown aetiology.
- A **syndrome/chronic condition plan/diagnosis** is a diagnosis that is associated with a group/cluster of other diagnoses (Alfaro-LeFevre, 2009).
- Currently six syndrome diagnoses are on the NANDA International list. *Risk for disuse syndrome* (poor mobility), for example, may be experienced by long-term bedridden patients. Groups of problems associated with this syndrome include *impaired physical mobility, risk for impaired tissue integrity, risk for activity intolerance, risk for constipation, risk for infection, risk for injury, risk for powerlessness, impaired gas exchange*, and so on (Nigam *et al.*, 2009).

Components of a NANDA Nursing Diagnosis

A nursing diagnoses has three components: (1) the problem and its definition, (2) the aetiology (cause) and (3) the defining characteristics. Each component serves a specific purpose.

Problem (Diagnostic Label) and Definition

The problem statement, or diagnostic label, describes a particular problem (each patient usually has several) and the patient's health status clearly and concisely in a few words. The purpose of the diagnostic label (problem) is to direct the formation of patient goals and desired outcomes. It will also guide nursing interventions.

To be clinically useful, problem/diagnostic labels need to be specific; when the word *specify* follows a NANDA label, the nurse states the area in which the problem occurs, for example, *deficient knowledge (medications)* or *deficient knowledge (dietary adjustments)*. Currently in many areas in the UK this is related to the initial problem, e.g. the patient has difficulty in breathing due to exacerbation of chronic obstructive pulmonary disease.

Further information or explanation/qualifiers are words that have been added (to some NANDA labels) to give additional meaning to the diagnostic statement and are frequently used in the UK, for example:

- **deficient** (inadequate in amount, quality or degree; not sufficient; incomplete)
- **impaired** (made worse, weakened, damaged, reduced, deteriorated)
- **decreased** (lesser in size, amount or degree)
- **ineffective** (not producing the desired effect)
- **compromised** (to make vulnerable to threat).

Each diagnostic label approved by NANDA carries a definition that clarifies its meaning. For example, the definition of the diagnostic label *activity intolerance* is shown in Table 10-6.

Aetiology (Cause) (Related Factors and Risk Factors)

The aetiology (causal) component of a nursing diagnosis identifies one or more probable causes of the health problem, gives direction to the required nursing care and enables the nurse to individualise the patient's care. As shown in Table 10-6, the probable causes of *activity intolerance* include sedentary life style, generalised weakness, and so on. Differentiating among possible causes in the nursing diagnosis is essential because each may require different nursing interventions. Table 10-7 provides examples of problems that have different aetiologies and therefore require different interventions.

Defining Characteristics

Defining characteristics are the group of signs and symptoms that indicate the presence of a particular diagnostic label. For actual nursing diagnoses, the defining characteristics are the patient's signs and symptoms. For risk nursing diagnoses, no subjective and objective signs are present. Thus the factors that

Table 10-6 Components of a Nursing Diagnosis Label

Diagnosis and definition	Aetiology/related factors	Defining characteristics
Activity intolerance	Bedrest or immobility	Verbal report of fatigue or weakness
Insufficient physiological or psychological energy to endure or complete required or desired daily activities	Generalised weakness	Abnormal heart rate or blood pressure response to activity
	Imbalance between oxygen supply/demand	ECG changes reflecting arrhythmias or Ischaemia
	Sedentary lifestyle	Exertional discomfort or dyspnoea

Source: *Nursing diagnoses-Definitions and classification, 2009-2011*. Copyright © 2009, 1994-2009 by NANDA International. Used by arrangement with Blackwell Publishing Limited, a company of John Wiley & Sons, Inc.

Table 10-7 Examples of Nursing Interventions to Address Different Aetiologies

Diagnostic label (problem)	Patient	Aetiology	Example of nursing interventions
Constipation	Kenneth Pennington	Long-term laxative use	Work with Mr Pennington to develop a plan for gradual withdrawal from the laxatives; teach components of a high-fibre diet.
	Emily Smith	Inactivity and insufficient fluid intake	Help Ms Smith develop an exercise regimen that she can follow at home; obtain information about her daily schedule and types of fluids she likes; help Ms Smith develop a plan for including sufficient amounts of fluids in her diet.
Ineffective breastfeeding	Jennifer Lowe	Breast engorgement	Teach Ms Lowe to massage her breasts before feeding; use hot packs or hot shower before nursing infant.
	Belinda Rossinger	Inexperience and lack of knowledge	Teach Ms Rossinger to feed infant on demand; show her how to be sure infant is sucking and swallowing; and demonstrate different holding positions for feedings.

cause the patient to be more than 'normally' vulnerable to the problem form the aetiology of a risk nursing diagnosis.

Differentiating Nursing Diagnoses from Medical Diagnoses

A nursing diagnosis is a statement of nursing judgement and refers to a condition that nurses are permitted to treat and/or manage. A medical diagnosis is made by a physician and refers to a condition that only a physician can treat. Medical diagnoses refer to disease processes – specific pathophysiological responses that are fairly uniform from one patient to another. In contrast, nursing diagnoses describe a patient's physical, sociocultural, psychological and spiritual responses to an illness or a health problem. See how these responses vary among individuals:

David Evans is a 17-year-old boy who following two seizures has been diagnosed with epilepsy. He finds this very difficult to come to terms with, and he gets very angry and frustrated, refuses counselling and takes his medication as and when he wants to. Every weekend he goes **binge drinking** *with his friends (as he is in denial), and inevitably ends up in the local accident and emergency department for treatment. David finds it very difficult to come to terms with his illness particularly when he feels he's at an age that he should be learning to drive the car and should be out enjoying himself with his friends every weekend, David feels that his personal identity, self-esteem and confidence is under threat.*

Jackie Williams is a 45-year-old woman who has had epilepsy from the age of four. Her epilepsy is well managed with medication and Jackie socialises and drinks in moderation. As Jackie has not had a seizure for over 20 years she is able to drive a car and has an active social life.

A patient's medical diagnosis remains the same for as long as the disease process is present, but nursing diagnoses change as the patient's responses change. David Evans's response to his illness may change over time to become more similar to that of Mrs Williams's.

Nurses have responsibilities related to both medical and nursing diagnoses. Nursing diagnoses relate to the nurse's independent functions, that is, the areas of healthcare that are unique to nursing and separate and distinct from medical management.

Nurses may not prescribe all the care for nursing diagnoses, but if the problem is a nursing diagnosis, the nurse can prescribe most of the interventions needed for prevention or resolution. For example, most patients with a nursing diagnosis of *pain* have medical prescriptions for analgesics, but many independent nursing interventions can also alleviate pain (e.g. music therapy, reading or teaching a patient to 'splint' an incision).

Differentiating Nursing Diagnoses from Collaborative Problems

A collaborative problem is a type of potential problem that nurses manage using both independent and physician-prescribed interventions. Independent nursing interventions for a collaborative problem focus mainly on monitoring the patient's condition and preventing development of the potential complication. Definitive treatment of the condition requires both medical and nursing interventions.

Collaborative problems tend to be present when a particular disease or treatment is present; that is, each disease or treatment has specific complications that are always associated with it. For example, a statement of collaborative problems is 'Potential complication of pneumonia: **atelectasis**, **respiratory failure**, pleural effusion, pericarditis and **meningitis**'.

Nursing diagnoses, by contrast, involve human responses, which vary greatly from one person to the next. Therefore, the same set of nursing diagnoses cannot be expected to occur with a particular disease or condition; moreover, a single nursing diagnosis may occur as a response to any number of diseases. For example, all patients who have had a hip replacement will

Table 10-8 Comparison of Nursing Diagnoses, Medical Diagnoses and Collaborative Problems

Category	Nursing diagnoses	Medical diagnoses	Collaborative problems
Example	*Activity intolerance* related to decreased cardiac output (Has restricted mobility for 48 hours following a myocardial infarction.)	Myocardial infarction	Potential complication of myocardial infarction: congestive heart failure
Description	Describe human responses to disease process or health problem; consist of a one-, two- or three-part statement, usually including problem and aetiology	Describe disease and pathology; do not consider other human responses; usually consist of not more than three words	Involve human responses – mainly physiologic complications of disease, tests or treatments; consist of a two-part statement of situation/pathophysiology and the potential complication
Orientation and responsibility for diagnosing	Oriented to the individual; nurses responsible for diagnosing	Oriented to pathology; physician responsible for diagnosing	Oriented to pathophysiology; nurses responsible for diagnosing
Treatment orders	Nurse orders most interventions to prevent and treat	Physician orders primary interventions to prevent and treat	Nurse collaborates with physician and other healthcare professionals to prevent and treat (require medical instruction) for definitive treatment
Nursing focus	Treat and prevent	Implement medical orders for treatment and monitor status of condition	Prevent and monitor for onset or status of condition
Nursing actions	Independent	Dependent (primarily)	Some independent actions, but primarily for monitoring and preventing
Duration	Can change frequently	Remains the same while disease is present	Present when disease or situation is present
Classification system	Classification system is developed and being used but is not universally accepted	Well-developed classification system accepted by the medical profession	No universally accepted classification system

have similar collaborative problems such as post-operative complications (e.g. haemorrhage, dislocation, pain) but not all patients who have had a hip replacement will have the nursing diagnoses. Some might experience constipation due to poor dietary intake, some will experience greater fluid loss from site of wound, some will have a positive cognitive attitude to mobility whereas others will not. Table 10-8 provides a comparison of nursing diagnoses, medical problems and collaborative problems.

THE DIAGNOSTIC PROCESS

The diagnostic process uses the critical-thinking skills of analysis and synthesis. Critical thinking is a cognitive process during which a person reviews data and considers explanations before forming an opinion. Analysis is the separation into components, that is, the breaking down of the whole into its parts. Synthesis is the opposite, that is, the putting together of parts into the whole.

The diagnostic process is used continuously by most nurses. An experienced nurse may enter a patient's room and immediately observe significant data and draw conclusions about the patient. As a result of attaining knowledge, skill and expertise in the practice setting, the expert nurse may seem to perform these mental processes automatically. Novice nurses, however, need guidelines to understand and formulate nursing diagnoses. The diagnostic process has three steps:

1 accurately analysing data;
2 identifying health problems, risks and strengths;
3 formulating diagnostic statements.

Analysing Data

In the diagnostic process, analysing involves the following steps:

1 Compare data against standards (identify significant cues).
2 Cluster cues (generate tentative theories).
3 Identify gaps and inconsistencies.

For experienced nurses, these activities occur continuously rather than sequentially.

Comparing Data with Standards

Nurses draw on knowledge and experience to compare patient data to standards and norms and identify significant and relevant cues. A standard or norm is a generally accepted measure, rule, model or pattern. The nurse uses a wide range of standards, such as growth and development patterns, normal vital signs and laboratory values. A cue is considered significant if it does any of the following (Gordon, 2002):

- Points to negative or positive change in a patient's health status or pattern. These may be positive or negative cues. For example, the patient states: 'I have recently experienced shortness of breath while climbing stairs' or 'I have not smoked for three months.'
- Varies from norms of the patient population. The patient's pattern may fit within cultural norms but vary from norms of the general society. The patient may consider a pattern – for example, the patient repeatedly has to check her handbag to see if her purse is in the handbag, which she does consistently during the interview process. This pattern, however, may not be productive and may require further exploration (e.g. obsessive compulsive disorder).
- Indicates a developmental delay. To identify significant cues, the nurse must be aware of the normal patterns and changes that occur as the person grows and develops. For example, by age nine months an infant is usually able to sit alone without support. The infant who has not accomplished this task needs further assessment for possible developmental delays.

Table 10-9 lists specific examples of patient cues and norms to which they may be compared.

Clustering or Information Gathering Cues

Data information gathering or clustering cues is a process of determining the relatedness of facts and determining whether any patterns are present, whether the data represent isolated incidents, and whether the data are significant. This is the beginning of synthesis.

The nurse may gather data inductively by combining data from different assessment areas to form a pattern and group the subjective and objective data into the appropriate categories. The latter is a deductive approach to data clustering, or pattern formation.

Experienced nurses may cluster data as they collect and interpret it, as evidenced in remarks or thoughts such as 'I'm getting a picture of . . .' or 'This cue doesn't fit the picture.' The novice nurse does not have the knowledge base or the clinical experience that aids in recognising cues. Thus the novice must take careful assessment notes, search data for abnormal cues and use all appropriate resources for comparing the patient's cues with the defining characteristics and aetiologic factors of the accepted nursing diagnoses.

Data clustering or information gathering involves making inferences about the data. The nurse interprets the possible meaning of the cues and labels the cue clusters with tentative diagnostic hypotheses.

Identifying Gaps and Inconsistencies in Data

Skilful assessment minimises gaps and inconsistencies in data. However, data analysis should include a final check to ensure that data are complete and correct.

Inconsistencies are conflicting data. Possible sources of conflicting data include measurement error, expectations and inconsistent or unreliable reports. For example, a nurse may learn from the nursing history that the patient reports not

Table 10-9 Comparing Cues to Standards and Norms

Type of cue	Patient cues	Standard/norm
Deviation from population norms	Height is 158cm (5 ft 2 in). Woman with small frame. Weighs 109kg.	Height and weight tables indicate that the 'ideal' weight for a woman 158cm (5 ft 2 in) with a small frame is 49–53kg.
Developmental delay	Child is 17 months old. Parents state child has not yet attempted to speak. Child laughs aloud and makes cooing sounds.	Children usually speak their first word by 10 to 12 months of age.
Changes in patient's usual health status	States, 'I'm just not hungry these days.' Ate only 15% of food on breakfast tray. Has lost 13kg in past three months.	Patient usually eats three balanced meals per day. Adults typically maintain stable weight.
Dysfunctional behaviour	Harry's mother reports that Harry has not left his room for two days. Harry is age 16. Harry has stopped attending school and has withdrawn from social contact.	Adolescents usually like to be with their peers; social group very important. Functional behaviour includes school attendance.
Changes in patient's usual behaviour	Ms Knightly reports that lately her husband angers easily. 'Yesterday he even yelled at the dog.' 'He just seems so tense.'	Mr Knightly is usually relaxed and easygoing. He is friendly and kind to animals.

having seen a doctor in 15 years, yet during the physical health examination he states, 'My doctor takes my blood pressure every year.' All inconsistencies must be clarified before a valid pattern can be established.

Identifying Health Problems, Risks and Strengths

After data are analysed, the nurse and patient can together identify strengths and problems. This is primarily a decision-making process as previously noted.

> **ACTIVITY 10-2**
>
> Discuss the role of the nurse when during the assessment process Mr Jones, who has frequent hospital admissions due to shortness of breath and chest infections, explains that he doesn't go to bed each night as he sits in his chair by the fireplace as it is nice and warm. In the diagnostic process can you differentiate the nurse's role from that of the doctor's and identify the collaborative care provided and provide a tentative diagnostic hypothesis.

Determining Problems and Risks

After grouping and clustering the data, the nurse and patient together identify problems that support tentative, actual risk and possible diagnoses. In addition the nurse must determine whether the patient's problem is a nursing diagnosis, medical diagnosis or collaborative problem (see Figure 10-6).

Determining Strengths

At this stage, the nurse and patient also establish the patient's strengths, resources and abilities to cope. Most people have a clearer perception of their problems or weaknesses than of their strengths and assets, which they often take for granted. By taking an inventory of strengths, the patient can develop a more well-rounded self-concept and self-image. Strengths can be an aid to mobilising health and regenerative processes.

A patient's strength might be weight that is within the normal range for age and height, thus enabling the patient to cope better with surgery. In another instance, a patient's strengths might be absence of allergies and being a non-smoker.

A patient's strengths can be found in the nursing assessment record (health, home life, education, recreation, exercise, work, family and friends, religious beliefs and sense of humour, for example), the health examination and the patient's records.

Formulating Diagnostic Statements

Most nursing diagnoses are written as two-part or three-part statements, but there are variations of these.

Basic Two-Part Statements

The basic two-part statement includes the following:

1 *Problem (P)*: statement of the patient's response (NANDA label/nursing model cluster).

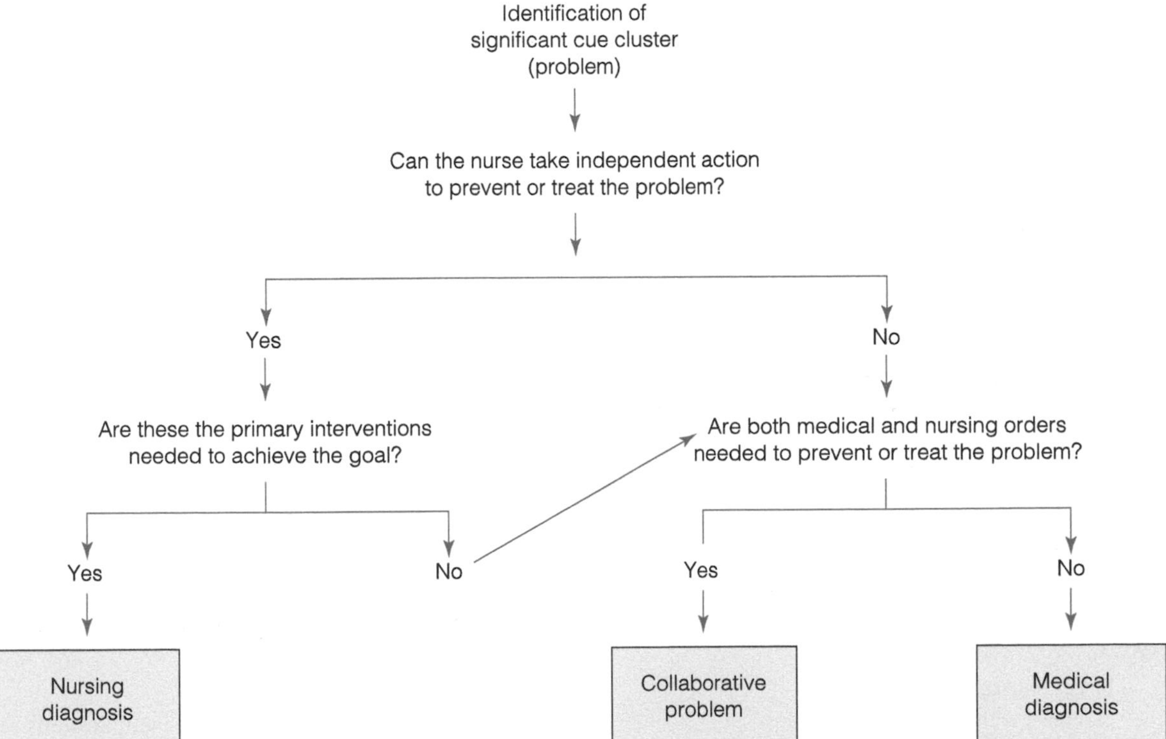

Figure 10-6 Decision tree for differentiating among nursing diagnoses, collaborative problems and medical diagnoses.

2 *Aetiology (E) (cause)*: factors contributing to or probable causes of the responses.

The two parts are joined by the words *related to* rather than *due to*. The phrase *due to* implies that one part causes or is responsible for the other part. By contrast, the phrase *related to* merely implies a relationship. Some examples of two-part nursing diagnoses are shown below.

BOX 10-3 Basic Two-Part Diagnostic Statement

Problem	Aetiology	Signs and symptoms
Increasing shortness of breath	related to	Chronic obstructive pulmonary disease
Continuous crying by 6-week-old baby	related to	Urinary tract infection

Basic Three-Part Statement

The basic three-part nursing diagnosis statement is called the PES format and includes the following:

1 *Problem (P)*: statement of the patient's response (NANDA label cluster/nursing model).
2 *Aetiology (E) (cause)*: factors contributing to or probable causes of the response (condition).
3 *Signs and symptoms (S)*: defining characteristics manifested by the patient.

Actual nursing diagnoses can be documented by using the three-part statement because the signs and symptoms have been identified. This format cannot be used for risk diagnoses because the patient does not have signs and symptoms of the diagnosis.

The PES format is especially recommended for beginning diagnosticians because the signs and symptoms validate why the diagnosis was chosen and make the problem statement more descriptive.

The disadvantage of the PES format is that it can create very long problem statements, thereby making the problem and aetiology (cause) unclear. However, because the signs and symptoms can be helpful in planning nursing interventions, they should be easily accessible. To promote access without long problem statements, the nurse can record the signs and symptoms in the nursing notes instead of on the care plan. Another possibility, recommended for students, is to list the signs and symptoms on the care plan below the nursing diagnosis. The signs and symptoms are easily accessible, and the problem (P) and aetiology (cause) (C) stand out clearly. For example:

Noncompliance (diabetic diet) related to unresolved anger about diagnosis as manifested by:

C - 'I forget to take my tablets.'
'I can't live without sugar in my food.'
P - Weight 98kg [gain of 4.5kg]
Blood pressure 190/100

One-Part Statements

Some diagnostic statements, such as wellness diagnoses (discharge planning) and syndrome (chronic condition) nursing diagnoses, consist of a NANDA label only. As the diagnostic labels are refined they tend to become more specific, so that nursing interventions can be derived from the label itself. Therefore, an aetiology may not be needed. For example, adding an aetiology to the label *rape-trauma syndrome* does not make the label any more descriptive or useful.

Variations of Basic Formats

Variations of the basic one-, two- and three-part statements include the following:

- Writing *unknown aetiology* when the defining characteristics are present but the nurse does not know the cause or contributing factors. One example is *noncompliance (medication regimen)* related to unknown aetiology.
- Using the phrase *complex factors* when there are too many aetiologic (cause) factors or when they are too complex to state in a brief phrase. The actual causes of chronic low self-esteem, for instance, may be long term and complex, as in the following nursing diagnosis: *chronic low self-esteem* related to complex factors.
- Using the word *possible* to describe either the problem or the aetiology (cause). When the nurse believes more data are needed about the patient's problem or the aetiology, the word *possible* is inserted. Examples are *possible low self-esteem* related to loss of job and rejection by family; *altered thought processes* possibly related to unfamiliar surroundings.
- Using *secondary to* divide the aetiology into two parts, thereby making the statement more descriptive and useful. The part following *secondary to* is often a pathophysiological or disease process, as in *risk for impaired skin integrity* related to decreased peripheral circulation secondary to diabetes.
- Adding a second part to the general response or NANDA label/model cluster to make it more precise. For example, the diagnosis *impaired skin integrity* does not indicate the location of the problem. To make this label more specific, the nurse can add a descriptor as follows: *impaired skin integrity (left lateral ankle)* related to decreased peripheral circulation.

Collaborative Problems

Carpenito (2009) suggests that all collaborative (multidisciplinary) problems begin with the diagnostic label *potential complication* (PC). Nurses should include in the diagnostic statement both the possible complication they are monitoring and the disease or treatment that is present to produce it. For example, if the patient has a head injury and could develop increased intracranial pressure, the nurses should write the following:

Potential complication of head injury: Increased intracranial pressure

When monitoring for a group of complications associated with a disease or pathology, the nurse states the disease and follows it with a list of the complications:

Potential complication of pregnancy-induced hypertension: seizures, foetal distress, pulmonary oedema, hepatic/renal failure, premature labour, CNS haemorrhage

Evaluating the Quality of the Diagnostic Statement

In addition to using the correct format, nurses must consider the content of their diagnostic statements. The statements should, for example, be accurate, concise, descriptive and specific. The nurse must always validate the diagnostic statements with the patient and compare the patient's signs and symptoms to the model used, the local health board policy or NANDA defining characteristics. For risk problems, the nurse compares the patient's risk factors to local health board policies or NANDA risk factors.

Avoiding Errors in Diagnostic Reasoning

Some error is inherent in any human undertaking and diagnosis is no exception. However, it is important that nurses make nursing diagnoses with a high level of accuracy. Nurses can avoid some common errors of reasoning by recognising them and applying the appropriate critical-thinking skills. Error can occur at any point in the diagnostic process: data collection, data interpretation and data clustering. The following suggestions help to minimise diagnostic error:

- **Verify.** Hypothesise possible explanations of the data, but realise that all diagnoses are only tentative until they are verified. Begin and end the diagnostic process by talking with the patient and family. When collecting data, ask them what their health problems are and what they believe the causes to be. At the end of the process, ask them to verify your diagnoses.
- **Build a good knowledge base and acquire clinical experience.** Nurses must apply knowledge from many different areas to recognise significant cues and patterns and generate hypotheses about the data. To name only a few, principles from chemistry, anatomy and pharmacology each help the nurse understand patient data in a different way.
- **Have a working knowledge of what is normal.** Nurses need to know the population norms for vital signs, laboratory tests, speech development, and so on. In addition, nurses must determine what is normal for a particular person, taking into account age, physical makeup, lifestyle, culture and the person's own perception of what is normal. For example, normal blood pressure for adults is in the range of 110/60 to 140/80. However, a nurse might obtain a reading of 90/50 that is perfectly normal for a particular patient. The nurse should compare findings to the patient's baseline when possible (see the weblink at the end of the chapter).
- **Consult resources.** Both novices and experienced nurses should consult appropriate resources whenever in doubt about a diagnosis. Professional literature, nursing colleagues and other professionals are all appropriate resources.
- **Base diagnoses on patterns.** That is, on behaviour over time – rather than on an isolated incident.
- **Improve critical-thinking skills.** These skills help the nurse to be aware of and avoid errors in thinking, such as overgeneralising, stereotyping, making unwarranted assumptions, and so on.

ONGOING DEVELOPMENT OF NURSING DIAGNOSES AND TERMINOLOGY

In 1997, NANDA changed the name of its official journal from *Nursing Diagnosis* to *Nursing Diagnosis: The International Journal of Nursing Language and Classification*. The subtitle emphasises that nursing diagnosis is part of a larger, developing system of standardised nursing language, worldwide. This system includes classifications of nursing interventions (NIC) and nursing outcomes (NOC) that are being developed by other research groups which are linked to the NANDA diagnostic labels, and in 2002 NANDA relaunched itself as NANDA International due to the more widespread interest in developments within the group.

While in the UK, due to the reluctance of nurse diagnosing, the models of nursing are used as the framework to manage care. However, the National Institute for Health and Clinical Excellence (NICE) provides guidance on the promotion of good health and the prevention and treatment of various health conditions (see the web link at the end of the chapter).

In 2007 SNOMED-CT® was purchased by International Health Terminology Standards Development Organisation (IHTSDO). SNOMED CT is a clinical terminology and stands for the Systematised Nomenclature of Medicine Clinical Terms. It is a common computerised language used by all computers in the NHS to facilitate communications between healthcare professionals in clear and unambiguous terms. It includes all the nursing terminologies recognised by the ANA, including the ICN's ICNP (which Scotland is beginning to use). It is rapidly becoming the global standard and is mandatory for use in the UK from 2015. It has a strong nursing network (led by Anne Casey of the UK), which continues to develop nursing terms. By acquiring the SNOMED-CT standard, the IHTSDO, which was established by a group of nine founding nations (Australia, Canada, Denmark, Lithuania, The Netherlands, New Zealand, Sweden, the USA and the UK), and its member countries, will help to ensure the continued maintenance and evolution of SNOMED-CT as well as its availability on an international scale (see the web link at the end of the chapter).

LIFESPAN CONSIDERATIONS

Mature Adults

Mature adults tend to have multiple problems with complex physical and psychosocial needs when they are ill. If the nurse has done a thorough, accurate assessment, nursing diagnoses can be selected to cover all problems and, at the same time, prioritise the special needs. For example, if a patient is admitted with severe congestive heart failure, prompt attention will be focused on *decreased cardiac output* and *excess fluid volume*, with interventions selected to improve these areas quickly. As these conditions improve, then other nursing diagnoses, such as *activity intolerance* (mobility) and *deficient knowledge* (communication) related to a new medication regime, might require more attention. They are all part of the same medical problem of congestive heart failure, but each nursing diagnosis has specific expected outcomes and nursing interventions. The patient's strengths should be an essential consideration in all phases of the nursing process.

PLANNING

Planning is a deliberative, individual, systematic phase of the nursing process that involves decision making and problem solving. In planning, the nurse refers to the patient's assessment data and diagnostic statements for direction in formulating patient individual healthcare goals and designing the nursing interventions required to prevent, reduce or eliminate the patient's health problems (see Figure 10-7). A nursing intervention is 'any treatment, based upon clinical judgement and knowledge, which a nurse performs to enhance patient outcomes' (McCloskey and Bulechek, 2008: xix). The product of the planning phase is a patient care plan.

While the nurse has responsibility for the care provided, it is important that the nurse, the patient and support persons work in collaboration with each other in order to assess, diagnose and plan the care provisions required. In a home setting, the patient's support people and caregivers are the ones who implement the plan of care; thus, its effectiveness depends largely on them.

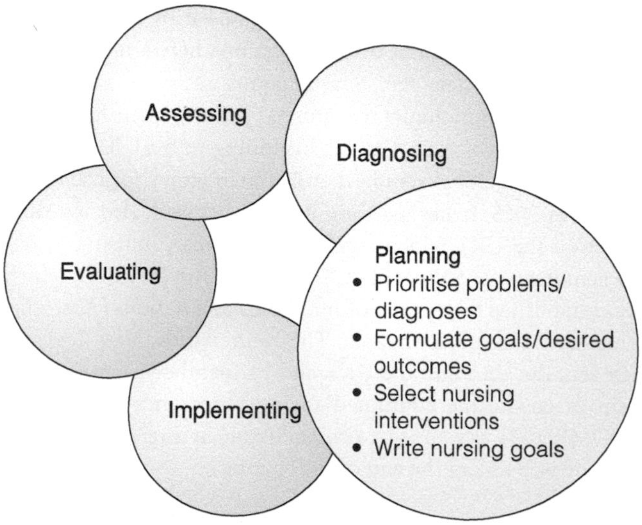

Assessing

Diagnosing

Planning
- Prioritise problems/ diagnoses
- Formulate goals/desired outcomes
- Select nursing interventions
- Write nursing goals

Evaluating

Implementing

Figure 10-7 Planning. The third phase of the nursing process in which the nurse and patient develop goals/desired outcomes and nursing interventions to prevent, reduce or alleviate the patient's health problems.

Types of Planning

Planning begins with the first patient contact and continues until the nurse–patient relationship ends, usually when the patient is discharged from a healthcare environment whether at home or in a hospital setting.

Initial Planning

The nurse who performs the admission assessment usually develops the initial comprehensive plan of care. This nurse has the benefit of the patient's body language as well as some intuitive kinds of information that are not available solely from the written database. Planning should be initiated as soon as possible after the initial assessment, especially due to shorter hospital stays.

Ongoing Planning

Ongoing planning is done by all nurses who work with the patient. As nurses obtain new information and evaluate the patient's responses to care, they can individualise the initial care plan further. Ongoing planning also occurs at the beginning of a shift as the nurse plans the care to be given that day. Using ongoing assessment data, the nurse carries out daily planning for the following purposes:

- To determine whether the patient's health status has changed.
- To set priorities for the patient's care during the shift.
- To decide which aspects of care needs more indepth focus during the day.
- To coordinate the nurse's activities so that more than one problem can be addressed at each patient contact.

Discharge Planning

Discharge planning, the process of anticipating and planning for needs after discharge, is a crucial part of comprehensive healthcare and should be addressed in each patient's care plan from the initial assessment on admission. Because the average stay of patients in acute care hospitals has become shorter, people are sometimes discharged still needing care. Although many patients are discharged to other agencies (e.g. long-term care facilities and nursing homes), such care is increasingly being delivered in the home and support provided by other agencies or acute response teams (ARTs). Effective discharge planning begins at first patient contact and involves comprehensive and ongoing assessment to obtain information about the patient's ongoing needs.

DEVELOPING NURSING CARE PLANS

The end product of the planning phase of the nursing process is a formal or informal plan of care. An *informal nursing care plan* is a strategy for action that exists in the nurse's mind. For example, the nurse may think, 'Mrs Lewis is very tired. I will need to reinforce her teaching after she is rested.' A *formal nursing care plan* is a written or computerised guide (e.g. Functional analysis in the care environment) (FACE) (Mental Health)) that organises information about the patient's care. The most obvious benefit of a formal written care plan is that it provides for continuity of care.

A *standardised care plan* is a formal plan that specifies the nursing care for groups of patients with common needs (e.g. all patients with myocardial infarction). An individualised care plan is tailored to meet the unique needs of a specific patient – needs that are not addressed by the standardised plan. It is important that all caregivers work towards the same outcomes and, if available, use approaches shown to be effective with a particular patient. Nurses also use the formal care plan for direction about what needs to be documented in patient progress notes and as a guide for delegating and assigning staff to care for patients. When nurses use the patient's nursing diagnoses to develop goals and nursing interventions, the result is a holistic, *individualised plan of care* that will meet the patient's unique needs.

Care plans include the actions nurses must take to address the patient's nursing diagnoses and produce the desired outcomes. The nurse begins the plan when the patient is admitted to the nursing care setting and constantly updates it throughout the patient's stay in response to changes in the patient's condition and evaluations of goal achievement. During the planning phase the nurse must (a) decide which of the patient's problems need individualised plans and which problems can be addressed by plans and routine care, and (b) write individualised desired outcomes and nursing goals for patient problems that require nursing attention beyond pre-planned, routine care.

The complete plan of care for a patient is made up of several different documents that (a) describe the routine care needed to meet basic needs (e.g. nutrition, hygiene such as bathing hair washing, etc.), (b) address the patient's nursing diagnoses and collaborative problems, and (c) specify nursing responsibilities in carrying out the medical plan of care (e.g. keeping the patient from eating or drinking before surgery; scheduling a laboratory test). A complete plan of care integrates dependent and independent nursing functions into a meaningful whole and provides a central source of patient information. Figure 10-8 illustrates the various documents that may be included in a nursing care plan.

Standardised Approaches to Care Planning

Most clinical environments have devised a variety of preprinted, standardised plans for providing essential nursing care to specified groups of patients who have certain needs in common (e.g. all patients with diabetes). Standards of care, standardised care plans, protocols, policies and procedures are developed and accepted by the nursing staff in order to (a) ensure that minimally acceptable standards are met and (b) promote efficient use of nurses' time by removing the need to author common activities that are done over and over for many of the patients on a nursing unit/ward.

Standards of care describe nursing actions for patients with similar medical conditions rather than individuals, and they describe achievable rather than ideal nursing care. They define the interventions for which nurses are held accountable; they do not contain medical interventions.

Standardised care plans are pre-printed guides for the nursing care of a patient who has a need that arises frequently in the clinical area (e.g. a specific nursing diagnosis or all nursing diagnoses associated with a particular medical condition). They are written from the perspective of what care the patient can expect. They should not be confused with standards of care; although the two have some similarities, they have important differences (see Figure 10-9 that shows a standardised care plan for *deficient fluid volume*). Standardised care plans:

- are kept with the patient's individualised care plan on the ward. When the patient is discharged, they become part of the permanent medical record;
- provide detailed interventions and contain additions or deletions from the standards of care;
- typically are written in the nursing process format:

  Problem ⇒ goals/desired outcomes ⇒ plan of care ⇒ Evaluation

- frequently include checklists, blank lines or empty spaces to allow the nurse to individualise goals and nursing interventions.

Like standards of care and standardised care plans, protocols/**care pathways** are pre-printed to indicate the actions commonly required for a particular group of patients. For example, the clinical environment may have a protocol for admitting a patient to the intensive care unit, for administering magnesium sulphate to a patient with pre-eclampsia or for caring for a patient receiving continuous epidural analgesia. Protocols may include both medical and nursing care and interventions.

Policies and procedures are developed to govern the handling of frequently occurring situations. For example, a hospital may have a policy specifying the number of visitors a patient may have. Some policies and procedures are similar to protocols

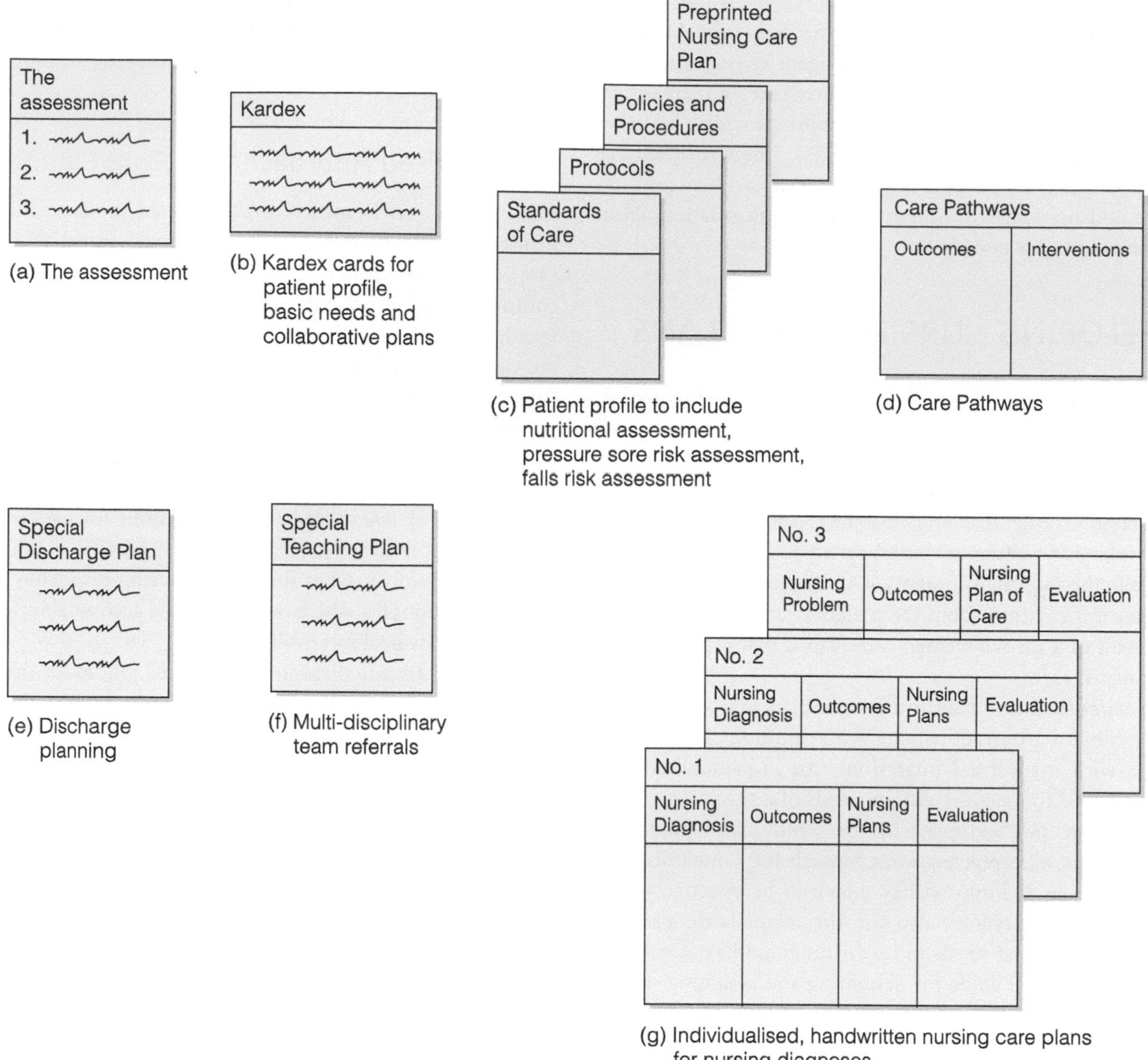

Figure 10-8 Documents that may be included in a complete patient care plan.
Source: Wilkinson, Judith M., *Nursing Process and Critical Thinking*, 3rd Edition, © 2001, pg 436. Reprinted by permission of Pearson Education, Inc, Upper Saddle River, NJ.

and specify what is to be done, for example, in the case of cardiac arrest. If a policy covers a situation pertinent to patient care, it is usually noted on the care plan (e.g. 'Make social service referral according to policy manual'). Policies are institutional records and do not become a part of the care plan or permanent record.

Regardless of whether care plans are handwritten, computerised or standardised, nursing care must be individualised to fit the unique needs of each patient. In practice, a care plan usually consists of both pre-printed and handwritten sections. The nurse uses standardised care plans for predictable, commonly occurring problems and handwrites an individual plan for unusual problems or problems needing special attention. For example, a standardised care plan for all 'patients with a medical diagnosis of pneumonia' would probably include a nursing diagnosis of *deficient fluid volume* and direct the nurse to assess the patient's hydration status.

Formats for Nursing Care Plans

Although formats differ from care setting to care setting, the care plan is often organised into four columns or categories: (a) nursing diagnoses, (b) goals/desired outcomes, (c) plan of care/nursing interventions and (d) evaluation. Some agencies use a three-column plan in which evaluation is done in the goals column or in the nurses' notes; others have a five-column plan that adds a column for assessment data preceding the nursing diagnosis column.

Aetiology	Desired Outcomes	Nursing Plan/Interventions (Identify Frequency)
✓Decreased oral intake	✓Urinary output > 30 ml/hr	✓Monitor intake and output q 1 h
✓Nausea	✓Urine specific gravity 1.005–1.025	✓Weigh daily
_Depression	✓Serum Na^+ normal	✓Monitor serum electrolyte levels X 1 or until normal
✓Fatigue, weakness	✓Mucous membranes moist	✓Check skin turgor and mucous membranes q 8 h
_Difficulty swallowing	✓Skin turgor good	✓Monitor temperature q 4 h
_Other:___	✓No weight loss	✓Administer prescribed IV therapy (Monitor according to protocol for Intravenous Therapy) 1000 ml D5 LR at 100 ml/hr
✓Excess fluid loss	✓8-hour intake = 400 ml oral	✓Offer oral liquids q 1 h Type clear, cold
✓Fever or increased metabolic rate	Other:	✓Instruct client regarding amount, type and schedule of fluid intake
✓Diaphoresis		✓Assess understanding of type of fluid loss; teach accordingly
✓Vomiting		✓Mouth care prn with mouthwash
_Diarrhoea		✓Institute measures to reduce fever (e.g. lower room temperature, remove bed covers, offer cold liquids)
_Burns		
_Other___		
Defining Characteristics		Other Nursing Orders: Monitor urine specific gravity q̄ shift
✓Insufficient intake		
✓Negative balance of intake and output		
✓Dry mucous membranes		
✓Poor skin turgor		
_Concentrated urine		
_Hypernatraemia		
✓Rapid, weak pulse		
_Falling B/P		
_Weight loss		

Plan initiated by: M. Medina RN **Date** 15-4-2011

Plan/outcomes evaluated___ **Date**___

Plan/outcomes evaluated___ **Date**___

Client: Joe Bloggs

Figure 10-9 A standardised care plan for the nursing diagnosis of Deficient Fluid Volume.

Computerised Care Plans

Computers are increasingly being used to create and store nursing care plans. The computer can generate both standardised and individualised care plans. Nurses access the patient's stored care plan from a centrally located terminal at the nurses' station or from terminals in patients' rooms. For an individualised plan the nurse chooses the appropriate diagnosis/problems from a menu suggested by the computer. The computer then lists possible goals and nursing interventions for those diagnoses/problems; the nurse chooses those appropriate for the patient and types in any additional goals and interventions or nursing actions not listed on the menu. The nurse can read the plan on the computer screen or print out an updated working copy.

Multidisciplinary (Collaborative) Care Plans/ Integrated Care Pathways

In 1994 England and Scotland explored the concept and benefits, etc. of ICPs and associations and groups were formed. In 1997 Integrated Care Pathways (ICP) were introduced in the UK following a visit to the US. They were also included in health legislation and the UK home countries then investigated further and developed their own strategy to implement ICPs into practice.

In Wales, for example, the Welsh Assembly Government has published a strategy that creates a world-class service for the 21st century (*Designed for life* in 2005) and central to this is the development of ICPs. A document, *Integrated care pathways: A guide to good practice* (2005) has been published by the National Leadership and Innovation Agency for Healthcare (NLIAH), an agency that works collaboratively with the National Health Service to improve services to patients ensuring that a world-class service is provided (see the web link at the end of the chapter).

In Scotland the Integrated Care Pathways Users Scotland (ICPUS) changed to the Scottish Pathways Association in May 2010 in order to develop and promote the work at a national level, following on from the publication of the *Quality improvement Scotland (QIS) standards for mental health ICPs* (see the web links at the end of the chapter).

A *multidisciplinary care plan* or *ICP* is a standardised plan that outlines the care required for patients with common, predictable – usually medical – conditions. Such plans are also referred to as *collaborative care plans*, or *critical or care pathways.* ICPs sequence the care that must be given on each day during the projected length of stay for the specific type of condition. Like the traditional nursing care plan, a multidisciplinary care plan can specify outcomes and nursing interventions to address patient problems (including nursing diagnosis/problems). However, it includes medical treatments to be performed by other healthcare providers as well.

The plan is usually organised with a column for each day, listing the interventions that should be carried out and the patient outcomes that should be achieved on that day. There are as many columns on the multidisciplinary care plan as the preset number of days allowed for the patients' diagnosis-related group (DRG). Multidisciplinary care plans do not include detailed nursing activities. They should be drawn from but do not replace standards of care and standardised care plans.

Guidelines for Writing Nursing Care Plans

The nurse should use the following guidelines when writing nursing care plans:

1 **Date and sign the plan.** The date the plan is written is essential for evaluation, review and future planning. The nurse's signature demonstrates accountability to the patient and to the nursing profession, since the effectiveness of nursing actions can be evaluated.
2 **Use category headings:** 'Plan of care' or 'Nursing Problems', 'Goals/Desired Outcomes', 'Nursing Interventions' and 'Evaluation'. Include a date for the evaluation of each goal.
3 **Use standardised medical or English terminology.** jargon and abbreviations should not be used. For example, write 'Turn and reposition the patient every two hours' rather than Turn and reposition 2h'. Or write 'Clean wound with normal saline twice a day, morning and evening' rather than 'Clean the patient's wound with n/s, bd am and pm'.
4 **Be specific.** Timing is very important when considering interventions so needs to be very clear.
5 **Be measurable.** For evaluation each intervention should be measurable. For example, if a patient has a wound it needs to be measured initially so that any reduction in size can be verified.
6 **Refer to procedure books or other sources of information rather than including all the steps on a written plan.** For example, write 'See unit procedure book for tracheostomy care,' or attach a standard nursing plan about such procedures as cardiac pacemaker care and pre-operative or post-operative care.
7 **Tailor the plan to the unique characteristics of the patient** by ensuring that the patient's choices, such as preferences about the times of care and the methods used, are included. This reinforces the patient's individuality and sense of control. For example, the written nursing intervention 'Please administer analgesia prior to wound dressing changes as per patient request' indicates that the patient's pain management was considered as were the individual needs of the patient.
8 **Ensure that the nursing plan incorporates health promotion in relation to primary, secondary and tertiary care.** For example, carrying out the intervention 'Provide limb exercises as prescribed by (physiotherapist) movements to lower limbs two hourly to prevent joint contractures and maintains muscle strength and joint mobility'.
9 **Ensure that the plan contains interventions for ongoing assessment of the patient** (e.g. assess cognitive behaviour of patient four hourly to identify any changes in behaviour).
10 **Include collaborative and coordination activities in the plan.** For example, the nurse may refer the patient to a dietician or physiotherapist for specific aspects of the patient's care.

11 **Include plans for the patient's discharge and home care needs.** It is often necessary to consult and make arrangements with the community nursing team, social worker and specific agencies that supply patient information and needed equipment. A complex discharge and transfer of care document may have to be completed.

THE PLANNING PROCESS

In the process of developing patient care plans, the nurse engages in the following activities:

- setting priorities;
- establishing patient goals/desired outcomes;
- selecting nursing interventions and activities;
- writing a nursing plan of care.

Setting Priorities

Priority setting is the process of establishing a preferential sequence for addressing the 'plan of care' or nursing interventions. The nurse and patient begin planning by deciding which aspect of care requires attention first, which second, and so on. Instead of rank-ordering care delivery, nurses can group them as having high, medium or low priority. Life-threatening problems, such as loss of respiratory or cardiac function, are designated as high priority. Health-threatening problems, such as acute illness and decreased coping ability, are assigned medium priority because they may result in delayed development or cause destructive physical or emotional changes. A low-priority problem is one that arises from normal developmental needs or that requires only minimal nursing support.

It is not necessary to resolve all high-priority nursing care provision before addressing others. The nurse may partially address a high-priority care requirement and then deal with a less acute care requirement. Furthermore, because patients usually have several problems, the nurse often deals with more than one requirement at a time.

Priorities change as the patient's responses, problems and therapies change. The nurse must consider a variety of factors when assigning priorities, including the following:

- **Patient's health values and beliefs:** Values concerning health may be more important to the nurse than to the patient. For example, a patient may believe being home for the children to be more urgent than a health problem. When there is such a difference of opinion, the patient and nurse should discuss it openly to resolve any conflict. However, in a life-threatening situation the nurse usually must take the initiative.
- **Patient's priorities:** Involving the patient in prioritising and care planning enhances cooperation. Sometimes, however, the patient's perception of what is important conflicts with the nurse's knowledge of potential problems or complications. For example, an elderly patient may not regard turning and repositioning in bed as important, preferring to be undisturbed. The nurse, however, aware of the potential complications of prolonged bed rest (e.g. muscle weakness and pressure sores), needs to inform the patient and carry out these necessary interventions.
- **Resources available to the nurse and patient:** Staffing, equipment or finances may be limited in a healthcare setting, then a problem may be given a lower priority than usual. Nurses in a home setting, for example, do not have the resources of a hospital. If the necessary resources are not available, the solution of that problem might need to be postponed, or the patient may need a referral. Patient resources, such as finances or coping ability, may also influence the setting of priorities. For example, a patient who is unemployed may defer dental treatment if not available via the NHS; a patient whose husband is terminally ill and dependent on her may feel unable to cope with nutritional guidance directed towards losing weight.
- **Urgency of the health problem:** Regardless of the framework used, life-threatening situations require that the nurse assign them high priority. Situations that affect the integrity of the patient, that is, those that could have a negative or destructive effect on the patient, also have high priority. Such health problems as drug abuse and radical alteration of self-concept due to amputation can be destructive both to the individual and to the family.
- **Medical treatment plan:** The priorities for treating health problems must be congruent with treatment by other health professionals. For example, a high priority for the patient might be to become mobile; however, if the medical treatment regimen calls for extended bed rest, then mobility must assume a lower priority in the nursing care plan. It is important to acknowledge that the nurse will defer teaching the patient mobility exercises in order to promote the overall well-being of the patient.

Establishing Patient Goals/Desired Outcomes

After establishing priorities, the nurse and patient set goals for each identified patient 'problem'. On a care plan the goals/desired outcomes describe, in terms of observable patient responses, what the nurse hopes to achieve by implementing the nursing interventions.

Some nursing literature differentiates the terms by defining goals as broad statements about the patient's status and desired outcomes as the more specific, observable criteria used to evaluate whether the goals have been met. For example:

Goal (broad)	Improved nutritional status.
Desired outcome (specific)	Gain 5kg by 25 April 2010.

When goals are stated broadly, as in this example, the care plan must include both goals and desired outcomes. They are sometimes combined into one statement linked as follows:

Improved nutritional status as evidenced by weight gain of 5kg by 25 April 2010.

Table 10-10 Deriving Desired Outcomes from Nursing Diagnoses

Nursing diagnosis/identified problem	Opposite healthy responses (goals)	Desired outcomes
Impaired physical mobility: inability to bear weight on left leg, related to inflammation of knee joint	Improved mobility Ability to bear weight on left leg	By end of the week walk to the end of the corridor. Stand without assistance by end of the month.
Ineffective airway clearance related to poor cough effort, secondary to incision pain and fear of damaging sutures	Effective airway clearance	No skin pallor or cyanosis by 12 hours post-operation. Within 24 hours after surgery, will demonstrate good cough effort.

Writing the broad, general goal first may help students to think of the specific outcomes that are needed, but the broad goal is just a starting point for planning. It is the specific, observable outcomes that must be written on the care plan and used to evaluate patient progress. Table 10-10 shows both broad goals and specific outcomes.

Purpose of Desired Outcomes/Goals

Desired outcomes/goals serve the following purposes:

- Provide direction for planning nursing interventions. Ideas for interventions come more easily if the desired outcomes state clearly and specifically what the nurse hopes to achieve.
- Serve as criteria for evaluating patient progress. Although developed in the planning step of the nursing process, desired outcomes serve as the criteria for judging the effectiveness of nursing interventions and patient progress at the evaluation stage.
- Enable the patient and nurse to determine when the problem has been resolved.
- Help motivate the patient and nurse by providing a sense of achievement. As goals are achieved, both patient and nurse can see that their efforts have been worthwhile. This provides motivation to continue following the plan, especially when difficult lifestyle changes need to be made.

BOX 10-4 Examples of Action Verbs

Apply	Assemble	Breathe	Choose	Compare
Define	Demonstrate	Describe	Differentiate	Discuss
Drink	Explain	Help	Identify	Inject
List	Move	Name	Prepare	Report
Select	Share	Sit	Sleep	State
Talk	Transfer	Turn	Verbalise	

Long-Term and Short-Term Goals

Goals may be short term or long term. A short-term goal might be 'Patient will raise right arm to shoulder height by Friday 25 April 2010.' In the same context, a long-term goal might be 'Patient will regain full use of right arm in six weeks.' Short-term goals are useful (a) for patients who require healthcare for a short time and (b) for those who are frustrated by long-term goals that seem difficult to attain and who need the satisfaction of achieving a short-term goal. In an acute care setting, much of the nurse's time is spent on the patient's immediate needs, so most goals are short term. However, patients in acute care settings also need long-term goals to guide planning for their discharge to their home or long-term care residence, especially in a managed care environment. Long-term goals are often used for patients who live at home and have chronic health problems and for patients in nursing homes, extended care facilities and rehabilitation centres.

Components of Goal/Desired Outcome Statements

Goal/desired outcome statements should usually have the following four components:

1. **Subject.** The subject – a noun – is the patient, any part of the patient or some attribute of the patient, such as the patient's pulse or urinary output. The subject is often omitted in goals; it is assumed that the subject is the patient unless indicated otherwise.
2. **Verb.** The verb specifies an action the patient is to perform, for example, what the patient is to do, learn or experience. Verbs that denote directly observable behaviours, such as *administer*, *show*, *walk*, must be used.
3. **Conditions or modifiers.** Conditions or modifiers may be added to the verb to explain the circumstances under which the behaviour is to be performed. They explain what, where, when or how. For example:
   - Walks with the help of a walking stick (how).
   - After attending two diabetic support group meetings, lists signs and symptoms of diabetes (when).
   - When at home, maintains weight at existing level (where).
   - Discusses food pyramid and recommended daily servings (what).

   Conditions need not be included if the criterion of performance clearly indicates what is expected.
4. **Criterion of desired performance.** The criterion indicates the standard by which a performance is evaluated or the level

Table 10-11 Components of Goals/Desired Outcomes

Subject	Verb	Conditions/modifiers	Criterion of desired performance
Patient	Drinks	2,500ml of fluid	daily (time)
Patient	Administers	correct insulin dose	using aseptic technique (quality standard)
Patient	Lists	three hazards of smoking (after reading literature)	(accuracy indicated by 'three hazards')
Patient	Recalls	five symptoms of diabetes before discharge	(accuracy indicated by 'five symptoms')
Patient	Walks	the length of the corridor without a walking stick	by date of discharge (time)
Patient	Measures	less than 10 inches in circumference	in 48 hours (time)
Patient	Performs	leg ROM exercises as taught	every 8 hours (time)
Patient	Identifies	foods high in salt from a prepared list	before discharge (time)
Patient	States	the purposes of his medications	before discharge (time)

at which the patient will perform the specified behaviour. These criteria may specify time or speed, accuracy, distance and quality. To establish a time-achievement criterion, the nurse needs to ask 'How long?' To establish an accuracy criterion, the nurse asks 'How well?' Similarly, the nurse asks 'How far?' and 'What is the expected standard?' to establish distance and quality criteria, respectively. Examples are:

- Weighs 75kg *by 2 June* (time).
- Lists *five out of six* signs of diabetes (accuracy).
- Walks to the local shop approximately *half a mile per day* (time and distance).
- Administers insulin *using aseptic technique* (quality).

Table 10-11 illustrates the format that should be used to write outcomes.

Guidelines for Writing Goals/Desired Outcomes

The following guidelines can help nurses write useful goals and desired outcomes:

- Write goals and outcomes in terms of patient responses, not nurse activities. Beginning each goal statement with *the patient* may help focus the goal on patient behaviours and responses. Avoid statements that start with *enable, facilitate, allow, let, permit* or similar verbs followed by the word *patient*. These verbs indicate what the nurse hopes to accomplish, not what the patient will do:
  - *Correct*: Patient will drink 100ml of water per hour (patient behaviour)
  - *Incorrect*: Maintain patient hydration (nursing action).
- Be sure that desired outcomes are realistic for the patient's capabilities, limitations and designated time span, if indicated. Limitations refer to finances, equipment, family support, social services, physical and mental condition and time. For example, the outcome 'Measures insulin accurately' may be unrealistic for a patient who has poor vision due to cataracts.
- Ensure that the goals and desired outcomes are compatible with the therapies of other professionals. For example, the outcome 'Will increase the time spent out of bed by 15 minutes each day' is not compatible with a doctor's prescribed therapy of bed rest.
- Make sure that each goal is derived from only one 'patient' health problem. For example, the goal 'The patient will increase the amount of nutrients ingested and show progress in the ability to feed self' is derived from two nursing diagnoses: *feeding self-care deficit* and *impaired nutrition: less than body requirements*. Keeping the goal statement related to only one diagnosis/problem facilitates evaluation of care by ensuring that planned nursing interventions are clearly related to the problem identified.
- Use observable, measurable terms for outcomes. Avoid words that are vague and require interpretation or judgement by the observer. For example, phrases such as *increase daily exercise* and *improve knowledge of nutrition* can mean different things to different people. If used in outcomes, these phrases can lead to disagreements about whether the outcome was met. These phrases may be suitable for a broad patient goal but are not sufficiently clear and specific to guide the nurse when evaluating patient responses.
- Make sure the patient considers the goals/desired outcomes important and values them. Some outcomes, such as those for problems related to self-esteem, parenting and communication, involve choices that are best made by the patient or in collaboration with the patient.

Some patients may know what they wish to accomplish with regard to their health problem; others may not know all the outcome possibilities. The nurse must actively listen to the patient to determine personal values, goals and desired outcomes in relation to current health concerns. Patients are usually motivated and expend the necessary energy to reach goals they consider important.

Selecting Nursing Interventions and Activities

Nursing interventions and activities are the actions that a nurse performs to achieve patient goals. The specific interventions chosen should focus on eliminating or reducing the aetiology of the nursing diagnosis/identified patient problem, which is the second clause of the diagnostic statement.

Types of Nursing Interventions

Nursing interventions are identified and written during the planning step of the nursing process; however, they are actually performed during the implementing step. Nursing interventions include both direct and indirect care, as well as nurse-initiated, medical-initiated and all members of the multidisciplinary team. Direct care is an intervention performed through interaction with the patient. Indirect care is an intervention performed away from but on behalf of the patient such as interdisciplinary collaboration or management of the care environment.

Independent interventions are those activities that nurses undertake on the basis of their knowledge and skills. They include physical care, ongoing assessment, emotional support and comfort, teaching, counselling, environmental management and making referrals to other healthcare professionals. McCloskey and Bulechek (2008) refer to these as *nurse-initiated treatments.* In performing an autonomous activity, the nurse determines that the patient requires certain nursing interventions; either carries these out or delegates them to other nursing personnel, and is accountable or answerable for the decision and the actions. An example of an independent action is planning and providing special mouth care for a patient after diagnosing/identifying *impaired oral mucous membranes.*

Dependent interventions are activities carried out according to specified routines. McCloskey and Bulechek (2008) call these *consultant-initiated treatments.* Consultant/doctor treatment commonly includes prescribed medications, intravenous therapy, diagnostic tests, treatments, diet and activity. The nurse is responsible for explaining, assessing the need for and administering the medical interventions. Nursing interventions may be written to individualise the medical treatment based on the patient's status.

Collaborative interventions are actions the nurse carries out in collaboration with other members of the multidisciplinary team, such as physiotherapists, social workers, dietitians and doctors. Collaborative nursing activities reflect the overlapping responsibilities of, and collegial relationships between, health personnel. For example, the doctor might recommend physiotherapy to teach the patient walking with crutches. The nurse would be responsible for informing the physiotherapy department and for coordinating the patient's care to include the physiotherapy sessions. When the patient returns to the ward, the nurse would assist the patient with their mobility (crutches) and collaborate with the physiotherapist to evaluate the patient's progress.

The amount of time the nurse spends in an independent versus a collaborative or dependent role varies according to the clinical area, type of institution and specific position of the nurse.

Considering the Consequences of Each Intervention

Usually several possible interventions can be identified for each nursing goal. The nurse's role is to choose those that are most likely to achieve the desired patient outcomes. The nurse begins by considering the risks and benefits of each intervention. An intervention may have more than one consequence. For example, 'Provide accurate information' could result in the following patient behaviours:

- increased anxiety
- decreased anxiety
- wish to talk with the doctor
- desire to leave the hospital
- relaxation.

Determining the consequences of each intervention requires nursing knowledge and experience. For example, the nurse's experience may suggest that providing information the night before the patient's surgery may increase the patient's worry and tension, whereas maintaining the usual rituals before sleep is more effective. The nurse might then consider providing information several days before surgery.

Criteria for Choosing Nursing Interventions

After considering the consequences of the alternative nursing interventions, the nurse chooses the appropriate ones for that patient. Although the nurse bases this decision on knowledge and experience, the patient's input is important.

The following criteria can help the nurse choose the best nursing interventions. The plan must be:

- Safe and appropriate for the individual's age, health and condition.
- Achievable with the resources available. For example, a district or community nurse might wish to include in the plan of care for an elderly patient to 'Check blood glucose daily'; but in order for that to occur, the patient must have intact sight, cognition and memory to carry this out independently, identify a family member that is able and willing to take on the responsibility or receive daily visits from a district/community nurse.
- Congruent with the patient's values, beliefs and culture.
- Congruent with other therapies (e.g. if the patient is not permitted food, the strategy of an evening snack must be deferred until health permits).
- Based on current up-to-date knowledge and the knowledge and experience of the nurse including knowledge from relevant sciences (i.e. based on a rationale).
- Within established standards of care as determined by law, both national and local policies (government, local health boards or trusts) or by professional governing bodies (e.g. Nursing and Midwifery Council or National Leadership Innovation Agency for Healthcare (NLIAH)). Many agencies have policies to guide the activities of health professionals and to safeguard patients. Rules for maintaining a safe environment and with standards, guidelines and policies that guide infection control practice to all healthcare staff, patients, relatives and all others.

Writing a Nursing Plan of Care

After choosing the appropriate nursing care, the nurse writes them on the care plan. Nursing careplans are instructions for the specific individualised activities the nurse performs to help the patient meet established healthcare goals.

Date

Nursing care provided is recorded on the care plans and are dated when they are written and reviewed regularly at intervals that depend on the individual's needs. In an intensive care unit, for example, the plan of care will be continually monitored and revised. In a community clinic, weekly or bi-weekly reviews may be indicated.

Action Verb

The action verb starts the intervention and must be precise. For example, 'Explain (to the patient) the actions of insulin' is a more precise statement than 'Teach (the patient) about insulin.' 'Measure and record ankle circumference daily at 0900 hrs' is more precise than 'Assess oedema of left ankle daily.' Sometimes a modifier for the verb can make the nursing care more precise. For example, 'patient to be nil by mouth from 06.00am on Tuesday 21.12.10 prior to **bronchoscopy**' is more precise than 'patient to be kept nil by mouth prior to bronchoscopy'.

Content

The content is the what and the where of the intervention. In the preceding order, 'bronchoscopy (a medical intervention)' and 'nil by mouth' state the what and where of the intervention. The content area in this example may also clarify whether any pre-medication should be taken at 06.00hrs.

Time Element

The time element answers when, how long or how often the nursing care provided is to occur. As per the examples above 'Nil by Mouth from midnight on 3 June 2010.'

Signature

The signature of the nurse planning the intervention shows the nurse's accountability and has legal significance, lack of signature or documentation suggests that the care has not been delivered.

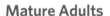

LIFESPAN CONSIDERATIONS

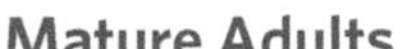

Mature Adults

When a patient receives extended care in a residential or nursing home, interventions and medications often remain the same day after day. It is important to review the care plan on a regular basis, because changes in the condition of the elderly may be subtle and go unnoticed. This applies to both changes of improvement or deterioration. Either one should receive attention so that appropriate revisions can be made in expected outcomes and interventions. Outcomes need to be realistic with consideration given to the patient's physical condition, emotional condition, support systems and mental status. Outcomes often have to be stated and expected to be completed in very small steps. For instance, a patient who has had a cerebrovascular accident may spend weeks learning to brush her own teeth or dress herself. When these small steps are successfully completed, it gives the patient a sense of accomplishment and motivation to continue working towards increasing self-care. This particular example also demonstrates the need to work collaboratively with other members of the multidisciplinary team, such as physiotherapists and occupational therapists, to develop the nursing care plan.

The nursing process is action oriented, patient focused and outcome directed. After developing a plan of care based on the assessing and diagnosing phases, the nurse implements the interventions and evaluates the desired outcomes. On the basis of this evaluation, the plan of care is either continued, modified or terminated. As in all phases of the nursing process, patients and support persons are encouraged to participate as much as possible.

IMPLEMENTING

In the nursing process, implementing is the phase in which the nurse implements the nursing interventions. Implementing consists of doing and documenting the activities that are the specific nursing actions needed to carry out the interventions. The nurse performs or delegates the nursing activities for the interventions that were developed in the planning step and then concludes the implementing step by recording nursing activities and the resulting patient responses.

Although the nurse may act on the patient's behalf (e.g. referring the patient to a district/community nurse for home care), professional standards support patient and family participation, as in all phases of the nursing process. The degree of participation depends on the patient's health status. For example, an unconscious man is unable to participate in his care and therefore needs to have care given to him. By contrast, a patient may require very little care from the nurse and carry out healthcare activities independently if they have good mobility.

Relationship of Implementing to Other Nursing Process Phases

The first three nursing process phases – assessing, diagnosing and planning – provide the basis for the nursing actions performed during the implementing step. In turn, the implementing phase provides the actual nursing activities and patient responses that are examined in the final phase, the evaluating phase. Using data acquired during assessment, the nurse can individualise the care given in the implementing phase, tailoring the interventions to fit a specific patient rather than applying them routinely to categories of patient (e.g. all patients with pneumonia).

While implementing nursing plans, the nurse continues to reassess the patient at every contact, gathering data about the patient's responses to the nursing activities and about any new problems that may develop. A nursing activity on the patient's care plan for *airway management* might read 'record four hourly respirations and oxygen saturation levels'. When performing this activity, the nurse is both carrying out the intervention (implementing) and performing an assessment.

Not every nursing action is directed by an intervention that follows from a nursing diagnosis/identified problem. Some routine nursing activities are, themselves, assessments. For example, all patient's require hygiene, nutrition and elimination. When assisting the patient with these, nurses carry out actions that may involve assessment. For example, while bathing an elderly patient, the nurse observes a reddened area on the patient's sacrum. Or, when emptying a urinary catheter bag, the nurse measures 200ml of strong-smelling, brown urine.

Implementing Skills

To implement the care plan successfully, nurses need cognitive, interpersonal and technical skills. These skills are distinct from one another; in practice, however, nurses use them in various combinations and with different emphasis, depending on the activity. For instance, when inserting a urinary catheter the nurse needs cognitive knowledge of the principles and steps of the procedure, interpersonal skills to inform and reassure the patient, and technical skill in draping the patient and manipulating the equipment.

The cognitive skills (intellectual skills) include problem solving, decision making, critical thinking and creativity. They are crucial to safe, intelligent nursing care. Interpersonal skills are all of the activities, verbal and nonverbal, people use when interacting directly with one another. The effectiveness of a nursing action often depends largely on the nurse's ability to communicate with others. The nurse uses therapeutic communication to understand the patient and in turn be understood. A nurse also needs to work effectively with others as a member of the healthcare team.

Interpersonal skills are necessary for all nursing activities: caring, comforting, advocating, referring, counselling and supporting are just a few. Interpersonal skills include conveying knowledge, attitudes, feelings, interest and appreciation of the patient's cultural values and lifestyle. Before nurses can be highly skilled in interpersonal relations, they must have self-awareness and sensitivity to others.

Technical skills are 'hands-on' skills such as manipulating equipment, giving injections and bandaging, moving, lifting and repositioning patients. These skills are also called tasks, procedures or **psychomotor** skills. The term *psychomotor* includes the interpersonal component, for example, the need to communicate with the patient.

Technical skills require knowledge and, frequently, manual dexterity. The number of technical skills expected of a nurse has greatly increased in recent years because of the increased use of technology, especially in acute care hospitals.

Process of Implementing

The process of implementing (see Figure 10-10) normally includes:

- reassessing the patient;
- determining the nurse's need for assistance;
- implementing the nursing interventions;
- supervising the delegated care;
- documenting nursing activities.

Reassessing the Patient

Just before implementing an intervention, the nurse must reassess the patient to make sure the intervention is still needed.

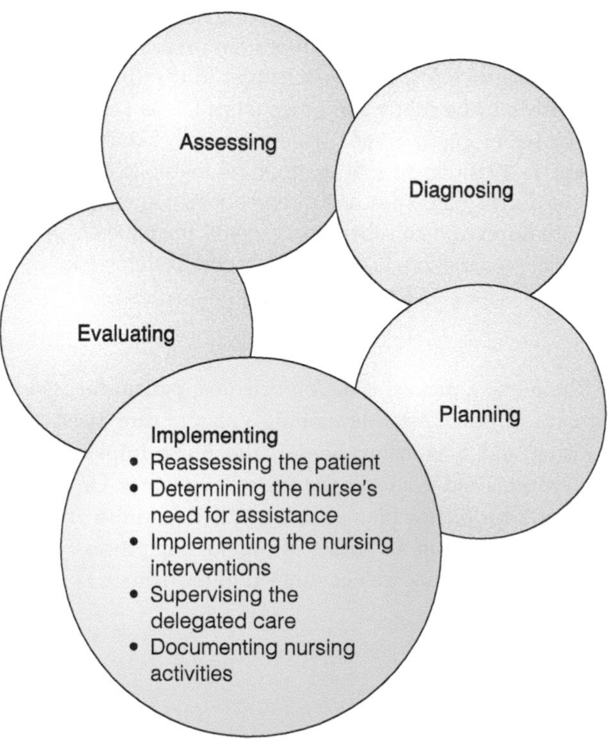

Figure 10-10 Implementing. The fourth phase of the nursing process, in which the nurse implements the nursing interventions and documents the care provided.

Even though an intervention is written on the care plan, the patient's condition may have changed. For example, John Jones has a nursing diagnosis of *disturbed sleep pattern* related to anxiety and unfamiliar surroundings. Overnight John has been observed and John has slept all night. This observation continues the following two nights with the same results, on reviewing the patient, the relaxation therapy planned for the following day has been cancelled.

New data may indicate a need to change the priorities of care or the nursing activities. For example, a nurse begins to teach Ms Webster, who has diabetes, how to give herself insulin injections. Shortly after beginning the teaching, the nurse realises that Ms Webster is not concentrating on the lesson. Subsequent discussion reveals that she is worried about her eyesight and fears she is going blind. Realising that the patient's level of stress is interfering with her learning, the nurse ends the lesson and makes arrangements for a doctor to examine the patient's eyes. The nurse also provides supportive communication to help alleviate the patient's stress.

Determining the Nurse's Need for Assistance

When implementing some nursing interventions, the nurse may require assistance for one of the following reasons:

- The nurse is unable to implement the nursing activity safely alone (e.g. when bathing an immobile patient who requires the use of a hoist).
- Assistance would reduce stress on the patient (e.g. turning a person who experiences acute pain when moved).
- The nurse lacks the knowledge or skills to implement a particular nursing activity (e.g. a nurse who is not familiar with a particular model of traction equipment needs assistance the first time it is applied).

Implementing the Nursing Interventions

It is important to explain to the patient what interventions will be done, what sensations to expect, what the patient is expected to do and what the expected outcome is. According to the Royal College of Nursing (2008) every NHS patient should have a guaranteed right to dignified care, supporting the report by the Healthcare Commission (2007) *Caring for Dignity – a national report on dignity in care for older people in hospital.* Dignity and privacy should always be maintained when interacting with a patient, for example by closing doors, pulling curtains or covering the patient. The number and kind of direct nursing interventions is almost unlimited. Nurses also coordinate patient care. This activity involves scheduling patient contacts with other departments (e.g. physiotherapists, occupational therapists, laboratory and radiographers) and serves as a liaison among the members of the multidisciplinary team.

When implementing interventions, nurses should follow these guidelines:

- Base nursing interventions on scientific knowledge, nursing research and professional standards of care (evidence-based practice) whenever possible. The nurse must be aware of the scientific rationale, as well as possible side-effects or complications, of all interventions. For example, a patient prefers to take an oral medication after meals; however, this medication is not absorbed well in the presence of food. Therefore, the nurse will need to explain why this preference cannot be honoured.
- Clearly understand the interventions to be implemented and question any that are not understood. The nurse is responsible for intelligent implementation of medical and nursing plans of care. This requires knowledge of each intervention, its purpose in the patient's plan of care, any contraindications (e.g. allergies) and changes in the patient's condition that may affect the care provided.
- Adapt activities to the individual patient. A patient's beliefs, values, age, health status and environment are factors that can affect the success of a nursing action. For example, the nurse determines that a patient chokes when swallowing pills, so consults with the doctor and pharmacist to change the prescription to a liquid form of the medication.
- Implement safe care. For example, when changing a sterile dressing, the nurse practises an aseptic technique to prevent infection; when giving a medication, the nurse administers the medication considering the 5 Rs: Right patient, Right route, Right dose, Right time and frequency and the Right Drug.
- Provide teaching, support and comfort. These independent nursing activities enhance the effectiveness of nursing care plans.
- Be holistic. The nurse must always view the patient as a whole and consider the patient's responses in that context.
- Respect the dignity of the patient and enhance the patient's self-esteem. Providing privacy and encouraging patients to make their own decisions are ways of respecting dignity and enhancing self-esteem.
- Encourage patients to participate actively in implementing the nursing interventions. Active participation enhances the patient's sense of independence and control. However, patients vary in the degree of participation they desire. Some want total involvement in their care, whereas others prefer little involvement. The amount of desired involvement may be related to the severity of the illness; the patient's culture; or the patient's fear, understanding of the illness and understanding of the intervention.

Supervising Delegated Care

Delegation of care to healthcare support workers or assistants, for example, is common practice but the nurse responsible for the patient's overall care must ensure that the activities have been implemented according to the care plan. Other caregivers may be required to communicate their activities to the nurse by documenting them on the patient record, reporting verbally or filling out a written form. The nurse validates and responds to any adverse findings or patient responses. This may involve modifying the nursing care plan.

Documenting Nursing Activities

After carrying out the nursing activities, the nurse completes the implementing phase by recording the interventions and patient responses in the nursing progress notes. These are a part of the permanent record for the patient.

Record keeping: Guidance for nurses and midwives (NMC, 2009a) states that:

> *Good record keeping, whether at an individual, team or organisational level, has many important functions. These include a range of clinical, administrative and educational uses such as:*
>
> - *helping to improve accountability*
> - *showing how decisions related to patient care were made*
> - *supporting the delivery of services*
> - *supporting effective clinical judgements and decisions*
> - *supporting patient care and communications*
> - *making continuity of care easier*
> - *providing documentary evidence of services delivered*
> - *promoting better communication and sharing of information between members of the multi-professional healthcare team*
> - *helping to identify risks, and enabling early detection of complications*
> - *supporting clinical audit, research, allocation of resources and performance planning, and*
> - *helping to address complaints or legal processes.*

The publication also informs nurses and midwives on the principles of good record keeping including, for example, confidentiality, accessibility, types of records and many others.

According to the NMC (2009a), the Data Protection Act 1998 defines a health record as 'consisting of information about the physical or mental health or condition of an identifiable individual made by or on behalf of a health professional in connection with the care of that individual'.

Nursing care must not be recorded in advance because the nurse may determine on reassessment of the patient that the intervention should not or cannot be implemented. For example, a nurse is authorised to inject 10mg of morphine sulphate subcutaneously to a patient, but the nurse finds that the patient's respiratory rate is 4 breaths per minute. This finding contraindicates the administration of morphine (a respiratory depressant). The nurse withholds the morphine and reports the patient's respiratory rate to the nurse in charge and doctor.

The nurse may record routine or recurring activities (e.g. mouth care) in the patient record at the end of a shift. In some instances, it is important to record a nursing intervention immediately after it is implemented. This is particularly true of the administration of medications and treatments because recorded data about a patient must be up to date, accurate and available to other nurses and healthcare professionals. Immediate recording helps safeguard the patient, for example, from receiving a duplicate dose of medication.

Nursing activities are communicated verbally as well as in writing. When a patient's health is changing rapidly, the charge nurse and/or the doctor may want to be kept up to date with verbal reports. Nurses also report patient status at a change of shift (handover) and on a patient's discharge to another area or home in person, via a voice recording or in writing.

EVALUATING

To evaluate is to judge or to appraise. Evaluating is the fifth and last phase of the nursing process. In this context, evaluating is a planned, ongoing, purposeful activity in which patients and healthcare professionals determine (a) the patient's progress toward achievement of goals/outcomes and (b) the effectiveness of the nursing care plan. Evaluation is an important aspect of the nursing process because conclusions drawn from the evaluation determine whether the nursing interventions should be terminated, continued or changed.

Evaluation is continuous. Evaluation undertaken during or immediately after implementing a nursing intervention enables the nurse to make on-the-spot modifications in an intervention. Evaluation performed at specified intervals (as appropriate to the individuals needs) shows the extent of progress towards goal achievement and enables the nurse to correct any deficiencies and modify the care plan as needed. Evaluation continues until the patient achieves the health goals or is discharged from nursing care. Evaluation at discharge includes the status of goal achievement and the patient's self-care abilities with regard to follow-up care. Most organisations have a special discharge record for this evaluation.

Through evaluating, nurses demonstrate responsibility and accountability for their actions, indicate interest in the results of the nursing activities and demonstrate a desire not to perpetuate ineffective actions but to adopt more effective ones.

Relationship of Evaluating to Other Nursing Process Phases

Successful evaluation depends on the effectiveness of the steps that precede it. Assessment data must be accurate and complete so that the nurse can formulate appropriate nursing interventions and desired outcomes. The desired outcomes must be stated concretely in behavioural terms if they are to be useful for evaluating patient responses. And finally, without the implementing phase in which the plan is put into action, there would be nothing to evaluate.

The evaluating and assessing phases overlap. As previously stated, assessment (data collection) is ongoing and continuous at every patient contact. However, data are collected for different purposes at different points in the nursing process. During the assessment phase the nurse collects data for the purpose of making diagnoses. During the evaluation step the nurse collects data for the purpose of comparing it to pre-selected goals and judging the effectiveness of the nursing care. The act of assessing (data collection) is the same; the differences lie in (a) when the data are collected and (b) how the data are used.

Process of Evaluating Patient Responses

Prior to evaluation, the nurse identifies the desired outcomes (indicators) that will be used to measure patient goal achievement. (This is done in the planning step.) Desired outcomes

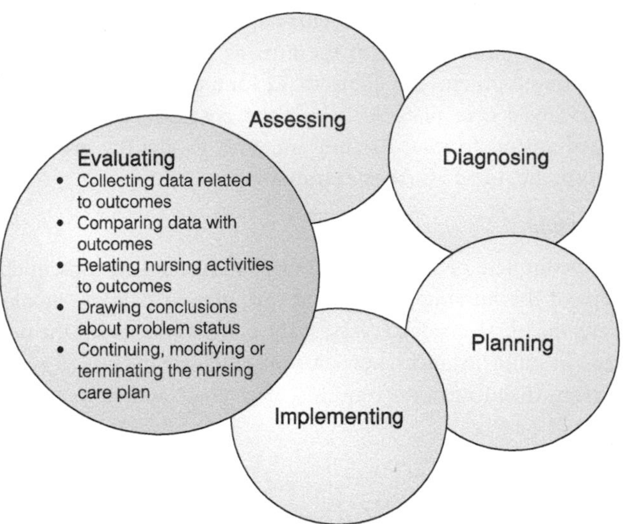

Figure 10-11 Evaluating. The final phase of the nursing process, in which the nurse determines the patient's progress towards goal achievement and the effectiveness of the nursing care plan. The plan may be continued, modified or terminated.

serve two purposes: they establish the kind of evaluative data that need to be collected and provide a standard against which the data are judged. For example, given the following expected outcomes, any nurse caring for the patient would know what data to collect:

- Daily fluid intake will not be less than 2,500ml.
- Urinary output will balance with fluid intake.
- **Residual urine** will be less than 100ml.

The evaluation process has five components (see Figure 10-11):

1 Collecting data related to the desired outcomes.
2 Comparing the data with outcomes.
3 Relating nursing activities to outcomes.
4 Drawing conclusions about problem status.
5 Continuing, modifying or discontinuing the nursing care plan.

Collecting Data

Using the clearly stated, precise and measurable desired outcomes as a guide, the nurse collects data so that conclusions can be drawn about whether goals have been met. It is usually necessary to collect both objective and subjective data.

Some data may require interpretation. An example of objective data requiring interpretation is the degree of tissue damage of a dehydrated patient or the degree of restlessness of a patient with pain. When objective data need interpretation, the nurse may obtain the views of other nurses to substantiate whether change has occurred. Examples of subjective data needing interpretation include complaints of nausea or pain by the patient. When interpreting subjective data, the nurse must rely upon either (a) the patient's statements (e.g. 'My pain is worse now than it was after breakfast') or (b) objective indicators of the subjective data, even though these indicators may require further interpretation (e.g. decreased restlessness, decreased pulse and respiratory rates, and relaxed facial muscles as indicators of pain relief). Data must be recorded concisely and accurately to facilitate the next part of the evaluating process.

Comparing the Data with Outcomes

If the first two parts of the evaluation process have been carried out effectively, it is relatively simple to determine whether a desired outcome has been met. Both the nurse and patient play an active role in comparing the patient's actual responses with the desired outcomes. Did the patient drink 3 litres of fluid in 24 hours? Did the patient walk unassisted the specified distance per day? When determining whether a goal has been achieved, the nurse can draw one of three possible conclusions:

- The goal was achieved; that is, the patient response is the same as the desired outcome.
- The goal was partially achieved; that is, either a short-term goal was achieved but the long-term goal was not, or the desired outcome was only partially attained.
- The goal was not achieved.

After determining whether a goal has been achieved, the nurse writes an evaluative statement on the care plan. An evaluation statement consists of two parts: a conclusion and supporting data. The conclusion is a statement that the goal/desired outcome was achieved, partially achieved or not achieved. The supporting data are the list of patient responses that support the conclusion, for example:

> Goal met: Oral intake 300ml more than output; skin integrity good; mucous membranes moist.

Relating Nursing Activities to Outcomes

The fourth aspect of the evaluating process is determining whether the nursing activities had any relation to the outcomes. It should never be assumed that a nursing activity was the cause of or the only factor in meeting, partially meeting or not meeting a goal. For example, Mr Alan Jones was a smoker who recently had suffered a myocardial infarction; as a smoker he recognised that he needed to give up smoking. When the nurse and patient drew up a care plan, one goal was 'for the patient to give up smoking by the end of the month'. A nursing strategy in the care plan was: 'To provide Mr Jones with all the information required to help Mr Jones give up smoking. Discuss the options that were available to help Mr Jones give up smoking and allow Mr Jones time to ask any questions.' Mr Jones was provided with written information so that he could read and absorb the information in his own time. Explanations were given on how to access nicotine patches, hypnosis, acupuncture or any other method that was Mr Jones's preferred choice. A follow up appointment was made with Mr Jones for the end of the month in the Cardiology clinic to assess his well-being and to record how Mr Jones was progressing with his smoking cessation. It was identified at the follow up appointment that Mr Jones had not smoked for over three weeks. While the nurse had provided all the information the actual activity was carried out by Mr Jones.

If the first possibility is found to be true, the nurse can safely judge that the nursing strategy 'Discuss and explain . . .' was effective in helping the patient give up smoking. The next step for the nurse is to collect data about what the patient actually did to give up smoking. It is important to establish the relationship (or lack thereof) of the nursing actions to the patient responses.

Drawing Conclusions about Problem Status

The nurse uses the judgements about goal achievement to determine whether the care plan was effective in resolving, reducing or preventing patient problems. When goals have been achieved the nurse can draw one of the following conclusions about the status of the patient's problem:

- The actual problem stated in the nursing diagnosis/goal has been resolved; or the potential problem is being prevented and the risk factors no longer exist. In these instances, the nurse documents that the goals have been achieved and discontinues the care for the problem.
- The potential problem stated in the nursing diagnosis/goal is being prevented, but the risk factors are still present. In this case, the nurse keeps the problem on the care plan.
- The actual problem still exists even though some goals are being met. For example, a desired outcome on a patient's care plan is 'Will drink 3 litres of fluid daily.' Even though the data may show this outcome has been achieved, other data (dry oral mucous membranes) may indicate that there is *deficient fluid volume*. Therefore, the nursing interventions must be continued even though this one goal was achieved, the problem has not been resolved.

When goals have been partially achieved or when goals have not been achieved, two conclusions may be drawn:

1 The care plan may need to be revised, since the problem is only partially resolved. The revisions may need to occur during assessing, diagnosing or planning phases, as well as implementing.
OR
2 The care plan does not need revision, because the patient merely needs more time to achieve the previously established goal(s). To make this decision, the nurse must assess why the goals are being only partially achieved, including whether the evaluation was conducted too soon.

Continuing, Modifying or Discontinuing the Nursing Care Plan

After drawing conclusions about the status of the patient's problems, the nurse modifies the care plan as indicated. Depending on local policy, modifications may be made by drawing a line through portions of the care plan, or marking portions using a highlighting pen, or writing 'Discontinued' and the date.

Whether or not goals were achieved, a number of decisions need to be made about continuing, modifying or discontinuing nursing care for each problem. Before making individual modifications, the nurse must first determine why the plan as a whole was not completely effective. This requires a review of the entire care plan and a critique of the nursing process steps involved in its development. See Table 10-12 for a checklist to use when reviewing a care plan. Although the checklist uses a closed-ended yes/no format, its only intent is to identify areas that require the nurse's further examination.

Assessing

An incomplete or incorrect database influences all subsequent steps of the nursing process and care plan. If data are incomplete, the nurse needs to reassess the patient and record the new data. In some instances, new data may indicate the need for new nursing diagnoses/interventions, new goals and new nursing plans of care.

Diagnosing

If the database is incomplete, new diagnostic statements/interventions may be required. If the database is complete, the nurse needs to analyse whether the problems were identified correctly and whether the nursing diagnoses are relevant to that database. After making judgements about problem status, the nurse revises or adds new diagnoses as needed to reflect the most recent patient data.

Planning: desired outcomes

If a nursing diagnosis is inaccurate, obviously the goal statement will need revision. If the nursing diagnosis is appropriate, the nurse then checks that the goals are realistic and attainable. Unrealistic goals require correction. The nurse should also determine whether priorities have changed and whether the patient still agrees with the priorities. Goals must also be written for any new nursing diagnoses.

Planning: nursing plan of care

The nurse investigates whether the plan of care was related to goal achievement and whether the best clinical decisions were made. Even when diagnoses and goals are appropriate, the nursing care selected may not have been the best ones to achieve the goal. The revised plan of care may reflect changes in the amount of nursing care the patient needs, scheduling changes, or rearrangement of nursing activities to group similar activities or to permit longer rest or activity periods for the patient. If new nursing diagnoses have been written, then new plans of care will also be necessary.

Implementing

Even if all sections of the care plan appear to be satisfactory, the manner in which the plan was implemented may have interfered with goal achievement. Before selecting new interventions, the nurse should check whether the nursing interventions were carried out. Other personnel may not have carried them out, either because the details were unclear or because they were unreasonable in terms of external constraints such as resources, staff and equipment.

After making the necessary modifications to the care plan, the nurse implements the modified plan and begins the nursing process cycle again.

Table 10-12 Evaluation Checklist

Assessing	Diagnosing	Planning	Implementing
____ Are data complete, accurate and validated? ____ Do new data require changes in the care plan?	____ Are nursing diagnoses relevant and accurate? ____ Are nursing diagnoses supported by the data? ____ Has problem status changed (i.e. potential, actual, risk)? ____ Are the diagnoses stated clearly and in correct format? ____ Have any nursing diagnoses been resolved?	**Desired outcomes** ____ Do new nursing diagnoses require new goals? ____ Are goals realistic? ____ Was enough time allowed for goal achievement? ____ Do the goals address all aspects of the problem? ____ Have patient priorities changed? **Nursing Plan of Care** ____ Do nursing care plans need to be written for new nursing diagnoses or new goals? ____ Does the plan of care relate to the stated goals? ____ Is there a rationale to justify each nursing instruction? ____ Are the care plans clear, specific and detailed? ____ Are new resources available? ____ Do the care plans address all aspects of the patient's goals? ____ Were the nursing orders actually carried out?	____ Was patient input obtained at each step of the nursing process? ____ Were goals and nursing interventions acceptable to the patient? ____ Did the caregivers have the knowledge and skill to perform the interventions correctly? ____ Were explanations given to the patient prior to implementing?

FUNDAMENTAL KEY SKILLS REQUIRED IN THE NURSING PROCESS

There are many skills that are fundamental to the effectiveness of the nursing process and ultimately in providing quality care to the patient examples of these are:

- critical thinking
- problem solving
- clinical judgement/decision making
- trial and error
- self-awareness/self-assessment
- reflection
- interpersonal skills
- collaboration/team working
- intuition/tacit knowledge.

Integral to the nursing process is critical thinking (see Figure 10-12).

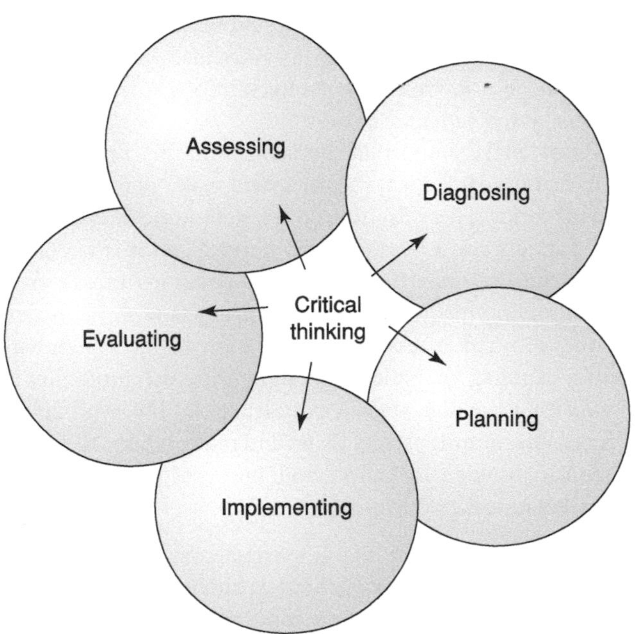

Figure 10-12 The five overlapping phases of the nursing process. Each phase depends on the accuracy of the preceding phase. Each phase involves critical thinking.

Critical Thinking

One key aspect of nursing is that nurses need to have a clear, logical and disciplined process to make appropriate decisions in the clinical environment. Bandman and Bandman (1995) define critical thinking as the 'rational examination of ideas, inferences, assumptions, principles, arguments, conclusions, issues, statements, beliefs and actions'. While Johnson and Webber (2010) state that critical thinking is intrinsic to the nursing process, problem solving, **critical analysis**, clinical judgement and reflection.

As previously noted the nursing process provides structure to collecting information from the patient, relatives or carers, but it is fundamental that the nurse gathering the information adopts a critical mind to assess, diagnose, plan, implement and evaluate the information provided. Thus, the information gathered from the individual is collaborated with the current evidence base, and national and local policies and guidelines to direct best patient care.

Nurses use critical-thinking skills in a variety of ways:

- Nurses use knowledge from other subjects and fields. Because nurses deal holistically with human responses, they must draw meaningful information from other subject areas (i.e. make interdisciplinary connections) in order to understand the meaning of patient data and to plan effective interventions. Nursing students take courses in the biological and social sciences and in the humanities so that they can acquire a strong foundation on which to build their nursing knowledge and skill. For example, the nurse might use knowledge from nutrition, physiology and physics to promote wound healing and prevent further injury to a patient with a pressure ulcer.
- Nurses deal with changes in stressful environments; they work in rapidly changing situations. Treatments, medications and technology change constantly, and a patient's condition may change from minute to minute. Routine actions may therefore not be adequate to deal with the situation at hand. Familiarity with the routine for giving medications, for example, does not help the nurse deal with a patient who is frightened of injections or with one who does not wish to take a medication. When unexpected situations arise, critical thinking enables the nurse to recognise important cues, respond quickly and adapt interventions to meet specific needs of the patient.
- Nurses make important decisions. In this ever-constant changing environment the nurse will make vital decisions of many kinds. These decisions often determine the well-being of patients and even their very survival, so it is important that the decisions be sound. The decisions can be from withholding medication, as it contradicts with the patient condition, risk assessments in relation to the safe moving and handling of patients, dealing with the protection of vulnerable adults (POVA), violence in the work place, infection control, staffing issues and many others. Nurses use critical thinking to collect and interpret the information needed to make decisions.

Creativity/innovation is an important component of critical thinking. When nurses incorporate creativity into their thinking, they are able to find unique solutions to unique problems. Innovation is thinking that results in the development of new ideas and products. Innovation in problem solving and decision making is the ability to develop and implement new and better solutions.

Innovation is required when the nurse encounters a new situation or a patient situation in which traditional interventions are not effective. For example, Wendy, a child nurse, is caring for five-year-old James, who has ineffective chest expansion due to respiratory problems. The physiotherapist has suggested incentive spirometry (a treatment device that promotes alveolar expansion). James is frightened by the equipment and tires quickly during the treatments. Wendy offers James a bottle of blowing bubbles and James enjoys blowing the bubbles. Wendy knows that the respiratory effort in blowing bubbles will promote alveolar expansion and suggests that James blow bubbles between incentive spirometry treatments.

Innovative thinkers must have knowledge of the problem. They must have assessed the present problem and be knowledgeable about the underlying facts and principles that apply. For example, in the previous situation, Wendy knows the anatomy and physiology of respiratory function and is aware of the purpose of incentive spirometry. She also understands paediatric growth and development. In trying to assist James, she builds on her knowledge and comes up with an innovative solution. Using innovation, nurses:

- generate many ideas rapidly;
- are generally flexible and natural; that is, they are able to change viewpoints or directions in thinking rapidly and easily;
- create original solutions to problems;
- tend to be independent and self-confident, even when under pressure;
- demonstrate individuality.

Skills in Critical Thinking

Complex mental processes such as analysis, problem solving and decision making require the use of cognitive critical-thinking skills. These skills include critical analysis, inductive and deductive reasoning, making valid inferences, differentiating facts from opinions, evaluating the credibility of information sources, clarifying concepts and recognising assumptions.

Critical analysis is the application of a set of questions to a particular situation or idea to determine essential information and ideas and discard superfluous information and ideas. The questions are not sequential steps; rather, they are a set of criteria for judging an idea. Not all questions will need to be applied to every situation, but one should be aware of all the questions in order to choose those questions appropriate to a given situation. Socrates (born about 470 BC) was a Greek philosopher who developed the Socratic method of posing a question and seeking an answer. Socratic questioning is a technique one can use to look beneath the surface, recognise and examine assumptions, search for inconsistencies, examine multiple points of view and differentiate what one knows from what one merely believes. Nurses can employ Socratic questioning when listening to an end-of-shift report/handover, reviewing a presenting history or progress notes, planning care or discussing a patient's care with colleagues.

Socratic questions

- Questions about the question (or problem).
- Is this question clear, understandable and correctly identified?
- Is this question important?
- Could this question be broken down into smaller parts?
- How might a staff nurse state this question?

Table 10-13 Differentiating Types of Statements

Statement	Description	Example
Facts	Can be verified through investigation	Blood pressure is affected by blood volume.
Inferences	Conclusions drawn from the facts, going beyond facts to make a statement about something not currently known	If blood volume is decreased (e.g. in haemorrhagic shock), the blood pressure will drop.
Judgements	Evaluation of facts or information that reflect values or other criteria; a type of opinion	It is harmful to the patient's health if the blood pressure drops too low.
Opinions	Beliefs formed over time and include judgements that may fit facts or be in error	Nursing intervention can assist in maintaining the patient's blood pressure within normal limits.

Questions about assumptions

- You seem to be assuming . . . ; is that so?
- What could you assume instead? Why?
- Does this assumption always hold true?

Questions about point of view

- You seem to be using the perspective of . . . Why?
- What would someone who disagrees with your perspective say?
- Can you see this any other way?

Questions about evidence and reasons

- What evidence do you have for that?
- Is there any reason to doubt that evidence?
- How do you know?
- What would change your mind?

Questions about implications and consequences

- What effect would that have?
- What is the probability that will actually happen?
- What are the alternatives?
- What are the implications of that?

Two other critical thinking skills are inductive and deductive reasoning. In **inductive reasoning**, generalisations are formed from a set of facts or observations. When viewed together, certain bits of information suggest a particular interpretation. For example, the nurse who observes that a patient has dry skin, poor skin elasticity, sunken eyes and dark amber urine may make the generalisation that the patient appears dehydrated. **Deductive reasoning**, by contrast, is reasoning from the general to the specific. The nurse starts with a conceptual framework – for example, Maslow's hierarchy of needs or a self-care framework – and makes descriptive interpretations of the patient's condition in relation to that framework. For example, the nurse who uses the needs framework might categorise data and define the patient's problem in terms of elimination, nutrition or protection needs.

In a more simplistic example, inductive reasoning is like looking at the pieces of a jigsaw puzzle and attempting to describe the whole (without seeing a picture of the completed puzzle). As the puzzler puts more and more pieces together, the whole picture becomes clearer. In deductive reasoning, the puzzler sees the whole picture (from the box cover) and puts the puzzle together by organising the pieces into border pieces, colours or some other grouping.

In critical thinking, the nurse also differentiates statements of fact, inference, judgement and opinion. Table 10-13 shows how these may be applied to a patient. Evaluating the credibility of information sources is an important step in critical thinking. Unfortunately, we cannot always believe what we read or are told. The nurse may need to ascertain the accuracy of information by checking other documents, with other informants or making a valued judgement.

Concepts are ideas or views representing things in the real world and their meanings, such as very hot water can cause a burn. Each person has developed their conceptualisations based on experience, input from others, study and other activities. To clearly comprehend a patient situation, the nurse and the patient must agree on the meaning of concept terms. For example, if the patient says to the nurse, 'I think I have a tumour,' the nurse needs to clarify what this word means to the patient – the medical definition of tumour (a solid mass) or the common lay meaning of cancer – before responding.

Applying Critical Thinking to Nursing Practice

Nurses function effectively some part of every day without thinking critically. Many small decisions are based primarily on habit with minimal thinking involved; examples include selecting what clothes to wear for work, choosing which route to take to work and deciding what to eat for lunch. Psychomotor skills in nursing often involve minimal thinking, such as operating a familiar piece of equipment. But the higher order skills of critical thinking are put into play as soon as a new idea is encountered or a less-than-routine decision must be made.

Critical thinking and problem solving are key aspect of the nursing process in order to sustain and improve patient care.

Problem Solving

In **problem solving**, the nurse obtains information that clarifies the nature of the problem and suggests possible solutions. The nurse then carefully evaluates the possible solutions and chooses the best one to implement. The situation is carefully monitored over time to ensure its initial and continued effectiveness. The nurse does not discard the other solutions but holds them in reserve in the event that the first solution is not effective. The nurse may also encounter a similar problem in a different patient situation where an alternative solution is determined to be the most effective. Therefore, problem solving for one situation contributes to the nurse's body of knowledge for problem solving in similar situations.

There are various approaches to problem solving. Commonly used are evidence based, the research process, the scientific/modified scientific method, intuition and trial and error.

Evidence-Based Practice

Evidence-based practice is an approach to care that integrates nursing experience and intuition with valid and current clinical research evidence. Evidence-based practice is about combining research, clinical intuition and knowledge and skills to identify the best possible solution for effective care of a patient. Evidence-based practice is a systematic approach to making decisions when there are no available answers. It is also about making good judgements in applying research evidence to patient care.

Research Process and Scientific/Modified Scientific Method

The **research process** is a formalised, logical, systematic approach to solving problems. The classic scientific method is most useful when the researcher is working in a controlled situation (e.g. a laboratory). Health professionals, often working with people in uncontrolled situations, require a modified approach to the scientific method for solving problems. For example, unlike experiments with animals, the effects of diet on health are complicated by a person's race, lifestyle and personal preferences. The person is able to choose what they eat whereas an animal on the whole will eat what it is given.

Table 10-14 compares the research process or scientific method with the modified scientific method. Critical thinking is important in all problem-solving processes as the nurse evaluates all potential solutions to a given problem and makes a decision to select the most appropriate solution for that situation.

Table 10-14 Comparison between the Research Process and the Modified Scientific Method

Research process (scientific method)	Modified scientific method
State a research question or problem.	Define the problem.
Define the purpose of or the rationale for the study.	
Review related literature.	Gather information.
Formulate hypotheses and defining variables.	Analyse the information.
Select a method to test hypotheses.	Develop solutions.
Select a population, sample and setting.	
Conduct a pilot study.	Make a decision.
Collect the data.	Implement the decision.
Analyse the data.	Evaluate the decision.
Communicate conclusions and implications.	

Intuition/Tacit Knowledge

Intuition/tacit knowledge is the understanding or learning of things without the conscious use of reasoning. It is also known as sixth sense, hunch, instinct, feeling or suspicion. As a problem-solving approach, intuition is viewed by some people as a form of guessing and, as such, an inappropriate basis for nursing decisions. However, others view intuition as an essential and legitimate aspect of clinical judgement acquired through knowledge and experience. The nurse must first have the knowledge base necessary to practise in the clinical area and then use that knowledge in clinical practice. Clinical experience allows the nurse to recognise cues and patterns and begin to reach correct conclusions.

Experience is important in improving intuition because the rapidity of the judgement depends on the nurse having seen similar patient situations many times before. Sometimes nurses use the words 'I had a feeling' to describe the critical-thinking element of considering evidence. These nurses are able to judge quickly which evidence is most important and to act on that limited evidence. Nurses in critical care often pay closer attention than usual to a patient when they sense that the patient's condition could change suddenly.

Although the intuitive method of problem solving is gaining recognition as part of nursing practice, it is not recommended for novices or students, however, because they usually lack the knowledge base and clinical experience on which to make a valid judgement, which is acknowledged in Benner's (2001) work on novice to expert.

Trial and Error

One way to solve problems is through trial and error, in which a number of approaches are tried until a solution is found. However, without considering alternatives systematically, one cannot know why the solution works. Trial-and-error methods in nursing care can be dangerous because the patient might suffer harm if an approach is inappropriate. However, nurses often use trial and error in the home setting where, due to logistics, equipment and patient lifestyle, hospital procedures cannot work as effectively (e.g. there may be no electrical supply convenient to a patient's continuous home oxygen).

Clinical Judgements and Decision Making

According to the Royal College of Nursing (2003), Nursing is . . .

> *The use of clinical judgement in the provision of care to enable people to improve, maintain, or recover health, to cope with health*

problems, and to achieve the best possible quality of life, whatever their disease or disability, until death.

Nurses make judgements/decisions in the course of solving problems, for example, in each step of the nursing process. Decision making, however, is also used in situations that do not involve problem solving. Nurses make value decisions (e.g. to keep patient information confidential); time management decisions (e.g. will call in pharmacy on her return from taking a patient to theatre); scheduling decisions (e.g. to assist the patient with hygiene needs before visiting hours); and priority decisions (e.g. which patient should be seen to first: the terminally ill patient waiting for pain control or the patient that is showing a super ventricular tachycardia on his cardiac telemetry?).

Decision making is a critical-thinking process for choosing the best actions to meet a desired goal. When faced with several patient needs at the same time, the nurse must prioritise and decide which need to action first. The nurse may (a) look at advantages and disadvantages of each option, (b) apply Maslow's hierarchy of needs (see Chapter 2), (c) consider which interventions can be delegated to others or (d) use another priority-setting framework. When a patient is trying to make a decision about what course of treatment to follow, the nurse may need to provide information or resources the patient can use in making a decision. Nurses must make decisions in their own personal and professional lives. For example, the nurse must decide whether to work in a hospital or community setting, whether to join a professional association/union and whether to carry individual personal professional liability insurance.

There are sequential steps to the decision-making process:

1 **Identify the purpose.** The nurse identifies why a decision is needed and what needs to be determined.
2 **Set the criteria.** When the nurse sets the criteria for decision making, three questions must be answered: What is the desired outcome? What needs to be preserved? and What needs to be avoided? For example, for a patient with pain, the criteria would be as follows:
   - What needs to be achieved? Relief of pain.
   - What needs to be preserved? Physical functioning, cognitive functioning, psychological functioning, patient comfort.
   - What needs to be avoided? Central nervous system depression, respiratory depression, nausea.
3 **Weight the criteria.** In this step, the decision maker sets priorities or ranks activities or services in order of importance from least important to most important as they relate to the specific situation. Because the weighting is specific to the situation, an activity may be ranked as most important in one situation and of less importance in another situation. For example, if a patient with pain has terminal cancer, pain relief may be more important than avoiding the side effects of the pain medication.
4 **Seek alternatives.** The decision maker identifies all possible ways to meet the criteria. In clinical situations, the alternatives may be selected from a range of nursing interventions or patient care strategies. Pain may be treated with oral, sub cutaneous or intra muscular medications as needed, or on a schedule, or without pharmacological intervention at all, instead using complementary alternative modalities (CAM), such as relaxation or distraction therapies.
5 **Examine alternatives.** The nurse analyses the alternatives to ensure that there is an objective rationale in relation to the established criteria for choosing one strategy over another. For pain that results from a procedure (such as removal of a foreign object), CAM may not be strong enough relief and oral medication may be effective but act too slowly, it is important to assess and consider all types of pain relief which could be intravenous narcotics or inhaled analgesic (such as analgesic gas/entonox) which may be the better choice.
6 **Project.** The nurse applies creative thinking and scepticism to determine what might go wrong as a result of a decision and develops plans to prevent, minimise or overcome any problems. If the intravenous narcotic is selected, decide what safety procedures need to be in place, for example, a narcotic antidote and supplemental oxygen being available promptly.
7 **Implement.** The decision plan is placed into action. The pain treatment is begun.
8 **Evaluate the outcome.** As with all nursing care, in evaluating, the nurse determines the effectiveness of the plan and whether the initial purpose was achieved. How does the patient rate the level of pain following the procedure?

The decision-making process and the nursing process share similarities and the nurse uses decision making in all steps of the nursing process. Table 10-15 compares these processes.

Developing Critical-Thinking Attitudes and Skills

After gaining an idea of what it means to think critically, solve problems and make decisions, nurses need to become aware

Table 10-15 Comparison Between the Nursing Process and the Decision-Making Process

Nursing process	Decision-making process*
Assess	Identify the purpose
Diagnose	
Plan	Set the criteria Weight the criteria Seek alternatives Examine alternatives Project
Implement	Implement
Evaluate	Evaluate the outcome

*The decision making process parallels the nursing process but is also used during each step of the process.

of their own thinking style and abilities. Acquiring critical-thinking skills and a critical attitude then becomes a matter of practice. Critical thinking is not an 'either-or' phenomenon; people develop and use it more or less effectively along a continuum. Some people make better evaluations than others; some people believe information from nearly any source; and still others seldom believe anything without carefully evaluating the credibility of the information. Critical thinking is not easy. Solving problems and making decisions is risky. Sometimes the outcome is not what was desired. With effort, however, everyone can achieve some level of critical thinking to become an effective problem solver and decision maker.

Self-Awareness/Self-Assessment

Self-awareness is the ability to examine one's behaviour, psychologically and physically, in relation to one's self in order to develop one's understanding of others' behaviour, psychological and physical 'being', and make sense of it. The ability to self-assess and be self-aware enables the nurse to avoid discrimination and examine behaviour, psychology and physical issues fairly and honestly.

The nurse should reflect on some of the attitudes that facilitate critical thinking, attitudes such as curiosity, fair-mindedness, humility, courage and perseverance. A nurse might benefit from a rigorous personal assessment to determine which attitudes they already possess and which need to be cultivated. This could also be done with a partner, as a group and/or as part of a clinical supervision programme. The nurse first determines which attitudes are held strongly and form a base for thinking, and which are held minimally or not at all. The nurse also needs to reflect (using reflective models) on situations where he or she made decisions that were later regretted and analyses thinking processes and attitudes or asks a trusted colleague to assess them. This will aid in personal growth and the development of skills. Identifying weak or vulnerable skills and attitudes is also important.

Reflection

The concept of reflection is not new, it can be traced as far back as Socrates well over 2000 years ago and more recently Lewin (1947), Kolb (1984) and Rolfe *et al.* (2001). Reflection is a tool by which development and integration of theory into practice challenges the technical-rational ideology espoused by the scientific method of problem solving, deduction and reasoning (Schon, 1983). Reflection is a way of examining your practice; reflect on your practice to explore whether your practice could be changed to enhance patient care. As according to Moon (2004) reflection is

> *. . . a process whereby we reflect in order to learn something, or we learn as a result of reflecting. Reflection is about professional development, and best practice. Schon (1987), an educationalist, identified two types of reflection: reflection-on-action and reflection-in-action.*

Reflection-in-action is when a practitioner reflects during an incident regardless of whether the incident is positive or negative. Reflection-on-action is when the practitioner reflects after the incident and looks back on the incident and explores possible different ways of practice. McBrien (2007) states that reflective practice closes the theory practice gap, stimulates personal and professional growth and ultimately improves patient care. For example, a student nurse observes a doctor breaking bad news to a patient, and recognises that the patient hasn't fully understood what the doctor has said. On reflection the student will explore the incident again and identify ways of how such a situation could be improved or avoided should it happen again.

Interpersonal Skills

Interpersonal skills or communication, or people skills as they are sometimes called, are skills that are used when we interact with others. Interpersonal skills are essential to nursing when communicating with the patient, family and other members of the healthcare team. Interpersonal skills incorporate professional attitudes such as nonjudgemental attitudes, perceptions and values. Good interpersonal skills can be, for example, effective when dealing with an aggressive patient or relative, or patients with a cognitive disability (e.g. Alzheimer's disease) or with a child that is misbehaving.

Collaboration Team Working

Effective teamwork relies heavily on good communication. Team work is working in collaboration with the patient, relatives and all members of the multidisciplinary team towards the same goal. Team work relies heavily on good people skills and a commitment to team approach, each member of the team brings in different knowledge and experiences that makes sense of the whole. Ownership and mutual trust and respect are essential components of team work. For team work to be effective there is an element of risk taking and constructive criticism. For example, Mrs Eileen Jeffrey is an 86-year-old woman who was admitted following a cerebrovascular accident. Following admission Mrs Jeffrey was assessed as having difficulty swallowing and with very limited movement on her left side. Mrs Jeffrey lived with her husband who was very keen to take her home as soon as possible. In order for Mrs Jeffreys to have a safe, well planned and supported discharge referrals were made to the dietician, physiotherapist, occupational therapist, social worker and discharge liaison nurse, and working collaboratively an effective discharge was established.

Tolerating Dissonance and Ambiguity

The nurse needs to make deliberate efforts to cultivate critical-thinking attitudes. For example, to develop fair-mindedness, one could deliberately seek out information that is in opposition to one's own views; this provides practice in understanding and learning to be open to other viewpoints such as cultural beliefs, etc.

It is a human tendency to seek out information that corresponds to one's previously held beliefs and to ignore evidence that may contradict cherished ideas. This perspective is true for both the nurse and the patient. The older generation may have great difficulty accepting the pervasiveness of technology, or that people do not stay in hospital as long as they did in the late 20th century, or that having a diagnosis of cancer does not always mean that one is going to die. However, new technology provides every individual with opportunities to research information regarding treatment and conditions and lifetime experiences of managing their 'conditions' often suggests that the patient may know better than the healthcare provider what will work well and be acceptable to them. Examples of these could be 'folklore' or alternative health treatments that have not been fully evaluated by the scientific community. To improve clinical practice nurses should increase their tolerance for ideas that contradict previously held beliefs and should practise suspending judgement.

Suspending judgement means tolerating ambiguity for a time. If an issue is complex, it may not be resolved quickly or neatly, and judgement should be postponed. For a while, the nurse will need to say, 'I don't know' and be comfortable with that answer until more is known. Although postponing judgement may not be feasible in emergency situations where fast action is required, it is usually feasible in other situations.

Creating Environments that Support Critical Thinking

A nurse cannot develop or maintain critical-thinking attitudes in a vacuum. Nurses in leadership positions must be particularly aware of the climate for thinking that they establish, and they must actively create a stimulating environment that encourages differences of opinion and fair examination of ideas and options. In order to deliver culturally competent care nurses must embrace exploration of the perspectives of persons from different ages, cultures, religions, socioeconomic levels and family structures. As leaders, nurses should encourage colleagues to examine evidence carefully before they come to conclusions, and to avoid 'group think', the tendency to defer unthinkingly to the will of the group.

LIFESPAN CONSIDERATIONS

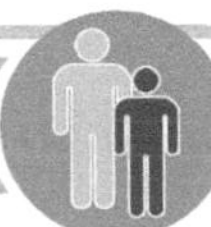

Longevity

While it is important to include patients in decision making and planning nursing care, it is especially difficult to do this when working with patients with impaired cognitive abilities, such as Alzheimer's disease. The goal should be to allow them to have as much control and input as possible, while keeping things simple and direct so they may be understood. Individuals with **thought disorders**, such as dementia, are usually unable to perform multiple tasks or even to think of more than one step at a time. Presenting and discussing issues at their level helps to maintain respect and dignity and allows them to participate in their own care for as long as possible. Multiple stimuli should be avoided when making decisions in this patient group, for example discussing care options during meal times which may lead to increased confusion and disorientation.

QUALITY OF NURSING CARE

Clinical governance is the system through which NHS organisations are accountable for continuously improving the quality of their services and safeguarding high standards of care, by creating an environment in which clinical excellence will flourish. Building on the document *A first class service: Quality in the new NHS* (DH, 1998) and the implementation of clinical governance in 1999/2000, further publications such as *Essence of Care: Benchmarks for promoting health* (DH, 2006) and *The Essence of Care: Patient-focused benchmarking for healthcare practitioners* (DH, 2003) demonstrate the importance that government place on healthcare and healthcare provision. The Essence of Care (EoC), first launched in 2001 and emerging from the 1999 nursing strategy 'Making a difference', formed the basis of a government strategy for improving the quality of care and has become an integral element of the clinical governance agenda.

According to the Department of Health (2001) in Northern Ireland: 'Essence of Care provides a structured and patient-centred approach to identifying best practice and setting standards for these fundamental aspects of care and highlights the importance of seeking patient and carer opinion. It acts as a tool for sharing and comparing practice, for developing action plans for improvement and audit, and for identifying education and training needs' (DH, 2001). *Essence of Care: Benchmarks for the fundamental aspects of care* (DH, 2010) provides a suite of benchmarks to drive forward best practice in delivering the fundamentals of care and improving the experience of people who use the services. Northern Ireland has developed further strategies in relation to quality and the well-being of healthcare provision documented in *A healthier future – a twenty-year vision for health and well-being in Northern Ireland 2005–2025* published by the Department of Health, Social Services and Public Safety (DHSSPS) in 2004.

The NHS Scotland Quality Strategy similarly emphasises the provision of 'high-quality, person-centred, clinically effective and safe healthcare services' (Scottish Government, 2010: 4) highlighting how these act as the key drivers for quality improvement.

The Strategy describes the priority areas for action and the improvement interventions required.

In Wales, building from *The Essence of Care* (2001) there have been key documents such as *Healthcare standards for Wales; making the connections designed for life* (2005) and the *Fundamentals of care* (2003), which describe healthcare as a commodity that is based on shared values. The latter document has been endorsed as it encompasses the whole range of health and social care settings throughout Wales and has included, for example, documents such as National Minimum Standards, National Service Frameworks, and National Institute of Clinical Excellence documents.

Occupational Standards and Professional Codes of Conduct

Nationally, the National Service Frameworks, NICE guidelines, and both national and local policies and guidelines ensure quality patient care. The British Thoracic Society, the Infection Prevention Society and the British Institute of Learning Disabilities are further examples of how quality is measured and improved within healthcare delivery.

EVALUATING NURSING CARE

In addition to delivering effective care, nurses are also involved in evaluating and modifying the overall quality of care given to groups of patients. Clinical governance is the 'umbrella' term for ensuring quality within the NHS and, for example, the Care Quality Commission is the independent regulator of health and social care in England. Throughout the UK evaluating nursing care is high on the agenda, and can be undertaken by, for example, nursing audit, peer review, patient surveys, benchmarking, etc.

Nursing Audit

An audit means the examination or review of records. A retrospective audit is the evaluation of a patient's record after discharge from a healthcare setting. A concurrent audit is the evaluation of a patient's healthcare while the patient is still receiving care within that environment. These evaluations use interviewing, direct observation of nursing care and review of clinical records to determine whether specific evaluative criteria have been met.

Peer Review

In nurse **peer review**, nurses functioning in the same capacity, that is as peers, appraise the quality of care or practice performed by other equally qualified nurses. The peer review is based on pre-established standards or criteria.

There are two types of peer reviews: individual and nursing audits. The individual peer review focuses on the performance of an individual nurse. The nursing audit focuses on evaluating nursing care through the review of records. The success of these audits depends on accurate documentation; auditors assume that if the data have not been recorded, the care has not been given.

Patient Surveys

User involvement is one of the key areas identified in clinical governance, therefore patient experiences are important tools in exploring how healthcare can be improved. The NHS Plan (2000) and the NHS Improvement Plan (2004) require each Trust in England to feed back on their experience of patient care. Patient surveys are one way of measuring the 'quality of care' experienced in healthcare whether as an in or out patient.

Benchmarking

Benchmarking is a process used to measure process and performance. It is a comparison method that is widely used. According to the Department of Health (2001) benchmarking enables practitioners to sit down and identify best practice, the changes necessary and deliver them. Benchmarking encourages team work and networking, and supports and guides innovative practice. Benchmarking is about getting the basics right and improving the patient experience.

CRITICAL REFLECTION

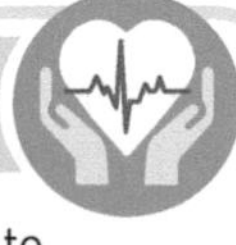

On reading this chapter you should be able to reflect and discuss the nursing process and a model of nursing when organising and planning the care of Ethel. Use the nursing process and the Roper, Logan and Tierney (RLT) model discussed in Chapter 9.

Maintaining a safe environment

- Ethel is confused (problem from assessment) due to possible urinary tract infection (diagnosis).
- Plan Ethel's care: to prevent her from any harm due to her confusion and for safe discharge, e.g. orientate her to time and place: reassure her at all times; talk to her in her preferred language; discuss with her any interventions, etc.
- Encourage fluids.
- Administer any prescribed medication (antibiotics).
- Discuss with Ethel and her daughter the possibility of referring Ethel to a social worker and occupational therapist.
- Refer to the discharge planning nurse.
- Implement the above plan of care.

Recheck - following the initial assessment, and results of tests (has the right diagnosis been made and is the plan of care appropriate?) and effective critical thinking (clinical judgement and decision making) should the current plan of care be continued?

Evaluate after 48 hours to assess whether Ethel's safety has been maintained and that a referral and plans for a safe discharge are in hand.

Communication

Ethel is confused and is aggressive due to possible urinary tract infection. The goal is to reduce confusion and aggression in 24 hours by good effective communication skills:

- Always introduce yourself to Ethel and approach her in a slow unhurried manner to alleviate any anxiety.
- Converse with Ethel in the tone, speed and language that is acceptable to her.
- Involve and include Ethel in any decision that is being considered or made for her care.
- Discuss and inform Ethel of the plan of care and fully consider the implications of her decision-making ability.

Maintain Ethel's dignity at all times by managing her care holistically.

Provide care for Ethel in a nonjudgemental manner and maintain respectability at all times.

Implement the above plan of care.

Recheck - evaluate after 24 hours to assess whether there is good, effective communication between the nurse and Ethel and that it has a positive influence on Ethel's care.

Eating and drinking

Ethel is reluctant to drink fluids due to her frequent visits to the bathroom. She needs to be encouraged to drink at least 2 litres of fluid in 24 hours:

- Discuss with Ethel the importance of drinking fluid.
- Provide Ethel with the fluids of her choice.
- Ensure that the temperature of the fluids are to Ethel's liking and tolerance.
- Record the amount taken on a fluid balance chart.
- Reassure Ethel that the fluid intake will aid her recovery.

Recheck - evaluate after 24 hours to assess whether Ethel has been able to drink 2 litres of fluid in the previous 24 hours.

Eliminating

Ethel visits the bathroom frequently to pass small amounts of urine. (During assessment it was noted that Ethel's normal pattern was 4-5 visits to the bathroom per day passing 'a pint jug full' of urine at each visit. For Ethel's normal pattern of eliminating to return to normal within four days of onset of antibiotic treatment:

- Save a midstream specimen of urine for culture and sensitivity and wait results.
- Reassure Ethel at all times that frequent visits to the bathroom are an important aspect of her treatment and not a 'bother' (possible patient perspective); maintain her dignity.
- Provide toilet facilities near to the Ethel.
- Depending on the results commence antibiotics as prescribed by a doctor.
- Monitor Ethel for any adverse side effects of antibiotics.
- Ensure that a call bell is within reach of Ethel so that she can call for the nurse when necessary.
- Ensure that hygiene needs are met.
- Implement the above care plan.

Recheck - evaluate that the amount of visits to the bathroom has been reduced and the volume of micturition has increased.

CHAPTER HIGHLIGHTS

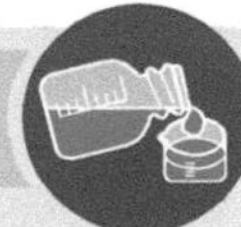

- The nursing process and the five stages incorporated within the nursing process were discussed.
- Good communication and interpersonal skills are fundamental to nursing care.
- When writing goals, time frames are very important to measure whether or not the goal has been achieved and assist in evaluation.
- Clear and appropriate goals, which are measurable and achievable to the patient, should be agreed.
- Critical thinking and decision making is fundamental to the nursing process and effective patient care.
- Audit is a valuable tool in the healthcare setting to evaluate standards of care and further develop the healthcare delivery system.
- Recognise that quality and assurance is an important aspect of healthcare provision.

ACTIVITY ANSWERS

ACTIVITY 10-1 The nursing process is a systematic, structured and methodical means of planning and providing nursing care. It aims to assess the patient holistically, physically, psychologically and socially in order to aid the nurse in making valid judgements and decisions through critical thinking to meet the needs of the individual and provide optimum care. The nursing process is cyclical, and the assessment process is ongoing and can be remodified at any time.

ACTIVITY 10-2 The nurse's role will follow the nursing process and a model of nursing in order to provide effective care to Mr Jones. However, the nurse will consider the issues in relation to Mr Jones's nonverbal communication and explore the possibility of Mr Jones not being able to climb the stairs to bed each night. The nurse will also explore the possibility that Mr Jones is unable to afford to heat the bedroom at night due to his financial situation. The nurse will then, following discussion with Mr Jones, refer Mr Jones to members of the multidisciplinary team. The doctor will follow the medical model and explore why Mr Jones has recurrent infections, and treat the symptoms.

REFERENCES

Alfaro-LeFevre, R. (2009) *Applying the nursing process: A step-by-step guide* (7th edn), Philadelphia/New York: Lippincott.

American Nurses Association (1998) *Standards of clinical nursing practice* (2nd edn), Kansas City, MO: Author.

Bandman, E. and Bandman, B. (1995) *Critical thinking in nursing* (2nd edn), Norwalk, Conn: Appleton and Lange.

Barrett, D., Wilson, B. and Woollands, A. (2008) *Care planning – a guide for nurses*, Harlow: Pearson Education.

Benner, P. (2001) *From novice to expert: Excellence and power in clinical nursing practice*, Menlo Park, CA: Addison-Wesley.

Carpenito, L.J. (2009) *Nursing diagnosis: Application to clinical practice* (13th edn), Philadelphia: Lippincott-Raven.

Commission for Healthcare Audit and Inspection (2007) *Caring for dignity – a national report on dignity in care for older people while in hospital.* London: Commission for Healthcare Audit and Inspection.

Department of Health (1998) *A first-class service: quality in the new NHS*, London: DH.

Department of Health (2000) *The NHS Plan: A plan for investment a plan for reform*, London: DH.

Department of Health (2001, 2003) *Essence of Care: Patient focused benchmarking for healthcare practitioners*, London: DH.

Department of Health (2004) *The NHS Improvement Plan: Putting people at the heart of public service*, London: DH.

Department of Health, Social Services and Public Safety (2004) *A healthier future: A twenty-year vision for health and well-being in Northern Ireland 2005–2025*, Northern Ireland: DHSSPS.

DH (2001) *The Essence of Care: Patient-focus benchmarking for healthcare practitioners*, Northern Ireland: DH.

DH (2010) *Essence of Care: Benchmarks for the fundamental aspects of care*, Northern Ireland: TSO.

Dougherty, L. and Lister, S. (2011) *The Royal Marsden Hospital manual of clinical nursing procedures* (7th edn), West Sussex: Wiley-Blackwell.

Gordon, M. (2002) *Manual of nursing diagnosis* (10th edn), St. Louis, MO: Mosby.

Hayes, S. and Llewellyn, Anne (2010) *The care process*, Exeter: Reflect Press.

Healthcare Commission (2007) *Caring for dignity*, London: Healthcare Commission.

International Council of Nurses (2010) *The nursing and social care interface.* Available from http://www.icn.ch/matters_nursing_social_care_interface.htm (Accessed on 05/02/2010.)

Johnson, D.E. (1959) 'A philosophy of nursing', *Nursing Outlook*, 7: 198–200.

Johnson, B.M. and Webber, P.B. (2010) *Introduction to theory and reasoning in nursing*, Philadelphia: Lippincott, Williams and Wilkins.

Joint Commission on Accreditation of Healthcare Organizations (2009) *Accreditation manual for hospitals*, available from http://www.jcrinc.com/Accreditation-Manuals/2010-Portable-Comprehensive-Accreditation-Manual-for-Hospitals-CAMH-The-Official-Handbook/1325/ (Accessed on 05/02/2009.)

Kolb, D.A. (1984) *Experiential learning experience as the source of learning and development*, New Jersey: Prentice Hall.

Lewin, K. (1947) 'Frontier in group dynamics: Social planning and action research', *Human Relations*, 1: 143–153.

McBrien, B. (2007) Learning from practice: Reflections from a critical incident', *Accident and Emergency Nursing*, 15(3): 128–133.

McCabe, C. and Timmins, F. (2006) *Communication skills for nursing practice*, Hampshire: Palgrave Macmillan.

McCloskey, J.C. and Bulechek, G.M. (eds) (2008) *Nursing interventions classification (NIC)* (5th edn), St. Louis, MO: Mosby.

Moon, J. (2004) 'Using effective learning to improve the impact of short courses and workshops', *Continuing Education in the Health Profession*, 24(1): 4–11.

NANDA International (2009) *NANDA nursing diagnoses: Definitions and classification 2009–2011*, Philadelphia: available from http://www.nanda.org/ (Accessed 05/02/2009.)

National Leadership and Innovation Agency for Healthcare (2005) Integrated care pathways: A guide to good practice, Llan. Wales: NLIAH.

Nigam, Y., Knight, J. and Jones, A. (2009) Effects of bedrest 3: Musculoskeletal and immune systems, skin and self perception, *Nursing Times*, 105(23): 18–22.

NMC (2008) *The NMC code of professional conduct: Standards for conduct, performance and ethics*, London: Nursing and Midwifery Council.

NMC (2009) *Guidance for the care of older people*, London: Nursing and Midwifery Council.

NMC (2009) *Record keeping: Guidance for nurses and midwives*, London: Nursing and Midwifery Council.

NMC (2010) *Standards for pre-registration nursing education*, London: NMC.

Orlando, I. (1961) *The dynamic nurse–patient relationship*, New York: Putnam.

Rolfe, G., Freshwater, D. and Jasper, M. (2001) *Critical reflection for nursing*, London: Palgrave.

Royal College of Nursing (2003) *Defining Nursing*, London: Royal College of Nursing.

Royal College of Nursing (2008) *Dignity at the heart of everything we do*, London: Royal College of Nursing.

Schon, D.A. (1983) *The reflective practitioner*, Basic Books, San Francisco: Harper Collins.

Schon, D.A. (1987) *Educating the reflective practitioner*, San Francisco: Jossey Bass.

Scottish Government (2010) *The healthcare quality strategy for NHS Scotland*, Edinburgh: NHS Scotland.

Welsh Assembly Government (2003) *Fundamentals of care*, Cardiff: WAG.

Welsh Assembly Government (2005) *Designed for life: Creating a world-class health and social care for wales in the 21st century*, Cardiff: WAG.

Welsh Assembly Government (2005) *Health care standards for wales*, Cardiff: WAG.

Wiedenbach, E. (1963) 'The helping art of nursing', *American Journal of Nursing*, 63(11): 54.

FURTHER RESOURCES

National Patient Safety Agency:
http://www.nrls.npsa.nhs.uk/resources/?EntryId45=59825

National Service Frameworks:
http://www.dh.gov.uk/en/Healthcare/index.htm

Electronic systems: http://www.connectingforhealth.nhs.uk/systemsandservices/data/snomed/snomed-ct.pdf

National Institute for Health and Clinical Excellence (NICE):
http://www.nice.org.uk

National Leadership and Innovation Agency for Healthcare (NLIAH): http://www.wales.nhs.uk/sitesplus/documents/829/integratedcarepathways.pdf

Integrated Care Pathways Users Scotland (ICPUS):
www.icpus.org.uk

Quality Improvement Scotland (QIS) Standards for Mental Health ICPs: www.icptoolkit.org

NMC: *Record keeping: Guidance for nurses and midwives* (2009a): http://www.nmc-uk.org/aDisplayDocument.aspx?DocumentID=6269

CHAPTER 11
PHYSICAL ASSESSMENT

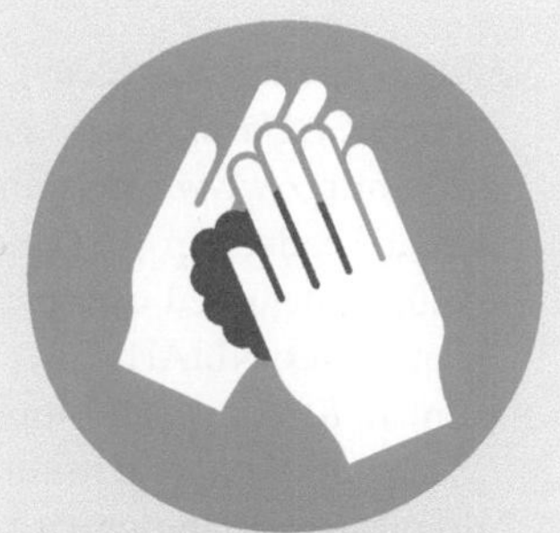

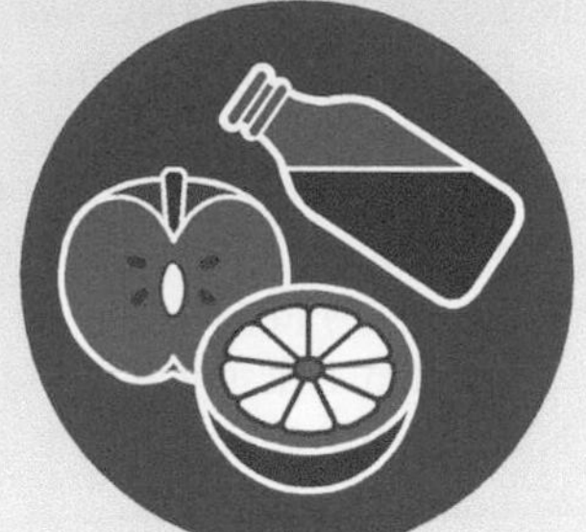

LEARNING OUTCOMES

After completing this chapter, you will be able to:

- Identify the purposes of the physical health examination.
- Explain the four methods of examining.
- Explain the significance of selected physical findings.
- Identify the steps in selected examination procedures.
- Describe suggested sequencing to conduct a physical health examination in an orderly fashion.
- Discuss variations in examination techniques appropriate for patients of different ages.

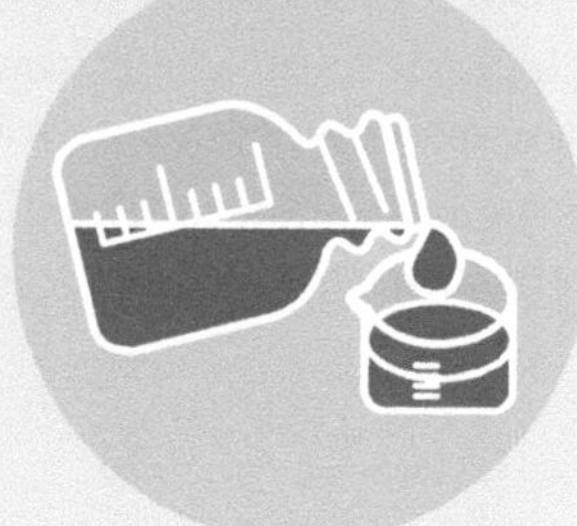

After reading this chapter you will be able to reflect on the nursing role in providing healthcare and health promotion to ensure that the patient is well informed, supported and assessed appropriately. It relates to **Essential Skills Clusters (NMC, 2010) 1–8**, as appropriate for each progression point.

Ensure that you really understand this chapter by logging on to your complimentary **MyNursingKit** at **www.pearsoned.co.uk/kozier**. Complete the self-assessment tests to check your progress and utilise further activities to practise and confirm your understanding.

CASE STUDY

You are working in the outpatients department and preparing the clinical environment for the morning clinic (a medical clinic). You note that there are two new referrals for the consultant that morning and therefore, in preparation for the patients, you visit their referral letters and medical notes to gain some insight into their conditions.

One of the patients is a Mr Frankburger who is 64 years old and lives with his wife. His general health has been well up until six months ago when he started presenting with slight tremors in his hands especially when at rest, some stiffness (rigidity) in his muscles when moving and frequent loss of balance causing falls. He visited his general practitioner who referred him to the medical consultant specialist for an opinion and further care management. Having worked with this consultant for a number of years you are aware of the physical examinations that she will undertake during the appointment and many of these she will have expected you to have already carried out, although some of them she will inevitably repeat just to confirm the findings.

After reading this chapter you will be able to prepare for Mr Frankburger's appointment, inform Mr Frankburger of the format of the appointment and what it will entail and prepare some of the documentation for further investigations.

INTRODUCTION

One of the major components of providing nursing care is an accurate examination/assessment. There are two types of examination/assessment; one form of examination is the health history taking which has been recognised and discussed in great depth in the previous chapter (Chapter 10), and a complete physical examination of the patient which is undertaken when a patient is admitted into your care. Both forms of examination are critical in order to provide a holistic and caring service to the patient.

A physical examination can either be a complete examination (the whole body), an examination of a system of the body (cardiovascular) or an examination of a body area (e.g. lungs when the patient presents with shortness of breath). Important to note is that the physical examination will be influenced by the age of the patient, the severity of the illness, the environment where the assessment takes place and the service provider's policies and procedures.

COMPLETE PHYSICAL ASSESSMENT

A complete physical examination is a systematic process starting at the head and proceeding downward to the toe (see *Box 11-1*). In most instances a physical examination of a patient will be undertaken by a doctor with the nurse's assistance, it is important that the nurse has a clear understanding of what a physical examination involves, how it aids diagnosis and provides accurate information on how patient care can be best managed. It is also important that the nurse is able to support and provide the patient with accurate information in order for the patient to be well informed and give informed consent on any or all aspects of the examination process.

The importance of physical examination is so that both the doctor and the nurse can:

- obtain baseline information in relation to the patient's functional abilities;
- support, supplement or counter the verbal information provided when the history is taken;
- aid both medical and nursing diagnosis and in the development of care planning;
- aid in the clinical judgement and decision-making process about the patient's functional status;
- evaluate the progress of the patient prior, during and following treatment;
- provide appropriate health education, health promotion and disease prevention information to the patient and their family.

BOX 11-1 Head-to-Toe Framework

- General assessment
- Vital signs
- Head
  - Hair, scalp, cranium, face
  - Eyes and vision
  - Ears and hearing
  - Nose and sinuses
  - Mouth and oropharynx
  - Cranial nerves
- Neck
  - Muscles
  - Lymph nodes
  - Trachea
  - Thyroid gland
  - Carotid arteries
  - Neck veins
- Upper extremities
  - Skin and nails
  - Muscle strength and tone
  - Joint range of motion
  - Brachial and radial pulses
  - Biceps tendon reflexes
  - Tendon reflexes

- Chest and back
  - Skin
  - Chest shape and size
  - Lungs
  - Heart
  - Spinal column
  - Breasts and axillae
- Abdomen
  - Skin
  - Abdominal sounds
  - Specific organs (e.g. liver, bladder)
  - Femoral pulses
- Genitals
  - Testicles
  - Vagina
  - Urethra
- Anus and rectum
- Lower extremities
  - Skin and toenails
  - Gait and balance
  - Joint range of motion
  - Popliteal, posterior tibial and pedal pulses
- Tendon and plantar reflexes

It is important to note that the format of the physical examination with children differs from that of adults. The examination of the ears, mouth, abdomen and genitals should be left to the end of the assessment as these are more intrusive, while the examination of the head, neck, heart and lungs are less so.

PREPARATION

During the physical examination it is important to prepare the environment and the patient. The less disruptions that occur will be respectful to the patient, maintain patient privacy and dignity, reduce anxiety and ensure the patient is as relaxed as possible prior to the examination. This in turn will possibly incur less discomfort for the patient.

It is important that the environment is well lit and warm enough for the patient to be comfortable during any stage of undress. A number of tools or equipment may be used to aid in the assessing process (see *Box 11-2*). The patient should be informed that they may be expected to change positions during the examination and the nurse should be aware of any patient limitations observed during the admission process and accommodate for these. It is important to cover any body areas that are not being examined as only those being examined should be left exposed.

Examinations of this type can be embarrassing for both the patients and any member of the multidisciplinary team. Effective communication is essential between all parties concerned in order for the examination to be undertaken with the minimum of discomfort while maintaining the privacy and dignity of the patient throughout.

There are four primary techniques used in the physical examination of a patient:

- inspection
- palpation
- percussion
- auscultation.

These techniques will be referred to throughout the chapter when discussing the examination of certain parts of the body.

Inspection is the technique of visual examination by using the sense of sight. As previously noted visual examination should be systematic, purposeful and rigorous. From observation the nurse can gather important information about the physical well-being of the patient. Often alcoholics will present with tremors (involuntary movements of the hand). The nurse can assess whether a patient is hypoxic by assessing whether the patient presents with rapid breathing and/or is cyanosed. Other senses can also be used during this 'inspection', e.g. the sense of smell and hearing. Inspection can also be combined with other techniques such as palpation.

Palpation is the examination of the body using the sense of touch. The pads of the fingers are used because their concentration of nerve endings makes them highly sensitive. Palpation can determine texture (e.g. of the hair); temperature (e.g. of a skin area); vibration (e.g. of a joint); position and size of organs or masses; distention (e.g. of the urinary bladder); pulsation; and the presence of pain upon pressure.

There are two types of palpation: light and deep. *Light* (superficial) *palpation* should always precede *deep palpation* because heavy pressure on the fingertips can dull the sense of touch. For light palpation, the nurse extends the dominant hand's fingers parallel to the skin surface and presses gently while moving the hand in a circle (see Figure 11-1). With light palpation, the skin is slightly depressed. If it is necessary to determine the details of a mass, the nurse presses lightly several times rather than holding the pressure.

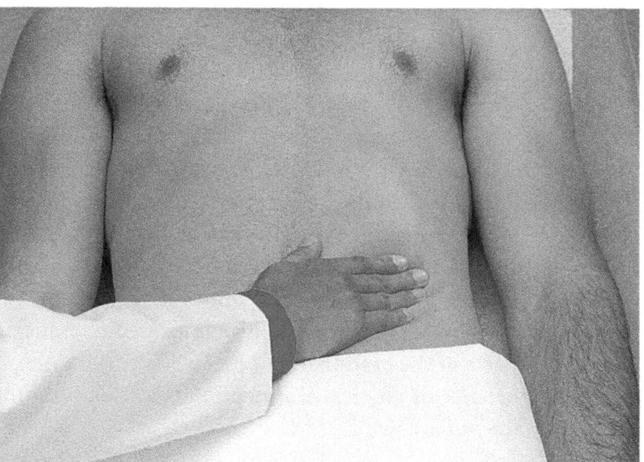

Figure 11-1 The position of the hand for light palpation.
Source: Pearson Education Ltd.

BOX 11-2 Assessment Tools and Diagnostic Equipment

- Gloves and apron
- Stethoscope
- Thermometer
- Tape measure
- Otoscope (for visualising the eardrum)
- Percussion hammer
- Wooden tongue depressors
- Blood test tubes
- Gauze swabs
- Specimen pots
- Lubricant gel
- Sphygmomanometer (for blood pressure)
- Oximeter (for oxygen saturation)
- Metric ruler
- Ophthalmoscope (to visualise interior of eye)
- Pen torch
- Weighing scales
- Vaginal speculum
- Vacutainer and needle
- Adhesive tape and dressing
- Electrocardiogram

Deep palpation is done by using both hands (see Figure 11-2). Deep palpation is done with extreme caution because pressure can damage internal organs. It is usually not indicated in patients who have acute abdominal pain or pain that is not yet diagnosed.

Percussion is the act of tapping parts of the body and listening to the sound or vibration that is made by that part of the body. There are two types of percussion: direct and indirect. In *direct* percussion the clinician taps one or two fingers against a body part (see Figure 11-3) using a rapid movement from the wrist. An example of using this technique is in the percussion of an adult's sinuses.

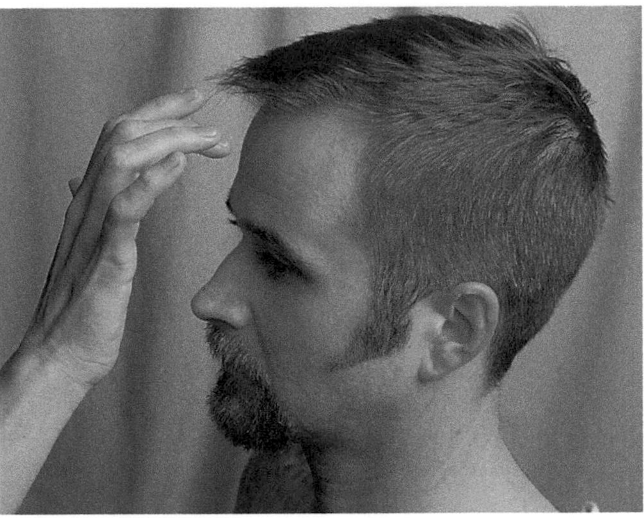

Figure 11-3 Direct percussion. Using one hand to strike the surface of the body.
Source: Pearson Education Ltd.

Indirect percussion, is using an object, e.g. finger, to aid in the examining process. In this technique, the middle finger of the nondominant hand is placed firmly on the patient's skin. Using the tip of the finger of the other hand (see Figure 11-4) and tapping the pleximeter (the middle finger of the hand resting on the patient's body) in rapid movements. The clinician listens to the sound and vibrations which will determine the size and shape of internal organs (e.g. liver and spleen) by establishing their boundaries. Percussion elicits five types of sound (see Table 11-1).

Auscultation is the listening of sounds produced within the body. There are two types of auscultation: *Direct* and *indirect*

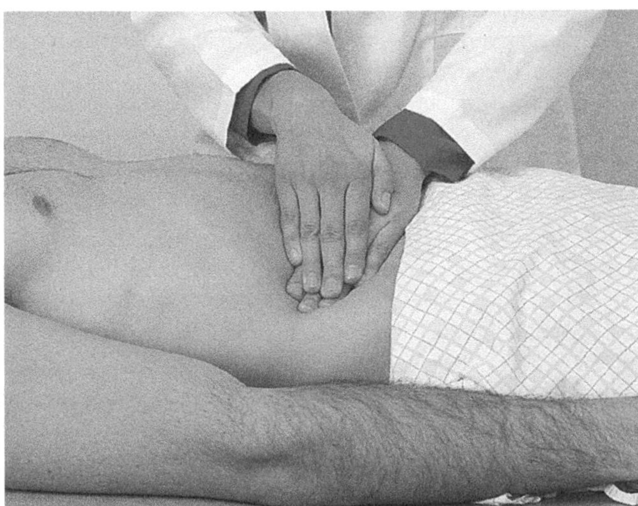

Figure 11-2 The position of the hands for deep bimanual palpation.
Source: Pearson Education Ltd.

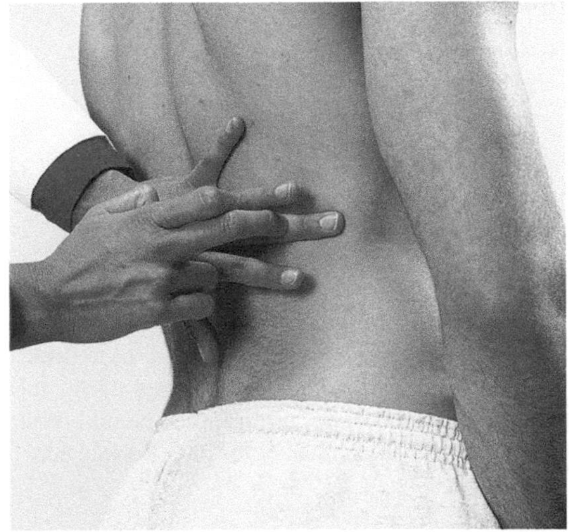

Figure 11-4 Indirect percussion. Using the finger of one hand to tap the finger of the other hand.
Source: Pearson Education Ltd.

Table 11-1 Percussion Sounds and Tones

Sound	Intensity	Pitch	Duration	Quality	Example of location
Flatness	Soft	High	Short	Extremely dull	This sound will indicate a normal bone or muscle
Dullness	Medium	Medium	Moderate	Thudlike	Indicates a normal liver or heart
Resonance	Loud	Low	Long	Hollow	Indicates a normal lung
Hyperresonance	Very loud	Very low	Very long	Booming	Indicates diseased lung or part of a lung
Tympany	Loud	High	Moderate	Musical	Stomach filled with gas (air).

auscultation. Direct auscultation is when the nurse will listen to the type of respiratory wheeze the patient makes. Indirect auscultation is referred to when the nurse uses a stethoscope to record a blood pressure or bowel sound.

GENERAL ASSESSMENT

Observation of the patient's general appearance and mental state, and measurement of baseline data such as vital signs, height and weight, is commonly regarded as a general assessment.

Appearance and Mental State

The general appearance and behaviour of an individual must be assessed considering the patient's culture, socioeconomic status, religion and current circumstances. For example, a person who has been informed that they have a terminal illness may appear depressed, which is understandable.

When assessing a patient's appearance and mental state, the following points should be considered:

- the patient's weight and height in relation to the patient's age, lifestyle and health;
- the patient's posture and gait, standing, sitting and walking;
- the patient's overall appearance including hygiene;
- the patient's body and breath (halitosis) odour;
- verbal and non-verbal signs of distress;
- patient's skin colour denoting ill health, e.g. jaundice or cyanosised or confused;
- the patient's coordination and posture;
- speech impediments;
- normal (for the patient) cognitive behaviour.

LIFESPAN CONSIDERATIONS

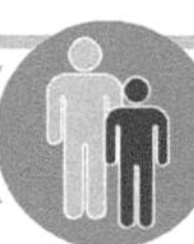

Infants

- Include measurement of head circumference until two years of age

Children

- Less intrusive examinations first.
- Use language that the child can understand.

Mature Adult

- Allow extra time for patients to answer questions.
- Adapt questioning techniques as appropriate for patients with hearing or visual limitations.
- Mature adults with osteoporosis can lose several inches in height. Be sure to document height and ask if they are aware of becoming shorter in height.
- When asking about weight loss, be specific about amount and time frame, for example, 'Have you lost more than five pounds in the last two months?'

Vital Signs

Vital signs are measured (a) to establish baseline data against which to compare future measurements and (b) to detect actual and potential health problems. See Chapter 15 for measurements of temperature, pulse, respirations, blood pressure and oxygen saturation. See Chapter 24 for pain assessment.

Height and Weight

The patient's height and weight are significant ways of providing information regarding the patient's well-being and nutritional status. The patient's weight will also aid medical diagnosis and calculating drug dosage. Patients are, for example, often weighed to assess whether the patient is in fluid retention to monitor the effects of the medication given.

In many clinical areas weighing patients is normal routine practice, and is undertaken on each admission. This is then used as a baseline for a new patient, and for use in continuing care as a method of assessing improvement or deterioration in the patient's condition.

It is important that patients wear clothes that are similar to those worn at each weighing and wet and saturated clothing

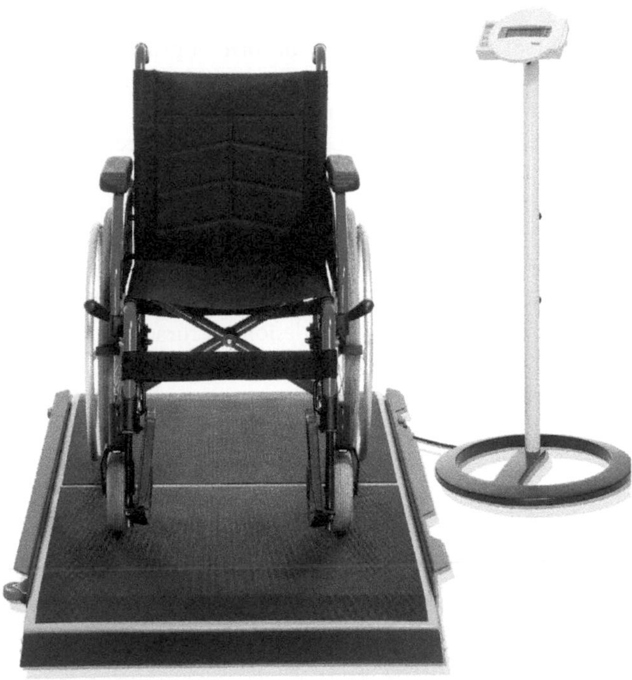

(a) Source: SECA Ltd.

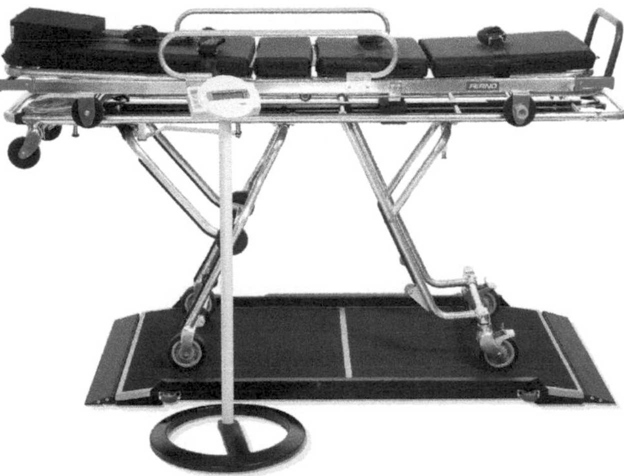

(b) Source: SECA Ltd.

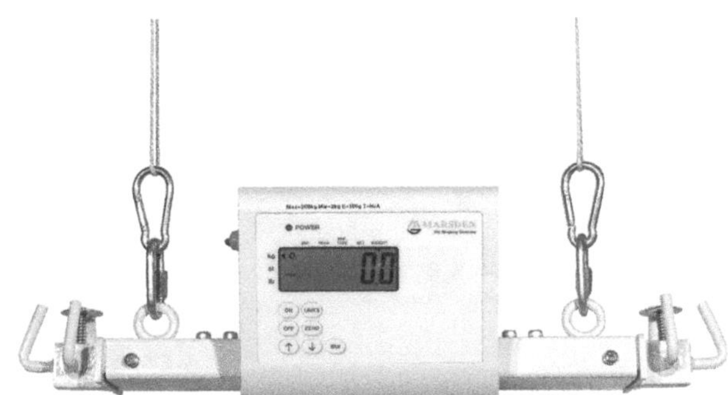

(c) Source: Marsden Weighing Machine Group Ltd.

Figure 11-5 (a) Wheelchair weighing scales; (b) Trolley or bed scales; (c) Hoist weighing scales.

should be changed. Ideally patient's weight should be recorded at the same time every day and using the same scale to ensure accuracy of readings.

When weighing a patient it is important to consider whether the patient is:

- able to stand unaided
- obese
- bedbound.

It is the nurse's responsibility that the appropriate and correct equipment is used to weigh the patient. There are many different types of scales to accommodate all different requirements which the nurse can consider (see Figure 11-5).

Height is measured using a measuring stick or wall chart and should be recorded as per local policy. Measuring the patient's height will give a good indication of the patient's dietary requirements and bone structure and disease.

THE INTEGUMENT (SKIN, HAIR AND NAILS)

The integument consists of the skin, hair and nails. Examination of the integument usually begins with a generalised inspection of the skin, hair and nails. Again, this is a systematic and rigorous examination which needs a good source of light, such as indirect natural daylight.

Skin

The initial general inspection of the skin examines its overall appearance. This will then allow the nurse to make clinical judgements on whether further, closer inspection is necessary. In some cases the nurse will also consider the olfactory sense to detect any unusual odours that are emanating from the patient. Often a patient is unaware of blisters or erosions that exist under skin flaps, etc. and it may take the nurse's sense of smell to detect these in the initial stage.

One of the first details that the nurse may notice is the **pallor** of the patient's skin. Pallor is the result of inadequate circulating blood or **haemoglobin** frequently identified by either a pale or ashen grey appearance. Pallor is not always easy to determine in darker skinned patients and often it is more readily noticeable in the buccal mucosa.

Cyanosis, a bluish tinge, is caused by an insufficient supply of oxygen in the blood system. It is often observed in the nail beds, lips and **buccal** mucosa. In dark-skinned patients, close inspection of the conjunctiva (the lining of the eyelids) and palms and soles may also show evidence of cyanosis.

Jaundice is a yellowish tinge in the mucous membrane of the skin or sclera of the eyes. Jaundice is caused by a high level of bilrubin in the blood. Nurses should take care not to confuse jaundice with the normal yellow pigmentation in the sclera of dark-skinned or black patients. If jaundice is suspected, the posterior part of the hard palate should also be inspected for a yellowish colour tone.

Erythema is a redness associated with a variety of rashes.

Dark-skinned patients have areas of lighter pigmentation, such as the palms, lips and nail beds. Localised areas of hyperpigmentation (increased pigmentation) and hypopigmentation (decreased pigmentation) may occur due to the changes in the distribution of melanin (the dark pigment) or in the function of the **melanocytes** in the **epidermis**. An example of hyperpigmentation is a birthmark, an example of hypopigmentation is vitiligo. **Vitiligo** is a chronic skin condition which causes depigmentation of patches of skin.

Other localised colour changes may indicate a problem such as oedema or a localised infection. **Oedema** is the presence of excess fluid, which often presents as a taut, shiny, swollen area that tends to blanch skin colour. Generalised oedema is usually an indication of an impaired circulation through the veins caused by cardiac dysfunction or abnormalities in the veins.

If a patient is dehydrated the skin elasticity is also poor. The skin will usually have a dry texture and the skin will lose its elasticity. Skin elasticity can be evaluated by gently squeezing the skin on the forearm or sternum (breastbone) between the thumb and the forefinger. Then release the skin. Normally the skin will spring back to its original shape but if it takes over 30 seconds to return to its original shape the skin has poor elasticity. Dry and scaly skin is often also seen. In contrast, oily or moist skin can be shiny, sticky or malodorous and can indicate a health concern, for example cardiac. Again the temperature of the skin will indicate if the patient is in **shock** or (multiple) organ shut down, or if there is infection or inflammation present.

Skin lesions can be classified into either a primary or secondary lesion. Primary skin lesions are new changes that may be in response to some external or internal changes in the skin (see Figure 11-6). Pressure sores are one form of primary lesion that should be identified and assessed and noted during physical examination. A breakdown in the skin should be swabbed (see Figure 11-7) to confirm the existence of an infection evident by signs of inflammation, fever, necrotic or **slough** (dead tissue) (see Figure 11-8) and/or pain. Secondary skin lesions are those that appear due to chronicity (long-term or reoccurring) trauma or infection. For example, a blister (primary lesion) may rupture and cause an erosion (secondary lesion). Nurses are responsible for describing skin lesions accurately in terms of location (e.g. face), distribution (body regions involved) and configuration (the arrangement or position of several lesions) as well as colour, shape, size, firmness, texture and characteristics of individual lesions.

CLINICAL ALERT

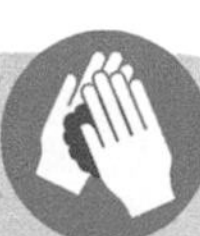

Too much sun can change the properties of a mole and develop it into a melanoma. Any changes should be assessed as a matter of urgency.

Of all the people diagnosed with melanoma in England and Wales, about 91 out of every 100 women (91%) and 78 out of 100 men (78%) will live for at least five years. This may be because women are more likely to see a doctor about their melanoma at an earlier stage, but the reason is not fully understood (Cancer Research UK, 2010).

LIFESPAN CONSIDERATIONS

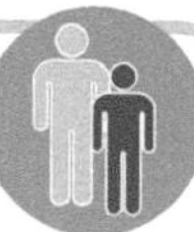

Assessing the Skin

Infants

- Newborns may be jaundiced for several weeks after birth.
- Newborns may have milia (whiteheads), small white nodules over the nose and face, and vernix caseosa (white cheesy, greasy material on the skin).
- In dark-skinned races, areas of hyperpigmentation may be found in the sacral area (bottom of the spine).
- If a rash is present, enquire in detail about immunisation history.
- Assess skin elasticity by pinching the skin on the abdomen.

Children

- In dark-skinned races, areas of hyperpigmentation may be found in the sacral area.
- As puberty approaches, skin may change in oiliness and acne may appear.
- If a rash is present, enquire in detail about immunisation history.

Mature Adults

- The skin loses its elasticity and has poor skin elasticity.
- The skin appears thin and translucent because of loss of **dermis** and subcutaneous fat.
- The skin is dry and flaky because sebaceous and sweat glands are less active. Dry skin is more prominent over the extremities.
- Due to the normal loss of peripheral skin elasticity in older adults, assess for hydration by checking skin elasticity over the sternum or clavicle.
- Flat tan to brown-coloured macules, referred to as *senile lentigines* or liver spots, are normally apparent on the back of the hand and other skin areas that are exposed to the sun.
- Warty lesions with irregularly shaped borders and a scaly surface often occur on the face, shoulders and trunk. These benign lesions begin as yellowish to tan and progress to a dark brown or black.

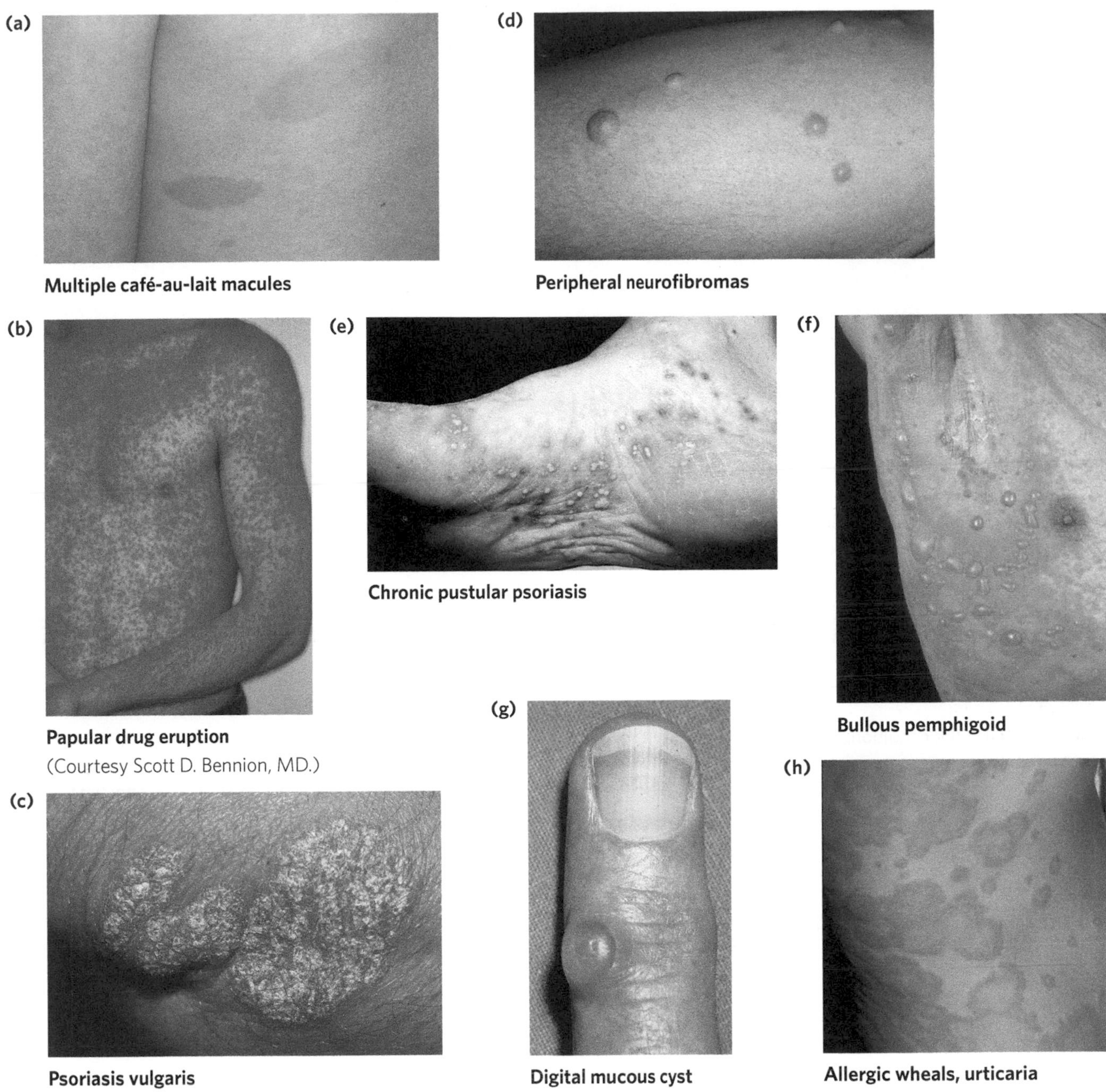

Figure 11-6 Primary skin lesions.

(a) Macule, Patch Flat, change in colour. Macules are 0.1–1cm in size and are confined to one area. Examples: freckles, measles, petechiae, flat moles. Patches are larger than 1cm and may have an irregular shape. Examples: port wine birthmark, vitiligo (white patches), rubella.

(b) Papule Circumscribed, solid elevation of skin. Papules are less than 1cm. Examples: warts, acne, pimples, elevated moles.

(c) Plaque Plaques are larger than 1cm. Examples: psoriasis, rubeola.

(d) Nodule, Tumour Elevated, solid, hard mass that extends deeper into the dermis than a papule. Nodules have a circumscribed border and are 0.5–2cm. Examples: squamous cell carcinoma, fibroma. Tumours are larger than 2cm and may have an irregular border. Examples: malignant melanoma, haemangioma.

(e) Pustule Vesicle or bulla filled with pus. Examples: acne vulgaris, impetigo.

(f) Vesicle, Bulla A circumscribed, round or oval, thin translucent mass filled with serous fluid or blood. Vesicles are less than 0.5cm. Examples: herpes simplex, early chickenpox, small burn blister. Bullae are larger than 0.5cm. Examples: large blister, second-degree burn, herpes simplex.

(g) Cyst A 1cm or larger, elevated, encapsulated, fluid-filled or semi-solid mass arising from the subcutaneous tissue or dermis. Examples: sebaceous and epidermoid cysts, chalazion of the eyelid.

(h) Wheal A reddened, localised collection of oedema fluid; irregular in shape. Size varies. Examples: hives, mosquito bites.

Source: (a)–(g) from *Dermatology Secrets in Colour*, 2nd edn, by J.E. Fitzpatrick and J.L. Aeling, 2001, Philadelphia: Hanley and Belfus, Inc.; (h) American Academy of Dermatology.

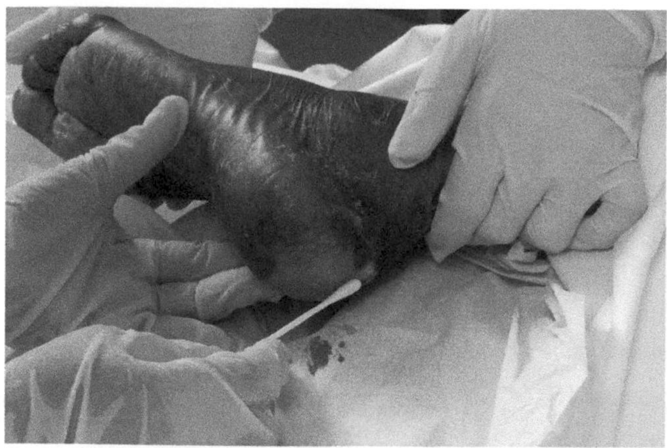

Figure 11-7 Wound swab.

Hair

Assessing a patient's hair should consider developmental and ethnic differences and will sometimes include its examination.

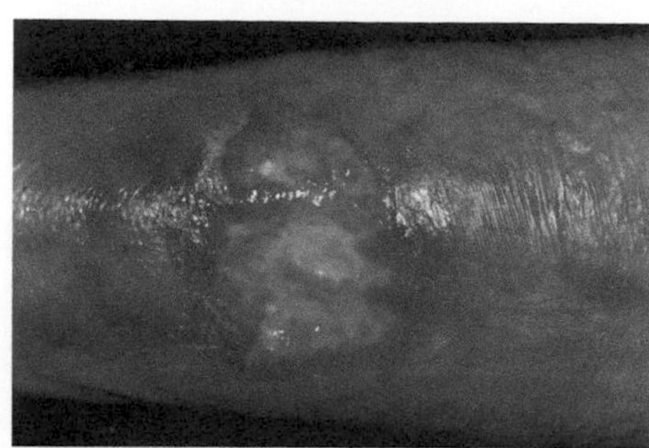

Figure 11-8 Sloughy wound

However, much of the information regarding the patient's hair can be collected by questioning.

Normal hair is resilient and evenly distributed. Some medical conditions, e.g. hypothyroidism, can cause thinning and brittle hair. While some medical treatment, i.e. chemotherapy, will cause hair loss (alopecia), or severe protein deficiency (kwashiorkor) may cause fading.

Procedure 11-1 describes how to assess the hair.

PROCEDURE 11-1 Assessing the Hair

Purpose

- To monitor the condition, texture and thickness of the patient's hair.
- Hair condition, quality and thickness will provide information on patient's general health and well may reflect an underlying medical condition, side effects of medication, poor diet etc.

Assessment

- The assessment must consider the patient's age, any underlying medical conditions, prescribed medication or any undergoing or recently completed treatments (e.g. chemotherapy).
- To identify any parasites, e.g. *Pediculus humanus capitis* (head louse) or eggs.

Planning

Patient's dignity and respect must be considered at all times. The Procedure should be carried out in privacy and confidentiality maintained. This may be best carried out when helping patients with their personal hygiene needs or when the patient is having their hair washed.

Equipment

- Examination gloves

Implementation

Performance

Follow local policy to ensure that you explain to the patient what you are going to do, why it is necessary and how they can cooperate. Obtain consent and maintain patient privacy and dignity and ensure that the appropriate local infection control procedures are observed. Enquire if the patient has any history of the following: recent use of hair dyes, rinses or curling or straightening preparations; recent chemotherapy (if alopecia is present); presence of disease, such as hypothyroidism, which can be associated with dry, brittle hair.

Assessment	Normal findings	Deviations from normal
1 Inspect the evenness of growth over the scalp.	Evenly distributed hair	Patches of hair loss (i.e. alopecia)
2 Inspect hair thickness or thinness.	Thick hair	Very thin hair (e.g. in hypothyroidism)
3 Inspect hair texture and oiliness.	Silky, resilient hair	Brittle hair (e.g. hypothyroidism); excessively oily or dry hair
4 Note presence of infections or infestations by parting the hair in several areas, checking behind the ears and along the hairline at the neck.	No infection or infestation	Flaking, sores, lice, nits (louse eggs) and ringworm
5 Inspect amount of body hair.	Variable	Hirsutism (abnormal hairiness) in women

Evaluation

- Report significant deviations from normal to medical staff.
- Document findings in the patient record using forms or checklists supplemented by narrative notes when appropriate.

Nails

Nails are made of keratin. Nails protect the nail beds and enhance sensations of the fingertips. The root of the nail is known as the germinal matrix which is hidden underneath the skin. The nails should be inspected for nail plate shape, angle between the nail and the nail bed, texture, colour and tissue intactness around the nails. The parts of the nail are shown in Figure 11-9.

The normal structure of the nails is a convex curve and is colourless. The angle between the nail and nail bed is normally about 160° (see Figure 11-10(a)). Abnormalities of the nail bed include the spoon shape (see Figure 11-10(b)) (nails curving upwards), **clubbing** (see Figure 11-10(c) and (d)) (the angle is ≥ 180°) or a horizontal depression of the nail caused by an injury or illness to the nail known as Beau's nail (see Figure 11-10(e)).

Due to the high vascular characteristic of the nail bed, a bluish or purple tint may indicate cyanosis and poor circulation is indicate if the nail bed is pale. A common inflammation surrounding the nail bed is paronychia. **Paronychia** is an inflammation of the surrounding tissues commonly known as an ingrowing toe nail.

A blanch test can sometimes be carried out to test the peripheral circulation. Normal nail bed capillaries blanch when pressed but quickly turn pink or their usual colour when pressure is released. Delay in the nail colour returning to normal can indicate circulatory problems.

Procedure 11-2 describes how to assess the nails.

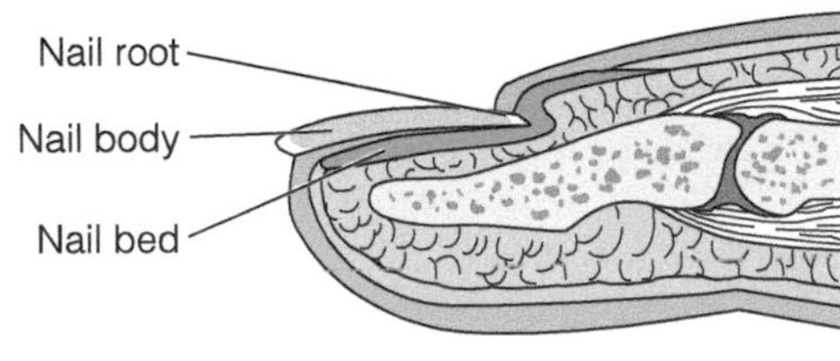

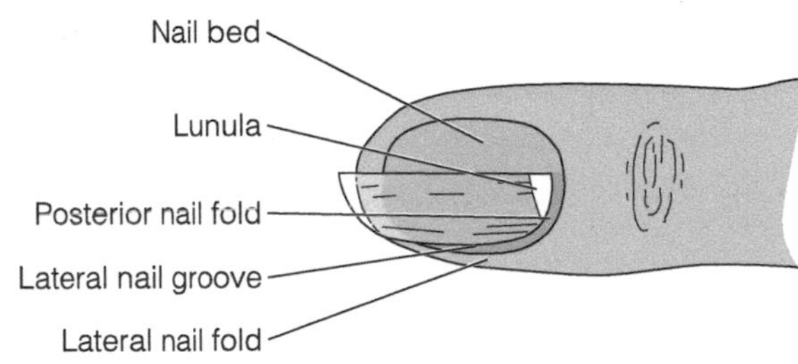

Figure 11-9 The parts of a nail.

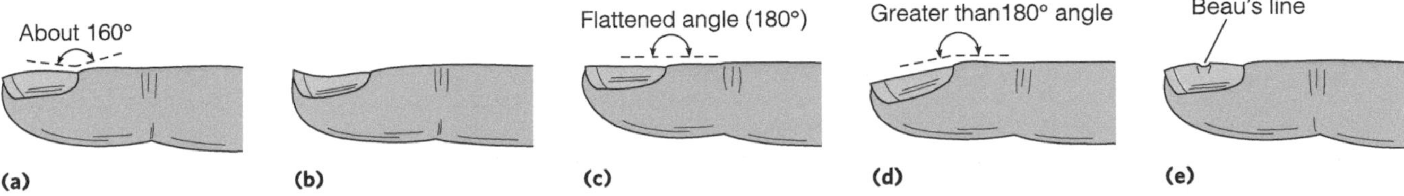

Figure 11-10 (a) A normal nail, showing the convex shape and the nail plate angle of about 160 degrees; (b) a spoon-shaped nail, which may be seen in patients with iron deficiency anaemia; (c) early clubbing; (d) late clubbing (may be caused by long-term oxygen lack); (e) Beau's line on nail (may result from severe injury or illness).

PROCEDURE 11-2 Assessing the Nails

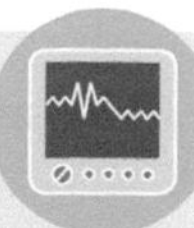

Purpose

- To examine the nails and identify any anomalies that can be seen from the visual examination (e.g. brittle nails, colour, shape, thickness, etc.).
- The examination of the nails may be an indication of any health and hygiene problems with the patient (e.g. clubbing).

Assessment

- Consider the age of the patient.
- Consider the medical history of the patient.

Planning

Equipment

- None

Implementation

Performance

Follow local policy to ensure that you explain to the patient what you are going to do, why it is necessary and how they can cooperate. Obtain consent and maintain patient privacy and dignity and ensure that the appropriate local infection control procedures are observed. Enquire if the patient has any history of the following: presence of diabetes mellitus, peripheral circulatory disease, previous injury or severe illness.

Assessment	Normal findings	Deviations from normal
1 Inspect fingernail plate shape to determine its curvature and angle.	Convex curvature; angle of nail plate about 160° (Figure 11-10(a))	Spoon nail (Figure 11-10(b)); clubbing (180° or greater) (Figure 11-10(c) and (d))
2 Inspect fingernail and toenail texture.	Smooth texture	Excessive thickness or thinness or presence of grooves or furrows; Beau's lines (Figure 11-10(e))
3 Inspect fingernail and toenail bed colour.	Highly vascular and pink in light-skinned patients; dark-skinned patients may have brown or black pigmentation in longitudinal streaks	Bluish or purplish tint (may reflect cyanosis); pallor (may reflect poor arterial circulation)
4 Inspect tissues surrounding nails.	Intact epidermis	Hangnails (triangular splits in the skin around the nail); paronychia (inflammation)
5 Perform branch test of capillary refill test. Press two or more nails between your thumb and index finger; look for blanching and return of pink colour to nail bed.	Prompt return of pink or usual colour (generally less than three seconds)	Delayed return of pink or usual colour (may indicate circulatory impairment)

Evaluation

- Perform a detailed follow-up examination of other individual systems based on findings that deviated from expected or normal for the patient. Relate findings to previous assessment data if available.
- Report significant deviations from normal to medical staff.
- Document findings in the patient record using forms or checklists supplemented by narrative notes when appropriate.

THE HEAD

Physical examination of the head includes inspection, palpation of the skull, face, eyes, ears, nose, sinuses, mouth and pharynx.

Skull and Face

A normal head size is referred to as normocephalic and each individual has an unique shape and size. Names of the bones in the head identify each specific area: frontal, parietal, occipital, mastoid process, mandible, maxilla and zygomatic (see Figure 11-11).

Medical disorders that present with oedema of the head due to kidney or cardiac disease can alter the shape of the head. Exophthalmoses (a protrusion of the eyeballs) can also be easily identified when examining the patient. The over-production of cortisol may develop Cushing's syndrome (an obese upper half of the body, a round face and swelling of the neck), and prolonged malnutrition can result in sunken eyes, cheeks and temples.

Procedure 11-3 describes how to assess the skull and face.

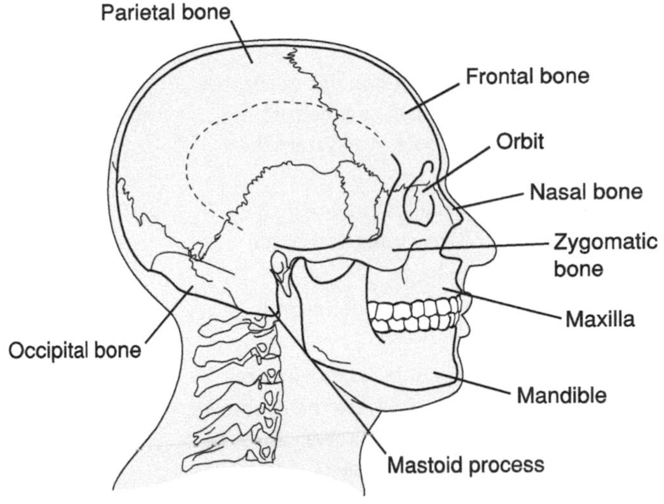

Figure 11-11 Bones of the head.

PROCEDURE 11-3 Assessing the Skull and Face

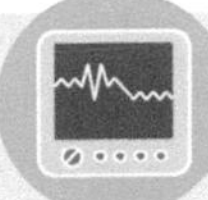

Purpose

- To examine the skull and face for symmetry and shape as this may be an indication of illness (e.g. renal or cardiac disease or endocrine disease).

Assessment

- The assessment should be undertaken during the initial assessment and medical history and age should be considered.

Planning

Equipment

- None

Implementation

Performance

Follow local policy to ensure that you explain to the patient what you are going to do, why it is necessary and how they can cooperate. Obtain consent and maintain patient privacy and dignity and ensure that the appropriate local infection control procedures are observed. Enquire if the patient has any history of the following: any past problems with lumps or bumps, itching, scaling or dandruff; any history of loss of consciousness, dizziness, seizures, headache, facial pain or injury; when and how any lumps occurred; length of time any other problem existed; any known cause of problem; associated symptoms, treatment and recurrences.

	Assessment	Normal findings	Deviations from normal
1	Inspect the skull for size, shape and symmetry	Rounded and symmetrical, with frontal, parietal and occipital prominences; smooth skull contour	Lack of symmetry; increased skull size with more prominent nose and forehead; longer mandible (may indicate excessive growth hormone or increased bone thickness)
2	Palpate the skull for nodules or masses, or depressions. Use a gentle rotating motion and palpate in a systematic manner.	Smooth, uniform consistency; absence of nodules or masses	Sebaceous cysts; local deformities from trauma
3	Inspect the facial features (e.g. symmetry of structures and of the distribution of hair).	Symmetric or slightly asymmetric facial features are normal	Increased facial hair; thinning of eyebrows; pronounced asymmetric features
4	Inspect the eyes for oedema and hollowness.		Oedema; sunken eyes
5	Note symmetry of facial movements. Ask the patient to elevate the eyebrows, frown or lower the eyebrows, close the eyes tightly, puff the cheeks, and smile and show the teeth.	Symmetric facial movements	Asymmetric facial movements (e.g. eye on affected side cannot close completely); drooping of lower eyelid and mouth; involuntary facial movements (i.e. tics or tremors); nerve palsy (paralysis)

Evaluation

- Perform a detailed follow-up examination of other systems based on findings that deviated from expected or normal for the patient. Relate findings to previous assessment data if available.
- Report significant deviations from normal to medical staff.
- Document findings in the patient notes.

LIFESPAN CONSIDERATIONS

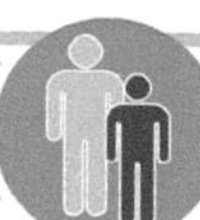

Assessing the Skull and Face

Infants

- Most newborns' heads are shaped according to the method of delivery for the first week.
- The posterior fontanelle (soft spot) usually closes by eight weeks but the anterior fontanelle may remain for up to 18 months.
- Voluntary head control should be present by about six months of age.

The Eyes and Vision

Many people consider vision the most important sense because it allows them to interact freely with their environment. Regular eye tests are advised to maintain optimum vision. In the UK eye testing is recommended biennially (every two years) unless eye conditions change or there is a medical indication for more frequent eye testing.

While many people wear eyeglasses or contact lenses due to conditions that require them – although laser treatment has reduced this number – current trends suggests that increasingly more people wear them to change or enhance the colour of their eyes. Some of the refractive malfunction of the lens of the eyes are myopia (shortsightedness), hyperopia (longsightedness) and astigmatism (an uneven curvature of the cornea). Testing visual acuity should be left to the expertise of an ophthalmologist but there are a couple of simple ways to determine whether a patient requires further investigation (see *Box 11-3*).

Examination of the eyes includes assessment of **visual acuity** (the degree of detail that can be seen from an image), ocular movement, **visual fields** (the area an individual can see when looking straight ahead), and external structures (see Figures 11-13 and 11-14).

Common inflammatory visual problems that may be encountered are conjunctivitis, dacryocystitis, hordeolum and iritis. Conjunctivitis (inflammation of the bulbar and palpebral

BOX 11-3 Assessing Distance Vision

Distance vision is usually tested if there is some indication that a patient's distance vision is affected. The most common cause of problems with distance vision is astigmatism (irregularly shaped cornea), which causes problems with seeing objects in the distance or objects that are placed close to the eye. Astigmatism can be the result of a progressive disease called keratoconus where the normally round cornea thins into a cone shape. To assess distance vision:

- Hold up an eye chart (see Figure 11-12) approximately 6 m from the patient.
- Ask the patient to cover their right eye and read the eye chart.
- Then do the same with the left eye covered.
- Finally, ask the patient to read the chart using both eyes.
- Record the readings of each eye and both eyes, i.e. the smallest line from which the person is able to read one-half or more of the letters.

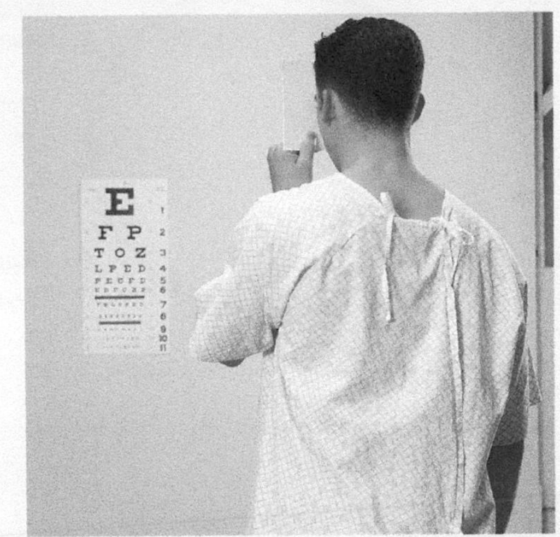

Figure 11-12 Testing distance vision using a Snellen chart.

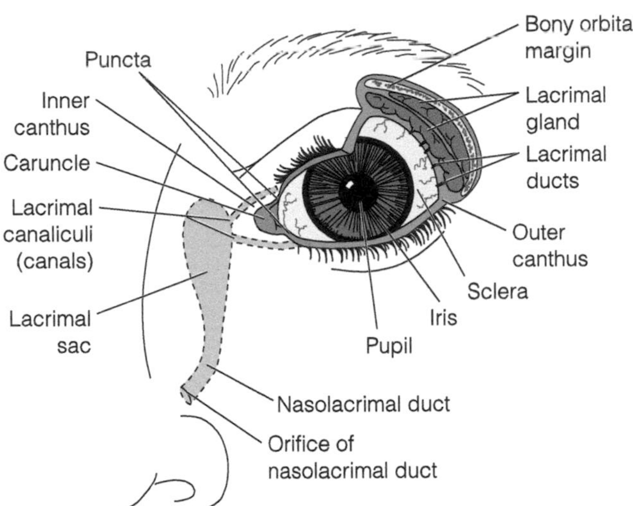

Figure 11-13 The external structures and lacrimal apparatus of the left eye.

conjunctiva) may be caused by foreign bodies, chemical agents, allergies, viruses or bacteria. Dacryocystitis is an inflammation of the lacrimal sac and is manifested by tearing and discharge of the nasolacrimal duct. Hordeolum (sty) is a swelling and tenderness of the hair follicle and glands. Iritis is an inflammation of the iris caused by infection.

Cataract is a clouding of the lens (NEI, 2010) which is most often related to ageing, although it can be a congenital condition or occur following radiation. The lens as shown in Figure 11-14 is a clear part of the eye that focuses light or an image onto the retina, and the lens lies behind the iris of the eye. The treatment is often new eyeglasses, anti-glare glasses or surgery.

Glaucoma is the disturbance of the circulation of normal fluid pressure behind the eye, which causes an increase in pressure within the eye and is the most frequent cause of blindness in people over 40. It is detected by the non-contact tonometry (NCT) test ('air puff' test) when measuring eye pressure. It is more often found in patients with familial history of glaucoma, many people over the age of 60 and often found in darker skinned people over 40 years old. The treatment is often medication, laser treatment or surgery.

It is important to note that normal appearances should be taken into consideration; the pupils should be, round, smooth borders, equal in size and appear black in colour. Enlarged or unequal pupils may indicate a problem with the eyes, for example enlarged eyes can be an indication of glaucoma, unequal pupils an indication of central nervous system disorder, and constricted pupils an inflammation of the iris or be drug induced. When assessing pupil reaction it is important to note the points in *Box 11-4*.

BOX 11-4 Assessing Pupil Reactions

Direct and Consensual Reaction to Light

- Partially darken the room.
- Ask the patient to look straight ahead.
- Using a pen torch and approaching from the side, shine a light on the pupil.
- Observe the response of the illuminated pupil. It should constrict (direct response).
- Shine the light on the pupil again, and observe the response of the other pupil. It should also constrict (consensual response).

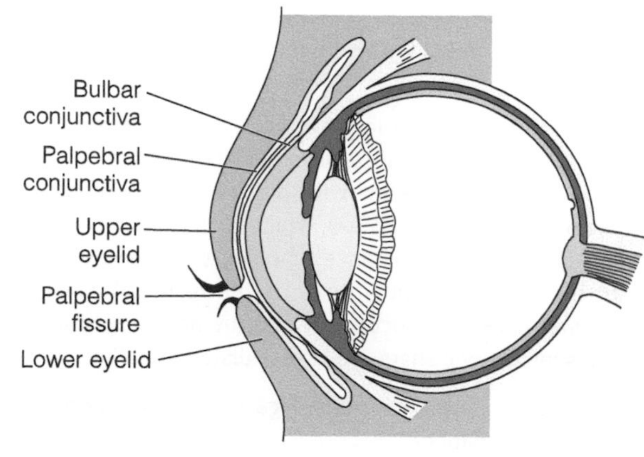

Figure 11-14 Anatomic structures of the right eye, lateral view.

Reaction to Accommodation

- Hold an object (a penlight or pencil) about 10cm from the bridge of the patient's nose.
- Ask the patient to look first at the top of the object and then at a distant object (e.g. the far wall) behind the penlight. Alternate the gaze from the near to the far object.
- Observe the pupil response. The pupils should constrict when looking at the near object and dilate when looking at the far object.
- Next, move the penlight or pencil towards the patient's nose. The pupils should converge. To record normal assessment of the pupils, use the abbreviation PEARL (pupils equal and reacting to light). All findings (see Figure 11-15) should be documented on the appropriate chart as per local policy.

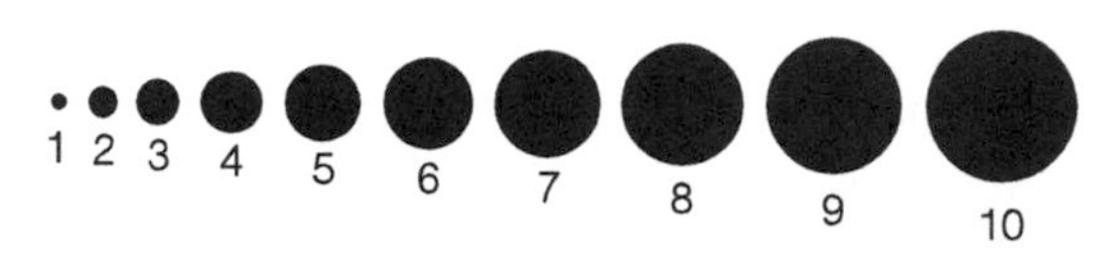

Figure 11-15 Variations in pupil diameters in millimetres.

The Ears and Hearing

Assessment of the ear includes direct inspection and palpation of the external ear, inspection of the remaining parts of the ear by an otoscope, and determination of auditory acuity.

The ear is made up of three parts; the external ear, middle ear and inner ear (see Figure 11-16). The external ear includes the pinna, the external auditory canal or outer ear, and the tympanic membrane or eardrum. The external ear canal is curved and is about 2.5cm long in the adult. It is covered with skin that has many fine hairs, glands and nerve endings. The glands secrete cerumen (earwax), which lubricates and protects the canal.

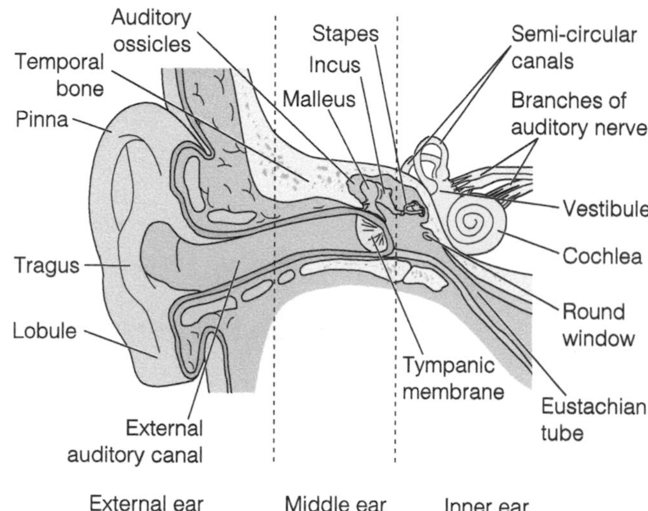

Figure 11-16 Anatomic structures of the external, middle and inner ear.

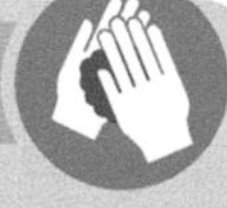

CLINICAL ALERT

The curvature of the external ear canal differs with age. In the infant and toddler, the canal has an upward curvature. By age three, the ear canal assumes the more downward curvature of adulthood, an important factor when examining the ear.

The middle ear is an air-filled cavity that starts at the tympanic membrane and contains three ossicles (bones of sound transmission): the malleus (hammer), which is the most easily seen, the incus (anvil) and the stapes (stirrups). The Eustachian tube, another part of the middle ear, connects the middle ear to the nasopharynx. The tube stabilises the air pressure between the external atmosphere and the middle ear, thus preventing rupture of the tympanic membrane and discomfort produced by marked pressure differences.

The inner ear contains the cochlea, a seashell-shaped structure essential for sound transmission and hearing, and the vestibule and semicircular canals, which contain the organs of equilibrium.

Sound is a complex process which is usually transmitted by air conduction or bone conduction.

The air transmission process is:

- a sound stimulus entering the external canal and travelling to the tympanic membrane;
- reaching the ossicles by the sound waves vibrating the tympanic membrane;
- the sound waves travelling from the ossicles to the opening of the inner ear;
- the cochlea accepting the sound vibrations;
- the stimulus transports to the auditory nerve and the cerebral cortex.

Bone sounds can be transmitted to the brain through the skull bones.

Hearing tests are usually performed by audiologist but it is the nurse's responsibility to identify patients who may have problems with their hearing. Also it is important to note that some trusts have a policy that states nurses should not perform otoscopic examinations due to potential damage to the external ear. Despite this there are a number of techniques that the nurse can use to assess the patient's ears and hearing. When assessing the ears and hearing *Procedure 11-4* should be followed.

PROCEDURE 11-4 Assessing the Ears and Hearing

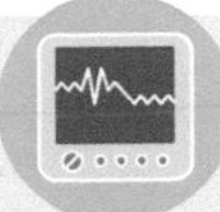

Purpose

- To assess for any breaks in the skin, any abnormal growths and hearing difficulties, and for early recognition if the patient is unable to hear or understand the information or questions being asked.

Assessment

- Provide a suitable environment in order to assess accurately.
- Prepare the equipment prior to the procedure.
- Consider the age and any underlying medical conditions that may affect the procedure.

Planning

Equipment

- Otoscope

Implementation

Performance

Follow local policy to ensure that you explain to the patient what you are going to do, why it is necessary and how they can cooperate. Obtain consent and maintain patient privacy and dignity and ensure that the appropriate local infection control procedures are observed. Enquire if the patient has any history of poor or loss of hearing or working with loud noises for long periods of time.

Assessment	Normal findings	Deviations from normal
1 Inspect the auricle (ear) for colour, size and position of the pinna (earlobe). The pinna should be the same colour as the face and of a similar size.	Colour same as face. Symmetrical Auricle aligned with outer canthus of eye.	Bluish colour may indicate cyanosis. Pallor may indicate frostbite. Redness may indicate infection. Asymmetry Low-set ears may indicate congenital abnormalities.
2 Palpate the pinna to test its texture, elasticity and areas of tenderness. The pinna should be mobile, firm and not tender.	Mobile, firm and not tender; pinna recoils after pulling the ear.	Lesions, flaky, scaly skin (seborrhoea), tenderness (infection).
3 Using an otoscope or with the naked eye inspect the external ear canal for cerumen (ear wax), skin lesions, pus and blood.	Distal third contains hair follicles and glands. Dry cerumen, greyish-tan colour or wet cerumen browny shades.	Redness and discharge. Scaling. Excessive cerumen obstructing canal.

4 Inspect the ear drum with an otoscope (as per local policy).	The ear drum should be semi-transparent and a pearly grey colour (see Figure 11-17). 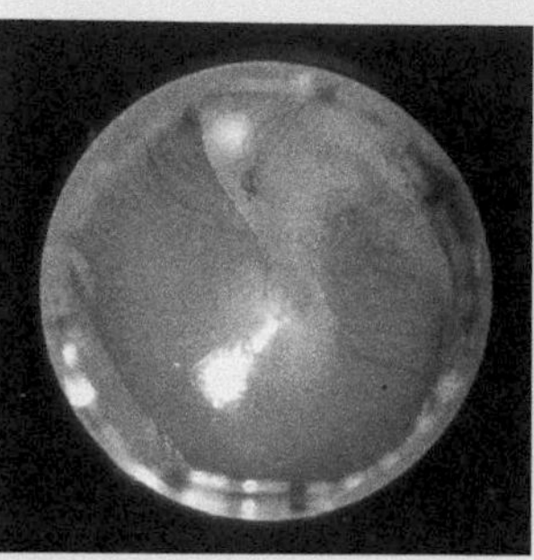 **Figure 11-17** Normal tympanic membrane.	Pink to red, some opacity. Yellow-amber. White. Blue or deep red. Dull surface.
5 Assess the patient's response to normal voice sounds, if patient has difficulty further tests should be considered and appropriate referrals made.	Normal voice tone and pitch.	Normal voice sound not audible.

Evaluation

- Document if there are any requests to repeat words or statements or if the patient leans towards the speaker.
- Report significant deviations from normal to medical staff.

LIFESPAN CONSIDERATIONS

Assessing the Ears and Hearing

Infants

- Assess overall hearing by ringing a bell from behind the infant or have the parent call the child's name to check for a response. At 3–4 months of age, the child will turn head and eyes towards the sound.

Children

- To inspect the external canal and tympanic membrane in children less than three years old, pull the pinna down and back. Insert the otoscope only 0.5–1cm.

Mature Adults

- The skin of the ear may appear dry and be less resilient because of the loss of connective tissue.
- Increased coarse and wire-like hair growth may grow on the external ear.
- The pinna increases in both width and length, and the earlobe elongates.
- Earwax tends to be drier.
- Hearing loss often occurs in mature adults.

Nose and Sinuses

The nasal passages are coated by a mucous membrane that consists of tiny hairy cells that protect the nasal canal, inhalation and gastric deposit from dust, bacteria and other particles. The nurse can easily inspect the nasal canal visually or more intensely with the use of a flashlight. Normally, the assessment of the nose includes inspection and palpation of the external nose, patency of the nasal cavities, and inspection of the nasal passages.

The nose should be inspected if there are any signs or symptoms that there may be a blockage or injury to the canal. The patient may also describe the inability to smell, and the nurse may test this by offering the patient something pungent to smell, which is carried out by asking the patient to close their eyes and identify the smell.

The patient may present with headaches, facial pain, reduced sense of smell, etc. which may indicate sinus problems. The nurse can also inspect and palpate the facial sinuses see Figure 11-18.

Procedure 11-5 describes how to assess the nose and sinuses.

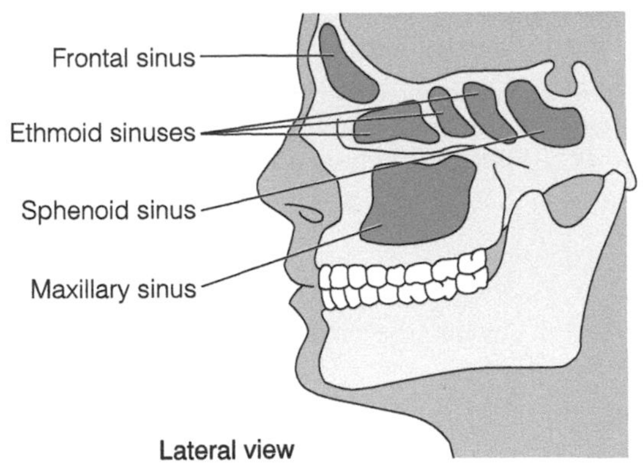

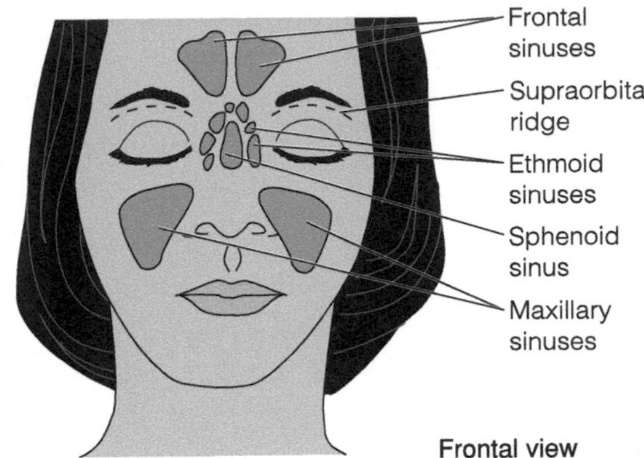

Figure 11-18 The facial sinuses.

PROCEDURE 11-5 Assessing the Nose and Sinuses

Purpose

- To identify any misalignment of the nose and note any foreign bodies or lesions embedded within the nasal canal, and examine mucosa for signs of infection.

Assessment

- Assess whether the patient is in pain and if there are any underlying medical conditions for the pain.
- Assess whether the patient needs any analgesia prior to the procedure.
- Examine and observe the patient for any breathing problems.
- Establish the most comfortable position for the patient.

Planning

Equipment

- Gloves
- Flashlight/penlight

Implementation

Performance

Follow local policy to ensure that you explain to the patient what you are going to do, why it is necessary and how they can cooperate. Obtain consent and maintain patient privacy and dignity and ensure that the appropriate local infection control procedures are observed. Enquire if the patient has any history of the following: allergies, difficulty breathing through the nose, sinus infections, injuries to nose or face, nosebleeds, any medications taken, any changes in sense of smell.

Assessment	Normal findings	Deviations from normal
Nose		
1 Inspect the external nose for any deviations in shape, size or colour, and flaring or discharge from the nostril (nares).	Symmetric and straight No discharge or flaring Uniform colour	If asymmetric, for example, this can be caused by trauma or injury (e.g. following a rugby injury when the player presents with either/or a bleeding nose, pain and a deviated nasal septum). Localised areas of redness.
2 Lightly palpate the external nose to determine any areas of tenderness, masses and displacements of bone and cartilage.	Not tender; no lesions	Tenderness on palpation.
3 Determine patency of both nasal cavities. Ask the patient to close the mouth, occlude one nostril, and breathe through the opposite nostril. Repeat the procedure to assess patency of the opposite nostril.	Air moves freely as the patient breathes through the nostrils	Air movement is restricted in one or both nostrils.

4 Inspect the nasal çavities using a flashlight.		
5 Observe for the presence of redness, swelling, growths and discharge.	Mucosa pink Clear, watery discharge No lesions	Mucosa red, oedematous Abnormal discharge (e.g. purulent). Presence of lesions (e.g. polyps).
6 Inspect the nasal septum between the nasal chambers.	Nasal septum intact and in midline	Septum deviated to the right or to the left.
Facial sinuses		
7 Palpate the maxillary and frontal sinuses for tenderness (see Figure 11-18).	Not tender	Tenderness in one or more sinuses.

Evaluation

- Perform a detailed follow-up examination of other systems based on findings that deviated from expected or normal for the patient. Relate findings to previous assessment data if available.
- Report significant deviations from normal to medical staff.
- Document findings in the patient notes.

Mouth and Oropharynx

The mouth and pharynx are composed of a number of structures: lips, inner and buccal mucosa, the tongue and floor of the mouth, teeth and gums, hard and soft palate, uvula, salivary glands, tonsillar pillars and tonsils. Anatomic structures of the mouth are shown in Figure 11-19.

The parotid, submandibular and sublingual glands are the three pairs of the salivary glands that empty into the mouth and their function is to moisten the mouth and begin the digestion of starches.

The teeth (fully developed by the age of 25) which are discussed in Chapter 17 and the mouth can be affected if not enough saliva is produced as it will create oral problems such as dental caries.

Dental caries (cavities) and periodontal disease (pyorrhea) are the most common problem associated with teeth. Plaque is an invisible film that sticks to the enamel surface of teeth. It consists of bacteria, saliva, epithelial cells and leukocytes. When plaque is unchecked, tartar (dental calculus) forms. Tartar is a visible, hard deposit of plaque and dead bacteria that forms at the gum lines. This will eventually disrupt bone tissue. Gingivitis is a peridontal disease presents with red, swollen gums, bleeding and receding gum lines.

Other problems nurses may see are glossitis (inflammation of the tongue), stomatitis (inflammation of the oral mucosa) and parotitis (inflammation of the parotid salivary gland). *Procedure 11-6* describes assessment of the mouth and oropharynx.

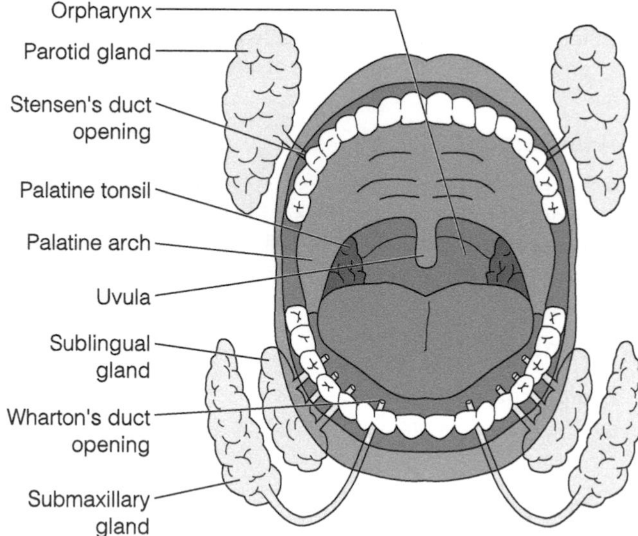

Figure 11-19 Anatomic structures of the mouth.

While in many cases the examination of teeth is the responsibility of an expert (e.g. a dentist) it is imperative that the nurse will examine and assess a patient's mouth for any signs of abnormalities or loose fitting dentures. Oral care is paramount and fundamental to the well-being of any individual in your care.

PROCEDURE 11-6 Assessing the Mouth and Oropharynx

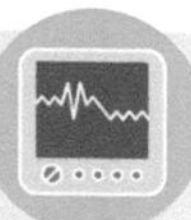

Purpose

- For early detection of any abnormalities within the oral orifice in order to promote the well-being of the patient.

Assessment

- The procedure should include a thorough examination of the mouth in order to assess the patient's ability to eat and communicate.
- The procedure should examine the tongue, gums, teeth, tongue and palate. Saliva and mucosa should be examined and any abnormalities reported and recorded.
- The assessment should consider the age and medical well-being of the patient.
- The environment where the procedure is going to be carried out.

Planning

If possible, arrange for the patient to sit with the head against a firm surface such as a headrest or examination table. This makes it easier for the patient to hold the head still during the examination.

Equipment

- Examination gloves
- Tongue depressor
- 2 × 2 gauze pads
- Flashlight or penlight

Implementation

Performance

Follow local policy to ensure that you explain to the patient what you are going to do, why it is necessary and how they can cooperate. Obtain consent and maintain patient privacy and dignity and ensure that the appropriate local infection control procedures are observed. Enquire if the patient has any history of the following: routine pattern of dental care, last visit to dentist; length of time ulcers or other lesions have been present; any denture discomfort; any medications patient is receiving.

Assessment	Normal findings	Deviations from normal
Lips and buccal mucosa		
1 Inspect the outer lips for symmetry of contour, colour and texture. Ask the patient to purse the lips as if to whistle.	Uniform pink colour (darker, e.g. bluish hue, in Mediterranean groups and dark-skinned patients) Soft, moist, smooth texture Symmetry of contour Ability to purse lips	Pallor; cyanosis Blisters; generalised or localised swelling. Inability to purse lips (indicative of facial nerve damage)
2 Inspect and palpate the inner lips and buccal mucosa for colour, moisture, texture and the presence of lesions.	Uniform pink colour (freckled brown pigmentation in dark-skinned patients) Moist, smooth, soft, glistening and elastic texture (drier oral mucosa in elderly due to decreased salivation)	Pallor. Excessive dryness Mucosal cysts; irritations from dentures; abrasions, ulcerations; nodules
Teeth and gums		
3 Inspect the teeth and gums while examining the inner lips and buccal mucosa.	32 adult teeth Smooth, white, shiny tooth enamel	Missing teeth; ill-fitting dentures Brown or black discoloration of the enamel (may indicate staining or the presence of caries)
	Pink gums (bluish or dark patches in dark-skinned patients)	Excessively red gums
	Moist, firm texture to gums	Spongy texture; bleeding; tenderness (may indicate periodontal disease)
	No retraction of gums (pulling away from the teeth)	Receding, atrophied gums; swelling that partially covers the teeth
4 Inspect the dentures. Ask the patient to remove complete or partial dentures. Inspect their condition, noting in particular broken or worn areas.	Smooth, intact dentures	Ill-fitting dentures; irritated and excoriated area under dentures
Tongue/floor of the mouth		
5 Inspect the surface of the tongue for position, colour and texture. Ask the patient to protrude the tongue.	Central position	Deviated from centre (may indicate damage to hypoglossal (12th cranial) nerve); excessive trembling

	Normal findings	Deviations from normal
	Pink colour (some brown pigmentation on tongue borders in dark-skinned patients); moist; slightly rough; thin whitish coating	Smooth red tongue (may indicate iron, vitamin B_{12} or vitamin B_3 deficiency)
		Dry, furry tongue (associated with fluid deficit)
	Smooth, lateral margins; no lesions Raised papillae (taste buds)	Nodes, ulcerations, discolorations (white or red areas); areas of tenderness
6 Inspect tongue movement. Ask the patient to roll the tongue upward and move it from side to side.	Moves freely; no tenderness	Restricted mobility
7 Inspect the base of the tongue and the mouth floor. Ask the patient to place the tip of the tongue against the roof of the mouth.	Smooth tongue base with prominent veins	Swelling, ulceration
Salivary glands		
8 Palpate the tongue and floor of the mouth for any nodules, lumps or excoriated areas.	Smooth with no palpable nodules	Swelling, nodules
9 Inspect salivary duct openings for any swelling or redness. See Figure 11-18.	Same as colour of buccal mucosa and floor of mouth	Inflammation (redness and swelling)
Palates and uvula		
10 Inspect the hard and soft palate for colour, shape, texture and the presence of bony prominences. Ask the patient to open the mouth wide and tilt the head backward. Then, depress tongue with a tongue blade as necessary, and use a penlight for appropriate visualisation.	Light pink, smooth, soft palate Lighter pink hard palate, more irregular texture	Discoloration (e.g. jaundice or pallor) Palates the same colour Irritations Bony growths (exostoses) growing from the hard palate
11 Inspect the uvula for position and mobility while examining the palates. To observe the uvula, ask the patient to say 'ah' so that the soft palate rises.	Positioned in midline of soft palate	Deviation to one side due to trauma or tumour.
Oropharynx and tonsils		
12 Inspect the oropharynx for colour and texture. Inspect one side at a time to avoid eliciting the gag reflex. To expose one side of the oropharynx, press a tongue blade against the tongue on the same side about halfway back while the patient tilts the head back and opens the mouth wide. Use a penlight for illumination, if needed.	Pink and smooth posterior wall	Reddened or oedematous (inflammation); presence of lesions, plaques or drainage
13 Inspect the tonsils (behind the fauces) for colour, discharge and size.	Pink and smooth No discharge Of normal size or not visible	Inflamed Presence of discharge Swollen
14 Elicit the gag reflex by pressing the posterior tongue with a tongue blade.	Present	Absent (may indicate problems with glossopharyngeal or vagus nerves)

Evaluation

- Perform a detailed follow-up examination of neurological and other systems based on findings that deviated from expected or normal for the patient. Relate findings to previous assessment data if available.
- Document findings in the patient notes.
- Report significant deviations from normal to medical staff.

LIFESPAN CONSIDERATIONS

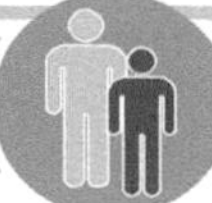

Assessing the Mouth and Oropharynx

Infants

- Inspect the palate for a cleft.

Children

- Tooth development should be appropriate for age.
- White spots on the teeth may indicate excessive fluoride ingestion.
- Drooling is common up to two years of age.
- The tonsils are normally larger in children than in adults and commonly extend beyond the palatine arch until the age of 11 or 12 years.

Mature Adults

- Decreased saliva production leads to dry oral mucosa.
- Some receding of the gums occurs, giving an appearance of increased toothiness.
- There may be a brownish pigmentation to the gums, especially in black people.
- Taste sensations diminish. Sweet and salty tastes are lost first.
- The teeth may show signs of staining, erosion, chipping and abrasions due to loss of dentin.
- Tooth loss occurs as a result of dental disease but is preventable with good dental hygiene.
- The gag reflex may be slightly sluggish.

THE NECK

Examination of the neck includes the muscles, lymph nodes, trachea, thyroid gland, carotid arteries and jugular veins (Figure 11-20). When the side of the neck is presented it can be divided into four sections:

1. Above – the lower part of the mandible and the imaginary line going from the mandible to the mastoid process (below the temporal bone).
2. Below – from the upper edge of the clavicle.
3. Front – the middle line of the neck.
4. Behind – the upper margin of the **trapezius** (see Figure 11-21).

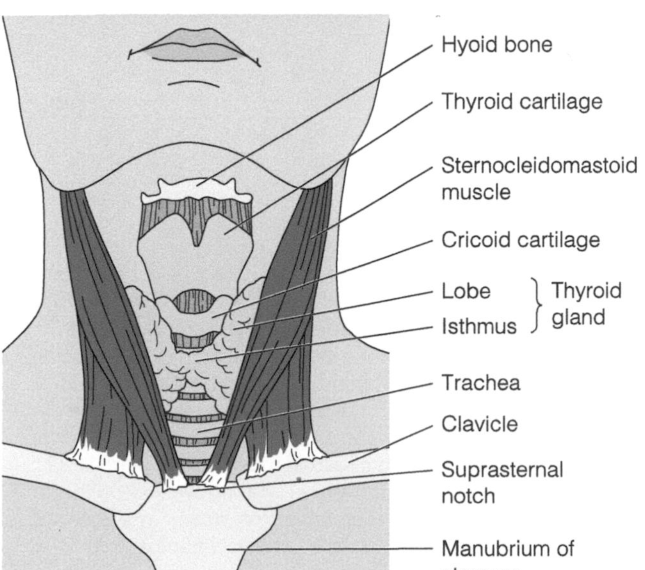

Figure 11-20 Structures of the neck.

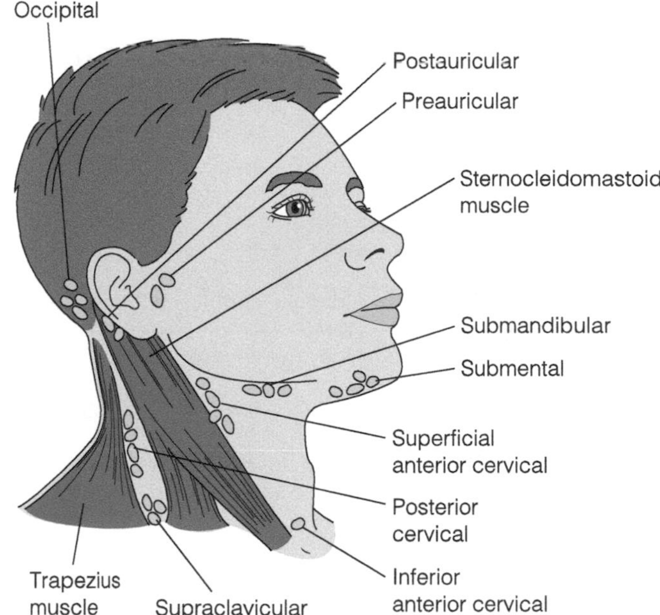

Figure 11-21 Lymph nodes of the neck.

The areas of the neck are defined by the sternocleidomastoid muscle which divides into two triangles, the anterior and posterior muscle either side of the neck. The anterior muscle contains the trachea, thyroid gland, anterior cervical nodes and the carotid artery. The posterior muscle contains the lymph nodes, and in human beings there are approximately 40 lymph nodes situated in the neck (see Table 11-2). The lymph nodes, referred to as *chains*, act as traps and filters and collect **lymph** (intestinal fluid) from the head and neck structures (see Figure 11-21). Swollen or inflamed lymph nodes are an early indicator of infection or a cancer due to their function within the immune system. There are between 500 and 700 lymph nodes found around the body with the most common areas being the neck, armpit or groin. Palpating the neck (see Figure 11-22) will often identify swollen lymph nodes or glands (more commonly known). During a neck examination of the lower frontal part of the neck may indicate a thyroid goitre and further tests may be required to confirm a diagnosis of hyperthyroidism.

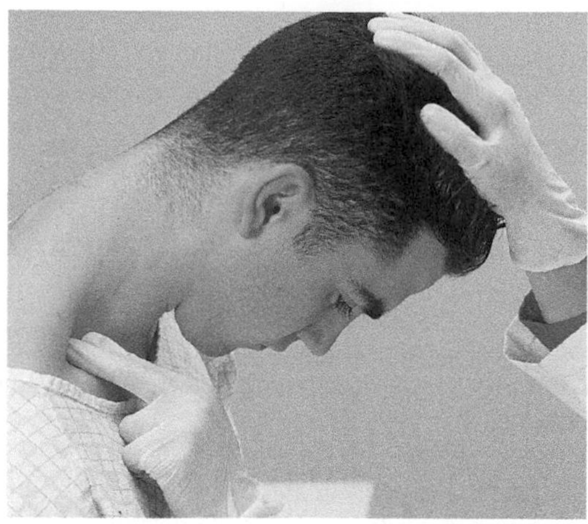

Figure 11-22 Palpating the supraclavicular lymph nodes.

ACTIVITY 11-1

During the admission and assessment process you note that the patient has a swelling at the lower frontal part of the neck. The patient appears to be unaware of the swelling. How would you manage the situation in the best interest for the well-being of the patient?

Table 11-2 Lymph Nodes of the Head and Neck

Node centre	Location	Part of the body drained of lymph
Head		
Occipital	At the posterior base of the skull	The occipital region of the scalp and the deep structures of the back of the neck
Postauricular (mastoid)	Behind the auricle of the ear or in front of the mastoid process	The parietal region of the head and part of the ear
Preauricular	In front of the tragus of the ear	The forehead and upper face
Floor of mouth		
Submandibular (submaxillary)	Along the medial border of the lower jaw, halfway between the angle of the jaw and the chin	The chin, upper lip, cheek, nose, teeth, eyelids, part of the tongue and the floor of the mouth
Submental	Behind the tip of the mandible in the midline, under the chin	The anterior third of the tongue, gums and floor of the mouth
Neck		
Superficial (anterior) cervical chain	Along the anterior to the sternocleidomastoid muscle	The skin and neck
Posterior cervical chain	Along the anterior aspect of the trapezius muscle	The posterior and lateral regions of the neck, occiput and mastoid
Deep cervical chain	Under the sternocleidomastoid muscle	The larynx, thyroid gland, trachea and upper part of the oesophagus
Supraclavicular	Above the clavicle, in the angle between the clavicle and the sternocleidomastoid muscle	The lateral regions of the neck and lungs

PRACTICE GUIDELINES

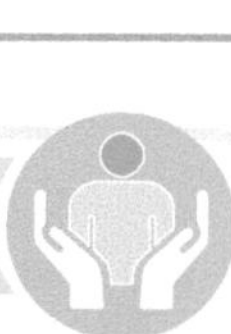

Palpating Neck Lymph Nodes

- Explain to the patient what you are going to do and how it will influence treatment.
- Obtain consent.
- Maintain patient dignity and privacy.
- Face the patient and bend the patient's head forward slightly or towards the side being examined to relax the soft tissue and muscles.
- Palpate the nodes using the pads of the fingers. Move the fingertips in a gentle rotating motion.
- When examining the submental and submandibular nodes, place the fingertips under the mandible on the side nearest the palpating hand, and pull the skin and subcutaneous tissue laterally over the mandibular surface so that the tissue rolls over the nodes.
- When palpating the supraclavicular nodes, have the patient bend the head forward to relax the tissues of the anterior neck and to relax the shoulders so that the clavicles drop. Use your hand nearest the side to be examined when facing the patient, i.e. your left hand for the patient's right nodes. Use your free hand to flex the patient's head forward if necessary. Hook your index and third fingers over the clavicle lateral to the sternocleidomastoid muscle (see Figure 11-22).
- When palpating the anterior cervical nodes and posterior cervical nodes, move your fingertips slowly in a forward circular motion against the sternocleidomastoid and trapezius muscles, respectively.
- To palpate the deep cervical nodes, bend or hook your fingers around the sternocleidomastoid muscle.

THE THORAX AND LUNGS

The thorax is the part of the body between the neck and the diaphragm, and encases the lungs. The lungs are the respiratory organs that are essential for human beings to breath and are discussed in greater detail in Chapter 16. Assessment of this system is critical. Changes in the respiratory system can come about slowly or quickly. In patients with chronic obstructive pulmonary disease (COPD), such as chronic bronchitis, emphysema and asthma, changes are frequently gradual.

An inspection of the shape and size of the thorax and lungs will indicate as to whether a patient is experiencing respiratory problems as, for example, some people with chronic respiratory problems tend to bend forward or even prop their arms on a support (e.g. bed table) to elevate the clavicle thus making breathing easier.

Chest Shape and Size

In adults, the thorax is normally oval in shape; any deviation from the 'norm' could indicate health problems. There are several deformities of the chest (see Figure 11-23), for example a pigeon chest (*pectus carinatum*) is a permanent deformity possibly caused by rickets, a funnel chest (*pectus excavatum*) is a congenital defect and a barrel chest is seen with patients with kyphosis and emphysema.

Breath Sounds

Abnormal breath sounds are the result of air passing through narrowed airways or airways filled with fluid or mucus, or when pleural linings are inflamed. Table 11-3 describes normal breath sounds. Sounds such as crackles (referred to as crepitations,

Table 11-3 Normal Breath Sounds

Type	Description	Location
Vesicular	Soft low pitched or 'gentle' sighing sounds	Over peripheral lung; best heard at base of lungs
Broncho-vesicular	Moderate-pitched 'blowing' sounds created by air moving through larger airway (bronchi)	Between the scapulae and lateral to the sternum at the first or second intercostals spaces.
Bronchial (tubular)	High-pitched, loud, 'harsh' sounds created by air moving through the trachea	Anteriorly over the trachea; not normally heard over lung tissue

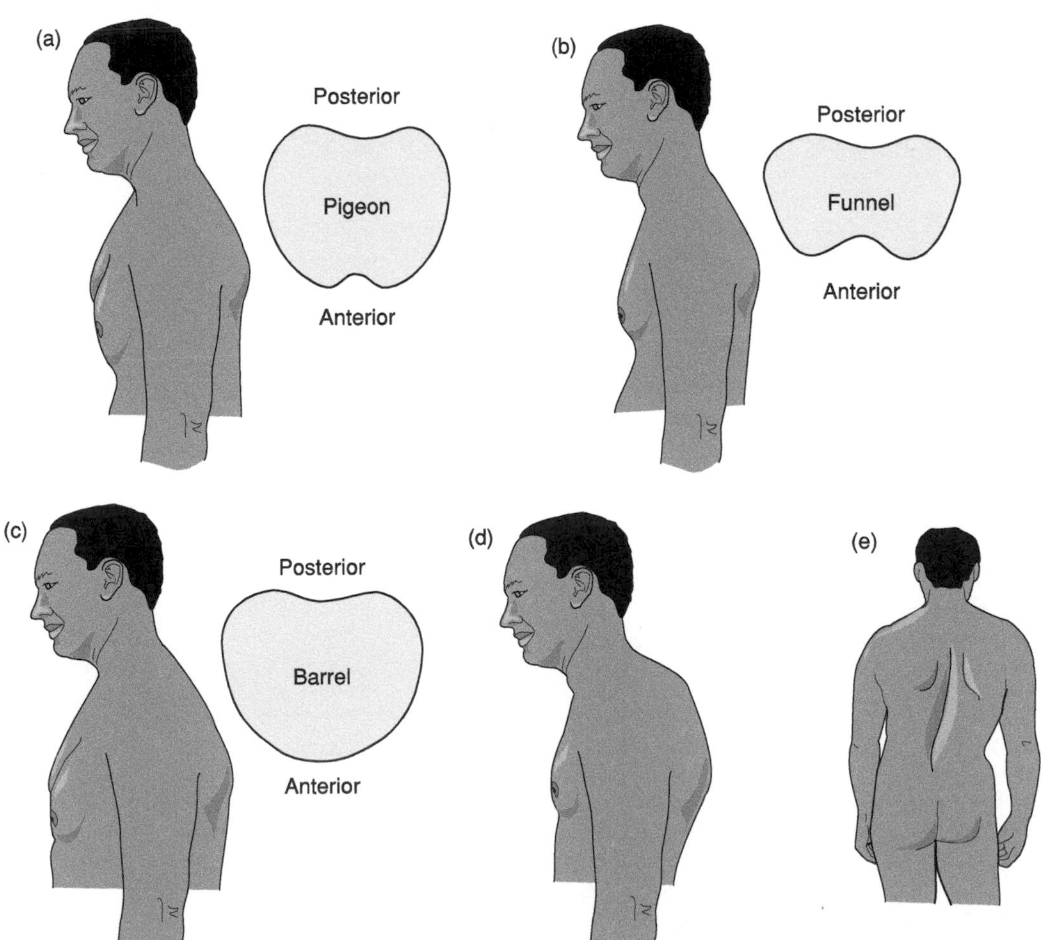

Figure 11-23 Chest deformities. (a) pigeon chest; (b) funnel chest; (c) barrel chest; (d) kyphosis; (e) scoliosis.

Table 11-4 Abnormal Breath Sounds

Name	Description	Cause	Location
Crackles (rales)	Fine crackling sounds. Sound can be simulated by rolling a lock of hair near the ear. Best heard on inspiration but can be heard on both inspiration and expiration. May not be cleared by coughing.	Air passing through fluid or mucus in any air passage. Course crackles can indicate chest infection or pneumonia.	Most commonly heard in the bases of the lower lung lobes.
Gurgles (rhonchi)	Continuous, low-pitched, coarse, gurgling, harsh, louder sounds with a moaning or snoring quality. Best heard on expiration but can be heard on both inspiration and expiration. May be altered by coughing.	Air passing through narrowed air passages as a result of secretions, swelling, tumours.	Loud sounds can be heard over most lung areas but predominate over the trachea and bronchi.
Friction rub	Superficial grating or creaking sounds heard during inspiration and expiration. Not relieved by coughing.	Rubbing together of inflamed pleural surfaces. Can be a sign of pleural effusion (collection of fluid between the pleural membranes).	Heard most often in areas of greatest thoracic expansion (e.g. lower anterior and lateral chest).
Wheeze	Continuous, high-pitched, squeaky musical sounds. Best heard on expiration. Not usually altered by coughing.	Air passing through a constricted bronchus as a result of secretions, swelling, tumours. A wheeze heard on expiration is a classic sign of asthma.	Heard over all lung fields.

gurgles, pleural friction rubs and wheezes) are often heard above normal breath sounds (see Table 11-4 for a description of these). Absence of breath sounds over some lung areas is also a significant finding, and is usually associated with collapsed and surgically removed lobes.

Assessment of the lungs and thorax includes all methods of examination: inspection, palpation, percussion and auscultation. *Procedure 11-7* describes how to assess the thorax and lungs.

PROCEDURE 11-7 Assessing the Thorax and Lungs

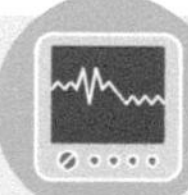

Purpose

- To examine the exterior respiratory system for early detection of any respiratory problems that may occur.

Assessment

- Ensure that the patient is in the correct position to enable the nurse to observe and record the information and accurate results and diagnosis to be made.
- Ensure that the environment is suitable for this type of examination.
- When respirations are being recorded try not to raise the patient's awareness to this as it can provide an incorrect reading.

Planning

For efficiency, the nurse usually examines the back of the patient's chest first, then the front of the chest. When examining the back or side of the chest the patient should be in a sitting position. A lying or sitting position may be preferred when examining the front of the chest.

Equipment

- Stethoscope

Implementation

Performance

Follow local policy to ensure that you explain to the patient what you are going to do, why it is necessary and how they can cooperate. Obtain consent and maintain patient privacy and dignity and ensure that the appropriate local infection control procedures are observed. Enquire if the patient has any history of the following: family history of illness, including cancer, allergies, tuberculosis; lifestyle habits such as smoking and occupational hazards (e.g. inhaling fumes); any medications being taken; current problems (e.g. swellings, coughs, wheezing and pain).

Assessment	Normal findings	Deviations from normal
1 Inspect the shape of the thorax from both back and side views.	The breathing from the back of the chest to the front (cross section) should be done symmetrically.	Barrel chest. Asymmetric.
2 Chest movement (front) should be observed and comparisons should be made between both sides of the chest.	Quiet, rhythmic and effortless respirations. Inhalation and exhalation should be carried out simultaneously with both sides of the chest walls symmetric during the whole process.	Patients in respiratory distress will use accessory muscles in the neck and shoulders to help them expand their lungs.
3 The colour of the patient's skin should be observed.	The skin should be the accepted skin colour for the patient.	Any bluish tint to the skin or mucous membranes indicates cyanosis.
4 Observe and monitor the patient's respiratory rate for one minute or longer, and record and report any abnormalities noted.	Adults normally breathe at a rate of between 12 and 20 breaths/minute. It is important to recognise that lifespan considerations should be deliberated as normal readings will differ depending on age.	See Chapter 16 for abnormal respiratory patterns.
5 Percuss the thorax and monitor and record sounds	Percussion notes resonate, except over scapula. Lowest point of resonance is at the diaphragm.	Asymmetry in percussion. Areas of dullness or flatness over lung tissue (associated with consolidation of lung tissue or a mass).
6 Ausculate the chest using the flat-disc diaphragm of the stethoscope (best for transmitting the high-pitched breath sounds). a. Use the systematic zigzag procedure used in percussion (see Figure 11-24). b. Ask the patient to take slow, deep breaths through the mouth. Listen at each point to the breath sounds during a complete inspiration and expiration. c. Compare findings at each point with the corresponding point on the opposite side of the chest.	Vesicular and bronchovesicular breath sounds (see Table 11-3). 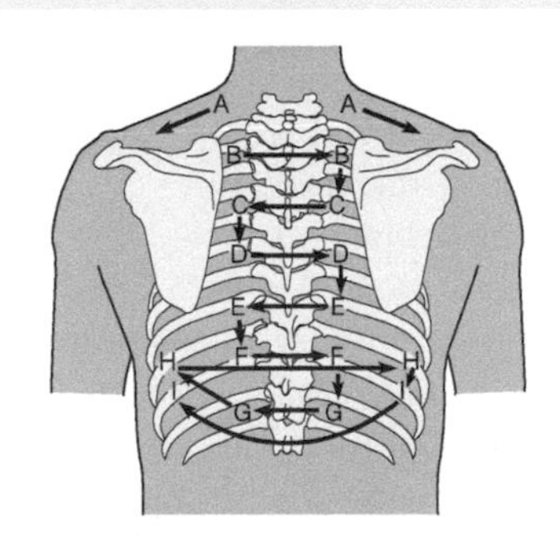 **Figure 11-24** Sequence for posterior chest percussion.	Abnormal breath sounds (e.g. crackles, rhonchi, wheeze, friction rub; see Table 11-4). Absence of breath sounds (associated with collapsed and surgically removed lung lobes).
Anterior thorax		
7 Repeat steps 1-6 for the anterior thorax.		

Evaluation

- Relate findings to previous assessment data if available. Report significant deviations from normal to the doctor.
- Document findings in the patient record using forms or checklists supplemented by narrative notes when appropriate.

LIFESPAN CONSIDERATIONS

Assessing the Thorax and Lungs

Infants

- The thorax is usually rounded.
- Ausculated sounds will be louder and harsher.
- Infants tend to breathe more abdominally than thoracically.

Children

- Children tend to breathe more abdominally than thoracically up to age six.

Mature Adults

- The thoracic curvature may be accentuated because of osteoporosis and changes in cartilage, resulting in collapse of the vertebrae. This can also compromise and decrease normal respiratory effort.
- Breathing rate and rhythm are unchanged at rest; the rate normally increases with exercise but may take longer to return to the pre-exercise rate.
- Expiration may require the use of accessory muscles.
- Cilia in the airways decrease in number and are less effective in removing mucus; older patients are therefore at greater risk for pulmonary infections.

CARDIOVASCULAR AND PERIPHERAL VASCULAR SYSTEMS

Heart

In the average adult, most of the heart lies behind and to the left of the sternum. A small portion (the right atrium) extends to the right of the sternum. The upper portion of the heart (atria) lies towards the back. The lower part of the heart (ventricles) points anteriorly. The apex (bottom) of the left ventricle actually touches the chest wall slightly below the left nipple. This point where the apex touches the anterior chest wall is known as the point of maximal impulse (PMI).

It is important to assess the heart by initially observing the appearance of the patient and noting, for example, the patient's colour and clubbing of fingers for hypoxia. Equally it is important to examine the precordium, the area of the chest overlying the heart, for the presence of abnormal pulsations or heaves or lifts. The term heave refers to the rise along the sterna wall with each heartbeat. It should be confirmed by palpation with the palm of the hand. Enlargement of the left ventricle produces a heave lateral to the apex, whereas enlargement of the right ventricle produces a heave at or near the sternum.

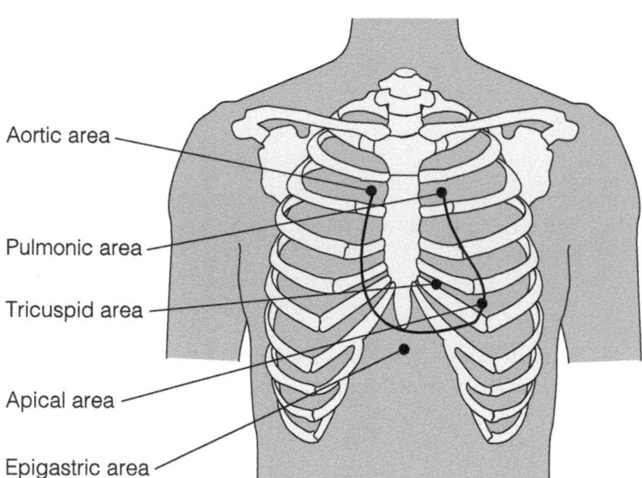

Figure 11-25 Anatomic sites of the precordium.

Ausculation is often used to hear heart sounds. The first two heart sounds heard are produced by closure of the valves of the heart. The first heart sound, S1, occurs when the atrioventricular (A–V) valves close when a dull, low-pitched sound described as 'lub' is heard via the stethoscope. After the ventricles empty their blood into the aorta and pulmonary arteries, the semilunar valves close, producing the second heart sound, S2, described as 'dub'. S_2 has a higher pitch than S_1 and is also shorter. These two sounds, S_1 and S_2 ('lub-dub'), occur within a second or less, depending on the heart rate. These heart sounds are audible anywhere in the precordium, but they are best heard over the aortic, pulmonic, tricuspid and apical areas (see Figure 11-25).

The experienced nurse may perceive extra heart sounds (S_3 and S_4) during diastole. Both sounds (S_3 and S_4) are low in pitch and heard best at the apical site, with the bell of the stethoscope, and with the patient lying on the left side. S_3 occurs early in diastole right after S_2 and sounds like 'lub-dub-*ee*' (S_1, S_2, S_3). It often disappears when the patient sits up. S_3 is normal in children and young adults. In mature adults, it may indicate heart failure. It occurs near the very end of diastole just before S_1 and creates the sound of '*dee*-lub-dub' (S_4, S_1, S_2). S_4 is rarely heard in healthy young adults. S_4 may be heard in many older patients and can be a sign of hypertension.

Palpation is another means of measuring for an apical pulse, often used when the doctor is concerned about the cardiac function and output of the heart (see Chapter 15).

Central Vessels

The carotid arteries supply oxygenated blood to the head and neck (see Figure 11-26). Because they are the only source of blood to the brain, prolonged occlusion (blockage) of these arteries can result in serious brain damage.

The carotid artery can be auscultated for a bruit, and if a bruit is found, the carotid artery is then palpated for a thrill. A bruit (a blowing or swishing sound) is created by turbulence of blood flow due either to a narrowed arterial lumen (space in the centre of an artery) (a common development in older people) or to a condition, such as **anaemia** or hyperthyroidism, which elevates cardiac output. A thrill, which frequently accompanies a bruit, is a vibrating sensation like the purring of a cat or water running through a hose. It, too, indicates turbulent blood flow due to arterial obstruction.

The jugular veins drain blood from the head and neck directly into the superior vena cava and right side of the heart. Normally the external jugular vein is superficial and may be visible, while the internal jugular vein may only be visible when the patient is lying flat. Right-sided heart failure may be indicated when there is evidence of bilateral jugular vein distention.

Procedure 11-8 describes how to assess the heart and central vessels.

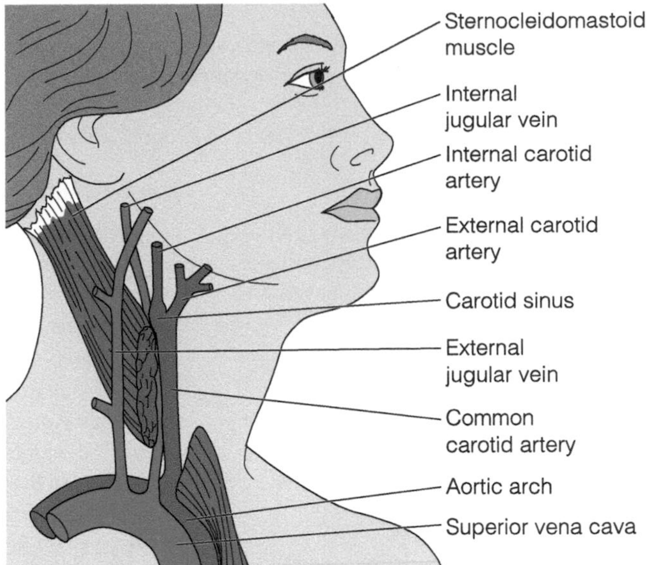

Figure 11-26 Arteries and veins of the right side of the neck.

PROCEDURE 11-8 Assessing the Heart and Central Vessels

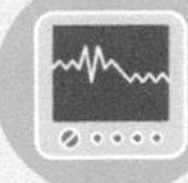

Purpose

- To monitor the function of the heart and for early detection of internal and external abnormalities of cardiac input and output.

Assessment

- Observe skin and the colour of the mucosa and for any clubbing of nails as they are an early indication of cardiac problems.
- Place the patient in a semi-recumbant position.

Planning

Heart examinations are usually performed while the patient is in a semi-recumbant position. The practitioner stands at the patient's right side, where palpation of the cardiac area is facilitated and optimal inspection allowed.

Equipment

- Stethoscope

Implementation

Performance

Follow local policy to ensure that you explain to the patient what you are going to do, why it is necessary and how they can cooperate. Obtain consent and maintain patient privacy and dignity and ensure that the appropriate local infection control procedures are observed. Enquire if the patient has any history of the following: family history of incidence and age of heart disease, high cholesterol levels, high blood pressure, stroke, obesity, congenital heart disease, arterial disease, hypertension and rheumatic fever; patient's past history of rheumatic fever, heart murmur, heart attack, varicosities or heart failure; present symptoms indicative of heart disease (e.g. fatigue, dyspnoea, orthopnea, oedema, cough, chest pain, palpitations, syncope, hypertension, wheezing, haemoptysis); presence of diseases that affect heart (e.g. obesity, diabetes, lung disease, endocrine disorders); lifestyle habits that are risk factors for cardiac disease (e.g. smoking, alcohol intake, eating and exercise patterns, areas and degree of stress perceived).

Assessment	Normal findings	Deviations from normal
1 Simultaneously inspect and palpate the precordium for the presence of abnormal pulsations or heaves.	No pulsations	
2 Auscultate the heart	S_1: Usually heard at all sites. Usually louder at apical area S_2: Usually heard at all sites. Usually louder at base of heart Systole: silent interval; slightly shorter duration than diastole at normal heart rate (60–90 beats/min) Diastole: silent interval; slightly longer duration than systole at normal heart rates S_3 in children and young adults S_4 in many older adults	Increased or decreased intensity Varying intensity with different beats Increased intensity at aortic area Increased intensity at pulmonic area Sharp-sounding ejection clicks S_3 in older adults S_4 may be a sign of hypertension
Jugular veins		
3 Inspect the jugular veins for distention while the patient is placed in a semi-Fowler's position (sitting up at a 30° to 45° angle), with the head supported on a small pillow.	Veins not visible (indicating right side of heart is functioning normally)	Veins visibly distended (indicating advanced cardiopulmonary disease)

Evaluation

- Perform a detailed follow-up examination based on findings that deviated from expected or normal for the patient. Relate findings to previous assessment data if available.
- Document findings in the patient record using forms or checklists supplemented by narrative notes when appropriate.
- Report significant deviations from normal to medical staff.

LIFESPAN CONSIDERATIONS

Assessing the Heart and Central Vessels

Children

- Heart sounds are louder because of the thinner chest wall.
- A third heart sound, best heard at the apex, is present in about one-third of all children.

Mature Adults

- If no disease is present, heart size remains the same size throughout life.
- Cardiac output and strength of contraction decrease with age.
- The heart rate returns to its resting rate more slowly after exertion than it did when the individual was younger.
- S_4 heart sound is considered normal in older adults.

Peripheral Vascular System

Assessing the peripheral vascular system includes measuring the blood pressure, palpating peripheral pulses, and inspecting the skin and tissues to determine perfusion (blood supply to an area) to the extremities. Certain aspects of peripheral vascular assessment are often incorporated into other parts of the assessment procedure. For example, blood pressure is usually measured at the beginning of the physical examination (see the section on assessing blood pressure in Chapter 15).

Procedure 11-9 describes how to assess the peripheral vascular system.

PROCEDURE 11-9 Assessing the Peripheral Vascular System

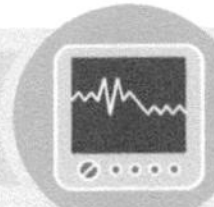

Purpose

- To monitor the cardiac output of the heart.

Assessment

- Appropriate environment.
- Patient's medical history.
- Underlying medical condition or treatment.

Planning

Equipment

- None

Implementation

Performance

Follow local policy to ensure that you explain to the patient what you are going to do, why it is necessary and how they can cooperate. Obtain consent and maintain patient privacy and dignity and ensure that the appropriate local infection control procedures are observed. Enquire if the patient has any history of the following: past history of heart disorders, varicosities, arterial disease and hypertension; lifestyle habits such as exercise patterns, activity patterns and tolerance, smoking and use of alcohol.

Assessment	Normal findings	Deviations from normal
Peripheral pulses		
1 Palpate the peripheral pulses (except the carotid pulse) on both sides of the patient's body individually, simultaneously, and systematically to determine the symmetry of the pulses.	Symmetric pulse readings	Asymmetric pulses readings. Absence of pulsation can indicate arterial spasm or occlusion. Decreased, weak, thready pulsations indicate impaired cardiac output (the amount of blood pumped out of the heart each minute). Increased pulse volume (may indicate hypertension, high cardiac output or circulatory overload).
Peripheral perfusion		
2 Inspect the skin of the hands and feet for colour, temperature, oedema and skin changes.	Skin colour pink	Cyanotic (venous insufficiency). Pallor that increases with limb elevation. Dusky red colour when limb is lowered (arterial insufficiency). Brown pigmentation around ankles (arterial or chronic venous insufficiency).
	Skin temperature not excessively warm or cold	Skin cool (arterial insufficiency).
	No oedema	Marked oedema (venous insufficiency). Mild oedema (arterial insufficiency).
	Skin texture resilient and moist	Skin thin and shiny or thick, waxy, shiny and fragile, with reduced hair and ulceration (venous or arterial insufficiency).
3 Assess the adequacy of arterial flow if arterial insufficiency is suspected.	Capillary refill test: immediate return of colour	Delayed return of colour (arterial insufficiency).

Evaluation

- Perform a detailed follow-up examination of the heart or central vessels, integument or other systems based on findings that deviated from expected or normal for the patient. Relate findings to previous assessment data if available.
- Document findings in the patient record using forms or checklists supplemented by narrative notes when appropriate.
- Report significant deviations from normal to medical staff.

When assessing the adequacy of an arterial blood flow capillary refill test the following should be considered:

- Squeeze the patient's fingernail and toenail between your fingers sufficiently to cause blanching.
- Release the pressure, and observe how quickly normal colour returns. Colour normally returns immediately.

LIFESPAN CONSIDERATIONS

Assessing the Peripheral Vascular System

Infants

- Palpation of the pulses in the lower extremities (particularly the femoral pulses) is essential to screen for coarctation (narrowing) of the aorta.

Mature Adults

- Peripheral vascular assessment should always include upper and lower extremities temperature, colour, pulses, oedema, skin integrity and sensation. Any differences in symmetry of these findings should be noted.
- Peripheral oedema is frequently observed and is most commonly the result of chronic venous insufficiency or low protein levels in the blood (hypoproteinaemia).

BREASTS AND AXILLAE

The breast is situated at the front of the chest. The breasts of both male and females have a raised nipple surrounded by a pigmented areola. The breast can be divided into two quadrants (see Figure 11-27): the upper quadrant contains the largest quantity of breast tissue, and the upper outer quadrant is where most breast tumours are located known as the *axillary tail of Spence* (see Figure 11-27).

The general structures of both male and female breasts are similar until puberty. In the female the breasts enlarge during puberty which may cause some pain (pain may also be experienced by some boys). The mammary glands are situated within the breasts and in adult females they are made of adipose tissue which gives the breast its shape and covers the 15–20 glandular lobes. Each lobe has a duct that has the ability to produce milk. Fibrocystic changes in the breast are benign, however regular examination of the breast is required for early detection of malignant tumours.

Both men and women should self examine themselves on a monthly basis. Examination of breast can be extremely stressful for the patient therefore the nurse must ensure that the patient's privacy and dignity are maintained throughout. Macmillan Cancer Support (2008) suggest that breast examination should not only be done routinely once a month but more irregularly so that the individual is aware of changes within their breast.

Macmillan Cancer Support (2008) state that when an individual is examining their breast they should look for:

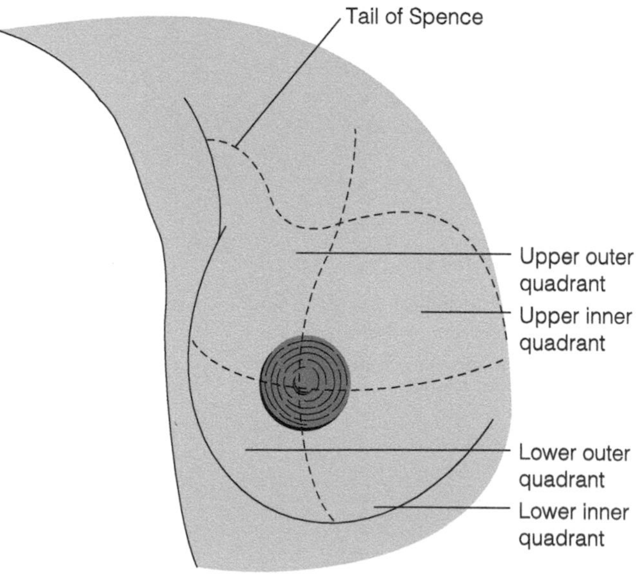

Figure 11-27 Four breast quadrants and the axillary tail of Spence.

- appearance – changes to outline or shape;
- lumps – new or thickening lumps, prominent lymph nodes (see Figure 11-28);
- feelings – discomfort or pain;
- nipple changes – bleeding, change of nipple position, rash and skin colour.

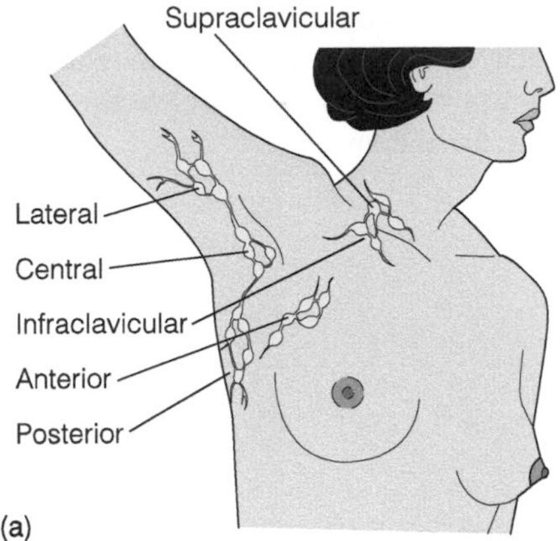

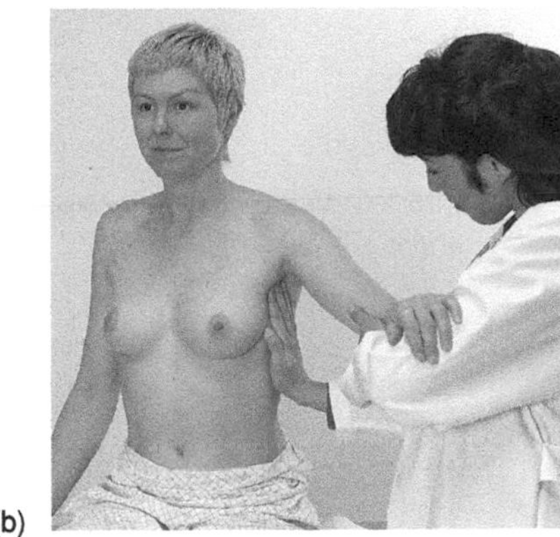

Figure 11-28 Location and palpation of the lymph nodes that drain the lateral breast. (a) Lymph nodes; (b) palpating the axilla.

It is a fundamental part of a nurse's role to educate and provide health promotion to patients in their care by openly discussing these issues with the patient provided they have given their consent.

ABDOMEN

The abdomen lies between the thorax and the pelvis. The abdomen is made up of the alimentary canal and it is where most of the absorption and digestion of food occurs. The abdomen consists of the liver, stomach transverse and descending colon, umbilicus small intestine ascending and sigmoid colon, bladder and pubic symphasis (see Figure 11-29).

The abdomen can be divided into four quarters; the right upper quadrant (*1*), left upper quadrant (*2*), right lower quadrant (*3*) and left lower quadrant (*4*). Specific organs or parts of organs lie in each abdominal quadrant.

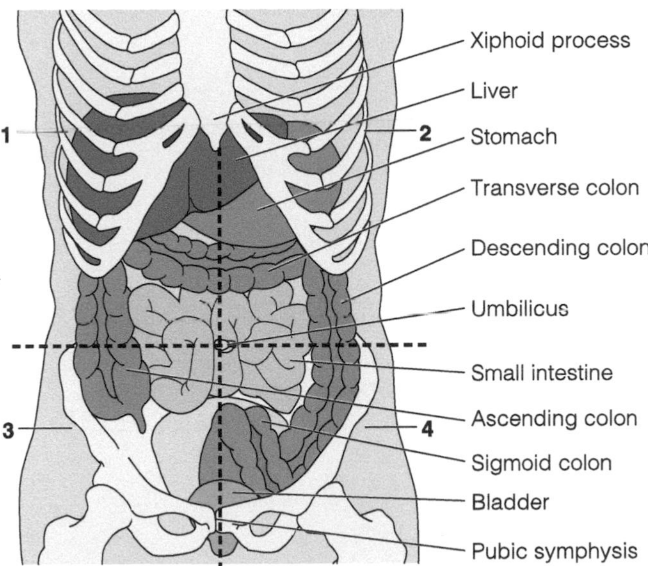

Figure 11-29 The four abdominal quadrants and the underlying organs: *1*, right upper quadrant; *2*, left upper quadrant; *3*, right lower quadrant; *4*, left lower quadrant.

BOX 11-5 Organs in the Four Abdominal Quadrants

Right upper quadrant

Liver	Gallbladder	Duodenum
Head of pancreas	Right adrenal gland	Upper lobe of right kidney
Hepatic flexure of colon	Section of ascending colon	Section of transverse colon

Right lower quadrant

Lower lobe of right kidney	Caecum	Appendix
Section of ascending colon	Right ovary	Right fallopian tube
Right ureter	Right spermatic cord	Part of uterus

Left upper quadrant

Left lobe of liver	Stomach	Spleen
Upper lobe of left kidney	Pancreas	Left adrenal gland
Splenic flexure of colon	Section of transverse colon	Section of descending colon

Left lower quadrant

Lower lobe of left kidney	Sigmoid colon	Section of descending colon
Left ovary	Left fallopian tube	Left ureter
Left spermatic cord	Part of uterus	

Assessment of the abdomen involves all four methods of examination (inspection, auscultation, palpation and percussion). When assessing the abdomen, the nurse performs inspection first, followed by auscultation, percussion and/or palpation. Auscultation is done before palpation and percussion because palpation and percussion cause movement or stimulation of the bowel, which can increase bowel motility and thus heighten bowel sounds, creating false results. *Procedure 11-10* describes how to assess the abdomen.

PROCEDURE 11-10 Assessing the Abdomen

Purpose

- To identify any external and or internal abnormalities within the abdominal wall and cavity.

Assessment

- Positioning of patient.
- Temperature of any equipment used.
- Environment.
- Level of pain if patient in pain.
- Whether a sample of urine is required for testing.
- Whether the patient is feeling nauseous.
- Religious or cultural beliefs.

Planning

- Ask the patient to urinate since an empty bladder makes the assessment more comfortable.
- Ensure that the room is warm since the patient will be exposed.

Equipment

- Examining light
- Tape measure
- Stethoscope

Implementation

Performance

Follow local policy to ensure that you explain to the patient what you are going to do, why it is necessary and how they can cooperate. Obtain consent and maintain patient privacy and dignity and ensure that the appropriate local infection control procedures are observed. Enquire if the patient has any history of the following: incidence of abdominal pain: its location, onset, sequence and chronology; its quality (description); its frequency; associated symptoms (e.g. nausea, vomiting, diarrhoea); bowel habits; incidence of constipation or diarrhoea (have patient describe what they mean by these terms); change in appetite, food intolerances and foods ingested in last 24 hours; specific signs and symptoms (e.g. heartburn, flatulence and/or belching, difficulty swallowing, haematemesis (vomiting blood), blood or mucus in stools, and aggravating and alleviating factors; previous problems and treatment (e.g. stomach ulcer, gallbladder surgery, history of jaundice).

Assist the patient to a **supine** position, with the arms placed comfortably at the sides. Place small pillows beneath the knees and the head to reduce tension in the abdominal muscles. Expose only the patient's abdomen from chest line to the pubic area to avoid chilling and shivering, which can tense the abdominal muscles.

Assessment	Normal findings	Deviations from normal
Inspection of the abdomen		
1 Inspect the abdomen for skin integrity (refer to the discussion of skin assessment, earlier in this chapter).	Unblemished skin Uniform colour	Presence of rash or other lesions Tense, glistening skin (may indicate ascites or oedema).
2 Inspect the abdomen for contour and symmetry:	Silver-white striae (stretch marks) or surgical scars	Purple striae (associated with Cushing's disease; a hormonal disorder resulting in upper body obesity which makes the skin fragile and prone to bruising)

• Observe the abdominal contour while standing at the patient's side when the patient is supine.	Flat, rounded (convex) or scaphoid (concave)	Distended
• Ask the patient to take a deep breath and to hold it *(makes an enlarged liver or spleen more obvious).*	No evidence of enlargement of liver or spleen	Evidence of enlargement of liver or spleen
• Assess the symmetry of contour while standing at the foot of the bed.	Symmetric contour	Asymmetric contour (e.g. localised protrusions around umbilicus, inguinal ligaments or scars (possible hernia or tumour)
• If distension is present, measure the abdominal girth by placing a tape around the abdomen at the level of the umbilicus (see Figure 11-30).		
3 Observe abdominal movements associated with respiration, peristalsis or aortic pulsations.	Symmetric movements caused by respiration. Visible peristalsis in very lean people. Aortic pulsations in thin persons at epigastric area.	Limited movement due to pain or disease process. Visible peristalsis in nonlean patients (with bowel obstruction). Marked aortic pulsations
Auscultation of the abdomen		
4 Auscultate the abdomen for bowel sounds.	Audible bowel sounds	Absent, hypoactive or hyperactive bowel sounds
Percussion of the abdomen		
5 Percuss several areas in each of the four quadrants to determine presence of tympany (gas in stomach and intestines) and dullness (decrease, absence or flatness of resonance over solid masses or fluid). Use a systematic pattern (see Figure 11-31).	Tympany over the stomach and gas-filled bowels; dullness, especially over the liver and spleen, or a full bladder	Large dull areas (associated with presence of fluid or a tumour)
Percussion of the liver		
6 Percuss the liver to determine its size.	6-12cm in the midclavicular line; 4-8cm at the midsternal line	Enlarged size (associated with liver disease)
Palpation of the abdomen		
7 Perform light palpation first to detect areas of tenderness and/or muscle guarding. Systematically explore all four quadrants. See below for palpation technique.	No tenderness; relaxed abdomen with smooth, consistent tension	Tenderness and hypersensitivity Superficial masses Localised areas of increased tension
8 Perform deep palpation over all four quadrants. See the *Practice Guidelines* below.	Tenderness may be present near xiphoid process, over caecum and over sigmoid colon	Generalised or localised areas of tenderness Mobile or fixed masses
Palpation of the liver		
9 Palpate the liver to detect enlargement and tenderness.	May not be palpable Border feels smooth	Enlarged (abnormal finding, even if liver is smooth and not tender) Smooth but tender; nodular or hard
Palpation of the bladder		
10 Palpate the area above the pubic symphysis if the patient's history indicates possible urinary retention (see Figure 11-32).	Not palpable	Distended and palpable as smooth, round, tense mass (indicates urinary retention)

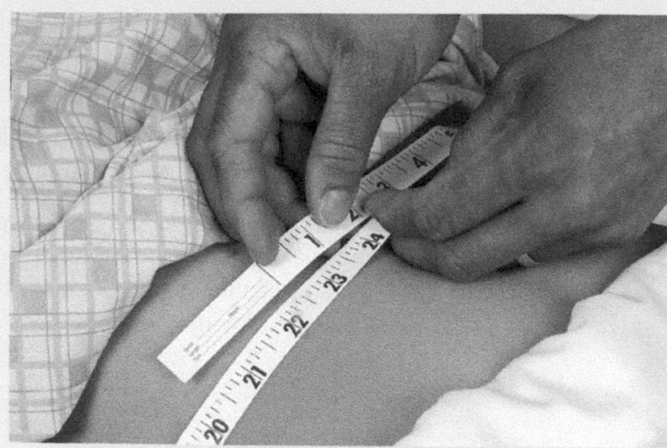
Figure 11-30 Measuring abdominal girth.

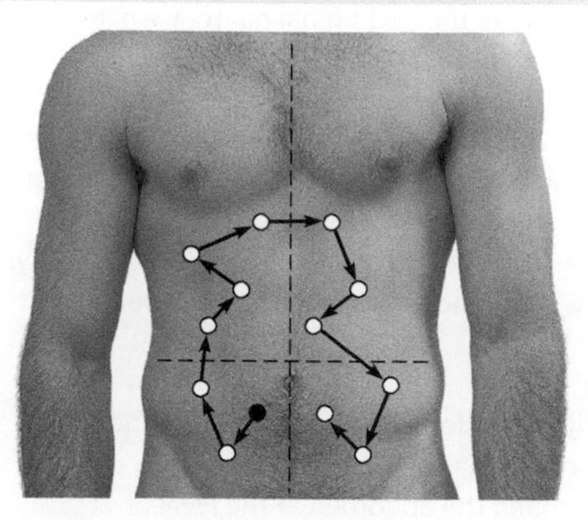
Figure 11-31 Systematic percussion sites for all four quadrants.

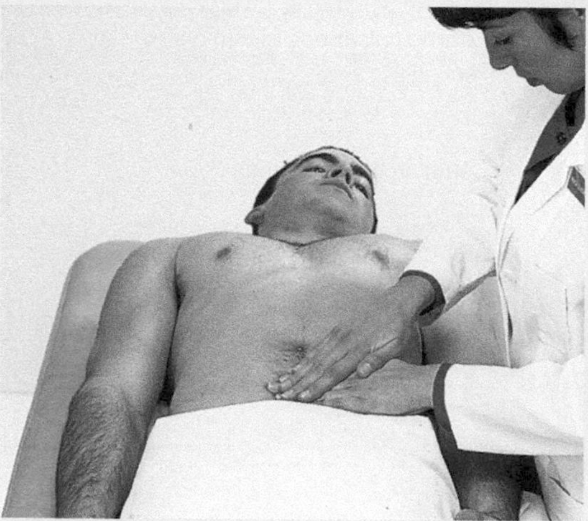
Figure 11-32 Palpating the bladder.

Evaluation

- Relate the findings of this examination to previous assessment data.
- Document findings in the patient record using forms or checklists supplemented by narrative notes when appropriate.
- Report any significant abnormalities to the medical staff.

PRACTICE GUIDELINES

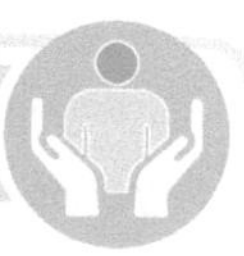

Auscultating the Abdomen

Warm the hands and the stethoscope diaphragms. Cold hands and a cold stethoscope may cause the patient to contract the abdominal muscles, and these contractions may be heard during auscultation.

For Bowel Sounds

- Explain the procedure to the patient and discuss the implications of the test to the patient.
- Obtain consent.
- Follow local policy and procedure and ensure infection control is managed.
- Maintain patient dignity and privacy.
- Use the flat-disc diaphragm. Intestinal sounds are relatively high pitched and best accentuated by the flat-disc diaphragm. Light pressure with the stethoscope is adequate.

- Ask when the patient last ate. Shortly after or long after eating, bowel sounds may normally increase. They are loudest when a meal is long overdue.

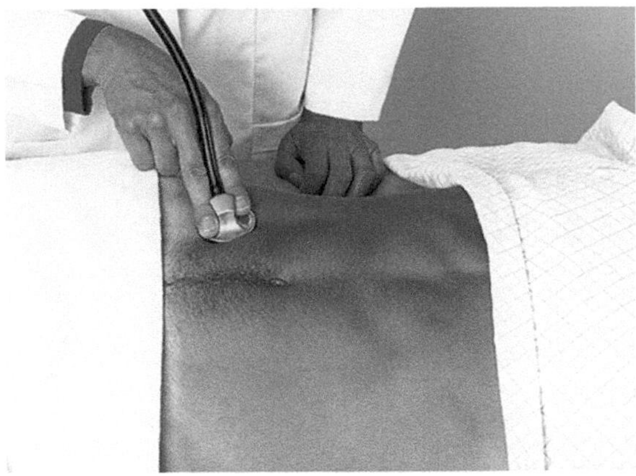

Figure 11-33 Auscultating the abdomen for bowel sounds.
Source: Pearson Education Ltd.

- Place the flat-disc diaphragm of the stethoscope in each of the four quadrants of the abdomen over all of the auscultatory sites shown in Figure 11-33.
- Listen for active bowel sounds - irregular gurgling noises occurring about every 5–20 seconds. The duration of a single sound may range from less than a second to more than several seconds.
- Normal bowel sounds are described as audible. Alterations in sounds are described as absent, hypoactive, i.e. extremely soft and infrequent (e.g. one per minute), or hyperactive/increased, i.e. high-pitched, loud, rushing sounds that occur frequently (e.g. every three seconds). True absence of sounds (none heard in 3-5 minutes) indicates a cessation of intestinal motility. Hypoactive sounds indicate decreased motility and are usually associated with manipulation of the bowel during surgery, inflammation, paralytic ileus (paralysis of the bowel) or late bowel obstruction. Hyperactive sounds indicate increased intestinal motility and are usually associated with diarrhoea, an early bowel obstruction or the use of laxatives.

PRACTICE GUIDELINES

Palpating the Abdomen

Palpation is used to detect tenderness, the presence of masses or distention, and the outline and position of abdominal organs (e.g. the liver, spleen and kidneys).

- Explain the procedure to the patient and discuss the implications of the procedure to the patient.
- Maintain infection control management throughout as per local policy.
- Obtain consent.
- Maintain patient privacy and dignity throughout.

Light Palpation

- Hold the palm of your hand slightly above the patient's abdomen, with your fingers parallel to the abdomen.
- Depress the abdominal wall lightly, about 1cm or to the depth of the subcutaneous tissue, with the pads of your fingers (see Figure 11-34).

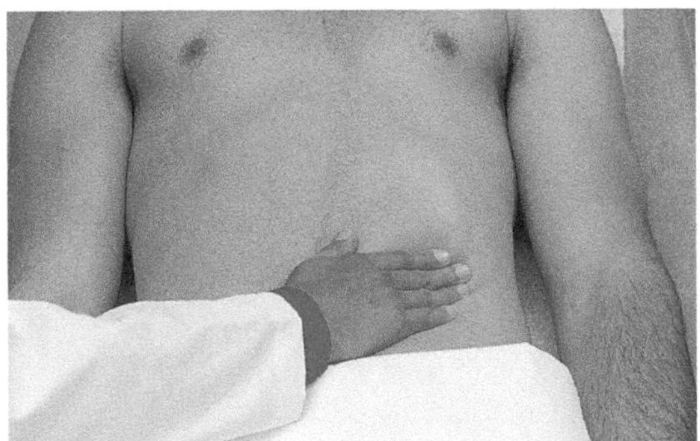

Figure 11-34 Light palpation of the abdomen.

- Move the finger pads in a slight circular motion.
- Note areas of tenderness or superficial pain, masses and muscle guarding. To determine areas of tenderness, ask the patient to tell you about them and watch for changes in the patient's facial expressions.

Deep Palpation

- Palpate sensitive areas last.
- Use the bimanual method of palpation discussed earlier in this chapter.
- Depress the abdominal wall about 4-5cm (see Figure 11-35).

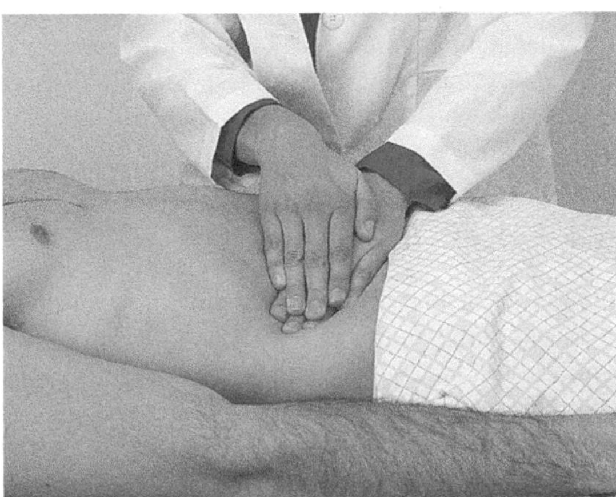

Figure 11-35 Deep palpation of the abdomen.

- Note masses and the structure of underlying contents. If a mass is present, determine its size, location, mobility, contour, consistency and tenderness.
- Check for rebound tenderness in areas where the patient complains of pain. With one hand, press slowly and deeply over the area indicated and then lift the hand quickly. If the patient does not complain of pain during the deep pressure but indicates pain at the release of the pressure, rebound tenderness is present. This can indicate peritoneal inflammation and should be reported to the medical staff immediately.

Source: Figures 11.34 and 11.35 © Pearson Education Ltd.

LIFESPAN CONSIDERATIONS

Assessing the Abdomen

Infants

- The abdomen of the newborn and infant is round.

Children

- Toddlers have a characteristic 'pot belly' appearance, which persists until about the fifth year.
- Children may not be able to pinpoint areas of tenderness; by observing facial expressions the examiner can determine areas of maximum tenderness.
- The liver is relatively larger than in adults. It can be palpated 1-2cm below the right costal margin.

Mature Adults

- The rounded abdomens of older adults are due to an increase in adipose tissue and a decrease in muscle tone.
- The abdominal wall is slacker and thinner, making palpation easier and more accurate than in younger patients.
- Faecal incontinence may occur in confused or neurologically impaired mature adults.
- Many older adults wrongly believe that the absence of a daily bowel movement signifies constipation.
- Decreased absorption of oral medications often occurs with ageing.

FEMALE GENITALS AND INGUINAL AREA

The examination and assessment of the female genitals and reproductive tract can often be embarrassing, emotional and unpleasant (for the patient), as often the lithotomy position needs to be taken. The inspection should include an examination of the inguinal lymph nodes and inspection and palpation of the external genitals (see below). Due to the nature of this examination it should only be undertaken by experienced nurses or those who have extended their role by further training.

Assessing the Female Genital Area

- Explain the procedure to the patient and inform them of the implications of the findings.
- Obtain consent.
- Maintain patient privacy and dignity at all times.
- Examine for the characteristic, amount and distribution of pubic hair.
- Inspect the skin of the pubic area for inflammation, swelling, rash, lesions and parasites. (Deeper and a fuller examination can be undertaken by separating the labia majora and labia minora.)
- Inspect the clitoris, uretharal orifice and vaginal orifice when separating the labia minora.
- Palpate the inguinal lymph nodes (see Figure 11-36) to note for enlargement or tenderness.
- Report any findings to appropriate expert.
- Document all findings in patient's notes.

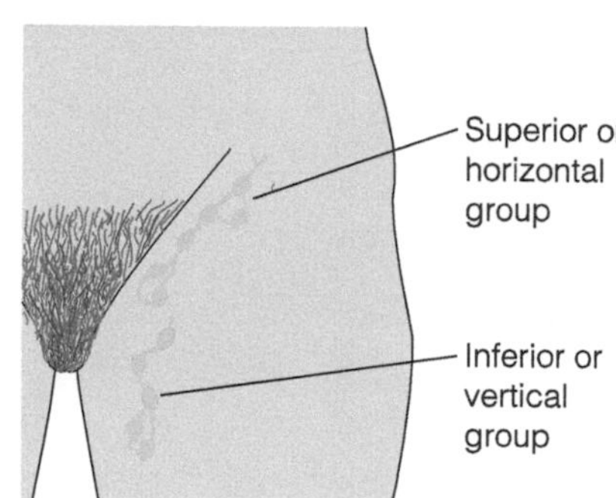

Figure 11-36 Lymph nodes of the groin area.

LIFESPAN CONSIDERATION

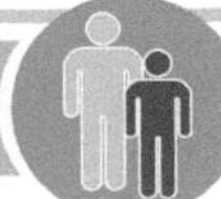

Female reproductive system

Infants

Some girls may be born without the enzyme 21-hydroxylase. Inwardly the girl will have all the female organs but outwardly will have male genitals.

Puberty/Teenager

At puberty the girls' breasts will start to grow. Pubic and armpit hair will grow. Body shape and odour alter. Emotions change. Menstruation starts.

Mature Adults

The menopause starts around the age of 50-52 which is defined as a woman who has not had a period for a year. Prior to the menopause (known as premenopausal) women experience hot flushes, night sweats and irritability. The menopause is the end of ovulation.

MALE GENITALS AND INGUINAL AREA

In adult men, complete examination should include assessment of the external genitals, the presence of any hernias and the prostate gland. As with women, nurses in some practice settings performing routine assessment of patients may assess only the external genitals. The male reproductive and urinary systems (see Figure 11-37) share the urethra, which is the passageway for both urine and semen. Therefore, in physical assessment of the male these two systems are frequently assessed together.

Most male patients accept examination by a female, especially if she is emotionally comfortable herself about performing it and does so in a professional and competent manner. The male patient is able to ask for a male practitioner if they would prefer this.

All male patients should be screened for the presence of inguinal or femoral hernias. A hernia is a protrusion of the intestine through the inguinal wall. The loop of bowel may even extend down to the scrotum.

Cancer of the prostate gland is the most common cancer in adult men and occurs primarily in men over age 50. Examination of the prostate gland is performed with the examination of the rectum and anus.

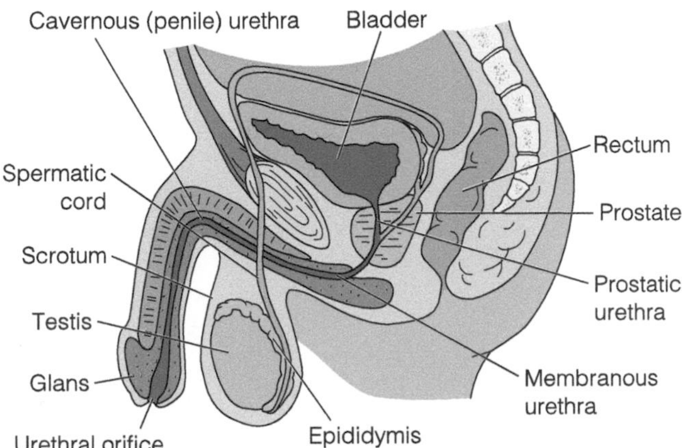

Figure 11-37 The male urogenital tract.

Testicular cancer is much rarer than prostate cancer and occurs primarily in young men aged 15–35. Testicular cancer is most commonly found on the anterior and lateral surfaces of the testes. As with women men should be encouraged to self-examine to detect any abnormal changes to their testes on a regular basis. Macmillan Cancer support advise that men should examine themselves after a warm bath or shower, check both testicles one at a time by holding the scrotum in their hands and rolling it from one side to the other, feeling for any abnormalities such as lumps or swelling.

Assessing the Male Genitals and Inguinal Area

- Explain the procedure to the patient and inform them of the implications of the findings.
- Obtain consent.
- Maintain patient privacy and dignity at all times.
- Examine for the characteristic, amount and distribution of pubic hair.
- Inspect the penile shaft and flans penis for lesions, nodules, swellings and inflammation.
- Inspect the urethral **meatus** for swelling, inflammation and discharge.
- Palpate the penis for tenderness, thickening and nodules.
- Inspect the scrotum for general size, appearance and symmetry.
- Palpate the scrotum to assess status of underlying testes, epididymis, and spermatic cord.
- Inspect both inguinal areas for bulges (standing if possible).
- Palpate any hernias.
- Report any findings to appropriate expert.
- Document all findings in the patient's notes.

Examination of the prostate gland is complex and should only be performed by nursing staff that have undergone appropriate training.

LIFESPAN CONSIDERATIONS

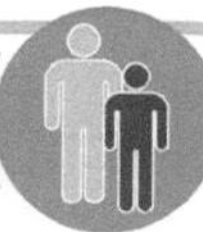

Assessing the Male Genitals and Inguinal Area

Infants

- The foreskin of the uncircumcised infant is normally tight the first two or three months of life and is not readily retractable.

Children

- The scrotum is usually palpated to determine whether testes are descended.

Mature Adults

- The penis decreases in size with age; the size and firmness of the testes decrease.
- Testosterone is produced in smaller amounts.
- Seminal fluid is reduced in amount and viscosity.
- Urinary frequency, **nocturia**, dribbling and problems with beginning and ending the stream are usually the result of prostatic enlargement.

RECTUM AND ANUS

Like examination of the genitals, the rectum and anus are only examined if there is an indication to do so and by a nurse who has undergone appropriate training. Usual symptoms that would require the nurse to examine the rectum and anus are history of haemarrhoids, rectal pain or a family history of colorectal cancer.

Assessing the Rectum and Anus

- Explain the procedure to the patient and inform them of the implications of the findings.
- Obtain consent.
- Maintain patient privacy and dignity at all times.
- Wash hands and apply gloves.
- Maintain infection control policy.
- Inspect the anus and surrounding tissue for colour, integrity and skin lesions.
- Inspect and palpate the anus for anal sphincter **tonicity**, nodules, mass and tenderness.
- Inspect your finger when withdrawing from rectum and anus for faeces.
- Report any findings to appropriate expert.
- Document all findings in patient's notes.

MUSCULOSKELETAL SYSTEM

The musculoskeletal system encompasses the muscles, bones and joints. The nurse usually assesses the musculoskeletal system for muscle strength, tone, size and symmetry of muscle development, and twitches and tremors.

Bones are assessed for normal form. Joints are assessed for tenderness, swelling, thickening, crepitation (the sound of bone grating on bone), presence of nodules and range of motion. Body posture is assessed for normal standing and sitting positions.

Procedure 11-11 describes how to assess the musculoskeletal system.

PROCEDURE 11-11 Assessing the Musculoskeletal System

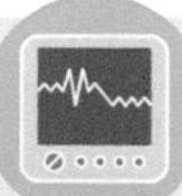

Purpose

- To assess the mobility of the patient.

Assessment

- Establish which part of the musculoskeletal system needs to be examined.
- Assess body posture.

Planning

Equipment

- None

Implementation

Performance

Follow local policy to ensure that you explain to the patient what you are going to do, why it is necessary and how they can cooperate. Obtain consent and maintain patient privacy and dignity and ensure that the appropriate local infection control procedures are observed. Enquire if the patient has any history of the following: presence of muscle pain: onset, location, character, associated phenomena (e.g. redness and swelling of joints), and aggravating and alleviating factors; any limitations to movement or inability to perform activities of daily living; previous sports injuries; any loss of function without pain.

Assessment	Normal findings	Deviations from normal
Muscles		
1 Inspect the muscles for size. Compare the muscles on one side of the body (e.g. of the arm, thigh and calf) to the same muscle on the other side. For any discrepancies, measure the muscles with a tape.	Equal size on both sides of body	Atrophy (a decrease in size) or hypertrophy (an increase in size)
2 Inspect the muscles and tendons for contractures (shortening).	No contractures	Malposition of body part (e.g. foot drop (foot flexed downward))
3 Inspect the muscles for twitches and tremors. Inspect any tremors of the hands and arms by having the patient hold the arms out in front of the body.	No twitches or tremors	Presence of twitches or tremor
4 Palpate muscles at rest to determine muscle tonicity (the normal condition of tension, or tone, of a muscle at rest).	Normally firm	Atonic (lacking tone)
5 Palpate muscles while the patient is active and passive for flaccidity, spasticity and smoothness of movement.	Smooth coordinated movements	Flaccidity (weakness or laxness) or spasticity (sudden involuntary muscle contraction)
6 Test muscle strength. See earlier tests. Compare the right side with the left side.	Equal strength on each body side	25% or less of normal strength
Bones		
7 Inspect the skeleton for normal structure and deformities.	No deformities	Bones misaligned
8 Palpate the bones to locate any areas of oedema or tenderness.	No tenderness or swelling	Presence of tenderness or swelling (may indicate fracture, neoplasms or osteoporosis)
Joints		
9 Inspect the joint for swelling.	No swelling	One or more swollen joints
Palpate each joint for tenderness, smoothness of movement, swelling, crepitation and presence of nodules.	No tenderness, swelling, crepitation or nodules Joints move smoothly	Presence of tenderness, swelling, crepitation or nodules
10 Assess joint range of motion.	Varies to some degree in accordance with person's genetic makeup and degree of physical activity	Limited range of motion in one or more joints
Ask the patient to move selected body parts.		

Evaluation

- Relate the findings of this examination to previous assessment data.
- Document findings in the patient record using forms or checklists supplemented by narrative notes when appropriate.
- Report any significant abnormalities to the medical staff.

Testing Muscle Strength

This can be done in a number of ways as follows:

- *Sternocleidomastoid.* Ask the patient to turn their head to one side against the resistance of your hand.
- *Trapezius.* Ask the patient to shrug their shoulders against the resistance of your hands.
- *Deltoid.* Ask the patient to raise their arms in the air and resist your attempts to push the arms down again.
- *Biceps.* Ask the patient to bend their arm at the elbow against resistance.
- *Triceps.* Ask the patient to bend their arm at the elbow and then attempt to straighten their arm against resistance.
- *Grip strength.* Ask the patient to grasp your fingers and resist your attempts to free your fingers.
- *Hip muscles.* Ask the patient to lie down and asking them to raise their legs one at a time against resistance.
- *Quadriceps.* Ask the patient to lie down and resist you trying to bend their knees.
- *Muscles of the ankles.* Ask the patient to resist your attempts to bend the foot upwards and downwards.

LIFESPAN CONSIDERATIONS

Assessing the Musculoskeletal System

Infants

- Newborns naturally return their arms and legs to the foetal position when extended and released.
- Check infants for developmental dysphasia of the hip (congenital dislocation) by examining for asymmetric **gluteal folds**, asymmetric abduction of the legs or apparent shortening of the femur.

Children

- Should be able to sit without support by eight months of age.
- **Pronation** of the feet, where the inner edge of the foot and the ankle are bent inwards, is common in children between 12 and 30 months of age.
- Genu varum (bowleg) is normal in children for one year after beginning to walk.

Mature Adults

- Muscle mass decreases progressively with age, but there are wide variations among different individuals.
- The bones become more fragile and osteoporosis leads to a loss of total bone mass. As a result, elderly people are predisposed to fractures and compressed vertebrae.
- In most mature people, osteoarthritic changes in the joints can be observed.

NEUROLOGICAL SYSTEM

A thorough neurological examination may take 1–3 hours; however, routine screening tests are usually done first. If the results of these tests raise questions, more extensive evaluations are made. Three major considerations determine the extent of a neurological exam: (a) the patient's main problems, (b) the patient's physical condition (i.e. level of consciousness and ability to ambulate), because many parts of the examination require movement and coordination of the extremities, and (c) the patient's willingness to participate and cooperate.

Examination of the neurological system includes assessment of (a) mental status including level of consciousness, (b) the cranial nerves, (c) reflexes, (d) motor function and (e) sensory function (see *Procedure 11-11*). Parts of the neurological assessment are performed throughout the health examination. For example, the nurse performs a large part of the mental status assessment during the taking of the history and when observing the patient's general appearance.

Mental Status

A general assessment of the mental state is normally undertaken during the initial meeting between the nurse and the patient. These functions include both intellectual functions and emotional functions. If problems with use of language, memory, concentration or thought processes are noted during the patient history, a more extensive examination is required during neurological assessment. Major areas of mental status assessment include language, orientation, memory and attention span and calculation.

Level of Consciousness

Loss of consciousness (LOC) can lie anywhere along a continuum from a state of alertness to coma. A fully alert patient responds to questions spontaneously; a comatose patient may not respond to verbal stimuli. The Glasgow Coma Scale was originally developed to predict recovery from a head injury; however, it is used by many professionals to assess LOC. It tests

Table 11-5 Levels of Consciousness: Glasgow Coma Scale

Faculty measured	Response	Score
Eye opening	Spontaneous	4
	To verbal command	3
	To pain	2
	No response	1
Motor response	To verbal command	6
	To localised pain	5
	Flexes and withdraws	4
	Flexes abnormally	3
	Extends abnormally	2
	No response	1
Verbal response	Oriented, converses	5
	Disoriented, converses	4
	Uses inappropriate words	3
	Makes incomprehensible sounds	2
	No response	1

in three major areas: eye response, motor response and verbal response. An assessment totalling 15 points indicates the patient is alert and completely oriented. A comatose patient scores 7 or less (see Table 11-5).

Cranial Nerves

The nurse needs to be aware of specific nerve functions and assessment methods for each cranial nerve to detect abnormalities (see Table 11-6). In some cases, each nerve is assessed; in other cases only selected nerve functions are evaluated. Cranial nerves are twelve nerves that emerge directly from the brain.

Reflexes

A **reflex** is an automatic response of the body to a stimulus. It is not voluntarily learned or conscious. Several reflexes are normally tested during the physical examination: (a) the biceps reflex, (b) the triceps reflex, (c) the brachioradialis reflex, (d) the patellar reflex, (e) the Achilles reflex and (f) the **plantar** (Babinski) reflex. (See *Procedure 11-12* for details of all these reflexes.)

Motor Function

Neurological assessment of the motor system examines the proprioception (sixth-sense perception of improvement, the position of the body, etc.) and cerebullar functions (posture and movement control and coordination). The structures involved in proprioceptors are the posterior columns of the spinal cord, the cerebellum and the vestibular apparatus in the labyrinth of the inner ear.

Sensory Function

Sensory functions include touch, pain, temperature, position and tactile discrimination. The first three are routinely tested. Generally, the face, arms, legs, hands and feet are tested for touch and pain, although all parts of the body can be tested. If the patient complains of numbness, peculiar sensations or paralysis, the nurse should check sensation more carefully. Abnormal responses to touch stimuli include loss of sensation (anaesthesia); more than normal sensation (hyperaesthesia); less than normal sensation (hypoaesthesia); or an abnormal sensation such as burning, pain or an electric shock (paraesthesia).

Procedure 11-12 describes how to assess the neurological system.

Table 11-6 Cranial Nerve Functions and Assessment Methods

Cranial nerve	Name	Type	Function	Assessment method
I	Olfactory	Sensory	Smell	Ask patient to close eyes and identify different mild aromas, such as coffee, vanilla, peanut butter, orange, lemon, lime, chocolate.
II	Optic	Sensory	Vision and visual fields	Ask patient to read Snellen chart (see Figure 11-12).
III	Oculomotor	Motor	Extraocular eye movement (EOM) movement of sphincter of pupil, movement of ciliary muscles of the lens	Assess six ocular movements of the eye and pupil reaction.
IV	Trochlear	Motor	EOM; specifically, moves eyeball downward and laterally	Assess the movement of each eye individually and then together.
V	Trigeminal Ophthalmic branch	Sensory	Sensation of cornea, skin of face and nasal mucosa	While patient looks upward, lightly touch lateral sclera of eye to elicit blink reflex. To test light sensation, have patient close eyes, wipe a wisp of cotton over patient's forehead and paranasal sinuses. To test deep sensation, use alternating blunt and sharp ends of a safety pin over same areas.

Table 11-6 (*continued*)

Cranial nerve	Name	Type	Function	Assessment method
	Maxillary branch	Sensory	Sensation of skin of face and anterior oral cavity (tongue and teeth)	Assess skin sensation as for ophthalmic branch above.
VI	Mandibular branch	Motor and sensory	Muscles of mastication; sensation of skin of face	Ask patient to clench teeth.
VII	Abducens	Motor	EOM; moves eyeball laterally	Assess directions of gaze.
VIII	Facial	Motor and sensory	Facial expression; taste (anterior two-thirds of tongue)	Ask patient to smile, raise the eyebrows, frown, puff out cheeks, close eyes tightly. Ask patient to identify various tastes placed on tip and sides of tongue: sugar (sweet), salt, lemon juice (sour) and quinine (bitter); identify areas of taste.
IX	Auditory Vestibular branch	Sensory	Equilibrium	Assessment methods are discussed with cerebellar functions (in next section).
X	Cochlear branch	Sensory	Hearing	Assess patient's ability to hear spoken word and vibrations of tuning fork.
XI	Glossopharyngeal	Motor and sensory	Swallowing ability, tongue movement, taste (posterior tongue)	Apply tastes on posterior tongue for identification. Ask patient to move tongue from side to side and up and down.
XII	Vagus	Motor and sensory	Sensation of pharynx and larynx; swallowing; vocal cord movement	Assessed with cranial nerve IX; assess patient's speech for hoarseness.
	Accessory	Motor	Head movement; shrugging of shoulders	Ask patient to shrug shoulders against resistance from your hands and turn head to side against resistance from your hand (repeat for other side).
	Hypoglossal	Motor	Protrusion of tongue; moves tongue up and down and side to side	Ask patient to protrude tongue at midline, then move it side to side.

PROCEDURE 11-12 Assessing the Neurological System

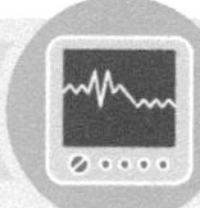

Purpose

- To assess both psychological and physical well-being of the patient.

Assessment

- Appropriate environment.
- Ensure confidentiality.
- Level of understanding and comprehension of patient.
- Language choice.

Planning

If possible, determine whether a screening or full neurological examination is indicated. This will affect the preparation of the patient, equipment and timing.

Equipment (Depending on Components of Examination)

- Percussion hammer
- Tongue depressors (one broken diagonally for testing pain sensation)
- Cotton wool to assess light-touch sensation

Implementation

Performance

Follow local policy to ensure that you explain to the patient what you are going to do, why it is necessary and how they can cooperate. Obtain consent and maintain patient privacy and dignity and ensure that the appropriate local infection control procedures are observed. Enquire if the patient has any history of the following: presence of pain in the head, back or extremities, as well as onset and aggravating and alleviating factors; disorientation to time, place or person; speech disorder; any history of loss of consciousness, fainting, convulsions, trauma, tingling or numbness, tremors or tics, limping, paralysis, uncontrolled muscle movements, loss of memory, mood swings, or problems with smell, vision, taste, touch or hearing.

Language

1 Establish the first language of choice for the patient.
2 Ask the patient to:
   - point to common objects and ask the patient to name them;
   - read some words and to match the printed and written words with pictures;
   - respond to simple verbal and written commands (e.g. 'point to your toes' or 'raise your left arm').

Orientation

3 Determine the patient's orientation to *time, place* and *person* by tactful questioning. Ask the patient for their home address, time of day, date, day of the week, duration of illness and names of family members. More direct questioning may be necessary for some people (e.g. 'Where are you now?' 'What day is it today?').

Memory

4 Listen for lapses in memory. Ask the patient about difficulty with memory. If problems are apparent, three categories of memory are tested: immediate recall, recent memory and remote memory.
5 To assess immediate recall:
   - Ask the patient to repeat a series of three digits, for example, 7-4-3, spoken slowly.
   - Gradually increase the number of digits, for example, 7-4-3-5, 7-4-3-5-6 and 7-4-3-5-6-7-2, until the patient fails to repeat the series correctly.
   - Start again with a series of three digits, but this time ask the patient to repeat them backward. The average person can repeat a series of five to eight digits in sequence and four to six digits in reverse order.
6 To assess recent memory:
   - Ask the patient to recall the recent events of the day, such as how the patient got to the clinic. This information must be validated, however.
   - Ask the patient to recall information given early in the interview (e.g. the name of a doctor).
   - Provide the patient with three facts to recall (e.g. a colour, an object, an address or a three-digit number), and ask the patient to repeat all three. Later in the interview, ask the patient to recall all three items.
7 To assess remote memory, ask the patient to describe a previous illness or surgery (e.g. five years ago) or a birthday or anniversary.

Attention span and calculation

8 Test the ability to concentrate or *attention span* by asking the patient to recite the alphabet or to count backward from 100. Test the ability to calculate by asking the patient to subtract 7 or 3 progressively from 100, i.e. 100, 93, 86, 79 or 100, 97, 94, 91 (referred to as *serial sevens* or *serial threes*). Normally, an adult can complete serial sevens test in about 90 seconds with three or fewer errors. Because educational level and language or cultural differences affect calculating ability, this test may be inappropriate for some people.

Level of consciousness

9 Apply the Glasgow Coma Scale: eye response, motor response and verbal response. An assessment totalling 15 points indicates the patient is alert and completely oriented. A comatosed patient would score 7 or less (see Table 11-5).

Cranial nerves

10 For the specific functions and assessment methods of each cranial nerve, see Table 11-6. Test each nerve not already being evaluated in another component of the health assessment.

Reflexes

11 Test reflexes using a percussion hammer, comparing one side of the body with the other to evaluate the symmetry of response.

Biceps reflex

12 The biceps reflex tests the spinal cord level C-5, C-6.
- Partially flex the patient's arm at the elbow, and rest the forearm over the thighs, placing the palm of the hand down.
- Place the thumb of your nondominant hand horizontally over the biceps tendon.
- Deliver a blow (slight downward thrust) with the percussion hammer to your thumb.
- Observe the normal slight **flexion** of the elbow, and feel the bicep's contraction through your thumb (see Figure 11-38(a)).

Triceps reflex

13 The triceps reflex tests the spinal cord level C-7, C-8.
- Flex the patient's arm at the elbow, and support it in the palm of your nondominant hand.
- Palpate the triceps tendon about 2-5cm above the elbow.
- Deliver a blow with the percussion hammer directly to the tendon (see Figure 11-38(b)).
- Observe the normal slight extension of the elbow.

Brachioradialis reflex

14 The brachioradialis reflex tests the spinal cord level C-3, C-6.
- Rest the patient's arm in a relaxed position on your forearm or on the patient's own leg.
- Deliver a blow with the percussion hammer directly on the radius 2-5cm above the wrist or the styloid process (the bony prominence on the thumb side of the wrist) (see Figure 11-38(c)).
- Observe the normal flexion and supination of the forearm (movement of the arm into a palm up position). The fingers of the hand may also extend slightly.

Patellar reflex

15 The patellar reflex tests the spinal cord level L-2, L-3, L-4:
- Ask the patient to sit on the edge of the examining table so that the legs hang freely.
- Locate the patellar tendon directly below the patella (kneecap).
- Deliver a blow with the percussion hammer directly to the tendon (see Figure 11-38(d)).
- Observe the normal extension or kicking out of the leg as the quadriceps muscle contracts.
- If no response occurs and you suspect the patient is not relaxed, ask the patient to interlock the fingers and pull. *This action often enhances relaxation so that a more accurate response is obtained.*

Achilles reflex

16 The Achilles reflex tests the spinal cord level S-1, S-2.
- With the patient in the same position as for the patellar reflex, slightly raise the upper part of the foot

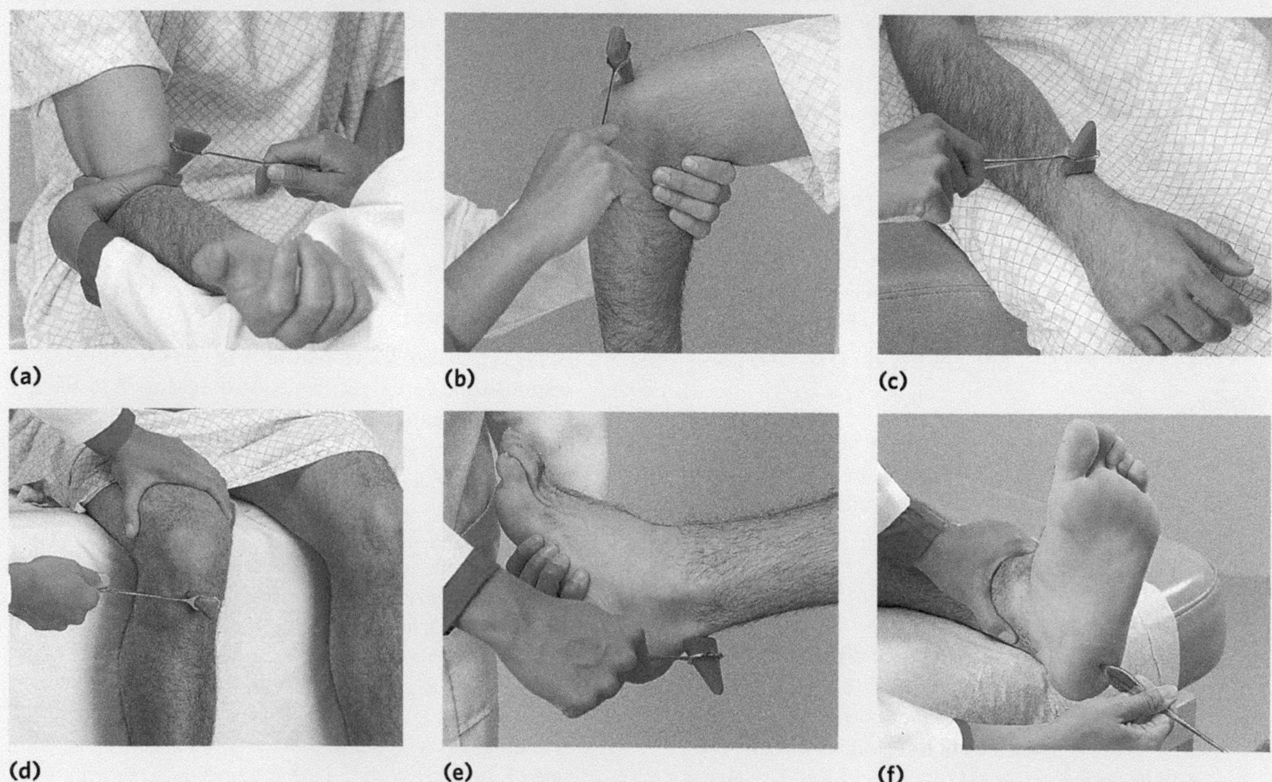

Figure 11-38 Testing reflexes: (a) the biceps reflex; (b) the triceps reflex; (c) the brachioradialis reflex; (d) the patellar reflex; (e) the Achilles reflex; (f) the plantar (Babinski) reflex.

Source: Pearson Education Ltd.

towards the shin (dorsiflexion) while supporting the foot lightly in the hand.

- Deliver a blow with the percussion hammer directly to the Achilles tendon just above the heel (see Figure 11-38(e)).
- Observe and feel the normal plantar flexion (downward jerk) of the foot.

Plantar (Babinski) reflex

17 The planter, or Babinski, reflex is superficial. It may be absent in adults without pathology or overridden by voluntary control:

- Use a moderately sharp object, such as the handle of the percussion hammer, a key or the dull end of a pin or applicator stick.
- Stroke the lateral border of the sole of the patient's foot, starting at the heel, continuing to the ball of the foot, and then proceeding across the ball of the foot towards the big toe (see Figure 11-38(f)).
- Observe the response. Normally, all five toes bend downward; this reaction is negative Babinski. In an abnormal Babinski response the toes spread outward and the big toe moves upward.

Motor function

Assessment	Normal findings	Deviations from normal
Walking gait		
Ask the patient to walk across the room and back, and assess the patient's gait.	Has upright posture and steady gait with opposing arm swing; walks unaided, maintaining balance	Has poor posture and unsteady, irregular, staggering gait with wide stance; bends legs only from hips; has rigid or no arm movements
Romberg test		
Ask the patient to stand with feet together and arms resting at the sides, first with eyes open, then closed. Stand close during this test *to prevent the patient from falling*.	*Negative Romberg*: may sway slightly but is able to maintain upright posture and foot stance	*Positive Romberg*: cannot maintain food balance; moves the feet apart to maintain stance. If patient cannot maintain balance with the eyes shut, patient may have sensory ataxia which is the loss of coordination when the eyes are closed. If balance cannot be maintained whether the eyes are open or shut, patient may have cerebellar ataxia (loss of coordination)
Standing on one foot with eyes closed		
Ask the patient to close the eyes and stand on one foot and then the other. Stand close to the patient during this test.	Maintains stance for at least five seconds	Cannot maintain stance for five seconds
Heel-toe walking		
Ask the patient to walk a straight line, placing the heel of one foot directly in front of the toes of the other foot.	Maintains heel-toe walking along a straight line (see Figure 11-39)	Assumes a wider foot gait to stay upright
Toe or heel walking		
Ask the patient to walk several steps on the toes and then on the heels.	Able to walk several steps on toes or heels	Cannot maintain balance on toes or heels
Finger-to-nose test		
Ask the patient to abduct and extend the arms at shoulder height and rapidly touch the nose alternately with one index finger and then the other. The patient repeats the test with the eyes closed if the test is performed easily.	Repeatedly and rhythmically touches the nose (see Figure 11-40)	Misses the nose or gives lazy response

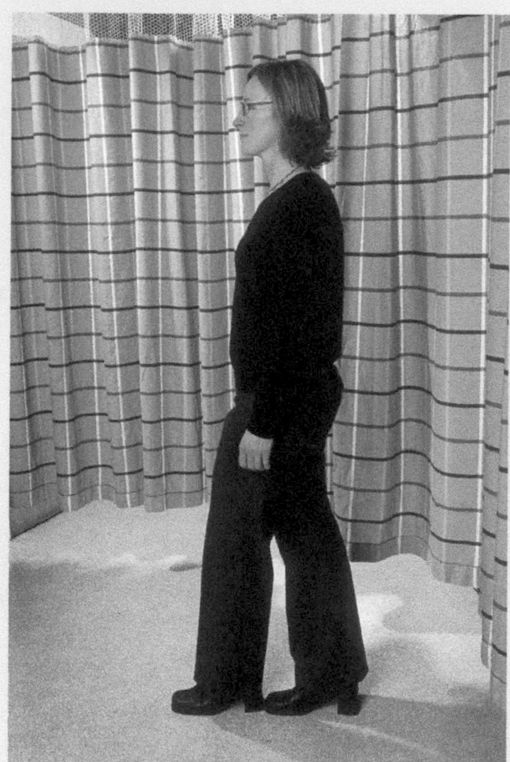

Figure 11-39 Heel-toe walking test.
Source: Pearson Education Ltd.

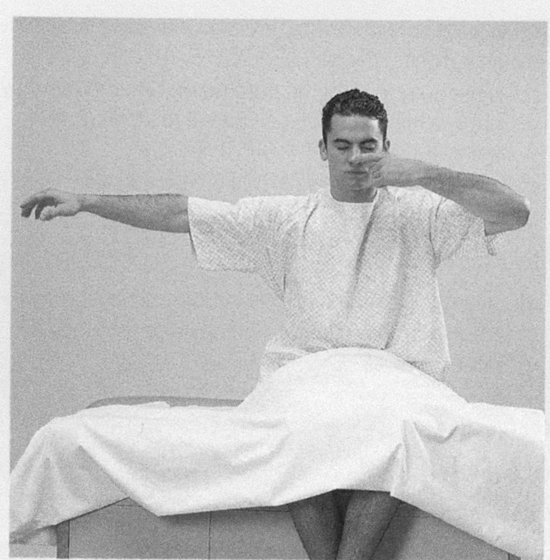

Figure 11-40 Finger-to-nose test.
Source: Pearson Education Ltd.

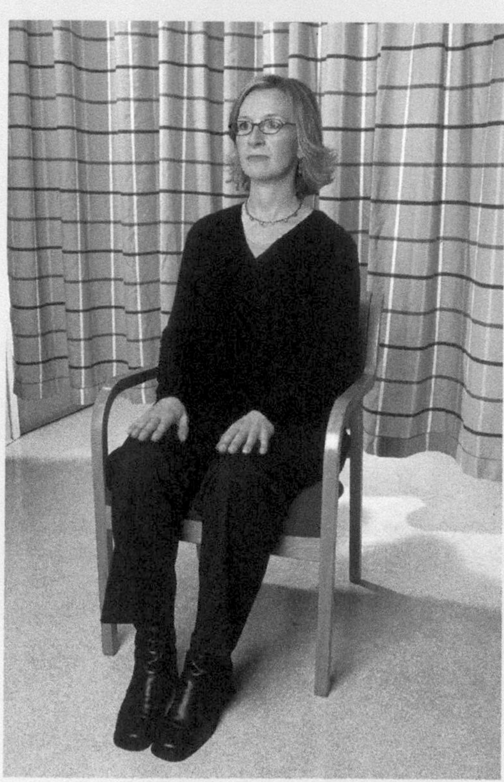

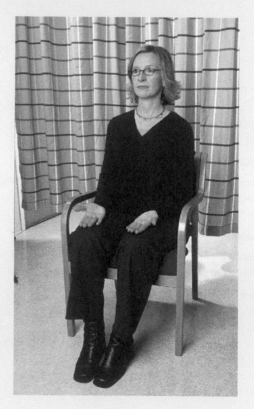

Figure 11-41 Alternating **pronation** and **supination** of hands-on-knees test.
Source: Pearson Education Ltd.

Alternating supination and pronation of hands on knees		
Ask the patient to pat both knees with the palms of both hands and then with the backs of the hands alternately at an ever-increasing rate.	Can alternately supinate and pronate hands at rapid pace (see Figure 11-41)	Performs with slow, clumsy movements and irregular timing; has difficulty alternating from supination to pronation
Finger to nose and to the nurse's finger		
Ask the patient to touch the nose and then your index finger, held at a distance at about 45cm, at a rapid and increasing rate.	Performs with coordination and rapidity (see Figure 11-42)	Misses the finger and moves slowly
Fingers to fingers		
Ask the patient to spread the arms broadly at shoulder height and then bring the fingers together at the midline, first with the eyes open and then closed, first slowly and then rapidly.	Performs with accuracy and rapidity (see Figure 11-43)	Moves slowly and is unable to touch fingers consistently
Fingers to thumb (same hand)		
Ask the patient to touch each finger of one hand to the thumb of the same hand as rapidly as possible. **Fine motor tests** for the lower extremities. Ask the patient to lie supine and to perform these tests.	Rapidly touches each finger to thumb with each hand (see Figure 11-44)	Cannot coordinate this fine discrete movement with either one or both hands
Heel down opposite shin		
Ask the patient to place the heel of one foot just below the opposite knee and run the heel down the shin to the foot. Repeat with the other foot. The patient may also use a sitting position for this test.	Demonstrates bilateral equal coordination (see Figure 11-45)	Has tremors or is awkward; heel moves off shin
Toe or ball of foot to the nurse's finger		
Ask the patient to touch your finger with the large toe of each foot.	Moves smoothly, with coordination (see Figure 11-46)	Misses your finger; cannot coordinate movement
Light-touch sensation. Compare the light-touch sensation of symmetric areas of the body. *Sensitivity to touch varies among different skin areas.* • Ask the patient to close the eyes and to respond by saying 'yes' or 'now' whenever the patient feels the cotton wisp touching the skin. • With a wisp of cotton, lightly touch one specific spot and then the same spot on the other side of the body. • Test areas on the forehead, cheek, hand, lower arm, abdomen, foot and lower leg. • Check a specific area of the limb first (i.e. the hand before the arm and the foot before the leg), because the sensory nerve may be assumed to be intact if sensation is felt at its most peripheral part. • Ask the patient to point to the spot where the touch was felt. This demonstrates whether the patient is able to determine	Light tickling or touch sensation	Anaesthesia, hyperaesthesia, hypoaesthesia and paraesthesia

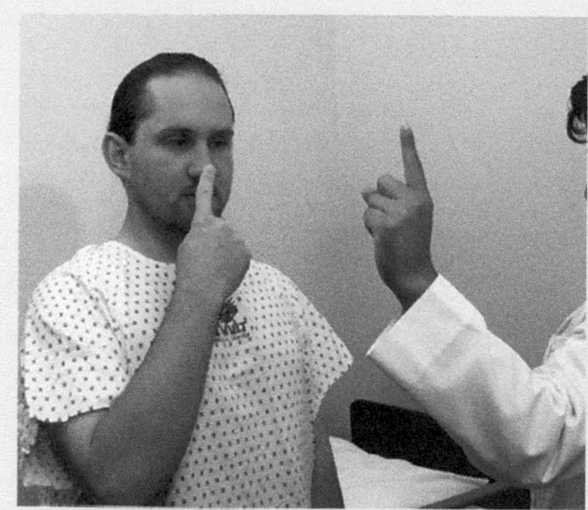

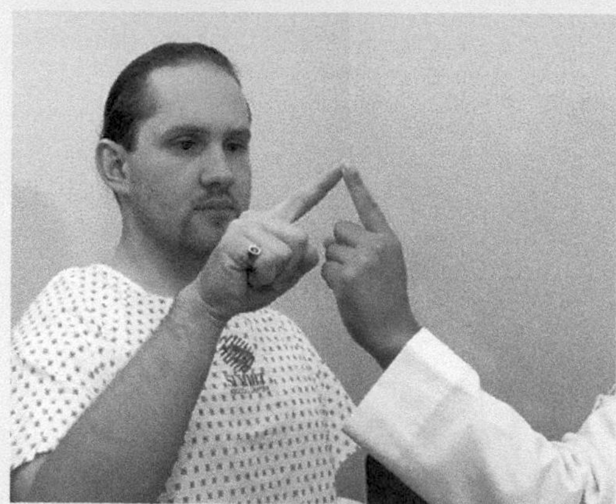

Figure 11-42 Finger to nose and to the nurse's finger test.

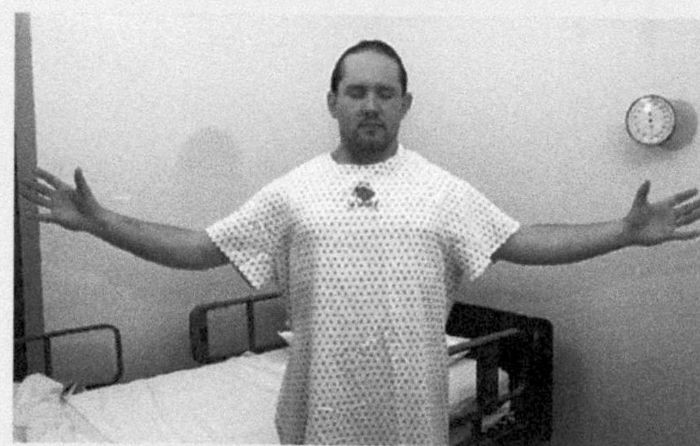

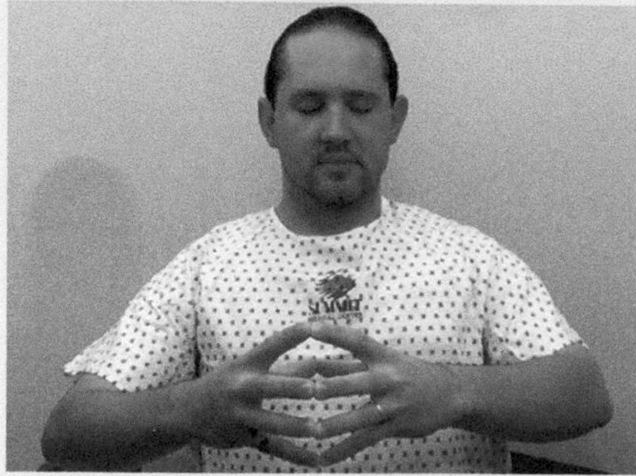

Figure 11-43 Fingers-to-fingers test.

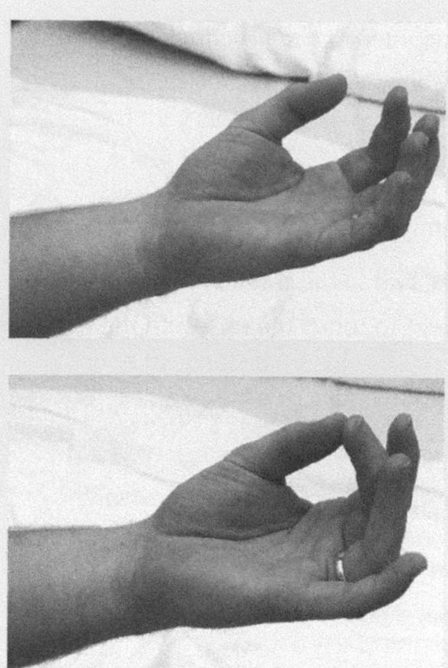

Figure 11-44 Fingers-to-thumb (same hand) test.

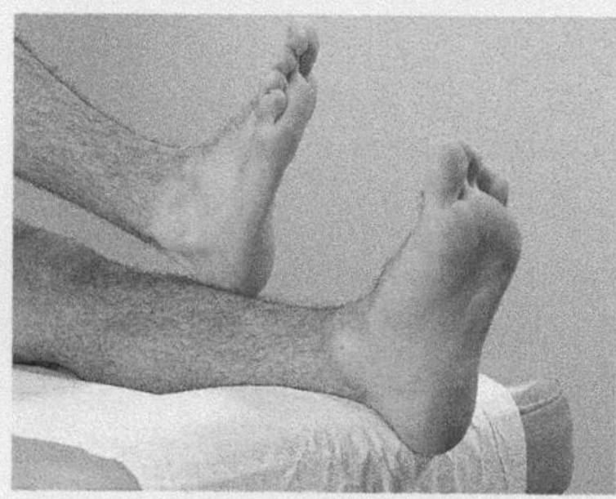

Figure 11-45 Heel down opposite shin test.

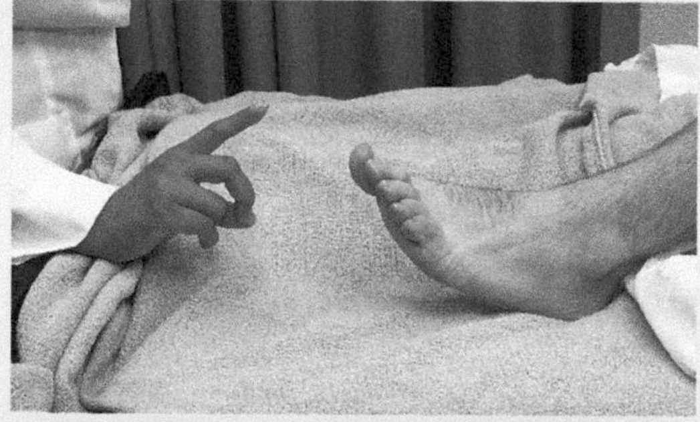

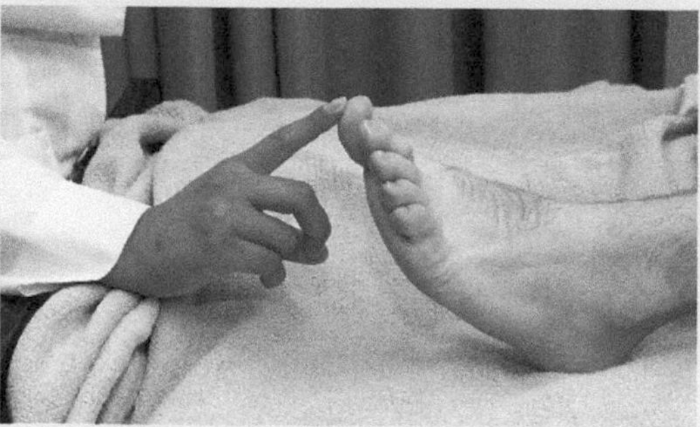

Figure 11-46 Toe or ball of foot to the nurse's finger test.

tactile location (point localisation), i.e. can accurately perceive where the patient was touched. • If areas of sensory dysfunction are found, determine the boundaries of sensation by testing responses about every 2.5cm in the area. Make a sketch of the sensory loss area for recording purposes.		
Pain sensation Assess pain sensation as follows: • Ask the patient to close the eyes and to say 'sharp', 'dull' or 'don't know' when the sharp or dull end of the broken tongue depressor is felt. • Alternately, use the sharp and dull end of a sterile pin or needle to lightly prick designated anatomic areas at random (e.g. hand, forearm, foot, lower leg, abdomen). The face is not tested in this manner. *Alternating the sharp and dull ends of the instrument more accurately evaluates the patient's response.* • Allow at least two seconds between each test to prevent summation effects of stimuli, i.e. several successive stimuli perceived as one stimulus.	Able to discriminate 'sharp' and 'dull' sensations.	Areas of reduced, heightened or absent sensation (map them out for recording purposes).
Temperature sensation is not routinely tested if pain sensation is found to be within normal limits. If pain sensation is not normal or is absent, testing sensitivity to temperature may prove more reliable. • Touch skin areas with test tubes filled with hot or cold water. • Have the patient respond by say saying 'hot', 'cold' or 'don't know'.	Able to discriminate between 'hot' and 'cold' sensations.	Areas of dulled or lost sensation (when sensations of pain are dulled, temperature sense is usually also impaired because distribution of these nerves over the body is similar).
Position or kinaesthetic sensation Commonly, the middle fingers and the large toes are tested for the kinaesthetic sensation (sense of position). • To test the fingers, support the patient's arm with one hand, and hold the patient's palm in the other. To test the toes, place the patient's heels on the examining table. • Ask the patient to close the eyes. • Grasp a middle finger or a big toe firmly between your thumb and index finger, and exert the same pressure on both sides of the finger or toe while moving it. • Move the finger or toe until it is up, down or straight out, and ask the patient to identify the position. • Use a series of brisk up-and-down movements before bringing the finger or toe suddenly to rest in one of the three positions.	Can readily determine the position of fingers and toes.	Unable to determine the position of one or more fingers or toes.

Tactile discrimination For all tests, the patient's eyes need to be closed.

One- and two-point discrimination

Alternately stimulate the skin with two pins simultaneously and then with one pin. Ask whether the patient feels one or two pinpricks.	Perception varies widely in adults over different parts of the body	Unable to sense whether one or two areas of the skin are being stimulated by pressure.

Evaluation

- Relate findings from previous assessment data.
- Document findings in the patient notes using appropriate tools supplemented by narrative notes.
- Report significant abnormalities to the medical staff.

LIFESPAN CONSIDERATIONS

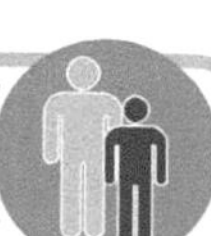

Assessing the Neurological System

Infants

- Reflexes commonly tested in newborns include the rooting reflex - when the baby's cheek is touched, the head turns towards that side; palmar grasp - the baby's fingers curl around an object; tonic neck reflex - when the baby is supine and the head is turned to one side, the arm and leg on that side extend while those on the opposite side flex (fencing position). Most of these disappear by six months of age.

Children

- Present the procedures as games whenever possible.
- Positive Babinski reflex is abnormal after the child ambulates or at age two.
- Note the child's ability to understand and follow directions.
- Assess immediate recall or recent memory by using names of cartoon characters. Normal recall in children is one less than age in years.
- Assess for signs of hyperactivity or abnormally short attention span.
- Should be able to walk backward by age two, balance on one foot for five seconds by age four, heel-toe walk by age five, and heel-toe walk backward by age six.
- Romberg test is appropriate over age three.

Mature Adults

- A full neurological assessment can be lengthy. Conduct in several sessions if indicated and cease the tests if the patient is noticeably fatigued.
- A decline in mental status is not a normal result of ageing. Changes are more the result of physical or psychological disorders (e.g. fever, fluid and electrolyte imbalances, medications). Acute, abrupt-onset mental status changes are usually caused by delirium. These changes are often reversible with treatment. Chronic subtle insidious mental health changes are usually caused by dementia and are usually irreversible.
- Intelligence and learning ability are unaltered with age. Many factors, however, inhibit learning (e.g. anxiety, illness, pain, cultural barrier).
- Short-term memory is often less efficient. Long-term memory is usually unaltered.
- As a person ages, reflex responses may become less intense.

CRITICAL REFLECTION

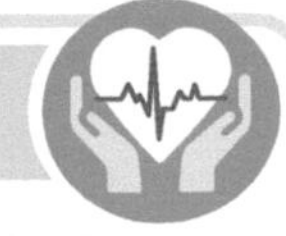

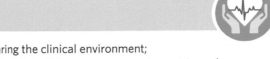

Let us revisit the case study on page 259. Reflecting on the signs and symptoms presented in the letter regarding Mr Frankburger, there are several diagnosis that you could consider. However, there are general physical examinations that would be required for most of these. In order to prepare for Mr Frankburger's visit to enable yourself as a nurse to 'inform' and prepare him for some of the examinations, identify the key physical examinations that are likely in Mr Frankburger's case that either you or the consultant might undertake. Suggested points for consideration are:

- preparing the clinical environment;
- ensuring that all the necessary equipment is ready;
- recording baseline observations;
- scales and height measures;
- tongue depressor;
- cotton wool;
- percussion hammer;
- gown and gloves;
- informing the patient and relative/carer;
- documentation;
- multidisciplinary team.

CHAPTER HIGHLIGHTS

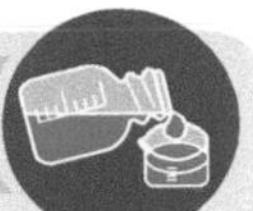

- The health examination is conducted to assess the function and integrity of the patient's body parts.
- The health examination may entail a complete head-to-toe assessment or individual assessment of a body system or body part.
- The health assessment is conducted in a systematic manner that requires the fewest position changes for the patient.
- Aspects of the physical assessment procedures should be incorporated in the assessment, intervention and evaluation phases of the nursing process.
- Data obtained in the physical health examination supplement, confirm or refute data obtained during the patient history.
- Patient history data help the nurse focus on specific aspects of the physical health examination.
- Data obtained in the physical health examination help the nurse establish nursing diagnoses, plan the patient's care and evaluate the outcomes of nursing care.
- Initial assessment findings provide baseline data about the patient's functional abilities against which subsequent assessment findings are compared.
- Skills in inspection, palpation, percussion and auscultation are required for the physical health examination. These skills are used in that order throughout the examination except during abdominal assessment, when auscultation follows inspection and precedes percussion and palpation.
- Knowledge of the normal structure and function of body parts and systems is an essential requisite to conducting physical assessment.

ACTIVITY ANSWERS

ACTIVITY 11.1 It is important when you are assessing a patient that you look and consider holistic care when managing a sick patient. Points to consider should be:

- Maintain respect, dignity and privacy of the patient.
- Discreetly question the patient about their general well-being in relation to pain, voice changes, difficulty in swallowing.
- Has the patient suffered with palpitations, tremors or weight loss?
- Anxiety or insomnia?
- Make baseline observations.
- Examine hair and eyes.
- Weigh patient.
- Check skin integrity.

REFERENCES

Cancer Research UK (2010) *Melanoma statistics and outlook*, London: The Information Standard.

Macmillan Cancer Support (2008) *Self-examination of breast*, London: Macmillan Cancer Support.

National Eye Institute (2010) *Facts about cataracts*, USA National Institute of Health.

NMC (2010) *Standards for pre-registration nursing education*, London: NMC.

FURTHER RESOURCES

For self-examination of testicles see
http://www.macmillan.org.uk/Cancerinformation/Cancertypes/Testes/Symptomsdiagnosis/Checkum.aspx

CHAPTER 12
INFECTION PREVENTION AND CONTROL

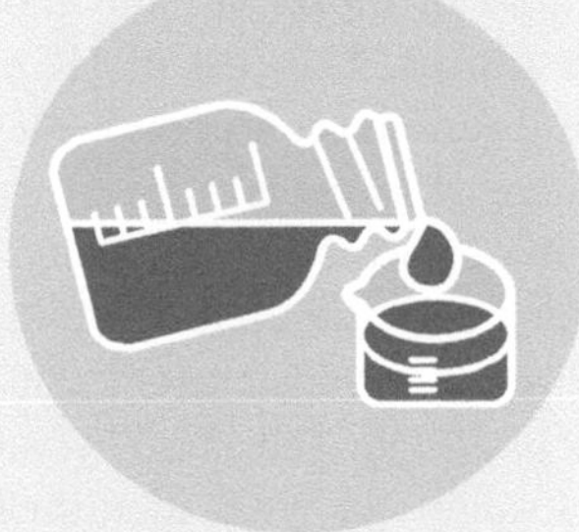

LEARNING OUTCOMES

After completing this chapter, you will be able to:

- Identify the risks posed by healthcare associated infections.
- Identify signs of localised and systemic infections.
- Identify factors influencing a micro-organism's capability to produce an infectious process.
- Identify anatomic and physiologic barriers that defend the body against micro-organisms.
- Discuss the key stages in the chain of infection.
- Identify measures that can break each link in the chain of infection.
- Correctly implement standard and transmission-based infection control practices, including hand hygiene, donning and removing personal protective equipment, decontamination, sharps management and patient isolation.
- Describe the steps to take in the event of an inoculation injury.

After reading this chapter you will be able to identify infection risks and utilise appropriate methods to promote infection prevention and control. The chapter incorporates the **Essential Skills Clusters (NMC, 2010) 21–26**, as appropriate for each progression point.

Ensure that you really understand this chapter by logging on to your complimentary **MyNursingKit** at **www.pearsoned.co.uk/kozier**. Complete the self-assessment tests to check your progress and utilise further activities to practise and confirm your understanding.

CASE STUDY

In March 2011 the BBC news website reported that one hospital in the UK was restricting visitors in a bid to control an outbreak of the vomiting and diarrhoea virus. With the virus affecting the community it was envisaged that reducing the number of visitors will help reduce the new cases of norovirus.

You are a nurse working on one of the wards which has patients with norovirus. What information are you going to give to visitors in order to reduce the risk of them acquiring the infection and of them potentially passing on the infection? (See end of chapter for suggestions.)

Source: BBC (2011) *Bournemouth hospital visiting ban lifted after virus*. Available at **http://www.bbc.co.uk/news/uk-england-dorset-12903738** (accessed 07 April 2011).

INTRODUCTION

Healthcare associated infections (HCAI) are classified as infections that are associated with the delivery of healthcare services. They occur in a variety of settings that healthcare takes place in, from an individual's home to an acute hospital. HCAI (e.g. MRSA (methicillin resistant *Staphylococcus aureus*); *Clostridium difficile*, *Mycobacterium tuberculosis*, *Escherichia coli* and norovirus) can either develop during a patient's stay in a clinical area or manifest after discharge. Some HCAI may also be acquired by healthcare personnel working in the facility and can cause significant illness and time lost from work.

The threat of HCAI remains a major worldwide concern (World Health Organization, 2007). HCAI are a substantial cause of morbidity and mortality while impacting on scarce resources. The cost of HCAI to the patient, the clinical area and funding sources is great. They extend hospitalisation time, increase patients' time away from work, cause disability and discomfort, and even result in loss of life. It is estimated that they cost the NHS £1 billion pounds annually while being directly responsible for 5,000 patient deaths annually (Plowman *et al.*, 1999). The Third Prevalence Survey of HCAI in UK Acute Hospitals in 2006 identified an infection prevalence rate of 7.6% in the UK and Republic of Ireland. Further analysis identified that the most common HCAI were gastro-intestinal, urinary tract and surgical site infections respectively (Smyth *et al.*, 2008).

In view of this challenge each of the UK's four devolved National Health Services have implemented strategies highlighting the importance of preventing and controlling infections (Department of Health, 2008; Department of Health, Social Services and Public Safety, 2006; Scottish Executive Health Department, 2004; Welsh Assembly Government, 2004; 2007). In addition to national strategies there are also evidence-based guidelines available for practitioners (Pratt *et al.*, 2007). In 2007 the Nursing and Midwifery Council (NMC) introduced Essential Skill Clusters for pre-registration nurse education. These Essential Skill Clusters are skills that are deemed essential for safe and competent practice. Infection prevention and control is included in these clusters and highlight the importance placed on infection prevention and control in nurse education.

The micro-organisms that cause HCAI can originate from the patients themselves (an **endogenous** source) or from the hospital environment, equipment and personnel (**exogenous** sources). Many HCAI appear to have endogenous sources. *Escherichia coli*, *Staphylococcus aureus* and enterococci are the most common bacterial infections although norovirus also tends to disrupt NHS services every year with outbreaks of diarrhoea and vomiting. A number of factors contribute to HCAI, and they can be acquired through the direct result of diagnostic or therapeutic procedures, such as bacteraemia that results from an intravascular line.

Not all HCAI infections are caused by procedures nor are all HCAI preventable, although we should always be aiming for this. Another factor contributing to the development of HCAI infections is the compromised host, that is, a patient whose normal defences have been lowered by surgery or illness. The hands of personnel are a common vehicle for the spread of micro-organisms and insufficient hand hygiene is thus an important factor contributing to the spread of HCAI.

CLINICAL ALERT

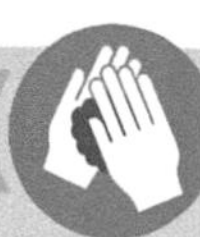

A person does not need to have an identified infection in order to pass potentially infective micro-organisms to another person. Even normal micro-organisms for one person can infect another person if they are able to breach the body's defences.

MICRO-ORGANISMS AND INFECTION

Nurses are directly involved in providing a biologically safe environment. Micro-organisms exist everywhere: in water, in soil, equipment and on body surfaces such as the skin, the intestinal tract and other areas open to the outside (e.g. the mouth, upper respiratory tract, vagina and lower urinary tract). Most micro-organisms are harmless, and some are even beneficial in that they perform essential functions in the body. Some micro-organisms found in the intestines (e.g. enterobacteria) produce substances called **bacteriocins**, which are lethal to related strains of bacteria. Others produce antibiotic-like substances and toxic metabolites that repress the growth of other micro-organisms.

Some micro-organisms are normal **resident flora** (the collective vegetation in a given area) in one part of the body, yet produce infection in another. For example, *Escherichia coli* is a normal inhabitant of the large intestine but a common cause of infection of the urinary tract. **Transient flora** are micro-organisms that are picked up from exogenous sources and live on the surface of the body for a short period of time. They are often associated with transmission of pathogenic micro-organisms on the hands of health professionals. Table 12-1 provides a list of common resident micro-organisms.

An **infection** is an invasion of body tissue by micro-organisms and their proliferation there which results in a host response (Fraise, 2009). Such a micro-organism is called an infectious agent. If the micro-organism produces no clinical evidence of disease, the infection is called asymptomatic or subclinical. Some subclinical infections can cause significant damage, for example, cytomegalovirus (CMV) infection in a pregnant woman can lead to significant disease in the unborn child.

Table 12-1 Examples of Common Resident Micro-organisms

Body area	Micro-organisms
Skin	*Staphylococcus epidermidis* *Propionibacterium acnes* *Staphylococcus aureus* *Corynebacterium xerosis*
Nasal passages	*Staphylococcus aureus* *Staphylococcus epidermidis*
Oropharynx	*Streptococcus pneumoniae*
Mouth	*Streptococcus mutans* *Lactobacillus* *Bacteroides* *Actinomyces*
Intestine	*Bacteroides* *Fusobacterium* *Eubacterium* *Lactobacillus* *Streptococcus* *Enterobacteriaceae* *Shigella* *Escherichia coli*
Urethral orifice	*Staphylococcus epidermidis*
Urethra (lower)	*Proteus*
Vagina	*Lactobacillus* *Bacteroides* *Clostridium* *Candida albicans*

Colonisation is the process by which strains of micro-organisms become resident flora. In this state, the micro-organisms may grow and multiply but do not cause disease. Infection occurs when newly introduced or resident micro-organisms succeed in invading a part of the body where the host's defence mechanisms are ineffective and the pathogen causes tissue damage. The infection becomes a disease when the signs and symptoms of the infection are unique and can be differentiated from other conditions. *Staphylococcus aureus* living normally on the skin can lead to significant disease if it gets into the persons' bloodstream.

Infections can be local or systemic. A local infection is limited to the specific part of the body where the micro-organisms remain. If the micro-organisms spread and damage different parts of the body, it is a systemic infection. When a culture of the person's blood reveals micro-organisms, the condition is called **bacteraemia**. When bacteraemia results in systemic infection, it is referred to as septicaemia. There are also acute or chronic infections. Acute infections generally appear suddenly or last a short time. A chronic infection may occur slowly, over a very long period, and may last months or years.

Micro-organisms vary in their **virulence** (i.e. their ability to produce disease). Micro-organisms also vary in the severity of the diseases they produce and their degree of communicability. For example, the common cold virus is more readily transmitted than the bacillus that causes leprosy (*Mycobacterium leprae*). If the infectious agent can be transmitted to an individual by direct or indirect contact, through a vector or vehicle, or as an airborne infection, the resulting condition is called a **communicable disease**.

Pathogenicity is the ability to produce disease; thus a pathogen is a micro-organism that causes disease. Many micro-organisms that are normally harmless can cause disease under certain circumstances. A 'true' pathogen causes disease or infection in a healthy individual. An opportunistic pathogen causes disease only in a susceptible individual.

Types of Micro-organisms Causing Infections

Four major categories of micro-organisms cause infection in humans: bacteria, viruses, fungi and parasites. Bacteria are by far the most common infection causing micro-organisms. Several hundred species can cause disease in humans and can live and be transported through air, water, food, soil, body tissues and fluids and inanimate objects. Most of the micro-organisms in Table 12-1 are bacteria. In the hospital setting there is a continued risk of micro-organisms becoming resistant to antibiotics. Three of the main resistant micro-organisms that are found in UK hospitals are resistant to certain groups of antibiotics and include MRSA, glycopeptide resistant enterococcus and the bacteria that can be grouped under the term Extended-Spectrum Beta-Lactamases (ESBL). ESBL are specific bacteria (*Klebsiella* and *E coli*) that are resistant to a group of antibiotics called cephalosporins. The resistant micro-organisms continue to challenge healthcare providers, emphasising the importance of optimal infection prevention and control practice.

Viruses consist primarily of nucleic acid and therefore must enter living cells in order to reproduce. Common virus families include norovirus, rhinovirus (causes the common cold), hepatitis, herpes and human immunodeficiency virus. Fungi include yeasts and moulds. *Candida albicans* is a yeast considered to be normal flora in the human vagina. Parasites live on other living organisms. They include protozoa such as the one that causes malaria, helminths (worms) and arthropods (mites, fleas, ticks).

BODY DEFENCES AGAINST INFECTION

Individuals normally have defences that protect the body from infection. These defences can be categorised as nonspecific and specific. Nonspecific defences protect the person against all micro-organisms, regardless of prior exposure. Specific (immune) defences, by contrast, are directed against identifiable infectious agents.

Nonspecific Defences

Nonspecific body defences include anatomical and physiological barriers, and the inflammatory response.

Anatomical and Physiological Barriers

Intact skin and mucous membranes are the body's first line of defence against micro-organisms. Unless the skin and mucosa become cracked and broken, they are an effective barrier against bacteria. Fungi can live on the skin, but they cannot penetrate it. The dryness of the skin also is a deterrent to bacteria. Bacteria are most plentiful in moist areas of the body, such as the perineum and axillae. Resident bacteria of the skin also prevent other bacteria from multiplying. They use up the available nourishment, and the end products of their metabolism inhibit other bacterial growth. Normal secretions make the skin slightly acidic; acidity also inhibits bacterial growth.

The nasal passages have a defensive function. As entering air follows the tortuous route of the passage, it comes in contact with moist mucous membranes and cilia. These trap micro-organisms, dust and foreign materials. The lungs have alveolar macrophages (large phagocytes). Phagocytes are cells that ingest micro-organisms, other cells and foreign particles.

Each body orifice also has protective mechanisms. The oral cavity regularly sheds mucosal epithelium to rid the mouth of colonisers. The flow of saliva and its partially buffering action help prevent infections. Saliva contains microbial inhibitors, such as lactoferrin, lysozyme and secretory IgA.

The eye is protected from infection by tears, which continually wash micro-organisms away and contain inhibiting lysozyme. The gastrointestinal tract also has defences against infection. The high acidity of the stomach normally prevents microbial growth. The resident flora of the large intestine help prevent the establishment of disease-producing micro-organisms. Peristalsis also tends to move microbes out of the body.

The vagina also has natural defences against infection. When puberty is reached, lactobacilli ferment sugars in the vaginal secretions, creating a vaginal pH of 3.5 to 4.5. This low pH inhibits the growth of many pathogenic micro-organisms. The entrance to the urethra normally harbours many micro-organisms. These include *Staphylococcus epidermidis* (from the skin) and *Escherichia coli* (from faeces). It is believed that the urine flow has a flushing and bacteriostatic action that keeps the bacteria from ascending the urethra. An intact mucosal surface also acts as a barrier.

Inflammatory Response

Inflammation is a local and nonspecific defensive response of the tissues to an injurious or infectious agent. It is an adaptive mechanism that destroys or dilutes the injurious agent, prevents further spread of the injury, and promotes the repair of damaged tissue. It is characterised by five signs: (a) pain, (b) swelling, (c) redness, (d) heat and (e) impaired function of the part, if the injury is severe. Commonly, words with the suffix *-itis* describe an inflammatory process. For example, *appendicitis* means inflammation of the appendix; *gastritis* means inflammation of the stomach.

CLINICAL ALERT

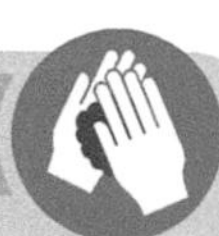

An easy way to remember the signs of inflammation are the rhyming Latin words: rubor (redness), tumor (swelling), colour/calor (heat), and dolor (pain).

Injurious agents can be categorised as physical agents, chemical agents and micro-organisms. *Physical agents* include mechanical objects causing trauma to tissues, excessive heat or cold, and radiation. *Chemical agents* include external irritants (e.g. strong **acids**, alkalis, poisons and irritating gases) and internal irritants (substances manufactured within the body such as excessive hydrochloric acid in the stomach). Micro-organisms include the broad groups of bacteria, viruses, fungi and parasites.

A series of dynamic events is commonly referred to as the three stages of the inflammatory response:

- *first stage*: vascular and cellular responses;
- *second stage*: **exudate** production;
- *third stage*: reparative phase.

Specific Defences

Specific defences of the body involve the immune system. An **antigen** is a substance that induces a state of sensitivity or immune responsiveness (**immunity**). If the proteins originate in a person's own body, the antigen is called an **autoantigen**.

The immune response has two components: antibody-mediated defences and cell-mediated defences. These two systems provide distinct but overlapping protection.

Table 12-2 Types of Immunity

Type	Antigen or antibody source	Duration
1 Active	Antibodies are produced by the body in response to an antigen.	Long
a. Natural	Antibodies are formed in the presence of active infection in the body.	Lifelong
b. Artificial	Antigens (vaccines or toxoids) are administered to stimulate antibody production.	Many years; the immunity must be reinforced by booster production.
2. Passive	Antibodies are produced by another source, animal or human.	Short
a. Natural	Antibodies are transferred naturally from an immune mother to her baby through the placenta or in colostrum.	6 months to 1 year
b. Artificial	Immune serum (antibody) from an animal or another human is injected.	2 to 3 weeks

Antibody-Mediated Defences

Another name for the *antibody-mediated defences* is **humoral immunity** (or **circulating immunity**) because these defences reside ultimately in the B lymphocytes and are mediated by antibodies produced by B cells. Antibodies, also called immunoglobulins, are part of the body's **plasma** proteins. The antibody-mediated responses defend primarily against the extracellular phases of bacterial and viral infections.

There are two major types of immunity: active and passive (see Table 12-2). In **active immunity**, the host produces antibodies in response to natural antigens (e.g. infectious micro-organisms) or artificial antigens (e.g. vaccines). B cells are activated when they recognise the antigen. They then differentiate into plasma cells, which secrete the antibodies, and serum proteins that bind specifically to the foreign substance and initiate a variety of elimination responses. The B cell may produce antibody molecules of five classes of immunoglobulins designated by letters and usually written as IgM, IgG, IgA, IgD and IgE. The presence of IgM in a laboratory analysis shows current infection. Before the antibody response can become effective, the phagocytic cells of the blood bind and ingest foreign substances. The rate of binding and **phagocytosis** increases if IgG antibodies (which indicate past infection and subsequent immunity) are present. With passive immunity (or acquired immunity), the host receives natural (e.g. from a nursing mother) or artificial (e.g. from an injection of immune serum) antibodies produced by another source.

Cell-Mediated Defences

The **cell-mediated** defences, or **cellular immunity**, occur through the T-cell system. On exposure to an antigen, the lymphoid tissues release large numbers of activated T cells into the lymph system. These T cells pass into the general circulation. There are three main groups of T cells: (a) helper T cells, which help in the functions of the immune system; (b) cytotoxic T cells, which attack and kill micro-organisms and sometimes the body's own cells; and (c) suppressor T cells, which can suppress the functions of the helper T cells and the cytotoxic T cells. When cell-mediated immunity is lost, as occurs with human immunodeficiency virus (HIV) infection, an individual is 'defenceless' against most viral, bacterial and fungal infections.

THE CHAIN OF INFECTION

The chain of infection illustrates the stages that need to be in place in order that transmission of a micro-organism can occur. Through understanding the chain we can identify where it can be broken to prevent transmission of infection. Six links make up the chain of infection (Figure 12-1): the micro-organism; the place where the organism naturally resides (reservoir); a portal of exit from the reservoir; a method (mode) of transmission; a portal of entry into a host; and the susceptibility of the host.

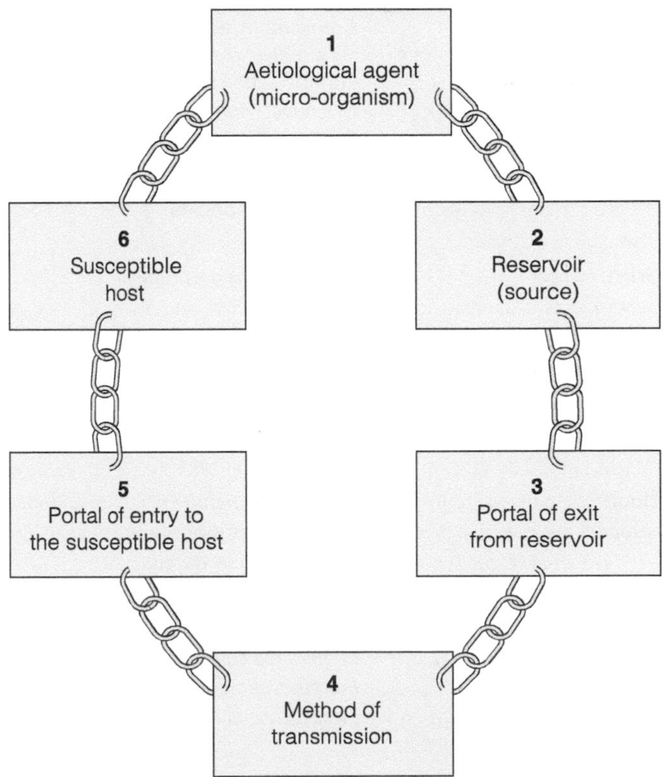

Figure 12-1 The chain of infection.

Micro-organism factors

The extent to which any micro-organism is capable of producing an infectious process depends on the number of micro-organisms present, the virulence and potency of the micro-organisms (pathogenicity), the ability of the micro-organisms to enter the body, the susceptibility of the host, and the ability of the micro-organisms to live in the host's body (see Table 12-3).

Some micro-organisms, such as the smallpox virus (now eradicated worldwide), have the ability to infect almost all susceptible people after exposure. By contrast, micro-organisms such as the tuberculosis bacillus infect a relatively small number of the population who are susceptible and exposed, usually people who are poorly nourished, who are living in crowded conditions, or whose immune systems are less competent (such as older adults or those with HIV or cancer).

Reservoir

There are many **reservoirs** or sources of micro-organisms. Common sources are other humans, the patient's own micro-organisms, plants, animals, clinical equipment or the general environment. People are the most common source of infection for others and for themselves (see Table 12-4). For example, the person with an influenza virus frequently spreads it to others.

Table 12-3 Healthcare Associated Infections

Most common micro-organisms	Potential causes
Urinary tract	
Escherichia coli	Improper catheterisation technique
Enterococcus species	Contamination of closed drainage system
Pseudomonas aeruginosa	Inadequate hand hygiene
Surgical sites	
Staphylococcus aureus (may be resistant)	Inadequate hand hygiene
Enterococcus species	Breakdown in peri-operative precautions
Pseudomonas aeruginosa	Improper dressing change technique
Bloodstream	
Coagulase-negative *staphylococci*	Inadequate hand hygiene
Staphylococcus aureus	Improper intravenous fluid, tubing and site care technique
Enterococcus species	
Pneumonia	
Staphylococcus aureus	Inadequate hand hygiene
Pseudomonas aeruginosa	Improper suctioning technique
Enterobacter species	

Table 12-4 Human Body Area Reservoirs, Common Infectious Micro-organisms and Portals of Exit

Body area	Common infectious organisms	Portals of exit
Respiratory tract	Parainfluenza virus *Mycobacterium tuberculosis* *Staphylococcus aureus*	Nose or mouth through sneezing, coughing, breathing or talking
Gastrointestinal tract	Hepatitis A virus *Salmonella* species Norovirus	Mouth: saliva, vomitus; anus: faeces; ostomies
Urinary tract	*Pseudomonas aeruginosa* *Escherichia coli* *Enterococci*	Urethral meatus and urinary diversion
Reproductive tract	*Neisseria gonorrhoeae* *Treponema pallidum* Herpes simplex virus type 2 Hepatitis B virus (HBV)	Vagina: vaginal discharge; Urinary meatus: semen, urine
Blood	Hepatitis B virus Human immunodeficiency virus (HIV) *Staphylococcus aureus* *Staphylococcus epidermidis*	Open wound, needle puncture site, any disruption of intact skin or mucous membrane surfaces
Tissue	*Staphylococcus aureus* *Escherichia coli* *Proteus* species *Streptococcus* beta-haemolytic A or B	Drainage from cut or wound

A carrier is a person or animal reservoir of a specific infectious agent that usually does not manifest any clinical signs of disease. The *Anopheles* mosquito reservoir carries the malaria parasite but is unaffected by it. The carrier state may also exist in individuals with a clinically recognisable disease such as the dog with rabies. Under either circumstance, the carrier state may be of short duration (temporary or transient carrier) or long duration (chronic carrier). Food, water and faeces also can be reservoirs.

Portal of Exit from Reservoir

Before an infection can establish itself in a host, the micro-organisms must leave the reservoir. Common human reservoirs and their associated portals of exit are summarised in Table 12-4.

Method of Transmission

After a micro-organism leaves its source or reservoir, it requires a means of transmission to reach another person or host through a receptive portal of entry. There are three mechanisms:

1 *Direct transmission.* Direct transmission involves immediate and direct transfer of micro-organisms from person to person through touching, biting, kissing or sexual intercourse. Droplet spread is also a form of direct transmission but can occur only if the source and the host are within a few metres of each other. Sneezing, coughing, spitting, singing or talking can project droplet spray into the conjunctiva or onto the mucous membranes of the eye, nose or mouth of another person.
2 *Indirect transmission.* Indirect transmission may be either vehicle-borne or vector-borne.
   - **Vehicle-borne transmission.** A *vehicle* is any substance that serves as an intermediate means to transport and introduce an infectious agent into a susceptible host through a suitable portal of entry. Fomites (inanimate materials or objects), such as handkerchiefs, toys, soiled clothes, cooking or eating utensils, and surgical instruments or dressings, can act as vehicles. Water, food, blood, serum and plasma are other vehicles. For example, food or water may become contaminated by a food handler who carries the hepatitis A virus. The food is then ingested by a susceptible host.
   - **Vector-borne transmission.** A *vector* is an animal or flying or crawling insect that serves as an intermediate means of transporting the infectious agent. Transmission may occur by injecting salivary fluid during biting or by depositing faeces or other materials on the skin through the bite wound or a traumatised skin area.
3 *Airborne transmission.* Airborne transmission may involve droplets or dust. Droplet nuclei, the residue of evaporated droplets emitted by an infected host such as someone with tuberculosis, can remain in the air for long periods. Dust particles containing the infectious agent can also become airborne. The material is transmitted by air currents to a suitable portal of entry, usually the respiratory tract, of another person.

Portal of Entry to the Susceptible Host

Before a person can become infected, micro-organisms must enter the body. The skin is a barrier to infectious agents; however, any break in the skin can readily serve as a portal of entry. Often, micro-organisms enter the body of the host by the same route they used to leave the source. Methods of entry include ingestion, inoculation, inhalation, transplacental and sexual.

Susceptible Host

A susceptible host is any person who is at risk for infection. A compromised host is a person 'at increased risk', an individual who for one or more reasons is more likely than others to acquire an infection. Impairment of the body's natural defences and a number of other factors can affect susceptibility to infection. Examples include age (the very young or the very old); patients receiving immune suppression treatment for cancer, chronic illness or following a successful organ transplant; and those with immune deficiency conditions.

FACTORS INCREASING SUSCEPTIBILITY TO INFECTION

Whether a micro-organism causes an infection depends on a number of factors already mentioned. One of the most important factors is host susceptibility, which is affected by age, heredity, level of stress, nutritional status, current medical therapy and pre-existing disease processes.

Age influences the risk of infection. Newborns and older adults have reduced defences against infection. With advancing age, the immune responses again become weak. Although there is still much to learn about ageing, it is known that immunity to infection decreases with advancing age. Infections are a major cause of death of newborns, who have immature immune systems and are protected only for the first two or three months by immunoglobulins passively received from the mother. Between one and three months of age, infants begin to synthesise their own immunoglobulins. Immunisations are usually started when children are at two months old, when the infant's immune system can respond. Childhood immunisation guidelines can change regularly so refer to the NHS immunisation website or the Department of Health for up to date information.

LIFESPAN CONSIDERATIONS

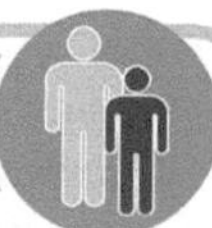

Older Adults

Normal ageing may predispose older adults to increased risk of infection and delayed healing. Organs and biochemical agents that are protective when a person is younger often change in structure and function with increasing age and then provide a decrease in their protective ability. Changes take place in the skin, respiratory tract, gastrointestinal system, kidneys and immune system. If unchallenged, these systems work well to maintain homoeostasis for the individual, but if compromised by stress, illness, infections, treatments or surgery, they find it difficult to keep up and therefore are not able to provide adequate protection. Special considerations for older adults are:

- Nutrition is often poor in older adults and certain components, especially adequate protein, are necessary to build up and maintain the immune system.
- Diabetes mellitus, which occurs more frequently in the elderly, increases the risk of infection and delayed healing by causing an alteration in nutrition and impaired peripheral circulation, which decreases the oxygen transport to the tissues.
- The immune system reacts slowly to the introduction of antigens, allowing the antigen to reproduce itself several times before it is recognised by the immune system. T-cell effectiveness is often decreased due to immaturity.
- The normal inflammatory response is delayed. This often causes atypical responses to infections with unusual presentations. Instead of displaying redness, swelling, and fever usually associated with infections, atypical symptoms such as confusion and disorientation, agitation, incontinence, falls, lethargy and general fatigue are often seen first.

Recognising these changes in older adults is important in early detection and treatment of infection and delayed healing. Nursing interventions to promote prevention are:

- Provide and teach ways to improve nutritional status.
- Use strict aseptic technique to decrease chance of infection.
- Provide information for older adults in relation to appropriate immunisations.
- Be alert to subtle atypical signs of infection and act quickly to diagnose and treat.

Heredity influences the development of infection in that some people have a genetic susceptibility to certain infections. For example, some may be deficient in serum immunoglobulins, which play a significant role in the internal defence mechanism of the body.

The nature, number and duration of physical and emotional stressors can influence susceptibility to infection. Stressors elevate blood cortisone. Prolonged elevation of blood cortisone decreases anti-inflammatory responses, depletes energy stores, leads to a state of exhaustion and decreases resistance to infection. For example, a person recovering from a major operation or injury is more likely to develop an infection than a healthy person.

Resistance to infection depends on adequate nutritional status. Because antibodies are proteins, the ability to synthesise antibodies may be impaired by inadequate nutrition, especially when protein reserves are depleted (e.g. as a result of injury, surgery or debilitating diseases).

Some medical therapies predispose a person to infection. For example, radiation treatments for cancer destroy not only cancerous cells but also some normal cells, thereby rendering them more vulnerable to infection. Some diagnostic procedures may also predispose the patient to an infection, especially when the skin is broken or sterile body cavities are penetrated during the procedure (venous catheterisation, wound drains, urinary catheterisation, surgery).

Certain medications also increase susceptibility to infection. Antineoplastic (anticancer) medications may depress bone marrow function, resulting in inadequate production of white blood cells necessary to combat infections. Anti-inflammatory medications, such as adrenal corticosteroids, inhibit the inflammatory response, an essential defence against infection. Even some antibiotics used to treat infections can have adverse effects. Antibiotics may kill resident flora, allowing the proliferation of strains that would not grow and multiply in the body under normal conditions (*Clostridium difficile*). Certain antibiotics can also induce resistance in some strains of micro-organisms.

Any disease that lessens the body's defences against infection places the patient at risk. Examples are chronic pulmonary disease, which impairs ciliary action and weakens the mucous barrier; peripheral vascular disease, which restricts blood flow; burns, which impair skin integrity; chronic or debilitating diseases, which deplete protein reserves; and such immune system diseases as leukaemia and aplastic anaemia, which alter the production of white blood cells. Diabetes mellitus is a major underlying disease predisposing patients to infection because compromised peripheral vascular status and increased serum glucose levels increase susceptibility.

SUPPORTING DEFENCES OF A SUSCEPTIBLE HOST

People are constantly in contact with micro-organisms in the environment. Normally a person's natural defences ward off the development of an infection. Susceptibility is the degree to which an individual can be affected, that is, the likelihood of a micro-organism causing an infection in that person. The following measures can reduce a person's susceptibility:

- *Hygiene.* Intact skin and mucous membranes are one barrier against micro-organisms entering the body. In addition, good oral care reduces the likelihood of an oral infection. Regular and thorough bathing and shampooing remove micro-organisms and dirt that can result in an infection.
- *Nutrition.* A balanced diet enhances the health of all body tissues, helps keep the skin intact and promotes the skin's ability to repel micro-organisms. Adequate nutrition enables tissues to maintain and rebuild themselves and helps keep the immune system functioning well.
- *Fluid.* Fluid intake permits fluid output that flushes out the bladder and urethra, removing micro-organisms that could cause an infection.
- *Rest and sleep.* Adequate rest and sleep are essential to health and to renewing energy.
- *Stress.* Excessive stress predisposes people to infections. Nurses can assist patients to learn stress-reducing techniques.
- *Immunisations.* The use of immunisations has dramatically decreased the incidence of infectious diseases. It is recommended that immunisations begin shortly after birth and be completed in early childhood except for boosters. Immunisations may be given by injection, inhalation, oral solutions or nasal sprays. They are frequently given in combination to minimise multiple injections. Because there are frequent changes to immunisation schedules, it is advisable to update immunisation schedules yearly.

There are immunisation programmes for high-risk groups such as healthcare personnel, older adults who are chronically ill and people travelling to foreign countries. For example, hepatitis B vaccine is recommended for all healthcare workers.

ASSESSMENT OF INFECTED PATIENTS

During the assessment phase of the nursing process, the nurse obtains the patient's history, conducts the physical assessment, and gathers laboratory data. Interpersonal skills including communication and observational skills are vital for effective assessment.

Patient History

During the patient history, the nurse assesses (a) the degree to which a patient is at risk of developing an infection and (b) any patient complaints suggesting the presence of an infection. The nurse needs to collect data regarding the factors influencing the development of infection; especially existing disease process, history of recurrent infections, current medications and therapeutic measures, current emotional stressors, nutritional status and history of immunisations.

Physiological Assessment

Signs and symptoms of an infection vary according to the body area involved. For example, sneezing, watery or mucoid discharge from the nose and nasal stuffiness commonly occur with an infection of the nose and sinuses; urinary frequency and possible cloudy or discoloured urine often occur with a urinary infection. Commonly the skin and mucous membranes are involved in a local infectious process, resulting in

- localised swelling;
- localised redness;
- pain or tenderness with palpation or movement;
- palpable heat at the infected area;
- loss of function of the body part affected, depending on the site and extent of involvement.

In addition, open wounds may exude drainage of various colours.

Signs of *systemic infection* include:

- fever;
- increased pulse and respiratory rate, if the fever is high;
- malaise and loss of energy;
- anorexia and, in some situations, nausea and vomiting;
- enlargement and tenderness of lymph nodes that drain the area of infection.

Laboratory Data

Laboratory data that indicate the presence of an infection include the following:

- elevated leukocyte (white blood cell or WBC) count;
- increases in specific types of leukocytes as revealed in the differential WBC count – specific types of white blood cells are increased or decreased in certain infections;
- elevated *erythrocyte sedimentation rate (ESR)* – red blood cells normally settle slowly, but the rate increases in the presence of an inflammatory process;
- urine, blood, sputum or other drainage cultures (laboratory cultivations of micro-organisms in a special growth medium) that indicate the presence of pathogenic micro-organisms.

PLANNING

The major goals for patients susceptible to infection are to:

- maintain or restore defences;
- avoid the spread of infectious micro-organisms;
- reduce or alleviate problems associated with the infection.

Desired outcomes depend on the individual patient's condition. Nursing strategies to meet the three broad goals stated above generally include using meticulous hand hygiene, standard and transmission based precautions and aseptic techniques to prevent the spread of potentially infectious micro-organisms, implementing measures to support the defences of a susceptible host, and teaching patients about protective measures to prevent infections and the spread of infectious agents when an infection is present.

Planning for Community Care

Patients being discharged following hospital care for an infection often require continued care to completely eliminate the infection or to adapt to a chronic state. In addition, such patients may be at increased risk for reinfection or development of an opportunistic infection following therapy for existing pathogens.

In preparation for discharge, the nurse needs to know the patient's and family's risks, needs, strengths and resources. The *Teaching: Community Care* box describes the specific assessment data required before establishing a discharge plan. Using the data gathered about the home situation, the nurse tailors the teaching plan for the patient and family (see the *Teaching: Wellness Care* box).

IMPLEMENTING

Whenever possible, the nurse implements strategies to prevent infection. If infection cannot be prevented, the nurse's goal is to control the spread of the infection within and between persons, and to treat the existing infection. In the sections that follow, specific infection prevention and control activities are described that interfere and disrupt the chain of infection to prevent and control transmission of infectious micro-organisms, and to promote care of the infected patient. These activities are summarised in Table 12-5.

TEACHING: COMMUNITY CARE

Environmental Management

- Discuss injury-proofing the home to prevent the possibility of further tissue injury (e.g. use of padding, handrails, removal of hazards).
- Explore ways to control the environmental temperature and airflow (especially if the patient has an airborne pathogen).
- Determine the advisability of visitors and family members in proximity to the patient.
- Describe ways to manipulate the bed, the room and other household facilities.

Infection Control

- Teach proper hand washing and related hygienic measures to all family members.
- Discuss food hygiene and cleaning.
- Ensure access to and proper use of gloves and other barriers as indicated by the type of infection or risk.
- Discuss the relationship between hygiene, rest, activity and nutrition in the chain of infection.
- Instruct about proper administration of medication.
- Instruct about cleaning reusable equipment and supplies.

Infection Protection

- Teach the patient and family members the signs and symptoms of infection, and when to contact a healthcare provider.
- Teach the patient and family members how to avoid infections.
- Suggest techniques for safe food preservation and preparation.
- Emphasise the need for proper immunisations of all family members.

Wound Care (if appropriate)

- Teach the patient and family the signs of wound healing and of wound infection.
- Explain the proper technique for changing the dressing and disposing of the soiled one.
- Delineate the factors that promote wound healing.

TEACHING: WELLNESS CARE

Preventing Infections in the Home

- Wash your hands before handling foods, before eating, after toileting, before and after any required home care treatment, and after touching any body substances (e.g. wound drainage).
- Keep your fingernails short, clean and well manicured to eliminate rough edges, which can harbour micro-organisms.
- Do not share personal care items: toothbrush, washcloths and towels.
- Wash raw fruits and vegetables before eating them.
- Refrigerate all opened and unpackaged foods.
- Clean used equipment with soap and water, and disinfect it with a chlorine bleach solution.
- Place contaminated dressings and other disposable items containing body fluids in moisture-proof clinical waste bags.
- Put used needles in a puncture-resistant sharps container.
- Clean obviously soiled linen separately from other laundry.
- Avoid coughing, sneezing or breathing directly on others. Cover the mouth and nose to prevent the transmission of airborne micro-organisms.
- Be aware of any signs or symptoms of an infection, and report these immediately to your healthcare contact person.
- Maintain a sufficient fluid intake to promote urine production and output. This helps flush the bladder and urethra of micro-organisms.

Table 12-5 Nursing Interventions that Break the Chain of Infection

Link	Interventions	Rationale
Micro-organism	Ensure that articles are correctly cleaned and disinfected or sterilised before use to eliminate micro-organisms.	Correct cleaning, disinfecting and sterilising reduce/eradicate micro-organisms.
	Educate patients and support persons about appropriate methods to clean, disinfect and sterilise articles.	Knowledge of ways to reduce or eliminate micro-organisms reduces the numbers of micro-organisms present and the likelihood of transmission.
Reservoir	Change dressings and bandages when they are soiled or wet.	Moist dressings are ideal environments for micro-organisms to grow and multiply.
	Assist patients to carry out appropriate skin and oral hygiene.	Hygienic measures reduce the numbers of resident and transient micro-organisms and the likelihood of infection.
	Dispose of damp, soiled linens appropriately.	Damp, soiled linens harbour more micro-organisms than dry linens.
	Dispose of faeces and urine in appropriate receptacles.	Urine and faeces in particular contain many micro-organisms.
	Ensure that all fluid containers, such as bedside water jugs and suction and drainage bottles, are covered or capped.	Prolonged exposure increases the risk of contamination and promotes microbial growth.
	Empty suction and drainage bottles at the end of each shift or before they become full, or according to local policy.	Drainage harbours micro-organisms that, if left for long periods, proliferate and can be transmitted to others.
Portal of exit from the reservoir	Avoid talking, coughing or sneezing over open wounds or sterile fields, and cover the mouth and nose when coughing and sneezing.	These measures limit the number of micro-organisms that escape from the respiratory tract.
Method of transmission	Perform hand hygiene before and after patient contact, after touching body substances, and before performing invasive procedures or touching open wounds.	Hand hygiene is an important means of controlling and preventing the transmission of micro-organisms.
	Instruct patients and support persons to perform hand hygiene before handling food or eating, after eliminating and after touching infectious material.	
	Wear gloves when handling secretions and excretions.	Gloves and gowns prevent soiling of the hands and clothing.
	Wear gowns/disposable plastic aprons if there is danger of soiling clothing with body substances.	
	Place discarded soiled materials in moisture-proof clinical waste bags.	Moisture-proof bags prevent the spread of micro-organisms to others.
	Hold used bedpans steadily to prevent spillage, and dispose of urine and faeces in appropriate receptacles.	Faeces in particular contain many micro-organisms.
	Initiate and implement aseptic precautions for all patients.	All patients may harbour potentially infectious micro-organisms that can be transmitted to others.
	Wear masks and eye protection when in close contact with patients who have infections transmitted by droplets from the respiratory tract.	Masks and eyewear reduce the spread of droplet-transmitted micro-organisms.
	Wear masks and eye protection when sprays of body fluid are possible (e.g. during irrigation procedures).	Masks and eye protection provide protection from micro-organisms in patients' body substances.
	Ensure equipment and environmental **decontamination** is carried out according to local policy.	Appropriate decontamination will reduce the risk of transmission of micro-organisms.

Table 12-5 (*continued*)

Link	Interventions	Rationale
Portal of entry to the susceptible host	Use aseptic technique for invasive procedures (e.g. injections, catheterisations).	Invasive procedures penetrate the body's natural protective barriers to micro-organisms.
	Use sterile technique when exposing open wounds or handling dressings.	Open wounds are vulnerable to microbial infection.
	Place used disposable needles and syringes in puncture-resistant sharps containers for disposal.	Injuries from needles contaminated by blood or body fluids from an infected patient or carrier are a primary cause of HBV, HCV and HIV transmission to healthcare workers.
	Provide all patients with their own personal care items.	People have less resistance to another person's micro-organisms than to their own.
Susceptible host	Maintain the integrity of the patient's skin and mucous membranes.	Intact skin and mucous membranes protect against infection.
	Ensure that the patient receives a balanced diet.	A balanced diet supplies proteins and vitamins necessary to build or maintain body tissues.
	Educate the public about the importance of immunisations.	Immunisations protect people against virulent infectious diseases.

EVALUATING OUTCOMES

Using data collected during care – vital signs, lung sounds, skin status, characteristics of urine or other drainage, laboratory blood values, and so on – the nurse judges whether patient outcomes have been achieved.

If outcomes are not achieved, the nurse may need to consider questions such as the following:

- Were appropriate measures implemented to prevent skin breakdown and lung infection?
- Was strict aseptic technique implemented for invasive procedures?
- Is there optimal compliance with standard/transmission based precautions?
- Are prescribed medications affecting the immune system?
- Is patient placement appropriate to reduce the risk of transmission of micro-organisms?
- Did the patient and family misunderstand or fail to comply with necessary instructions?

PREVENTING AND CONTROLLING HCAI

HCAI can be prevented and controlled by making the patient less vulnerable to infection through reducing intrinsic and extrinsic risk factors, interrupting the means of transmission and isolating the source of the infectious micro-organisms. These will help break the chain of infection. The key concept underpinning the prevention and control of infection are standard precautions.

Standard Precautions

Meticulous use of infection prevention and control precautions is necessary to prevent transmission of potentially infectious micro-organisms. Many HCAI can be prevented and controlled using standard precautions. Standard precautions are the foundation of effective infection prevention and control management and are the minimum precautions necessary to reduce exposure to or transmission of micro-organisms from patients with or without known infections. They must be used by all staff on all occasions in every setting. Standard precautions are a development of universal precautions and are endorsed for use in the UK (Pratt *et al.*, 2007). They are based on a set of principles that can reduce the risk of exposure to and transmission of micro-organisms.

The underpinning principle of standard precautions is that since it is impossible to identify every patient with an infection, all body fluids, secretions, excretions, broken skin and mucous membranes are treated as potentially infectious. So taking appropriate precautions at all times will reduce the risk of infection for patients and staff. Standard precautions advocate that health professionals, in all settings, regard all patients as high risk and categorise procedures into low, medium and high risk based on likelihood of exposure to blood and/or body fluids, secretions, excretions, broken skin and mucous membranes. So it is the procedure that is risk assessed and not the patient (Gould and Booker, 2008). It is important to maintain high standards at all times in order to provide protection and consistency (Cutter and Gammon, 2007). Standard precautions can be supplemented by transmission-based precautions when caring for patients with infections that are transmitted through certain routes (see page 336).

Standard precautions include:

- hand hygiene;
- personal protective equipment (PPE);
- prevention of exposure to blood and body fluids;
- management of blood and body fluid spillages;
- decontamination of equipment;
- patient placement (Isolation);
- linen and waste management.

These will be discussed throughout the remainder of the chapter.

In addition to standard precautions the nurse also implements other precautions when performing many specific therapies. The following are some examples:

- Use strict aseptic technique when performing any invasive procedure (e.g. suctioning an airway or inserting a urinary catheter) and when changing surgical dressings.
- Change intravenous tubing according to local policy (e.g. every 48 to 72 hours).
- Check all sterile supplies for expiration date and intact packaging.
- Prevent urinary infections by maintaining a closed urinary drainage system with a downhill flow of urine. Provide regular catheter care, and clean the perineal area with soap and water. Keep the drainage bag and spout off the floor.
- Implement measures to prevent impaired skin integrity and to prevent accumulation of secretions in the lungs (e.g. encourage the patient to move, cough and breathe deeply at least every two hours).
- Use transmission-based precautions in conjunction with standard precautions when caring for patients with suspected or known infections.

There are also other initiatives that are key in the fight to prevent and control HCAI. These include food hygiene regulations, infection surveillance, staffing levels and bed occupancy levels, staff education, antibiotic stewardship, audit, immunisation and also the many initiatives that have been instigated to help educate and motivate staff into improving their infection prevention and control practice. These are outside the scope of this chapter but there will be some relevant web addresses at the end of the chapter where further information can be found.

Hand Hygiene

Hand hygiene is the single most important infection prevention and control intervention. It is important in every setting where healthcare is delivered. Any patient may harbour micro-organisms that are currently harmless to the patient yet potentially harmful to another person or to the same patient if they find a portal of entry. It is important that health professionals perform hand hygiene at the following critical times, as identified by the World Health Organization (2009) in their 'Five Moments for Hand Hygiene'. They identify that hand hygiene should be performed: (1) before touching a patient, (2) before a clean/aseptic technique, (3) after body fluid exposure risk, (4) after touching a patient and (5) after touching patients' surrounds (WHO, 2009).

It is also important that patients perform or are assisted with hand hygiene after they have been to the toilet, after the hands have come in contact with any body substances, such as sputum or drainage from a wound and before and after meal times as a minimum.

From the WHO's five moments of hand hygiene it is easy to identify the importance of hand hygiene at the point of care. It is the moment when the highest likelihood of transmission of micro-organisms from the hands of healthcare workers to patients and from patients to healthcare workers exists. Hand hygiene must be performed even if gloves have been worn and it will often need to be performed between different tasks on the same patient (Welsh Healthcare Associated Infection Programme, 2009).

There are three levels of hand hygiene of which the first two will be discussed in this chapter. Level 1 refers to social hand hygiene, which is hand washing with general liquid soap and water or application of alcohol hand rub (70% concentration) if hands are physically clean. It aims to render the hands physically clean and to remove micro-organisms picked up during social activities (transient micro-organisms).

Level 2 refers to hygienic hand hygiene and is used before and after any aseptic technique, after contact with infected patients, and after contact with blood and body fluids. It aims to remove or destroy transient micro-organisms and to provide a residual effect which reduces resident micro-organisms which normally live on the skin (Welsh Healthcare Associated Infection Programme, 2009). An approved antiseptic hand cleanser should be used as identified in your local policy. Alcohol hand rub may also be applied after hand washing with plain liquid soap to achieve hygienic hand hygiene. For surgical scrub (level 3) please refer to the local policy of your clinical establishment. Figures 12-2 and 12-3 and Procedure 12-1 demonstrate correct hand hygiene procedure for hand washing and application of alcohol hand rub.

Alcohol-Based Hand Rubs

Alcohol hand rub (70% concentration) is used for decontamination of physically clean hands. This means hands that are free from organic matter, including dust, dirt, vomit, pus, faeces, urine and blood. It is used for social hand hygiene when the hands are physically clean and also for hygienic hand hygiene after first washing with liquid soap. The amount used should be as per manufacturer's recommendations and should be massaged into the hands using a technique that covers all areas (see Figure 12-3).

The process is complete when the gel has evaporated and the hands are completely dry. It is ideal to use in between patients/activities as long as the hands are physically clean and may increase healthcare worker's adherence to hand hygiene (Bischoff *et al.*, 2000).

Where applicable and after a local risk assessment, alcohol gel should be made available at the point-of-patient contact. Caution must be taken in relation to the flammability of alcohol-based products and also the potential for ingestion (Welsh Healthcare Associated Infection Programme, 2009).

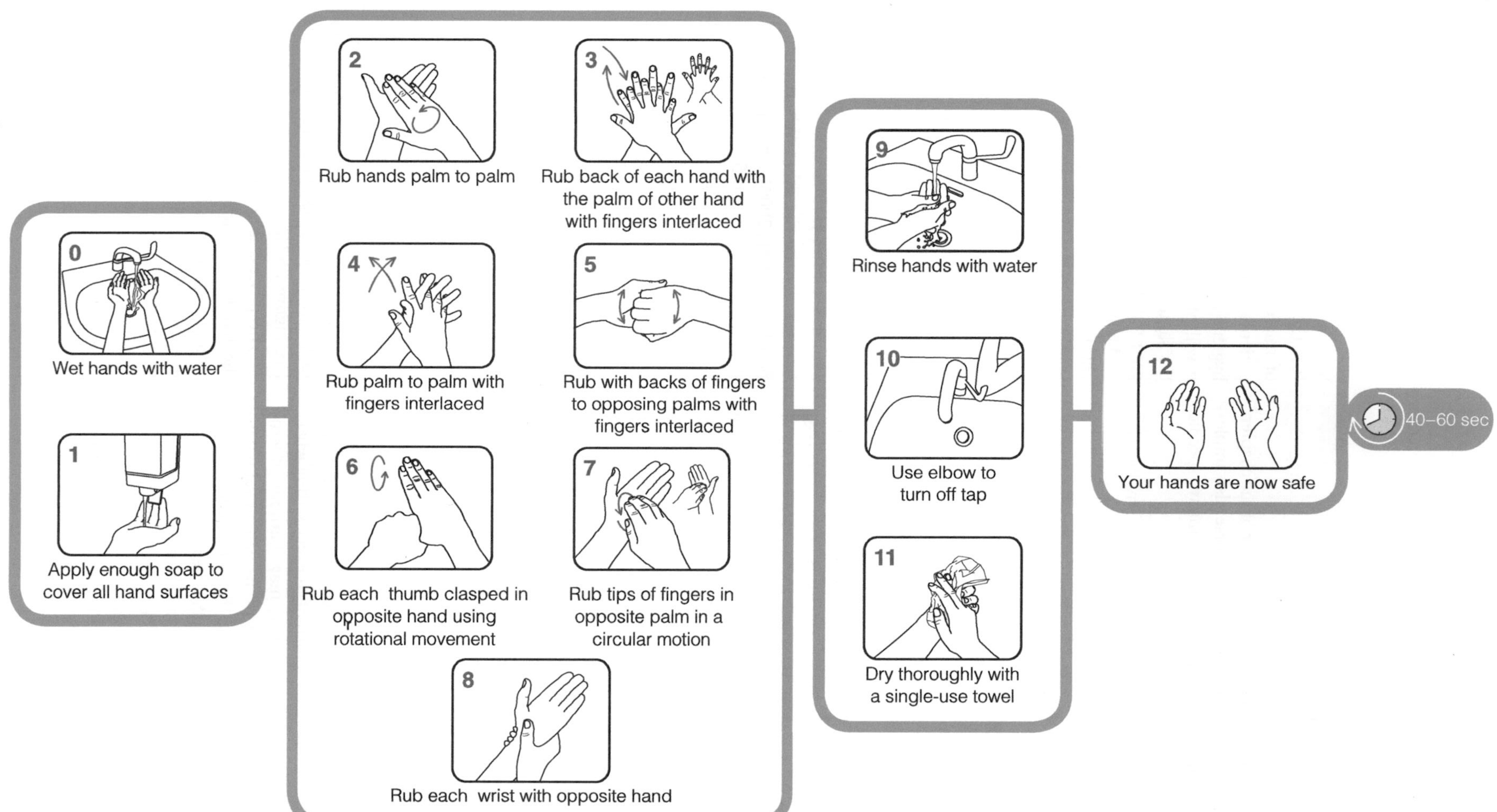
0
Wet hands with water
1
Apply enough soap to cover all hand surfaces
2
Rub hands palm to palm
3
Rub back of each hand with the palm of other hand with fingers interlaced
4
Rub palm to palm with fingers interlaced
5
Rub with backs of fingers to opposing palms with fingers interlaced
6
Rub each thumb clasped in opposite hand using rotational movement
7
Rub tips of fingers in opposite palm in a circular motion
8
Rub each wrist with opposite hand
9
Rinse hands with water
10
Use elbow to turn off tap
11
Dry thoroughly with a single-use towel
12
Your hands are now safe
40–60 sec

Figure 12-2 Guide to hand washing.
Source: How to handwash?, **www.npsa.nhs.uk/cleanyourhands**

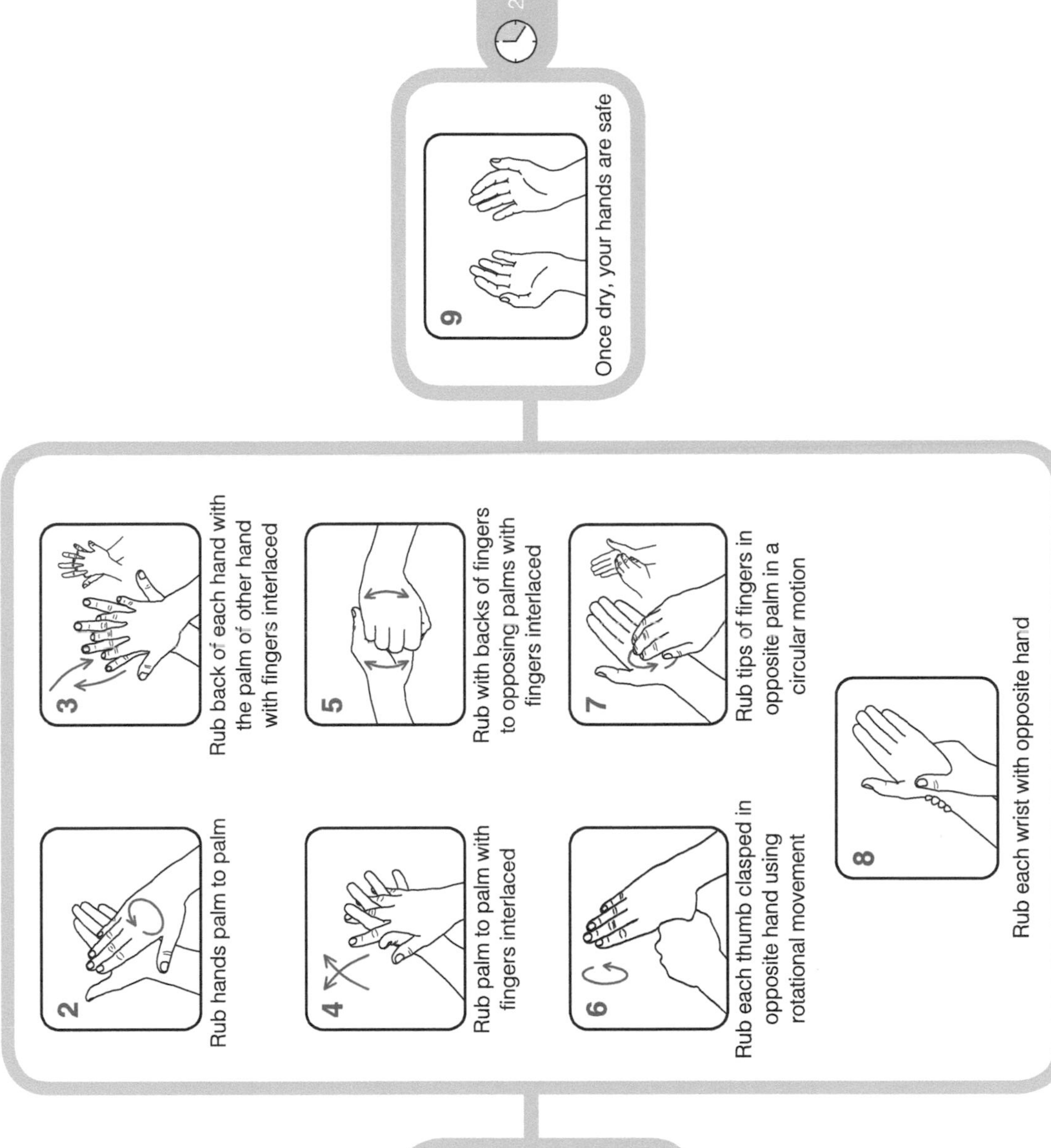

1a
1b
Apply a small amount (about 3ml) of the product in a cupped hand, covering all surfaces
2
Rub hands palm to palm
3
Rub back of each hand with the palm of other hand with fingers interlaced
4
Rub palm to palm with fingers interlaced
5
Rub with backs of fingers to opposing palms with fingers interlaced
6
Rub each thumb clasped in opposite hand using rotational movement
7
Rub tips of fingers in opposite palm in a circular motion
8
Rub each wrist with opposite hand
9
Once dry, your hands are safe
20–30 sec

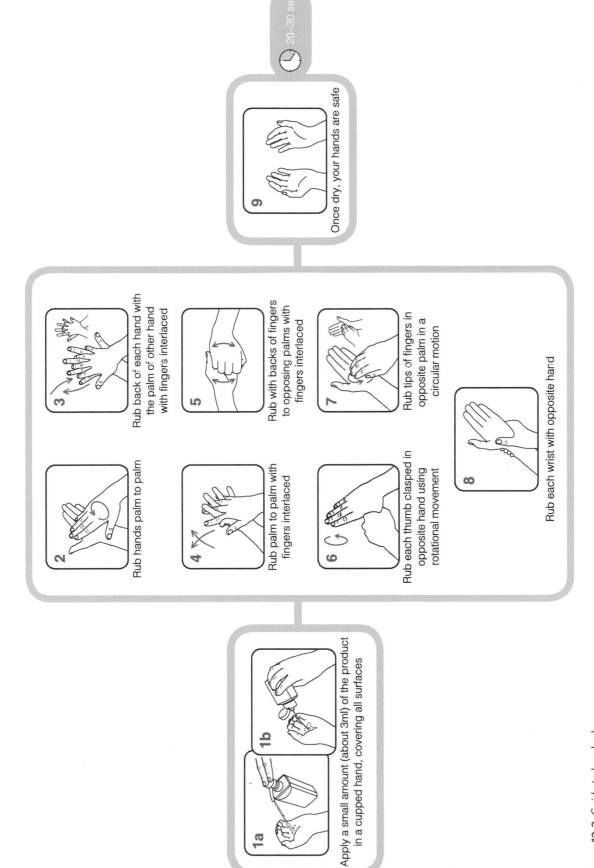

Figure 12-3 Guide to hand rub.
Source: How to handwash?, **www.npsa.nhs.uk/cleanyourhands**

CLINICAL ALERT

Alcohol gel is a highly effective hand hygiene agent for most micro-organisms but it is not effective against spore-forming organisms (e.g. *Clostridium difficile*) and its use is disputed against non-enveloped viruses (norovirus). So when caring for patients who may have these infections ensure that hand washing is performed although alcohol gel can then be applied once the hands are washed.

Hand hygiene principles

Ensure jackets/coats/wristwatches are removed, and wrists and forearms are exposed. Nails should be kept short. Short natural nails are less likely to harbour micro-organisms, scratch a patient or puncture gloves. Artificial nails and/or nail polish must not be worn. Remove all jewellery. Micro-organisms can lodge in the settings of jewellery and under rings. Removal facilitates proper cleaning of the hands and arms (only plain band rings may be worn, but these should be removed in order to perform optimal hand hygiene). All cuts and abrasions on hands and arms should be covered with a waterproof dressing.

Procedure 12-1 describes proper handwashing techniques.

PROCEDURE 12-1 Handwashing

Purposes

- To reduce the number of micro-organisms on the hands
- To reduce the risk of transmission of micro-organisms to patients
- To reduce the risk of cross-contamination among patients
- To reduce the risk of transmission of infectious organisms to oneself

Assessment

Assess

- Presence of factors increasing susceptibility to infection
- Use of immunosuppressive medications
- Recent diagnostic procedures or treatments that penetrated the skin or a body cavity
- Current nutritional status
- Signs and symptoms indicating the presence of an infection:
- Localised signs, such as swelling, redness, pain or tenderness with palpation or movement, palpable heat at site, loss of function of affected body part, presence of exudate
- Systemic indications, such as fever, increased pulse and respiratory rates, lack of energy, anorexia, enlarged lymph nodes

Planning

Determine the location of running water and soap or soap substitutes.

Equipment

- Soap
- Warm running water
- Disposable paper towels
- Alcohol gel (if performing hygienic hand hygiene)

Implementation

Preparation

Assess the hands.

Nails should be kept short. *Short, natural nails are less likely to harbour micro-organisms, scratch a patient or puncture gloves.*

Remove all jewellery. *Micro-organisms can lodge in the settings of jewellery and under rings. Removal facilitates proper cleaning of the hands and arms.*

Check hands for breaks in the skin, such as hangnails or cuts. *A nurse who has open sores may require a clinical placement with decreased risk for transmission of infectious organisms.*

Performance

1 Follow local policy to ensure that you explain to the patient what you are going to do, why it is necessary and how they can cooperate. Obtain consent and maintain patient privacy and dignity and ensure that the appropriate local infection control procedures are observed.

2 Turn on the water, and adjust the flow.
There are several common types of tap controls: hand-operated handles; elbow controls (move these with the elbows instead of the hands); infrared controls (motion in front of the sensor causes water to start and stop flowing

automatically). Adjust the flow so that the water is warm. Warm water removes less of the protective oil of the skin than hot water.

3 Wet the hands thoroughly by holding them under the running water, and apply the chosen agent to the hands (about 2 to 4ml, plain liquid soap for social, antiseptic for hygienic).
4 Thoroughly wash and rinse the hands (see Figure 12-2). Ensure a good lather is achieved and use firm, rubbing and circular movements to wash the hands. Ensure all areas of the hands are covered, including the wrists and forearms if applicable. Pay particular attention to fingertips, thumbs and the area between the fingers. Hands should be vigorously rubbed and the whole process should take between 40-60 seconds. Hands (and forearms where applicable) should be rinsed well under running water. The physical action of washing and rinsing hands is essential as different solutions will have different activity against micro-organisms.
5 Turn off the water. Turn taps off using elbows if applicable, otherwise use a new paper towel to grasp a hand-operated control. This prevents you from picking up micro-organisms from the tap handles.
6 Thoroughly dry the hands and arms with a paper towel. Moist skin becomes chapped readily which can then harbour bacteria. Damp hands readily pick up and transfer certain types of bacteria.
7 Dispose of the paper towels using the foot pedal on the bin, ensuring that hands are not recontaminated in the process by touching the bin lid, the environment or yourself.

If carrying out hygienic hand decontamination using plain liquid soap, apply alcohol hand rub as recommended by the manufacturers. Ensure all areas of the hand are covered and the hands are completely dry, through evaporation, before carrying on with your duties (see Figure 12-3).

Evaluation

There is no traditional evaluation of the effectiveness of the individual nurse's handwashing/hand hygiene. Institutional infection control departments monitor the occurrence of patient infections and investigate those situations in which healthcare providers are implicated in the transmission of infectious organisms. Audit and feedback is also used to assess the hand hygiene frequency, technique and appropriateness of health professionals. Research has repeatedly shown the positive impact of careful hand hygiene on patient health associated with prevention of infection. Common areas missed during hand hygiene include the backs of the hands, web spaces between fingers and fingernails. Therefore it is important to pay attention to these areas.

CRITICAL REFLECTION

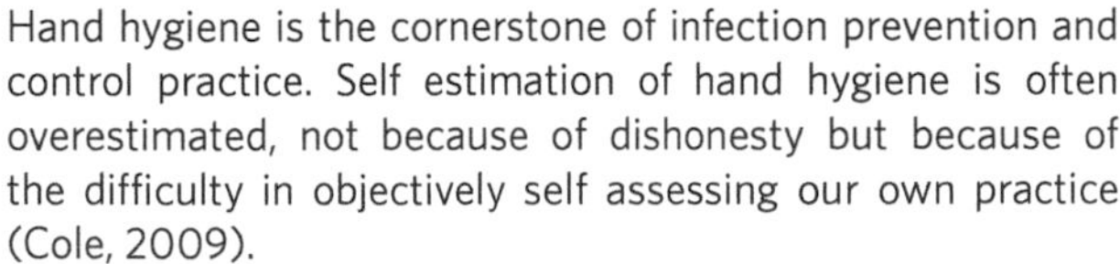

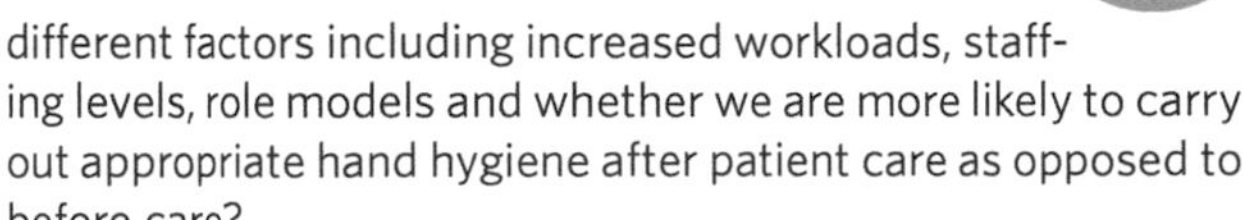

Hand hygiene is the cornerstone of infection prevention and control practice. Self estimation of hand hygiene is often overestimated, not because of dishonesty but because of the difficulty in objectively self assessing our own practice (Cole, 2009).

Cole (2009) advocates reflection as a means of identifying both our strengths and the areas that need improving in relation to hand hygiene. Through keeping a reflective diary or a note book it is possible to reflect on our hand hygiene performance over the course of a clinical period. Reflection will assist us in identifying instances when our performance is sub-optimal. It will help identify if we are influenced by different factors including increased workloads, staffing levels, role models and whether we are more likely to carry out appropriate hand hygiene after patient care as opposed to before care?

Through reflection we can identify these barriers to hand hygiene and analyse why this happens. This will help us understand what we need to do in order to overcome these obstacles and improve our hand hygiene practice. *During your next clinical opportunity keep a note of your hand hygiene practice and reflect on it using a reflective framework. From your analysis and findings identify an action plan to improve your practice.*

SKIN CARE

When skin is damaged bacterial counts increase. Any damaged skin must be covered with an impermeable waterproof dressing. Hands must be wet before applying soap and thoroughly rinsed and dried after washing. The application of hand cream can help protect the hands from damage, but communal jars/tubes of hand cream must not be used. Staff who suffer a reaction to any of the hand hygiene products used in the establishment or who develop any skin condition affecting their hands should report the concern to their manager or to the Occupational Health Department.

RESEARCH NOTE

Will a Soap-and-Water Alternative Increase Compliance with Handwashing?

Alcohol-based hand gels are available to the general public and to healthcare institutions as a substitute for soap-and-water handwashing of physically clean hands. However, limited research has been conducted on the effectiveness of these gels from the perspectives of their ability to kill micro-organisms, affect handwashing frequency or impact on skin condition. In a study by Earl *et al.* (2001), researchers designed three phases to specifically address the question of frequency of handwashing by nurses, physicians and ancillary personnel (technicians and therapists) in two intensive care units.

In phase I, prior to any intervention, the number of opportunities to wash hands was compared to actual compliance with handwashing over four weeks. In phase II, alcohol gel dispensers were installed inside and outside of patient rooms and both opportunities and occurrences for handwashing with either soap and water or gel were counted for four weeks. Phase III examined opportunities and occurrences for handwashing between 10 and 14 weeks after installation of the dispensers.

The results were as follows: phase I, 39.6% compliance; phase II, 52.6%; phase III, 57%. The highest rates of compliance were by ancillary personnel, followed by nursing staff and then physicians. The alcohol gel was used instead of soap about 50%-60% of the time. Although total amount of required time (including walking to the sinks) was not determined, less actual time was spent in hand hygiene with gel in phase III (7.5 seconds) than with soap and water in phase I (9.4 seconds).

Implications

Although the gel dispensers succeeded in increasing the percentage of compliance with hand hygiene, the researchers expressed concern that the final rate was still only about 60% of the incidences requiring hand hygiene. However, the gel did take less time and was most likely more effective than the inadequate nine-second soap use. The authors recognised weaknesses in the study, including the common Hawthorne effect. This effect states that the participants' behaviour may change purely by knowing that a study is being conducted. In this case, the healthcare providers may have paid more attention to hand hygiene than they would have had the study not been performed. In addition, it is not possible to extrapolate these results to other institutions and types of care units.

However, this study is an important example of the need to assess, intervene and reassess effectiveness of procedures designed to increase the safety and health of both providers and patients. The study could easily be replicated in other settings and the results expanded to include other variables such as cost and true time savings.

Source: based on 'Improved Rates of Compliance with Hand Antisepsis Guidelines: A Three-Phase Observational Study,' by M.L. Earl, M.M. Jackson and L.S. Rickman, 2001, *American Journal of Nursing*, 101(3), pp. 26-33.

PERSONAL PROTECTIVE EQUIPMENT (PPE)

PPE is a key component of standard precautions and is used to reduce the potential exposure to infective agents and material thereby protecting both the patient and the member of staff (Clark *et al.*, 2002). All healthcare practitioners should choose PPE after carrying out a risk assessment in relation to the risk of transmission of micro-organisms to the patient, and the risk of contamination of healthcare practitioners clothing and skin by patients' blood, body fluids, secretions and excretions (Pratt *et al.*, 2007).

PPE should be appropriate and fit for purpose, accessible and available. It does not cancel out the need for hand hygiene or should not become a source of contamination (Health Protection Scotland (HPS), 2009a).

The key components of PPE are:

- gloves (sterile and non sterile)
- gowns
- aprons
- masks
- goggles
- visors

(Clark *et al.*, 2002).

Gloves

Gloves are a single-use item and neither powdered or polythene gloves should be used in the clinical area. The decision to use sterile or nonsterile is based on a risk assessment of whether there will be contact with susceptible sites or clinical devices. They should be put on immediately before an episode of patient contact and removed as soon as the activity is completed (HPS, 2009a).

Gloves are worn for the following reasons. They protect the hands when the nurse is likely to handle any body substances, for example, blood, urine, faeces, sputum, mucous membranes and non intact skin. They reduce the likelihood of nurses transmitting their own endogenous micro-organisms to individuals receiving care. Nurses who have open sores or cuts on the hands must wear gloves for protection in addition to applying an impermeable dressing to the broken area. Gloves reduce the chance that the nurse's hands will transmit micro-organisms from one patient to another (Pratt *et al.*, 2007).

In all situations, gloves are changed between patient contacts. The hands are washed each time gloves are removed for two primary reasons: (a) the gloves may have imperfections or be damaged during wearing so that they could allow micro-organism entry and (b) the hands may become contaminated during glove removal.

Many of the gloves used in infection prevention and control are made of latex rubber, as are various other items used in healthcare (catheters, blood pressure cuffs, rubber sheets, intravenous tubing, stockings and adhesive bandages). Because of the frequent use of gloves, patients with chronic illnesses and healthcare workers have increasingly reported allergic reactions to latex. Latex gloves lubricated by powder or cornstarch are particularly allergenic because the latex allergen adheres to the powder, which is aerosolised during glove use and inhaled by the user. Latex gloves that are labelled 'hypoallergenic' still contain measurable latex and should not be used by or on persons with known latex sensitivity. Recent studies show some level of latex allergy in 6% to 17% of healthcare personnel (Corbin, 2002). The people at greatest risk for developing latex allergies are those with other allergic conditions and those who have had frequent or long-term exposure to latex.

Latex allergies can be either local or systemic and may take the form of dermatitis, urticaria (hives), asthma or anaphylaxis. Patients and healthcare workers should be assessed for possible allergies through a thorough history taking and screening. Ask patients if they have had any adverse reactions to items such as balloons, condoms or dishwashing or utility gloves. Strategies to avoid sensitisation or exposure to latex include use of nonlatex products, nonlatex barriers between latex products and the skin, and gloves that are unpowdered or washed before use. People with significant allergies should have no contact with latex products. Latex alternatives must be provided.

Procedure 12-2 describes application and removal of PPE including gloves.

PROCEDURE 12-2 Donning and Removing Personal Protective Equipment (Gloves, Gown, Mask, Eyewear)

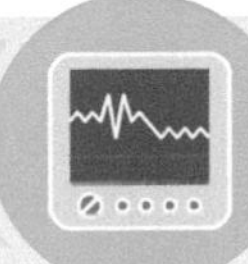

Purposes

To protect healthcare workers and patients from transmission of potentially infective materials.

Assessment

Consider which activities will be required while the nurse is in the patient's room at this time. *This will determine which personal protective equipment is required.*

Planning

- Application and removal of personal protective equipment can be time consuming. Arrange for the care of your other patients if indicated.
- Determine which supplies are present within the patient's room and which must be brought with you.
- Consider if special handling is indicated for removal of any specimens or other materials from the room.

Equipment

As indicated according to which activities will be performed. Ensure that extra supplies are easily available.

- Apron/gown
- Mask/respirator
- Eye protection
- Gloves

Implementation

Preparation

See *Procedure 12-1* for preparation for handwashing. Remove or secure all loose items such as nametags or jewellery.

Performance

1 Follow local policy to ensure that you explain to the patient what you are going to do, why it is necessary and how they can cooperate. Obtain consent and maintain patient privacy and dignity and ensure that the appropriate local infection control procedures are observed.

2 Don a clean apron or gown. Pick up a clean apron/gown, and allow it to unfold in front of you without allowing it to touch any area soiled with body substances.
Slide the arms and the hands through the sleeves (if a gown). Fasten the ties at the neck to keep the gown in place.

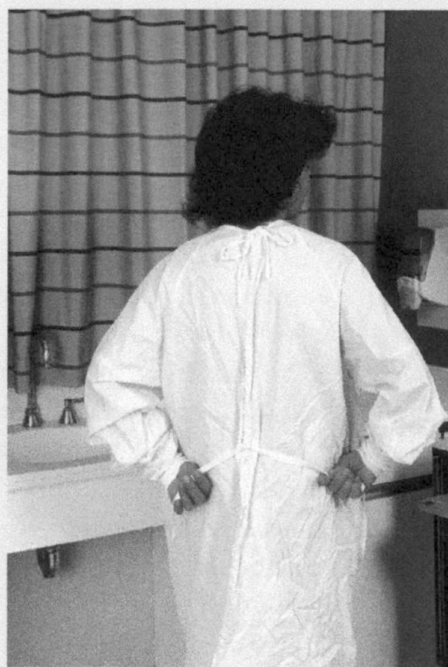

Figure 12-4 Overlapping the gown at the back to cover the nurse's uniform.

3 Overlap the gown at the back as much as possible, and fasten the waist ties or belt (see Figure 12-4). Overlapping securely covers the uniform at the back. Waist ties keep the apron/gown from falling away from the body and prevent inadvertent soiling of the uniform.
4 Don the face mask. (Refer to local policy for tight fitting particulate respirator.)
   - Locate the top edge of the mask. The mask usually has a narrow metal strip along the edge. Place the upper edge of the mask over the bridge of the nose, and secure ties or elastic bands at middle of head and neck. If glasses are worn, fit the upper edge of the mask under the glasses. *With the edge of the mask under the glasses, clouding of the glasses is less likely to occur.* Secure the lower edge of the mask under the chin (see Figure 12-5). *To be effective, a mask must cover both the nose and the mouth, because air moves in and out of both.*
   - If the mask has a metal strip, adjust this firmly over the bridge of the nose. A secure fit prevents both the escape and the inhalation of micro-organisms around the edges of the mask and the fogging of eyeglasses.
   - Wear the mask only once, and do not wear any mask longer than the manufacturer recommends or once it becomes wet or soiled. *A mask should be used only once because it becomes ineffective when moist.*
   - Do not leave a used face mask hanging around the neck.
5 Don protective eyewear (goggles or visor) if it is not combined with the face mask.
6 Don clean disposable gloves. No special technique is required, if you are wearing a gown, pull the gloves up to cover the cuffs of the gown. If you are not wearing a gown, pull the gloves up to cover the wrists (if using sterile gloves refer to *Procedure 12-3*).

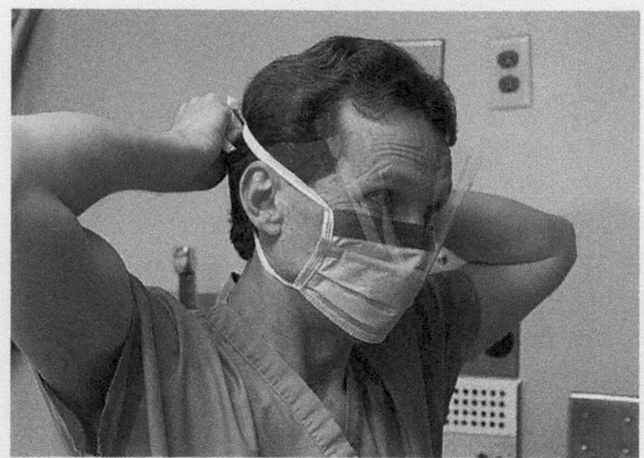

Figure 12-5 A facemask and eye protection covering the nose, mouth and eyes.

7 To remove soiled personal protective equipment, remove the gloves first since they are the most soiled. Remove the first glove by grasping it on its palmar surface just below the cuff, taking care to touch only glove to glove (see Figure 12-6). *This keeps the soiled parts of the used gloves from touching the skin of the wrist or hand.*
   - Pull the first glove completely off by inverting or rolling the glove inside out.
   - Continue to hold the inverted removed glove by the fingers of the remaining gloved hand. Place the first two fingers of the bare hand inside the cuff of the second glove (see Figure 12-7). Pull the second glove off to the fingers by turning it inside out. This pulls the first glove inside the second glove. The soiled part of the glove is folded to the inside to reduce the chance of transferring any micro-organisms by direct contact.

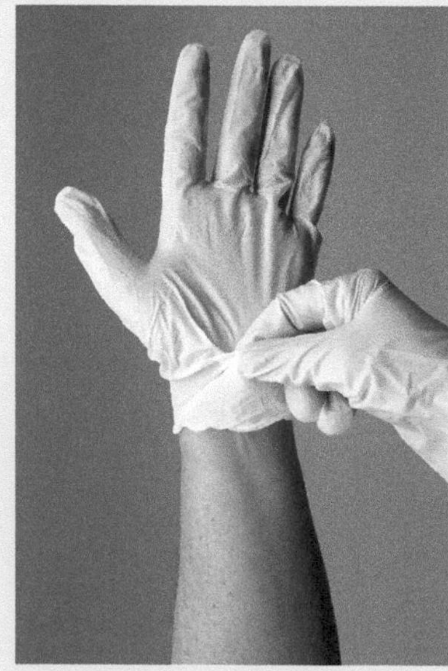

Figure 12-6 Plucking the palmar surface below the cuff of a contaminated glove.

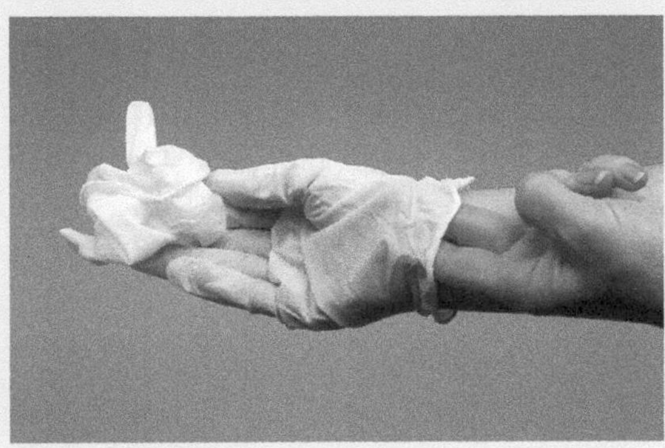

Figure 12-7 Inserting fingers to remove the second contaminated glove.
Source: Pearson Education Ltd.

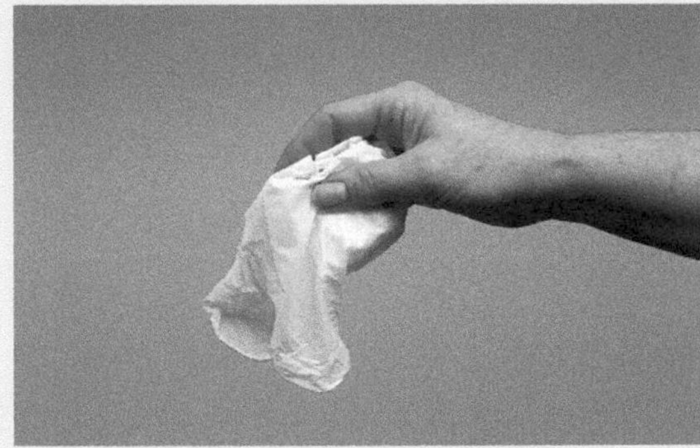

Figure 12-8 Holding contaminated gloves, which are inside out.
Source: Pearson Education Ltd.

Using the bare hand, continue to remove the gloves, which are now inside out, and dispose of appropriately (see Figure 12-8).

8 Assume the gown/apron front are contaminated. Unfasten or break ties and pull gown/apron away from the neck and shoulders, touching the inside of gown only. Turn the gown inside out and fold or roll into a bundle and discard appropriately (HPS, 2009b).

9 Assume the goggles/visor is contaminated and handle by head band or ear pieces. Discard appropriately.

10 Remove the mask. Assume the front of mask/respirator is contaminated. Untie or break bottom ties, followed by top ties or elastic and remove by handling ties only. Discard appropriately.

11 Perform hand hygiene immediately. If at any time you feel you have compromised your safety when removing PPE then perform hand hygiene before proceeding to the next stage. Do not rush the removal stage as it is possible to contaminate yourself by handling the PPE inappropriately.

Evaluation

- Conduct any follow-up indicated during your care of the patient.
- Ensure that an adequate supply of equipment is available for the next healthcare provider.

Gowns and Aprons

Aprons are single-use items and should be worn when there is the potential for close contact with the patient, materials or equipment and when there is a risk that clothing may become contaminated with pathogenic micro-organisms or blood, body fluid, secretions or excretions (Pratt *et al.*, 2007). If there is an extensive risk of contamination then full body fluid repellent gowns must be worn. They must be changed between each patient contact and must not be reused.

Masks

Masks are worn to reduce the risk for transmission of micro-organisms by the droplet and airborne routes, and by splatters of body substances. Masks may be worn under the following conditions:

- By those close to the patient if the infection is transmitted by large-particle aerosols (droplets). Large-particle aerosols are transmitted by close contact and generally travel short distances (about 1m).
- By all persons entering the room if the infection is transmitted by small-particle aerosols (droplet nuclei). Small-particle aerosols remain suspended in the air and thus travel greater distances by air. Special respirators that provide a tighter face seal and better filtration may be used for certain infections. It is important that staff are fit tested and trained to use the mask/respirator before it is used in the clinical environment.

Various types of masks differ in their filtration effectiveness and fit. Single-use disposable surgical masks are effective for use while the nurse provides care to most patients but should be changed if they become wet or soiled. These masks are discarded in the waste container after use. Disposable particulate respirators of different types may be effective for droplet transmission, splatters and airborne micro-organisms. If unsure then refer to local policy or contact your local infection prevention and control team for advice. Guidelines for donning and removing face masks are shown in *Procedure 12-2*.

Eyewear

Protective eyewear (goggles, glasses or face shields) and masks may be indicated in situations where body substances may splatter the face (see *Procedure 12-2*). If the nurse wears prescription glasses, goggles may be worn over the glasses. The protective eyewear must extend around the sides of the glasses in order to provide all round protection.

Sterile Gloves

Sterile gloves may be donned by the open method or the closed method. The open method is used most frequently outside of the operating department. Sterile gloves are worn during many procedures to maintain the sterility of equipment and to protect a patient's wound.

Sterile gloves are packaged with a cuff of about 5cm and with the palms facing upward when the package is opened. The package usually indicates the size of the glove.

Procedure 12-3 describes how to don and remove sterile gloves by the open method.

PROCEDURE 12-3 Donning and Removing Sterile Gloves (Open Method)

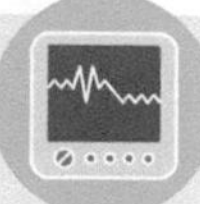

Purposes

- To enable the nurse to handle or touch sterile objects freely without contaminating them.
- To prevent transmission of potentially infective micro-organisms from the nurse's hands to patients at high risk for infection.

Assessment

- Review the patient's record and orders to determine exactly what procedure will be performed that requires sterile gloves.
- Check the patient record and ask about latex allergies.

Planning

- Think through the procedure, planning which steps need to be completed before the gloves can be applied. Determine what additional supplies are needed to perform the procedure for this patient. Always have an extra pair of sterile gloves available.

Equipment

- Packages of sterile gloves

Implementation

Preparation

Ensure the sterility of the package of gloves by checking the expiry date and ensuring the package is intact.

Performance

1 Follow local policy to ensure that you explain to the patient what you are going to do, why it is necessary and how they can cooperate. Obtain consent and maintain patient privacy and dignity and ensure that the appropriate local infection control procedures are observed.

2 Open the package of sterile gloves. Place the package of gloves on a clean, dry surface. Any moisture on the surface could contaminate the gloves.
Some gloves are packed in an inner as well as an outer package. Open the outer package without contaminating the gloves or the inner package.
Remove the inner package from the outer package.
Open the inner package according to the manufacturer's directions. Some manufacturers provide a numbered sequence for opening the flaps and folded tabs to grasp for opening the flaps. If no tabs are provided, pluck the flap so that the fingers do not touch the inner surfaces. *The inner surfaces, which are next to the sterile gloves, will remain sterile.*

3 Put the first glove on the dominant hand. If the gloves are packaged so that they lie side by side, grasp the glove for the dominant hand by its folded cuff edge (on the palmar side) with the thumb and first finger of the nondominant hand. Touch only the inside of the cuff (see Figure 12-9). *The hands are not sterile. By touching only the inside of the glove, the nurse avoids contaminating the outside.*
Alternatively, if the gloves are packaged one on top of the other, grasp the cuff of the top glove as above, using the opposite hand. Insert the dominant hand into the glove and pull the glove on. Keep the thumb of the inserted hand against the palm of the hand during insertion (see Figure 12-10). *If the thumb is kept against the palm, it is less likely to contaminate the outside of the glove.* Leave the cuff turned down.

4 Put the second glove on the nondominant hand. Pick up the other glove with the sterile gloved hand, inserting the gloved fingers under the cuff and holding the gloved

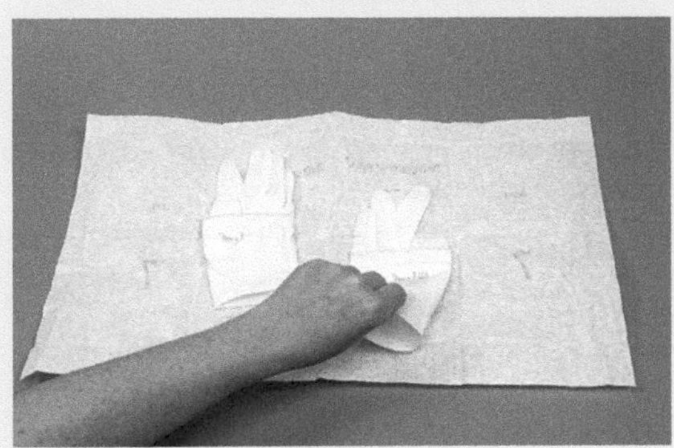

Figure 12-9 Picking up the first sterile glove.

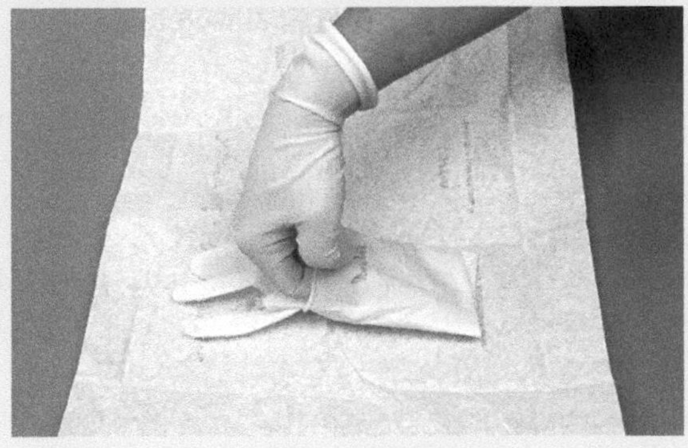

Figure 12-11 Picking up the second sterile glove.

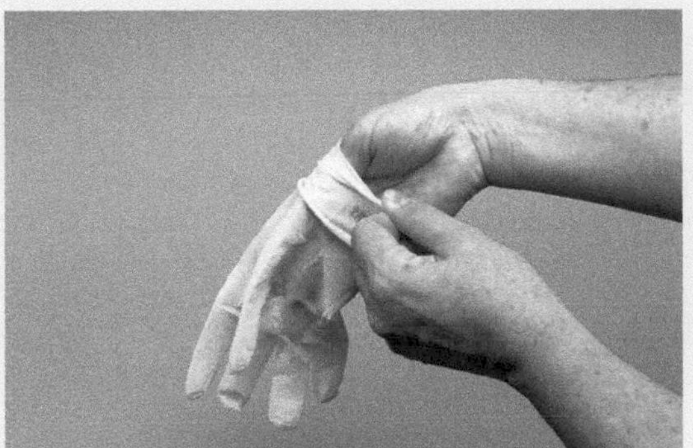

Figure 12-10 Putting on the first sterile glove.

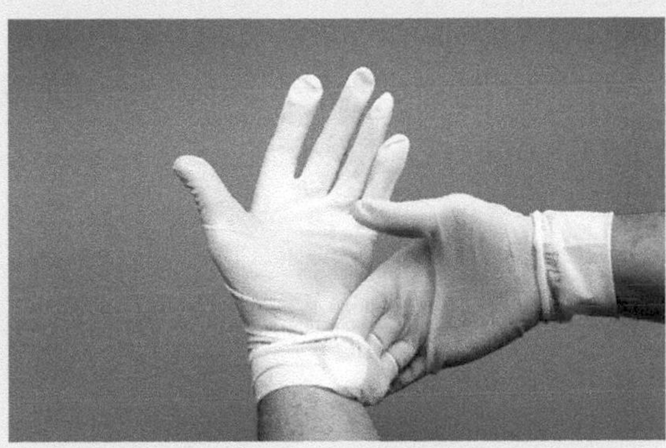

Figure 12-12 Putting on the second sterile glove.

thumb close to the gloved palm (see Figure 12-11). *This helps prevent accidental contamination of the glove by the bare hand.* Pull on the second glove carefully. Hold the thumb of the gloved first hand as far as possible from the palm (see Figure 12-12). *In this position, the thumb is less likely to touch the arm and become contaminated.* Adjust each glove so that it fits smoothly, and carefully pull the cuffs up by sliding the fingers under the cuffs.

5 Remove and dispose of used gloves. There is no special technique for removing sterile gloves. If they are soiled with secretions, remove them by turning them inside out. See removal of disposable gloves in *Procedure 12-2*. Document that an aseptic technique was used in the performance of the procedure.

Evaluation

- Conduct any follow-up indicated during your care of the patient.
- Ensure that adequate numbers and types of sterile supplies are available for the next healthcare provider.

PREVENTION OF OCCUPATIONAL EXPOSURE TO BLOOD AND BODY FLUIDS

In addition to other actions and precautions discussed in this chapter, significant emphasis is placed on avoiding injury due to sharp instruments, measures to be taken in case of exposure to bloodborne pathogens and communication about biohazards to employees. Inoculation injuries are any injury that follows after contact with a sharp instrument or splashing of blood or body fluids onto mucous membranes or nonintact skin.

Sharps are any items that are able to penetrate or cut the skin or mucous membranes (Gould and Brooker, 2008). They include needles, razors, **ampoules**, stitch cutters, scalpel blades and lancets.

There are three major modes of transmission of infectious materials that can pose a risk to health professionals in the clinical setting:

1 Puncture wounds from contaminated needles or other sharps.
2 Skin contact, which allows infectious fluids to enter through wounds and broken or damaged skin.
3 Mucous membrane contact, which allows infectious fluids to enter through mucous membranes of the eyes, mouth and nose.

Complying with standard precautions and avoiding carelessness in the clinical area will place the caregiver at significantly less risk for injury. The chance of a healthcare worker becoming infected following percutaneous exposure to pathogens has been estimated as between 6% to 30% for hepatitis B, 1.8% to 3% for hepatitis C and 0.3% for HIV (Department of Health, 1998). Measures to be taken in case of possible exposure to blood or body fluids is outlined in the *Practice Guidelines* below.

Staff should adhere to the following principles when handling sharps:

- All staff are responsible for the safe disposal of sharps that they have used.
- Avoid using sharps whenever possible.
- Do not pass sharps between staff.
- Do not resheath needles or bend or break them.
- Do not remove needle from barrel of syringe.
- Dispose of sharps immediately at the point of use into an approved sharps container.
- Use the correct size bin that complies with current regulations.
- Do not overfill the bin.
- Never try and retrieve any item from a sharps bin or attempt to empty the bin.
- Keep out of the reach of children and confused adults.
- Secure and tag correctly when three quarters full and store in a secure place ready for collection.
- Know and follow the Inoculation Injury Policy.

CLINICAL ALERT

Nurses should consider in advance whether or not they would want prophylaxis for HIV exposure since this must be started within one hour of exposure.

PRACTICE GUIDELINES

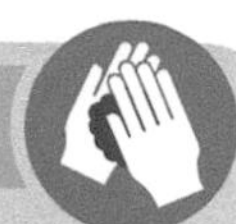

Steps to Follow after Exposure to Blood or Body Fluids

For a puncture/laceration:

- Encourage bleeding by gently squeezing the affected part under running water.
- Wash thoroughly with soap and water.
- Cover with a waterproof dressing.

Splashes to eyes, mouth and nose:

- Rinse thoroughly with plenty of water or saline for five to ten minutes.

Then:

- Make a note of the name of the patient (if known).
- Report the incident immediately to appropriate personnel within the clinical area and complete incident report form.
- Report to occupational health or accident and emergency depending on local policy, within a hour.

MANAGEMENT OF SPILLAGES OF BLOOD OR BODY FLUIDS

Blood and body fluid spillages must be dealt with immediately. They may provide a reservoir for infection as well as being a general health and safety risk. PPE should be worn when carrying out the task and hand hygiene performed when the PPE is removed. Gould and Brooker (2008) identified the following procedure when dealing with spillages. The *Practice Guidelines* below demonstrate the steps to take when faced with a spillage of blood or body fluids.

PRACTICE GUIDELINES

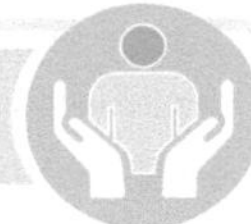

Steps to Follow when there is a Spillage of Blood or Body Fluids

- Ensure PPE is worn.
- Either use a 1% hypochlorite solution (10,000 parts per million, ppm) or chlorine releasing granules.
- If using granules cover spillage with them and leave for two minutes.
- If using hypochlorite solution cover spillage with paper towels to absorb the spillage and then cover with the solution and leave for two minutes.
- Scoop up the debris into a clinical waste bag.
- Clean the area with water and detergent.
- Remove PPE and perform hand hygiene.

Spillages of urine or vomit

Chlorine-releasing agents or hypochlorite solutions **must not** be used directly on spills of urine or vomit, as it can cause the release of chlorine gas.

- Wear appropriate PPE.
- Contain and absorb the spill (e.g. using disposable paper towels).
- Carefully clean the area removing all solid matter (if vomit) and absorbing all liquid (if urine), e.g. with disposable paper towels.
- Wash the area with warm water and a general purpose detergent using disposable paper towels and then dry the area.
- Wipe over the dry area with a solution 0.1% hypochlorite solution (1000 ppm) and let it dry. If the urine or vomit was blood-stained, a solution of 1% hypochlorite (10,000 ppm) should be used.
- Scoop up the debris into a clinical waste bag.
- Remove PPE and perform hand hygiene.

DECONTAMINATION OF EQUIPMENT

In order to reduce the risk of infection and help break the chain of infection it is vital that all equipment that has been used is decontaminated appropriately. Manufacturers' instructions should always be followed in conjunction with the local infection control policy. Nurses should be familiar with the cleaning, disinfecting and sterilising protocols of the clinical area in which they practise and should be prepared to teach patients and family members appropriate techniques for home care.

In order to understand how medical devices should be decontaminated it is important to be aware of the following three classifications. *Reusable equipment* is a device that can be decontaminated and reprocessed for repeated use. *Single patient* use refers to a device that may be used more than once on the same patient and can undergo reprocessing.

Single use equipment is a medical device that is intended to be used on an individual patient during a single procedure then discarded. It is not intended to be reprocessed and used on another patient (Medicines and Healthcare Products Regulatory Agency, 2006). Reuse can result in cross infection, endotoxin reaction and patient injury. If a single-use item is reused then an individual may be legally liable for the safe performance of the device. Single use equipment is denoted by the single use symbol (see Figure 12-13).

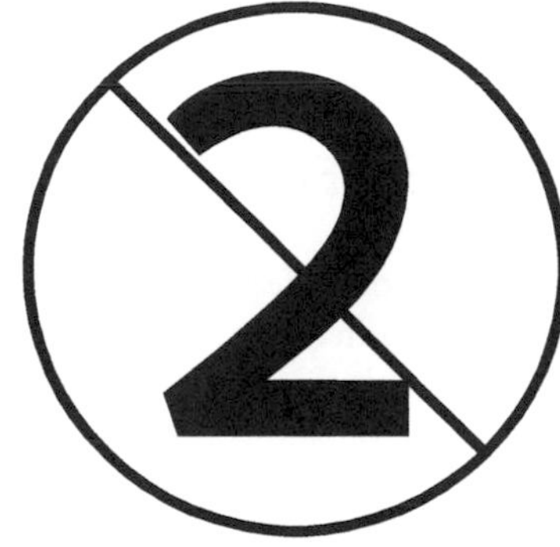

Figure 12-13 Single use symbol.
Source: www.npsa.nhs.uk/easysiteweb/gatewaylink.aspx?akld=24926

There are three levels of decontamination: cleaning, disinfection and sterilisation.

Cleaning

Cleanliness inhibits the growth of micro-organisms. It is the physical removal of organic matter and micro-organisms using detergent and water and is vital for items that are used on intact skin. When cleaning visibly soiled objects nurses must always wear PPE to avoid direct contact with infectious micro-organisms. It is important to use a rigorous method in order to remove any physical waste. Cleaning must be performed before disinfection or sterilisation.

Disinfection

This is a process that aims to reduce micro-organisms to a level where they are no longer harmful. It does not always destroy bacterial spores. Disinfection can be achieved through using chemicals or moist heat. It is used for equipment that is contaminated with micro-organisms and for equipment that has been used on mucous membranes.

When disinfecting articles, nurses need to follow local policy and consider the following:

- The type and number of infectious organisms. Some micro-organisms are readily destroyed, whereas others require longer contact with the disinfectant.
- The recommended concentration of the disinfectant and the duration of contact.
- The temperature of the environment. Most disinfectants are intended for use at room temperature.
- The presence of soap. Some disinfectants are ineffective in the presence of soap or detergent.
- The presence of organic materials. The presence of saliva, blood, pus or excretions can readily inactivate many disinfectants.
- The surface areas to be treated. The disinfecting agent must come into contact with all surfaces and areas.

Sterilising

Sterilisation is a process that destroys all micro-organisms, including spores and viruses. It is used for equipment that is used in high risk procedures. Sterilisation is often carried out in specialist sterile service units where stringent quality control is implemented.

If you are unsure how to decontaminate a piece of clinical equipment then either refer to the local decontamination policy or contact the infection prevention and control team for advice.

PATIENT PLACEMENT (ISOLATION)

Patient placement/isolation refers to measures designed to prevent the spread of infections or potentially infectious micro-organisms to health personnel, patients and visitors. Various infection prevention and control precautions are used to decrease the risk of transmission of micro-organisms in hospitals. Isolation can be divided into source isolation and protective isolation.

Source isolation is used when a patient has a known or suspected infection and there is the need to prevent transmission to other patients. It utilises standard precautions and transmission-based precautions (see below) in conjunction with the physical separation of the patient from non-infected patients. This can be achieved through using single rooms or in some cases through cohorting of patients with the same infection. The placing of patients in source isolation can act as a prompt to staff to practice optimum infection prevention and control. It is important to refer to local policy in order to identify the correct precautions to take when a patient is placed in isolation as procedures may differ depending on how the micro-organism is transmitted. It is also important to know when to discontinue isolation.

Protective isolation is implemented to protect immunocompromised patients who may be susceptible to acquiring infections from other patients. Immunocompromised patients (those highly susceptible to infection) are also often infected by their own micro-organisms, by micro-organisms on the inadequately washed hands of healthcare personnel, and by non-sterile items (food, water, air and patient-care equipment). Patients who are severely compromised include those who:

- have diseases, such as leukaemia, that depress the patient's resistance to infectious organisms;
- have extensive skin impairments, such as severe dermatitis or major burns, which cannot be effectively covered with dressings.

GENERAL PRINCIPLES OF ISOLATION

Initiation of practices to prevent the transmission of micro-organisms is generally a nursing responsibility and is based on a comprehensive assessment of the patient. This assessment takes into account the status of the patient's normal defence mechanisms, the patient's ability to implement necessary precautions and the source and mode of transmission of the infectious agent. Based on this risk assessment the nurse then decides what type of isolation needs to be implemented based on their knowledge of transmission-based precautions. In all patient situations *nurses must perform hand hygiene before and after giving care.*

It is important that supplies of PPE are available at the entrance to the isolation room and that it is donned prior to entering the room. PPE must be changed and hand hygiene carried out between different care activities on the same patient. PPE must also be removed, when leaving the isolation room, safely disposed of and hand hygiene performed (HPS, 2009b).

Linen used within the isolation area may be contaminated and should be disposed of in an alginate bag at the point of use and not carried loosely down the ward. It should then be placed in the appropriate linen bag and labelled as per local policy. Waste should also be managed in line with policy and PPE should be worn when dealing with both followed by hand hygiene.

The environment should be free from clutter and cleaned regularly with an appropriate disinfectant and its frequency may need to be increased. Patient equipment (thermometer, blood pressure monitor, and commode) should be allocated to individual patients and decontaminated before removal from the room. Terminal cleaning of the environment and equipment should be performed when the patient is removed from isolation.

Transmission-Based Precautions

Transmission-based precautions are designed for patients known or suspected to be infected with highly transmissible or epidemiologically important micro-organisms. They are used in conjunction with standard precautions to interrupt transmission in hospitals.

There are three types of transmission-based precautions:

- contact pecautions
- droplet precautions
- airborne precautions.

These may be combined for diseases that have multiple routes of transmission. When used either singly or in combination, they are to be used in addition to standard precautions (Siegel *et al.*, 2007).

Contact precautions are required when caring for patients with a known or suspected infection. They are used in conjunction with standard precautions and are used to prevent transmission of organisms spread via the direct or indirect route. Micro-organisms spread through contact include norovirus, MRSA and *C difficile.* A risk assessment will be required to identify what precautions will need to be taken and will often involve patient source isolation.

Droplet precautions are used to reduce the risk of transmission of infections via the droplet route. Micro-organisms that can be spread through this route include influenza and meningococcal disease. Droplet transmission relates to the transfer of large droplets from the respiratory tract of an infected individual onto the mucous membranes (nose, mouth and eyes) of another person. Droplets are relatively heavy and thought to only travel up to one metre when they are expelled. Because of this a risk assessment will need to be performed to identify whether you will need to wear a face mask and eye protection in addition to apron and gloves and other standard precautions (HPS, 2009b).

Airborne precautions are again used in conjunction with standard precautions and are designed to reduce the risk of transmission of organisms that are spread by small respiratory particles. Common airborne micro-organisms include *Mycobacterium tuberculosis*, measles and chickenpox. It is imperative that the correct precautions are instigated to prevent transmission. Face protection will be necessary which may involve fit testing and training in the use of specialist respiratory masks. If you are unsure of what type of precautions are required, seek advice from the infection prevention and control team and local policy.

For all precautions it is important to teach patients and visitors the importance of hand and respiratory hygiene. Respiratory hygiene will involve the use of tissues that cover both the mouth and the nose when coughing or sneezing and the disposal of them in the nearest waste bin. Hands must then immediately be washed to prevent possible transmission. Hands should be kept away from the mouth, eyes and nose (HPS, 2009b).

TRANSPORTING PATIENTS WITH INFECTIONS

Transporting patients with infections outside their own rooms is avoided unless absolutely necessary. If a patient must be moved, the nurse implements appropriate precautions and measures to prevent contamination of the environment. For example, the nurse ensures that any draining wound is securely covered or places a surgical mask on the patient who has an airborne infection. In addition, the nurse notifies personnel at the receiving area of any infection risk so that they can maintain necessary precautions.

PSYCHOSOCIAL NEEDS OF ISOLATION PATIENTS

Patients requiring isolation precautions can develop several problems as a result of the separation from others and of the special precautions taken in their care. Two of the most common are sensory deprivation and decreased self-esteem related to feelings of inferiority. *Sensory deprivation* occurs when the environment lacks normal stimuli for the patient, for example communication with others. Nurses should therefore be alert to common clinical signs of sensory deprivation: boredom, inactivity, slowness of thought, daydreaming, increased sleeping, thought disorganisation, anxiety, hallucinations and panic.

A patient's *feeling of inferiority* can be due to the perception of the infection itself or to the required precautions. Many people place a high value on cleanliness, and the idea of being 'soiled', 'contaminated' or 'dirty' can give patients the feeling that they are at fault and substandard. Although this is obviously not true, the infected persons may feel 'not as good' as others and blame themselves.

Nurses need to provide care that prevents these two problems or deals with them positively. Nursing interventions include the following:

- Assess the individual's need for stimulation.
- Initiate measures to help meet the need, including regular communication with the patient and diversionary activities, such as toys for a child and books, television or radio for an adult; provide a variety of foods to stimulate the patient's sense of taste; stimulate the patient's visual sense by providing a view or an activity to watch.
- Explain the infection and the associated procedures to help patients and their visitors to understand and accept the situation.
- Demonstrate warm, accepting behaviour. Avoid conveying to the patient any sense of annoyance about the precautions or any feelings of revulsion about the infection.
- Do not use stricter precautions than are indicated by the diagnosis or the patient's condition.
- Discontinue isolation as soon as it is safe to do so.

Standard precautions should be used for all patients, regardless of infectious status. Sometimes these will be combined with transmission precautions for certain micro-organisms. Compliance with these are vital in order to prevent and control infection and to ensure patient and staff safety.

ROLE OF THE INFECTION PREVENTION AND CONTROL NURSE

All healthcare organisations must have multidisciplinary infection control committees. Representatives from the medical and nursing staff, clinical laboratory, cleaning maintenance, catering and patient care areas should be included. An important member of this committee is the infection prevention and control nurse. This nurse is specially trained to be knowledgeable about the latest research and practices in preventing, detecting and controlling infections.

All infections are reported to the nurse in a manner that allows for recording and analysis. This data can assist in improving infection prevention and control practices. In addition, the infection prevention and control nurse will be involved in employee education, surveillance of infections and audit. If you are unsure of any infection prevention and control practice or procedure then the infection prevention and control team should be contacted for advice.

Now that you have read this chapter you should have an understanding of the chain of infection, our bodies' defences and standard and transmission-based precautions. Using this knowledge return to the chain of infection (Figure 12-1) and work your way through each stage of the chain. Identify what interventions can be used to 'break the chain' for specific micro-organisms that are transmitted via different routes.

ACTIVITY 12-1

Mr Jones is a 72-year-old man who is independent and lives alone. He was active and healthy until about two weeks ago, at which time he developed a persistent upper respiratory infection. Because he had difficulty in obtaining and preparing foods, he has become very weak. He finally went to see the GP who admitted Mr Jones to the acute medical ward for shortness of breath, productive cough, dehydration and nutritional deficiency. The GP suspects pneumonia.

Referring back to the chapter, what data supports Mr Jones's increased risk of such an infection? What other information or assessment data would be helpful to you when planning care for Mr Jones? You recognise that standard precautions are instituted for all hospitalised patients. Explain why the use of such precautions may not prevent the spread of Mr Jones's respiratory infection to other susceptible patients. What can you do to prevent the spread of Mr Jones's infection to other hospitalised patients and at the same time prevent him from getting infections from other patients? You observe a member of staff providing direct care to Mr Jones and then proceeding to leave without performing hand hygiene. What should you do? (Refer to end of chapter for suggestions.)

CHAPTER HIGHLIGHTS

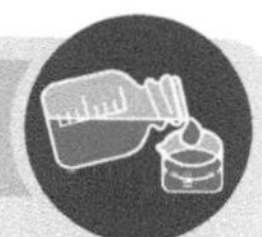

- Micro-organisms are everywhere. Most are harmless and some are beneficial; however, many can cause infection in susceptible persons.
- Effective control of infectious disease is an international, national, community and individual responsibility.
- The incidence of healthcare associated infections is significant. Major sites for these infections are the respiratory and urinary tracts, the bloodstream and wounds.
- Factors that contribute to HCAI risks are invasive procedures, medical therapies, the existence of a large number of susceptible persons, inappropriate use of antibiotics, and insufficient hand hygiene.
- An infection can develop if the links in the chain of infection - infectious agent, reservoir, portal of exit, mode of transmission, portal of entry and susceptible host - are not interrupted.
- Intact skin and mucous membranes are the body's first line of defence against micro-organisms.
- Some normal body flora release bacteriocins and antibiotic-like substances that inhibit microbial growth and destroy foreign bacteria.
- Some body secretions (e.g. saliva and tears) contain enzymes that act as antibacterial agents.
- The inflammatory response limits physical, chemical and microbial injury and promotes repair of injured tissue.
- Immunity is the specific resistance of the body to infectious agents.
- Acquired immunity is active or passive and in either case may be naturally or artificially induced.
- Especially at risk of acquiring an infection are the very young or old; those with poor nutritional status, a deficiency of serum immunoglobulins, multiple stressors, insufficient immunisations or an existing disease process; and those receiving certain medical therapies.
- Preventing infections in healthy or ill persons and preventing the transmission of micro-organisms from infected patients to others are major nursing functions.
- The nurse must be knowledgeable about sources and modes of transmission of micro-organisms.
- Micro-organisms are invisible, and nurses have an ethical obligation to ensure that appropriate standard and transmission-based precautions are taken to protect patients, support people and health personnel, including themselves.
- All healthcare providers must apply appropriate personal protective equipment according to the risk of exposure to potentially infective materials.
- Should a healthcare worker be exposed to substances with high risk of transmitting blood-borne pathogens, post-exposure practices and consideration of prophylactic treatment must be followed immediately.
- Hand hygiene is the single most important infection prevention and control practice.

CRITICAL REFLECTION

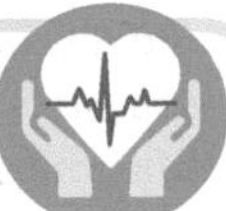

Considerations for norovirus case study on page 312 include the following:

- Discourage anyone who is unwell from visiting and also the very young and the very old.
- No one must visit if they are symptomatic of the virus themselves and they must wait until they are asymptomatic for 48–72 hours, depending on local policy, before visiting.
- Advise visitors not to bring food into hospital.
- Advise visitors that after visiting the affected ward not to go and visit another patient on any other ward.
- Encourage visitors to perform hand hygiene before and after visiting.
- Ensure the visitor is aware of where to get further information.
- Ensure standard and transmission precautions are implemented in line with local policy.

ACTIVITY ANSWERS

ACTIVITY 12-1 Mr Jones may have been at an increased risk of infection due to life span changes. The older person is at a greater risk of aquiring infections. There is also the possibility that he has not yet had his pneumococcal immunisation. The nursing process could be used as a tool to assess, plan, implement and evaluate care for Mr Jones. In conjunction with this laboratory data will contribute to the care provided. A sputum specimen should be sent for culture and sensitivity and a full blood count should be taken. The results of the sputum specimen will identify the causative micro-organism and ensure that appropriate anti-microbial drugs are prescribed. The patient would also need an x-ray.

Standard precautions may not be enough to prevent the spread of this infection, due to it being transmitted through the droplet route. So in order to protect other patients from infection Mr Jones may be placed in source isolation and droplet transmission precautions taken in conjunction with standard precautions. This will involve a risk assessment to identify what face protection is needed. Through implementing source isolation and using standard and transmission precautions, Mr Jones's infection will be prevented from spreading because the links of the chain of infection will have been broken. If there is a break down in these precautions then the micro-organism may be transmitted to other patients. In view of this all healthcare staff are accountable in ensuring that optimal procedures are followed by all staff. So if someone is observed not complying with these precautions then they should be challenged appropriately using tact and diplomacy, in order to protect the other patients.

REFERENCES

Bischoff, W.E., Reynolds, T.M., Sessler, C.N., Edmond, M.B. and Wenzel, R.P. (2000) 'Handwashing compliance by healthcare workers: The impact of introducing an accessible, alcohol-based hand antiseptic', *Archives of Internal Medicine*, 160, 1017–1021.

Clark, L., Smith, W. and Young, L. (2002) *Protective clothing: Principles and guidance*, London: Infection Control Nurses Association.

Cole, M. (2009) 'Exploring the hand hygiene compliance of student nurses: A case of flawed self assessment', *Nurse Education Today*, 29, 380–388.

Corbin, D.E. (2002) 'Latex allergy and dermatitis', *Occupational Health and Safety*, 71(1), 36, 38, 89.

Cutter, J. and Gammon, J. (2007) 'Review of standard precautions and sharps management in the community', *British Journal of Community Nursing*, 12(2), 54–60.

Department of Health (1998) *Guidance for clinical healthcare workers: Protection against infection with blood-borne viruses. Recommendations of the expert advisory group on AIDS and the advisory group on hepatitis*, DH: London.

Department of Health (2008) *Clean, safe care: Reducing infections and saving lives*, DH: London.

Department of Health, Social Services and Public Safety (2006) *Changing the culture: An action plan for the prevention and control of HCAI in Northern Ireland*, DHSSPS: Belfast.

Earl, M.E., Jackson, M.M. and Rickman, L.S. (2001) 'Improved rates of compliance with hand antisepsis guidelines: A three-phase observational study', *American Journal of Nursing*, 101(3), 26–33.

Fraise, A. (2009) 'Introduction', in Fraise, P.F. and Bradley, C. (eds) *Ayliffe's control of healthcare-associated infection* (5th edn), Hodder Armold: London, 3–12.

Gould, D. and Brooker, C. (2008) *Infection prevention and control: Applied microbiology for healthcare* (2nd edn), Palgrave Macmillan: Basingstoke.

Health Protection Scotland (2009a) *Personal protective equipment policy and procedure.* Available at http://www.documents.hps.scot.nhs.uk/hai/infection-control/sicp/ppe/mic-p-ppe-2009-02.pdf (Accessed 26 April 2010).

Health Protection Scotland (2009b) *Transmission based precautions policy.* Available at http://www.documents.hps.scot.nhs.uk/hai/infection-control/transmission-based-precautions/mic-p-tbp-2009-04.pdf (Accessed 12 July 2010).

Medicines and Healthcare Products Regulatory Agency (2006) *Single use medical devices: Implications and consequences of reuse DB2006(04)*, MHRA: London.

NMC Nursing and Midwifery Council (2010) *Standards for pre-registration nursing education*, London: NMC.

Plowman, R.P., Graves, N., Griffin, M., Roberts, J.A., Swan, A.V., Cookson, B.C. and Taylor, L. (1999) *The socioeconomic burden of hospital acquired infection*, Public Health Laboratory Service: London.

Pratt, R.J., Pellowe, C.M., Wilson, J.A., Loveday, T.R., Harper, R.J., Jones, S.R.L.J., McDougall, C., Wilcox, M.H. epic 2 (2007) *National evidence-based guidelines for the prevention of healthcare associated infection in NHS hospitals.* Available at http://www.epic.tvu.ac.uk/epic/notice.html (Accessed 19 May 2010).

Scottish Executive Health Department (2004) *The NHS Scotland code of practice for the local management of hygiene and healthcare associated infection*, SEHD: Edinburgh.

Siegel, J.D., Rhinehart, E., Jackson, M., Chiarello, L., the Healthcare Infection Control Practices Advisory Committee (2007) *Guideline for isolation precautions: Preventing transmission of infectious agents in healthcare settings.* Available at http://www.cdc.gov/ncidod/dhqp/pdf/isolation2007.pdf (Accessed 10 July 2009).

Smyth, E.T.M., McIlvenny, G., Enstone, J.E., Emmerson, A.M., Humphreys, H., Fitzpatrick, F., Davies, E., Newcombe, R.G. and Spencer, R.C., on behalf of the Hospital Infection Society Prevalence Survey Steering Group (2008) 'Four country healthcare associated infection prevalence survey 2006: Overview of the results', *Journal of Hospital Infection*, 69(3), 230–248.

Welsh Assembly Government (2004) *Healthcare associated infections – a strategy for hospitals in Wales*, WAG: Cardiff.

Welsh Assembly Government (2007) *Healthcare associated infections – a community strategy for Wales.* WAG: Cardiff.

Welsh Healthcare Associated Infection Programme (2009) *Infection Prevention Model Policy/Procedure 2, Hand Hygiene Policy and Procedure.* Available at http://www.wales.nhs.uk/sites3/Documents/379/PHW_HandPolicy_20091006_V1.pdf (Accessed 4 May 2010).

World Health Organization (2007) *The world health report 2007: A safer future*, WHO: Geneva.

World Health Organization (2009) *WHO guidelines on hand hygiene in healthcare*, WHO: Geneva.

FURTHER RESOURCES

Weblinks

Department of Health
http://www.dh.gov.uk/

Health Protection Scotland
http://www.hps.scot.nhs.uk/

National Resource for Infection Control
http://www.nric.org.uk/

Welsh Healthcare Associated Infection Programme
http://www.wales.nhs.uk/sites3/home.cfm?orgid=379

CHAPTER 13

MOVING AND HANDLING: PROMOTING THE SAFETY OF THE PATIENT AND THE NURSE

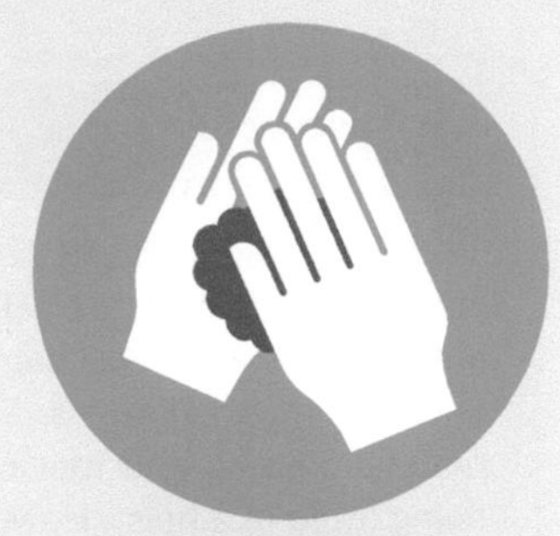

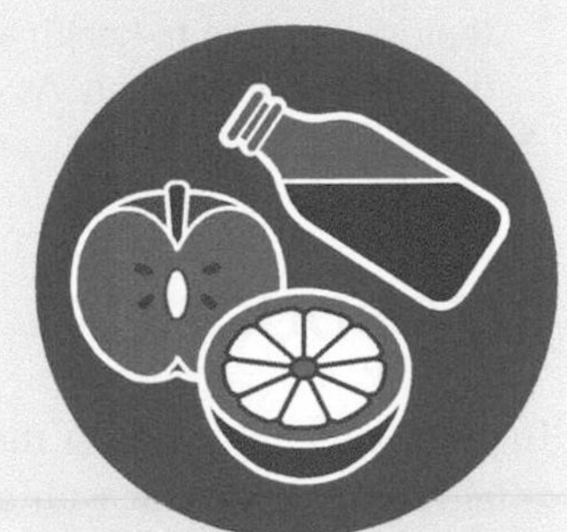

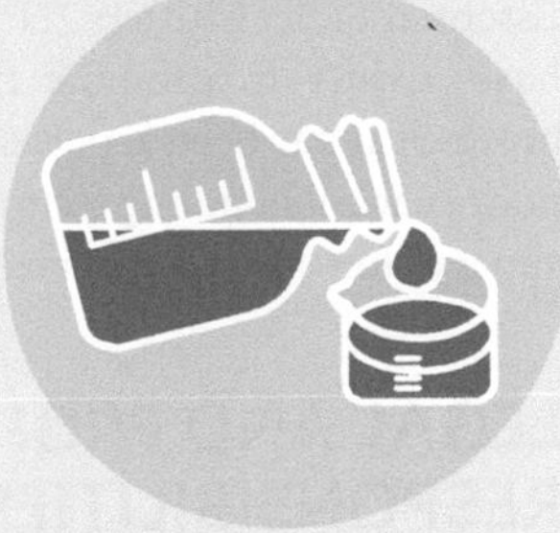

LEARNING OUTCOMES

After completing this chapter, you will be able to:

- Discuss the implications of manual handling in practice.
- Discuss the regulations that control manual handling.
- Discuss the professional responsibilities when handling a patient.
- Identify the four emergency situations when a person can be manually lifted.
- Identify the components of the spine.
- Discuss the principles of safer handling.
- Perform a risk assessment when handling a patient or object.
- Describe how to lift an inanimate object.
- Describe a range of handling manoeuvres.

By the end of this chapter you will be able to understand the legal and moral implications of manual handling in nursing practice. It relates to **Essential Skills Clusters (NMC, 2010) 1, 2, 3, 5, 6, 8–13, 15–20**, as appropriate for each progression point.

Ensure that you really understand this chapter by logging on to your complimentary **MyNursingKit** at **www.pearsoned.co.uk/kozier**. Complete the self-assessment tests to check your progress and utilise further activities to practise and confirm your understanding.

CASE STUDY

Two sisters aged 26 and 22 years, with profound physical and learning disabilities, are being cared for at home by their parents and social service home carers as they are unable to do anything for themselves. Some of the care needed involves manually lifting and moving the sisters as they do not like being lifted in a hoist. However, the local council has decided that in response to health and safety requirements it is introducing a no lifting ban. As a result, the council is refusing to employ carers to look after the sisters in their own home and have decided to place the sisters in a care home. The local council has even refused the sisters' parents' offer to pay for the home carers, resulting in the parents having to care for their daughters. The family therefore decide to take the council to the high court.

This is an actual manual handling case, *A & B, X & Y* v *East Sussex County Council* (2003).

INTRODUCTION

In 2004, back injuries cost the National Health Service (NHS) £400 million each year with one in four nurses having to take time off work as a result of a back injury (Department of Health, 2004). Unison has estimated that approximately 3600 nurses are forced to retire each year as a result of back injuries (NHS Employers, 2009). Such statistics have prompted the NHS and social services to prioritise moving and handling.

However, it is not just the healthcare professional that is at risk of injury. Cornish and Jones (2010) suggests that patients too are at risk of injury from inappropriate handling techniques. Indeed, Smith (2005) states that poor manual handling techniques can lead to patients suffering pain and discomfort leading to muscle contractions and respiratory problems. The Essential Skills Clusters (NMC, 2010) clearly state that nurses have a duty to promote the patient's comfort and dignity, however it has been reported that many nurses continue to use poor manual handling techniques, blaming staff shortages, poor supervision and inadequate provision of handling equipment.

LEGAL AND PROFESSIONAL RESPONSIBILITIES

The law within the UK with regard to the moving and handling of patients has two clear goals: first to prevent injury and second to compensate the handler when an injury occurs. The no manual lifting policy implemented by East Sussex County Council was imposed to protect their employees from injury and to avoid having to pay compensation if injuries occurred. However, the law must also consider the patient's needs and their human rights (discussed later in the chapter). This has and continues to be a 'balancing act' within law.

Accident Prevention

The Health and Safety at Work Act 1974 (abbreviated to HSWA 74) clearly states that an employer must ensure the health, safety and welfare at work of its employees, as far as it is reasonably practicable. This means that the employer has a duty to provide safe equipment, information, training and instruction of health and safety issues, for example fire training, and also provide the employee with a healthy working environment, for example no smoking environments. However it is important to note that the employee also has a duty to take reasonable care of their own health and safety.

The term 'reasonably practicable' means that the employer's duty is not absolute. If the benefit is minimal and the cost is considerable the employer may not have to comply with the duty. However, if the employer fails to meet the duty when it is reasonably practical to do so, it may face either criminal prosecution from the Health and Safety Executive (HSE) or a civil suit from its employee.

The judgment made in the case of *A & B, X & Y* v *East Sussex County Council* (2003) EWHC 167 (Admin) held that although it is important to protect the rights of the employees, the local authority should also have considered the two sisters' rights. This would involve very careful and balanced decision making but would not mean that the rights of the two sisters should override the rights of the carers or that the rights of the carers should override the rights of the sisters. However, the court conceded that it may mean that the carers might have to work with higher, but not unacceptable, levels of risk.

In addition to HSWA 74 other regulations help to regulate the issue of manual handling in the workplace. The Manual Handling Operations Regulations 1992, as amended by the Health and Safety Miscellaneous Amendments Regulations 2002 (MHOR 92) sets very specific duties for the employer in relation to manual handling in the workplace (see *Box 13-1*), while the Provision and Use of Work Equipment Regulations 1992 (PUWER) aims to prevent or control the risk to an individual's health and safety from work equipment such as photocopiers, hoists, etc. and sets out a number of requirements that the employer must adhere to (see *Box 13-2*). The Lifting Operations and Lifting Equipment Regulations 1998 (LOLER) (see *Box 13-3*), on the other hand, regulates lifting equipment used in the workplace and like PUWER it sets out requirements that the employer must adhere to. Any breach by the employer under any or all of these regulations can result in criminal prosecution.

It is the LOLER regulations that East Sussex County Council were trying to uphold. In addition to accident prevention, the council was trying to avoid paying compensation to any injured employees caring for the sisters.

BOX 13-1 Manual Handling Operations Regulations 1992 (MHOR 92)

The basic duties of the employer include:

- Hazardous manual handling should be avoided if reasonably practicable.
- Make a suitable and sufficient assessment of any hazardous manual handling which cannot be avoided.
- Reduce the risk of injury so far as is reasonably practicable.
- Provide information about the load and centre of weight.
- Any assessment must be reviewed if there are significant changes.

BOX 13-2 The Provision and Use of Work Equipment Regulations 1992 (PUWER)

Regulates work equipment such as hoists which must be:

- Suitable for their intended use.
- Safe for use, maintained in a safe condition and inspected to ensure they are safe for use.
- Used only by people who have had adequate information, instruction and training.
- Accompanied by suitable safety measures such as instructions, warnings and markings.

BOX 13-3 The Lifting Operations and Lifting Equipment Regulations 1998 (LOLER)

These regulations require that lifting equipment is:

- Strong and stable enough for its use and is marked with safe working loads, i.e. the weight that can safely be lifted with the equipment.
- Positioned and installed to minimise any risks.
- Used safely by competent personnel who have planned its use and have organised the lifting task.
- Inspected regularly by competent persons.

Source: Health and Safety Executive (1998) Simple Guide to the Lifting Operations and Lifting Equipment Regulations 1998, Caerphilly, Wales: HSE.

Compensation for the Injured Handler

HSWA 74 and the Manual Handling Operations Regulations (MHOR, 1992) and HSWA 74 clearly set out the employer's duties (see *Box 13-1* earlier), but a breach of these duties does not automatically entitle the injured handler to compensation. Nevertheless, common law, a uniform set of laws derived from custom and practice of judges, places duties on the employer to take reasonable care regarding the safety of its employees and to ensure that they are not placed under any unnecessary risk. In addition to this, the employer is also responsible for the negligence of the employees even when the employer is not at fault. This is known as **vicarious liability**.

Despite HSWA 74 stating that a breach of duties does not entitle the injured handler to compensation, the introduction of new regulations – the Management of Health and Safety at Work and Fire Precautions (Workplace) (Amendment) Regulations 2003 does entitle the injured handler to claim compensation if the employer has failed to comply with the Management of Health and Safety at Work Regulations 1999 (MHSWR).

In order to claim compensation for an alleged failure to comply with MHSWR 99, the injured handler must also prove that the injury sustained was due to the failure. This requires that the injured handler has expert medical evidence that unequivocally proves that the injury was due to the failure.

Employee Duties

It is not only the employer who has duties to the employee; the employee has duties that they must comply with. If injured, failure to comply with these duties could result in a reduction in the amount of compensation awarded, if successful.

These duties sometimes provide healthcare professionals with manual handling dilemmas. Where the employer has not complied with the obligations under MHOR 92 and the employee is put in the position of coping with inappropriate equipment, inadequate training and poor staffing levels, then when presented with a situation where a patient has to be moved does the healthcare professional have the right to refuse? It could be argued that a request to move or handle a patient in circumstances that could cause injury and where it is reasonably practical to avoid that risk is an unlawful order. However, healthcare professionals have a duty of care to meet the needs of patients. According to Griffith and Stevens (2003), lecturers with a background in law and manual handling, this may mean that the healthcare professional may be required to manually handle a patient even if there is a risk of injury to the handler. But does this breach their professional responsibilities?

Professional Responsibilities

Nurses and midwives are accountable to the Nursing and Midwifery Council (NMC), which aims to protect the public by setting and maintaining professional standards. As a result, all nurses and midwives are subject to the NMC's 'Code of Professional Conduct' (2008), a set of standards aimed at informing the professions and the public of the standard of professional conduct expected from a nurse or midwife. The Code (NMC, 2008) stipulates that the nurse must adhere to the following when caring for patients:

- Respect the patient as an individual.
- Obtain consent before any treatment or care is given.

- Protect confidential information.
- Collaborate with those in your care.
- Cooperate with others in the team.
- Maintain professional knowledge and competence.
- Be open and honest, act with integrity and uphold the reputation of your profession.
- Act to identify and minimise risk to patients.

These standards state that all nurses and midwives must adhere to the laws of the country in which they are practising. This is important when considering manual handling as the law clearly states that employers have a duty to ensure the health and safety of their employees as far as is reasonably practicable and that employees have a reciprocating duty. This means that nurses have a duty to take reasonable care of their own health and safety. However, in the past, nurses have been brought before the NMC and UK Central Council (UKCC), the predecessor of the NMC, to face allegations of professional misconduct for refusing to lift patients.

One such case found a nurse facing the UKCC for refusing to perform an unsafe lift and accused of conduct unbefitting a registered nurse (*U.K.C.C.* v *Lalis Lillian Grant* (as reported in the *Nursing Standard*, 18 February 1989). In this case, the nurse was found not guilty of professional misconduct. The guidance of the UKCC was that any refusal to manually handle a patient should be fully documented, clearly stating the reasons for the decision made (Smith, 2005).

ACTIVITY 13-1

When you are on placement, consider where moving and handling legislation affects working practices.

HUMAN RIGHTS

Everyone, including patients and health and social care workers, is protected by the Human Rights Act 1998. Human rights are the rights all individuals have just because they are human beings. These rights not only affect matters of life and death, like freedom from torture and killing, but also affect the individual's rights in everyday life: what they can say and do, their beliefs, their right to a fair trial along with other similar fundamental rights (see *Box 13-4*).

The case of *A & B, X & Y* v *East Sussex County Council* centred on the human rights of the two sisters. The specific issues highlighted in this case were:

- moving in a hoist appeared to cause the sisters distress;
- when bathing, the sisters slipped down in the bath and went under the water;
- swimming was difficult as the sisters needed to be lifted into the water;
- the sisters could not be taken shopping as they would have to be lifted to be toileted.

Specifically it was argued that using mechanical lifts to move the sisters in all situations breached their human rights. This argument was supported by the Disability Rights Commission, who stated that East Sussex County Council's policy regarding manual lifting should not restrict the sisters' rights to autonomy, privacy or dignity.

However, it is important to state that it is not only the sisters who had rights, the carers too had rights that needed to be upheld. A balance needed to be struck between the rights of the sisters to treatment respecting personal dignity and not to be deprived of valuable activities, and the rights of the carer not to be exposed to undue risk of physical harm. However, the RCN guidance had advised that 'manual lifting of patients is to be eliminated in all but exceptional or life-threatening situations' (RCN, 2003):

- if a person is threatened by bomb or bullet;
- if a person is threatened by fire;
- if a person is threatened with drowning;
- if a person is in a collapsing building.

BOX 13-4 The Human Rights Act 1998

The main provisions set out by the Human Rights Act are:

Right

Right to life
Prohibition of torture
Prohibition of slavery
Right to liberty and security
Right to a fair trial
No punishment without law

Right to respect for private and family life
Freedom of thought, conscience and religion
Freedom of expression
Freedom of assembly and association
Right to marry
Prohibition of discrimination

Protection of property
Right to education
Right to free elections
Abolition of the death penalty

Issues arising from the right

Abortion; availability of life-saving treatments; euthanasia
Respecting the dignity of vulnerable people
Slavery was effectively abolished in 1774
Detention of the mentally ill
Right to legal representation; right to silence
Criminal law must be certain and an offence at the time it was committed
Care orders; fertility treatment
Certain employment practices
Restrictions on the media with regard to privacy

Right to belong to a trade union
Arranged marriages; same-sex marriages
Prohibits discrimination on the grounds of race, colour, sex, language, religion, political opinion, national or social origin or any other status
Planning; access to environmental information
School exclusions; special educational needs
Right to vote
No person should be put to death for a crime committed

The Human Rights Act 1998 also prohibits torture, inhuman or degrading treatment, but what constitutes this is 'a matter of fact and degree in each case' (Griffith and Stevens, 2003). Thus, to refuse to manually handle or lift a patient who is at risk of developing pressures sores, if the patient refused to be moved in any other way (e.g. by using a hoist) would breach the human rights of the patient and thereby may be seen as unlawful.

In the *East Sussex County Council* case the judge made a number of important observations, including:

- manual lifting is an inherent feature of caring for the disabled;
- a blanket ban on manual lifting is likely to be unlawful;
- all lifts required to maintain a person's dignity and quality of life must be performed somehow;
- a significant amount of manual handling may be required to facilitate a disabled person's right to participate in community life.

The judgment made in this case is rather complex and has been interpreted differently by opposing parties. The Disability Rights Commission, an independent body established to end discrimination and promote equality for disabled people, who supported the sisters, felt the judgment heralded a victory for them and disabled people as it meant that the sisters could be manually lifted in certain circumstances. However, the actual judgment was that the carers would be expected to lift the sisters once each day. This means that they could be manually lifted into the bath, for example, but could not be lifted out of the bath and therefore would need to be hoisted or moved by some other means.

Since the judgment did state that in certain circumstances the carers would be expected to lift the sisters it is important to consider some of the principles of safe handling of people.

RESEARCH NOTE

Factors Affecting Compliance with Moving and Handling Policy: Student Nurses' Views and Experiences

Using a qualitative approach, Cornish and Jones (2010) set out to explore student nurses' reports of their experience of adhering to moving and handling policies in clinical practice. Focus groups, questionnaires and unstructured interviews were used. The results of the study appeared to centre around examples of poor practice, with students reporting that they were being actively encouraged to participate in poor practice. It also found that students required further support in order to enable them to comply with current moving and handling policies.

Source: based on Cornish, J. and Jones, A. (2010) 'Factors affecting compliance with moving and handling policy: Student nurses' views and experiences', *Nurse Education in Practice*, 10: 96–100.

THE SPINE

The spine or vertebral column extends from the base of the skull to the pelvis and is made up of 33 individual bones or vertebrae. These individual bones give the spine strength and flexibility. The 33 vertebrae are divided into regions:

- seven cervical (neck) vertebrae
- twelve thoracic (chest) vertebrae
- five lumbar (lower back) vertebrae
- five sacrum and four **coccyx**, which are fused together (see Figure 13-1).

Each of the vertebrae is linked together by facet joints. These joints allow the vertebrae to move against one another and give the spine its flexibility. The facets are the bony prominences that meet between each vertebra. There are two facet joints between each pair of vertebrae (see Figure 13-2) that extend and flex over one another.

One quarter of the spine's length is made up by the intervertebral discs, which are fibrocartilaginous cushions and act as shock absorbers for the spine protecting the brain, vertebrae and nerves. Intervertebral discs are nonvascular and therefore depend on the end plates of each of the vertebra for nutrients. The discs allow for movement within the spine. It is damage to these discs that cause most back pain. This condition is commonly referred to as 'a slipped disc' or prolapsed disc. This is where the disc slips out of position (see Figure 13-3).

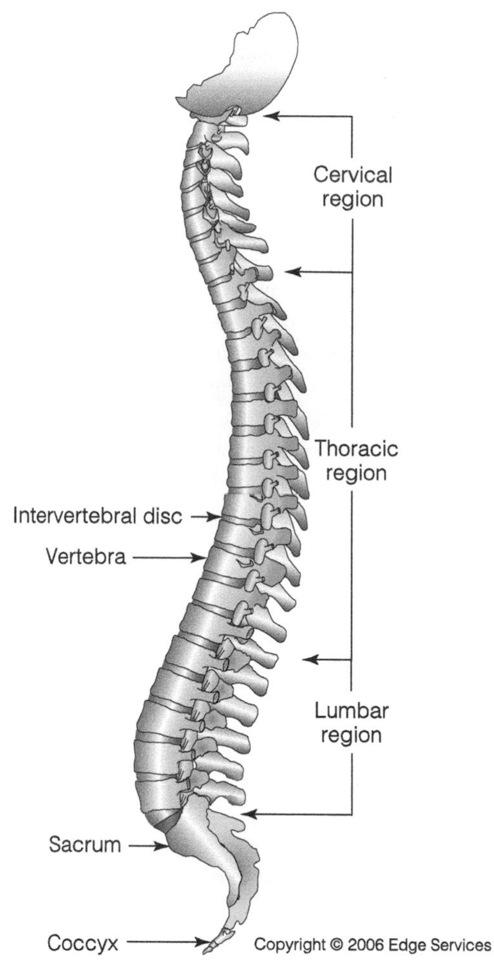

Figure 13-1 The spine.

Source: Manual handling illustrations © EDGE Services (2006) reproduced by kind permission of EDGE Services - The Manual Handling Training Co. Ltd (01904 677853) sourced from People Handling and Risk Assessment Key Trainer's Certificate course materials.

The views expressed in this text book, generally and with specific reference to manual handling, do not necessarily reflect the views, approach, company policies or course content of training programmes of EDGE Services - The Manual Handling Training Co. Ltd.

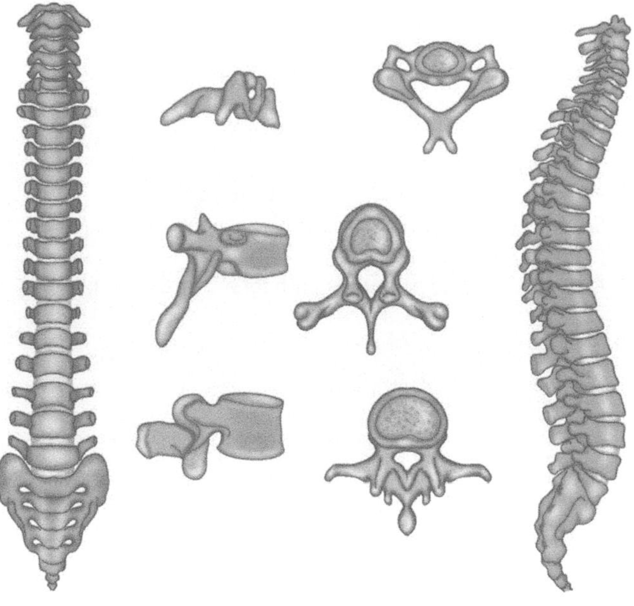

Figure 13-2 Facet joints of spine.

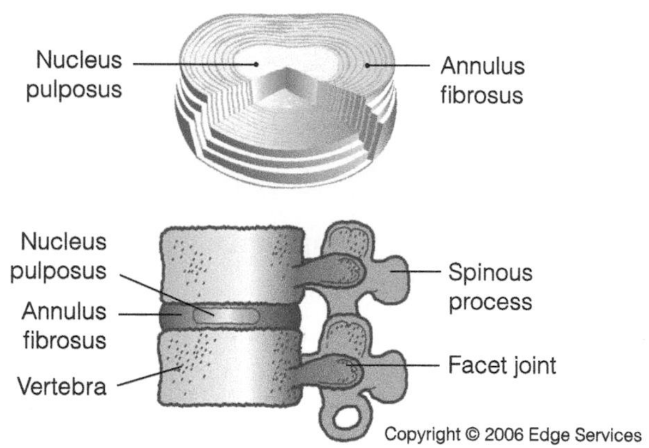

Figure 13-3 Prolapsed intervertebral disc.

Source: Manual handling illustrations © EDGE Services (2006) reproduced by kind permission of EDGE Services - The Manual Handling Training Co. Ltd (01904 677853) sourced from People Handling and Risk Assessment Key Trainer's Certificate course materials.

The views expressed in this text book, generally and with specific reference to manual handling, do not necessarily reflect the views, approach, company policies or course content of training programmes of EDGE Services - The Manual Handling Training Co. Ltd.

Each disc is made up of an annulus fibrosus and a nucleus pulposus (see Figure 13-4). The annulus fibrosus is made up of concentric circles of **collagen** that connects to the vertebral end plates, and can be likened to a car tyre and encapsulates the nucleus pulposus. The nucleus pulposus contains a gel-like substance that resists compression.

Although the vertebral column is strong and flexible, it still requires support from a number of muscles and ligaments. In fact there are over 30 muscles that support the spine giving it stability and allowing for mobility (see Table 13-1).

The purpose of the vertebral column is two-fold; it gives us mobility, flexibility and allows us to stand up but also acts as a protective casing for the spinal cord, which passes down through the middle of the vertebral column in the spinal canal (see Figure 13-5). The spinal nerves branch off at each level of the vertebral column and carry nerve impulses to and from various parts of the body.

Although the spine is relatively robust, back pain is the most common cause of absence from work in the UK. In 2008–09 a survey performed by the Health and Safety Executive (HSE) (2010) found that 42% of the UK's workforce self-reported back pain. Many believe that back pain is caused by one specific incident but this is rarely the case. Indeed most back pain is cause by an accumulation of damage over many years as a result of six possible factors:

- poor posture – how we stand and sit;
- poor body mechanics – how we use our body to pull, lift or push objects;

Table 13-1 Spinal Muscles

Cervical muscles	Function
Sternocleidomastoid	Extends and rotates head, flexes vertebral column
Scalenus	Flexes and rotates neck
Spinalis Cervicis	Extends and rotates head
Spinalis Capitus	Extends and rotates head
Semispinalis Cervicis	Extends and rotates vertebral column
Semispinalis Capitus	Rotates head and pulls backward
Splenius Cervicis	Extends vertebral column
Longus Colli Cervicis	Flexes cervical vertebrae
Longus Capitus	Flexes head
Rectus Capitus Anterior	Flexes head
Rectus Capitus Lateralis	Bends head laterally
Iliocostalis Cervicis	Extends cervical vertebrae
Longissimus Cervicis	Extends cervical vertebrae
Longissimus Capitus	Rotates head and pulls backward
Rectus Capitus Posterior Major	Extends and rotates head
Rectus Capitus Posterior Minor	Extends head
Obliquus Capitus Inferior	Rotates atlas
Obliquus Capitus Superior	Extends and bends head laterally
Thoracic muscles	**Function**
Longissimus Thoracis	Extension, lateral flexion of vertebral column, rib rotation
Iliocostalis Thoracis	Extension, lateral flexion of vertebral column, rib rotation
Spinalis Thoracis	Extends vertebral column
Semispinalis Thoracis	Extends and rotates vertebral column
Rotatores Thoracis	Extends and rotates vertebral column
Lumbar muscles	**Function**
Psoas Major	Flexes thigh at hip joint and vertebral column
Intertransversarii Lateralis	Lateral flexion of vertebral column
Quadratus Lumborum	Lateral flexion of vertebral column
Interspinales	Extends vertebral column
Intertransversarii Mediales	Lateral flexion of vertebral column
Multifidus	Extends and rotates vertebral column
Longissimus Lumborum	Extends and rotates vertebral column
Iliocostalis Lumborum	Extension, lateral flexion of vertebral column, rib rotation

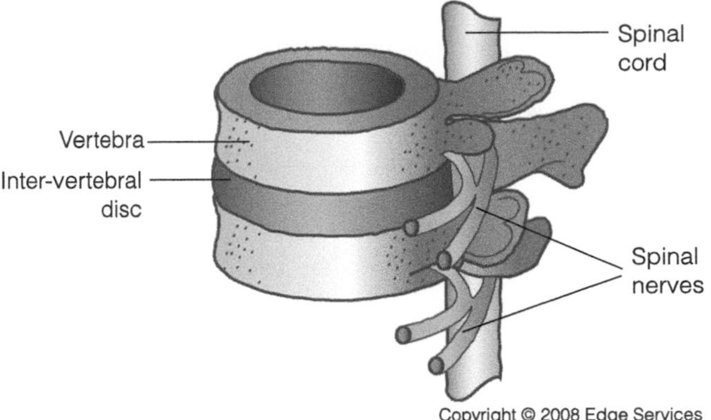

Figure 13-4 Intervertebral disc.

Source: Manual handling illustrations © EDGE Services (2008) reproduced by kind permission of EDGE Services - The Manual Handling Training Co. Ltd (01904 677853) sourced from People Handling and Risk Assessment Key Trainer's Certificate course materials.

The views expressed in this text book, generally and with specific reference to manual handling, do not necessarily reflect the views, approach, company policies or course content of training programmes of EDGE Services - The Manual Handling Training Co. Ltd.

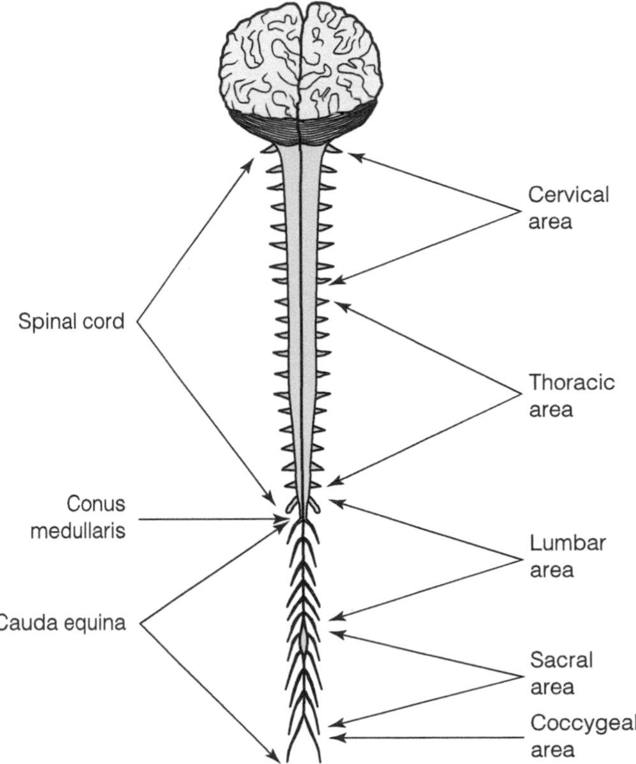

Figure 13-5 The spinal cord.

- the way we live and work – repetitive motions (e.g. shopping, lifting a child, sitting for too long and not being able to relax);
- loss of flexibility – stiffening up, unable to have a full range of movement;
- poor physical condition – loss of stamina and strength;
- age – weakens the spine.

Usually damage to the spine has already occurred before pain is felt. However a painful episode can be triggered by something as simple as a sneeze or twisting to put shopping into a trolley or bending down to put a patient's slippers on. But what do you do if you suffer with back pain? A recent Welsh strategy for tackling absence from work due to back pain suggests:

- *Staying active - back muscles weaken if they are not used.*
- *Take control - do not allow the pain to control your life, continue as if normal and take regular analgesia if needed.*
- *Stay in control - by keeping active as usually the pain will subside.*

(Welshbacks, 2006)

In order to prevent back injury there are a number of principles that should be adhered to – these are termed the principles of biomechanics.

PRINCIPLES OF BIOMECHANICS

Biomechanics is the study of the mechanics of living organisms and ranges from the inner workings of the cell to the development of bones and muscles. An understanding of the basic principles of biomechanics is important as they can help prevent damage to the spine.

There are three main principles of biomechanics that are important when considering moving patients or objects. They are:

- centre of gravity
- stable base
- keeping external levers short.

Principle 1 - Using the Centre of Gravity

Everything has a centre of gravity. The centre of gravity is where the total mass or weight of the object is concentrated. For uniform objects such as a brick, the centre of gravity will always be in the middle of the object (see Figure 13-6).

The human body also has a centre of gravity but unlike the brick whose dimensions remain constant, the human body changes its dimensions at will from sitting to standing, from crouching to lying. When standing upright the centre of gravity is usually situated around the navel (belly button) (see Figure 13-7).

The lower the centre of gravity is to the floor the more stable the body is, such as when we are on all fours. The higher the centre of gravity the less stable the body becomes, such as when the arms are raised above the head.

If the centre of gravity is within the body, stability is increased and it is easier to move. However, if the centre of gravity is outside the body, the body is less stable and more difficult to move. For instance when sitting all the way back in a chair the centre of gravity is outside the body, standing from this position is difficult (see Figure 13-8). However, if we sit forward in the chair

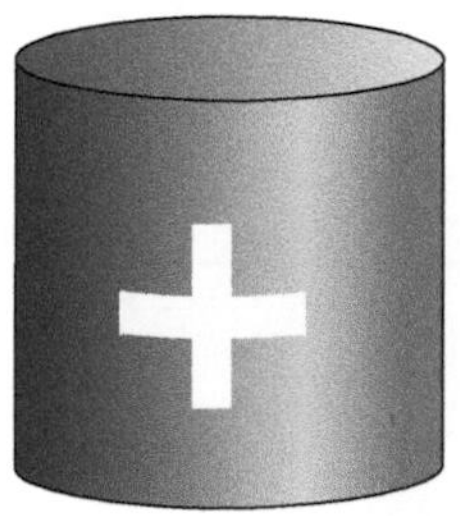
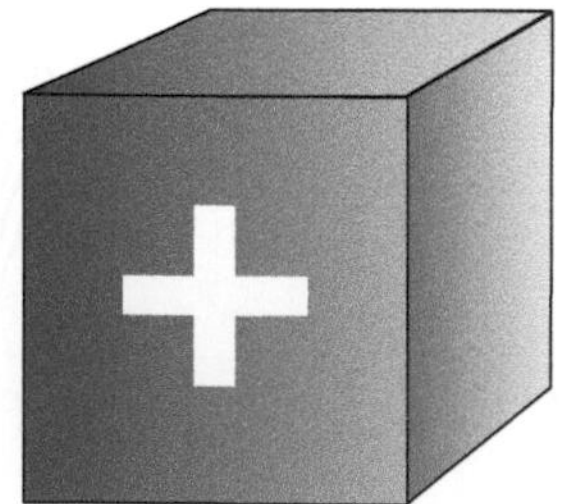

Figure 13-6 Uniform objects centre of gravity.

Source: Manual handling illustrations © EDGE Services (2006) reproduced by kind permission of EDGE Services - The Manual Handling Training Co. Ltd (01904 677853) sourced from People Handling and Risk Assessment Key Trainer's Certificate course materials.

The views expressed in this text book, generally and with specific reference to manual handling, do not necessarily reflect the views, approach, company policies or course content of training programmes of EDGE Services - The Manual Handling Training Co. Ltd.

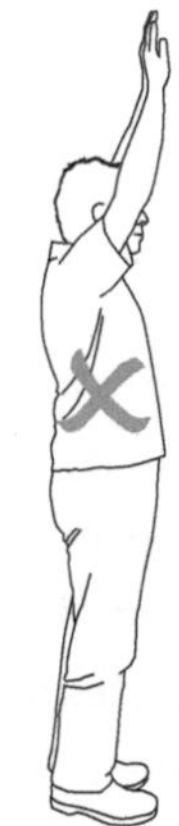

Figure 13-7 Centre of gravity of a human.

Source: Manual handling illustrations © EDGE Services (2010) reproduced by kind permission of EDGE Services - The Manual Handling Training Co. Ltd (01904 677853) sourced from People Handling and Risk Assessment Key Trainer's Certificate course materials.

The views expressed in this text book, generally and with specific reference to manual handling, do not necessarily reflect the views, approach, company policies or course content of training programmes of EDGE Services - The Manual Handling Training Co. Ltd.

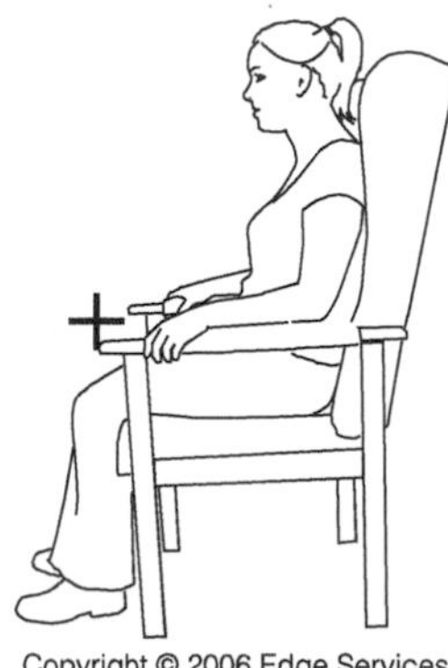

Figure 13-8 Centre of gravity outside the body making it difficult to stand.

Source: Manual handling illustrations © EDGE Services (2006) reproduced by kind permission of EDGE Services - The Manual Handling Training Co. Ltd (01904 677853) sourced from People Handling and Risk Assessment Key Trainer's Certificate course materials.

The views expressed in this text book, generally and with specific reference to manual handling, do not necessarily reflect the views, approach, company policies or course content of training programmes of EDGE Services - The Manual Handling Training Co. Ltd.

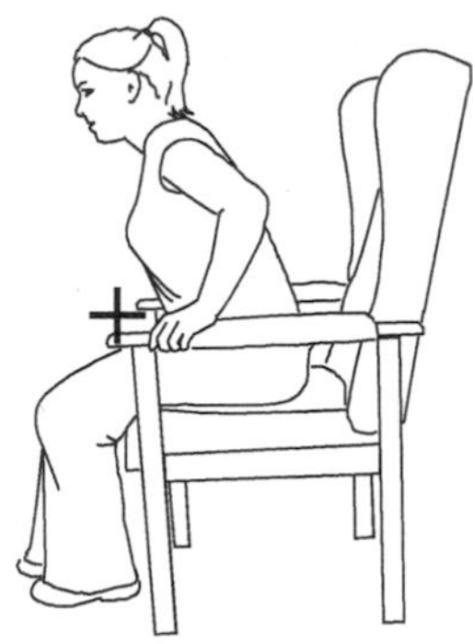

Figure 13-9 Leaning forward brings the centre of gravity closer to the body.

Source: Manual handling illustrations © EDGE Services (2006) reproduced by kind permission of EDGE Services - The Manual Handling Training Co. Ltd (01904 677853) sourced from People Handling and Risk Assessment Key Trainer's Certificate course materials.

The views expressed in this text book, generally and with specific reference to manual handling, do not necessarily reflect the views, approach, company policies or course content of training programmes of EDGE Services - The Manual Handling Training Co. Ltd.

the centre of gravity comes closer to the body making it easier to stand (see Figure 13-9).

Principle 2 - Using a Stable Base

When standing, the feet and the area between them acts as the base of support for the body (see Figure 13.10). In order to remain stable the line of gravity should be within the base of support. Humans tend to be more stable when their feet are placed shoulder width apart and knees slightly bent (which brings the centre of gravity closer to the floor) (see Figure 13-11).

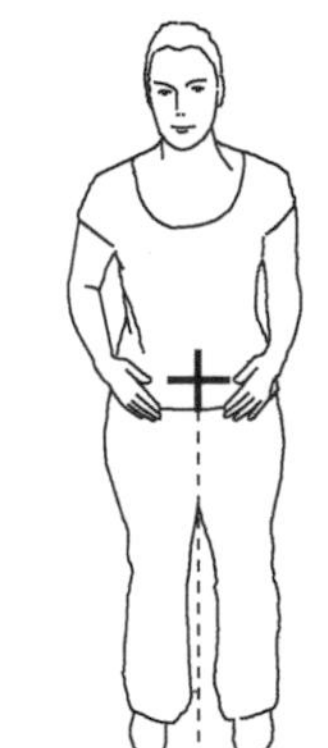

Figure 13-10 Knees slightly bent and feet shoulder width apart provides stability.

Source: Manual handling illustrations © EDGE Services (2006) reproduced by kind permission of EDGE Services - The Manual Handling Training Co. Ltd (01904 677853) sourced from People Handling and Risk Assessment Key Trainer's Certificate course materials.

The views expressed in this text book, generally and with specific reference to manual handling, do not necessarily reflect the views, approach, company policies or course content of training programmes of EDGE Services - The Manual Handling Training Co. Ltd.

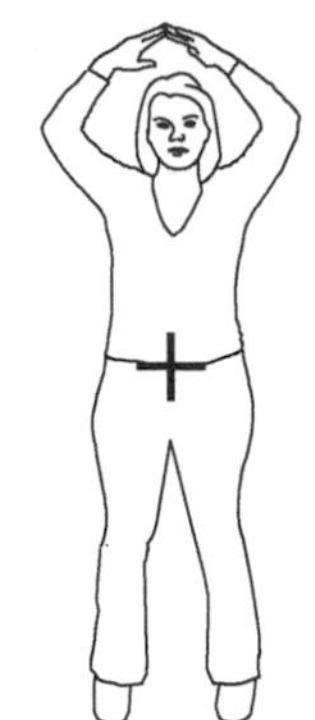

Figure 13-11 Centre of gravity of a human.

Source: Manual handling illustrations © EDGE Services (2006) reproduced by kind permission of EDGE Services - The Manual Handling Training Co. Ltd (01904 677853) sourced from People Handling and Risk Assessment Key Trainer's Certificate course materials.

The views expressed in this text book, generally and with specific reference to manual handling, do not necessarily reflect the views, approach, company policies or course content of training programmes of EDGE Services - The Manual Handling Training Co. Ltd.

Principle 3 - Keeping the External Levers Short

The term 'external levers' in manual handling refers to the arms. These need to be kept as short as possible: therefore keeping the load (weight) closer to the body ultimately brings the centre of gravity closer to the body, resulting in added stability.

If we consider a person leaning forward to lift an object as in Figure 13-12, a common position that many of us adopt, then the centre of gravity moves outside of the body, which causes instability. In order to keep the body as stable as possible the muscles and ligaments of the back are put under a great deal of

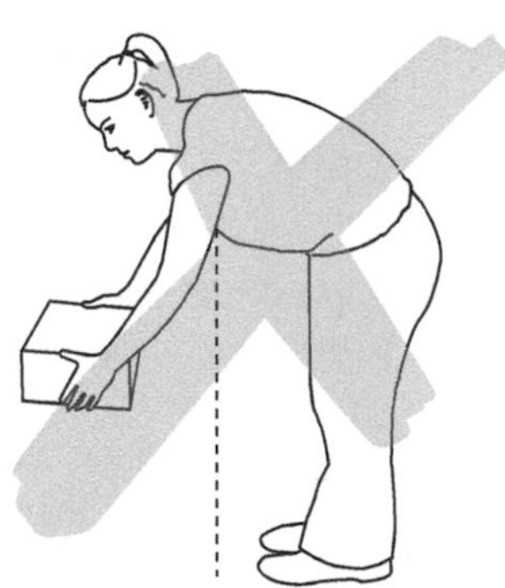

Figure 13-12 Bending forward causes instability and increased tension in the muscles of the back.

Source: Manual handling illustrations © EDGE Services (2006) reproduced by kind permission of EDGE Services - The Manual Handling Training Co. Ltd (01904 677853) sourced from People Handling and Risk Assessment Key Trainer's Certificate course materials.

The views expressed in this text book, generally and with specific reference to manual handling, do not necessarily reflect the views, approach, company policies or course content of training programmes.

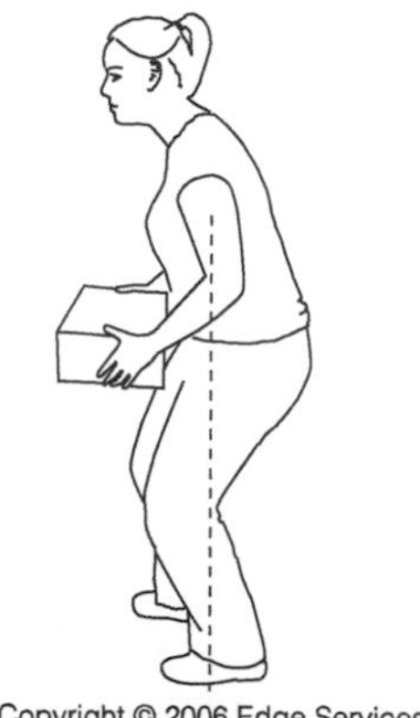

Figure 13-13 Keeping the arms short, knees bent and feet a shoulder width apart reduces the tension on the muscles of the back.

Source: Manual handling illustrations © EDGE Services (2006) reproduced by kind permission of EDGE Services - The Manual Handling Training Co. Ltd (01904 677853) sourced from People Handling and Risk Assessment Key Trainer's Certificate course materials.

The views expressed in this text book, generally and with specific reference to manual handling, do not necessarily reflect the views, approach, company policies or course content of training programmes of EDGE Services - The Manual Handling Training Co. Ltd.

stress. If the person were to stay in this position for long the muscles would become fatigued. If the person then lifts the object they will find it extremely difficult as only minor muscles are available for the manoeuvre. Basically in this position the person is at increased risk of injury.

Therefore to prevent injury, keep the arms short and close to the body, and bend the knees with the feet slightly apart (see Figure 13-13). This keeps the centre of gravity within the body resulting in stability.

These three principles to safer handling can then be applied to moving and handling any object including patients. However, before contemplating moving an object or person there is one more point to consider: risk assessment.

RISK ASSESSMENT

The Manual Handling Operations Regulations 1992, as discussed earlier, set out some clear guidelines for the manual handling of an object or person (see Figure 13-14). As part of these guidelines, MHOR 92 clearly states that manual handling should be avoided but if it cannot then the hazards and risks associated with the handling should be fully assessed.

A hazard is the potential to cause harm, for example, lifting a person on your own has the potential to cause you harm (i.e. back injury) while a risk is the likelihood and severity of that harm occurring. So, for the previous example, it is highly likely that you would injure your back if you were to lift a person on your own and that injury could actually cause you to have persistent long-term back pain.

In order to risk assess a manual handling procedure we need to consider the following:

Avoid
Wherever possible avoid manually handling anything
Assess
the hazards and risks of the procedure
Reduce
the risk of injury to all of the people involved
Review
the risk assessments regularly to ensure they are effective
Manual handling situation

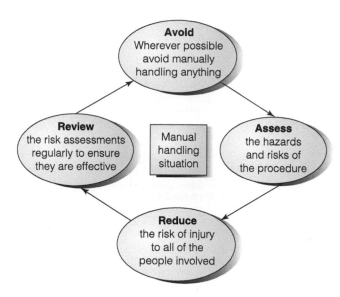

Figure 13-14 Manual Handling Operations Regulations 1992 requirements.

- Task: What you are doing. Does it involve stooping, bending, twisting, reaching upwards, carrying long distances, etc?
- Individual: Are you capable of moving the object? Are you pregnant? Do you have an injury that could prevent you from performing the task? Are you overweight? Do you have the necessary knowledge? Have you had appropriate training?
- Load: Is it heavy, bulky, unwieldy? Do you know its weight? (see Figure 13-15) Is it hot, cold or sharp?
- Environment: Are there slippery floors, variations in levels? Are there leads, equipment in the way? Are the conditions hot, cold or humid?

The acronym TILE, can be quickly and easily used informally to risk assess a manual handling procedure and can also be used for more formal documented risk assessments as undertaken in many hospital and home environments by nurses.

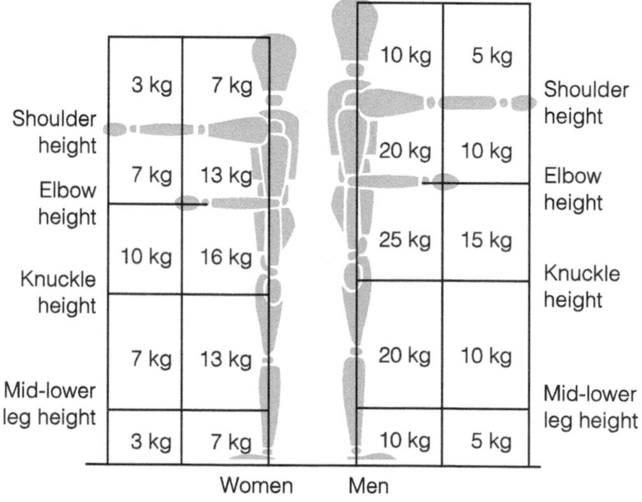

Figure 13-15 The Health and Safety Executive's Guidelines for Handling Loads.

TEACHING: COMMUNITY CARE

In the community setting manual handling assessment should be carried out by the district nursing sister, who should have undergone appropriate training. Where possible the amount of local (or individual) assessments should be minimised by producing generic assessments where appropriate (RCN, 2003). These generic assessments should serve as a guide for those performing particular manoeuvres with patients. Some examples of generic assessments include (RCN, 2003):

- bed to chair/commode/toilet transfers;
- patients who have a history of falls;
- bathing;
- floor coverings (hoisting on carpets/slippery bathroom floors);
- difficulties in using hoists, e.g. carpets, lack of space;
- in/out of car;
- babies in high-sided cots;
- handling supplies (packages/boxes) at a health centre.

HANDLING AN INANIMATE LOAD

It is probably a misconception that the only handling a nurse does is that of patient handling, but it is far more likely that a nurse will handle inanimate objects such as intravenous fluid boxes, beds, lockers and chairs. Nurses also have personal lives where they lift shopping from a trolley into the boot of a car or unload a washing machine and carry the heavy basket to the tumble dryer. Therefore it is important that the nurse applies the principles of safe manual handling to all aspects of their life. The *Practice Guidelines* below considers the safe lifting of a box from the floor to a shelf.

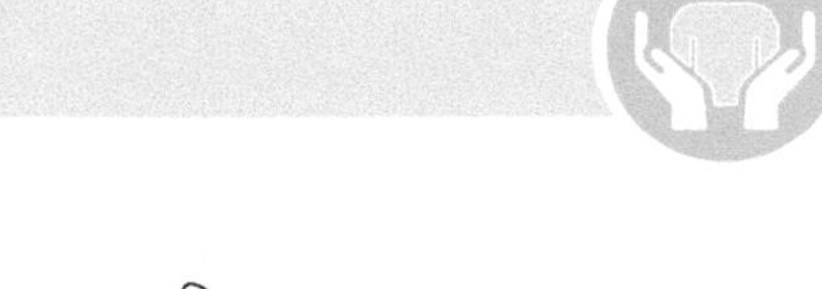

PRACTICE GUIDELINES

Lifting a Box from the Floor to a Shelf

First risk assess the manoeuvre using TILE. (See Figure 13-16.)

- **T** - Do I need to lift this box? Where do you want to move the item? Does moving the box require bending or stooping? Does the manoeuvre involve long carrying distances? What could I do to reduce the risk of injury, e.g. can I move the box by some other means such as using a hoist or trolley?
- **I** - Am I capable of lifting this box? Am I in good health at the moment?
- **L** - How do I know I can lift this weight? What does the box contain? Can the contents be moved individually?
- **E** - Are the floors slippery? Are there any potential hazards such as other people, furniture, leads and cables?

If you feel that it is safe to proceed after doing the risk assessment, you need to consider your approach to the lift, in particular the positioning of your feet. Place your feet apart ensuring that you are in a stable position. Put your leading foot forward. (See Figure 13-17.)

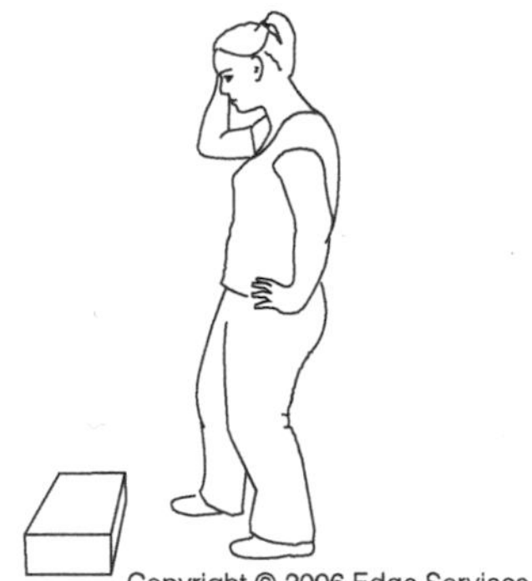

Figure 13-16 Risk assess the manoeuvre before starting.

Source: Manual handling illustrations © EDGE Services (2006) reproduced by kind permission of EDGE Services - The Manual Handling Training Co. Ltd (01904 677853) sourced from People Handling and Risk Assessment Key Trainer's Certificate course materials.

The views expressed in this text book, generally and with specific reference to manual handling, do not necessarily reflect the views, approach, company policies or course content of training programmes of EDGE Services - The Manual Handling Training Co. Ltd.

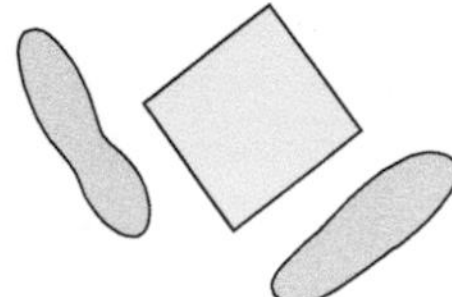

Figure 13-17 Put your leading foot forward.

Your knees should be bent but you should not be kneeling on the floor. Your arms should be between the legs, and shoulders should be in line with your hips. Hands should maintain a secure grip on the box. Remember to keep the natural curves of the spine. (See Figure 13-18.)

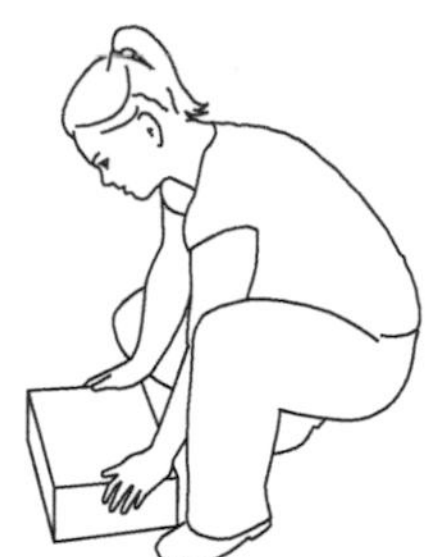

Figure 13-18 Bend the knees, keep your arm between your legs and securely grip the box.

Source: Manual handling illustrations © EDGE Services (2006) reproduced by kind permission of EDGE Services - The Manual Handling Training Co. Ltd (01904 677853) sourced from People Handling and Risk Assessment Key Trainer's Certificate course materials.

The views expressed in this text book, generally and with specific reference to manual handling, do not necessarily reflect the views, approach, company policies or course content of training programmes of EDGE Services - The Manual Handling Training Co. Ltd.

When you are ready to lift, lead with your head, that is keep your head up, looking where you are going. Then raise your body lifting the box smoothly without any jarring. (See Figure 13-19.)

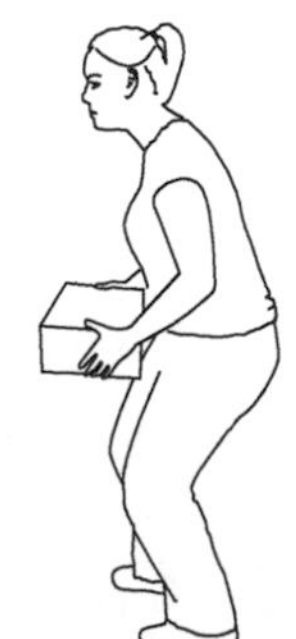

Figure 13-19 Lead with your head and raise the box smoothly.

Source: Manual handling illustrations © EDGE Services (2006) reproduced by kind permission of EDGE Services - The Manual Handling Training Co. Ltd (01904 677853) sourced from People Handling and Risk Assessment Key Trainer's Certificate course materials.

The views expressed in this text book, generally and with specific reference to manual handling, do not necessarily reflect the views, approach, company policies or course content of training programmes of EDGE Services - The Manual Handling Training Co. Ltd.

Keep the load as close to the body as possible. Remember not to twist or turn your body. If you need to change direction use your feet. (See Figure 13-20.)

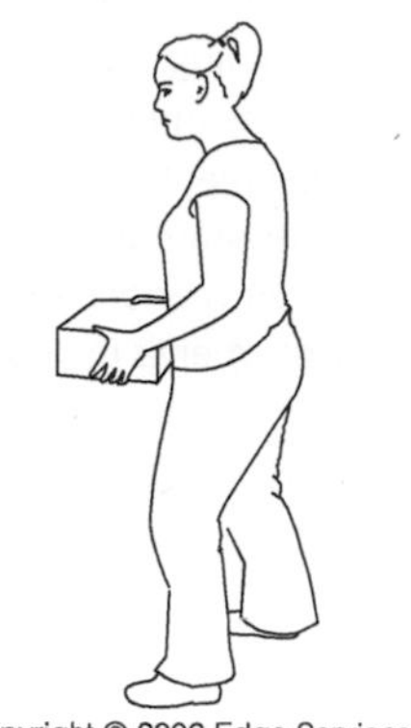

Figure 13-20 Keep the load close to the body.

Source: Manual handling illustrations © EDGE Services (2006) reproduced by kind permission of EDGE Services - The Manual Handling Training Co. Ltd (01904 677853) sourced from People Handling and Risk Assessment Key Trainer's Certificate course materials.

The views expressed in this text book, generally and with specific reference to manual handling, do not necessarily reflect the views, approach, company policies or course content of training programmes of EDGE Services - The Manual Handling Training Co. Ltd.

When you reach the shelf, place the box down as close to your body as possible, you can then move the box to the desired position once it is on the shelf. (See Figure 13-21.)

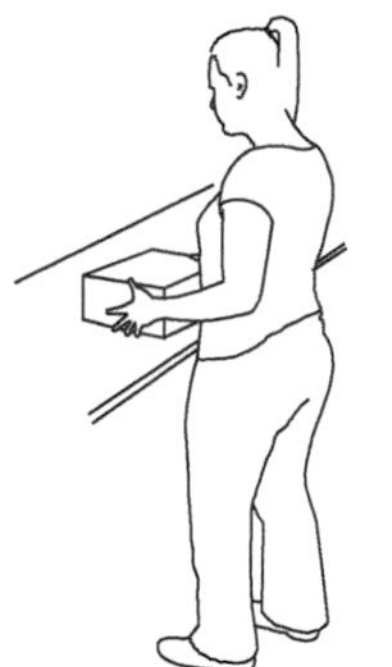

Figure 13-21 Place the box on the shelf and readjust its position if needed.

Source: Manual handling illustrations © EDGE Services (2006) reproduced by kind permission of EDGE Services - The Manual Handling Training Co. Ltd (01904 677853) sourced from People Handling and Risk Assessment Key Trainer's Certificate course materials.

The views expressed in this text book, generally and with specific reference to manual handling, do not necessarily reflect the views, approach, company policies or course content of training programmes of EDGE Services - The Manual Handling Training Co. Ltd.

PATIENT HANDLING

Handling patients is a key component of the nurse's role. The nurse needs to be aware of the legal and professional responsibilities surrounding handling patients in order to have a clear understanding of the implications of such a task.

The principles of safer handling and biomechanics – risk assessment, using the centre of gravity, stable base, keeping external levers short – apply to both inanimate objects and people. According to the RCN (2002), when nursing small children and babies it would be impossible to eradicate lifting but in these circumstances the nurse should apply commonsense and prevent injury to themselves by taking measures such as choosing the correct cot for the weight of the child.

The following procedures (*Procedures 13-1* to *13-12*) demonstrate how to perform particular handling tasks using the principles of safer handling. Many handling tasks involve more than one nurse or nursing assistant and in these cases it is important that one of the nurses acts as team leader in order that the task be undertaken smoothly.

PROCEDURE 13-1 Moving a Person from Sitting to Standing

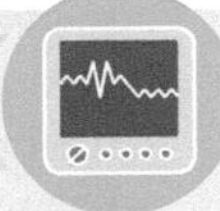

Purpose

- To promote a sense of well-being
- To check and/or relieve pressure areas and maintain skin integrity
- To aid the recovery of the patient
- To stimulate circulation

Assessment

Assess

- Risk assess the procedure using TILE.
- The patient's ability to stand by assessing mobility, strength and ability to understand (see *Practice Guidelines* on page 354).
- Fatigue.
- Presence of pain and need for adjunctive measures (e.g. an analgesic) before standing the patient.

Planning

- Plan the procedure with any assistants including the patient (*promotes concordance*).
- Encourage the patient to do as much as possible for themselves (*increasing mobility aids recovery and rehabilitation*).
- Gather any equipment that may be needed.
- Ensure patient is properly dressed (*ensures the patient's dignity is maintained*).
- Ensure the patient is wearing appropriate footwear or is barefooted (*ill fitting shoes, slippers or feet in stockings can lead to falls*).

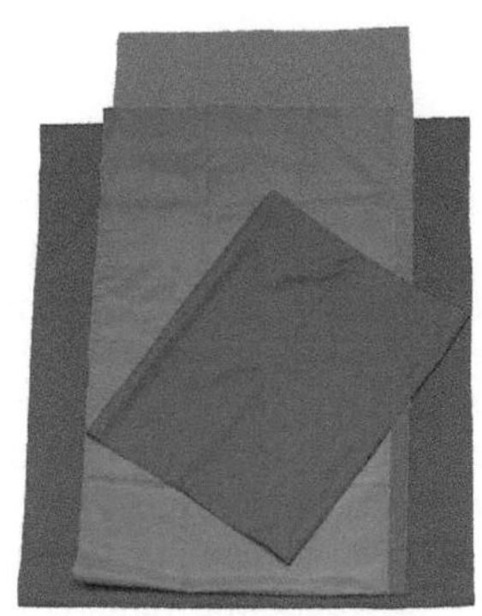

Figure 13-22 Tubular slide sheets.
Source: MEDesign Ltd.

Equipment

- Tubular slide sheets (see Figure 13-22)
- Flexi disc (see Figure 13-23)
- Handling belt (see Figure 13-24)

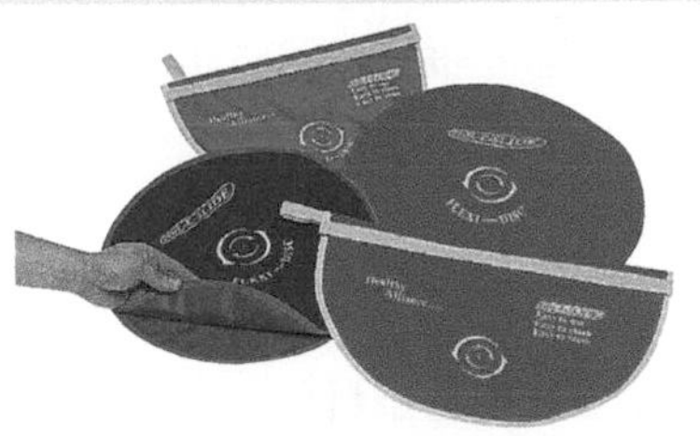

Figure 13-23 Flexi disc. Phil-e-slide patient handling system.
Source: Ergo Ike Ltd. **www.phil-e-slide-uk.com**

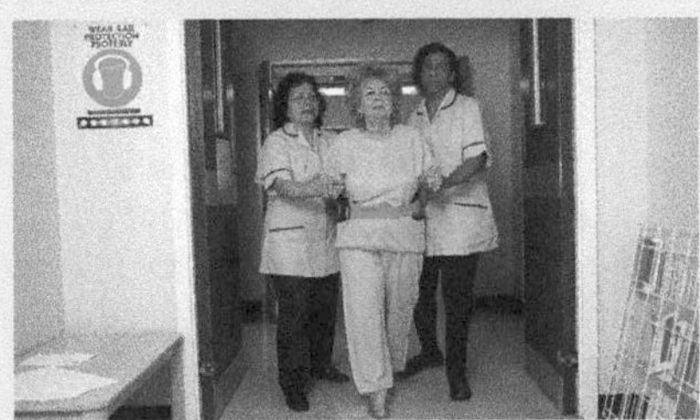

Figure 13-24 Handling belt.
Source: Mediscan.

Implementation

Performance

1 Follow local policy to ensure that you explain to the patient what you are going to do, why it is necessary and how they can cooperate. Obtain consent and maintain patient privacy and dignity and ensure that the appropriate local infection control procedures are observed.
2 If the patient is being returned to bed ensure that the bed is prepared and at the correct height for the patient with the head of the bed tilted up.
3 The patient needs to lean forward with their head over their knees, usually placing the hand on the arms of the chair will help stabilise the patient (see Figure 13-25). *To move their centre of gravity and make it easier to move the patient.*
4 Encourage the patient to move forward in the chair by walking on the cheeks of their bottom.
5 If the patient is unable to do this then you may consider using tubular slide sheets, which should be placed underneath the patient.
6 If you do use slide sheets then you must adhere to the safety guidelines for their use (see the *Practice Guidelines* on page 355).
7 Once the patient is towards the front of the chair the feet need to be positioned slightly apart or in a walk stance position and positioned posterior to the knees. *To stabilise the patient.*
8 When ready to stand, the patient should gain momentum by leaning back, then forward in a rocking motion while pushing down on the arms of the chair. The nurse can say 'Ready, steady, stand' to help the coordination of the movement. *To gain momentum and improve patient concordance.*

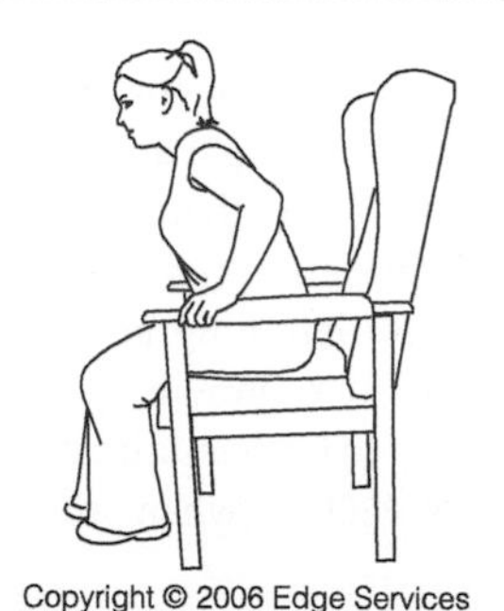

Figure 13-25 Leaning forward and putting their hands on the arms of the chair or on their knees stabilises the patient.
Source: Manual handling illustrations © EDGE Services (2006) reproduced by kind permission of EDGE Services - The Manual Handling Training Co. Ltd (01904 677853) sourced from People Handling and Risk Assessment Key Trainer's Certificate course materials.
The views expressed in this text book, generally and with specific reference to manual handling, do not necessarily reflect the views, approach, company policies or course content of training programmes of EDGE Services - The Manual Handling Training Co. Ltd.

9 For reassurance, the nurse can place their hands on the patient's shoulder or can use a handling belt, ensuring that they do not lift the patient or bend or stoop during the procedure. *To reassure the patient.*
10 Once standing the patient can then turn if needed to the bed or if they are unable to do this the nurse can use the Flexi Disc on the floor to turn the patient towards the bed or chair.

Evaluation

- Note the patient's tolerance of the procedure (e.g. respiratory rate and effort, pulse rate, behaviour, cooperation).
- Document procedure and findings in the nursing notes.

PRACTICE GUIDELINES

Assessing a Patient's Mobility, Strength and Understanding

Before performing the following, the nurse must gain consent from the patient:

- Ask the patient when they moved last and how they felt.
- Ask the patient if they can feel their hands, arms, feet and legs. *This checks understanding and sensation.*
- Apply pressure to the patient's knee by placing your hand on their knee then ask the patient to lift their knee; repeat for other knee. *The patient should be able to lift both knees with equal strength.*
- Place your hand on top of the patient's foot and ask the patient to lift their foot off the floor or bed. *The patient should be able to lift both feet with equal strength.*
- Ask the patient to place their hands on the arms of the chair and lift themselves off the chair slightly. *The patient should be able to lift themselves slightly off the chair.*
- Ask the patient to squeeze your hand tightly with their left hand, repeat with right hand. The patient should be able to squeeze equally with both hands. *This checks understanding, sensation and strength.*
- Explain to the patient what the manoeuvre involves and ask the patient to repeat the requirements. *This checks understanding.*
- If in any doubt at any stage do not move the patient.

PRACTICE GUIDELINES

Slide Sheets

- Slide sheets are made from specialised flexible fabric that has been designed to reduce friction during handling procedures.
- There are different types of slide sheets made by a number of different companies.
- The main types are tubular slide sheets and flat slide sheets.
- Tubular slide sheets are tubes of fabric that have a low friction inner surface (usually shiny surface) which slides over itself and can be used for the seated patient or a patient who is lying down.
- Flat sheets are sheets of fabric that have a low friction surface. These must be used in pairs unless advised by the manufacturer. When using in pairs, the low friction surfaces must be next to one another (shiny surface to shiny surface).

Safety While Using Slide Sheets

- Because of the slippery nature of the slide sheets they may not be suitable for all handling procedures with all patients. Assess the individual situation and patient before using.
- If the low friction surfaces are not together, this can cause added stress on the nurse's back and potentially cause injury.
- You must receive training before using slide sheets as with all manual handling equipment.
- Once used, do not put the slide sheet on the floor as it is a slipping hazard.
- Slide sheets should be for single patient use.
- Most slide sheets can be washed when soiled and between patients.
- Disposable slide sheets are for single patient use and then should be disposed of.

Removing Tubular Slide Sheets

- Place your hand between the layers of the tubular sheet.
- Grasp the opposite corner and pull the tube inside out in the direction you have just moved the patient: so if you have moved the patient up the bed you should pull to the top of the bed.

Removing Flat Slide Sheets

- Place your hand between the two layers of the sheets.
- Grasp the opposite corner bottom sheet and pull it over the top of itself (shiny surface to shiny surface) in the direction you have just moved the patient (see Figure 13-26).
- Grasp the opposite corner of the top sheet and pull it under itself (shiny surface to shiny surface) in the direction you have just moved the patient.

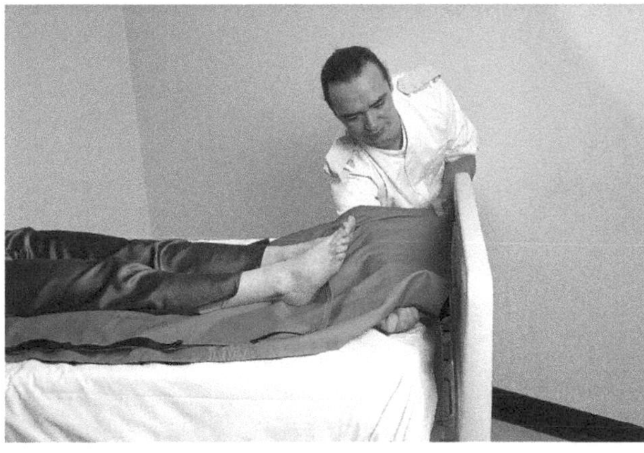

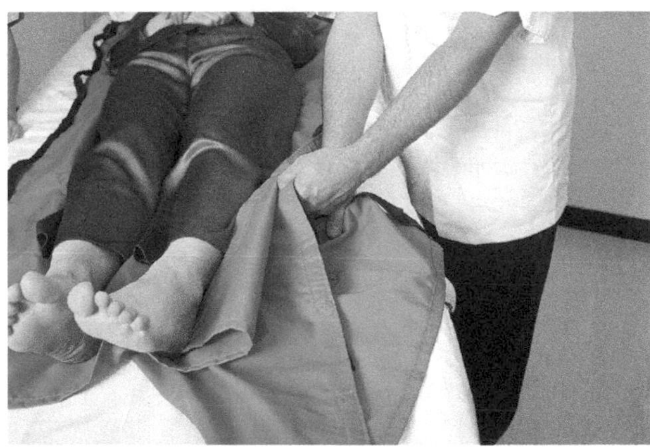

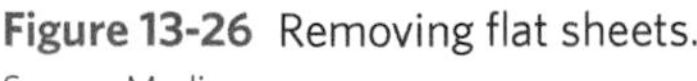

Figure 13-26 Removing flat sheets.
Source: Mediscan.

PROCEDURE 13-2 Moving a Person from a Lying Position to Standing

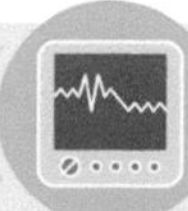

Purpose

- To promote a sense of well-being
- To check and/or relieve pressure areas and maintain skin integrity
- To aid the recovery of the patient
- To stimulate circulation

Assessment

Assess

- Risk assess the procedure using TILE.
- The patient's ability to stand by assessing mobility, strength and ability to understand (see *Practice Guidelines* on page 354).
- Fatigue.
- Presence of pain and need for adjunctive measures (e.g. an analgesic) before standing the patient.

Planning

- Plan the procedure with any assistants including the patient (*promotes concordance*).
- Encourage the patient to do as much as possible for themselves (*increasing mobility aids recovery and rehabilitation*).
- Gather any equipment that may be needed.
- Ensure patient is properly dressed (*ensures the patient's dignity is maintained*).
- Ensure the patient is wearing appropriate footwear or is barefooted (*ill fitting shoes, slippers or feet in stockings can lead to falls*).

Equipment

- Tubular slide sheets (see Figure 13-22)
- Flexi disc (see Figure 13-23)
- Handling belt (see Figure 13-24)

Implementation

Performance

1 Follow local policy to ensure that you explain to the patient what you are going to do, why it is necessary and how they can cooperate. Obtain consent and maintain patient privacy and dignity and ensure that the appropriate local infection control procedures are observed.

2 Prepare the patient and the environment. *To ensure the safety of the patient/nurse.*

3 If the patient is to sit in a chair ensure this is correctly positioned.

4 The patient needs to roll themselves onto their side or be assisted on to their side by the nurse and their assistants (see *Procedure 13-5*). *To position the patient ready to manoeuvre.*

5 The patient should then be encouraged to push the uppermost part of the arm onto the bed so they are able to lift their head and trunk (see Figure 13-27).

6 The opposite arm can then be used to take their weight and raise the trunk.

7 If the patient then swings their legs over the edge of the bed the pelvis will become vertical and help the patient into a sitting position. *To gain momentum.*

8 If the patient is unable to swing their legs over the edge of the bed then you may consider using tubular slide sheets, which should be placed underneath the patient's legs. If you do use slide sheets then you must adhere to the safety guidelines for their use (see *Practice Guidelines* on page 355).

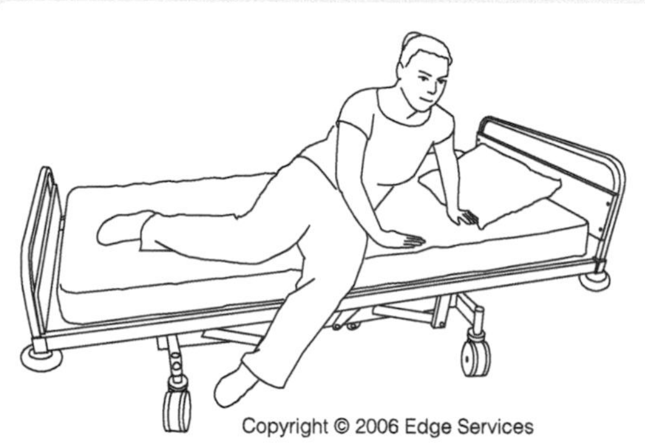

Figure 13-27 Encourage the patient to push up from the bed using their arms.

Source: Manual handling illustrations © EDGE Services (2006) reproduced by kind permission of EDGE Services - The Manual Handling Training Co. Ltd (01904 677853) sourced from People Handling and Risk Assessment Key Trainer's Certificate course materials.

The views expressed in this text book, generally and with specific reference to manual handling, do not necessarily reflect the views, approach, company policies or course content of training programmes of EDGE Services - The Manual Handling Training Co. Ltd.

9 Once the patient is on the edge of the bed they should be encouraged to stabilise themselves by positioning their arms on either side of their hips (see Figure 13-28).
10 To stand, the patient's feet need to be positioned slightly apart or in a walk stance position and positioned posterior to the knees.
11 When ready to stand, the patient should gain momentum by leaning back, then forward in a rocking motion while pushing down on the bed. *To gain momentum and promote concordance.*
12 The nurse can say 'Ready, steady, stand' to help the coordination of the movement.
13 For reassurance, the nurse can place their hands on the patient's shoulder or can use a handling belt, ensuring that they do not lift the patient or bend or stoop during the procedure.
14 Once standing the patient can then turn if needed to the chair or if they are unable to do this the nurse can use the flexi disc on the floor to turn the patient towards the bed or chair.

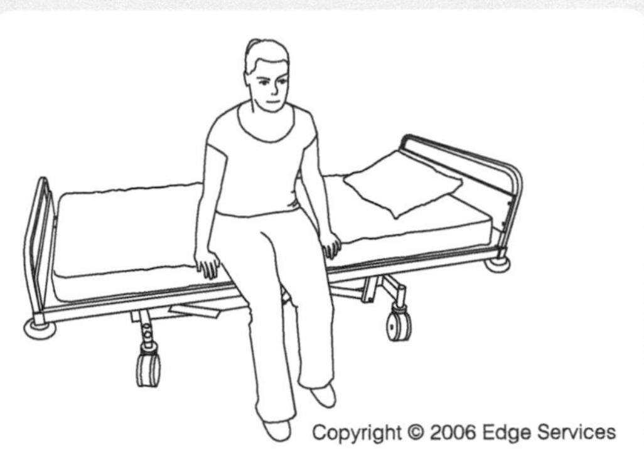

Figure 13-28 Encourage the patient to place their hands on the bed to stabilise themselves.

Source: Manual handling illustrations © EDGE Services (2006) reproduced by kind permission of EDGE Services - The Manual Handling Training Co. Ltd (01904 677853) sourced from People Handling and Risk Assessment Key Trainer's Certificate course materials.

The views expressed in this text book, generally and with specific reference to manual handling, do not necessarily reflect the views, approach, company policies or course conte nt of training programmes of EDGE Services - The Manual Handling Training Co. Ltd.

Evaluation

- Note the patient's tolerance of the procedure (e.g. respiratory rate and effort, pulse rate, behaviour, cooperation).
- Document procedure and findings in the nursing notes.

PROCEDURE 13-3 Moving a Person from the Floor to Sitting or Standing

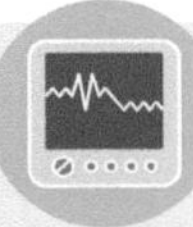

Purpose

- To raise the fallen patient
- To aid the recovery of the patient

Assessment

Assess

- Risk assess the procedure using TILE.
- The patient's ability to stand by assessing mobility, strength and ability to understand (see the *Practice Guidelines* on page 354).
- Fatigue.
- Presence of pain and need for adjunctive measures (e.g. an analgesic) before standing the patient.
- Any medical injuries as a result of the fall.

Planning

- Plan the procedure with any assistants including the patient (*promotes concordance*).
- Encourage the patient to do as much as possible for themselves (*increasing mobility aids recovery and rehabilitation*).
- Gather any equipment that may be needed.
- Ensure patient is properly dressed (*ensures the patient's dignity is maintained*).
- Ensure the patient is wearing appropriate footwear or is barefooted (*ill-fitting shoes, slippers or feet in stockings can lead to falls*).

Equipment

- Two chairs

Implementation

Performance

1 Follow local policy to ensure that you explain to the patient what you are going to do, why it is necessary and how they can cooperate. Obtain consent and maintain patient privacy and dignity and ensure that the appropriate local infection control procedures are observed.

2 Prepare the patient and the environment. *To ensure safety of patient/nurse.*

3 If the patient is being returned to bed ensure that the bed is prepared and at the correct height for the patient with the head of the bed tilted up.

4 Ask the patient to roll onto their side or assist them onto their side.

5 Once on their side ask them to place both their hands on the floor and push their head and trunk off the floor (see Figure 13-29).

6 The patient then can position themselves on 'all fours'. If needed they can rest in this position (see Figure 13-30).

7 Place a chair in front of the patient and ask the patient to pull themselves up onto it (see Figure 13-31).

8 Once standing another chair can be positioned behind them in order for them to sit down (see Figure 13-32).

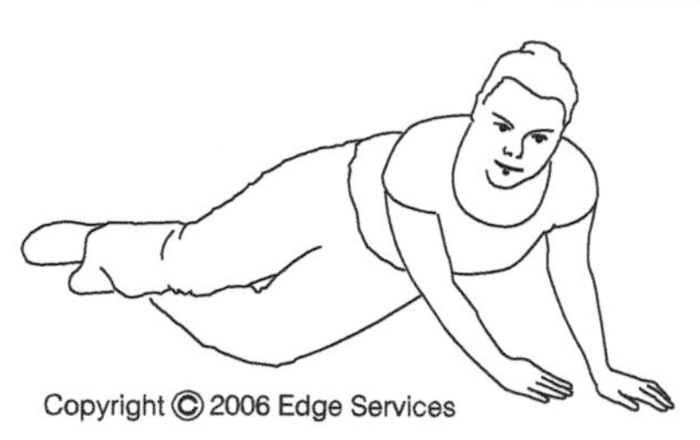

Figure 13-29 Encourage the patient to push up from the floor using their arms.

Source: Manual handling illustrations © EDGE Services (2006) reproduced by kind permission of EDGE Services - The Manual Handling Training Co. Ltd (01904 677853) sourced from People Handling and Risk Assessment Key Trainer's Certificate course materials.

The views expressed in this text book, generally and with specific reference to manual handling, do not necessarily reflect the views, approach, company policies or course content of training programmes of EDGE Services - The Manual Handling Training Co. Ltd.

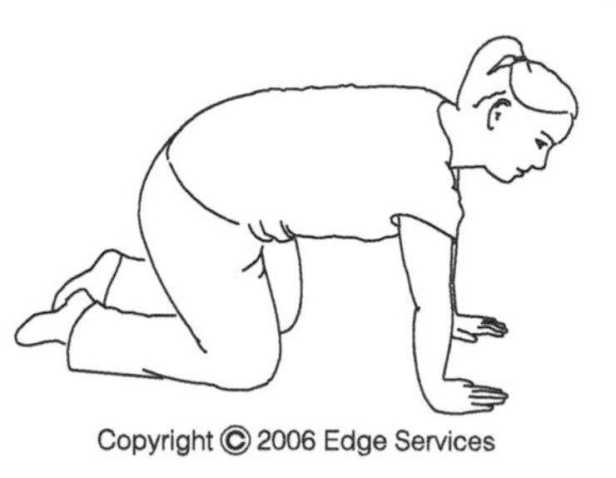

Figure 13-30 The patient can rest on all fours.

Source: Manual handling illustrations © EDGE Services (2006) reproduced by kind permission of EDGE Services - The Manual Handling Training Co. Ltd (01904 677853) sourced from People Handling and Risk Assessment Key Trainer's Certificate course materials.

The views expressed in this text book, generally and with specific reference to manual handling, do not necessarily reflect the views, approach, company policies or course content of training programmes of EDGE Services - The Manual Handling Training Co. Ltd.

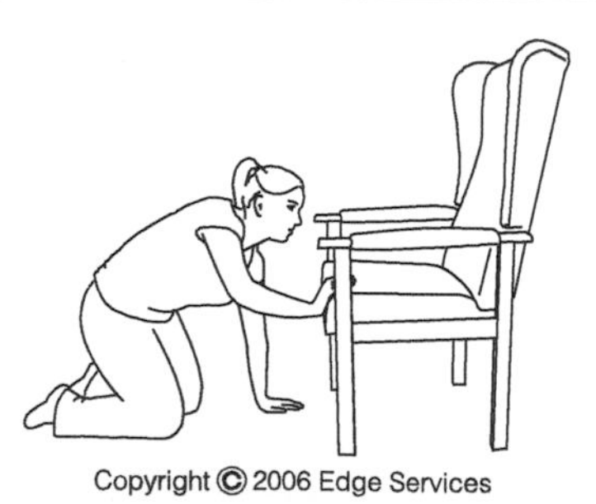

Figure 13-31 Place a chair in front of the patient so they can pull themselves up.

Source: Manual handling illustrations © EDGE Services (2006) reproduced by kind permission of EDGE Services - The Manual Handling Training Co. Ltd (01904 677853) sourced from People Handling and Risk Assessment Key Trainer's Certificate course materials.

The views expressed in this text book, generally and with specific reference to manual handling, do not necessarily reflect the views, approach, company policies or course content of training programmes of EDGE Services - The Manual Handling Training Co. Ltd.

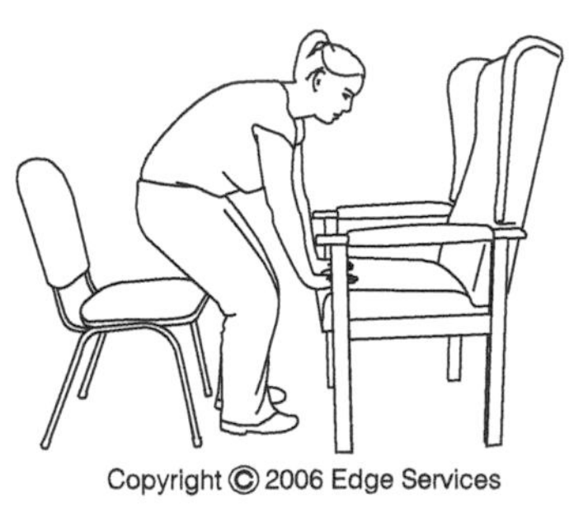

Figure 13-32 Place another chair behind so they can sit down.

Source: Manual handling illustrations © EDGE Services (2006) reproduced by kind permission of EDGE Services - The Manual Handling Training Co. Ltd (01904 677853) sourced from People Handling and Risk Assessment Key Trainer's Certificate course materials.

The views expressed in this text book, generally and with specific reference to manual handling, do not necessarily reflect the views, approach, company policies or course content of training programmes of EDGE Services - The Manual Handling Training Co. Ltd.

Evaluation

- Note the patient's tolerance of the procedure (e.g. respiratory rate and effort, pulse rate, behaviour, cooperation).
- Note any injuries.
- Document procedure and findings in the nursing notes.

PROCEDURE 13-4 Assisting a Patient to Walk

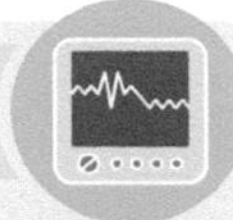

Purpose

- To promote a sense of well-being
- To aid the recovery of the patient
- To stimulate circulation

Assessment

Assess

- Risk assess the procedure using TILE.
- The patient's ability to walk by assessing mobility, strength and ability to understand (see the *Practice Guidelines* on page 354).
- Fatigue.
- Presence of pain and need for adjunctive measures (e.g. an analgesic) before walking the patient.

Planning

- Plan the procedure with any assistants including the patient (*promotes concordance*).
- Ensure patient is properly dressed (*ensures the patient's dignity is maintained*).
- Ensure the patient is wearing appropriate footwear or is barefooted (*ill-fitting shoes, slippers or feet in stockings can lead to falls*).

Equipment

- No equipment needed

Implementation

Performance

1. Follow local policy to ensure that you explain to the patient what you are going to do, why it is necessary and how they can cooperate. Obtain consent and maintain patient privacy and dignity and ensure that the appropriate local infection control procedures are observed.
2. Prepare the patient and the environment.
3. Stand to the side of the patient, half a step behind them.
4. Ask the patient to place their hand in your furthest hand using a palm-to-palm grip (see Figure 13-33). *To allow breakaway if needed.*
5. The nurse's closest hand can be placed on the patient's back. *To reassure the patient.*
6. The nurse can then walk with the patient at the patient's pace.

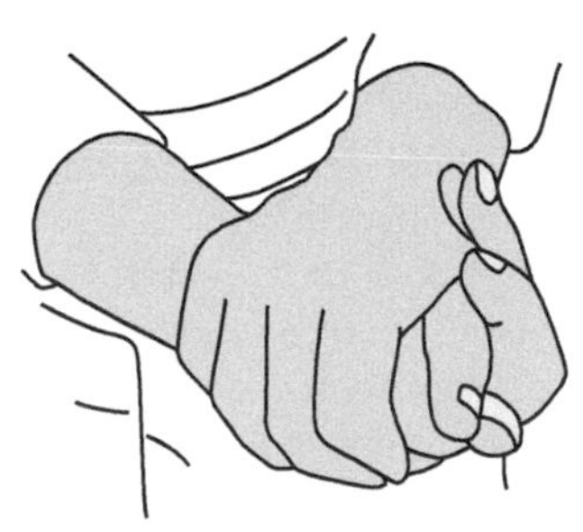

Figure 13-33 Palm-to-palm grip avoiding thumb hold.

7. If needed another nurse or nursing assistant can push a wheelchair behind the patient in case they need to rest. *To reassure the patient and to offer rests if required.*

Evaluation

- Note the patient's tolerance of the procedure (e.g. respiratory rate and effort, pulse rate, behaviour, cooperation).
- Document procedure and findings in the nursing notes.

PROCEDURE 13-5 Turning a Patient in Bed and Positioning in a 30° Tilt

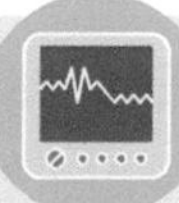

Purpose

- To promote a sense of well-being
- To check and/or relieve pressure areas and maintain skin integrity
- To reposition the patient
- To aid the recovery of the patient
- To stimulate circulation

Assessment

Assess

- Risk assess the procedure using TILE.
- The patient's haemodynamic stability.
- Fatigue.
- Presence of pain and need for adjunctive measures (e.g. an analgesic) before turning the patient.

Planning

- Plan the procedure with any assistants including the patient (*promotes concordance*).
- Encourage the patient to do as much as possible for themselves (*increasing mobility aids recovery and rehabilitation*).
- Gather any equipment that may be needed.
- Ensure dignity is maintained by drawing curtains, and closing windows and doors.

Equipment

- Two or three pillows

Implementation

Performance

1 Follow local policy to ensure that you explain to the patient what you are going to do, why it is necessary and how they can cooperate. Obtain consent and maintain patient privacy and dignity and ensure that the appropriate local infection control procedures are observed.
2 Prepare the patient and the environment. *To ensure the safety of the patient/nurse.*
3 Usually one or two nurses or nursing assistants are required to turn a patient in bed.
4 The nurses should position themselves at the heaviest parts of the patient, which is usually the trunk and upper legs. *To stabilise the patient.*
5 The bed should be positioned so that all involved in moving the patient are comfortable. *To promote safe working practices.*
6 Position the patient to aid moving (see Figure 13-34).
7 The nurse closest to the patient's head should place one hand on the patient's shoulder and one on their hip. While the other nurse should place one hand on the patient's hip and the other should be used to guide the legs over. No pressure should be applied to the knee joint as this can cause injury to the patient.

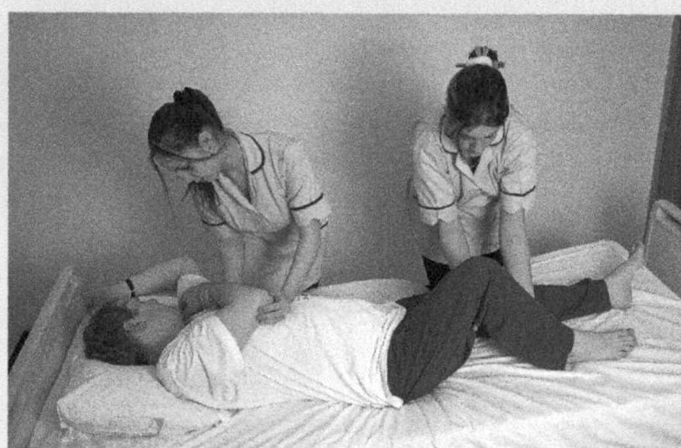

Figure 13-34 Position the patient in bed ready to roll. Head turned to the direction of the roll, opposite arm across chest and opposite leg bent.
Source: Mediscan.

8 When ready to move the patient the team leader should say 'Ready, steady, roll'. The nurses will then roll the patient. *To promote patient concordance.*
9 Once over on their side, pillows can be placed behind the patient and between the patient's knees. *To stabilise the patient.*
10 The patient should then be rested back onto the pillows.
11 The same process can be used for changing sheets and checking pressure areas.

Evaluation

- Note the patient's tolerance of the procedure (e.g. respiratory rate and effort, pulse rate, behaviour, cooperation).
- Document procedure and findings in the nursing notes.

PROCEDURE 13-6 Moving a Supine Patient Up and Down the Bed

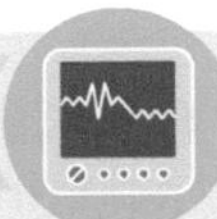

Purpose

- To promote a sense of well-being
- To reposition the patient
- To aid the recovery of the patient
- To stimulate circulation and respiratory function

Assessment

Assess

- Risk assess the procedure using TILE.
- The patient's haemodynamic stability.
- Fatigue.
- Presence of pain and need for adjunctive measures (e.g. an analgesic) before moving the patient.

Planning

- Plan the procedure with any assistants including the patient (*promotes concordance*).
- Encourage the patient to do as much as possible for themselves (*increasing mobility aids recovery and rehabilitation*).
- Gather any equipment that may be needed.
- Ensure dignity is maintained by drawing curtains and closing windows and doors.

Equipment

- Flat slide sheets

Implementation

Performance

1. Follow local policy to ensure that you explain to the patient what you are going to do, why it is necessary and how they can cooperate. Obtain consent and maintain patient privacy and dignity and ensure that the appropriate local infection control procedures are observed.
2. Prepare the patient and the environment. *To ensure safety of patient/nurse.*
3. Ask the patient to turn onto their side or assist the patient to roll (see Procedure 13-5). *To move the patient's centre of gravity and aid manoeuvring of the patient.*
4. Position the flat sheets under the patient, ensuring they are positioned correctly (see the *Practice Guidelines* on page 355).
5. Roll the patient back onto their back and ensure that the slide sheets are pulled through.
6. Tilt the bed in the direction you wish the patient to move.
7. Push or pull the patient up or down the bed.
8. Reposition the bed and remove the flat slide sheets (see the *Practice Guidelines* on page 355).

Evaluation

- Note the patient's tolerance of the procedure (e.g. respiratory rate and effort, pulse rate, behaviour, cooperation).
- Document procedure and findings in the nursing notes.

PROCEDURE 13-7 Transferring a Patient from Bed to Bed/Trolley with the Patient in a Lying Position

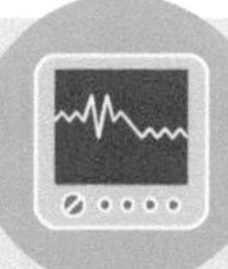

Purpose

- To move the patient to a more suitable bed or mattress
- To transfer the patient to or from theatre

Assessment

Assess

- Risk assess the procedure using TILE.
- The patient's haemodynamic stability.
- Fatigue.
- Presence of pain and need for adjunctive measures (e.g. an analgesic) before standing the patient.

Planning

- Plan the procedure with any assistants including the patient (*promotes concordance*).
- Encourage the patient to do as much as possible for themselves (*increasing mobility aids recovery and rehabilitation*).
- Gather any equipment that may be needed.
- Ensure dignity is maintained by drawing curtains and closing windows and doors.

Equipment

Lateral transfer aid (see Figure 13-35)

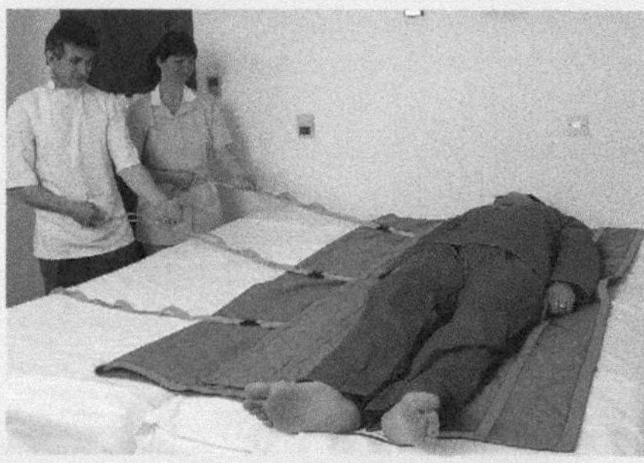

Figure 13-35 Lateral transfer aid. Phil-e-slide patient handling system.
Source: Ergo Ike Ltd. **www.phil-e-slide-uk.com**

Implementation

Performance

1 Follow local policy to ensure that you explain to the patient what you are going to do, why it is necessary and how they can cooperate. Obtain consent and maintain patient privacy and dignity and ensure that the appropriate local infection control procedures are observed.
2 Prepare the patient and the environment. *To ensure the safety of the patient/nurse.*
3 A minimum of two healthcare staff are required for this move depending on the size of the patient and haemodynamic stability.
4 The nurse should ask the patient to roll away from the other bed/trolley or should be assisted to roll (see *Procedure 13-5*). *To aid insertion of the lateral transfer aid.*
5 Once the patient is over on their side the nurse can position the lateral transfer aid under the patient.
6 The patient can then be rolled back on to the bed and the other bed or trolley can then be positioned next to and slightly lower than the bed the patient is on. Ensure the brakes are on each of the beds. *To work with gravity.*
7 Ask the patient to place their hands across their chest or down by their sides. *To ensure the safety of the patient.*
8 Once ready to transfer the team leader can say 'Ready, steady, slide', the nurses will then hand over hand pull the patient across from one bed to the other (see Figure 13-35). *To promote concordance.*
9 Once the patient is on the other bed or trolley the lateral transfer aid can be removed.
10 The patient can then be made comfortable on the bed or trolley.

Evaluation

- Note the patient's tolerance of the procedure (e.g. respiratory rate and effort, pulse rate, behaviour, cooperation).
- Document procedure and findings in the nursing notes.

PROCEDURE 13-8 Transferring a Patient from Bed to Chair in a Seated Position

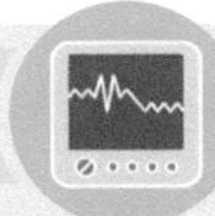

Purpose

- To promote a sense of well-being
- To reposition the patient
- To aid the recovery of the patient
- To stimulate circulation

Assessment

Assess

- Risk assess the procedure using TILE
- The patient's ability by assessing mobility, strength and ability to understand (see the *Practice Guidelines* on page 354)
- Fatigue
- Presence of pain and need for adjunctive measures (e.g. an analgesic) before moving the patient

Planning

- Plan the procedure with any assistants including the patient (*promotes concordance*)
- Encourage the patient to do as much as possible for themselves (*increasing mobility aids recovery and rehabilitation*)
- Gather any equipment that may be needed
- Ensure dignity is maintained by drawing curtains, and closing windows and doors

Equipment

- Curved or straight seated transfer aid (see Figure 13-36)
- Bed ladder if needed (see Figure 13-37)

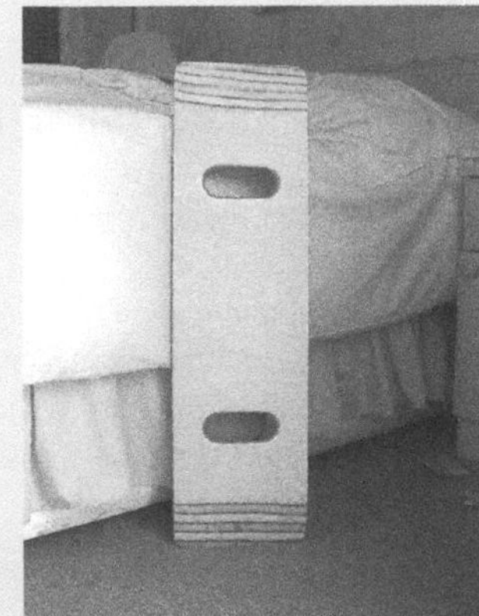

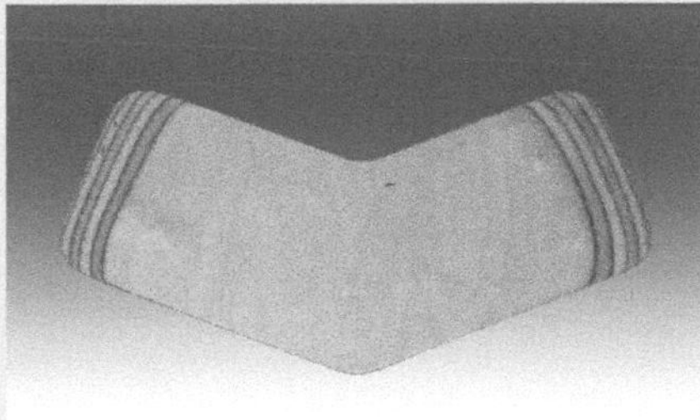

Figure 13-36 Straight and curved seated lateral transfer aids.
Source: MEDesign Ltd.

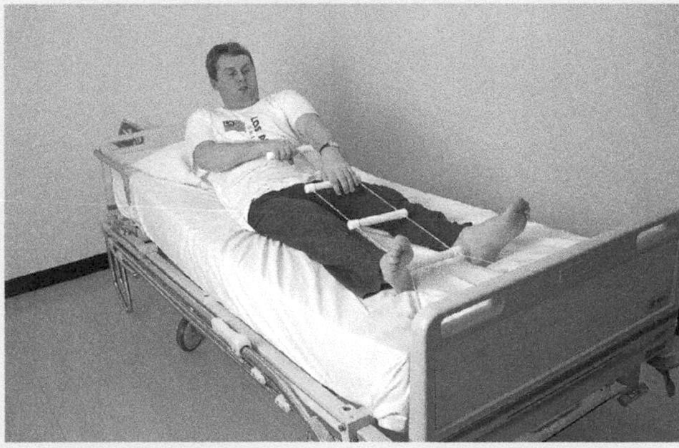

Figure 13-37 Bed ladder.
Source: Mediscan.

Implementation

Performance

1. Follow local policy to ensure that you explain to the patient what you are going to do, why it is necessary and how they can cooperate. Obtain consent and maintain patient privacy and dignity and ensure that the appropriate local infection control procedures are observed.
2. Prepare the patient and the environment. *To ensure the safety of the patient/nurse.*
3. Ask the patient to get into a seated position or assist them into a seated position using the bed or a bed ladder.
4. If the chair has arms that can be lowered a straight seated transfer board is needed with the chair positioned directly next to the bed (see Figure 13-38). *To aid transfer of the patient.*
5. Place the transfer aid under the patient's buttock ensuring that the board bridges the gap between the bed and chair.
6. Instruct the patient *not* to put their hands under the end of the board as this can cause injury. Instead tell the patient to use the handles provided or place their hand flat on the transfer aid. *To ensure the safety of the patient.*
7. The patient may then begin to slide themselves across between the bed and chair. *To empower the patient.*

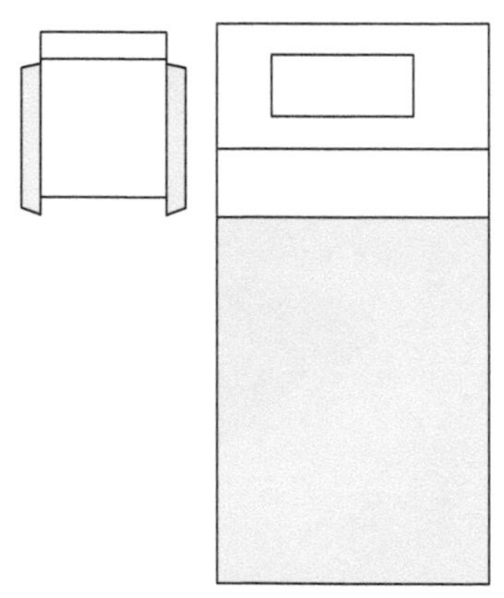

Figure 13-38 Place the chair next to the bed.

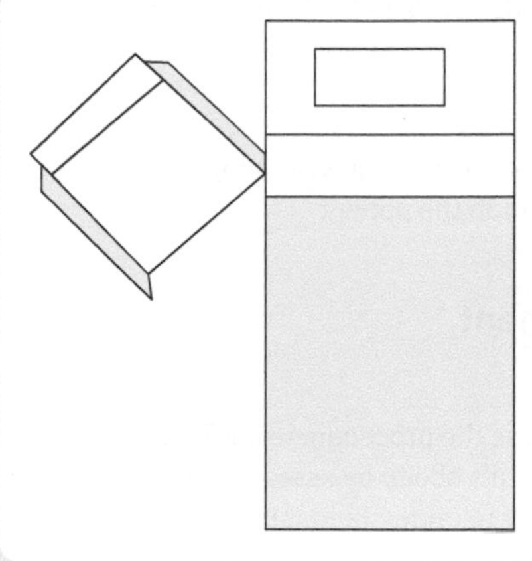

Figure 13-39 If the chair does not have arms that lower then place the chair at a 45° angle to the bed.

8. If using a normal arm chair, it will need to be positioned at an angle for transferring using a curved seated transfer aid (see Figure 13-39).
9. The patient may need to bring themselves to the edge of the bed in order to slide across when using the curved transfer aid.
10. Once across onto the chair ensure the patient is comfortable.
11. If the patient has a tendency to slide forward or slump in the chair they may need to use a one-way slide sheet (see Figure 13-40) which allows them to slide back in the chair but does not allow them to slide forward in the chair.

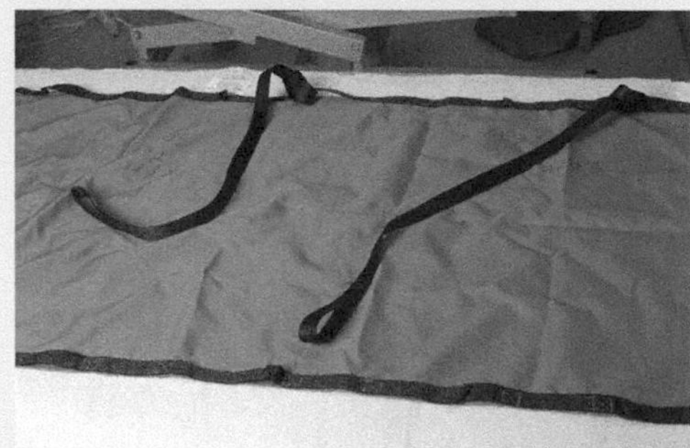

Figure 13-40 One-way slide sheet.
Source: Mediscan.

Evaluation

- Note the patient's tolerance of the procedure (e.g. respiratory rate and effort, pulse rate, behaviour, cooperation).
- Document procedure and findings in the nursing notes.

PROCEDURE 13-9 Hoisting a Patient from Bed to Chair

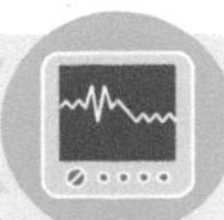

Purpose

- To promote a sense of well-being
- To reposition the patient
- To aid the recovery of the patient
- To stimulate circulation

Assessment

Assess

- Risk assess the procedure using TILE
- The patient's ability by assessing mobility, strength and ability to understand (see the *Practice Guidelines* on page 354)
- Fatigue
- Presence of pain and need for adjunctive measures (e.g. an analgesic) before hoisting the patient

Planning

- Plan the procedure with any assistants including the patient (*promotes concordance*).
- Encourage the patient to do as much as possible for themselves (*increasing mobility aids recovery and rehabilitation*).
- Gather any equipment that may be needed.
- Ensure dignity is maintained by drawing curtains and closing windows and doors.

Equipment

- Suitable hoist (see Figure 13-41)
- Suitable sling for the hoist and patient (see Figure 13-42)

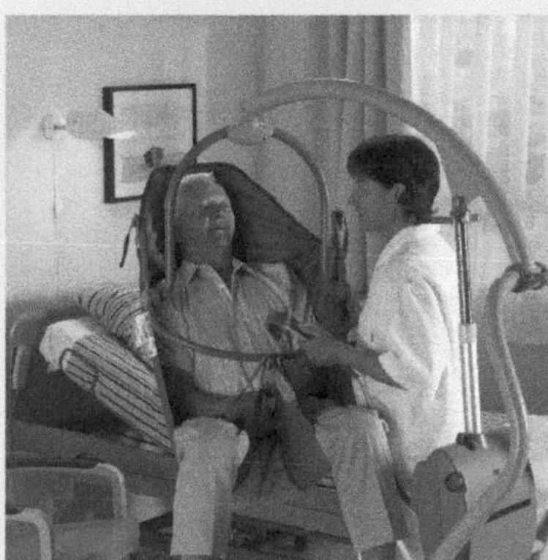

Figure 13-41 Hoist that lifts the whole body.
Source: ARJO MED AB Ltd.

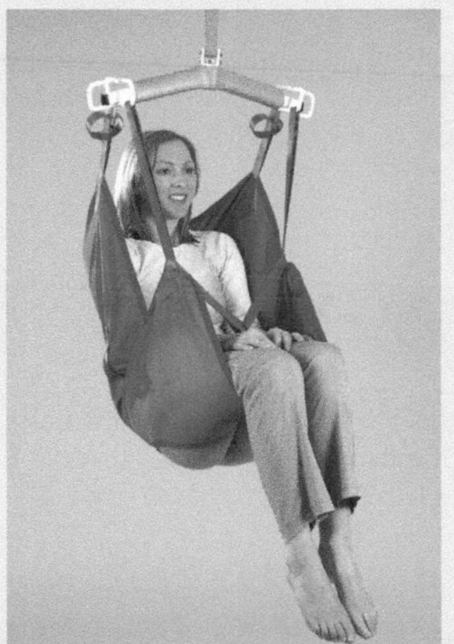

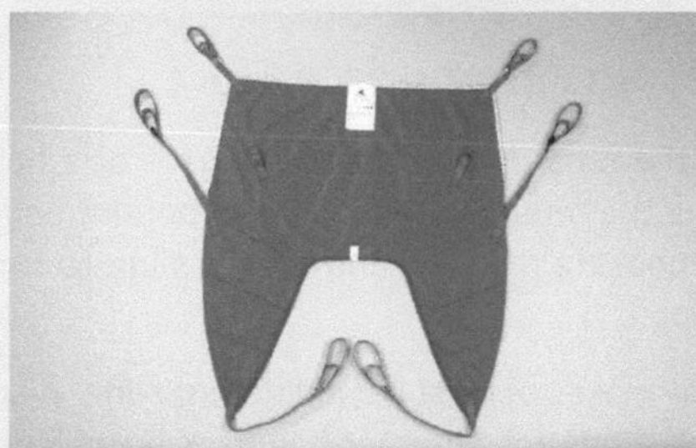

Figure 13-42 Universal sling.
Source: Hoist and Shower Chair Company Ltd.

Implementation

Performance

1 Follow local policy to ensure that you explain to the patient what you are going to do, why it is necessary and how they can cooperate. Obtain consent and maintain patient privacy and dignity and ensure that the appropriate local infection control procedures are observed.

2 Prepare the patient and the environment. *To ensure the safety of the patient/nurse.*
3 Ask the patient to roll onto their side or assist them to roll (see *Procedure 13-5*).
4 Place the appropriate sling (see the *Practice Guidelines* below) under the patient and ask the patient to roll back onto their back.
5 Position the hoist over the patient (make sure the brakes are off on the hoist), lower and attach the sling to the hoist (see the *Practice Guidelines* on page 367).
6 If the patient is competent and the hoist has a remote control, then the patient can control the lift. *To empower the patient and promote recovery and rehabilitation.*
7 Raise the patient slightly off the bed and check that the hoist is comfortable for the patient.
8 The patient can then be raised further but only enough so that they are able to clear the bed.
9 The hoist can then be moved so that the patient is over the chair.
10 Again if competent the patient can lower themselves into the chair.
11 Ensure the patient is right in the back of the chair.
12 Sometimes tilting the chair can help to position the patient correctly in the chair.
13 Once in the chair the sling can be removed.
14 Ensure that the patient is comfortable before leaving the patient.

Evaluation

- Note the patient's tolerance of the procedure (e.g. respiratory rate and effort, pulse rate, behaviour, cooperation).
- Document procedure and findings in the nursing notes.

CLINICAL ALERT

With hoists that lift the whole person, the hoist has to find its centre of gravity. If the brakes are put on the hoist when lifting, it is liable to fall over as it cannot find its centre of gravity.

PRACTICE GUIDELINES

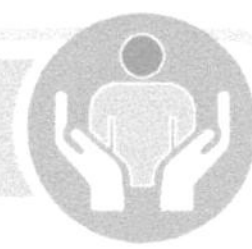

Choosing an Appropriate Sling

Slings are the most important component of a hoist system as a sling is the interface between the patient and the hoist. So when choosing the type and size of sling to use consider the following:

- Different makes of hoist have different sling. Also there are different slings for different handling procedures such as for bathing and toileting.
- Check the label of the sling to ensure that it is appropriate sling for the type of hoist you are using.
- Check the safe working load of the sling (maximum weight that the sling will lift) usually found on the label.
- Check that the safe working load of the sling is less than the safe working load of the hoist, the maximum weight that can be lifted would be the weight denoted on the sling.
- The sling should not be soiled and if so slings usually can be washed.
- All attachments of the sling should be checked to ensure that they are in good working order. If there are signs of fraying or damage to the sling do not use it.

Sizing Slings

- Slings are usually colour coded for sizing. However, it is important to note that different companies use different colours for different sizes: for example, yellow may denote small size with one company but with another may denote medium size.
- The sling should fit comfortably around the patient: too big and the patient may feel that they are going to fall out; too small and the patient may find it uncomfortable.
- Specific sizing will depend on the type of sling used but generally you need to measure the sling against the patient's back to ensure that there is enough length from shoulder to buttocks and from arm to arm across the back.

You must receive training on the use of hoists and their slings.

PRACTICE GUIDELINES

Safe Use of a Hoist

Hoist Checks

- Check that the hoist is the type needed for the handling procedure: for example, for standing a patient a stand aid hoist is needed.
- Check the safe working load of the hoist.
- Check when it was serviced last (usually a sticker on the frame of the hoist).
- Check that it looks in good working order.
- If it is dirty it can be cleaned with soap and water or alcohol wipes.
- Check that the battery is charged, if not change or charge it.
- Check that the mechanism works.
- Check that all attachments are in working order and attached properly.
- Check the brakes are in good working order.
- Check the wheels of the hoist run smoothly.

Using the Hoist

- When using a hoist act confidently, as this will reduce the patient's fear.
- When lowering the jig or cross bar of the hoist to attach the sling ensure that it does not hit the patient.
- Raise the hoist smoothly; do not stop and start the lift as this can frighten the patient.
- The maximum distance that a hoist should be pushed is 10 metres, less if it is over carpeted flooring.

Training must be received before using a hoist.

PROCEDURE 13-10 Using a Stand Aid Hoist to Move a Patient

Purpose

- To promote a sense of well-being
- To reposition the patient
- To aid the recovery of the patient
- To stimulate circulation

Assessment

Assess

- Risk assess the procedure using TILE
- The patient's ability to stand by assessing mobility, strength and ability to understand (see *Practice Guidelines* on page 354)
- Fatigue
- Presence of pain and need for adjunctive measures (e.g. an analgesic) before standing the patient

Planning

- Plan the procedure including the patient (*promotes concordance*)
- Encourage the patient to do as much as possible for themselves (*increasing mobility aids recovery and rehabilitation*)
- Gather any equipment that may be needed
- Ensure dignity is maintained by drawing curtains and closing windows and doors

Equipment

- Suitable stand aid hoist (see Figure 13-43)
- Suitable sling for the hoist and patient

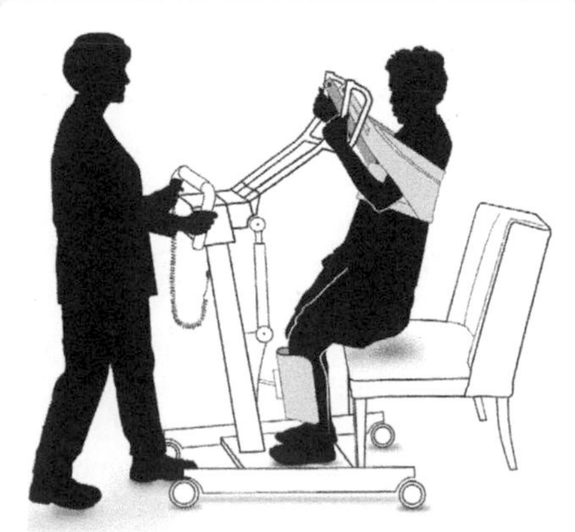

Figure 13-43 Stand aid hoist.

Implementation

Performance

1 Follow local policy to ensure that you explain to the patient what you are going to do, why it is necessary and how they can cooperate. Obtain consent and maintain patient privacy and dignity and ensure that the appropriate local infection control procedures are observed.

2 Prepare the patient and the environment. *To ensure the safety of the patient/nurse.*

3 Place the appropriate sling (see *Practice Guidelines* on page 366) under the patient.

4 Position the hoist over the patient (make sure the brakes are on), lower and attach the sling to the hoist (see the *Practice Guidelines* on page 367).

5 Ask the patient to place their feet on the platform of the hoist and push their knees into the knee braces of the hoist.

6 If the patient is competent and the hoist has a remote control, then the patient can control the lift. *To empower the patient and promote recovery and rehabilitation.*

7 Raise the patient slightly off the chair and check that the sling is comfortable for the patient.

8 The patient can then be raised further so they are standing in the hoist.

9 The hoist's brakes can then be removed and the patient moved to the desired location.

10 Once at the desired location, the patient can be lowered and the sling and hoist removed.

11 Ensure that the patient is comfortable before leaving the patient.

Evaluation

- Note the patient's tolerance of the procedure (e.g. respiratory rate and effort, pulse rate, behaviour, cooperation).
- Document procedure and findings in the nursing notes.

ACTIVITY 13-2

Reflect on how you would react if a qualified nurse asked you to assist in a moving and handling procedure that contravened safe working practice. Why would you react in this way? What knowledge would underpin this reaction?

CLINICAL ALERT

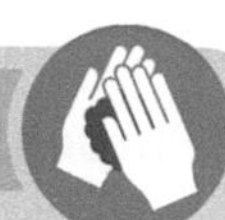

For stand aid hoists the brakes must be left on when lifting the patient because the centre of gravity for the hoist will be the person's legs.

CRITICAL REFLECTION

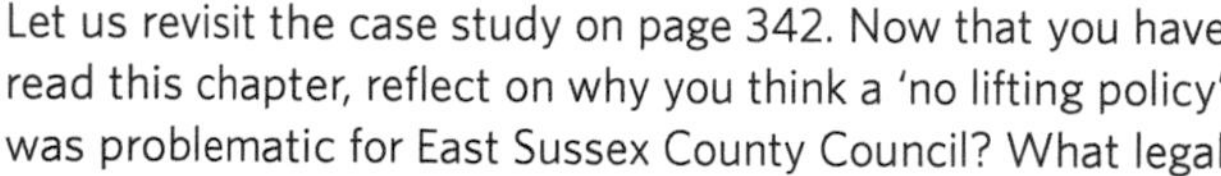

Let us revisit the case study on page 342. Now that you have read this chapter, reflect on why you think a 'no lifting policy' was problematic for East Sussex County Council? What legal and professional responsibilities would prevent a 'no lifting policy' being implemented?

CHAPTER HIGHLIGHTS

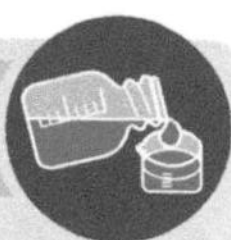

- Back injuries cost the NHS £400 million each year with one in four nurses having to take time off work as a result of a back injury.
- The law within the UK with regard to the moving and handling of patients has two clear goals: first to prevent injury and second to compensate the handler when an injury occurs.

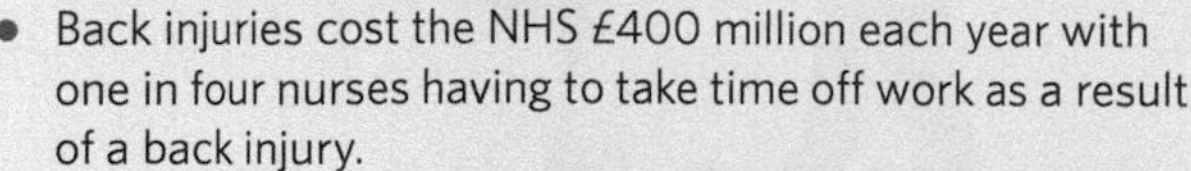

- The Health and Safety at Work Act 1974 clearly states that an employer must ensure the health, safety and welfare at work of its employees, as far as it is reasonably practicable.
- However, it is important to note that the employee also has a duty to take reasonable care of their own health and safety.

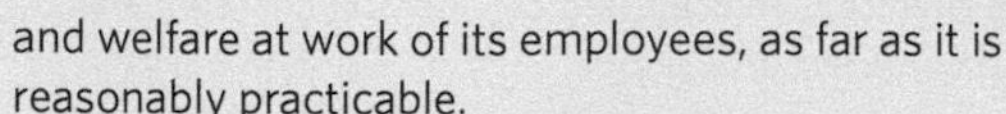

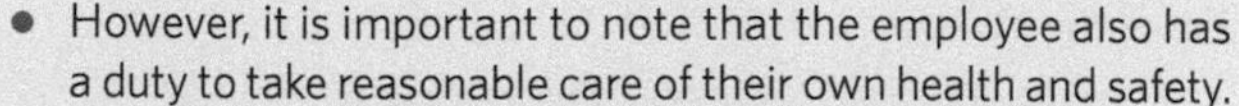

- The Manual Handling Operations Regulations 1992 (MHOR 92), as amended by the Health and Safety Miscellaneous Amendments Regulations 2002, sets very specific duties for the employer in relation to manual handling in the workplace.

- The Provision and Use of Work Equipment Regulations 1992 (PUWER) aims to prevent or control the risk to an individual's health and safety from work equipment such as photocopiers, hoists, etc. and sets out a number of requirements that the employer must adhere to.
- The Lifting Operations and Lifting Equipment Regulations 1998 (LOLER), on the other hand, regulates lifting equipment used in the workplace and like PUWER it sets out requirements that the employer must adhere to.
- Any breach by the employer under any or all of these regulations can result in criminal prosecution.
- Everyone, including patients and health and social care workers, is protected by the Human Rights Act 1998.
- The spine or vertebral column extends from the base of the skull to the pelvis and is made up of 33 individual bones or vertebrae.
- An understanding of basic principles of biomechanics is important as this can help prevent damage to the spine.
- A hazard is the potential to cause harm, for example, lifting a person on your own has the potential to cause you harm that is back injury.
- A risk is the likelihood and severity of that harm occurring. The acronym TILE can be quickly and easily used to informally risk assess a manual handling procedure and can also be used for more formal documented risk assessments as used in many hospital and home environments by nurses.

ACTIVITY ANSWERS

ACTIVITY 13-1 In the clinical environment you are likely to see the following:

- Training (e.g. fire training, intravenous pump training, manual handling training).
- Provision of manual handling equipment that is maintained and serviced regularly.
- Instructions on equipment (e.g. hoists).
- Signs on wet floors.
- LOLER and PUWER checks on hoists.
- Heavy equipment/consumables kept at waist height (e.g. intravenous fluid boxes).
- Fire doors.
- Safe working load labels on equipment (e.g. beds).

See how many others you can find.

ACTIVITY 13-2 Your personal reflection should have considered the following:

- Your duty to care for the patient.
- Your responsibility to abide by the NMC (2008) Code of Professional Conduct.
- The patient and your own human rights.
- The RCN guidance on Moving and Handling Patients.

REFERENCES

Cornish, J. and Jones, A. (2010) 'Factors affecting compliance with moving and handling policy: Student nurses' views and experiences', *Nurse Education in Practice*, 10: 96–100.

Department of Health (2004) *The manager's guide: Back in work campaign*, London: Crown Copyright.

Griffith, R. and Stevens, M. (2003) 'Manual handling and the lawfulness of no-lift policies', *Nursing Standard*, 18(21): 39–43.

Health and Safety Executive (1998) *Simple guide to the lifting operations and lifting equipment regulations 1998*, Caerphilly: HSE.

Health and Safety Executive (2010) *Self-reported worker-related illness and workplace injuries in 2008/09: Results from the Labour Force Survey*, Caerphilly: HSE.

NHS Employers (2009) *Back in work: Introduction and key messages*, London: NHS Employers.

NMC (2008) *The Code: Standards of conduct, performance and ethics for nurses and midwives*, London: NMC.

NMC (2010) *Standards for pre-registration nursing education*, London: NMC.

RCN (2002) *Code of practice for patient handling*, London: RCN.

RCN (2003) *Manual handling assessments in hospitals and the community: An RCN guide*, London: RCN.

Smith, J. (ed.) (2005) *The guide to the handling of people*, Middlesex: Backcare.

Welshbacks (2006) *Don't take back pain lying down*, Cardiff: NHS Wales. Available from **http://www.welshbacks.com** (Accessed on 7/12/2006).

FURTHER RESOURCES

For the full text of Acts and Regulations mentioned in this chapter see **www.legislation.hmso.gov.uk.**

CHAPTER 14
MOBILITY, REST AND SLEEP

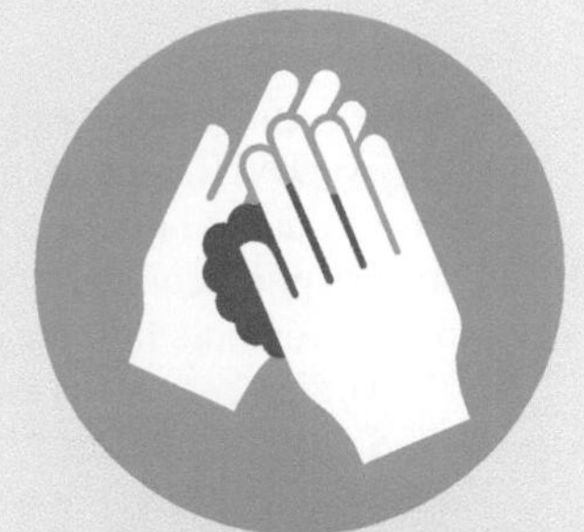

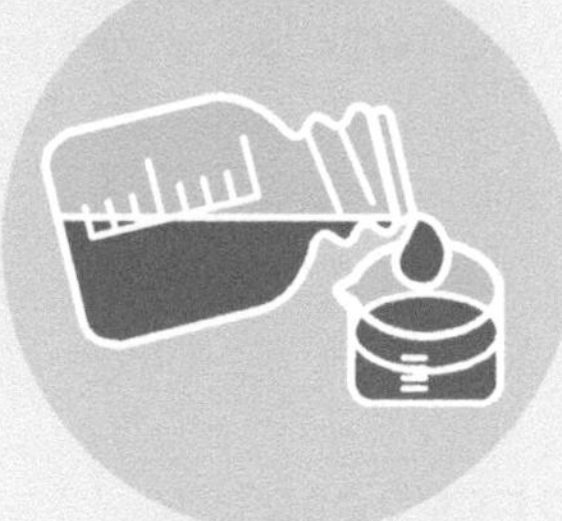

LEARNING OUTCOMES

After completing this chapter, you will be able to:

- Describe four basic elements of normal movement.
- Differentiate isotonic, isometric, isokinetic, aerobic and anaerobic exercise.
- Compare the effects of exercise and immobility on body systems.
- Identify factors influencing a person's body alignment and activity.
- Assess activity-exercise pattern, alignment, mobility capabilities and limitations, activity tolerance and potential problems related to immobility.
- Develop nursing outcomes and interventions related to activity, exercise and mobility problems.
- Explain the functions and the physiology of sleep.
- Identify the characteristics of NREM and REM sleep.
- Identify the four stages of NREM sleep.
- Describe variations in sleep patterns throughout the life span.
- Identify factors that affect normal sleep.
- Describe common sleep disorders.
- Identify the components of a sleep pattern assessment.
- Develop nursing diagnoses, outcomes and nursing interventions related to sleep problems.
- Describe interventions that promote normal sleep.

After reading this chapter you will be able to reflect on the nursing role in providing healthcare relating to mobility, rest and sleep; assess and provide accurate information and any pain management required. It relates to **Essential Skills Clusters (NMC, 2010) Sections 1, 2, 6, 8, 35, 36, 39**, as appropriate for each progression point.

Ensure that you really understand this chapter by logging on to your complimentary **MyNursingKit** at **www.pearsoned.co.uk/kozier**. Complete the self-assessment tests to check your progress and utilise further activities to practise and confirm your understanding.

CASE STUDY

Working on a Saturday late shift in the Accident and Emergency department you admit Richard who following an x-ray was diagnosed with a fractured tibia. The consultant on call has requested a long leg plaster cast for Richard with a follow up appointment in a week's time. Richard is a 25-year-old rugby player and sustained his injury whilst playing rugby. He is a physically fit young man and plays in a forward position so his upper body strength is good. The plaster technician on duty is very busy (Saturday late afternoon) with sporting injuries and has asked you to manage Richard's care after he has completed putting on the cast.

Following the initial assessment when information was gathered it is your responsibility to ensure that Richard is discharged safely and has been provided with all the relevant information to maintain his well-being.

INTRODUCTION

Mobility (in this context) is referred to as the ability to move freely, easily, rhythmically and purposefully in the environment, and is an essential part of living. People must move to protect themselves from trauma and to meet their basic needs. Mobility is vital to independence; a fully immobilised person is as vulnerable and dependent as an infant.

An *activity-exercise pattern* refers to a person's routine of exercise, activity, leisure and recreation. It includes (a) activities of daily living (ADLs) that require energy expenditure such as hygiene, cooking, shopping, eating, working and home maintenance, and (b) the type, quality and quantity of exercise, including sports (Gordon, 2007).

People often define their health and physical fitness by their activity because mental well-being and the effectiveness of body functioning depend largely on their mobility status. For example, when a person is upright, the lungs expand more easily, intestinal activity (peristalsis) is more effective and the kidneys are able to empty completely. In addition, motion is essential for proper functioning of bones and muscles.

The ability to move also influences self-esteem and body image. For most people, self-esteem depends on a sense of independence and a feeling of usefulness or being needed. People with mobility impairments may feel helpless and burdensome to others. Body image can be altered by paralysis, amputations or any motor impairment. The reaction of others to impaired mobility can also alter self-esteem and body image significantly.

NORMAL MOVEMENT

Normal movement and stability are the result of an intact musculoskeletal system, an intact nervous system and intact inner ear structures responsible for equilibrium.

Body movement requires coordinated muscle activity and neurological integration. It involves four basic elements: body alignment (posture), joint mobility, balance and coordinated movement.

Alignment and Posture

Proper body alignment and posture bring body parts into position in a manner that promotes optimal balance and maximal body function whether the patient is standing, sitting or lying down. A person maintains balance as long as the line of gravity (an imaginary vertical line drawn through the body's centre of gravity) passes through the *centre of gravity* (the point at which all of the body's mass is centred) and the *base of support* (the foundation on which the body rests). In humans, the usual line of gravity begins at the top of the head and falls between the shoulders, through the trunk, slightly anterior to the sacrum, and between the weight-bearing joints and base of support (see Figure 14-1). For a person in the upright position, the centre of gravity is located in the centre of the pelvis approximately midway between the umbilicus and the symphysis pubis. For greatest balance and stability, a standing adult must centre body weight symmetrically along the line of gravity. Greater stability and balance are provided in a sitting or lying position than in a standing position. The feet of the chair or bed form a considerably wider base of support, the centre of gravity is lower and the line of gravity is less mobile.

When the body is well aligned, strain on the joints, muscles, tendons or ligaments is minimised and internal structures and organs are supported. People are usually unaware of the functions of the skeletal muscles that maintain body posture. These muscles function almost continuously, making tiny adjustments that enable an erect or seated posture despite the endless downward pull of gravity. The extensor muscles, often referred to as the *antigravity muscles*, carry the major load.

Proper body alignment enhances lung expansion and promotes efficient circulatory, renal and gastrointestinal functions. A person's posture is one criterion for assessing general health, physical fitness and attractiveness. Posture reflects the mood, self-esteem and personality of an individual.

Joint Mobility

Joints are the functional units of the musculoskeletal system. The bones of the skeleton articulate at the joints and most of the skeletal muscles attach to the two bones at the joint.

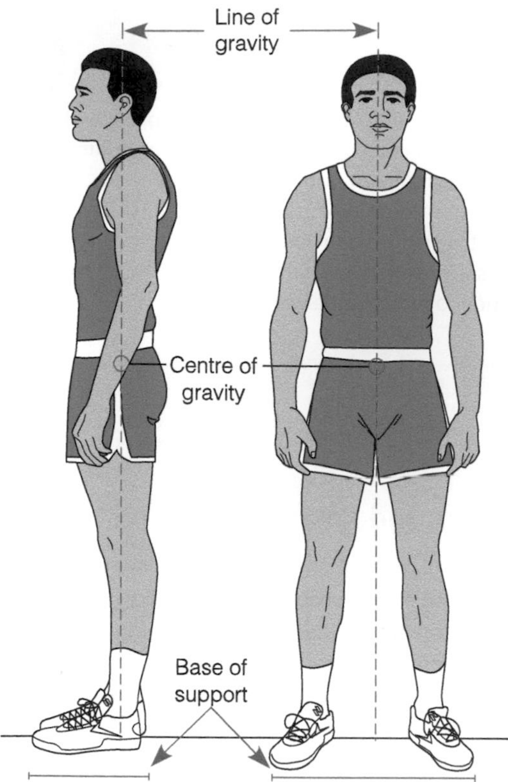

Figure 14-1 The centre of gravity and the line of gravity influence standing alignment.

Table 14-1 Types of Joint Movements

Movement	Action
Flexion	Decreasing the angle of the joint (e.g. bending the elbow)
Extension	Increasing the angle of the joint (e.g. straightening the arm at the elbow)
Hyperextension	Further extension or straightening of a joint (e.g. bending the head backward)
Abduction	Movement of the bone away from the midline of the body
Adduction	Movement of the bone towards the midline of the body
Rotation	Movement of the bone around its central axis
Circumduction	Movement of the distal part of the bone in a circle while the **proximal** end remains fixed
Eversion	Turning the sole of the foot outward by moving the ankle joint
Inversion	Turning the sole of the foot inward by moving the ankle joint
Pronation	Moving the bones of the forearm so that the palm of the hand faces downward when held in front of the body
Supination	Moving the bones of the forearm so that the palm of the hand faces upward when held in front of the body

These muscles are categorised according to the type of joint movement they produce on contraction. Muscles are therefore called flexors, extensors, internal rotators and the like. The flexor muscles are stronger than the extensor muscles. Thus, when a person is inactive, the joints are pulled into a flexed (bent) position. If this tendency is not counteracted with exercise and position changes, the muscles permanently shorten, and the joint becomes fixed in a flexed position. Types of joint movement are shown in Table 14-1.

The *range of motion (ROM)* of a joint is the maximum movement that is possible for that joint. Joint range of motion varies from individual to individual and is determined by genetic makeup, developmental patterns, the presence or absence of disease and the amount of physical activity in which the person normally engages. Table 14-2 shows the various joint movements and the usual ranges of motion.

Balance

The mechanisms involved in maintaining balance and posture are complex. Mechanisms of equilibrium (sense of balance) respond, frequently without our awareness, to various head movements. The equilibrium sense depends on informational inputs from the labyrinth (inner ear), vision (vestibulo-ocular input) and from stretch receptors of muscles and tendons (vestibulospinal input). The labyrinth consists of the cochlea, vestibule and semicircular canals. The cochlea is concerned with hearing and the vestibule and semicircular canals with equilibrium. Under normal conditions the equilibrium receptors in the semicircular canals and vestibule, collectively called the vestibular apparatus, send signals to the brain that initiate reflexes needed to make required changes in position. The receptors, hairlike cells, respond to displacement of the head in any direction. When the head moves, the fluid flow within the vestibule and semicircular canals stimulates sensory hair cells. Information from these balance receptors goes directly to reflex centres in the brain stem rather than to the cerebral cortex as with other special senses. This enables fast reflexive responses to body imbalance.

Coordinated Movement

Balanced, smooth, purposeful movement is the result of proper functioning of the cerebral cortex, cerebellum and basal ganglia. The cerebral cortex initiates voluntary motor activity, the cerebellum coordinates the motor activities of movement, and the basal ganglia maintain posture. The cerebral cortex operates movements, not muscles. The cortex, for example, may direct the arm to pick up a cup of coffee. The cerebellum, which operates below the level of consciousness, blends and coordinates the muscles involved in voluntary movement. It does not direct the movement but translates the 'instructions' from the cerebral cortex into detailed actions by the many different muscles in the hand, arm and shoulder. When a patient's cerebellum is injured, movements become clumsy, unsure and uncoordinated.

Table 14-2 Selected Joint Movements

Body part - type of joint/movement	Normal range	Illustration
Neck - pivot joint		
Flexion. Move the head from the upright midline position forward, so that the chin rests on the chest (see Figure 14-2).	415° from midline	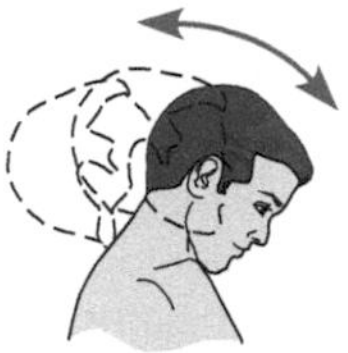
Extension. Move the head from the flexed position to the upright position (Figure 14-2).	45° from midline	Figure 14-2
Hyperextension. Move the head from the upright position back as far as possible (Figure 14-2).	45° from midline	
Lateral flexion. Move the head laterally to the right and left shoulders (see Figure 14-3).	40° from midline	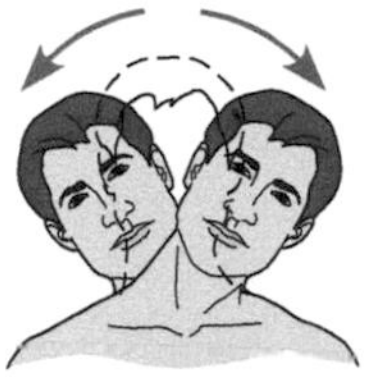 Figure 14-3
Rotation. Turn the face as far as possible to the right and left (see Figure 14-4).	70° from midline	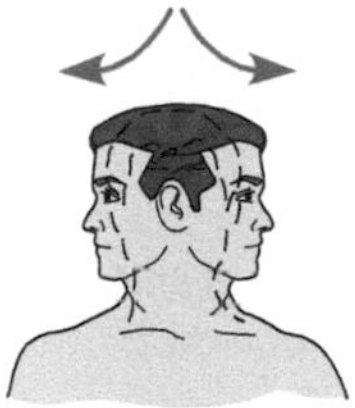 Figure 14-4
Shoulder - ball-and-socket joint		
Flexion. Raise each arm from a position by the side forward and upward to a position beside the head (see Figure 14-5).	180° from the side	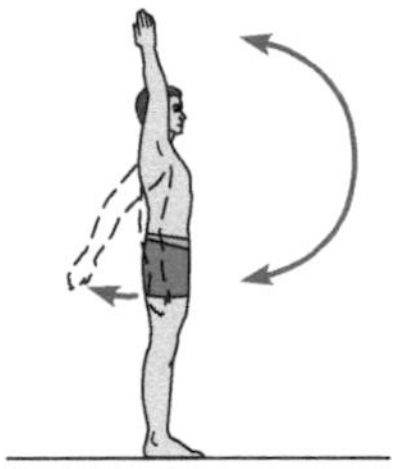
Extension. Move each arm from a vertical position beside the head forward and down to a resting position at the side of the body (Figure 14-5).	180° from vertical position beside the head	
Hyperextension. Move each arm from a resting side position to behind the body (Figure 14-5).	50° from side position	Figure 14-5
Abduction. Move each arm laterally from a resting position at the sides to a side position above the head, palm of the hand away from the head (see Figure 14-6).	180°	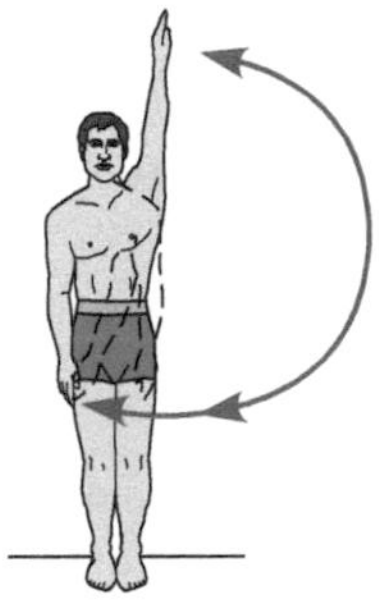
Adduction (anterior). Move each arm from a position at the sides across the front of the body as far as possible (see Figure 14-6). The elbow may be straight or bent.	50°	Figure 14-6
Circumduction. Move each arm forward, up, back and down in a full circle (see Figure 14-7).	360°	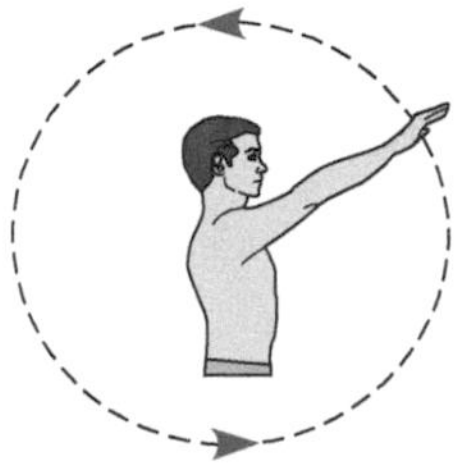 Figure 14-7

Table 14-2 (*continued*)

Body part - type of joint/movement	Normal range	Illustration
External rotation. With each arm held out to the side at shoulder level and the elbow bent to a right angle, fingers pointing down, move the arm upward so that the fingers point up (see Figure 14-8).	90°	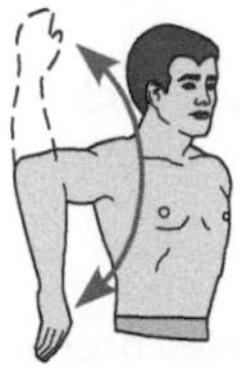
Internal rotation. With each arm held out to the side at shoulder level and the elbow bent to a right angle, fingers pointing up, bring the arm forward and down so that the fingers point down (Figure 14-8).	90°	Figure 14-8
Elbow - hinge joint		
Flexion. Bring each lower arm forward and upward so that the hand is at the shoulder (see Figure 14-9).	150°	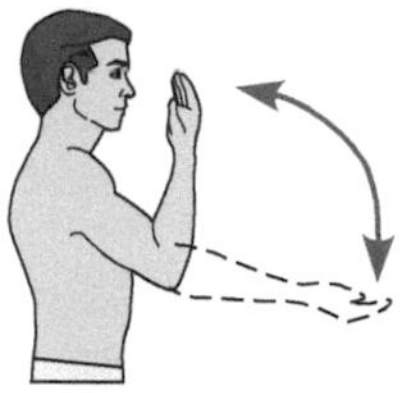
Extension. Bring each lower arm forward and downward, straightening the arm (Figure 14-9).	150°	Figure 14-9
Rotation for supination. Turn each hand and forearm so that the palm is facing upward (see Figure 14-10).	70° to 90°	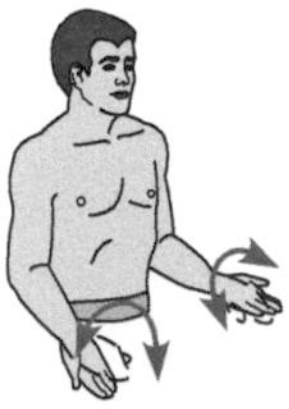
Rotation for pronation. Turn each hand and forearm so that the palm is facing downward (Figure 14-10).	70° to 90°	Figure 14-10
Wrist - condyloid joint		
Flexion. Bring the fingers of each hand towards the inner aspect of the forearm (see Figure 14-11).	80° to 90°	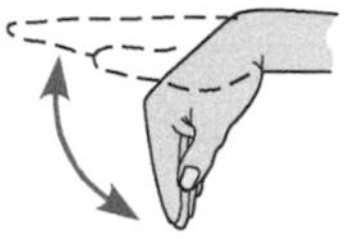
Extension. Straighten each hand to the same plane as the arm (Figure 14-11).	80° to 90°	Figure 14-11
Hyperextension. Bend the fingers of each hand back as far as possible (see Figure 14-12).	70° to 90°	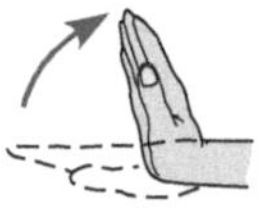 Figure 14-12
Radial flexion (abduction). Bend each wrist laterally towards the thumb side with hand supinated (see Figure 14-13).	0° to 20°	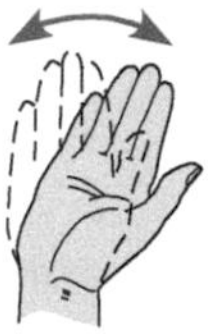
Ulnar flexion (adduction). Bend each wrist laterally towards the fifth finger with the hand supinated (Figure 14-13).	30° to 50°	Figure 14-13
Hand and fingers: metacarpophalangeal joints - condyloid; interphalangeal joints - hinge		
Flexion. Make a fist with each hand (see Figure 14-14).	90°	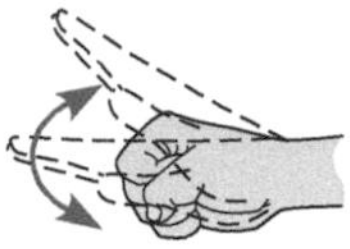
Extension. Straighten the fingers of each hand (Figure 14-14).	90°	Figure 14-14
Hyperextension. Bend the fingers of each hand back as far as possible (Figure 14-14).	30°	
Abduction. Spread the fingers of each hand apart (see Figure 14-15).	20°	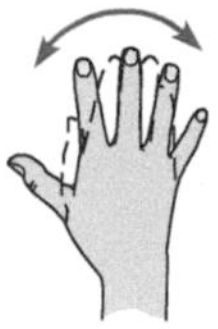
Adduction. Bring the fingers of each hand together (Figure 14-15).	20°	Figure 14-15

Table 14-2 *(continued)*

Body part – type of joint/movement	Normal range	Illustration
Thumb – saddle joint		
Flexion. Move each thumb across the palmar surface of the hand towards the fifth finger (see Figure 14-16).	90°	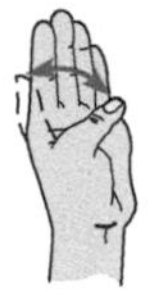
Extension. Move each thumb away from the hand (Figure 14-16).	90°	Figure 14-16
Abduction. Extend each thumb laterally (see Figure 14-17).	30°	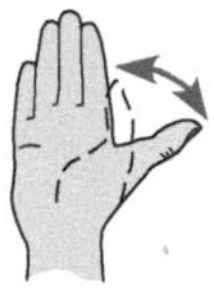
Adduction. Move each thumb back to the hand (Figure 14-17).	30°	Figure 14-17
Opposition. Touch each thumb to the top of each finger of the same hand. The thumb joint movements involved are abduction, rotation and flexion (see Figure 14-18).		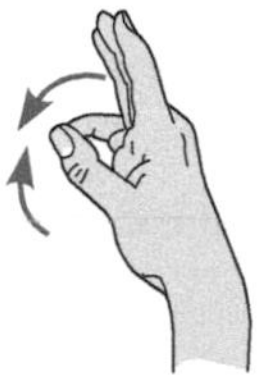 Figure 14-18
Hip – ball-and-socket joint		
Flexion. Move each leg forward and upward. The knee may be extended or flexed (see Figure 14-19).	Knee extended, 90°; knee flexed, 120°	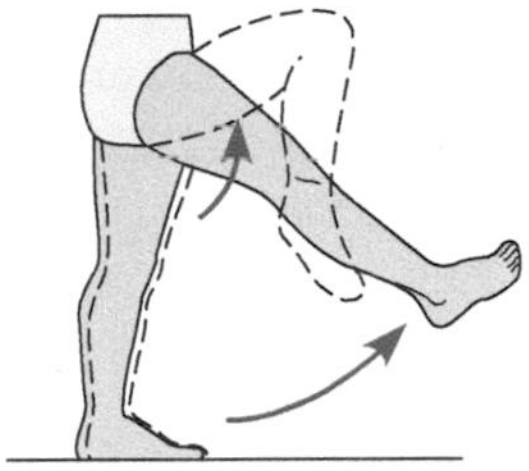 Figure 14-19
Extension. Move each leg back beside the other (see Figure 14-20).	90° to 120°	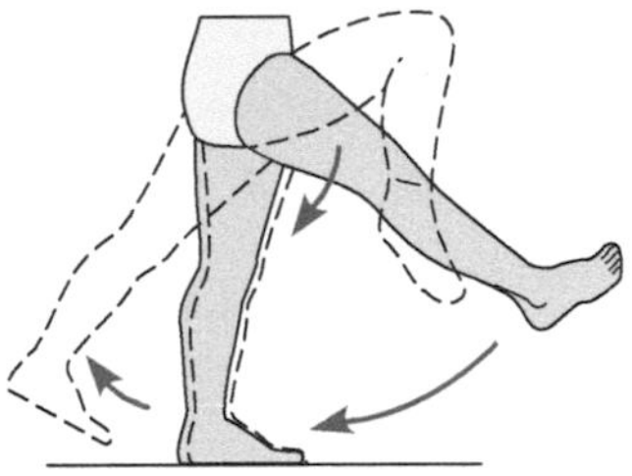
Hyperextension. Move each leg back behind the body (Figure 14-20).	30° to 50°	Figure 14-20
Abduction. Move each leg out to the side (see Figure 14-21).	45° to 50°	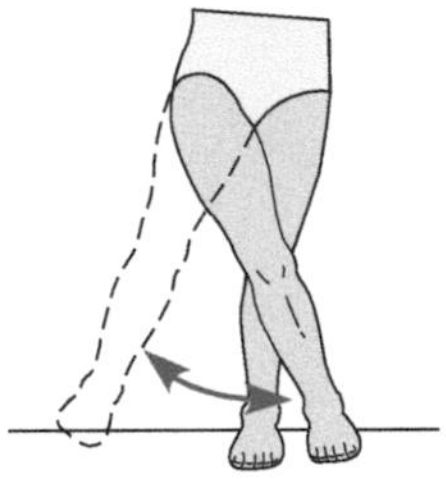
Adduction. Move each leg back to the other leg and beyond in front of it (Figure 14-21).	20° to 30° beyond other leg	Figure 14-21
Circumduction. Move each leg backward, up, to the side and down in a circle (see Figure 14-22).	360°	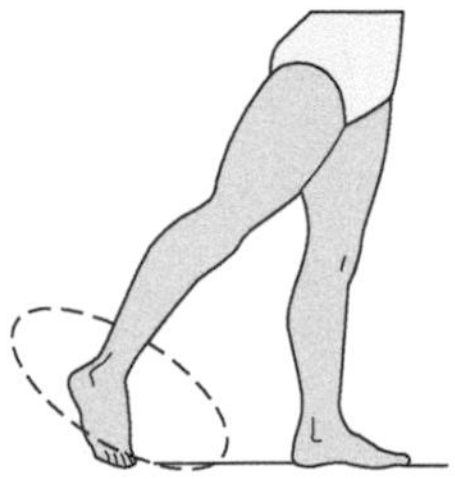 Figure 14-22

Table 14-2 *(continued)*

Body part - type of joint/movement	Normal range	Illustration
Internal rotation. Turn each foot and leg inward so that the toes point as far as possible towards the other leg (see Figure 14-23).	90°	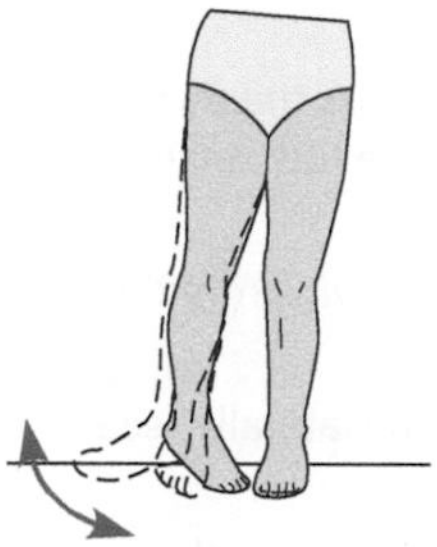
External rotation. Turn each foot and leg outward so that the toes point as far as possible away from the other leg (Figure 14-23).	90°	Figure 14-23
Knee - hinge joint		
Flexion. Bend each leg, bringing the heel towards the back of the thigh (see Figure 14-24).	120° to 130°	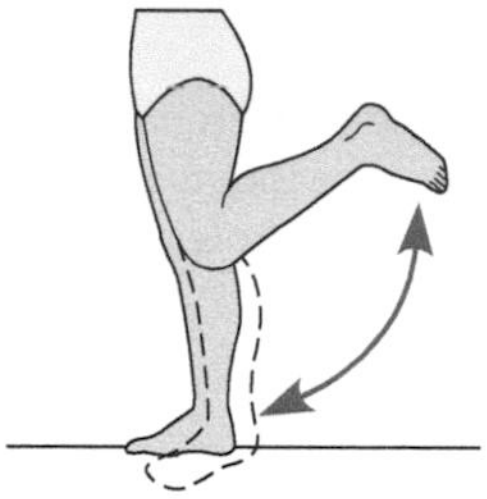
Extension. Straighten each leg, returning the foot to its position beside the other foot (Figure 14-24).	120° to 130°	Figure 14-24
Ankle - hinge joint		
Extension (plantar flexion). Point the toes of each foot downward (see Figure 14-25).	45° to 50°	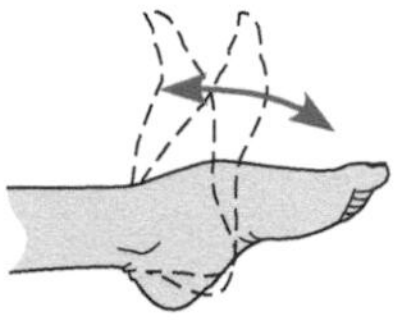
Flexion (dorsiflexion). Point the toes of each foot upward (Figure 14-25).	20°	Figure 14-25
Foot - gliding		
Eversion. Turn the sole of each foot laterally (see Figure 14-26).	5°	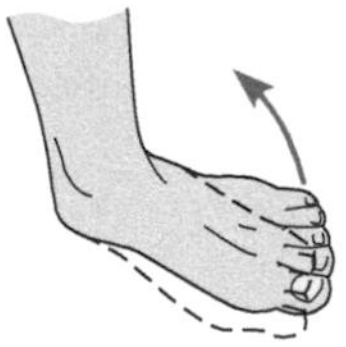
Inversion. Turn the sole of each foot medially (Figure 14-26).	5°	Figure 14-26
Toes: interphalangeal joints - hinge; metatarsophalangeal joints - hinge; intertarsal joints - gliding		
Flexion. Curl the toe joints of each foot downward (see Figure 14-27).	35° to 60°	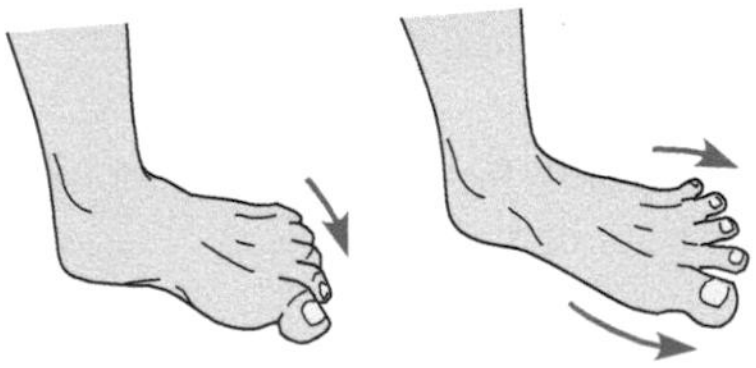
Extension. Straighten the toes of each foot (Figure 14-27).	35° to 60°	Figure 14-27
Trunk - gliding joint		
Flexion. Bend the trunk towards the toes (see Figure 14-28).	70° to 90°	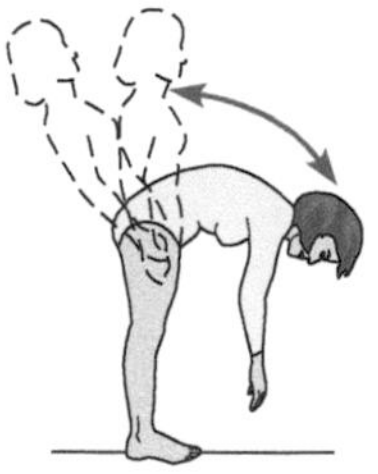
Extension. Straighten the trunk from a flexed position (Figure 14-28).		
Hyperextension. Bend the trunk backward (Figure 14-28).	20° to 30°	Figure 14-28

Table 14-2 *(continued)*

Body part - type of joint/movement	Normal range	Illustration
Lateral flexion. Bend the trunk to the right and to the left (see Figure 14-29).	35° on each side	Figure 14-29
Rotation. Turn the upper part of the body from side to side (see Figure 14-30).	30° to 45°	Figure 14-30

EXERCISE

Exercise and physical activity may be defined as:

- *Physical activity* is bodily movement produced by skeletal muscles that requires energy expenditure and produces progressive health benefits.
- *Exercise* is a type of physical activity defined as a planned, structured and repetitive bodily movement done to improve or maintain one or more components of physical fitness.

People participate in exercise programmes to decrease risk factors for cardiovascular disease and to increase their health and well-being. *Activity tolerance* is the type and amount of exercise or daily living activities an individual is able to perform without experiencing adverse effects.

TEACHING: WELLNESS CARE

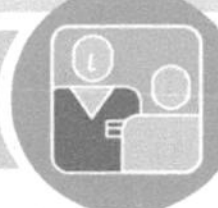

Guidelines for Physical Activity

5–17 years old For children and young people of this age group physical activity includes play, games, sports, transportation, recreation, physical education or planned exercise, in the context of family, school and community activities. In order to improve cardiorespiratory and muscular fitness, bone health, cardiovascular and metabolic health biomarkers and reduced symptoms of anxiety and depression, the following are recommended:

1 Children and young people aged 5–17 years old should accumulate at least 60 minutes of moderate- to vigorous-intensity physical activity daily.
2 Physical activity of amounts greater than 60 minutes daily will provide additional health benefits.
3 Most of daily physical activity should be aerobic. Vigorous-intensity activities should be incorporated, including those that strengthen muscle and bone, at least three times per week.

18–64 years old For adults of this age group, physical activity includes recreational or leisure-time physical activity, transportation (e.g. walking or cycling), occupational (i.e. work), household chores, play, games, sports or planned exercise, in the context of daily, family and community activities. In order to improve cardiorespiratory and muscular fitness, bone health and reduce the risk of NCDs and depression the following are recommended:

1 Adults aged 18–64 years should do at least 150 minutes of moderate-intensity aerobic physical activity throughout the week, or do at least 75 minutes of vigorous-intensity aerobic physical activity throughout the week, or an equivalent combination of moderate- and vigorous-intensity activity.
2 Aerobic activity should be performed in bouts of at least 10 minutes duration.

3 For additional health benefits, adults should increase their moderate-intensity aerobic physical activity to 300 minutes per week, or engage in 150 minutes of vigorous-intensity aerobic physical activity per week, or an equivalent combination of moderate- and vigorous-intensity activity.
4 Muscle-strengthening activities should be done involving major muscle groups on 2 or more days a week.

65 years old and above For adults of this age group, physical activity includes recreational or leisure-time physical activity, transportation (e.g. walking or cycling), occupational (if the person is still engaged in work), household chores, play, games, sports or planned exercise, in the context of daily, family and community activities. In order to improve cardiorespiratory and muscular fitness, bone and functional health, and reduce the risk of NCDs, depression and cognitive decline, the following are recommended:

1 Adults aged 65 years and above should do at least 150 minutes of moderate-intensity aerobic physical activity throughout the week, or do at least 75 minutes of vigorous-intensity aerobic physical activity throughout the week, or an equivalent combination of moderate- and vigorous-intensity activity.
2 Aerobic activity should be performed in bouts of at least 10 minutes duration.
3 For additional health benefits, adults aged 65 years and above should increase their moderate-intensity aerobic physical activity to 300 minutes per week, or engage in 150 minutes of vigorous-intensity aerobic physical activity per week, or an equivalent combination of moderate- and vigorous-intensity activity.
4 Adults of this age group with poor mobility should perform physical activity to enhance balance and prevent falls on 3 or more days per week.
5 Muscle-strengthening activities should be done involving major muscle groups, on 2 or more days a week.
6 When adults of this age group cannot do the recommended amounts of physical activity due to health conditions, they should be as physically active as their abilities and conditions allow. Overall, across all the age groups, the benefits of implementing the above recommendations, and of being physically active, outweigh the harms. At the recommended level of 150 minutes per week of moderate-intensity activity, musculoskeletal injury rates appear to be uncommon. In a population-based approach, in order to decrease the risks of musculoskeletal injuries, it would be appropriate to encourage a moderate start with gradual progress to higher levels of physical activity.

Source: *Global Recommendations on Physical Activity for Health* (WHO, 2010).

Types of Exercise

Exercise involves the active contraction and relaxation of muscles. Exercises can be classified according to the type of muscle contraction (isotonic, isometric or isokinetic) and according to the source of energy (aerobic or anaerobic).

Isotonic (dynamic) exercises are those in which the muscle shortens to produce muscle contraction and active movement. Most physical conditioning exercises – running, walking, swimming, cycling and other such activities – are isotonic, as are activities of daily living (ADL) and active range of movement (ROM) exercises (those initiated by the individual). Examples of isotonic bed exercises are pushing or pulling against a stationary object, using a trapeze to lift the body off the bed, lifting the buttocks off the bed by pushing with the hands against the mattress, and pushing the body to a sitting position.

Isotonic exercises increase muscle tone, mass and strength, and maintain joint flexibility and circulation. During isotonic exercise, both heart rate and cardiac output quicken to increase blood flow to all parts of the body. Little or no change in blood pressure occurs.

Isometric (static or setting) exercises are those in which there is a change in muscle tension but there is no change in muscle length and no muscle or joint movement. These exercises involve exerting pressure against a solid object and are useful for strengthening abdominal, gluteal and quadriceps muscles used in ambulation; for maintaining strength in immobilised muscles in casts or traction; and for endurance training. Examples of isometric bed exercise would be extending the leg in a supine position, tensing the thigh muscles, and pressing the knee against the bed, holding it for several seconds. These are often called quadriceps (or quad) sets.

Isometric exercises produce a moderate increase in heart rate and cardiac output, but no appreciable increase in blood flow to other parts of the body.

Isokinetic (resistive) exercises involve muscle contraction or tension against resistance; thus, they can be either isotonic or isometric. During isokinetic exercises, the person moves (isotonic) or tenses (isometric) against resistance. Special machines or devices provide the resistance to the movement. These exercises are used in physical conditioning and are often done to build up certain muscle groups; for example, the pectorals (chest muscles) may be increased in size and strength by lifting weights.

Aerobic exercise is activity during which the amount of oxygen taken in the body is greater than that used to perform the activity. Aerobic exercises use large muscle groups, are performed continuously and are rhythmic in nature. Examples are walking, jogging, running, bicycling, dancing, cross-country skiing, skipping, rowing, swimming and skating. Aerobic exercises improve cardiovascular conditioning and physical fitness.

Intensity of exercise can be measured in two ways:

1 *Target heart rate.* With this system, the goal is to work up to and sustain a target heart rate during exercise, based on the person's age. To determine the target heart rate, first calculate

the person's maximum heart rate by subtracting their current age in years from 220. Then obtain the target heart rate by taking 60% to 85% of the maximum. At least 60% of maximum heart rate is the recommended intensity. Because heart rates are so variable among individuals, the tests that follow are replacing this measure.

2 *Talk test.* This test is easier to implement and keeps most people at 60% of maximum heart rate or more. When exercising, the person should be able to carry on a conversation even with some laboured breathing. However, exercise intensity should be increased if the person can carry on with unlimited unlaboured discussion.

Anaerobic exercise involves activity in which the muscles cannot draw out enough oxygen from the bloodstream, and anaerobic pathways are used to provide additional energy for a short time. This type of exercise is used in endurance training for athletes.

Benefits of Exercise

Regular exercise is essential for healthy functioning of major body systems. The benefits of exercise on these systems follow.

Musculoskeletal System

The size, shape, tone and strength of muscles (including the heart muscle) are maintained with mild exercise and increased with strenuous exercise. With strenuous exercise, muscles hypertrophy (enlarge), and the efficiency of muscular contraction increases. Hypertrophy is commonly seen in the arm muscles of a tennis player, the leg muscles of a skater, and the arm and hand muscles of a plumber.

Exercise increases joint flexibility and range of motion. Bone density is maintained through weight-bearing. The stress of weight-bearing maintains a balance between osteoblasts (bone-building cells) and osteoclasts (bone-resorption and breakdown cells).

Cardiovascular System

Adequate exercise increases the heart rate, the strength of heart muscle contraction, and the blood supply to the heart and muscles. Cardiac output (the amount of blood pumped by the heart) increases as much as 30 l/min. Normal cardiac output is 5 l/min.

Respiratory System

Ventilation (air circulating into and out of the lungs) increases. In strenuous exercise, the intake of oxygen increases to as much as 20 times normal intake. Normal ventilation is about 5 or 6 l/min. Adequate exercise also prevents pooling of secretions in the bronchi and bronchioles, decreases breathing effort and improves diaphragmatic excursion.

Gastrointestinal System

Exercise improves the appetite and increases gastrointestinal tract tone, facilitating **peristalsis**.

Metabolic System

Exercise elevates the metabolic rate, thus increasing the production of body heat and waste products and **calorie** use. During strenuous exercise, the metabolic rate can increase to as much as 20 times the normal rate. Exercise increases the use of **triglycerides** and **fatty acids**, resulting in a reduced level of serum triglycerides and cholesterol. Exercise also enhances the effectiveness of insulin, lowering blood sugar. In diabetics, exercise can reduce their need for injecting supplemental insulin.

Urinary System

As adequate exercise promotes efficient blood flow, the body excretes wastes more effectively. In addition, stasis (stagnation) of urine in the bladder is usually prevented.

Psychoneurological System

Exercise produces a sense of well-being and improves tolerance to stress. It may also improve self-concept by reducing depression and improving one's body image. Energy level increases and quality of sleep is enhanced.

FACTORS AFFECTING BODY ALIGNMENT AND ACTIVITY

A number of factors affect an individual's body alignment, mobility and daily activity level. These include growth and development, physical health, mental health, nutrition, personal values and attitudes, and certain external factors.

Growth and Development

A person's age and musculoskeletal and nervous system development affect posture, body proportions, body mass, body movements and reflexes. Newborn movements are reflexive and random. All extremities are generally flexed but can be passively moved through a full range of motion. The feet are usually inverted but can be passively everted. As the neurological system matures, control over movement progresses during the first year. Gross motor development precedes fine motor skills, that is to say a child learns to walk before they can tie a shoe lace. Gross motor development occurs in a head-to-toe fashion, that is, progression from head control, to crawling, to pulling up to a standing position, to standing, and to walking, usually after the first birthday. Initially, walking involves a wide stance and unsteady gait, thus the term toddler. From ages 1–5 years, both gross and fine motor skills are refined. For example, pre-schoolers master riding a tricycle, dancing, running, jumping, using crayons to draw, fastening or using zippers, and brushing their teeth.

From 6–12 years, refinement of motor skills continues and exercise patterns for later life are generally determined. Many schools provide physical education and competitive sports programmes to enhance physical activity. Posture in school-age children is excellent, often the best during one's lifetime. In adolescence, growth spurts may result in awkwardness that can be manifested in posture. Postural habits formed during adolescence often persist into adulthood.

Adults between 20 and 40 years of age generally have few physical changes affecting mobility with the exception of pregnant women. Pregnancy alters centre of gravity, affects balance, and reduces exercise tolerance. As age advances, muscle tone and bone density decrease, joints lose flexibility, reaction time slows and bone mass decreases, particularly in women who have osteoporosis. Osteoporosis is a condition in which the bones become brittle and fragile due to calcium depletion. Osteoporosis is common in older women and primarily affects the weight-bearing joints of the lower extremities and the back, causing compression fractures of the vertebrae and hip fractures. All of these changes affect older adults' posture, gait and balance. Posture becomes forward leaning and stooped, which shifts the centre of gravity forward. To compensate for this shift, the knees flex slightly for support and the base of support is widened. Gait becomes wide based, short stepped and shuffling.

Physical Health

Mobility and activity tolerance are affected by any disorder that impairs the ability of the nervous system, musculoskeletal system, cardiovascular system, respiratory system and vestibular apparatus. Congenital problems such as hip dysplasia, spina bifida, cerebral palsy and the muscular dystrophies affect motor functioning. Disorders of the nervous system such as Parkinson's disease, multiple sclerosis, central nervous system tumours, cerebrovascular accidents (strokes), infectious processes (e.g. meningitis) and head and spinal cord injuries can leave muscle groups weakened, paralysed, spastic (with too much muscle tone) or flaccid (without muscle tone). Musculoskeletal disorders affecting mobility include strains, sprains, fractures, joint dislocations, amputations and joint replacements. Inner ear infections and dizziness can impair balance.

Many other acute and chronic illnesses that limit the supply of oxygen and nutrients needed for muscle contraction and movement can seriously affect activity tolerance. Examples include chronic obstructive lung disease, anaemia, congestive heart failure and angina.

Mental Health

Mental or affective disorders such as depression or chronic stress may affect a person's desire to move. The depressed person may lack enthusiasm for taking part in any activity and may even lack energy for usual hygiene practices. Lack of visible energy is seen in a slumped posture with head bowed. By contrast, happy, confident people usually stand erect. Chronic stress can deplete the body's energy reserves to the point that fatigue discourages the desire to exercise, even though exercise can energise the person and facilitate coping.

Nutrition

Both undernutrition and overnutrition can influence body alignment and mobility. Poorly nourished people may have muscle weakness and fatigue. Vitamin D deficiency causes bone deformity during growth. Inadequate calcium intake increases the risk of osteoporosis. Obesity can distort movement and can adversely affect posture and balance.

Personal Values and Attitudes

Whether people value regular exercise is often the result of family influence. In families that incorporate regular exercise in their daily routine or spend time together in activities, children learn to value physical activity. Sedentary families, on the other hand, participate in sports only as spectators, and this lifestyle is often transmitted to their children. Values about physical appearance also influence some people's participation in regular exercise. People who value a muscular build or physical attractiveness may participate in regular exercise programmes to produce the appearance they desire. Choice of physical activity or type of exercise is also influenced by values. Choices may be influenced by geographic location and cultural role expectations.

External Factors

Many external factors affect a person's mobility. Excessively high temperature and high humidity discourage activity, whereas comfortable temperature and humidity are conducive to activity. The availability of recreational facilities also influences activity; for example, lack of money may prohibit an individual from joining an exercise club or gymnasium. Neighbourhood safety promotes outdoor activity, whereas an unsafe environment discourages people from going outdoors. Adolescents, in particular, may spend many hours sitting at computers, watching television or playing video games rather than going outside to visit friends or to exercise.

Prescribed Limitations

Limitations to movement may be medically prescribed for some health problems. To promote healing, devices such as casts, braces, splints and traction are often used to immobilise body parts. Individuals who are short of breath may be advised not to walk up stairs. Bed rest may be the therapeutic choice for certain patients, for example, to relieve oedema, to reduce metabolic and oxygen needs, to promote tissue repair or to decrease pain.

The term bed rest varies in meaning to some extent. In some environments bed rest means strict confinement to bed or complete bed rest. Others may allow the patient to use a bedside commode or go to the bathroom. Nurses need to familiarise themselves with the meaning of bed rest in their practice setting.

EFFECTS OF IMMOBILITY

Individuals who have inactive lifestyles or who are faced with inactivity because of illness or injury are at risk of many problems that can affect major body systems. Whether immobility causes any problems often depends on the duration of the inactivity, the patient's health status and the patient's sensory awareness. The most obvious signs of prolonged immobility are often manifested in the musculoskeletal system. Individuals experience a significant decrease in muscular strength and agility whenever they do not maintain a moderate amount of physical activity. In addition, immobility adversely affects the cardiovascular, respiratory, metabolic, urinary and psycho-neurological systems. Nurses need to understand these effects and encourage patient movement as much as possible. Early ambulation after illness or surgery is an essential measure to prevent complications. Potential effects of immobility on body systems follow.

Musculoskeletal System

- *Disuse osteoporosis.* Without the stress of weight-bearing activity, the bones demineralise. They are depleted chiefly of calcium, which gives the bones strength and density. Regardless of the amount of calcium in a person's diet, the demineralisation process, known as *osteoporosis*, continues with immobility. The bones become spongy and may gradually deform and fracture easily.
- *Disuse atrophy.* Unused muscles atrophy (decrease in size), losing most of their strength and normal function.
- *Contractures.* When the muscle fibres are not able to shorten and lengthen, eventually a contracture (permanent shortening of the muscle) forms, limiting joint mobility. This process eventually involves the tendons, ligaments and joint capsules; it is irreversible except by surgical intervention. Joint deformities such as foot drop (see Figure 14-31) and external hip rotation occur when a stronger muscle dominates the opposite muscle.
- *Stiffness and pain in the joints.* Without movement, the collagen (connective) tissues at the joint become ankylosed (permanently immobile). In addition, as the bones demineralise, excess calcium may deposit in the joints, contributing to stiffness and pain.

Cardiovascular System

- *Diminished cardiac reserve.* Decreased mobility creates an imbalance in the autonomic nervous system, resulting in a preponderance of sympathetic activity over cholinergic activity that increases heart rate. Rapid heart rate reduces diastolic pressure, coronary blood flow and the capacity of the heart to respond to any metabolic demands above the basal levels. Because of this diminished cardiac reserve, the immobilised person may experience tachycardia with even minimal exertion.

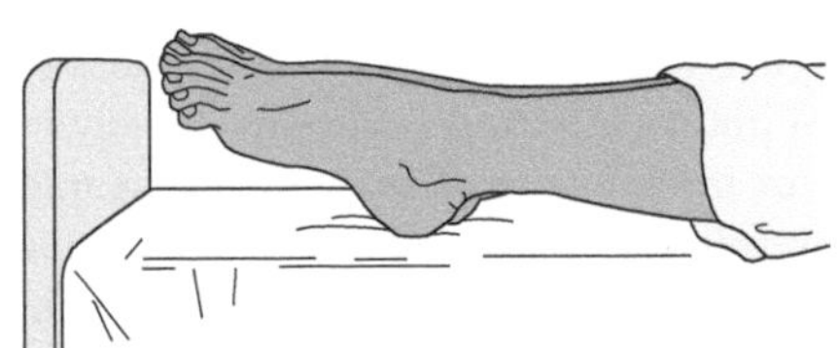

Figure 14-31 Plantar flexion contracture (foot drop).

- *Increased use of the Valsalva manoeuvre.* The Valsalva manoeuvre refers to holding the breath and straining against a closed glottis. For example, patients tend to hold their breath when attempting to move up in a bed or sit on a bedpan. This builds up sufficient pressure on the large veins in the thorax to interfere with the return blood flow to the heart and coronary arteries. When the individual exhales and the glottis again opens, pressure is suddenly released and a surge of blood flows to the heart. Tachycardia and cardiac arrhythmias can result if the patient has cardiac disease.
- *Orthostatic (postural) hypotension.* Orthostatic hypotension is a common result of immobilisation. Under normal conditions, sympathetic nervous system activity causes automatic vasoconstriction in the blood vessels in the lower half of the body when a mobile person changes from a horizontal to a vertical posture. Vasoconstriction prevents pooling of the blood in the legs and effectively maintains central blood pressure to ensure adequate perfusion of the heart and brain. During any prolonged immobility, this reflex becomes dormant. When the immobile person attempts to sit or stand, this reconstricting mechanism fails to function properly in spite of increased adrenalin output. The blood pools in the lower extremities, and central blood pressure drops. Cerebral perfusion is seriously compromised, and the person feels dizzy or light headed and may even faint. This sequence is usually accompanied by a sudden and marked increase in heart rate, the body's effort to protect the brain from an inadequate blood supply.
- *Venous vasodilation and stasis.* The skeletal muscles of an active person contract with each movement, compressing the blood vessels in those muscles and helping to pump the blood back to the heart against gravity. The tiny valves in the leg veins aid in venous return to the heart by preventing backward flow of blood and pooling. In an immobile person, the skeletal muscles do not contract sufficiently, and the muscles atrophy. The skeletal muscles can no longer assist in pumping blood back to the heart against gravity. Blood pools in the leg veins, causing vasodilatation and engorgement. The valves in the veins can no longer work effectively to prevent backward flow of blood and pooling (see Figure 14-32). This phenomenon is known as incompetent valves. As the blood continues to pool in the veins, its greater volume increases venous blood pressure, which can become much higher than that exerted by the tissues surrounding the vessel.
- *Dependent oedema.* When the venous pressure is sufficiently great, some of the serous part of the blood is forced out of the blood vessel into the interstitial spaces surrounding the blood vessel, causing oedema. Oedema is most common in parts of the body positioned below the heart. Dependent oedema is most likely to occur around the sacrum or heels of a patient who sits up in bed or in the feet and lower legs of a patient who sits in a chair. Oedema further impedes venous return of blood to the heart, causing more pooling and more oedema. Oedematous tissue is uncomfortable and more susceptible to injury than normal tissue.

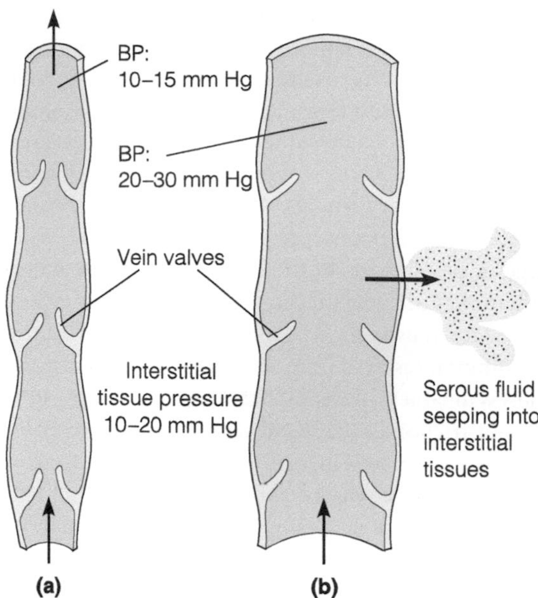

Figure 14-32 Leg veins: (a) in a mobile person; (b) in an immobile person.

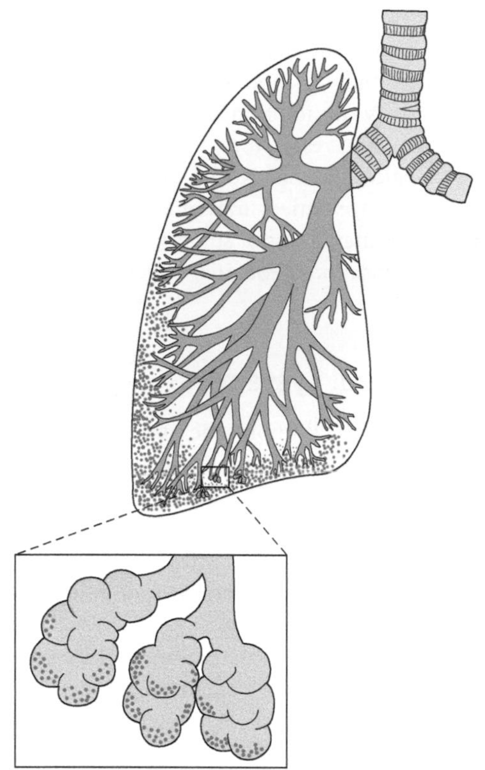

Figure 14-33 Pooling of secretions in the lungs of an immobile person.

- *Thrombus formation.* Three factors collectively predispose a patient to the formation of a thrombophlebitis (a clot that is loosely attached to an inflamed vein wall): impaired venous return to the heart, hypercoagulability of the blood, and injury to a vessel wall.

A thrombus (clot) is particularly dangerous if it breaks loose from the vein wall to enter the general circulation as an embolus (an object that has moved from its place of origin, causing obstruction to circulation elsewhere). Large emboli that enter the pulmonary circulation may occlude the vessels that nourish the lungs to cause an infarcted (dead) area of the lung. If the infarcted area is large, pulmonary function may be seriously compromised, or death may ensue. Emboli travelling to the coronary vessels or brain can produce a similarly dangerous outcome.

Respiratory System

- *Decreased respiratory movement.* In a recumbent, immobile patient, ventilation of the lungs is passively altered. The body presses against the rigid bed and curtails chest movement. The abdominal organs push against the diaphragm, restricting lung movement and making it difficult to expand the lungs fully. An immobile recumbent person rarely sighs, partly because overall muscle atrophy also affects the respiratory muscles and partly because there is no stimulus of activity. Without these periodic stretching movements, the cartilaginous intercostal joints may become fixed in an expiratory phase of respiration, further limiting the potential for maximal ventilation. These changes produce shallow respirations and reduce vital capacity (the maximum amount of air that can be exhaled after a maximum inhalation).
- *Pooling of respiratory secretions.* Secretions of the respiratory tract are normally expelled by changing positions or posture and by coughing. Inactivity allows secretions to pool by gravity (see Figure 14-33), interfering with the normal diffusion of oxygen and carbon dioxide in the alveoli. The ability to cough up secretions may also be hindered by loss of respiratory muscle tone, dehydration (which thickens secretions) or sedatives that depress the cough reflex. Poor oxygenation and retention of carbon dioxide in the blood can, if allowed to continue, predispose the person to **respiratory acidosis**, a potentially lethal disorder.
- *Atelectasis.* When ventilation is decreased, pooled secretions may accumulate in a dependent area of a bronchiole and effectively block it. Because of changes in regional blood flow, bed rest decreases the amount of **surfactant** produced. (Surfactant enables the alveoli to remain open.) The combination of decreased surfactant and blockage of a bronchiole with mucus can cause atelectasis (the collapse of a lobe or of an entire lung) distal to the mucous blockage. Immobile elderly, post-operative patients are at greatest risk of atelectasis.
- *Hypostatic pneumonia.* Pooled secretions provide excellent media for bacterial growth. Under these conditions, a minor upper respiratory infection can evolve rapidly into a severe infection of the lower respiratory tract. Pneumonia caused by static respiratory secretions can severely impair oxygen–carbon dioxide exchange in the alveoli and is a fairly common cause of death among weakened, immobile persons, especially heavy smokers.

Metabolic System

- *Decreased metabolic rate.* **Metabolism** refers to the sum of all the physical and chemical processes by which living substance is formed and maintained and by which energy is made available for use by the body. The basal metabolic rate is the minimal energy expended for the maintenance of these processes, expressed in calories per hour per square metre of body surface. In immobile patients, the basal metabolic rate and gastrointestinal motility and secretions of various digestive glands decrease as the energy requirements of the body decrease.
- *Negative nitrogen balance.* In an active person, a balance exists between protein synthesis (anabolism) and protein breakdown (catabolism). Immobility creates a marked imbalance, and the catabolic processes exceed the anabolic processes. Catabolised muscle mass releases nitrogen. Over time, more nitrogen is excreted than is ingested, producing a negative nitrogen balance. The negative nitrogen balance represents a depletion of protein stores that are essential for building muscle tissue and for wound healing.
- *Anorexia.* Loss of appetite (**anorexia**) occurs because of the decreased metabolic rate and the increased catabolism that accompany immobility. Reduced caloric intake is usually a response to the decreased energy requirements of the inactive person. If protein intake is reduced, the nitrogen imbalance may become more pronounced, sometimes so severely that malnutrition ensues.
- *Negative calcium balance.* A negative calcium balance occurs as a direct result of immobility. Greater amounts of calcium are extracted from bone than can be replaced. The absence of weight-bearing and of stress on the musculoskeletal structures is the direct cause of the calcium loss from bones. Weight-bearing and stress are also required for calcium to be replaced in bone.

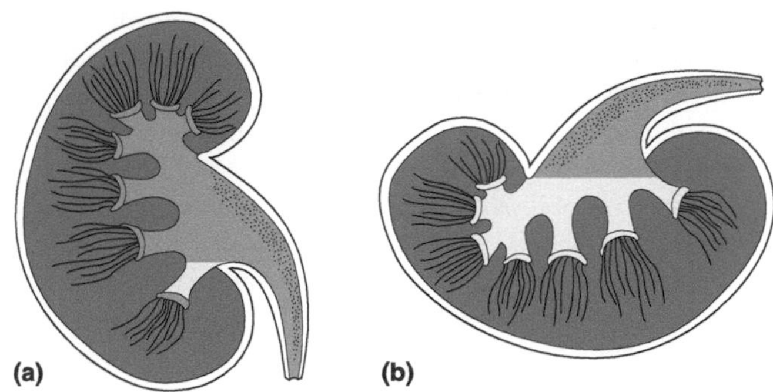

Figure 14-34 Pooling of urine in the kidney: (a) The patient is in an upright position; (b) the patient is in a back-lying position.

Urinary System

- *Urinary stasis.* In a mobile person, gravity plays an important role in the emptying of the kidneys and the bladder. The shape and position of the kidneys and active kidney contractions are important in completely emptying the urine from the calyces, renal pelvis and ureters (see Figure 14-34(a)). The shape and position of the urinary bladder (the **detrusor muscle**) and active bladder contractions are also important in achieving complete emptying (see Figure 14-35(a)).
- When the person remains in a horizontal position, gravity impedes the emptying of urine from the kidneys and the urinary bladder. To urinate, the person who is supine (in a back-lying position) must push upward, against gravity (Figures 14-34(b) and 14-35(b)). The renal pelvis may fill with urine before it is pushed into the ureters. Emptying is not as complete, and urinary stasis (stoppage or slowdown of flow) occurs after a few days of bed rest. Because of the overall decrease in muscle tone during immobilisation, including the tone of the detrusor muscle, bladder emptying is further compromised.

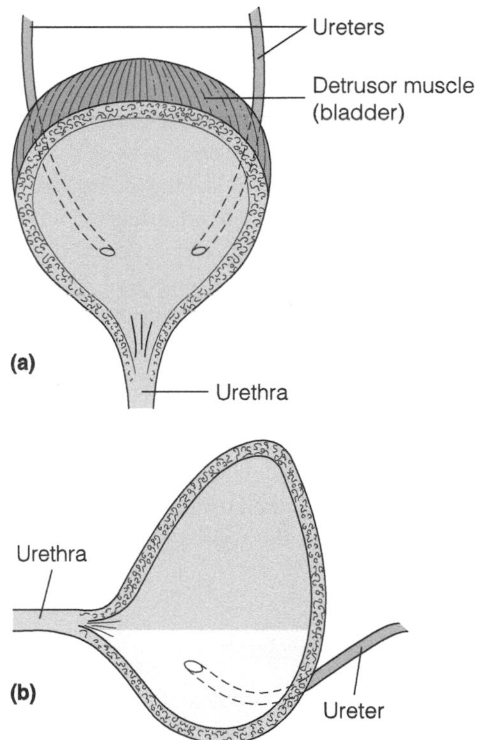

Figure 14-35 Pooling of urine in the urinary bladder: (a) The patient is in an upright position; (b) the patient is in a back-lying position.

- *Renal calculi.* In a mobile person, calcium in the urine remains dissolved because calcium and citric acid are balanced in an appropriately acid urine. With immobility and the resulting excessive amounts of calcium in the urine, this balance is no longer maintained. The urine becomes more alkaline, and the calcium salts precipitate out as crystals to form renal calculi (stones). In an immobile person in a horizontal position, the renal pelvis filled with stagnant, alkaline urine is an ideal location for calculi to form. The stones usually develop in the renal pelvis and pass through the ureters into the bladder. As the stones pass along the long, narrow ureters, they cause extreme pain and bleeding and can sometimes obstruct the urinary tract.

- *Urinary retention.* The immobile person may suffer from **urinary retention** (accumulation of urine in the bladder), bladder distention and, occasionally, urinary incontinence (involuntary urination). The decreased muscle tone of the urinary bladder inhibits its ability to empty completely, and the immobilised person is unable to relax the perineal muscles sufficiently to urinate. The discomfort of using a bedpan or urinal, the embarrassment and lack of privacy associated with this function, and the unnatural position for urination combine to make it difficult for the patient to relax the perineal muscles sufficiently to urinate while lying in bed.

  When urination is not possible, the bladder gradually becomes distended with urine. The bladder may stretch excessively, eventually inhibiting the urge to void. When bladder distention is considerable, some involuntary urinary 'dribbling' may occur (retention with overflow). This does not relieve the urinary distention, because most of the stagnant urine remains in the bladder.
- *Urinary infection.* Static urine provides an excellent medium for bacterial growth. The flushing action of normal, frequent urination is absent, and urinary distention often causes minute tears in the bladder mucosa, allowing infectious organisms to enter. The increased alkalinity of the urine caused by the hypercalcuria supports bacterial growth. The organism most commonly causing urinary tract infections is *Escherichia coli*, which normally resides in the colon. The normally sterile urinary tract may be contaminated by improper perineal care, the use of an indwelling urinary catheter or occasionally urinary reflux (backward flow). During reflux, contaminated urine from an overly distended bladder backs up into the renal pelvis to contaminate the kidney pelvis as well.

Gastrointestinal System

Constipation is a frequent problem for immobilised people because of decreased peristalsis and colon motility. The overall skeletal muscle weakness affects the abdominal and perineal muscles used in defecation. When the stool becomes very hard, more strength is required to expel it. The immobile person may lack this strength.

The bedfast person's unnatural and uncomfortable position on the bedpan does not facilitate elimination. The backward-leaning posture does not promote effective use of the muscles used in defecation. Some people are reluctant to use the bedpan in the presence of others. The embarrassment, lack of privacy, dependence on others to assist with the bedpan, and disruption of normal bowel habits may cause the individual to postpone or ignore the urge for elimination. Repeated postponement eventually suppresses the urge and weakens the defecation reflex.

Some persons may make excessive use of the Valsalva manoeuvere by straining at stool in an attempt to expel the hard stool. This effort dangerously increases intra-abdominal and intrathoracic pressures and places undue stress on the heart and circulatory system.

ACTIVITY 14-1

From the information provided, can you identify the life span consideration of the changes in physical activity necessary to maintain the well-being of an individual?

Integumentary System

Reduced skin elasticity. The skin can atrophy as a result of prolonged immobility. Shifts in body fluids between the fluid compartments can affect the consistency and health of the **dermis** and subcutaneous tissues in dependent parts of the body, eventually causing a gradual loss in skin elasticity.

Skin breakdown. Normal blood circulation relies on muscle activity. Immobility impedes circulation and diminishes the supply of nutrients to specific areas. As a result, skin breakdown and formation of pressure ulcers can occur.

Psychoneurological System

People who are unable to carry out the usual activities related to their roles (e.g. as breadwinner, husband, mother or athlete) become aware of an increased dependence on others. These factors lower the person's self-esteem. Frustration and the decrease in self-esteem may in turn provoke exaggerated emotional reactions. Emotional reactions vary considerably. Some individuals become apathetic and withdrawn, some regress and some become angry and aggressive.

Because the immobilised person's participation in life becomes much narrower and the variety of stimuli decreases, the person's perception of time intervals deteriorates. Problem-solving and decision-making abilities may deteriorate as a result of lack of intellectual stimulation and the stress of the illness and immobility. In addition, the loss of control over events can cause anxiety.

Immobility can impair the social and motor development of young children.

ASSESSING MOBILITY

Assessment relative to a patient's activity and exercise includes a patient history and a physical assessment of body alignment, gait, appearance and movement of joints, capabilities and limitations for movement, muscle mass and strength, activity tolerance, problems related to immobility and physical fitness. This physical assessment is usually completed by a physiotherapist.

The nurse collects information from the patient, from other nurses and from the patient's records. The examination and history are important sources of information about disabilities affecting the patient's mobility and activity status, such as contractures, oedema, pain in the extremities or generalised fatigue.

Patient History

Gathering the patient's details regarding their mobility and exercise history is usually part of the comprehensive patient history and includes daily activity level, activity tolerance, type and frequency of exercise, factors affecting mobility and effects of immobility. If the individual indicates a recent pattern change or difficulties with mobility, a more detailed history is required. This detailed history should include the specific nature of the problem, when it first began and its frequency, its causes if known, how the problem affects daily living, what the patient is doing to cope with the problem, and whether these methods have been effective. Examples of interview questions to elicit this data are shown in the *Assessment Interview*.

ASSESSMENT INTERVIEW

Activity and Exercise

Daily Activity Level

- What activities do you carry out during a routine day?
- Are you able to carry out the following tasks independently?
  - Eating
  - Dressing/grooming
  - Bathing
  - Toileting
  - Ambulating
  - Using a wheelchair
  - Transferring in and out of bed, bath and car
  - Cooking
  - House cleaning
  - Shopping
- Where problems exist in your ability to carry out such tasks:
  (i) Would you rate yourself as partially or totally dependent?
  (ii) How is the task achieved (by family, friend, agency or use of specialised equipment)?
- If it is a child:
  - Is the child developing as expected for his or her age?
  - Have you any concerns regarding the child's development?

Activity Tolerance

- How much and what types of activities make you tired?
- Do you ever experience dizziness, shortness of breath, marked increase in respiratory rate or other problems following mild or moderate activity?

Exercise

- What type of exercise do you carry out to enhance your physical fitness?
- What is the frequency and length of this exercise session?
- Do you believe exercise is beneficial to your health? Explain.

Factors Affecting Mobility

- *Environmental factors.* Do stairs, lack of railings or other assistive devices, or an unsafe neighbourhood impede your mobility or exercise regimen?
- *Health problems.* Do any of the following health problems affect your muscle strength or endurance: heart disease, lung disease, stroke, cancer, neuromuscular problems, musculoskeletal problems, visual or mental impairments, trauma or pain?
- *Financial factors.* Are your finances adequate to obtain equipment or other aids that you require to enhance your mobility?

Physical Examination

The physical examination is initially undertaken by the nurse and completed by a physiotherapist if there are any abnormalities or concerns identified. The assessment focuses on mobility and exercise emphasises body alignment, gait, appearance and movement of joints, capabilities and limitations for movement, muscle mass and strength, and activity tolerance.

Body Alignment

Assessment of body alignment includes an inspection of the individual while they stand. The purpose of body alignment assessment is to identify:

- normal developmental variations in posture;
- posture and learning needs to maintain good posture;
- factors contributing to poor posture, such as fatigue or low self-esteem;
- muscle weakness or other motor impairments.

To assess alignment, the nurse inspects the patient from lateral (see Figure 14-36(a)), anterior and posterior perspectives. From the anterior and posterior views, the practitioner should observe whether:

- the shoulders and hips are level;
- the toes point forward;
- the spine is straight, not curved to either side.

The 'slumped' posture (Figure 14-36(b)) is the most common problem that occurs when people stand. The neck is flexed far forward, the abdomen protrudes, the pelvis is thrust forward to create lordosis (an exaggerated inward curvature of the lumbar spine), and the knees are hyperextended. Low back pain and fatigue occur quickly in people with poor posture.

Gait

The characteristic pattern of a person's gait (walk) is assessed to determine the patient's mobility and risk for injury due to

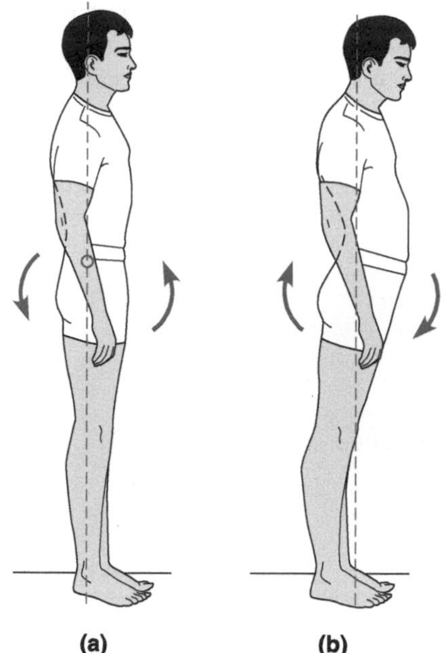

Figure 14-36 A standing person with (a) good trunk alignment; (b) poor trunk alignment. The arrows indicate the direction in which the pelvis is tilted.

falling. Two phases of normal gait are stance and swing (see Figure 14-37). When one leg is in the swing phase, the other is in the stance phase. In the *stance phase*, (a) the heel of one foot strikes the ground, and (b) body weight is spread over the ball of that foot while the other heel pushes off and leaves the ground. In the *swing phase*, the leg from behind moves in front of the body.

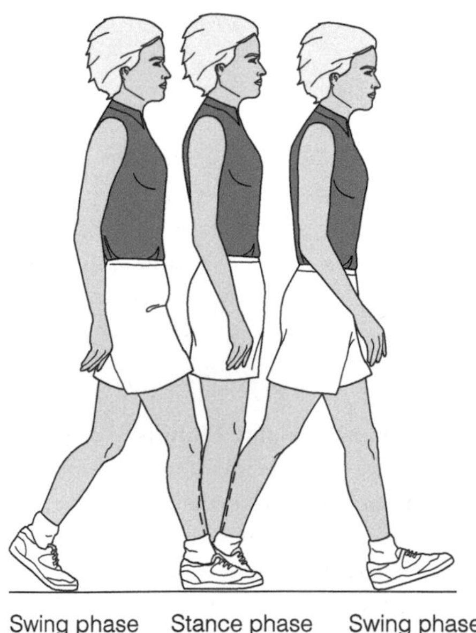

Figure 14-37 The stance and swing phases of a normal gait.

The practitioner assesses gait as the individual walks into the room or asks the individual to walk a distance of 10 metres down a hallway and observes for the following:

- Head is erect, gaze is straight ahead and vertebral column is upright.
- Heel strikes the ground before the toe.
- Feet are dorsiflexed in the swing phase.
- Arm opposite the swing-through foot moves forward at the same time.
- Gait is smooth, coordinated and rhythmic, with even weight borne on each foot; it produces minimal body swing from side to side and directs movement straight ahead; and it starts and stops with ease.

The practitioner may also assess pace (the number of steps taken per minute). A normal walking pace is 70–100 steps per minute. The pace of an older person may slow to about 40 steps per minute.

The nurse should also note the individual for a prosthesis or assistive device, such as a walking stick or frame. For an individual who uses assistive aids, the practitioner assesses gait without the device and compares the assisted and unassisted gaits.

Appearance and Movement of Joints

Physical examination of the joints involves inspection, palpation, assessment of range of active motion, and if active motion is not possible, assessment of range of passive motion. The nurse should assess the following:

- Any joint swelling or redness, which could indicate the presence of an injury or an inflammation.
- Any deformity, such as a bony enlargement or contracture, and symmetry of involvement.
- The muscle development associated with each joint and the relative size and symmetry of the muscles on each side of the body.
- Any reported or palpable tenderness.
- Crepitation (palpable or audible crackling or grating sensation produced by joint motion).
- Increased temperature over the joint. Palpate the joint using the backs of the fingers and compare the temperature with that of the symmetric joint.
- The degree of joint movement. Ask the patient to move selected body parts as shown in Table 14-2. If indicated, measure the extent of movement with a goniometer, a device that measures the angle of the joint in degrees.

Assessment of range of motion should not be unduly fatiguing, and the joint movements need to be performed smoothly, slowly and rhythmically. No joint should be forced. Uneven, jerky movement and forcing can injure the joint and its surrounding muscles and ligaments.

Capabilities and Limitations for Movement

The nurse needs to obtain data that may indicate hindrances or restrictions to the patient's movement and the need for assistance, including the following:

- How the patient's illness influences the ability to move and whether the patient's health contraindicates any exertion, position or movement.
- Encumbrances to movement, such as an intravenous line in place or a heavy cast.
- Mental alertness and ability to follow directions. Check whether the patient is receiving medications that hinder the ability to walk safely. Narcotics, sedatives, tranquillisers and some antihistamines cause drowsiness, dizziness, weakness and orthostatic hypotension.
- Balance and coordination.
- Presence of orthostatic hypotension before transfers. Specifically, assess for any increase in pulse rate, marked fall in blood pressure, dizziness, lightheadedness and dimming of vision when the patient moves from a supine to a vertical posture.
- Degree of comfort. People who have pain may not want to move and can require an analgesic before they are moved.
- Vision. Is it adequate to prevent falls?

The nurse also assesses the amount of assistance the individual requires for the following:

- Moving in the bed. In particular, observe for the amount of assistance the patient requires for turning:
  (a) from a supine position to a lateral position;
  (b) from a lateral position on one side to a lateral position on the other;
  (c) from a supine position to a sitting position in bed.
- Rising from a lying position to a sitting position on the edge of the bed. Healthy people can normally rise without support from the arms.
- Rising from a chair to a standing position. Normally this can be done without pushing with the arms.
- Coordination and balance. Determine the patient's abilities to hold the body erect, to bear weight and keep balance in a standing position either on one leg or both to take steps, and to push off from a chair or bed.

Muscle Mass and Strength

Before the patient undertakes a change in position or attempts to ambulate, it is essential that the nurse assesses the patient's strength and ability to move. Providing appropriate assistance lowers the risk of muscle strain and body injury to both the patient and nurse. Assessment of upper extremity strength is especially important for patients who use ambulation aids, such as walking frames and crutches.

Activity Tolerance

By determining an appropriate activity level for an individual, the nurse can predict whether the individual has the strength and endurance to participate in activities that require similar expenditures of energy. This assessment is useful in encouraging increasing independence in people who (a) have a cardiovascular or respiratory disability, (b) have been completely immobilised for a prolonged period, (c) have decreased muscle mass or a musculoskeletal disorder, (d) have experienced inadequate sleep, (e) have experienced pain or (f) are depressed, anxious or unmotivated.

The most useful measures in predicting activity tolerance are heart rate, strength and rhythm; respiratory rate, depth and rhythm; and blood pressure. These data are obtained at the following times:

- before the activity starts (baseline data), while the patient is at rest;
- during the activity;
- immediately after the activity stops;
- three minutes after the activity has stopped and the patient has rested.

The activity should be stopped immediately in the event of any physiological change indicating the activity is too strenuous or prolonged for the patient. These changes include the following:

- sudden facial pallor;
- feelings of dizziness or weakness;
- change in level of consciousness;
- heart rate or respiratory rate that significantly exceeds baseline or pre-established levels;
- change in heart or respiratory rhythm from regular to irregular;
- weakening of the pulse;
- dyspnoea, shortness of breath or chest pain;
- diastolic blood pressure change of 10mm Hg or more.

If, however, the patient tolerates the activity well, and if heart rate returns to baseline levels within five minutes after the activity ceases, the activity is considered safe. This activity, then, can serve as a standard for predicting the tolerance for similar activities.

Problems Related to Immobility

When collecting data pertaining to the problems of immobility, the practitioner uses the assessment methods of inspection, palpation and auscultation; checks results of laboratory tests; and takes measurements, including body weight, fluid intake and fluid output. Specific techniques for assessing immobility problems and abnormal assessment findings related to the complications of immobility are listed in Table 14-3.

It is extremely important to obtain and record baseline assessment data soon after the individual first becomes immobile. These baseline data serve as the standard against which all data collected throughout the period of immobilisation are compared.

Because a major nursing responsibility is to prevent the complications of immobility, the nurse needs to identify patients at risk of developing such complications before problems arise. Individuals at risk include those who (a) are poorly nourished; (b) have decreased sensitivity to pain, temperature or pressure; (c) have existing cardiovascular, pulmonary or neuromuscular problems; and (d) have altered level of consciousness.

Table 14-3 Assessing Problems of Immobility

Assessment	Problem
Musculoskeletal system	
Measure arm and leg circumferences	Decreased circumference due to decreased muscle mass
Palpate and observe body joints	Stiffness or pain in joints
Take goniometric measurements of joint ROM	Decreased joint ROM, joint contractures
Cardiovascular system	
Auscultate the heart	Increased heart rate
Measure blood pressure	Orthostatic hypotension
Palpate and observe sacrum, legs and feet	Peripheral dependent oedema, increased peripheral vein engorgement
Palpate peripheral	Weak peripheral pulses
Measure calf muscle circumferences	Oedema
Observe calf muscle for redness, tenderness and swelling	Thrombophlebitis
Respiratory system	
Observe chest movements	Asymmetric chest movements, dyspnoea
Auscultate chest	Diminished breath sounds, crackles, wheezes and increased respiratory rate
Metabolic system	
Measure height and weight	Weight loss due to muscle atrophy and loss of subcutaneous fat
Palpate skin	Generalised oedema due to low blood protein levels
Urinary system	
Measure fluid intake and output	Dehydration
Inspect urine	Cloudy, dark urine; high **specific gravity**
Palpate urinary bladder	Distended urinary bladder due to urinary retention
Gastrointestinal system	
Observe stool	Hard, dry, small stool
Auscultate bowel sounds	Decreased bowel sounds due to decreased intestinal motility
Integumentary system	
Inspect skin	Break in skin integrity

PLANNING

As part of planning, the nurse is responsible for identifying those patients who need assistance with body alignment and determining the degree of assistance they need. The nurse must be sensitive to the patient's need to function as independently as possible yet provide assistance when the patient needs it.

Most patients require some nursing guidance and assistance to learn about, achieve and maintain proper body mechanics. The nurse should also plan to teach patients applicable skills. For example, a patient with a back injury needs to learn how to get out of bed safely and comfortably, a patient with an injured leg needs to learn how to transfer from bed to wheelchair safely, and a patient with a newly acquired walker needs to learn how to use it safely. Nurses along with other members of the multidisciplinary team often teach family members or caregivers safe moving, lifting and transfer techniques in the home setting (see Chapter 13).

The goals established for a patient will vary according to the diagnosis and defining characteristics related to each individual. Examples of overall goals for patients with actual or potential problems related to mobility or activity follow.

The patient will have:

- increased tolerance for physical activity;
- restored or improved capability to ambulate and/or participate in activities of daily living;
- absence of injury from falling or improper use of body mechanics;
- enhanced physical fitness;
- absence of any complications associated with immobility;
- improved social, emotional and intellectual well-being.

Planning for Care in the Community

Patients who have been hospitalised for activity or mobility problems often need continued care in the home. In preparation for discharge, the nurse needs to determine the patient's actual and potential health problems, strengths and resources. The Community Care Considerations describe the specific assessment data required before establishing a discharge plan for individuals with mobility or activity problems. A major aspect of discharge planning involves instructional needs of the patient and family.

COMMUNITY CARE CONSIDERATIONS

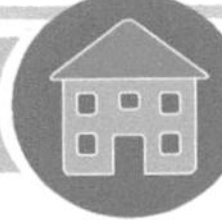

Mobility and Activity Problems

Patient and Environment

- Capabilities or tolerance for required and desired activities: self-care (feeding, bathing, toileting, dressing, grooming, home maintenance, shopping, cooking); recreational activities
- Mobility aids required: stick, walking frame, crutches, wheelchair, transfer boards
- Equipment required if immobilised: special bed, side rails, pressure-reducing mattress
- Current level of knowledge: body mechanics for use of mobility aids; specific exercises prescribed
- Home mobility hazard appraisal: adequacy of lighting; presence of handrails; safety of pathways and stairs; congested areas; unanchored rugs, mats or electrical wires, and any other obstacles to safe movement; structural adjustments needed for wheelchair access

Family or Caregiver

- Caregiver availability, skills and willingness: primary people able to assist patient with self-care, movement, shopping, and so on; physical and emotional status to assist with care; learning needs
- Family role changes and coping: effect on financial status, parenting and spousal roles, social roles
- Availability of caregiver support: other support people available for occasional duties such as shopping, transportation, housekeeping, cooking, budgeting, respite care

Community

- Resources: availability and familiarity with sources of medical equipment, financial assistance, homemaker services, hygienic care; Meals on Wheels; spiritual counsellors and visitors; sources of respite for caregiver

TEACHING: COMMUNITY CARE

Activity and Exercise

Maintaining Musculoskeletal Function

- Teach in conjunction with the physiotherapist the systematic performance of passive or assistive ROM exercises to maintain joint mobility.
- As appropriate, demonstrate the proper way to perform isotonic, isometric or isokinetic exercises to maintain muscle mass and tone (collaborate with the physical therapist about these). Incorporate ADLs into exercise programme if appropriate.
- Provide a written schedule for the type, frequency and duration of exercises; encourage the use of a progress graph or chart to facilitate adherence with the therapy.
- Offer a mobility schedule.
- Instruct in the availability of assistive mobility devices and correct use of them.
- Discuss pain control measures required before exercise.

Preventing Injury

- Teach safe transfer and ambulation techniques.
- Discuss safety measures to avoid falls (e.g. locking wheelchairs, wearing appropriate footwear, using rubber tips on crutches, keeping the environment safe and using mechanical aids such as raised toilet seat, grab bars, urinal and bedpan or commode to facilitate toileting).
- Teach the use of proper body mechanics.
- Teach ways to prevent postural hypotension.

Managing Energy to Prevent Fatigue

- Discuss activity and rest patterns and develop a plan as indicated; intersperse rest periods with activity periods.
- Discuss ways to minimise fatigue such as performing activities more slowly and for shorter periods, resting more often and using more assistance as required.
- Provide information about available resources to help with ADLs and home maintenance management.
- Teach ways to increase energy (e.g. increasing intake of high-energy foods, ensuring adequate rest and sleep, controlling pain).
- Teach techniques to monitor activity tolerance as appropriate.

Referrals

- Provide appropriate information about accessing community resources: home care agencies, sources of equipment, and so on.

IMPLEMENTING

Nursing strategies to maintain or promote body alignment and mobility involve positioning patients appropriately, moving and handling patients, providing ROM exercises, ambulating patients with or without mechanical aids, and strategies to prevent the complications of immobility. Whenever positioning, moving, handling and ambulating patients, nurses must always use proper body mechanics to avoid musculoskeletal strain and injury (see Chapter 13).

Positioning Patients

Positioning a patient in good body alignment and changing the position regularly and systematically are essential aspects of nursing practice. Individuals who can move easily, automatically reposition themselves for comfort. Such people generally require minimal positioning assistance from nurses, other than guidance about ways to maintain body alignment and to exercise their joints. However, people who are weak, frail, in pain, paralysed or unconscious rely on nurses to provide or assist with position changes. For all patients, it is important to assess the skin and provide skin care before and after a position change.

Any position, correct or incorrect, can be detrimental if maintained for a prolonged period. Frequent change of position helps to prevent muscle discomfort, undue pressure resulting in pressure ulcers, damage to superficial nerves and blood vessels, and contractures. Position changes also maintain muscle tone and stimulate postural reflexes.

When the individual is not able to move independently or assist with moving, the preferred method is to have two or more people move or turn the patient (see Chapter 13). Appropriate assistance reduces the risk of muscle strain and body injury to both the patient and nurse.

When positioning patients in bed, the nurse can do a number of things to ensure proper alignment and promote comfort and safety:

- Use an appropriate mattress following a risk assessment (as per local policy).
- Make sure the mattress is firm and level yet has enough give to fill in and support natural body curvatures. A sagging mattress, a mattress that is too soft or an underfilled waterbed used over a prolonged period can contribute to the development of hip flexion contractures and low back strain and pain. It is particularly important in the home setting to inspect the mattress for support.
- Ensure that the bed is clean and dry. Wrinkled or damp sheets increase the risk of pressure ulcer formation. Make sure extremities can move freely whenever possible. For example, the top bedclothes need to be loose enough for the patient to move the feet.
- Only use support devices in specified areas as per local policy and according to the patient's medical requirements. Use only those support devices needed to maintain alignment and to prevent stress on the individual's muscles and joints. If the person is capable of movement, too many devices limit mobility and increase the potential for muscle weakness and atrophy. Common alignment problems that can be corrected with support devices include the following:
  - flexion of the neck
  - internal rotation of the shoulder
  - adduction of the shoulder
  - flexion of the wrist
  - anterior convexity of the lumbar spine
  - external rotation of the hips
  - hyperextension of the knees
  - plantar flexion of the ankle.

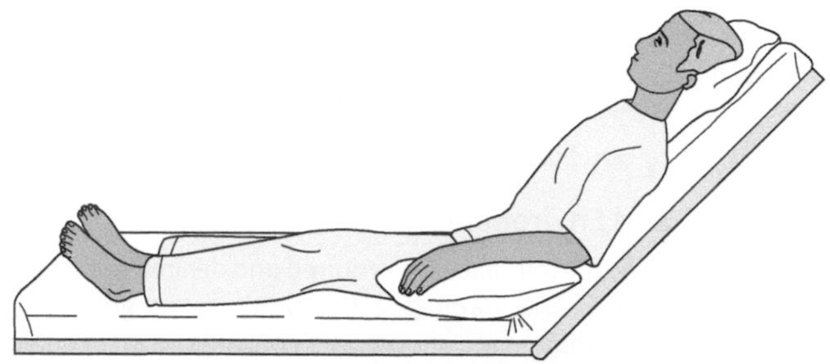

Figure 14-38 Low-Fowler's (semi-Fowler's) position (supported). Note that arm support is omitted in this instance. The amount of support depends on the needs of the individual patient.

- Avoid placing one body part, particularly one with bony prominences, directly on top of another body part. Excessive pressure can damage veins and predispose the patient to thrombus formation. Pressure against the popliteal space may damage nerves and blood vessels in this area.
- Plan a systematic 24-hour schedule for position changes.
- Sometimes a person who appears well aligned may be experiencing real discomfort. Both appearance, in relation to alignment criteria, and comfort are important in achieving effective alignment.

Fowler's Position

Fowler's position, or a semi-sitting position, is a bed position in which the head and trunk are raised 45–90 degrees. In low-Fowler's or semi-Fowler's position (see Figure 14-38), the head and trunk are raised 15–45 degrees; in high-Fowler's position, the head and trunk are raised 90 degrees. In this position, the knees may or may not be flexed.

Fowler's position is the position of choice for people who have difficulty breathing and for some people with heart problems. When the patient is in this position, gravity pulls the diaphragm downward, allowing greater chest expansion and lung ventilation.

A common error nurses make when aligning patients in Fowler's position is placing an overly large pillow or more than one pillow behind the patient's head. This promotes the development of neck flexion contractures. If a patient desires several head pillows, the nurse should encourage the patient to rest without a pillow for several hours each day to extend the neck fully and counteract the effects of poor neck alignment.

Orthopnoeic Position

In the **orthopnoeic position**, the individual sits either in bed or on the side of the bed with an overbed table across the lap (see Figure 14-39). This position facilitates respiration by allowing maximum chest expansion. It is particularly helpful to patients who have problems exhaling, because they can press the lower part of the chest against the edge of the overbed table.

Dorsal Recumbent Position

In the **dorsal** recumbent (back-lying) position (see Figure 14-40), the patient's head and shoulders are slightly elevated on a small pillow. In some areas, the terms *dorsal recumbent* and *supine* are

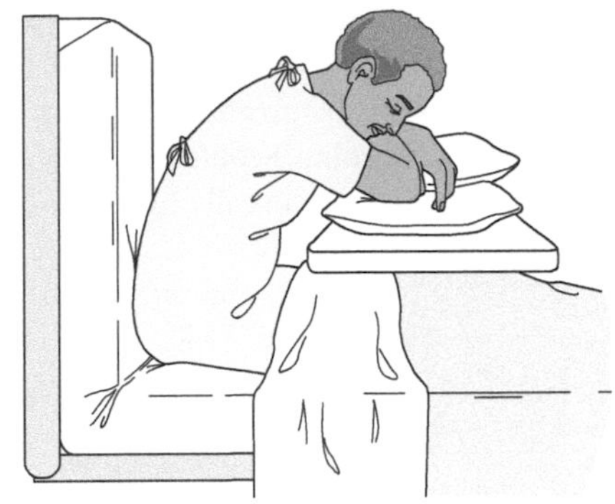

Figure 14-39 Orthopnoeic position.

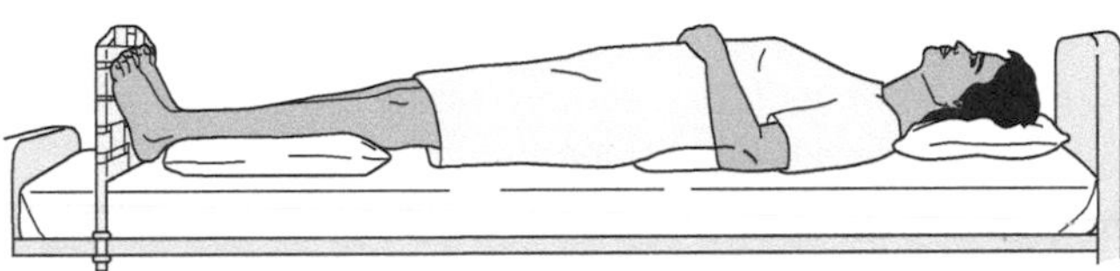

Figure 14-40 Dorsal recumbent position (supported).

used interchangeably; strictly speaking, however, in the supine or dorsal position the head and shoulders are not elevated. In both positions, the patient's forearms may be elevated on pillows or placed at the patient's sides. Supports are similar in both positions, except for the head pillow. The dorsal recumbent position is used to provide comfort and to facilitate healing following certain procedures or anaesthetics (e.g. spinal).

Prone Position

In the prone position, the patient lies on the abdomen with the head turned to one side (see Figure 14-41). The hips are not flexed. Both children and adults often sleep in this position, sometimes with one or both arms flexed over their heads. This position has several advantages. It is the only bed position that allows full extension of the hip and knee joints. When used periodically, the prone position helps to prevent flexion contractures of the hips and knees, thereby counteracting a problem caused by all other bed positions. The prone position also promotes drainage from the mouth and is especially useful for unconscious patients or those recovering from surgery of the mouth or throat.

The prone position poses some distinct disadvantages. The pull of gravity on the trunk produces a marked lordosis in most people, and the neck is rotated laterally to a significant degree. For this reason, the prone position may not be recommended for people with problems of the cervical or lumbar spine. This position also causes plantar flexion. Some patients with cardiac or respiratory problems find the prone position confining and suffocating because chest expansion is inhibited during respirations. The prone position should be used only when the patient's back is correctly aligned, only for short periods, and only for people with no evidence of spinal abnormalities.

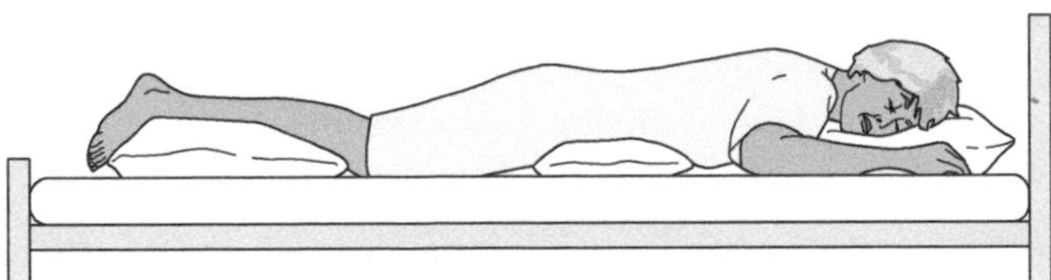

Figure 14-41 Prone position (supported).

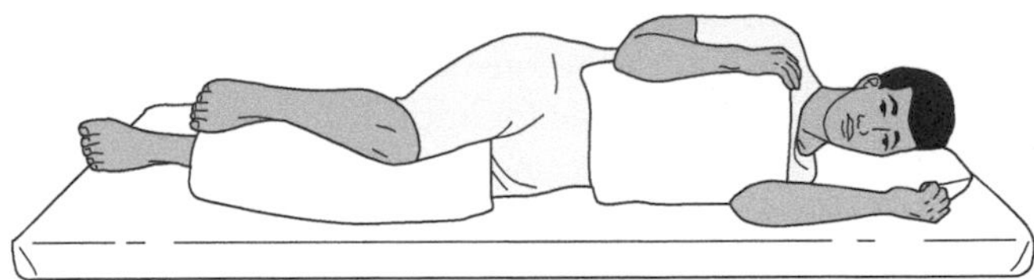

Figure 14-42 Lateral position (supported).

Lateral Position

In the lateral (side-lying) position (see Figure 14-42), the person lies on one side of the body. Flexing the top hip and knee and placing this leg in front of the body creates a wider, triangular base of support and achieves greater stability. The greater the flexion of the top hip and knee, the greater the stability and balance in this position. This flexion reduces lordosis and promotes good back alignment. For this reason, the lateral position is good for resting and sleeping patients. The lateral position helps to relieve pressure on the sacrum and heels in people who sit for much of the day or who are confined to bed and rest in Fowler's or dorsal recumbent positions much of the time. In the lateral position, most of the body's weight is borne by the lateral aspect of the lower scapula, the lateral aspect of the ilium and the greater trochanter of the femur. People who have sensory or motor deficits on one side of the body usually find that lying on the uninvolved side is more comfortable.

Sims' Position

In Sims' (semiprone) position (see Figure 14-43), the individual assumes a posture halfway between the lateral and the prone positions. The lower arm is positioned behind the patient, and the upper arm is flexed at the shoulder and the elbow. Both legs

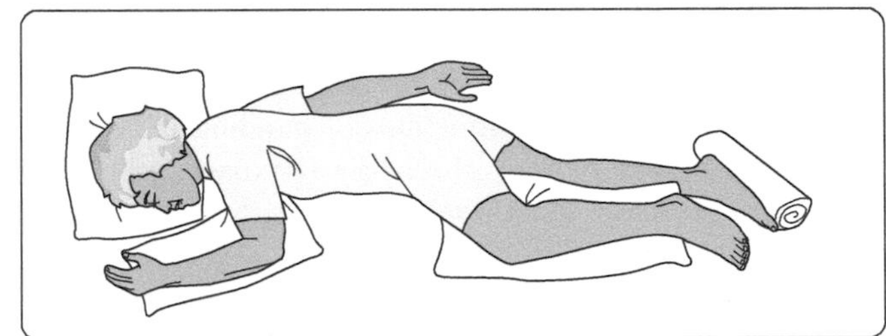

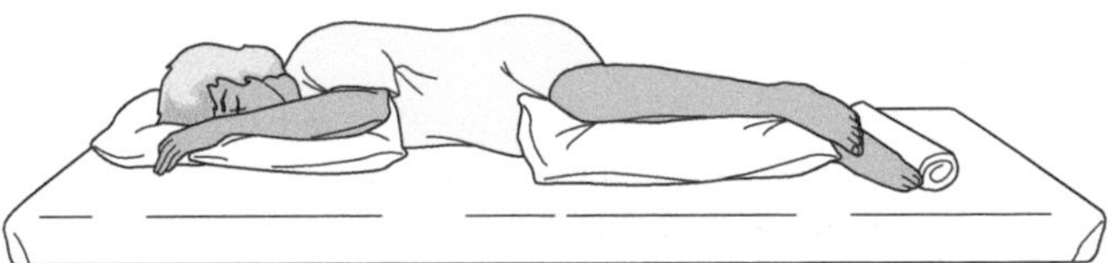

Figure 14-43 Sims' position (supported).

are flexed in front of the patient. The upper leg is more acutely flexed at both the hip and the knee than is the lower one.

Sims' position may be used for unconscious patients because it facilitates drainage from the mouth and prevents aspiration of fluids. It is also used for paralysed individuals because it reduces pressure over the sacrum and greater trochanter of the hip. It is often used for patients receiving enemas and occasionally for those undergoing examinations or treatments of the perineal area. Many people, especially pregnant women, find Sims' position comfortable for sleeping. People with sensory or motor deficits on one side of the body usually find that lying on the uninvolved side is more comfortable.

LIFESPAN CONSIDERATIONS

Positioning Patients

Infants

- Position infants on their back for sleep (NHS, 2010).

Children

- Carefully inspect the dependent skin surfaces of all infants and children confined to bed at least three times in each 24-hour period.

Mature Adults

- Decreased subcutaneous fat and thinning of the skin place elders at risk for skin breakdown. Repositioning at least every two hours helps reduce pressure on bony prominences and avoids skin trauma.
- In patients who have had cerebrovascular accidents (strokes), there is a risk of shoulder displacement on the paralysed side from improper moving or repositioning techniques. Use care when moving, positioning in bed and transferring.

Range of Movement (ROM) Exercises

When people are ill, they may need to perform ROM exercises until they can regain their normal activity levels. Active ROM exercises are isotonic exercises in which the individual moves each joint in the body through its complete range of movement, maximally stretching all muscle groups within each plane over the joint. These exercises maintain or increase muscle strength and endurance and help to maintain cardio-respiratory function in an immobilised individual. They also prevent deterioration of joint capsules, ankylosis and contractures.

Full ROM does not occur spontaneously in the immobilised individual who independently achieves ADLs, moves about in bed, transfers between bed and wheelchair or chair or ambulates a short distance, because only a few muscle groups are maximally stretched during these activities. Although the patient may successfully achieve some active ROM movements of the upper extremities while combing the hair, bathing and dressing, the immobilised patient is very unlikely to achieve any active ROM movements of the lower extremities when these are not used in the normal functions of standing and walking about. For this reason, most wheelchair and many ambulatory patients need active ROM exercises until they regain their normal activity levels.

At first, the nurse may need to teach the patient to perform the needed ROM exercises; eventually, the patient may be able to accomplish these independently. Instructions for the patient performing active ROM exercises are shown in the *Teaching: patient care.*

During passive ROM exercises, another person moves each of the patient's joints through its complete range of movement, maximally stretching all muscle groups within each plane over each joint. Because the individual does not contract the muscles, passive ROM exercises are of no value in maintaining muscle strength but are useful in maintaining joint flexibility. For this reason, passive ROM exercises should be performed only when the patient is unable to accomplish the movements actively.

Passive ROM exercises should be accomplished for each movement of the arms, legs and neck that the individual is unable to achieve actively. As with active ROM exercises, passive ROM exercises should be accomplished to the point of slight resistance, but not beyond, and never to the point of discomfort. The movements should be systematic, and the same sequence should be followed during each exercise session. Each exercise should consist of three repetitions, and the series of exercises should be done twice daily. Performing one series of exercises along with the bath is helpful. Passive ROM exercises are accomplished most effectively when the individual lies supine in bed. General guidelines for providing passive exercises are shown in the *Practice Guidelines* on page 393.

During active-assistive ROM exercises, the patient uses a stronger, opposite arm or leg to move each of the joints of a limb incapable of active motion. The patient learns to support and move the weak arm or leg with the strong arm or leg as far as possible. Then the nurse continues the movement passively to its maximal degree. This activity increases active movement on the strong side of the patient's body and maintains joint flexibility on the weak side. Such exercise is especially useful for stroke victims who are hemiplegic (paralysed on one-half of the body).

Functional joint flexibility is also maintained in the performance of ADLs. The following are examples:

- Eating, shaving, grooming and bathing exercise the elbow (flexion and extension) and shoulder (abduction).

- Activities requiring fine motor skills, such as writing and eating, exercise the fingers (flexion, extension, adduction, abduction) and the thumb (opposition).
- Walking exercises the shoulders (flexion, extension), hip (flexion, extension, hyperextension), knee (flexion, extension) and ankle (plantar flexion and dorsiflexion).
- Reaching for articles exercises the shoulders (flexion, extension and perhaps slight abduction or adduction).
- Dressing involves many joint movements.

Ambulating Patients

Ambulation (the act of walking) is a function that most people take for granted. However, when people are ill they are often confined to bed and are thus nonambulatory. The longer individuals are in bed, the more difficulty they have walking.

TEACHING: PATIENT CARE

Active ROM Exercises

- Perform each ROM exercise as taught to the point of slight resistance, but not beyond, and never to the point of discomfort.
- Perform the movements systematically, using the same sequence during each session.
- Perform each exercise three times.
- Perform each series of exercises twice daily.

Mature Adults

- For mature adults, it is not essential to achieve full range of motion in all joints. Instead, emphasise achieving a sufficient range of motion to carry out ADLs, such as walking, dressing, combing hair, showering and preparing a meal.

PRACTICE GUIDELINES

Providing Passive ROM Exercises

- Ensure that the individual understands the reason for doing ROM exercises.
- Obtain consent.
- If there is a possibility of hand swelling, make sure rings are removed.
- Maintain patient dignity and privacy.
- Clothe the patient in a loose gown, and cover the body with a bath blanket.
- Use correct body mechanics when providing ROM exercise to avoid muscle strain or injury to both yourself and the patient.
- Position the bed at an appropriate height.
- Expose only the limb being exercised to avoid embarrassing the patient.
- Support the patient's limbs above and below the joint as needed to prevent muscle strain or injury (see Figure 14-44). This may also be done by cupping joints in the palm of your hand or cradling limbs along your forearm (see Figure 14-45). If a joint is painful (e.g. arthritic), support the limb in the muscular areas above and below the joint.
- Use a firm, comfortable grip when handling the limb.

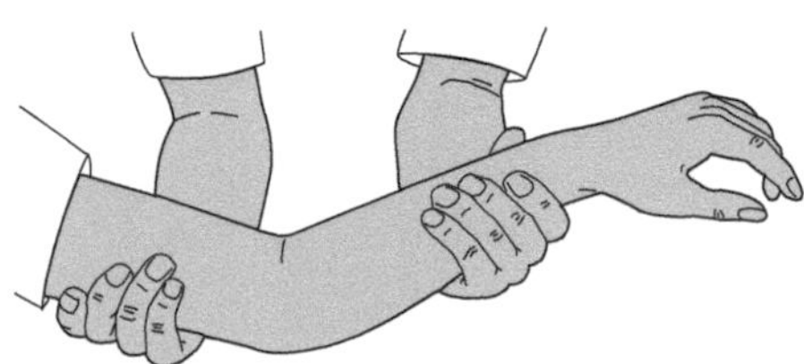

Figure 14-44 Supporting a limb above and below the joint for passive exercise.

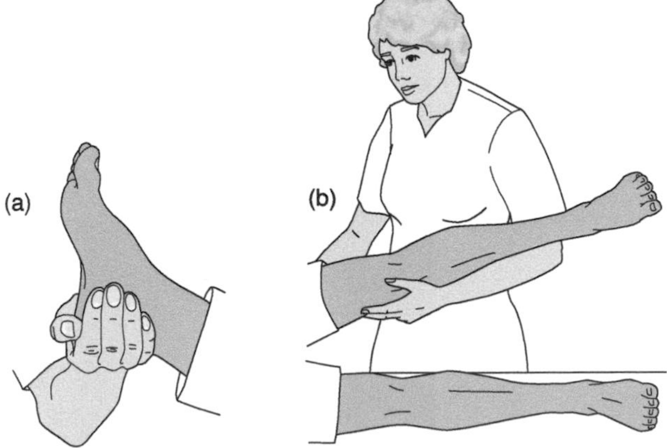

Figure 14-45 Holding limbs for support during passive exercise: (a) cupping; (b) cradling.

Preambulatory Exercises

Patients who have been in bed for long periods often need a plan of muscle tone exercises to strengthen the muscles used for walking before attempting to walk. One of the most important muscle groups is the quadriceps femoris, which extends the knee and flexes the thigh. This group is also important for elevating the legs, for example, for walking upstairs. These exercises are frequently called quadriceps drills or sets. To strengthen these muscles, the patient consciously tenses them, drawing the kneecap upward and inward. The patient pushes the popliteal space of the knee against the bed surface, relaxing the heels on the bed surface (see Figure 14-46). On the count of 1, the muscles are tensed; they are held during the counts of 2, 3, 4; and they are relaxed at the count of 5. The exercise should be done within the patient's tolerance, that is, without fatiguing the muscles. Carried out several times an hour during waking hours, this simple exercise significantly strengthens the muscles used for walking.

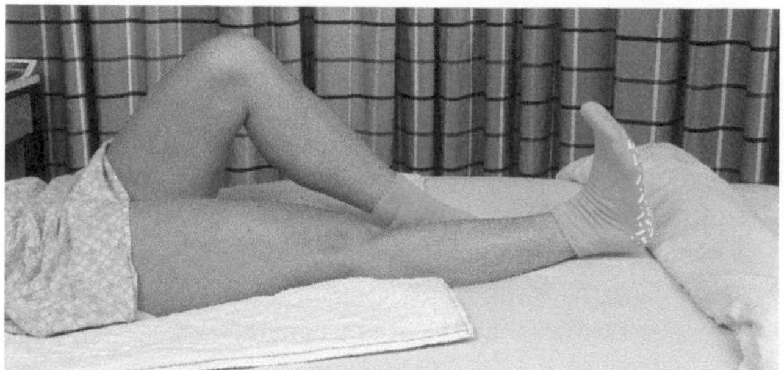

Figure 14-46 Tensing the quadriceps femoris muscles before ambulation.
Source: Pearson Education Ltd.

Assisting Patients to Ambulate

Patients who have been immobilised for even a few days may require assistance with ambulation. The amount of assistance will depend on the individual's condition, including age, health status and length of inactivity. Assistance may mean walking alongside the patient while providing physical support or providing instruction to the patient about the use of assistive devices such as a stick, walking frame or crutches.

Some patients experience postural (orthostatic) hypo-tension on assuming a vertical position from a lying position and may need information about ways to control this problem (see *Teaching: Patient Care*). The patient may exhibit some or all of the following symptoms: pallor, diaphoresis, nausea, tachycardia and dizziness. If any of these are present, the patient should be assisted to a supine position in bed and closely assessed.

TEACHING: PATIENT CARE

Controlling Postural Hypotension

- Rest with the head of the bed elevated 18-26cm (8-12 inches). This position makes the position change on rising less severe.
- Avoid sudden changes in position. Arise from bed in three stages:
  (a) Sit up in bed for one minute.
  (b) Sit on the side of the bed with legs dangling for one minute.
  (c) Stand with care, holding onto the edge of the bed or another nonmovable object for one minute.
- Never bend down all the way to the floor or stand up too quickly after stooping.
- Postpone activities such as shaving and hair grooming for at least one hour after rising.
- Be aware that the symptoms of hypotension are most severe at the following times:
  (a) 30-60 minutes after a heavy meal.
  (b) 1-2 hours after taking an antihypertension medication.
- Get out of a warm bath very slowly, because high temperatures can lead to venous pooling.
- Use a passive movement to improve circulation in the lower extremities. Even mild leg conditioning can strengthen muscle tone and enhance circulation.
- Refrain from any strenuous activity that results in holding the breath and bearing down. This Valsalva manoeuvere slows the heart rate, leading to subsequent lowering of blood pressure.

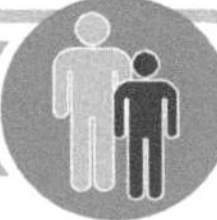

LIFESPAN CONSIDERATIONS

Assisting the Patient to Ambulate

Mature Adults

- Enquire how the patient has ambulated previously and modify assistance accordingly.
- Move the body parts smoothly, slowly and rhythmically. Jerky movements cause discomfort and, possibly, injury. Fast movements can cause spasticity (sudden, prolonged involuntary muscle contraction) or rigidity (stiffness or inflexibility).
- Avoid moving or forcing a body part beyond the existing range of motion. Muscle strain, pain and injury can result. This is particularly important for people with flaccid (limp) paralysis, whose muscles can be stretched and joints dislocated without their awareness.
- If muscle spasticity occurs during movement, stop the movement temporarily, but continue to apply slow, gentle pressure on the part until the muscle relaxes; then proceed with the motion.
- If a contracture is present, apply slow firm pressure, without causing pain, to stretch the muscle fibres.
- If rigidity occurs, apply pressure against the rigidity and continue the exercise slowly.
- Avoid hypertension of joints in older adults if joints are arthritic.
- Use the exercises as an opportunity to also assess skin condition.

Even one or two days of bed rest can make a person feel weak, unsteady and shaky when first getting out of bed. A patient, who has had surgery, is elderly or has been immobilised for a longer time will feel more pronounced weakness. The potential problems of immobility are far less likely to occur when patients become ambulatory as soon as possible. The nurse can assist patients to prepare for ambulation by helping them become as independent as possible while in bed. Nurses should encourage individuals to perform ADLs, maintain good body alignment and carry out active ROM exercises to the maximum degree possible yet within the limitations imposed by their illness and recovery programme.

Bear in mind the following:

- Take into account a decrease in speed, strength, resistance to fatigue, reaction time and coordination due to a decrease in nerve conduction.
- Be cautious when using a transfer belt with a patient with osteoporosis. Too much pressure from the belt can increase the risk of vertebral compression fractures.
- If assistive devices, such as a walker or walking stick are used, make sure patients are supervised in the beginning to learn the proper method of using them. Crutches may be much more difficult for mature adults due to decreased upper body strength.
- Be alert to signs of activity intolerance, especially in mature adults with cardiac and lung problems.
- Set small goals and increase slowly to build endurance, strength and flexibility.
- Be aware of any fall risks the mature adult may have, such as:
  - effects of medications;
  - neurological disorders;
  - environmental hazards;
  - orthostatic hypotension.
- In mature adults, the body's responses return to normal more slowly. For instance, an increase in heart rate from exercise may stay elevated for hours before returning to normal.

Using Mechanical Aids for Walking

Mechanical aids for ambulation include walking sticks, walking frames and crutches.

Walking Sticks

Two types of stick are commonly used today: the standard straight-legged stick and the quad device, which has four feet and provides the most support (see Figure 14-47). Stick tips should have rubber caps to improve traction and prevent

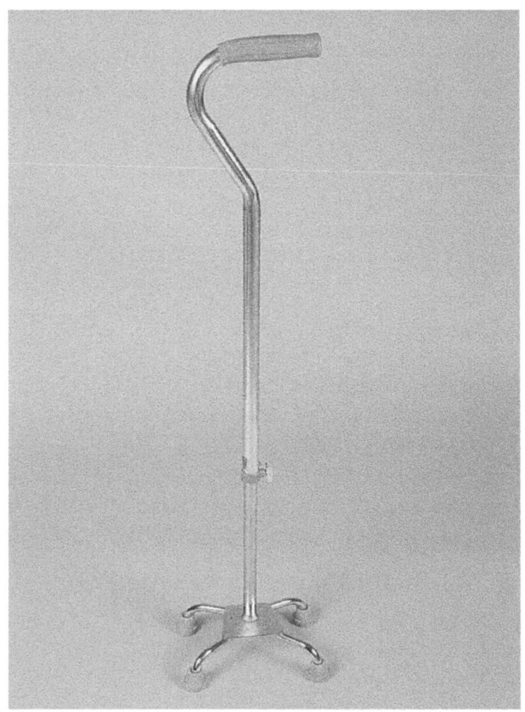

Figure 14-47 A quad device.
Source: ARJO MED AB Ltd.

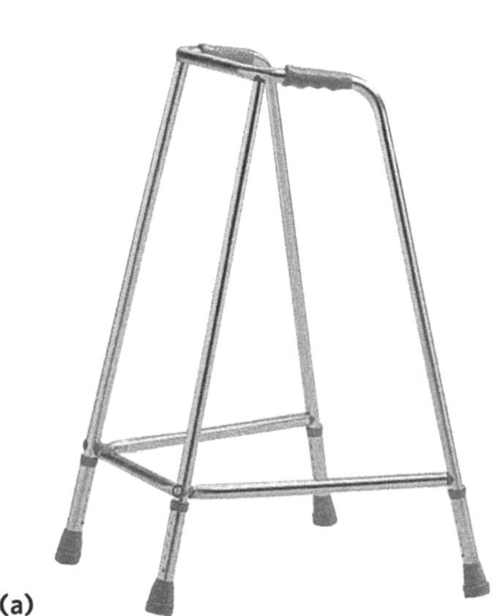

(a)

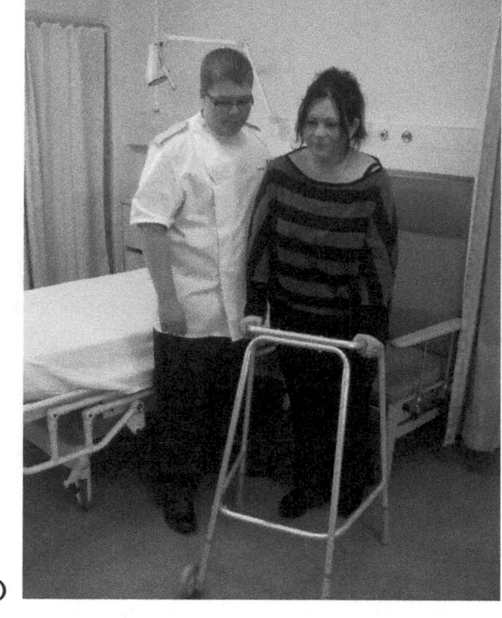

(b)

Figure 14-48 (a) standard walker; (b) two-wheeled walker.

slipping. The standard length is 91cm long; some aluminium sticks can be adjusted from 56–97cm and should be adjusted to the patient's own needs. The length should permit the elbow to be slightly flexed. Individuals may use either one or two sticks, depending on how much support they require, and their physical ability to use two sticks.

Walking Frames

Walking frames are mechanical devices for ambulatory individuals who need more support than a stick provides. Walking frames come in many different shapes and sizes, with devices suited to individual needs. The standard type is made of polished aluminium. It has four legs with rubber tips and plastic hand grips (see Figure 14-48). Many walking frames have adjustable legs.

The standard frame needs to be picked up to be used. The patient therefore requires partial strength in both hands and wrists, strong elbow extensors and strong shoulder depressors. The individual also needs the ability to bear at least partial weight on both legs.

TEACHING: PATIENT CARE

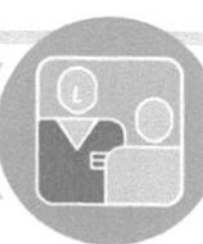

Using Walking Sticks

- Hold the stick with the hand on the stronger side of the body to provide maximum support and appropriate body alignment when walking.
- Position the tip of a standard stick (and the nearest tip of other stick) about 15cm to the side and 15cm in front of the near foot, so that the elbow is slightly flexed.

When Maximum Support is Required

- Move the stick forward about 30cm or a distance that is comfortable while the body weight is borne by both legs (see Figure 14-49(a)).
- Then move the affected (weak) leg forward to the stick while the weight is borne by the stick and stronger leg (see Figure 14-49(b)).

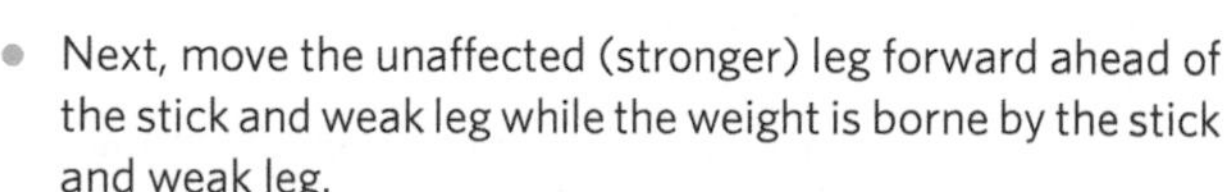

- Next, move the unaffected (stronger) leg forward ahead of the stick and weak leg while the weight is borne by the stick and weak leg.
- Repeat the steps. This pattern of moving provides at least two points of support on the floor at all times.

As You Become Stronger and Require Less Support

- Move the stick and weak leg forward at the same time, while the weight is borne by the stronger leg (see Figure 14-50(a)).
- Move the stronger leg forward; while the weight is borne by the stick and the weak leg (see Figure 14-50(b)).

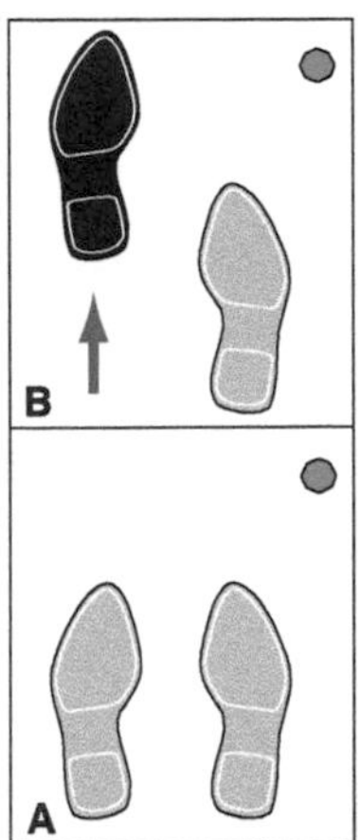

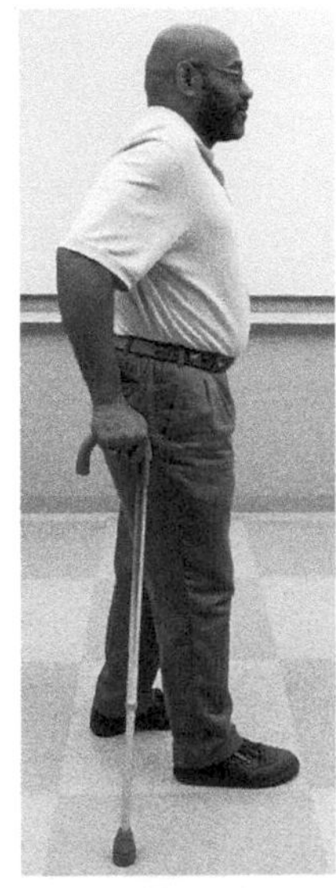

Figure 14-49 Steps involved in using a stick to provide maximum support.
Source: Pearson Education Ltd.

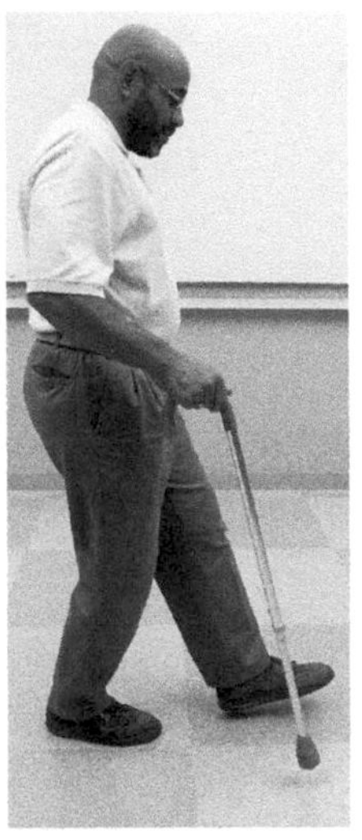

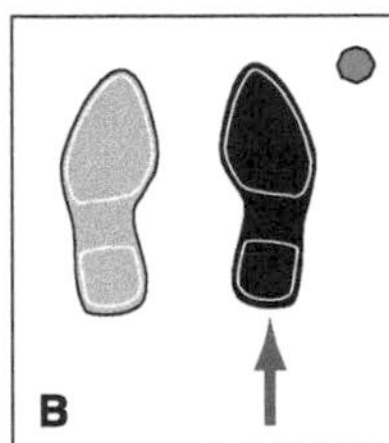

Figure 14-50 Steps involved in using a stick when less than maximum support is required.
Source: Pearson Education Ltd.

TEACHING: PATIENT CARE

Using Walking Frames

When Maximum Support is Required

- Move the walker ahead about 15cm while your body weight is borne by both legs.
- Then move the right foot up to the walker while your body weight is borne by the left leg and both arms.
- Next, move the left foot up to the right foot while your body weight is borne by the right leg and both arms.

If One Leg is Weaker than the Other

- Move the walker and the weak leg ahead together about 15cm while your weight is borne by the stronger leg.
- Then move the stronger leg ahead while your weight is borne by the affected leg and both arms.

Four-wheeled and two-wheeled models of walkers (roller walkers) do not need to be picked up to be moved, but they are less stable than the standard walker is. They are used by patients who are too weak or unstable to pick up and move the walker with each step. Some roller walkers have a seat at the back so the patient can sit down to rest when desired. An adaptation of the standard and four-wheeled walker is one that has two tips and two wheels. This type provides more stability than the four-wheeled model yet still permits the patient to keep the walker in contact with the ground all the time. The patient tilts the walker towards the body, lifting the tips while the wheels remain on the ground, and then pushes the walker forward.

The nurse may need to adjust the height of a patient's walker so that the hand bar is just below the patient's waist and the patient's elbows are slightly flexed. This position helps the patient assume a more normal stance. A walker that is too low causes the patient to stoop; one that is too high makes the patient stretch and reach.

Crutches

Crutches may be a temporary need for some people and a permanent one for others. Sometimes individuals are discouraged when they attempt crutch walking. Patients confined to bed are often unaware of weakness that becomes apparent when they try to stand or walk. Patients realise that they can no longer take balance for granted when they must cope with the weight of a heavy cast or a paralysed limb. Frequently, progress may be slower than the patient anticipated. Encouragement from the nurse and the setting of realistic goals are especially important.

There are several kinds of crutches. The most frequently used are the adjustable forearm crutch, the arthritic crutch or the children's quad crutch (see Figure 14-51). All crutches require suction tips, usually made of rubber, which help to prevent slipping on a floor surface.

In crutch walking, the patient's weight is borne by the muscles of the shoulder girdle and the upper extremities. Before beginning crutch walking, exercises that strengthen the upper arms and hands are recommended.

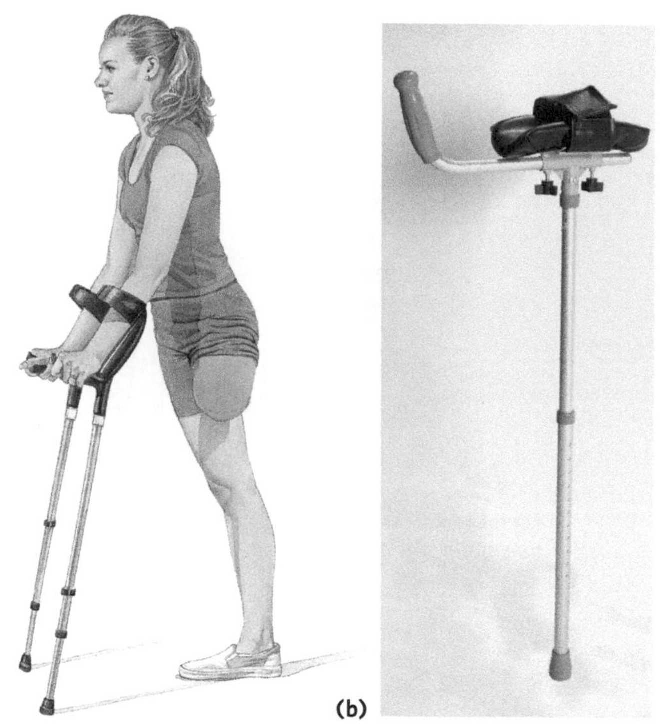

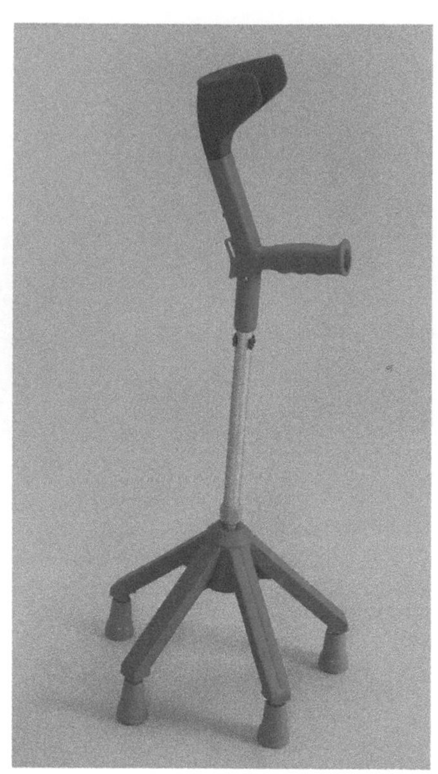

Figure 14-51 Types of crutches: (a) forearm; (b) arthritic; (c) children's quad crutch.
Source: (a) courtesy of the Krames Staywell Company; (b) and (c) © Patterson Medical Ltd.

TEACHING: PATIENT CARE

Using Crutches

- Follow the plan of exercises developed for you to strengthen your arm muscles before beginning crutch walking.
- Have a healthcare professional establish the correct length for your crutches and the correct placement of the hand-pieces. Crutches that are too long force your shoulders upward and make it difficult for you to push your body off the ground. Crutches that are too short will make you hunch over and develop an improper body stance.
- Maintain an erect posture as much as possible to prevent strain on muscles and joints and to maintain balance.
- Each step taken with crutches should be a comfortable distance for you. It is wise to start with a small rather than a large step.
- Inspect the crutch tips regularly, and replace them if worn.
- Keep the crutch tips dry and clean to maintain their surface friction. If the tips become wet, dry them well before use.
- Wear a shoe with a low heel that grips the floor. Rubber soles decrease the chances of slipping. Adjust shoelaces so they cannot come untied or reach the floor where they might catch on the crutches. Consider shoes with alternate forms of closure (e.g. Velcro), especially if you cannot easily bend to tie laces. Slip-on shoes are acceptable only if they are snug and the heel does not come loose when the foot is bent.

Measuring Patients for Crutches

When nurses measure patients for the forearm crutch, it is most important to obtain the correct length for the crutches and the correct placement of the hand piece.

To determine the correct placement of the hand bar:

1 The patient stands upright and supports the body weight by the hand grips of the crutches.
2 The nurse measures the height from the elbow crease to a point 15cm out from the side of the heel. This is the height that the crutches should be set.
3 The forearm piece should be measured 2.5cm from the elbow crease to a clenched fist. This section of the crutch should be adjusted accordingly.
4 The nurse should ensure that the cuff is adjusted so that it does not fall off the forearm.

Crutch Gaits

The crutch gait is the gait a person assumes on crutches by alternating body weight on one or both legs and the crutches. Five standard crutch gaits are the four-point gait, three-point gait, two-point gait, swing-to gait and swing-through gait. The gait used depends on the following individual factors: (a) the ability to take steps, (b) the ability to bear weight and keep balance in a standing position on both legs or only one, and (c) the ability to hold the body erect.

Patients also need instruction about how to get into and out of chairs and go up and down stairs safely. All of these crutch skills are best taught before the patient is discharged and preferably before the patient has surgery. This teaching is usually undertaken by an experienced clinician, e.g. a nurse, plaster technician or physiotherapist.

Crutch Stance (Tripod Position)

Before crutch walking is attempted, the patient needs to learn facts about posture and balance. The proper standing position with crutches is called the tripod (triangle) position (see Figure 14-52). The crutches are placed about 15cm in front of the feet and out laterally about 15cm, creating a wide base of support. The feet are slightly apart. A tall person requires a wider base than a short person does. Hips and knees are extended, the back is straight, and the head is held straight and high. There should be no hunch to the shoulders and thus no weight borne by the axillae. The elbows are extended sufficiently to allow weight-bearing on the hands. If the patient is unsteady, the nurse places a walking belt around the patient's waist and grasps the belt from above, not from below. A fall can be prevented more effectively if the belt is held from above.

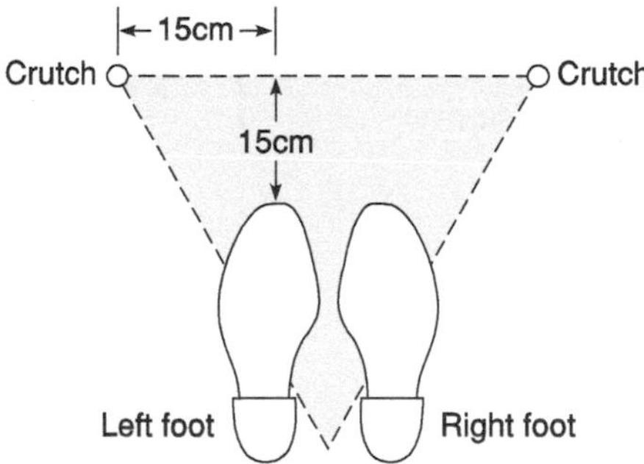

Figure 14-52 The tripod position.

Four-point Alternate Gait

This is the most elementary and safest gait, providing at least three points of support at all times, but it requires coordination. Patients can use it when walking in crowds because it does not require much space. To use this gait, the patient needs to be able to bear weight on both legs (see Figure 14-53, reading from bottom to top). The nurse asks the patient to:

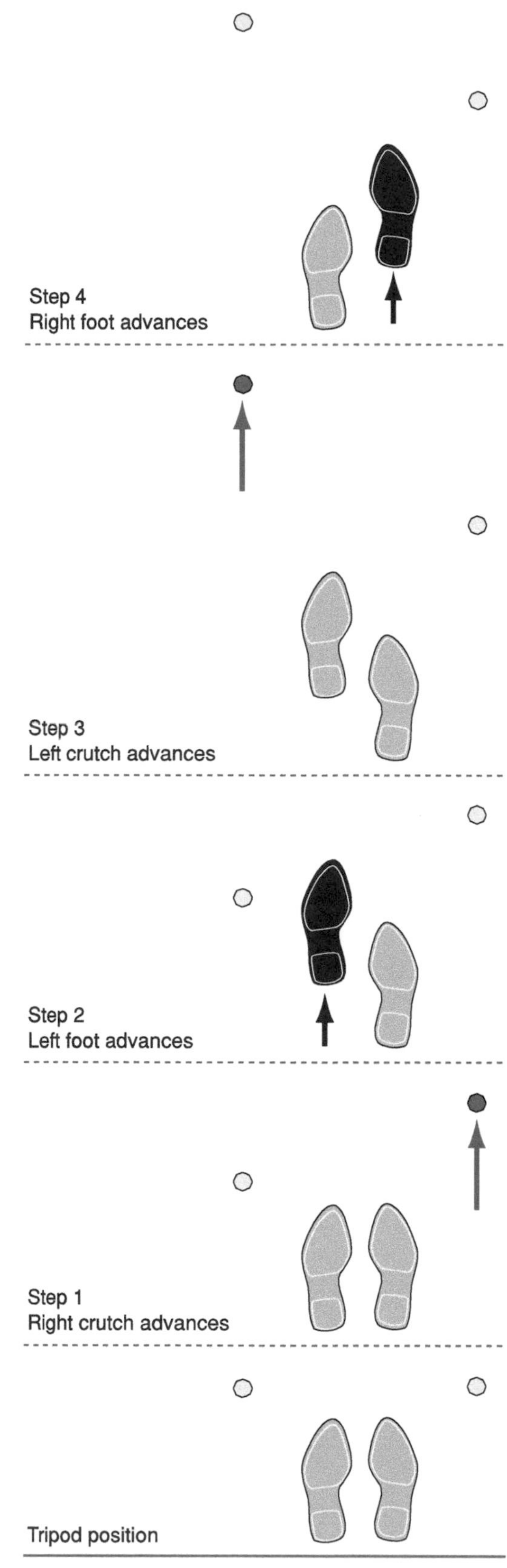

Figure 14-53 The four-point alternate crutch gait.

1 Move the right crutch ahead a suitable distance, such as 10–15cm.
2 Move the left front foot forward, preferably to the level of the left crutch.
3 Move the left crutch forward.
4 Move the right foot forward.

Three-point Gait

To use this gait, the patient must be able to bear the entire body weight on the unaffected leg. The two crutches and the unaffected leg bear weight alternately (see Figure 14-54, reading from bottom to top). The nurse asks the patient to:

1 Move both crutches and the weaker leg forward.
2 Move the stronger leg forward.

Two-point Alternate Gait

This gait is faster than the four-point gait. It requires more balance because only two points support the body at one time; it also requires at least partial weight-bearing on each foot. In this gait, arm movements with the crutches are similar to the arm movements during normal walking (see Figure 14-55, reading from bottom to top). The nurse asks the patient to:

1 Move the left crutch and the right foot forward together.
2 Move the right crutch and the left foot ahead together.

Swing-to Gait

The swing gaits are used by patients with paralysis of the legs and hips. Prolonged use of these gaits results in atrophy of the unused muscles. The swing-to gait is the easier of these two gaits. The nurse asks the patient to:

1 Move both crutches ahead together.
2 Lift body weight by the arms and swing to the crutches.

Swing-through Gait

This gait requires considerable skill, strength and coordination. The nurse asks the patient to:

1 Move both crutches forward together.
2 Lift body weight by the arms and swing through and beyond the crutch.

Getting into a Chair

Chairs that have armrests and are secure or braced against a wall are essential for patients using crutches. For this procedure, the nurse instructs the patient to:

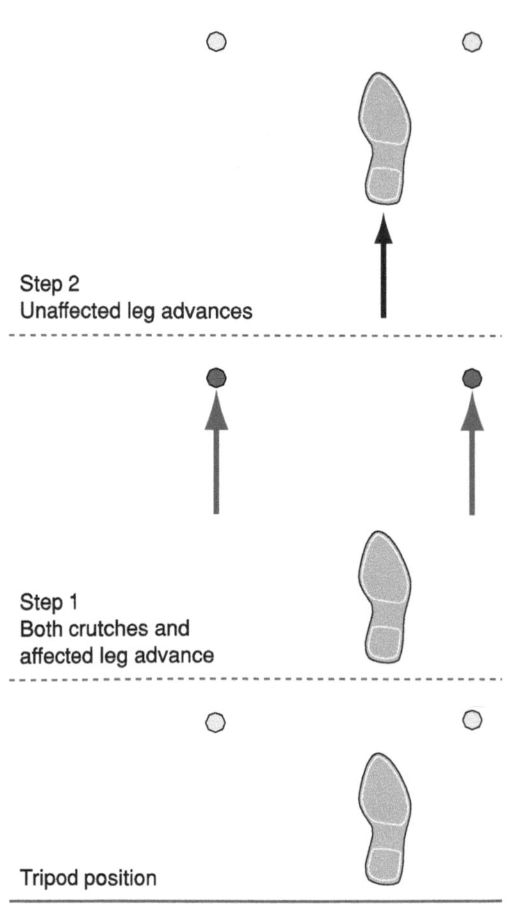

Figure 14-54 The three-point crutch gait.

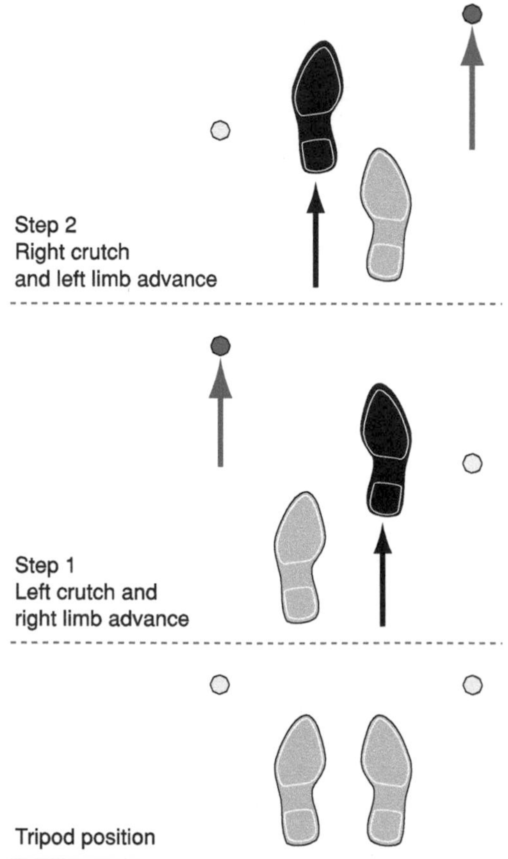

Figure 14-55 The two-point alternate crutch gait.

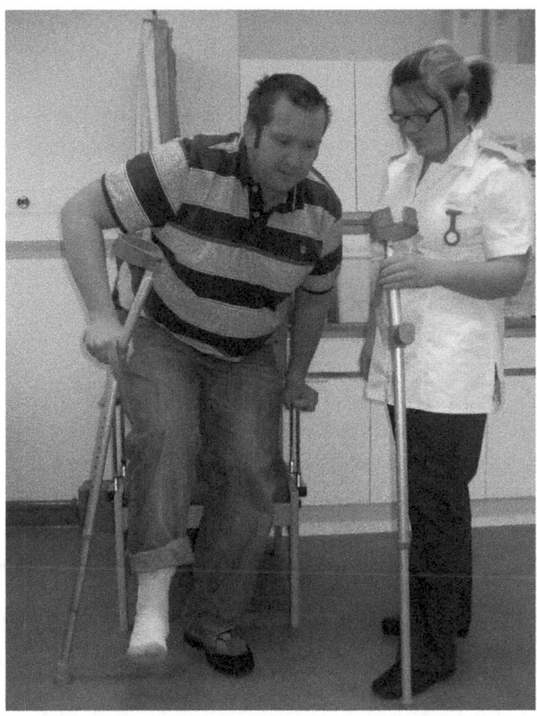

Figure 14-56 A patient using crutches getting into a chair.
Source: Heulwen Morgan-Samuel.

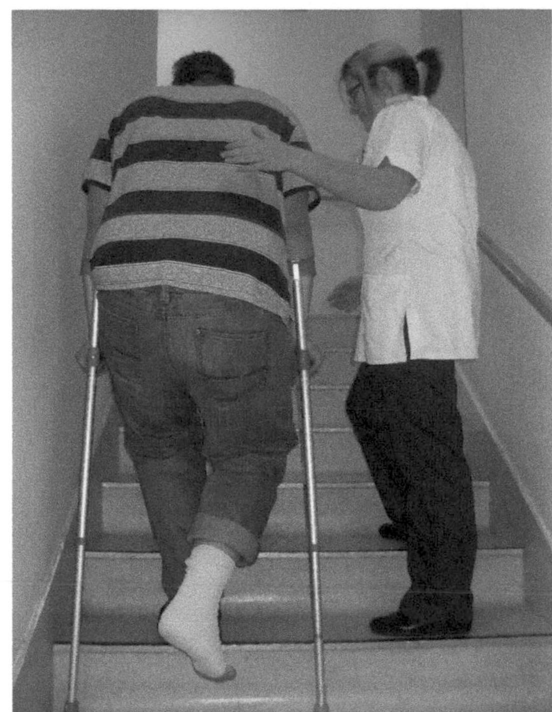

Figure 14-57 Climbing stairs: placing weight on the crutches while first moving the unaffected leg onto a step.
Source: Heulwen Morgan-Samuel.

1 Stand with the back of the unaffected leg centred against the chair. The chair helps support the patient during the next steps.
2 Transfer the crutches to the hand on the affected side and hold the crutches by the hand bars. The patient grasps the arm of the chair with the hand on the unaffected side (see Figure 14-56). This allows the patient to support the body weight on the arms and the unaffected leg.
3 Lean forward, flex the knees and hips, and lower into the chair.

Getting Out of a Chair

For this procedure, the nurse instructs the patient to:

1 Move forward to the edge of the chair and place the unaffected leg slightly under or at the edge of the chair. This position helps the patient stand up from the chair and achieve their balance, since the unaffected leg is supported against the edge of the chair.
2 Grasp the crutches by the hand bars in the hand on the affected side, and grasp the arm of the chair by the hand on the unaffected side. The body weight is placed on the crutches and the hand on the armrest to support the unaffected leg when the patient rises to stand.
3 Push down on the crutches and the chair armrest while elevating the body out of the chair.
4 Assume the tripod position before moving.

Going Up Stairs

For this procedure, the nurse stands behind the patient and slightly to the affected side if needed. The nurse instructs the patient to:

1 Assume the tripod position at the bottom of the stairs.
2 Transfer the body weight to the crutches and move the unaffected leg onto the step (see Figure 14-57).
3 Transfer the body weight to the unaffected leg on the step and move the crutches and affected leg up to the step. The affected leg is always supported by the crutches.
4 Repeat steps 2 and 3 until the patient reaches the top of the stairs.

Going Down Stairs

For this procedure, the nurse stands one step below the patient on the affected side if needed. The nurse instructs the patient to:

1 Assume the tripod position at the top of the stairs.
2 Shift the body weight to the unaffected leg, and move the crutches and affected leg down onto the next step (see Figure 14-58).
3 Transfer the body weight to the crutches, and move the unaffected leg to that step. The affected leg is always supported by the crutches.
4 Repeat steps 2 and 3 until the patient reaches the bottom of the stairs.

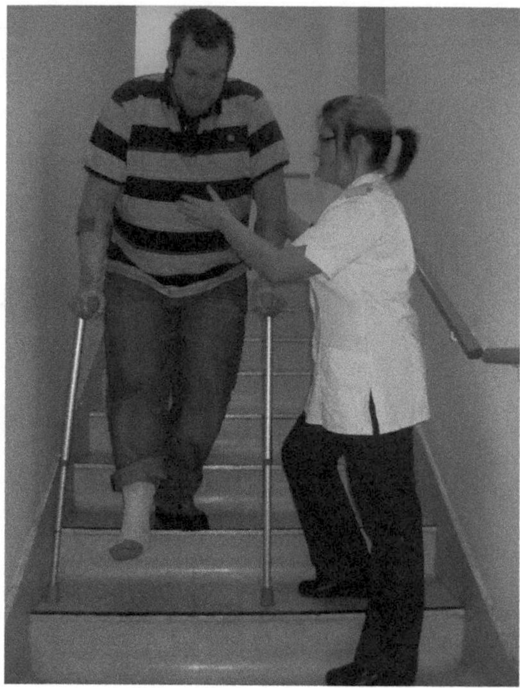

Figure 14-58 Descending stairs: moving the crutches and affected leg to the next step.
Source: Heulwen Morgan-Samuel.

EVALUATING

The goals established during the planning phase are evaluated according to specific desired outcomes, also established in that phase.

If outcomes are not achieved, the nurse, patient and support person if appropriate need to explore the reasons before modifying the care plan. For example, the following questions may be considered if an immobilised patient fails to maintain muscle mass and tone and joint mobility:

- Has the patient's physical or mental condition changed motivation to perform required exercise?
- Were appropriate range-of-motion exercises implemented?
- Was the patient encouraged to participate in self-care activities as much as possible?
- Was the patient encouraged to make as many decisions as possible when developing a daily activity plan and to express concerns?
- Did the nurse provide appropriate supervision and monitoring?
- Was the patient's diet adequate to provide appropriate nourishment for energy requirements?

REST AND SLEEP

Rest and sleep are essential for health and important following any strenuous activities. People who are ill frequently require more rest and sleep than usual. Often, debilitated individuals expend excessive amounts of energy to regain health or perform the activities of daily living. As a result, such people experience increased and frequent fatigue and need extra rest and sleep. Rest restores a person's energy, allowing the individual to resume optimal functioning. When people are deprived of rest, they are often irritable, depressed and tired, and they may have poor control over their emotions. Providing a restful environment for patients is an important function of nurses.

The meaning of rest and the need for rest vary among individuals. Rest implies calmness, relaxation without emotional stress and freedom from anxiety. Therefore, rest does not always imply inactivity; in fact, some people find certain activities such as walking in fresh air restful. When rest is prescribed for a patient, both nurse and patient must know whether the patient is to be inactive and whether that inactivity involves the whole body or a body part (e.g. an arm).

Sleep is a basic human need; it is a universal biological process common to all people. Historically, sleep was considered a state of unconsciousness. More recently, sleep has come to be considered an altered state of consciousness in which the individual's perception of and reaction to the environment are decreased. Sleep is characterised by minimal physical activity, variable levels of consciousness, changes in the body's physiological processes and decreased responsiveness to external stimuli. Some environmental stimuli, such as a smoke detector alarm, will usually awaken a sleeper, whereas other noises will not. It appears that individuals respond to meaningful stimuli while sleeping and selectively disregard unmeaningful stimuli.

PHYSIOLOGY OF SLEEP

The cyclic nature of sleep is thought to be controlled by centres located in the lower part of the brain. These centres actively inhibit wakefulness, thus causing sleep.

Circadian Rhythms

Biorhythms (rhythmic biological clocks) exist in plants, animals and humans. In humans, these are controlled from within the body and synchronised with environmental factors, such as light and darkness, gravity and electromagnetic stimuli. The most familiar biorhythm is the circadian rhythm. The term circadian is from the Latin *circa dies*, meaning 'about a day'.

Sleep is a complex biological rhythm. When a person's biological clock coincides with sleepwake patterns, the person is said to be in circadian synchronisation; that is, the person is awake when the physiological and psychological rhythms are most active and is asleep when the physiological and psychological rhythms are most inactive.

Circadian regularity begins by the third week of life and may be inherited. Babies are awake most often in the early morning and the late afternoon. After four months of age, infants enter a 24-hour cycle in which they sleep mostly during the night. By the end of the fifth or sixth month, infants' sleep wake patterns are almost like those of adults.

Stages of Sleep

The electroencephalogram (EEG) provides a good picture of what occurs during sleep. Electrodes are placed on various parts of the sleeper's scalp. The electrodes transmit electric energy from the cerebral cortex to pens that record the brain waves on graph paper.

Two types of sleep have been identified: NREM (non-REM) sleep and REM (rapid eye movement) sleep.

NREM Sleep

NREM sleep is also referred to as slow-wave sleep because the brain waves of a sleeper are slower than the alpha and beta waves of a person who is awake or alert. Most sleep during a night is NREM sleep. It is a deep, restful sleep and brings a decrease in some physiological functions. Basically, all metabolic process including vital signs, metabolism and muscle action slow.

NREM sleep is divided into four stages. *Stage I* is the stage of very light sleep. During this stage, the person feels drowsy and relaxed, the eyes roll from side to side, and the heart and respiratory rates drop slightly. The sleeper can be readily awakened and this stage lasts only a few minutes.

Stage II is the stage of light sleep during which body processes continue to slow down. The eyes are generally still, the heart and respiratory rates decrease slightly, and body temperature falls. Stage II lasts only about 10–15 minutes but constitutes 40–45% of total sleep.

During *Stage III*, the heart and respiratory rates, as well as other body processes, slow further because of the domination of the parasympathetic nervous system. The sleeper becomes more difficult to arouse. The person is not disturbed by sensory stimuli, the skeletal muscles are very relaxed, reflexes are diminished and snoring may occur.

Stage IV signals deep sleep, called delta sleep. The sleeper's heart and respiratory rates drop 20–30% below those exhibited during waking hours. The sleeper is very relaxed, rarely moves and is difficult to arouse. Stage IV is thought to restore the body physically. During this stage, the eyes usually roll, and some dreaming occurs.

REM Sleep

REM sleep usually recurs about every 90 minutes and lasts 5–30 minutes. REM sleep is not as restful as NREM sleep, and most dreams take place during REM sleep. Furthermore, these dreams are usually remembered; that is, they are consolidated in the memory.

During REM sleep, the brain is highly active, and brain metabolism may increase as much as 20%. This type of sleep is also called paradoxical sleep because it seems a paradox that sleep can take place simultaneously with this type of brain activity. In this phase, the sleeper may be difficult to arouse or may wake spontaneously, muscle tone is depressed, gastric secretions increase, and heart and respiratory rates often are irregular.

Sleep Cycles

During a sleep cycle, people pass through NREM and REM sleep, the complete cycle usually lasting about 1½ hours in adults. In the first sleep cycle, a sleeper passes through all of the first three NREM stages in a total of about 20–30 minutes. Then, Stage IV may last about 30 minutes. After Stage IV NREM, the sleep passes back through Stages III and II over about 20 minutes. Thereafter, the first REM stage occurs, lasting about 10 minutes, completing the first sleep cycle. The usual sleeper experiences four to six cycles of sleep during 7–8 hours (see Figure 14-59). The sleeper who is awakened during any stage must begin anew at Stage I NREM sleep and proceed through all the stages to REM sleep.

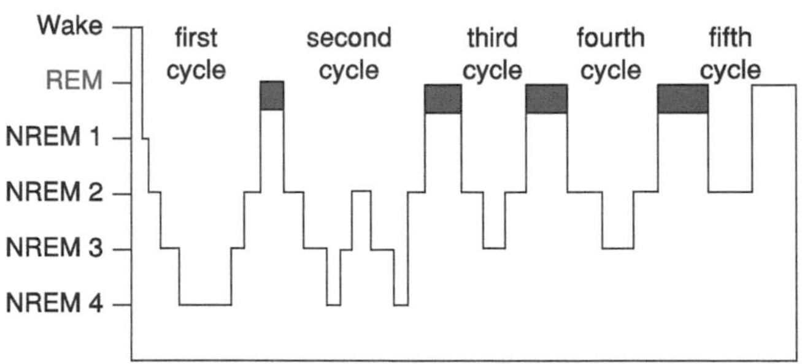

Figure 14-59 Time spent in REM and non-REM stages of sleep cycles.

The duration of NREM stages and REM sleep varies throughout the sleep period. As the night progresses, the sleeper becomes less tired and spends less time in Stages III and IV of NREM sleep. REM sleep increases and dreams tend to lengthen. If the sleeper is very tired, REM cycles are often short – for example, five minutes instead of 20 – during the early portion of sleep. Before sleep ends, periods of near wakefulness occur, and Stages I and II NREM sleep and REM sleep predominate.

FUNCTIONS OF SLEEP

The effects of sleep on the body are not completely understood. Sleep exerts physiological effects on both the nervous system and other body structures. Sleep in some way restores normal levels of activity and normal balance among parts of the nervous system. Sleep is also necessary for protein synthesis, which allows repair processes to occur.

The role of sleep in psychological well-being is best noticed by the deterioration in mental functioning related to sleep loss. Persons with inadequate amounts of sleep tend to become emotionally irritable, have poor concentration and experience difficulty making decisions.

NORMAL SLEEP PATTERNS AND REQUIREMENTS

It has been suggested that maintaining a regular sleep wake rhythm is more important than the number of hours actually slept. Some people, for example, can function well on as little as five hours of sleep each night. Re-establishing the sleep/wake rhythm (e.g. after the disruption of surgery) is an important aspect of nursing.

Newborns

Newborns sleep 16–18 hours a day, usually divided into about seven sleep periods. NREM sleep is characterised by regular respirations, closed eyes and the absence of body and eye movements. REM sleep has rapid eye movements that are observable through closed lids, body movement and irregular respirations. Most of the sleep time is spent in Stages III and IV of NREM sleep. Nearly 50% of sleep is REM.

Infants

Some infants sleep as long as 22 hours a day, others 12–14 hours a day. About 20–30% of sleep is REM sleep. At first, infants awaken every three or four hours, eat and then go back to sleep. Periods of wakefulness gradually increase during the first months. By four months, most infants sleep through the night and establish a pattern of daytime naps that varies among individuals. They generally awaken early in the morning, however. At the end of the first year, an infant usually takes one or two naps per day and sleeps about 14 of every 24 hours.

About half of the infant's sleep time is spent in light sleep. During light sleep, the infant exhibits a great deal of activity, such as movement, gurgles and coughing. Parents need to ascertain that infants are truly awake before picking them up for feeding and changing. Many infants begin waking up again in the middle of the night between five and nine months of age. For parents who find this behaviour a problem, the nurse needs to assess the infant's total sleep pattern and compare it with the parents' sleep schedule. Parents need reassurance that there is no one correct way to handle this situation. The best solution is one that provides a continuous healthy environment for both the infant and the parents.

Toddlers

The sleep requirements of toddlers decrease to 10–12 hours per day. About 20–30% is REM sleep. Most still need an afternoon nap, but the need for midmorning naps gradually decreases. The toddler's normal sleep/wake cycle is usually established by age two or three. The toddler may exhibit a great deal of resistance to going to bed. Parents need assurance that if the child has had adequate attention from them during the day, maintaining a consistent approach with respect to bedtime will promote good sleep habits for the entire family. The child who awakens at night may be afraid of the dark or have experienced night terrors or nightmares.

Pre-schoolers

The pre-school child usually requires 11–12 hours of sleep per night, particularly if the child is in pre-school. Sleep needs fluctuate in relation to activity and growth spurts. Many children of this age dislike bedtime and resist by requesting another story, game or television programme. The four- to five-year-old may become restless and irritable if sleep requirements are not met. A nap or quiet time during the day may be needed to restore energy levels.

Children in this age group still require bedtime rituals. Parents can help children who resist bedtime by warning them that bedtime is approaching and by continuing to use the same firm and consistent approach suggested for the toddler. Pre-school children wake up frequently at night. REM sleep is still 20–30% higher than for adults; however, Stage I sleep is less.

School-age Children

The school-age child sleeps 8–12 hours a night without daytime naps. The eight-year-old requires at least 10 hours of sleep each night. As the child approaches 11 or 12 years of age, less sleep is required and bedtime may be as late as 10 pm. The REM sleep of children at this age is reduced to about 20%. Although some children still experience night awakenings due to nightmares, this problem continues to decrease with age.

Adolescents

Most adolescents require 8–10 hours of sleep each night to prevent undue fatigue and susceptibility to infections. A change in sleep pattern is common in adolescence. Children who once were early risers begin to sleep late in the mornings and occasionally take afternoon naps. The reason for daytime sleeping is not fully understood, but it is possibly a result of physical maturity and reduced nocturnal sleep. Sleep at this age is about 20% REM.

During adolescence, boys begin to experience nocturnal emissions (orgasm and emission of semen during sleep), known as 'wet dreams', several times each month. Boys need to be informed about this normal development to prevent embarrassment and fear.

Young Adults

The sleep/wake cycle is very important to young adults. They usually have an active lifestyle, and are thought to require 7–8 hours of sleep each night but may do well on less.

Middle-aged Adults

Middle-aged adults generally maintain the sleep pattern established at a younger age. They usually sleep 6–8 hours per night. About 20% is REM sleep. The numbers of arousals from sleep increases and the amount of Stage IV sleep begins to decrease.

Mature Adults

The mature adult sleeps about six hours a night. About 20–25% is REM sleep. Stage IV sleep is markedly decreased and in some instances absent. The first REM period is longer. Many older adults awaken more often during the night and it often takes them longer to go back to sleep. Because of the change in Stage IV sleep, older people have less restorative sleep (see *Lifespan Considerations*).

Some mature adults may be said to have *Sundowner's syndrome*. Although not a sleep disorder directly, it refers to a confusional state that tends to appear at dusk (thus the name) and may happen because of a change in circadian rhythms (changes in the sleep/wake cycle), decreased sensory stimulation at the end of the day or a mental condition such as Alzheimer's disease.

FACTORS AFFECTING SLEEP

Both the quality and the quantity of sleep are affected by a number of factors. *Quality of sleep* refers to the individual's ability to stay asleep and to get appropriate amounts of REM and NREM sleep. *Quantity of sleep* is the total time the individual sleeps.

Illness

Illness that causes pain or physical distress can result in sleep problems. People who are ill require more sleep than normal, and the normal rhythm of sleep and wakefulness is often disturbed. People deprived of REM sleep subsequently spend more sleep time than normal in this stage.

Respiratory conditions can disturb an individual's sleep. Shortness of breath often makes sleep difficult, and people who have nasal congestion or sinus drainage may have trouble breathing and hence may find it difficult to sleep.

People who have gastric or duodenal ulcers may find their sleep disturbed because of pain, often a result of the increased gastric secretions that occur during REM sleep.

LIFESPAN CONSIDERATIONS

Mature Adults

The quality of sleep is often diminished in mature adults. Some of the leading factors that often are influential in sleep disturbances are:

- side-effects of medications;
- gastric reflux disease;
- respiratory and circulatory disorders, which may cause breathing problems or discomfort;
- pain from arthritis, increased stiffness, or impaired immobility;
- nocturia;
- depression;
- loss of life partner and/or close friends;
- disruptions of bedtime rituals/routines when a person is hospitalised or institutionalised;
- confusion related to delirium or dementia.

Interventions to promote sleep and rest can help enhance the rejuvenation and renewal that sleep provides. Rituals and routines that become the rhythm of one's life and have been performed for years are often disrupted by being hospitalised or institutionalised. The following interventions can help promote sleep and rest is follows:

- Maintain usual bedtime ritual, or develop a new one with the individual that will encourage relaxation or sleep, such as music, relaxation techniques and warm drinks.
- Be sure their environment is warm and safe, especially if they get out of bed during the night.
- Provide comfort measures, such as analgesics if indicated, and proper positioning.
- Enhance the sense of safety and security by checking on patients frequently and making sure that the call bell is within reach.
- If lack of sleep is caused by medications or certain health conditions, work on specific interventions related to these problems.
- Evaluate the situation and find out what the rest and sleep disturbances mean to the patient. They may not perceive sleeplessness to be a serious problem, but will just do other activities and sleep when tired.

Certain endocrine disturbances can also affect sleep. Hyperthyroidism lengthens presleep time, making it difficult for a patient to fall asleep. Hypothyroidism, conversely, decreases Stage IV sleep. Women with low levels of oestrogen often report excessive fatigue. In addition, they may experience sleep disruptions due, in part, to the discomfort associated with hot flushes or night sweats that can occur with reduced oestrogen levels.

Elevated body temperatures can cause some reduction in Stages III and IV NREM sleep and REM sleep.

The need to urinate during the night also disrupts sleep, and people who awaken at night to urinate sometimes have difficulty getting back to sleep.

Environment

Environment can promote or hinder sleep. Any change – for example, noise in the environment – can inhibit sleep. The absence of usual stimuli or the presence of unfamiliar stimuli can prevent people from sleeping. Stage I sleep is the lightest and Stages III and IV the deepest; as a result, louder noises are needed to awaken a person in Stages III and IV. However, over time people can be habituated to a noise so that the level has less effect.

Discomfort from environmental temperature and lack of ventilation can affect sleep. Light levels can be another factor.

A person accustomed to darkness while sleeping may find it difficult to sleep in the light.

Fatigue

It is thought that a person who is moderately fatigued usually has a restful sleep. Fatigue also affects a person's sleep pattern. The more tired the person is, the shorter the first period of paradoxical (REM) sleep. As the person rests, the REM periods become longer.

Lifestyle

A person who does shift work and changes shifts frequently must arrange activities to be ready to sleep at the right time. Moderate exercise usually is conducive to sleep, but excessive exercise can delay sleep. The person's ability to relax before retiring is an important factor affecting the ability to fall asleep.

Emotional Stress

Anxiety and depression frequently disturb sleep. A person preoccupied with personal problems may be unable to relax sufficiently to get to sleep. Anxiety increases the norepinephrine blood levels through stimulation of the sympathetic nervous system. This chemical change results in less Stage IV NREM and REM sleep and more stage changes and awakenings.

Stimulants and Alcohol

Caffeine-containing beverages act as stimulants of the central nervous system, thus interfering with sleep. People who drink an excessive amount of alcohol often find their sleep disturbed. Excessive alcohol disrupts REM sleep, although it may hasten the onset of sleep. While making up for lost REM sleep after some of the effects of the alcohol have worn off, people often experience nightmares. The alcohol-tolerant person may be unable to sleep well and become irritable as a result.

Diet

Weight loss has been associated with reduced total sleep time as well as broken sleep and earlier awakening. Weight gain, on the other hand, seems to be associated with an increase in total sleep time, less broken sleep and later waking. Dietary L-tryptophan – found, for example, in cheese and milk – may induce sleep, a fact that might explain why warm milk helps some people get to sleep.

Smoking

Nicotine has a stimulating effect on the body, and smokers often have more difficulty falling asleep than nonsmokers do. Smokers are usually easily aroused and often describe themselves as light sleepers. By refraining from smoking after the evening meal, the person usually sleeps better; moreover, many former smokers report that their sleeping patterns improved once they stopped smoking.

Motivation

The desire to stay awake can often overcome a person's fatigue. For example, a tired person can probably stay alert while attending an interesting concert. When a person is bored and is not motivated to stay awake, by contrast, sleep often readily ensues.

Medications

Some medications affect the quality of sleep. Hypnotics can interfere with Stages III and IV NREM sleep and suppress REM sleep. Beta-blockers have been known to cause insomnia and nightmares. Narcotics, such as morphine, which is known to suppress REM sleep and to cause frequent awakenings and drowsiness. Tranquillisers interfere with REM sleep. Amphetamines and antidepressants decrease REM sleep abnormally. A patient withdrawing from any of these drugs gets much more REM sleep than usual and as a result may experience upsetting nightmares.

COMMON SLEEP DISORDERS

Knowledge of common sleep disorders helps nurses obtain and recognise pertinent data. Sleep disorders may be categorised as parasomnias, primary disorders and secondary disorders.

Parasomnias

A **parasomnia** is behaviour that may interfere with sleep or that occurs during sleep. The *International Classification of Sleep Disorders* (American Sleep Disorders Association, 2005) subdivides parasomnias into arousal disorders (e.g. sleepwalking, sleep terrors), sleep wake transition disorders (e.g. sleep talking), parasomnias associated with REM sleep (e.g. nightmares) and others (e.g. bruxism). Examples of parasomnias are:

- *Bruxism.* Usually occurring during Stage II NREM sleep, this clenching and grinding of the teeth can eventually erode dental crowns and cause teeth to come loose.
- *Nocturnal enuresis.* Bed-wetting during sleep can occur in children over three years old. More males than females are affected. It often occurs 1–2 hours after falling asleep, when rousing from NREM Stages III to IV.
- *Nocturnal erections.* Nocturnal erections and emissions occur during REM sleep. They begin during adolescence and do not present a sleep problem.
- *Periodic limb movements disorder (PLMD).* In this condition, the legs jerk twice or three times per minute during sleep and is most common among older adults. This kicking motion can wake the individual and result in poor sleep. The condition may be treated with medications such as those otherwise used for Parkinson's disease. PLMD differs from restless leg syndrome (RLS), which occurs whenever the person is at rest, not just at night when sleeping. RLS may occur during pregnancy or be due to other medical problems that can be treated.
- *Sleeptalking.* Talking during sleep occurs during NREM sleep before REM sleep. It rarely presents a problem to the person unless it becomes troublesome to others.

- *Somnambulism*. Somnambulism (sleepwalking) occurs during Stages III and IV of NREM sleep. It is episodic and usually occurs 1–2 hours after falling asleep. Sleepwalkers tend not to notice dangers (e.g. stairs) and often need to be protected from injury.

Primary Sleep Disorders

Primary sleep disorders are those in which the person's sleep problem is the main disorder. These disorders include insomnia, hypersomnia, narcolepsy, sleep apnoea and sleep deprivation.

Insomnia

Insomnia, the most common sleep disorder, is the inability to obtain an adequate amount or quality of sleep. People suffering from insomnia do not feel refreshed on arising. There are three types of insomnia:

1 difficulty in falling asleep (initial insomnia);
2 difficulty in staying asleep because of frequent or prolonged waking (intermittent or maintenance insomnia);
3 early morning or premature waking (terminal insomnia).

Insomnia can result from physical discomfort but more often is a result of mental overstimulation due to anxiety. People who become habituated to drugs or who drink large quantities of alcohol are likely to have insomnia.

Treatment for insomnia frequently requires the patient to develop new behaviour patterns that induce sleep. The usefulness of sleeping medications is questionable. Such medications do not deal with the cause of the problem and their prolonged use can create drug dependencies.

Hypersomnia

Hypersomnia, the opposite of insomnia, is excessive sleep, particularly in the daytime. The afflicted person often sleeps until noon and takes many naps during the day. Hypersomnia can be caused by medical conditions, for example, central nervous system damage and certain kidney, liver or metabolic disorders, such as diabetic acidosis and hypothyroidism. In some instances, a person uses hypersomnia as a coping mechanism to avoid facing the responsibilities of the day.

Narcolepsy

Narcolepsy – from the Greek *narco*, meaning 'numbness' and *lepsis*, meaning 'seizure' – is a sudden wave of overwhelming sleepiness that occurs during the day; thus, it is referred to as a 'sleep attack'. Its cause is unknown, although it is believed to be a lack of the chemical hypocretin in the central nervous system that regulates sleep. Onset of symptoms tends to occur between ages 15 and 30. In narcoleptic attacks, sleep starts with the REM phase. Even though people who have narcolepsy sleep well at night, they nod off several times a day even when conversing with someone or driving a car. Narcolepsy historically has been controlled by central nervous system stimulants and antidepressants.

Sleep Apnoea

Sleep apnoea is the periodic cessation of breathing during sleep. This disorder needs to be assessed by a sleep expert, but it is often suspected when the person has loud snoring, frequent nocturnal awakenings, excessive daytime sleepiness, insomnia, morning headaches, intellectual deterioration, irritability or other personality changes, and physiological changes such as hypertension and cardiac **arrhythmias**. It is most frequent in men over 50 and in postmenopausal women.

The periods of apnoea, which last from 10 seconds to two minutes, occur during REM or NREM sleep. Frequency of episodes ranges from 50–600 per night. These apnoeic episodes drain the person of energy and lead to excessive daytime sleepiness.

Three common types of sleep apnoea are obstructive apnoea, central apnoea and mixed apnoea. Obstructive apnoea occurs when the structures of the pharynx or oral cavity block the flow of air. The person continues to try to breathe; that is, the chest and abdominal muscles move. The movements of the diaphragm become stronger and stronger until the obstruction is removed. Enlarged tonsils, a deviated nasal septum, nasal polyps and obesity predispose the individual to obstructive apnoea.

Central apnoea is thought to involve a defect in the respiratory centre of the brain. All actions involved in breathing, such as chest movement and airflow, cease. Patients who have brain stem injuries and muscular dystrophy, for example, often have central sleep apnoea. At this time, there is no available treatment. Mixed apnoea is a combination of central apnoea and obstructive apnoea.

An episode of sleep apnoea usually begins with snoring; thereafter, breathing ceases, followed by marked snorting as breathing resumes. Towards the end of each apnoeic episode, increased carbon dioxide levels in the blood cause the individual to wake.

Treatment for sleep apnoea can be directed at the cause of the apnoea. For example, enlarged tonsils may be removed. Other surgical procedures, including laser removal of excess tissue in the pharynx, reduce or eliminate snoring and may be effective in relieving the apnoea. In other cases, the use of a nasal continuous positive airway pressure (CPAP) device at night is effective in maintaining an open airway.

Sleep apnoea profoundly affects a person's work or school performance. In addition, prolonged sleep apnoea can cause a sharp rise in blood pressure and may lead to cardiac arrest. Over time, apnoeic episodes can cause cardiac arrhythmias, pulmonary hypertension and subsequent left-sided heart failure.

CLINICAL ALERT

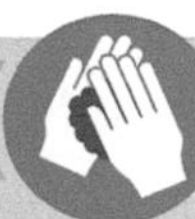

Partners of patients with sleep apnoea may become aware of the problem because they hear snoring that stops during the apnoea period and then restarts. Surgical removal of tonsils or other tissue in the pharynx, if not the cause of the sleep apnoea, can actually worsen the situation by removing the snoring and, thus, the warning that apnoea is occurring.

Table 14-4 Types, Causes and Signs of Sleep Deprivation

Type	Causes	Clinical signs
REM deprivation	Alcohol, barbiturates, shift work, jet lag, extended ICU hospitalisation, morphine	Excitability, restlessness, irritability and increased sensitivity to pain Confusion and suspiciousness Emotional instability
NREM deprivation	All the above plus diazepam (Valium), flurazepam hydrochloride, hypothyroidism, depression, respiratory distress disorders, sleep apnoea and age (common in the elderly)	Withdrawal, apathy, hypo-responsiveness Feeling physically uncomfortable Lack of facial expression Speech deterioration Excessive sleepiness
Both REM and NREM deprivation	As above	Decreased reasoning ability (judgement) and ability to concentrate Inattentiveness Marked fatigue: blurred vision, itchy eyes, nausea, headache Difficulty performing activities of daily living Lack of memory, mental confusion, visual or auditory hallucinations, illusions

Sleep Deprivation

A prolonged disturbance in amount, quality and consistency of sleep can lead to a syndrome referred to as sleep deprivation. This is not a sleep disorder in itself but a result of sleep disturbances. It produces a variety of physiological and behavioural symptoms, the severity of which depends on the degree of the deprivation. Two major types of sleep deprivation are REM deprivation and NREM deprivation. A combination of the two increases the severity of symptoms. Table 14-4 shows the causes and clinical signs of sleep deprivation.

Secondary Sleep Disorders

Secondary sleep disorders are sleep disturbances caused by other clinical conditions. They may be associated with mental, neurological or other conditions. Examples of conditions causing secondary sleep disorders include depression, alcoholism, dementia, Parkinsonism, thyroid dysfunction, chronic obstructive pulmonary disease and peptic ulcer disease.

ASSESSING PATIENT'S SLEEP

Assessment relative to a patient's sleep includes a sleep history, a sleep diary, a physical assessment, a review of diagnostic studies and a partner's observations regarding the patient's sleep pattern.

Sleep History

A brief general sleep history, which is usually part of the comprehensive patient history, is obtained for all patients on admission. This enables the nurse to incorporate the patient's needs and preferences in the plan of care. A general sleep history includes the following:

- Usual sleeping pattern, specifically sleeping and waking times; hours of undisturbed sleep; quality of or satisfaction with sleep (e.g. effect on energy level for daily functioning); and time and duration of naps.
- Bedtime rituals performed to help the person fall asleep (e.g. a glass of hot fluid, reading or other method of relaxing, and special equipment or positioning aids).
- Use of sleep medication and other drugs. Sleep can be disturbed by a variety of drugs, such as stimulants or steroids, if they are taken close to bedtime. Hypnotics and sedating antidepressants may cause excessive daytime sleepiness.
- Sleep environment (e.g. dark room, cool or warm temperature, noise level, night-light).
- Recent changes in sleep patterns or difficulties in sleeping.

If the patient indicates a recent pattern change or difficulties in sleeping, a more detailed history is required. This detailed history should explore the exact nature of the problem and its cause, when it first began and its frequency, how it affects daily living, what the patient is doing to cope with the problem, and whether these methods have been effective. Questions the nurse might ask the patient with a sleeping disturbance are shown in the *Assessment Interview* below.

Sleep Diary

Sometimes patients with a sleeping problem can provide more precise information if they keep a written record of their sleep pattern and the habits associated with it. Such a sleep diary or log can be kept by patients who are sleeping at home and should be maintained for at least a week. A sleep diary may include all or selected aspects of the following information that pertain to the patient's specific problem:

- total number of sleep hours per day;
- activities performed 2–3 hours before bedtime (type, duration and time);
- bedtime rituals (e.g. ingestion of food, fluid or medication) before going to bed;

- time of (a) going to bed, (b) trying to fall asleep, (c) falling asleep (approximate), (d) any instances of waking up and duration of these periods and (e) waking up in the morning;
- any worries that the patient believes may affect sleep;
- factors that the patient believes have a positive or negative effect on sleep.

ASSESSMENT INTERVIEW

Sleep Disturbances

- How would you describe your sleeping problem? What changes have occurred in your sleeping pattern? How often does this happen?
- Do you have difficulty falling asleep?
- Do you wake up often during the night? If so, how often?
- Do you wake up earlier in the morning than you would like and have difficulty falling back to sleep?
- How do you feel when you wake up in the morning?
- Do you sleep more than usual? If so, how often do you sleep?
- Do you have periods of overwhelming tiredness? If so, when does this happen?
- Have you ever suddenly fallen asleep in the middle of a daytime activity? If so, has any muscle weakness or paralysis occurred?
- Has anyone ever told you that you snore, walk in your sleep, talk in your sleep, or stop breathing for a while when sleeping?
- What have you been doing to deal with this sleeping problem? Does it help?
- What do you think might be causing this problem? Do you have any medical condition that might be causing you to sleep more (or less)? Are you receiving medications for an illness that might alter your sleeping pattern? Are you experiencing any stressful or upsetting events or conflicts that may be affecting your sleep?
- How is your sleeping problem affecting you?

Keeping such a diary may become stressful for some patients and further affect their sleep. The nurse needs to advise the patient to obtain the assistance of a bed partner in keeping the diary or to discontinue the diary if it presents a problem. When a diary is completed, the nurse and patient can develop flow charts or graphs that will assist in organising the data and identifying the specific problem.

Physical Assessment

Examination of the patient includes observation of the patient's facial appearance, behaviour and energy level. Darkened areas around the eyes, puffy eyelids, reddened conjunctiva, glazed or dull-appearing eyes and limited facial expression are indicative of sleep insufficiency. Behaviours such as irritability, restlessness, inattentiveness, slowed speech, slumped posture, hand tremor, yawning, rubbing the eyes, withdrawal, confusion and uncoordination are also suggestive of sleep problems. Lack of energy may be noted by observing whether the patient appears physically weak, lethargic or fatigued.

In addition, the nurse assesses whether the patient has a deviated nasal septum, enlarged neck or is obese. These findings may be associated with obstructive sleep apnoea or snoring.

Diagnostic Studies

Sleep is measured objectively in a sleep disorder laboratory by polysomnography: an electroencephalogram (EEG), electromyogram (EMG) and electro-oculogram (EOG) are recorded simultaneously. Electrodes are placed on the centre of the scalp to record brain waves (EEG), on the outer canthus of each eye to record eye movement (EOG) and on the chin muscles to record the structural electromyogram (EMG). The following may also be monitored, depending on findings of the initial interview: respiratory effort and airflow, ECG, leg movements and oxygen saturation. Oxygen saturation is determined by monitoring with a pulse oximeter, a light-sensitive electric cell that attaches to the ear or a finger. Oxygen saturation and ECG assessments are of particular importance if sleep apnoea is suspected. Through polysomnography, the patient's activity (movements, struggling, noisy respirations) during sleep can be assessed. Such activity of which the patient is unaware may be the cause of arousal during sleep.

PLANNING

The major goal for patients with sleep disturbances are to maintain (or develop) a sleeping pattern that provides sufficient energy for daily activities. Other goals may relate to enhancing the patient's feeling of well-being or improving the quality (as opposed to the quantity) of the patient's sleep. The nurse plans specific nursing interventions to reach the goal based on the aetiology of each nursing problem. These interventions may include reducing environmental distractions, promoting bedtime rituals, providing comfort measures, scheduling nursing care to provide for uninterrupted sleep periods, and teaching stress reduction, relaxation techniques or ways to develop good sleep habits.

IMPLEMENTING

Nursing interventions to enhance the quantity and quality of patients' sleep involve largely non-pharmacological measures. These involve health teaching about sleep habits, support of bedtime rituals, the provision of a restful environment, specific measures to promote comfort and relaxation, and essential considerations about the use of sleep medications.

For hospitalised patients, sleep problems are often related to the hospital environment or their illness. Assisting the patient to sleep in such instances can be challenging to a nurse, often involving scheduling activities, administering analgesics and providing a supportive environment. Explanations and a supportive relationship are essential for the fearful or anxious patient.

Patient Teaching

Healthy individuals need to learn the importance of rest and sleep in maintaining active and productive lifestyles. They need to learn (a) the conditions that promote sleep and those that interfere with sleep, (b) safe use of sleep medications, (c) effects of other prescribed medications on sleep, and (d) effects of their disease states on sleep. Patient teaching for promoting sleep is shown in *Teaching: Wellness Care.*

Supporting Bedtime Rituals

Most people are accustomed to bedtime rituals or pre-sleep routines that are conducive to comfort and relaxation. Altering or eliminating such routines can affect an individual's sleep. Common pre-bedtime activities of adults include an evening stroll, listening to music, watching television, taking a soothing bath and praying. Children, too, are socialised into pre-sleep routines such as a bedtime story, holding onto a favourite toy or blanket, and kissing everyone goodnight. Sleep is also usually preceded by hygienic routines, such as washing the face and hands (or bathing), brushing the teeth and voiding.

In institutional settings, nurses can provide similar bedtime rituals – assisting with a hand and face wash, hot drink, plumping of pillows and providing extra blankets as needed. Conversing about accomplishments of the day or enjoyable events such as visits from friends can also help to relax patients and bring peace of mind.

Creating a Restful Environment

All people need a sleeping environment with minimal noise, a comfortable room temperature, appropriate ventilation and appropriate lighting. Although most people prefer a darkened environment, a low light source may provide comfort for children or those in a strange environment. Infants and children need a quiet room usually separate from the parents' room, a light or warm blanket as appropriate, and a location away from open windows or drafts.

TEACHING: WELLNESS CARE

Promoting Rest and Sleep

Sleep Pattern

- Establish a regular bedtime and wake-up time for all days of the week to prevent disruptions in your biological rhythm. Eliminate lengthy naps, or if a daytime nap is necessary, take it at the same time each day and limit the time to 30 minutes, preferably once a day.
- Get adequate exercise during the day to reduce stress, but avoid excessive physical exertion two hours before bedtime.
- Avoid dealing with office work or family problems before bedtime.
- Establish a regular routine before sleep such as reading, listening to soft music, taking a warm bath or doing some other quiet activity you enjoy.
- When you are unable to sleep, pursue some relaxing activity until you feel drowsy.
- If you have trouble falling asleep, get up and pursue nonstrenuous activity until you feel sleepy.
- Use the bed mainly for sleep, so that you associate it with sleep.

Environment

- Ensure appropriate lighting, temperature and ventilation.
- Keep noise to a minimum; block out extraneous noise as necessary with soft music.

Diet

- Avoid heavy meals three hours before bedtime.
- Avoid alcohol and caffeine-containing foods and beverages (coffee, tea, chocolate) at least four hours before bedtime. Caffeine can interfere with sleep and both caffeine and alcohol act as diuretics, creating the need to void during sleep time.
- Decrease fluid intake 2–4 hours before sleep if necessary to avoid the need to use the bathroom during sleeping hours.
- If a bedtime snack is necessary, consume only light carbohydrates or a milk drink. Heavy or spicy foods can cause gastrointestinal upsets that disturb sleep.

Medications

- Use sleeping medications only as a last resort. Use over-the-counter medications sparingly because many contain antihistamines that cause daytime drowsiness.
- Take analgesics before bedtime to relieve aches and pains.
- Consult with your healthcare provider about adjusting other medications that may cause insomnia.

Environmental distractions such as environmental noises and staff communication noise are particularly troublesome for hospitalised patients. Environmental noises include the sound, telephones and call lights/buzzers; doors closing; elevator chimes; furniture squeaking; and linen trolleys being wheeled through corridors. Staff communication is a major factor creating noise, particularly at staff change of shift.

To create a restful environment, the nurse needs to reduce environmental distractions, reduce sleep interruptions, ensure a safe environment and provide a room temperature that is satisfactory to the patient. Some interventions to reduce environmental distractions, especially noise, may be practised.

The environment must also be safe so that the patient can relax. People who are unaccustomed to narrow hospital beds may feel more secure with side rails. Providing the patient with a night lamp and/or call bell may also help.

Promoting Comfort and Relaxation

Comfort measures are essential to help the patient fall asleep and stay asleep, especially if the effects of the person's illness interfere with sleep. A concerned, caring attitude, along with the following interventions, can significantly promote patient comfort and sleep:

- Provide loose-fitting nightwear.
- Assist patients with hygienic routines.
- Make sure the bed linen is smooth, clean and dry.
- Assist or encourage the patient to void before bedtime.
- Position dependent patients appropriately to aid muscle relaxation, and provide supportive devices to protect pressure areas.
- Schedule medications, especially diuretics, to prevent nocturnal awakenings.
- For patients who have pain, administer analgesics 30 minutes before sleep.
- Listen to the patient's concerns and deal with problems as they arise.

Emotional stress obviously interferes with a person's ability to relax, rest and sleep, and inability to sleep further aggravates feelings of tension. Sleep rarely occurs until a person is relaxed. Relaxation techniques can be encouraged as part of the nightly routine. Slow, deep breathing for a few minutes followed by slow, rhythmic contraction and relaxation of muscles can alleviate tension and induce calm. Imagery, meditation and yoga can also be taught.

Enhancing Sleep with Medications

Sleep medications often prescribed on a prn (as-needed) basis for patients include the sedative-hypnotics, which induce sleep, and anti-anxiety drugs or tranquillisers, which decrease anxiety and tension. When prn sleep medications are prescribed in institutional settings, the nurse is responsible for making decisions with the patient about when to administer them. These medications should be administered only with complete knowledge of their actions and effects and only when indicated. Whenever possible, nonpharmacological interventions to induce and maintain sleep, discussed earlier, are the preferred interventions.

Both nurses and patients need to be aware of the actions, effects, and risks of the specific medication prescribed. Although medications vary in their activity and effects, considerations include the following:

Sedative-hypnotic medications produce a general central nervous system (CNS) depression and an unnatural sleep; REM or NREM sleep is altered to some extent and daytime drowsiness and a morning hangover effect may occur.

- Anti-anxiety medications decrease levels of arousal by facilitating the action of neurons in the CNS that suppress responsiveness to stimulation. These medications are contraindicated in pregnant women because of their associated risk of congenital anomalies, and in nursing mothers because the medication is excreted in breast milk.
- Sleep medications vary in their onset and duration of action and will impair waking function as long as they are chemically active. Some medication effects can last many hours beyond the time that the patient's perceptions of daytime drowsiness and impaired psychomotor skills have disappeared. Patients need to be cautioned about such effects and about driving or handling machinery while the drug is in their system.
- Sleep medications affect REM sleep more than NREM sleep. Patients need to be informed that one or two nights of increased dreaming (REM rebound) are usual after the drug is discontinued.
- Initial doses of medications should be low and increases added gradually, depending on the patient's response. Mature adults, in particular, are susceptible to side-effects because of their metabolic changes; they need to be closely monitored for changes in mental alertness and coordination. Patients need to be instructed to take the smallest effective dose and then only for a few nights or intermittently as required.
- Regular use of any sleep medication can lead to tolerance over time (e.g. four weeks) and rebound insomnia. In some instances, this may lead patients to increase the dosage. Patients must be cautioned about developing a pattern of drug dependency.
- Abrupt cessation of barbiturate sedative-hypnotics can create withdrawal symptoms such as restlessness, tremors, weakness, insomnia, increased heart rate, seizures, convulsions and even death. Long-term users need to taper withdrawal by about 25–30% weekly.

EVALUATING

Using data collected during care and the desired outcomes developed during the planning stage as a guide, the nurse judges whether patient goals and outcomes have been achieved. Data collection may include (a) observations of the duration of the patient's sleep and the presence of signs of REM and NREM sleep and (b) questions about how the patient feels on awakening, or about the effectiveness of specific interventions such as the use of relaxation techniques, adherence to a consistent sleep wake cycle or the ingestion of milk products before bedtime.

If the desired outcomes are not achieved, the nurse, patient and support people if appropriate should explore the reasons, which may include answers to the following questions:

- Were etiological factors correctly identified?
- Has the patient's physical condition or medication therapy changed?

- Did the patient comply with instructions about establishing a regular sleep wake pattern?
- Did the patient avoid ingesting caffeine?
- Did the patient participate in stimulating daytime activities to avoid excessive daytime naps?
- Were all possible measures taken to provide a restful environment for the patient?
- Were bedtime rituals supported?
- Were the comfort and relaxation measures effective?

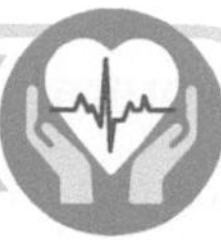

CRITICAL REFLECTION

On reading this chapter you should now be able to understand the importance of ensuring that Richard is discharged home safely. Reflect back on the information provided within this chapter and using the nursing process discuss the plan of care that would ensure that Richard is discharged safely into the community. Some points to consider within your reflection are as follows:

- physical and cognitive assessment - range of movements
- height, weight, gait
- education (e.g. management and moving with crutches)

CHAPTER HIGHLIGHTS

- The ability to move freely, easily and purposefully in the environment is essential for people to meet their basic needs.
- Purposeful coordinated movement of the body relies on the integrated functioning of the musculoskeletal system, the nervous system and the vestibular apparatus of the inner ear.
- Body movement involves four basic elements: body alignment, joint mobility, balance and coordinated movement.
- People maintain alignment and balance when the line of gravity passes through the centre of gravity and the base of support.
- The broader the base of support and the lower the centre of gravity, the greater the stability and balance achieved.
- Exercise is physical activity performed to maintain muscle tone and joint mobility, to enhance physiologic functioning of body systems and to improve physical fitness. Activity tolerance is the type and amount of exercise or daily living activities an individual is able to perform without experiencing adverse effects.
- Exercise is classified as either isotonic, isometric or isokinetic and as either aerobic or anaerobic.
- Many factors influence body alignment and activity. These include growth and development, physical health, mental health, personal values and attitudes, and prescribed limitations to movement.
- Immobility affects almost every body organ and system adversely; complications also include psychosocial problems. Exercise, by contrast, provides many benefits to the same body organs and systems.
- Problems of immobility include disuse osteoporosis and atrophy; contractures; diminished cardiac reserve; orthostatic hypotension; venous stasis, oedema and thrombus formation; decreased respiratory movement and pooling of secretions; decreased metabolic rate and negative nitrogen balance; urinary stasis, retention and infection; constipation; and varying emotional reactions.
- The nurse has responsibilities (a) to prevent the complications of immobility and reduce the severity of any problems resulting from immobility and (b) to design exercise programmes for patients that promote wellness.
- Assessment relative to a patient's mobility and exercise includes a nursing assessment and physical examination of body alignment, gait, joint appearance and movement, capabilities and limitations for movement, muscle mass and strength, activity tolerance, and problems related to immobility.
- A mobility and exercise history includes daily activity level, activity tolerance, type and frequency of exercise, and factors affecting mobility.
- Body mechanics is the efficient, coordinated and safe use of the body to move objects and carry out the activities of daily living.
- Preambulatory exercises that strengthen the muscles for walking are essential for patients who have been immobilised for a prolonged period.
- Sleep is a naturally occurring altered state of consciousness in which a person's perception and reaction to the environment are decreased.
- Rest and sleep are restorative, protective and energy conserving.
- The sleep cycle is controlled by specialised areas in the brain stem and is affected by the individual's circadian rhythm.
- During a normal night's sleep, an adult has four to six sleep cycles, each with NREM (quiet sleep) and REM (rapid eye movement) sleep.
- REM sleep recurs about every 90 minutes, is less restful than NREM sleep and is often associated with dreaming.

- Many factors can affect sleep, including illness, environment, fatigue, lifestyle, emotional stress, stimulants and alcohol, diet, smoking, motivation and medications.
- Common sleep disorders include parasomnias (such as bruxism, nocturnal enuresis, sleeptalking and somnambulism), insomnia, hypersomnia, narcolepsy, sleep apnoea and sleep deprivation.
- Assessment of an individual's sleep includes obtaining a sleep history, reviewing a sleep diary, and conducting a physical examination to detect signs of sleep deprivation.
- Nursing responsibilities to help patients sleep include (a) teaching patients ways to enhance sleep and rest, (b) supporting bedtime rituals, (c) creating a restful environment, (d) promoting comfort and relaxation, and (e) using prescribed sleep medications.
- Nonpharmacological interventions to induce and maintain sleep are always the preferred interventions.

ACTIVITY ANSWERS

ACTIVITY 14-1

- The lifespan of an adult is from birth to death and during this lifespan consideration and attention should be paid to both intrinsic and extrinsic factors that can affect physical activity in any way.
- In relation to physical activity there are many physical activities that are affected by physical, medical and other influences (e.g. physical activity is influenced by the individual's age and mobility, cognitive activity is influenced by age, understanding and comprehension while medical history is essential to understanding the physical activity of an individual. Many of these can be assessed during admission or observed at each visit.

REFERENCES

American Sleep Disorders Association (2005) *The international classification of sleep disorders: Diagnostic and coding manual* (2nd edn), Westchester, Ill.: American Academy of Sleep Medicine.

Gordon, M. (2007) *Manual of nursing diagnosis* (11th edn), Sudbury, MA, London: Jones and Bartlett.

NHS (2010) *NHS Choices – Sudden infant death syndrome*, London: NHS.

World Health Organization (2010) *Global recommendations on physical activity for health*, Switzerland: World Health Organization.

FURTHER RESOURCES

http://www.who.int/dietphysicalactivity/pa/en/index.html

CHAPTER 15

VITAL SIGNS

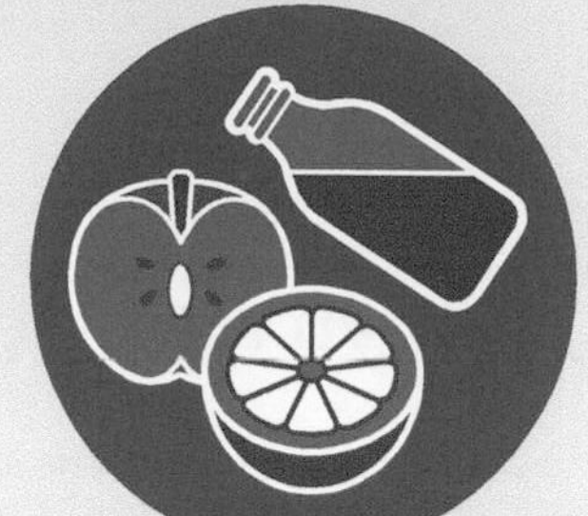

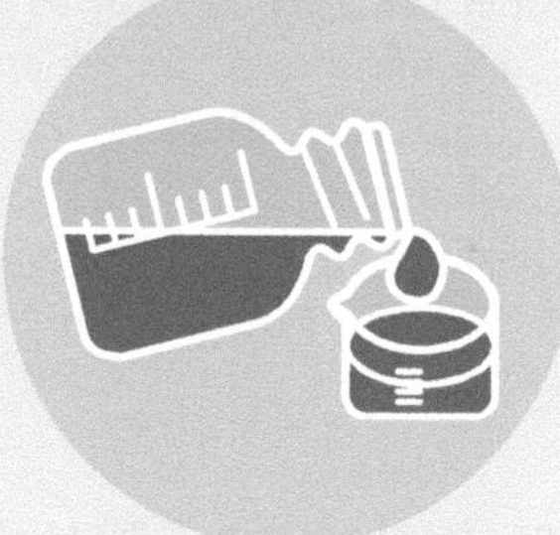

LEARNING OUTCOMES

After completing this chapter, you will be able to:

- Describe factors that affect the vital signs and accurate measurement of them.
- Identify the normal ranges for each vital sign.
- Identify the variations in normal body temperature, pulse, respirations and blood pressure that occur from infancy to old age.
- Compare oral, tympanic, rectal and axillary methods of measuring body temperature.
- Describe appropriate nursing care for alterations in body temperature.
- List the characteristics that should be included when assessing pulses.
- Explain how to measure the apical pulse and the apical-radial pulse.
- Describe the mechanics of breathing and the mechanisms that control respirations.
- Identify the components of a respiratory assessment.
- Differentiate systolic from diastolic blood pressure.
- Describe five phases of Korotkoff's sounds.
- Describe various methods and sites used to measure blood pressure.
- Discuss measurement of blood oxygenation using pulse oximetry.
- Discuss the relevance of lifespan considerations when taking and recording vital signs in relation to risk and patient safety.
- Demonstrate the importance of effective communication with both the patient and clinicians.

After reading this chapter you will be able to reflect on the nursing role in the unwell patient by clinical observation and recording of vital signs. Clearly understanding the difference between normal and abnormal readings relevant to age, sex and other internal and external factors. The chapter relates to **Essential Skills Clusters (NMC, 2010) 1, 2, 3, 4, 5, 6, 7 and 12**, as appropriate for each progression point.

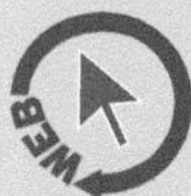

Ensure that you really understand this chapter by logging on to your complimentary **MyNursingKit** at **www.pearsoned.co.uk/kozier**. Complete the self-assessment tests to check your progress and utilise further activities to practise and confirm your understanding.

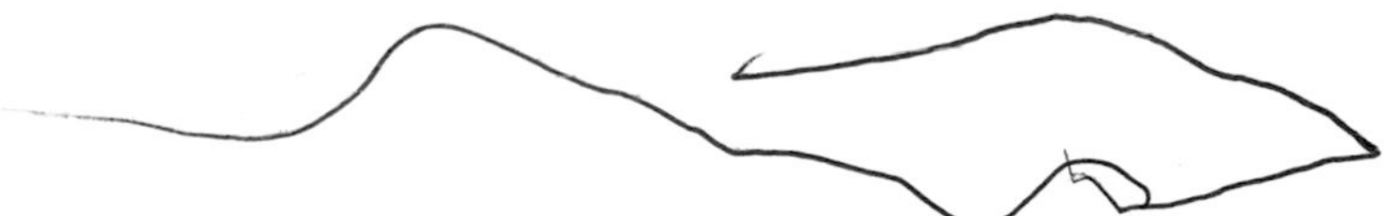

CASE STUDY

Abdullah is a 75-year-old gentleman who has been admitted to your care following several episodes of falling and confusion at home. His wife Bushra has been very concerned about him lately and has asked him to visit his GP on several occasions. However, following a home visit, Abdullah's GP has requested that Abdullah is admitted to hospital for an assessment as he has found that his blood pressure was 95/60 and his oxygen saturation levels were 85%. Both his respiratory and pulse rate are also elevated at this point. Abdullah is confused and has no concept of date or time and is demonstrating verbal signs of slight aggression.

INTRODUCTION

Vital signs are the physiological measures nurses record in clinical situations to assess the clinical status of patients in their care and to monitor for changes. The vital signs include body temperature, pulse, respirations and blood pressure and increasingly, pulse oximetry, or oxygen sats as they are more colloquially referred to, which are a measurement of the amount of oxygen the blood is carrying. These signs, which should be looked at in total, are checked to monitor the functions of the body. The signs reflect changes in function that otherwise might not be observed. Monitoring a patient's vital signs should not be an automatic or routine procedure; it should be a thoughtful, scientific assessment. Vital signs, which should be evaluated with reference to the patient's present and prior health status, are compared to the patient's usual 'base line' (if known) and accepted normal standards (see Table 15-1).

When and how often to assess a specific patient's vital signs are chiefly nursing judgements, depending on the patient's health status. It is important to recognise that many hospitals or healthcare organisations have policies and guidelines that are specific in the time and duration of recording vital signs, e.g. post surgery, during chemotherapy treatments, etc. However, this important role of the nurse often relies on clinical observation, judgement and often intuition. Examples of times to assess vital signs are:

- When the patient initially presents themselves to a clinical area or during the initial visit to the patient's home or care home to obtain baseline data.
- When a patient has a change in health status or reports symptoms such as chest pain or feeling hot, dizzy or faint.
- Before and after surgical intervention or an invasive procedure.
- Before and/or after the administration of a medication that could affect the respiratory or cardiovascular systems; for example, before giving a digitalis preparation (Digoxin).
- Before and after any nursing intervention that could affect the vital signs (e.g. mobilising a patient who has been on bed rest).

The taking and recording of these routine vital signs is more often carried out by a non-registered or student nurse. Therefore, it is important that the nurse is confident that the delegated person has the knowledge and skills to record and document this information accurately. The delegated person, e.g. student nurse, must also be aware that the findings should be reported to the registered nurse if the patient presents with readings that are outside the normal for that person. There are many different types of charts to record this information and many healthcare organisations now have a risk assessment included on the charts that easily identifies any changes in patient condition, e.g. the modified early warning score (MEWS).

CLINICAL ALERT

Normal vital signs change with age, sex, weight, exercise tolerance and condition, and the ones illustrated in Table 15-1 may vary slightly from other tables.

Table 15-1 Variations in Normal Vital Signs by Age

Age	Oral temperature in degrees celsius	Pulse (average and ranges)	Respirations (average and ranges)	Blood pressure (mm Hg)
Newborns	36.8 (axillary)	130 (80-180)	35 (30-80)	73/55
1 year	36.8 (axillary)	120 (80-140)	30 (20-40)	90/55
5-8 years	37	100 (75-120)	20 (15-25)	95/57
10 years	37	70 (50-90)	19 (15-25)	102/62
Teen	37	75 (50-90)	18 (15-20)	120/80
Adult	37	80 (60-100)	16 (12-20)	120/80
Older adult (>70 years)	37	70 (60-100)	16 (15-20)	Possible increased diastolic

BODY TEMPERATURE

Body temperature reflects the balance between the heat produced and the heat lost from the body, measured in heat units called *degrees*. There are two kinds of body temperature: core temperature and surface temperature. **Core temperature** is the temperature of the deep tissues of the body, such as the abdominal cavity and pelvic cavity. It remains relatively constant. The normal core body temperature is a range of temperatures (see Figure 15-1). The surface temperature is the temperature of the skin, the subcutaneous tissue and fat. It, by contrast, rises and falls in response to the environment.

The body continually produces heat as a by-product of metabolism. When the amount of heat produced by the body equals the amount of heat lost, the person is in heat balance (see Figure 15-2).

A number of factors affect the body's heat production. The most important are these five:

1 *Basal metabolic rate.* The basal metabolic rate (BMR) is the rate of energy utilisation in the body required to maintain essential activities such as breathing. Metabolic rates decrease with age. In general, the younger the person, the higher the BMR (Marieb, 2010).
2 *Muscle activity.* Muscle activity, including shivering, increases the metabolic rate.
3 *Thyroxine output.* Increased thyroxine output increases the rate of cellular metabolism throughout the body. This effect is called chemical thermogenesis, the stimulation of heat production in the body through increased cellular metabolism.
4 *Epinephrine, norepinephrine and sympathetic stimulation.* These hormones immediately increase the rate of cellular metabolism in many body tissues. Epinephrine (adrenaline) and norepinephrine (noradrenaline) directly affect liver and muscle cells, thereby increasing cellular metabolism.

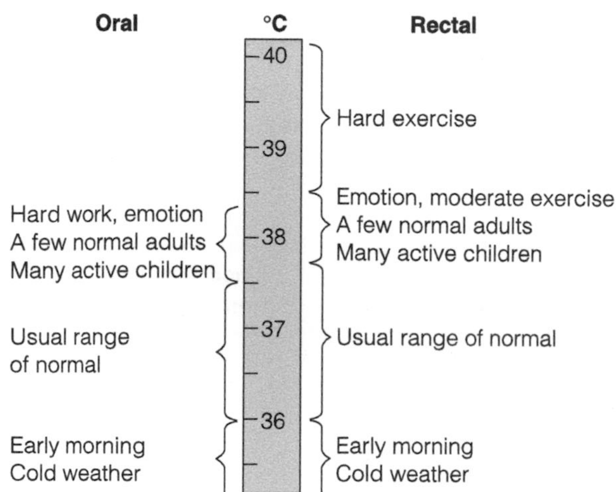

Figure 15-1 Estimated ranges of body temperatures in normal persons.

Source: adapted from *Fever and the Regulation of Body Temperature*, by E.F. DuBois, 1948, Springfield, IL: Charles C. Thomas. Reprinted with permission.

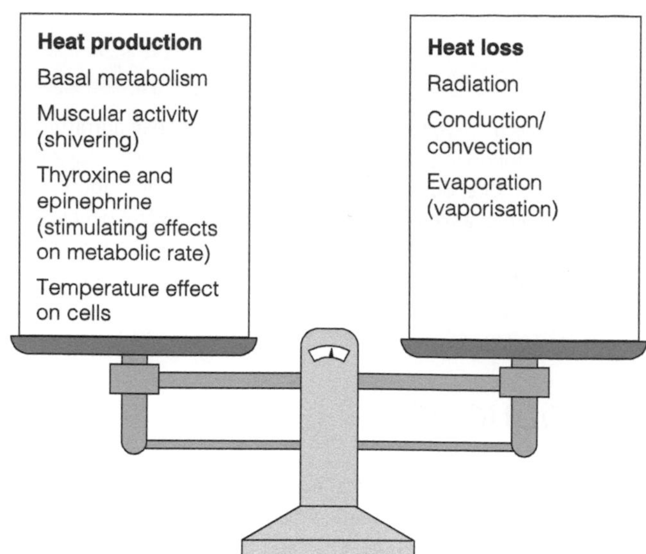

Figure 15-2 As long as heat production and heat loss are properly balanced, body temperature remains constant. Factors contributing to heat production (and temperature rise) are shown on the left side of the scale; those contributing to heat loss (and temperature fall) are shown on the right side of the scale.

Source: adapted from *Human Anatomy and Physiology*, 8th edn (p. 953), by E.N. Marieb, 2010, Menlo Park, CA: Benjamin/Cummings. Reprinted with permission.

5 *Fever.* Fever increases the cellular metabolic rate and thus increases the body's temperature further.

Heat is lost from the body through radiation, conduction, convection and vaporisation. **Radiation** is the transfer of heat from the surface of one object to the surface of another without contact between the two objects, mostly in the form of infrared rays. For example, radiation accounts for 60% of the heat lost by a nude person standing in a room at normal room temperature (Guyton, 2006).

Conduction is the transfer of heat from one molecule to a molecule of lower temperature. Conductive transfer cannot take place without contact between the molecules and normally accounts for minimal heat loss except, for example, when a body is immersed in cold water. The amount of heat transferred depends on the temperature difference and the amount and duration of the contact.

Convection is the dispersion of heat by air currents. The body usually has a small amount of warm air adjacent to it. This warm air rises and is replaced by cooler air, and so people always lose a small amount of heat through convection.

Vaporisation is continuous evaporation of moisture from the respiratory tract and from the mucosa of the mouth and from the skin. This continuous and unnoticed water loss is called **insensible fluid loss**, and the accompanying heat loss is called insensible heat loss. Insensible heat loss accounts for about 10% of basal heat loss. When the body temperature increases, vaporisation accounts for greater heat loss.

Regulation of Body Temperature

The system that regulates body temperature has three main parts: sensors in the peripheral body shell and in the body core, an integrator in the hypothalamus, and an effector system that adjusts the production and loss of heat. Most sensors or sensory receptors are in the skin. The skin has more receptors for cold than warmth. Therefore, skin sensors detect cold more efficiently than warmth.

When the skin becomes chilled over the entire body, three physiologic processes to increase the body temperature take place:

1 Shivering increases heat production.
2 Sweating is inhibited to decrease heat loss.
3 Vasoconstriction decreases heat loss.

The hypothalamic integrator, the centre that controls the core temperature, is located in the preoptic area of the hypothalamus. When the sensors in the hypothalamus detect heat, they send out signals intended to reduce the temperature, that is, to decrease heat production and increase heat loss. When the cold sensors are stimulated, signals are sent out to increase heat production and decrease heat loss.

The signals from the cold-sensitive receptors of the hypothalamus initiate effectors, such as vasoconstriction, shivering and the release of epinephrine, which increases cellular metabolism and hence heat production. When the warmth-sensitive receptors in the hypothalamus are stimulated, the effector system sends out signals that initiate sweating and peripheral vasodilatation. Also, when this system is stimulated, the person consciously makes appropriate adjustments, such as putting on additional clothing in response to cold or turning on a fan in response to heat.

Factors Affecting Body Temperature

Nurses should be aware of the factors that can affect a patient's body temperature so that they can recognise normal temperature variations and understand the significance of body temperature measurements that deviate from normal. Among the factors that affect body temperature are the following:

- *Age.* The infant is greatly influenced by the temperature of the environment and must be protected from extreme changes. Children's temperatures continue to be more variable than those of adults until puberty. Many older people, particularly those over 75 years old, are at risk of hypothermia (temperatures below 36°C) for a variety of reasons, such as inadequate diet, loss of subcutaneous fat, lack of activity and reduced thermoregulatory efficiency. Older people are also particularly sensitive to extremes in the environmental temperature due to decreased thermoregulatory controls.
- *Diurnal variations (circadian rhythms).* Body temperatures normally change throughout the day, varying as much as 1.0°C between the early morning and the late afternoon. The point of highest body temperature is usually reached between 20.00 and 24.00 hours (8.00 pm and midnight), and

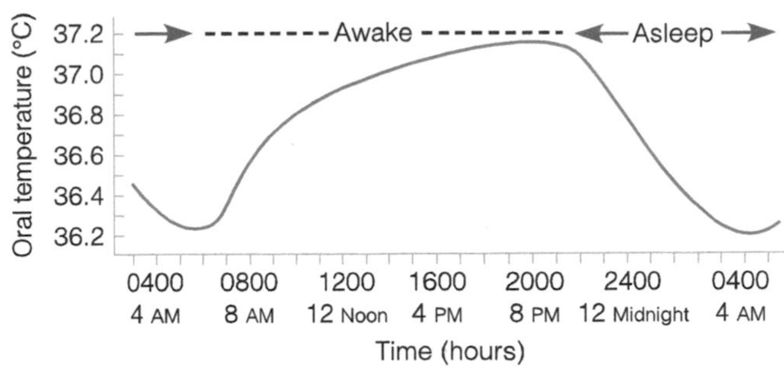

Figure 15-3 Range of oral temperatures during 24 hours for a healthy young adult.

the lowest point is reached during sleep between 04.00 and 06.00 hours (4.00 and 6.00 am) (see Figure 15-3).
- *Exercise.* Hard work or strenuous exercise can increase body temperature to as high as 38.3 to 40°C measured rectally.
- *Hormones.* Women usually experience more hormone fluctuations than men. In women, progesterone secretion at the time of ovulation raises body temperature by about 0.3 to 0.6°C above basal temperature (Ladewig *et al.*, 1998).
- *Stress.* Stimulation of the sympathetic nervous system can increase the production of epinephrine and norepinephrine, thereby increasing metabolic activity and heat production. Nurses may anticipate that a highly stressed or anxious patient could have an elevated body temperature for that reason.
- *Environment.* Extremes in environmental temperatures can affect a person's temperature regulatory systems. If the temperature is assessed in a very warm room and the body temperature cannot be modified by convection, conduction or radiation, the temperature will be elevated. Similarly, if the patient has been outside in extremely cold weather without suitable clothing, the body temperature may be low.

Alterations in Body Temperature

There are two primary alterations in body temperature: pyrexia and hypothermia.

Pyrexia

A body temperature above the usual range is called **pyrexia**, hyperthermia or (in lay terms) fever. A very high temperature, such as 41°C, is called hyperpyrexia. The patient who has a raised temperature is referred to as febrile; the one who has not is afebrile.

Four common types of pyrexia are intermittent, remittent, relapsing and constant. During an intermittent pyrexia, the body temperature alternates at regular intervals between periods of raised and periods of normal or subnormal temperatures. During a remittent pyrexia, a wide range of temperature fluctuations (more than 2°C) occurs over the 24-hour period, all of which are above normal. In a relapsing pyrexia, short febrile periods of a few days are interspersed with periods of one or two days of normal temperature. During a constant pyrexia, the body temperature fluctuates (minimally) but always remains above normal. A temperature that rises to pyrexia level rapidly following a normal temperature and then returns to normal within a few hours is called a spiked 'temperature'.

The clinical signs of fever vary with the onset, course and abatement stages of the fever. These signs occur as a result of changes in the set point of the temperature control mechanism regulated by the hypothalamus. Under normal conditions, whenever the core temperature rises above 37°C, the rate of heat *loss* is increased, resulting in a fall in temperature towards the set-point level. Conversely, when the core temperature falls below 37°C, the rate of heat *production* is increased, resulting in a rise in temperature towards the set point.

The clinical signs of a raised temperature are:

- Onset (cold or chill stage)
  - increased heart rate
  - increased respiratory rate and depth
  - shivering
  - pallid, cold skin
  - complaints of feeling cold
  - cyanotic nail beds
  - 'goose pimples' appearance of the skin
  - cessation of sweating
- Course
  - absence of chills
  - skin that feels warm
  - photosensitivity
  - glassy-eyed appearance
  - increased pulse and respiratory rates
  - increased thirst
  - mild to severe dehydration
  - drowsiness, restlessness, delirium or convulsions
  - herpetic lesions of the mouth
  - loss of appetite (if the fever is prolonged)
  - loss of appetite (if the fever is prolonged)
  - malaise, weakness and aching muscles
- **Deferescence (temperature abatement)**
  - skin that appears flushed and feels warm
  - sweating
  - decreased shivering
  - possible dehydration

During a raised temperature the set point of the hypothalamic thermostat changes suddenly from the normal level to a higher than normal value (e.g. 39.5°C) as a result of the effects of tissue destruction, pyrogenic substances or dehydration on the hypothalamus. Although the set point changes rapidly, the core body temperature (i.e. the blood temperature) reaches this new set point only after several hours. During this interval, the usual heat production responses that cause elevation of the body temperature occur: chills, feeling of coldness, cold skin due to vasoconstriction, and shivering.

When the core temperature reaches the new set point, the person feels neither cold nor hot and no longer experiences chills. Depending on the degree of temperature elevation, other signs may occur during the course of the pyrexia. Very high temperatures, such as 41 to 42°C, damage the cells throughout the body, particularly in the brain where destruction of neuronal cells is irreversible. Damage to the liver, kidneys and other body organs can also be great enough to disrupt functioning and eventually cause death.

When the cause of the high temperature is suddenly removed, the set point of the hypothalamic thermostat is suddenly reduced to a lower value, perhaps even back to the original normal level. In this instance, the hypothalamus now attempts to lower the temperature to 37°C, and the usual heat loss responses causing a reduction of the body temperature occur: excessive sweating and a hot, flushed skin due to sudden vasodilatation. This sudden change of events is known as the *crisis*, the *flush* or the *defervescent (abatement) stage* of a pyrexic condition.

Nursing interventions for a patient who has a pyrexia are designed to support the body's normal physiological processes, provide comfort and prevent complications (see *Practice Guidelines*). During the course of pyrexias, the nurse needs to monitor the patient's vital signs closely.

Nursing measures during the chill phase are designed to help the patient decrease heat loss. At this time, the body's physiological processes are attempting to raise the core temperature to the new set-point temperature. During the flush or crisis phase, the body processes are attempting to lower the core temperature to the reduced or normal set-point temperature. At this time, the nurse takes measures to increase heat loss and decrease heat production.

PRACTICE GUIDELINES

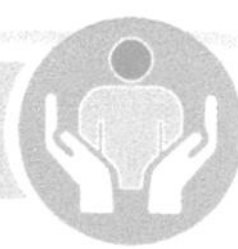

Nursing Interventions for Pyrexial Patients

- Monitor vital signs.
- Assess skin colour and temperature.
- Monitor white blood cell count, and relevant laboratory reports for indications of infection or dehydration.
- Remove excess blankets when the patient feels warm, but provide extra warmth when the patient feels chilled.
- Provide adequate nutrition and fluids (e.g. 2,500–3,000ml per day) to meet the increased metabolic demands and prevent dehydration.
- Measure intake and output accurately.
- Reduce physical activity to limit heat production, especially during the flush stage.
- Administer antipyretics (drugs that reduce the level of temperature such as Paracetamol) as prescribed.
- Provide oral hygiene to keep the mucous membranes moist.
- Provide a tepid sponge bath to increase heat loss through conduction.
- Provide dry clothing and bed linen.

Hypothermia

Hypothermia is a core body temperature below the lower limit of normal. The three physiological mechanisms of hypothermia are (a) excessive heat loss, (b) inadequate heat production to counteract heat loss and (c) impaired hypothalamic thermoregulation.

Hypothermia may be accidental or induced. Accidental hypothermia can occur as a result of (a) exposure to a cold environment, (b) immersion in cold water and (c) lack of adequate clothing, shelter or heat. In older people the problem can be compounded by a decreased metabolic rate and the use of sedatives. Downing (2009) lists the clinical signs of mild, moderate and severe hypothermia as:

- Mild 32–35°C (temperature)
  - shivering
  - cold to touch
  - lethargy
  - pallor
- Moderate 30–32°C
  - uncontrollable shivering
  - altered consciousness level
  - weakness
- Severe >30°C
  - not shivering
  - dilated pupils
  - muscle rigidity
  - unconscious
  - cardiac arrest may occur.

Managing hypothermia involves removing the patient from the cold and rewarming the patient's body. For the patient with mild hypothermia, the body is rewarmed by applying blankets; for the patient with severe hypothermia, a rewarming blanket (an electronically controlled blanket that provides a specified temperature either via direct heat or warm air) is applied and warm intravenous fluids may be given. Wet clothing, which increases heat loss because of the high conductivity of water, should be replaced with dry clothing. Nursing interventions for patients who have hypothermia are given in the *Practice Guidelines*.

PRACTICE GUIDELINES

Nursing Interventions for Patients with Hypothermia

- Provide a warm environment.
- Remove wet clothes and provide dry clothing.
- Apply warm blankets and warm environment.
- Keep limbs close to body.
- Cover the patient's head to reduce heat loss.
- Supply warm oral or intravenous fluids depending on consciousness level and medical contraindications.
- If mobile encourage mobility.
- Apply warming pads.
- Establish IV access (if IV fluids administered do not infuse cold fluids - room temperature).
- Depending on severity may need to be catheterised.
- Cardiac and pulse oximetry monitoring.
- Regular observations.

Induced hypothermia is the deliberate lowering of the body temperature to decrease the need for oxygen by the body tissues. Induced hypothermia can involve the whole body or a body part. It is sometimes indicated prior to surgical intervention (e.g. cardiac and brain surgery).

Assessing Body Temperature

The four most common sites for measuring body temperature are oral, rectal, axillary and the tympanic membrane(ear) forehead and core, and normal temperature ranges vary slightly with each site (see Figure 15-4). Each of the sites has advantages and disadvantages (see Table 15-2).

The body temperature is frequently measured *orally*. This method reflects changing body temperature more quickly than the rectal method. If a patient has been taking cold or hot food or fluids or smoking, the nurse should wait 30 minutes before taking the temperature orally to ensure that the temperature of the mouth is not affected by the temperature of the food, fluid or warm smoke.

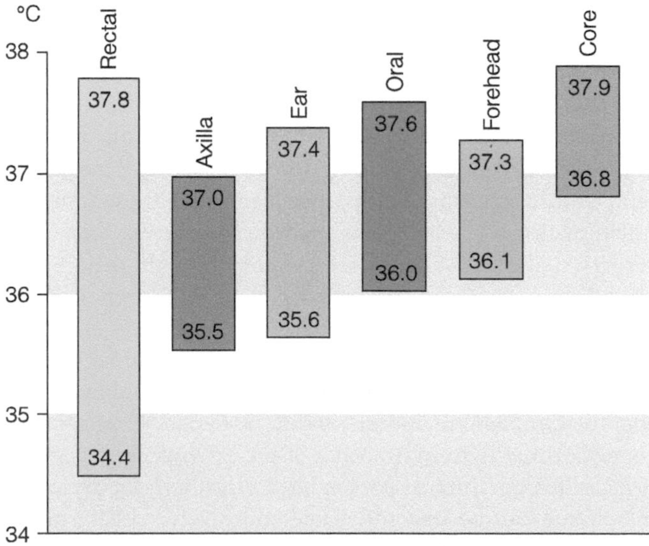

Figure 15-4 Normal temperature ranges for measurement sites.
Source: adapted from Crawford *et al.*, 2005.

Table 15-2 Advantages and Disadvantages of Four Sites for Body Temperature Measurement

Site	Advantages	Disadvantages
Oral	Accessible and convenient	Glass thermometers can break if bitten
		Inaccurate if patient has just ingested hot or cold food or fluid or smoked
		Could injure the mouth following oral surgery
Rectal	Reliable measurement	Inconvenient and more unpleasant for patients; difficult for patient who cannot turn to the side
		Could injure the rectum following rectal surgery
		A rectal glass thermometer does not respond to changes in arterial temperatures as quickly as an oral thermometer, a fact that may be potentially dangerous for febrile patients because misleading information may be acquired
		Presence of stool may interfere with thermometer placement. If the stool is soft, the thermometer may be embedded in stool rather than against the wall of the rectum
		(No longer used routinely for reasons of safety)
Axillary (in the arm pit)	Safe and noninvasive	The thermometer must be left in place a long time to obtain an accurate measurement
Tympanic membrane	Readily accessible; reflects the core temperature. Very fast	Can be uncomfortable and involves risk of injuring the membrane if the probe is inserted too far
		Repeated measurements may vary. Right and left measurements can differ
		Presence of cerumen/ear wax can affect the reading

Rectal temperature readings are considered to be very accurate although used less frequently due to the easier oral route. In some clinical areas, taking temperatures rectally is not advised for patients with myocardial infarction. It is believed that inserting a rectal thermometer can produce vagal stimulation, which in turn can cause myocardial damage. However, not all authorities share this belief. Rectal temperatures are contraindicated for patients who are undergoing rectal surgery, have diarrhoea or diseases of the rectum, are immuno-suppressed, have a clotting disorder or have significant **haemorrhoids**.

The axilla is the preferred site for measuring temperature in newborns because it is accessible and offers no possibility of rectal perforation. However, some research indicates that the axillary method is inaccurate when assessing a pyrexia (Bindler and Ball, 2003). Nurses should check local policy and protocol when taking the temperature of newborns, infants, toddlers and children. Adult patients for whom the axillary method of temperature assessment is appropriate include those with oral inflammation or wired jaws, patients recovering from oral surgery, patients who cannot breathe through their noses, irrational or confused patients, and patients for whom other temperature sites are contraindicated.

The *tympanic membrane*, or nearby tissue in the ear canal, is another site for core body temperature. Like the sublingual oral site, the tympanic membrane has an abundant arterial blood supply, primarily from branches of the external carotid artery. Because temperature sensors applied directly to the tympanic membrane can be uncomfortable and involve risk of membrane injury or perforation, noninvasive infrared thermometers are now used. Electronic tympanic thermometers are found extensively in both inpatient/client hospital and primary care settings.

In addition to the four common sites for measuring temperature, the forehead may also be used using a chemical thermometer. Forehead temperature measurements are most useful for infants and children where a more invasive measurement is not necessary. If the forehead indicates a temperature elevation, a glass or electronic thermometer should be used to obtain a more accurate measurement.

ACTIVITY 15-1

Julian is a 79-year-old gentleman who has dementia. He was missing from the nursing home yesterday and was found in the early hours of this morning having been out most of the night. The doctor has asked for his respirations, pulse, temperature and blood pressure to be recorded hourly, and the nurse in charge has asked you to monitor his temperature half hourly. Reflect, explore and rationalise why Julian needs his temperature recorded so often and how you would record it.

Types of Thermometers

Traditionally, body temperatures were measured using *mercury-in-glass thermometers*. However, over the last 20 years, due to the hazards of using the glass mercury thermometers, they have been removed from practice and indeed the marketing of this type of thermometer has been restricted following a directive from the European Council (MHRA, 2010). Development of systems to replace the glass mercury thermometer in practice has led to several options and, according to Davie and Amoore (2010), there are many devices currently used in the United Kingdom:

- chemical thermometers;
- electronic contact thermometers;
- infrared sensing thermometers;
- temperature-sensitive tape;
- non-touch temporal artery thermometers.

Chemical thermometers

Chemical thermometers use liquid crystal dots or bars or heat-sensitive tape or patches applied to the forehead which change colour to indicate temperature. Some of these are single use and others may be reused several times. The chemical thermometers are predominantly used for oral and axilla readings (see Figure 15-5) (Frommelt *et al.*, 2008).

Electronic contact thermometers

Electronic contact thermometers use thermistor properties to indirectly measure temperature. They are most often used orally or per axilla and have a disposable cover over the probe which can be thrown away after each use. Most devices will be a single probe device. Some have two probes, in which case a red probe is used to record a rectal temperature (see Figure 15-6).

Infrared thermometers (tympanic thermometers)

Infrared (tympanic) thermometers (see Figure 15-7) sense body heat in the form of infrared energy given off by a heat source from the ear canal and tympanic membrane. The optical sensor of the thermometer probe converts thermal energy into electrical energy which will produce a temperature reading (Crawford *et al.*, 2006). The infrared thermometer makes no contact with the tympanic membrane and the probes are protected by a throwaway cover that can be disposed of as per local board or Trust's policy.

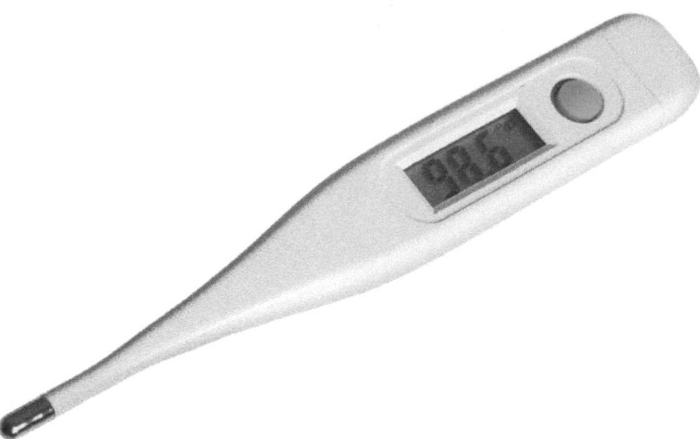

Figure 15-6 Electronic contact thermometer.
Source: Alamy Images.

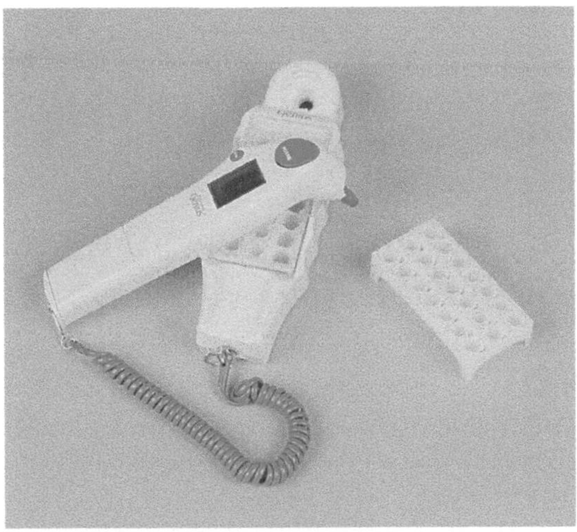

Figure 15-7 An infrared (tympanic) thermometer used to measure the tympanic membrane temperature.
Source: Pearson Education Ltd.

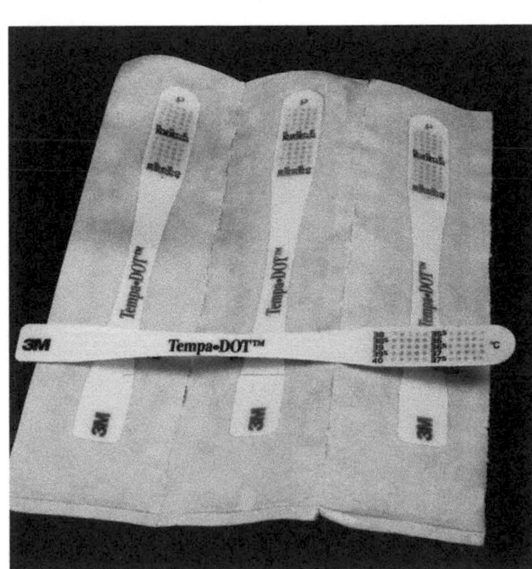

Figure 15-5 A chemical thermometer.
Source: Simon Evans/Photographers Direct.

Temperature-sensitive tape

Temperature-sensitive tape (e.g. temporal artery thermometers) may also be used to obtain a general indication of body surface temperature. It does not indicate the core temperature. The tape contains liquid crystals that change colour according to temperature. When applied to the skin, usually of the forehead or abdomen, the temperature digits on the tape respond by changing colour (see Figure 15-8). The skin area should be dry. After the length of time specified by the manufacturer (e.g. 15 seconds), a colour appears on the tape. This method is particularly useful at home and for infants whose temperatures are to be monitored.

Non-Touch Temporal Artery Thermometers

Non-touch temporal artery thermometers are thermometers which are held above the body surface and use a tracker system to record the temperature (see Figure 15-9).

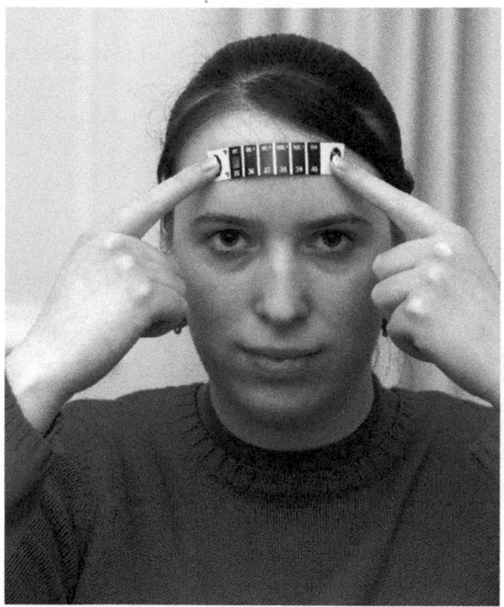

Figure 15-8 A temperature-sensitive skin tape.
Source: Art Directors and TRIP Photo Library.

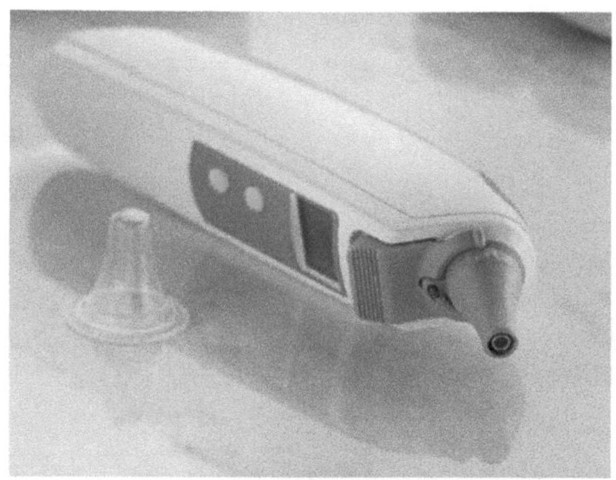

Figure 15-9 Non-touch temporal artery thermometer.
Source: Alamy Images.

The steps in assessing body temperature are given in *Procedure 15-1* and instructions on thermometer placement in the *Practice Guidelines.*

PROCEDURE 15-1 Assessing Body Temperature

Purposes

- To establish baseline data for subsequent evaluation
- To identify whether the patient's temperature is within normal range
- To determine changes in the patient's temperature in response to specific therapies (e.g. antipyretic medication, immunosuppressive therapy, invasive procedure)
- To monitor patients at risk for imbalanced body temperature (e.g. patients at risk for infection or diagnosis of infection; those who have been exposed to temperature extremes)

Assessment

Assess

- Clinical signs of pyrexia
- Clinical signs of hypothermia
- Site most appropriate for measurement
- Factors that may alter body temperature

Planning

Equipment

- Thermometer
- Thermometer sheath or cover
- Water-soluble lubricant for a rectal temperature (if required)
- Disposable gloves
- Towel for axillary temperature
- Tissues/wipes

Implementation

Preparation

Check that all equipment is functioning normally. Ensure that the thermometer used has been recently calibrated and maintained (otherwise false readings may occur).

Performance

1 Follow local policy to ensure that you explain to the patient what you are going to do, why it is necessary and how they can cooperate. Obtain consent and maintain patient

privacy and dignity and ensure that the appropriate local infection control procedures are observed.

2 Ensure that the thermometer is in the right mode for the site that the reading is to be taken from (i.e. oral, rectal etc)

3 Place the patient in the appropriate position (e.g. lateral position for inserting a rectal thermometer).

4 Place the thermometer (see *Practice Guidelines* on page 424):
   - Apply a protective sheath or probe cover if appropriate.
   - Lubricate a rectal thermometer.

5 Wait the appropriate amount of time, as directed by manufacturers. Electronic and tympanic thermometers will indicate that the reading is complete through a light or tone.

6 Remove the thermometer and discard the cover as per local board or Trust's policy.

7 Read the temperature - if the temperature is obviously too high, too low or inconsistent with the patient's condition, recheck it with a thermometer known to be functioning properly.

8 Clean the thermometer in accordance with local infection control policy.

9 Document the temperature on the patient's observation chart which will vary from area to area (e.g. see Figure 15-10). A rectal temperature may be recorded with an 'R' next to the value or with the mark on a graphic sheet circled. An axillary temperature may be recorded with PA or marked on a graphic sheet with an X.

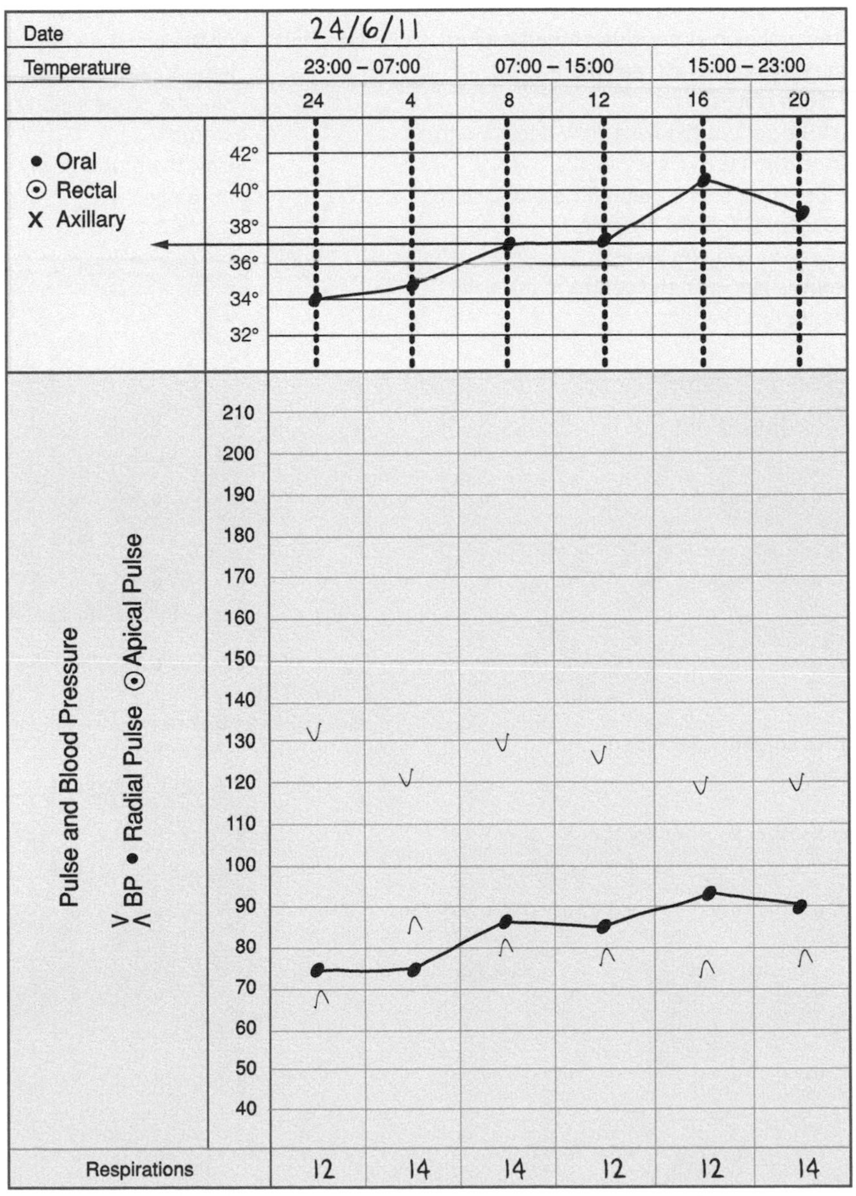

Figure 15-10 Vital signs chart.

Evaluation

- Compare the temperature measurement to baseline data, normal range for age of patient, and patient's previous temperatures. Assess and evaluate the reading considering time of day and any additional influencing factors and other vital signs.
- Conduct appropriate follow-up such as notifying the medical staff, administering a medication or adjusting the patient's environment. This includes teaching the patient how to lower an elevated temperature through actions such as increasing fluid intake, coughing and deep breathing, or removing heavy coverings.

PRACTICE GUIDELINES

Thermometer Placement

Oral	Place the probe on either side of the frenulum underneath the tongue (see Figure 15-11).
Rectal	Apply clean gloves. Instruct the patient to take a slow deep breath during insertion (see Figure 15-12). Never force the thermometer if resistance is felt. Insert 3.5 cm (1½ inch) in adults.
Axillary	Pat the axilla dry if very moist. The probe is placed in the centre of the axilla (see Figure 15-13).
Tympanic	Pull the pinna slightly upward and backward (see Figure 15-14). Point the probe slightly anteriorly, towards the eardrum. Insert the probe slowly using a circular motion until snug.

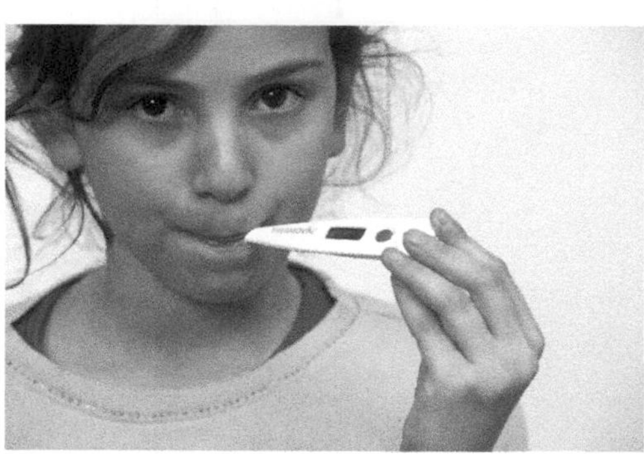

Figure 15-11 Oral thermometer placement.
Source: Science Photo Library Ltd.

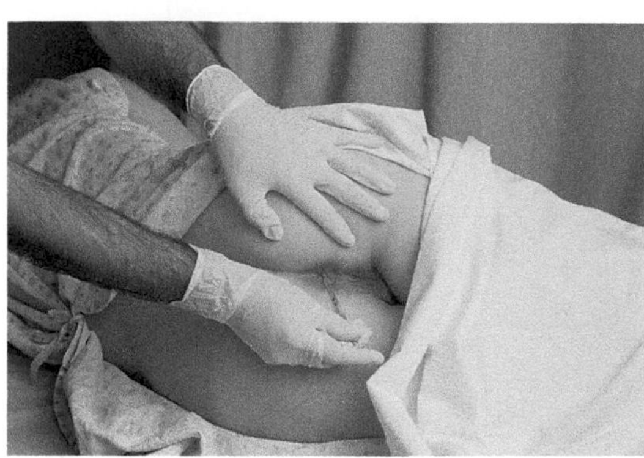

Figure 15-12 Inserting a rectal thermometer.
Source: Elena Dorfmann.

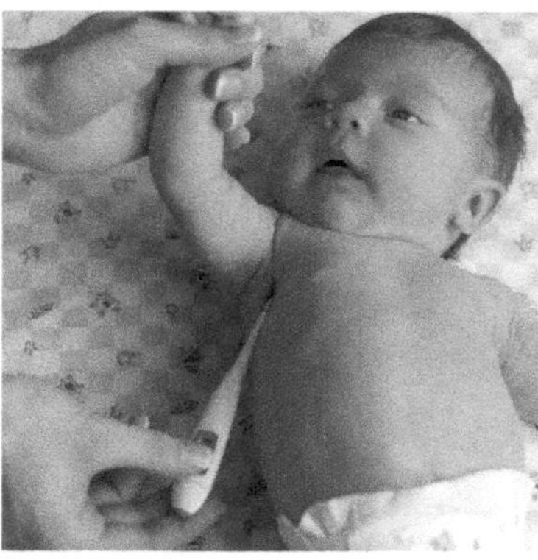

Figure 15-13 Placing the bulb of the thermometer in the centre of the axilla.
Source: Corbis/Radius Images.

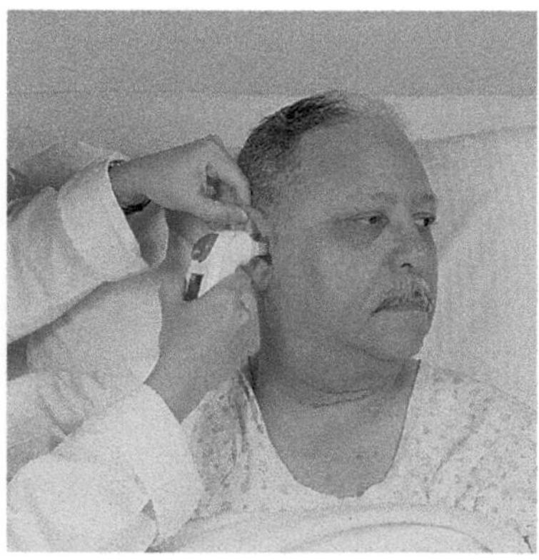

Figure 15-14 Pull the pinna of the ear up and back while inserting the tympanic thermometer.
Source: Jenny Thomas.

CLINICAL ALERT

- Muller *et al.* (2008) carried out a study on the comparisons made during recording of axillary and rectal temperatures in neonates. The conclusion was that the mean difference between axillary and rectal temperature showed a wide variation.
- NICE recommends the use of infrared tympanic thermometers in children between 4 weeks and 5 years old (NICE, 2007).

LIFESPAN CONSIDERATIONS

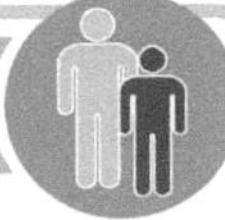

Temperature

Infants

- The choice of route is important when used with neonates as axillary routes are not always accurate.

Children

- Avoid the tympanic route for children with an ear infection.

Mature Adults

- Mature adults' temperatures tend to be lower than those of middle-age adults.
- Mature adults' temperatures are strongly influenced by both environmental and internal temperature changes. Their thermoregulation control processes are not as efficient as when they are younger and they are at higher risk for both hypothermia and hyperthermia.
- Mature adults can develop significant build up of ear cerumen/wax that may interfere with tympanic thermometer readings.
- Mature adults are more likely to have haemorrhoids. Inspect the anus before taking a rectal temperature.
- Mature adults' temperatures may not be a valid indication of the seriousness of the pathology of a disease. They may have pneumonia or a urinary tract infection and have only a slight temperature elevation. Other symptoms, such as confusion and restlessness, may be displayed and need follow-up to determine if there is an underlying process.

PULSE

The **pulse** is a wave of blood created by contraction of the left ventricle of the heart. Generally the pulse wave represents the stroke volume output and the amount of blood that enters the arteries with each ventricular contraction. Compliance of the arteries is their ability to contract and expand. When a person's arteries lose their elasticity, as can happen in old age, greater pressure is required to pump the blood into the arteries.

Cardiac output is the volume of blood pumped into the arteries by the heart and equals the result of the stroke volume (SV) times the heart rate (HR) per minute. For example, 65 ml × 70 beats per minute = 4.55 l per minute. When an adult is resting, the heart pumps about 5 litres of blood each minute.

In a healthy person, the pulse reflects the heartbeat; that is, the pulse rate is the same as the rate of the ventricular contractions of the heart. However, in some types of cardiovascular disease, the heartbeat and pulse rates can differ. For example, a patient's heart may produce very weak or small pulse waves that are not detectable in a peripheral pulse far from the heart. In these instances, the nurse should assess the heartbeat and the peripheral pulse. A **peripheral pulse** is a pulse located away from the heart, for example, in the foot, wrist or neck. The **apical pulse**, in contrast, is a central pulse; that is, it is located at the apex of the heart.

Factors Affecting the Pulse

The rate of the pulse is expressed in beats per minute (BPM). A pulse rate varies according to a number of factors. The nurse should consider each of the following factors when assessing a patient's pulse:

- *Age.* As age increases, the pulse rate gradually decreases. See Table 15-1 on page 415 for specific variations in pulse rates from birth to adulthood.
- *Gender.* After puberty, the average male's pulse rate is slightly lower than the female's.
- *Exercise.* The pulse rate normally increases with activity. The rate of increase in the professional athlete is often less than in the average person because of greater cardiac size, strength and efficiency.
- *Pyrexia.* The pulse rate increases (a) in response to the lowered blood pressure that results from peripheral vasodilatation associated with elevated body temperature and (b) because of the increased metabolic rate.
- *Medications.* Some medications decrease the pulse rate, and others increase it. For example, cardiotonics (e.g. digitalis preparations – Digoxin) decrease the heart rate, whereas epinephrine/adrenaline increases it.
- *Hypovolaemia.* Loss of blood from the vascular system normally increases pulse rate. In adults the loss of circulating

volume results in an adjustment of the heart rate to increase blood pressure as the body compensates for the lost blood volume. Adults can usually lose up to 10% of their normal circulating volume without adverse effects.

- *Stress.* In response to stress, sympathetic nervous stimulation increases the overall activity of the heart. Stress increases the rate as well as the force of the heartbeat. Fear and anxiety as well as the perception of severe pain stimulate the sympathetic system.
- *Position changes.* When a person is sitting or standing, blood usually pools in dependent vessels of the venous system. Pooling results in a transient decrease in the venous blood return to the heart and a subsequent reduction in blood pressure and increase in heart rate.
- *Pathology.* Certain diseases such as some heart conditions or those that impair oxygenation can alter the resting pulse rate.

CLINICAL ALERT

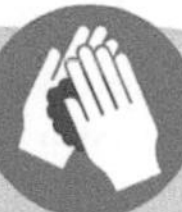

Never press both carotids at the same time because this can cause a reflex drop in blood pressure or pulse rate.

Pulse Sites

A pulse may be measured in nine sites (see Figure 15-15).

1 Temporal, where the temporal artery passes over the temporal bone of the head. The site is superior (above) and lateral to (away from the midline of) the eye.
2 Carotid, at the side of the neck where the carotid artery runs between the trachea and the sternocleidomastoid muscle.
3 Apical, at the apex of the heart. In an adult this is located on the left side of the chest, about 8cm to the left of the sternum (breastbone) and at the fourth, fifth or sixth intercostal space (area between the ribs). For a child seven to nine years of age, the apical pulse is located at the fourth or fifth intercostal spaces. Before four years of age it is left of the midclavicular line (MCL); between four and six years, it is at the MCL (see Figure 15-16).
4 Brachial, at the inner aspect of the biceps muscle of the arm or medially in the antecubital space.
5 Radial, where the radial artery runs along the radial bone, on the thumb side of the inner aspect of the wrist.
6 Femoral, where the femoral artery passes alongside the inguinal ligament.
7 Popliteal, where the popliteal artery passes behind the knee.
8 Posterior tibial, on the medial surface of the ankle where the posterior tibial artery passes behind the medial **malleolus**.
9 Pedal (dorsalis pedis), where the dorsalis pedis artery passes over the bones of the foot, on an imaginary line drawn from the middle of the ankle to the space between the big and second toes. The radial site is most commonly used in adults. It is easily found in most people and readily accessible. Some reasons for use of each site are given in Table 15-3.

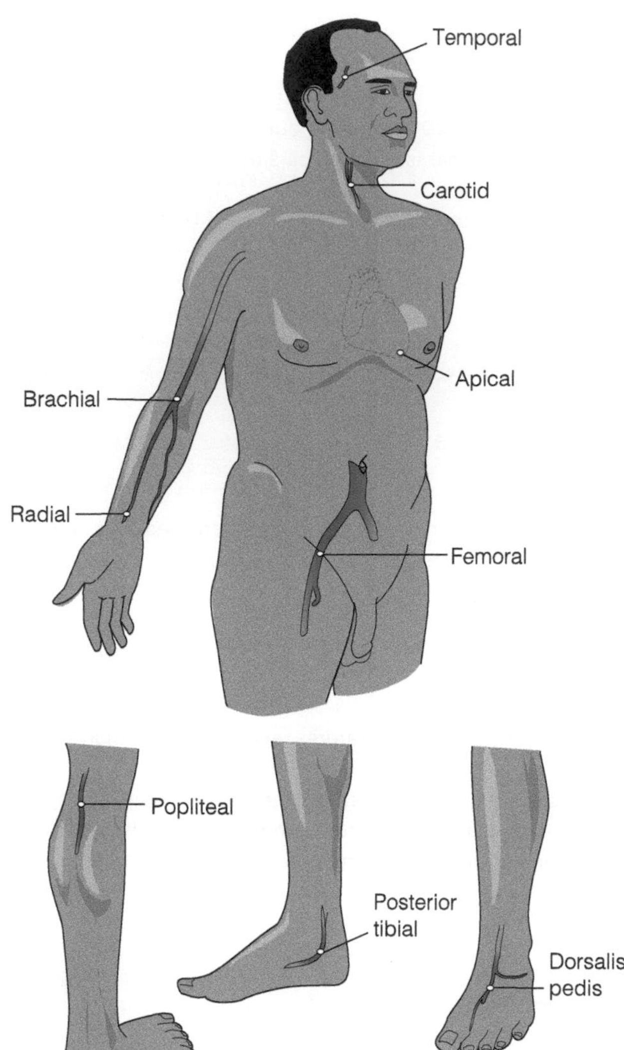

Figure 15-15 Nine sites for assessing pulse.

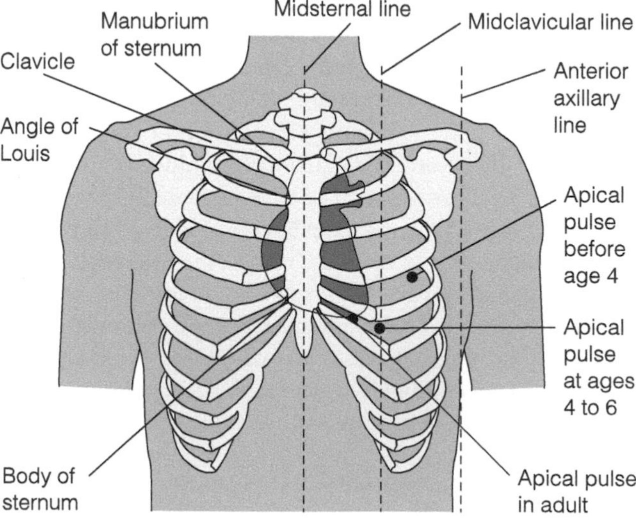

Figure 15-16 Location of the apical pulse for a child under four years, a child four to six years, and an adult.

Table 15-3 Reasons for Using Specific Pulse Site

Pulse site	Reasons for use
Radial	Readily accessible
Temporal	Used when radial pulse is not accessible
Carotid	Used in cases of cardiac arrest Used to determine circulation to the brain
Apical	Routinely used for infants and children up to three years of age Used to determine discrepancies with radial pulse Used in conjunction with some medications
Brachial	Used to measure blood pressure Used during cardiac arrest for infants
Femoral	Used in cases of cardiac arrest Used for infants and children Used to determine circulation to a leg
Popliteal	Used to determine circulation to the lower leg
Posterior tibial	Used to determine circulation to the foot
Pedal	Used to determine circulation to the foot

Assessing the Pulse

A pulse is commonly assessed by palpation (feeling) or auscultation (hearing). The middle three fingertips are used for palpating all pulse sites except the apex of the heart. A stethoscope is used for assessing apical pulses and foetal heart tones. A Doppler ultrasound stethoscope (DUS; see Figure 15-17) is used for pulses that are difficult to assess. The DUS headset has earpieces similar to standard stethoscope earpieces, but it has a long cord attached to a volume-controlled audio unit and an ultrasound transducer. The DUS detects movement of red blood cells through a blood vessel. In contrast to the conventional stethoscope, it excludes environmental sounds.

A pulse is normally palpated by applying moderate pressure with the three middle fingers of the hand. The pads on the most distal aspects of the finger are the most sensitive areas for detecting a pulse. With excessive pressure one can obliterate a pulse, whereas with too little pressure one may not be able to detect it. Before the nurse assesses the resting pulse, the patient should assume a comfortable position. The nurse should also be aware of the following:

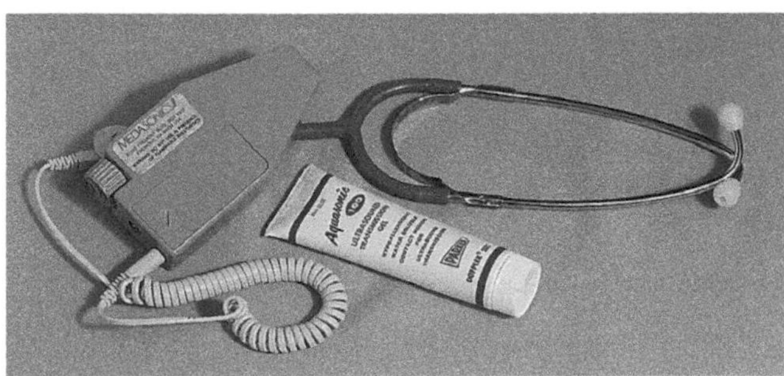

Figure 15-17 A Doppler ultrasound stethoscope (DUS).
Source: Pearson Education Ltd.

- Any medication that could affect the heart rate.
- Whether the patient has been physically active. If so, wait 10–15 minutes until the patient has rested and the pulse has slowed to its usual rate.
- Any baseline data about the normal heart rate for the patient. For example, a physically fit athlete may have a heart rate below 60 BPM.
- Whether the patient should assume a particular position (e.g. sitting). In some patients, the rate changes with the position because of changes in blood flow volume and autonomic nervous system activity.

When assessing the pulse, the nurse collects the following data: the rate, rhythm, volume, arterial wall elasticity and presence or absence of bilateral equality. An excessively fast heart rate (e.g. over 100 BPM in an adult) is referred to as **tachycardia**. A heart rate in an adult of 60 BPM or less is called **bradycardia**. If a patient has either tachycardia or bradycardia, the apical pulse should be assessed.

The pulse rhythm is the pattern of the beats and the intervals between the beats. Equal time elapses between beats of a normal pulse. A pulse with an irregular rhythm is referred to as a dysrhythmia or arrhythmia. It may consist of random, irregular beats or a predictable pattern of irregular beats. When a dysrhythmia is detected, the apical pulse should be assessed. An electrocardiogram (ECG) is necessary to define the dysrhythmia further.

Pulse volume, also called the pulse strength or amplitude, refers to the force of blood with each beat. Usually, the pulse volume is the same with each beat. It can range from absent to bounding. A normal pulse can be felt with moderate pressure of the fingers and can be obliterated with greater pressure. A forceful or full blood volume that is obliterated only with difficulty is called a full or bounding pulse. A pulse that is readily obliterated with pressure from the fingers is referred to as weak, feeble or thready.

The elasticity of the arterial wall reflects its expansibility or its deformities. A healthy, normal artery feels straight, smooth, soft and pliable. Older people often have inelastic arteries that feel twisted (tortuous) and irregular upon palpation.

When assessing a peripheral pulse to determine the adequacy of blood flow to a particular area of the body, the nurse should also assess the corresponding pulse on the other side of the body. The second assessment gives the nurse data with which to compare the pulses. For example, when assessing the blood flow to the right foot, the nurse assesses the right dorsalis pedis pulse and then the left dorsalis pedis pulse. If the patient's right and left pulses are the same, the patient's dorsalis pedis pulses are bilaterally equal.

Procedure 15-2 provides guidelines for assessing a peripheral pulse, *Procedure 15-3* for an apical pulse and *Procedure 15-4* for an apical-radial pulse.

PROCEDURE 15-2 Assessing a Peripheral Pulse

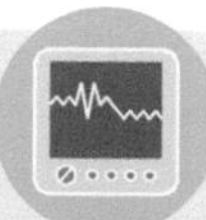

Purposes

- To establish baseline data for subsequent evaluation
- To identify whether the pulse rate is within normal range
- To determine whether the pulse rhythm is regular and the pulse volume is appropriate
- To compare the equality of corresponding peripheral pulses on each side of the body
- To monitor and assess changes in the patient's health status
- To monitor patients at risk for pulse alterations (e.g. those with a history of heart disease or experiencing cardiac arrhythmias, haemorrhage, acute pain, infusion of large volumes of fluids, pyrexia)

Assessment

Assess

- Clinical signs of cardiovascular alterations, other than pulse rate, rhythm or volume (e.g. dyspnoea [difficult respirations], fatigue, pallor, cyanosis [bluish discoloration of skin and mucous membranes], palpitations, syncope [fainting], impaired peripheral tissue perfusion as evidenced by skin discoloration and cool temperature)
- Factors that may alter pulse rate (e.g. emotional status and activity level)
- Site most appropriate for assessment

Planning

Equipment

- Watch with a second hand or indicator
- If using a DUS, the transducer probe, the stethoscope headset, transmission gel and tissues/wipes

Implementation

Preparation

If using a DUS, check that the equipment is calibrated and maintained as per manufacturer's policy.

Performance

1 Follow local policy to ensure that you explain to the patient what you are going to do, why it is necessary and how they can cooperate. Obtain consent and maintain patient privacy and dignity and ensure that the appropriate local infection control procedures are observed.

2 Select the pulse point. Normally, the radial pulse is taken, unless it cannot be exposed or circulation to another body area is to be assessed.

3 Assist the patient to a comfortable resting position. When the radial pulse is assessed, with the palm facing downward, the patient's arm can rest alongside the body or the forearm can rest at a 90-degree angle across the chest. For the patient who can sit, the forearm can rest across the thigh, with the palm of the hand facing downward or inward.

4 Palpate and count the pulse. Place two or three middle fingertips lightly and squarely over the pulse point (see Figure 15-18). *Using the thumb is contraindicated because the thumb has a pulse that the nurse could mistake for the patient's pulse.*
   - Count for one minute. An irregular pulse also requires taking the apical pulse.

5 Assess the pulse rhythm and volume.
   - Assess the pulse rhythm by noting the pattern of the intervals between the beats. A normal pulse has equal time periods between beats.
   - Assess the pulse volume. A normal pulse can be felt with moderate pressure, and the pressure is equal with each beat. A forceful pulse volume is full; an easily obliterated pulse is weak.

6 Document the pulse rate, rhythm and volume and your actions in patient observations chart. Also record pertinent related data such as variation in pulse rate compared to normal for the patient and abnormal skin colour and skin temperature in the nurse's notes, and report any variances of readings to appropriate colleague or doctor.

Variation: using a DUS

- If used, plug the stethoscope headset into one of the two output jacks located next to the volume control. DUS units

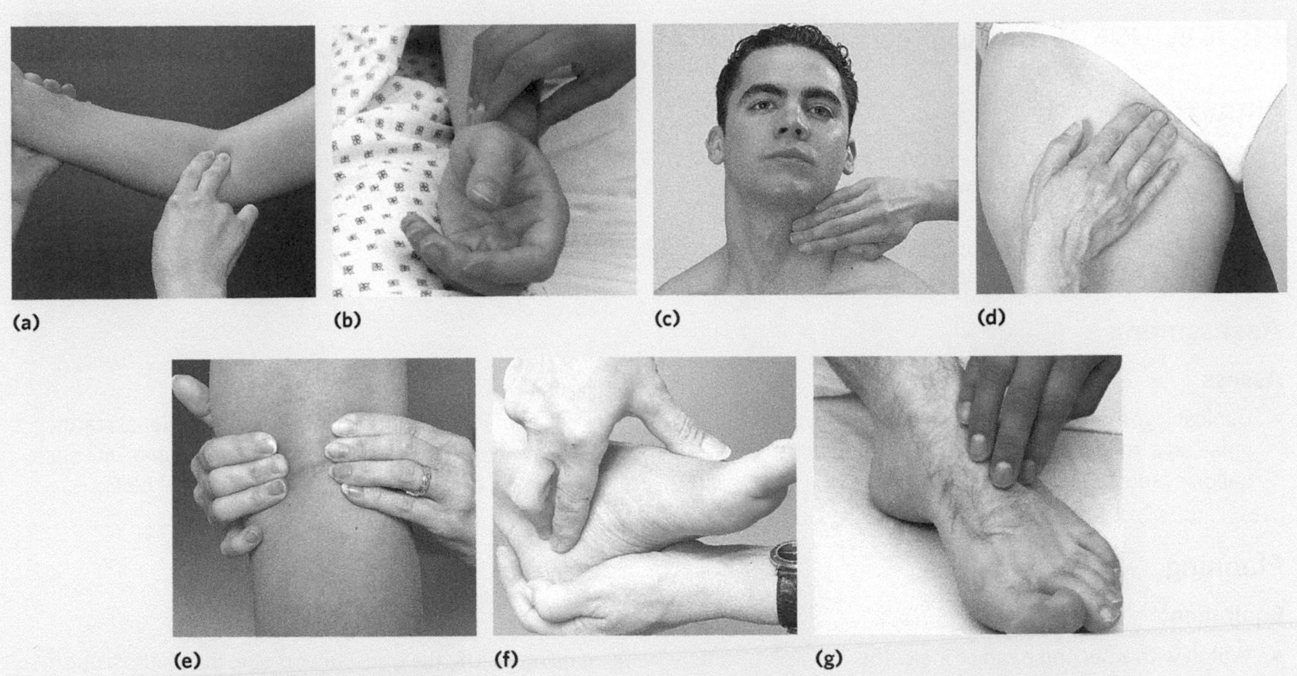

Figure 15-18 Assessing the pulses: (a) brachial; (b) radial; (c) carotid; (d) femoral; (e) popliteal; (f) posterior tibial; and (g) pedal (dorsalis pedis).
Source: Pearson Education Ltd.

may have two jacks so that a second person can listen to the signals.

- Apply transmission gel either to the probe at the narrow end of the plastic case housing of the transducer, or to the patient's skin. *Ultrasound beams do not travel well through air. The gel makes an airtight seal, which then promotes optimal ultrasound wave transmission.*
- Press the 'on' button.
- Hold the probe against the skin over the pulse site. Use a light pressure, and keep the probe in contact with the skin (see Figure 15-19). *Too much pressure can stop the blood flow and obliterate the signal.*
- Adjust the volume if necessary. Distinguish artery sounds from vein sounds. The artery sound (signal) is distinctively pulsating and has a pumping quality. The venous sound is intermittent and varies with respirations. Both artery and vein sounds are heard simultaneously through the DUS because major arteries and veins are situated close together throughout the body. If arterial sounds cannot be easily heard, then reposition the probe.
- After assessing the pulse, remove all gel from the probe to prevent damage to its surface. Clean the transducer with aqueous solutions. *Alcohol or other disinfectants may damage the face of the transducer. Remove all gel from the patient.*

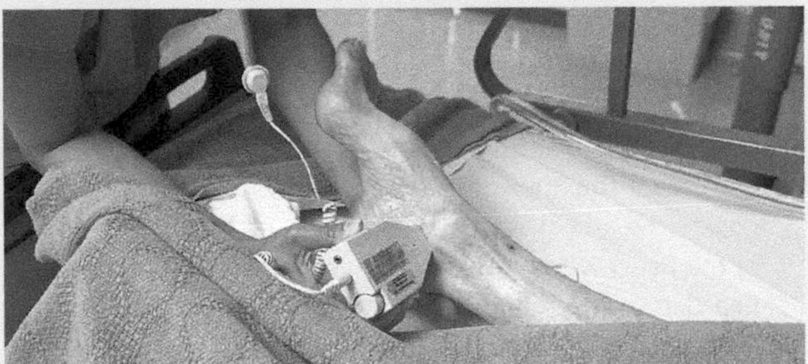

Figure 15-19 Using a (Doppler) ultrasound stethoscope to assess the posterior tibial pulse.
Source: Pearson Education Ltd.

Evaluation

- Compare the pulse rate to baseline data or normal range for age of patient.
- Relate pulse rate and volume to other vital signs; pulse rhythm and volume to baseline data and health status.
- If assessing peripheral pulses, evaluate equality, rate and volume in corresponding extremities.
- Conduct appropriate follow-up such as notifying the medical staff or administering medication.

PROCEDURE 15-3 Assessing an Apical Pulse

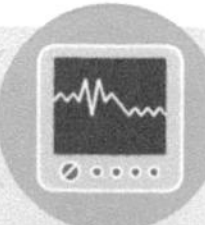

Purposes

- To obtain the heart rate of newborns, infants and children 2–3 years old or of an adult with an irregular peripheral pulse
- To establish baseline data for subsequent evaluation
- To determine whether the cardiac rate is within normal range and the rhythm is regular
- To monitor patients with cardiac disease and those receiving medications to improve heart action

Assessment

Assess

- Clinical signs of cardiovascular alterations, other than pulse rate, rhythm or volume (e.g. dyspnoea, fatigue, pallor, cyanosis, syncope)
- Factors that may alter pulse rate (e.g. emotional status, activity level, and medications that affect heart rate such as digoxin, beta blockers or calcium channel blockers)

Planning

Equipment

- Watch with a second hand or indicator
- Stethoscope
- Antiseptic wipes
- If using a DUS, the transducer probe, the stethoscope headset, transmission gel and tissues/wipes

Implementation

Preparation

If using a DUS, check that the equipment is calibrated and maintained as per manufacturer's policy.

Performance

1 Follow local policy to ensure that you explain to the patient what you are going to do, why it is necessary and how they can cooperate. Obtain consent and maintain patient privacy and dignity and ensure that the appropriate local infection control procedures are observed.

2 Position the patient appropriately in a comfortable supine position or in a sitting position. Expose the area of the chest over the apex of the heart.

3 Locate the apical impulse. This is the point over the apex of the heart where the apical pulse can be most clearly heard. It is also referred to as the point of maximal impulse (PMI).
   - Palpate the angle of Louis (the angle between the manubrium, the top of the sternum and the body of the sternum). It is palpated just below the suprasternal notch and is felt as a prominence (see Figure 15-16 on page 426).
   - Slide your index finger just to the left of the patient's sternum and palpate the second intercostal space.
   - Place your middle or next finger in the third intercostal space, and continue palpating downward until you locate the fifth intercostal space.
   - Move your index finger laterally along the fifth intercostal space towards the MCL. Normally, the apical impulse is palpable at or just medial to the MCL (see Figure 15-16).

4 Auscultate and count heartbeats.
   - Use appropriate wipes to clean the earpieces and diaphragm of the stethoscope after use (as per local policy). The diaphragm needs to be cleaned and disinfected if soiled with body substances and before and after each use.
   - Warm the diaphragm of the stethoscope by holding it in the palm of the hand for a moment. The metal of the diaphragm is usually cold and can startle the patient when placed immediately on the chest.
   - Insert the earpieces of the stethoscope into your ears in the direction of the ear canals, or slightly forward, *to facilitate hearing.*

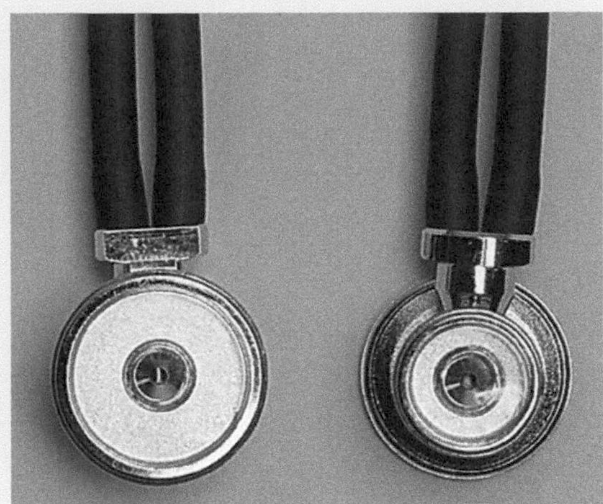

Figure 15-20 Close-up of a flat-disc amplifier (left) and a bell amplifier (right).
Source: Barts and The London NHS Trust.

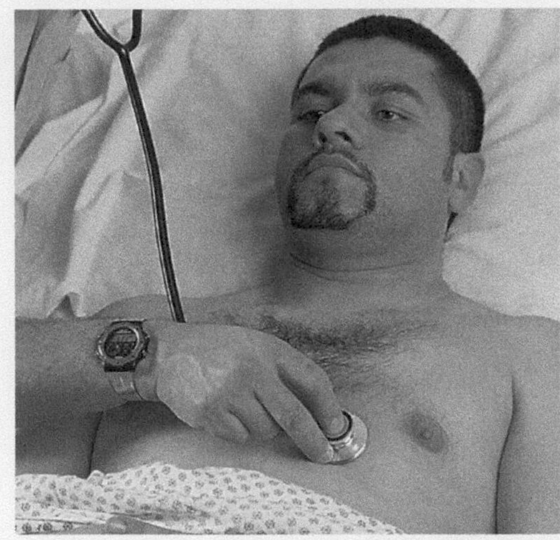

Figure 15-21 Taking an apical pulse using the flat disc of the stethoscope. Note how the amplifier is held against the chest.
Source: Barts and The London NHS Trust.

- Tap your finger lightly on the diaphragm *to be sure it is the active side of the head.* If necessary, rotate the head to select the diaphragm side (see Figure 15-20).
- Place the diaphragm of the stethoscope over the apical impulse and listen for the normal S1 and S2 heart sounds, which are heard as 'lub-dub' (see Figure 15-21). *The heartbeat is normally loudest over the apex of the heart.* Each lub-dub is counted as one heartbeat. *The two heart sounds are produced by closure of the valves of the heart. The S1 heart sound (lub) occurs when the atrioventricular valves close after the ventricles have been sufficiently filled. The S2 heart sound (dub) occurs when the semilunar valves close after the ventricles empty.*
- The heartbeat should be counted for 60 seconds (1 minute).
- Assess the rhythm of the heartbeat by noting the pattern of intervals between the beats. A normal pulse has equal time periods between beats.
- Assess the strengths (volume) of the heartbeat. Normally, the heartbeats are equal in strength and can be described as strong or weak.

5 Document the pulse site, rate, rhythm and volume and your actions in the patient observation chart. Also record pertinent related data such as variation in pulse rate compared to normal for the patient and abnormal skin colour and skin temperature.

Evaluation

- Relate pulse rate to other vital signs; pulse rhythm to baseline data and health status.
- Report to the medical staff any abnormal findings such as irregular rhythm, and reduced ability to hear the heartbeat, pallor, cyanosis, dyspnoea, tachycardia or bradycardia.
- Conduct appropriate follow-up such as administering medication prescribed based on apical heart rate.

Apical Pulse Assessment

Assessment of the apical pulse is indicated for patients whose peripheral pulse is irregular or unavailable as well as for patients with known cardiovascular, pulmonary and renal diseases. It is commonly assessed prior to administering medications that affect heart rate. The apical site is also used to assess the pulse for neonates, infants and children up to 2–3 years old.

Apical-Radial Pulse Assessment

An apical-radial pulse may need to be assessed for patients with certain cardiovascular disorders. Normally, the apical and radial rates are identical. An apical pulse rate greater than a radial pulse rate can indicate that the thrust of the blood from the heart is too feeble for the wave to be felt at the peripheral pulse site, or it can indicate that vascular disease is preventing impulses from being transmitted. Any discrepancy between the two pulse rates is called a pulse deficit and needs to be reported promptly. In no instance is the radial pulse greater than the apical pulse.

An apical-radial pulse can be taken by two nurses or one nurse, although the two-nurse technique may be more accurate. *Procedure 15-4* outlines the steps for assessing an apical-radial pulse.

PROCEDURE 15-4 Assessing an Apical-Radial Pulse

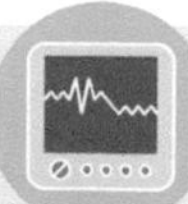

Purpose

- To determine adequacy of peripheral circulation or presence of pulse deficit

Assessment

Assess

- Clinical signs of hypovolaemic shock (hypotension, pallor, cyanosis and cold, clammy skin)
- Cardiac dysfunction

Planning

Equipment

- Watch with a second hand or indicator
- Stethoscope
- Appropriate wipes

Implementation

Preparation

If using the two-nurse technique ensure that the other nurse is available at this time.

Performance

1 Follow local policy to ensure that you explain to the patient what you are going to do, why it is necessary and how they can cooperate. Obtain consent and maintain patient privacy and dignity and ensure that the appropriate local infection control procedures are observed.

2 Position the patient appropriately. Assist the patient to assume the position described for taking the apical pulse. Position the patient appropriately in a comfortable supine position or to a sitting position. Expose the area of the chest over the apex of the heart. If previous measurements were taken, determine what position the patient assumed, and use the same position. *This ensures an accurate comparative measurement.*

3 Locate the apical and radial pulse sites. In the two-nurse technique, one nurse locates the apical impulse by palpation or with the stethoscope while the other nurse palpates the radial pulse site (see *Procedures 15-2* and *15-3*).

4 Count the apical and radial pulse rates.

Two-nurse technique

- Place the watch where both nurses can see it. The nurse who is taking the radial pulse may hold the watch.
- Decide on a time to begin counting. A time when the second hand is on 12, 3, 6 or 9 or an even number on digital clocks is usually selected. The nurse taking the radial pulse says 'Start' at the same time. *This ensures that simultaneous counts are taken.*
- Each nurse counts the pulse rate for 60 seconds. Both nurses end the count when the nurse taking the radial pulse says 'Stop'. *A full 60-second count is necessary for accurate assessment of any discrepancies between the two pulse sites.*
- The nurse who assesses the apical rate also assesses the apical pulse rhythm and volume (i.e. whether the heartbeat is strong or weak). If the pulse is irregular, note whether the irregular beats come at random or at predictable times.
- The nurse assessing the radial pulse rate also assesses the radial pulse rhythm and volume.

One-nurse technique

- Assess the apical pulse for 60 seconds.
- Assess the radial pulse for 60 seconds.

5 Document the apical and radial (AR) pulse rates, rhythm, volume and any pulse deficit on the patient observation chart. Also record related data such as variation in pulse rate compared to normal for the patient and other pertinent observations, such as pallor, cyanosis or dyspnoea.

Evaluation

- Relate pulse rate and rhythm to other vital signs, to baseline data and to general health status.
- Report to the medical staff any changes from previous measurements or any discrepancy between the two pulses.
- Conduct appropriate follow-up such as administering medication or other actions to be taken for a discrepancy in the AR pulse rates.

LIFESPAN CONSIDERATIONS

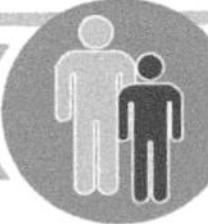

Pulse

Infants

- Use the apical pulse for the heart rate of newborns, infants and children 2–3 years old to establish baseline data for subsequent evaluation, to determine whether the cardiac rate is within normal range, and to determine if the rhythm is regular.
- Place a baby in a supine position. Crying and physical activity will increase the pulse rate. For this reason, take the apical pulse rate of infants and small children before assessing body temperatures.
- Locate the apical pulse in the fourth intercostal space, lateral to the midclavicular line during infancy.
- Brachial, popliteal and femoral pulses may be palpated. Due to a normally low blood pressure and rapid heart rate, infants' other distal pulses may be hard to feel.

Children

- To take a peripheral pulse, position the child comfortably in the adult's arms or have the adult remain close by. This may decrease anxiety and yield more accurate results.
- To assess the apical pulse, assist a young child to a comfortable supine or sitting position.
- Demonstrate the procedure to the child using a stuffed animal or doll, and allow the child to handle the stethoscope before beginning the procedure. This will decrease anxiety and promote cooperation.
- The apex of the heart is normally located in the fourth intercostal space in young children; fifth intercostal space in children seven years of age and over.
- Locate the apical impulse along the fourth intercostal space, between the MCL and the anterior axillary line (see Figure 15-16 on page 426).

Mature Adults

- If the patient has severe hand or arm tremors, the radial pulse may be difficult to count.
- Cardiac changes in older adults, such as decrease in cardiac output, sclerotic changes to heart valves and dysarhythmias often indicate that obtaining an apical pulse will be more accurate.
- Mature adults often have decreased peripheral circulation so that pedal pulses should also be checked for regularity, volume and symmetry.

RESPIRATIONS

Respiration is the act of breathing. External respiration refers to the interchange of oxygen and carbon dioxide between the alveoli of the lungs and the pulmonary blood. Internal respiration, by contrast, takes place throughout the body; it is the interchange of these same gases between the circulating blood and the cells of the body tissues.

Inhalation or inspiration refers to the intake of air into the lungs. Exhalation or expiration refers to breathing out or the movement of gases from the lungs to the atmosphere. **Ventilation** is also used to refer to the movement of air in and out of the lungs.

There are basically two types of breathing: costal (thoracic) breathing and diaphragmatic (abdominal) breathing. Costal breathing involves the external intercostal muscles and other accessory muscles, such as the sternocleidomastoid muscles. It can be observed by the movement of the chest upward and outward. By contrast, diaphragmatic breathing involves the contraction and relaxation of the diaphragm, and it is observed by the movement of the abdomen, which occurs as a result of the diaphragm's contraction and downward movement.

Mechanics and Regulation of Breathing

During *inhalation*, the following processes normally occur (see Figure 15-22): The diaphragm contracts (flattens), the ribs move upward and outward, and the sternum moves outward, thus enlarging the thorax and permitting the lungs to expand. During *exhalation* (see Figure 15-23), the diaphragm relaxes, the ribs move downward and inward, and the sternum moves inward, thus decreasing the size of the thorax as the lungs are compressed. Normally breathing is carried out automatically and effortlessly. A normal adult inspiration lasts 1–1.5 seconds, and an expiration lasts 2–3 seconds.

Respiration is controlled by (a) respiratory centres in the medulla oblongata and the pons of the brain and (b) by chemoreceptors located centrally in the medulla and peripherally in the carotid and aortic bodies. These centres and receptors respond to changes in the concentrations of oxygen (O_2), carbon dioxide (CO_2) and hydrogen (H^+) in the arterial blood.

Assessing Respirations

Resting respirations should be assessed when the patient is relaxed because exercise affects respirations, increasing their

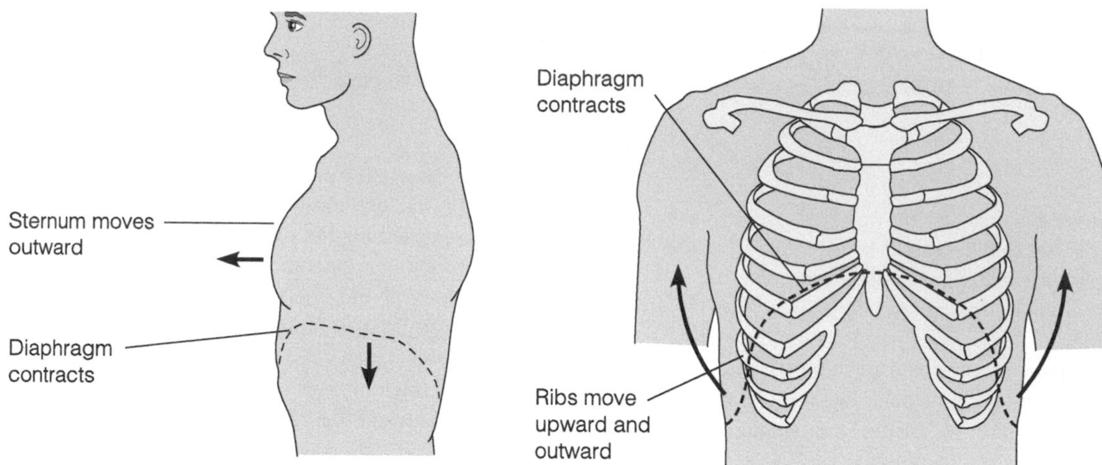

Figure 15-22 Respiratory inhalation, *Left*: lateral view; *Right*: anterior view.

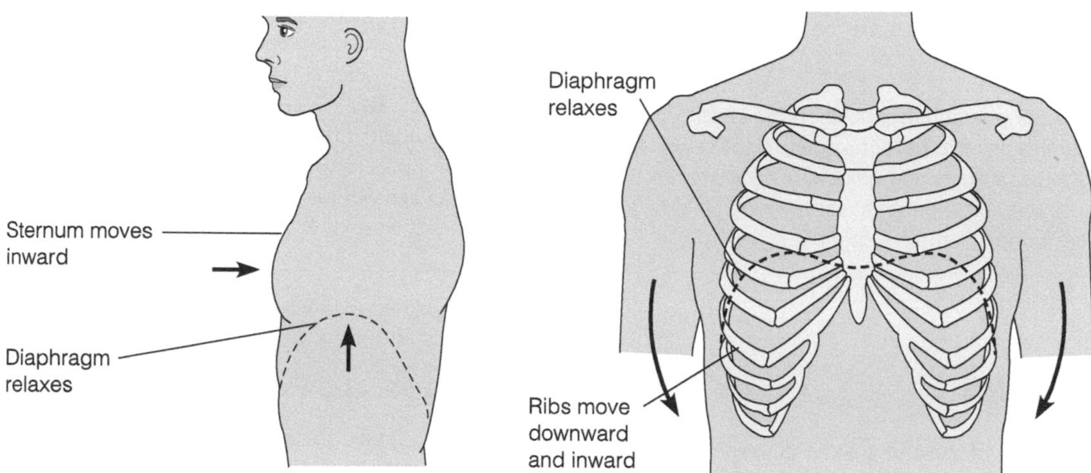

Figure 15-23 Respiratory exhalation. *Left:* lateral view; *Right:* anterior view.

rate and depth. Anxiety is likely to affect respiratory rate and depth as well. Respirations may also need to be assessed after exercise to identify the patient's tolerance to activity. Before assessing a patient's respirations, a nurse should be aware of the following:

- the patient's normal breathing pattern;
- the influence of the patient's health problems on respirations;
- any medications or therapies that might affect respirations;
- the relationship of the patient's respirations to cardiovascular function;
- anxiety due to the approach of a nurse or doctor.

The rate, depth, rhythm and quality and effectiveness of respirations should be assessed.

The *respiratory rate* is normally described in breaths per minute. Breathing that is normal in rate and depth is called eupnoea. Abnormally slow respirations are referred to as **bradypnoea**, and abnormally fast respirations are called **tachypnoea** or polypnoea. **Apnoea** is the absence of breathing. For the respiratory rates for different age groups, see Table 15-1 on page 415.

Factors Affecting Respirations

Several factors influence respiratory rate; those that increase the rate include exercise (increases metabolism), stress (readies the body for 'fight or flight'), increased environmental temperature and lowered oxygen concentration at increased altitudes. Factors that may decrease the respiratory rate include decreased environmental temperature, certain medications (e.g. narcotics) and increased intracranial pressure.

The *depth* of a person's respirations can be established by watching the movement of the chest. Respiratory depth is generally described as normal, deep or shallow. *Deep respirations* are those in which a large volume of air is inhaled and exhaled, inflating most of the lungs. *Shallow respirations* involve the exchange of a small volume of air and often the minimal use of lung tissue. During a normal inspiration and expiration, an adult takes in about 500ml of air. This volume is called the tidal volume.

Body position also affects the amount of air that can be inhaled. People in a supine position experience two physiological processes that suppress respiration: an increase in the volume of blood inside the thoracic cavity and compression of the chest. Consequently, patients lying on their back have poorer lung aeration, which predisposes them to the stasis of fluids and subsequent infection. Certain medications also affect the respiratory depth. For example, narcotics such as morphine and large doses of barbiturates (hypnotic drug or sedation drugs) depress the respiratory centres in the brain, thereby depressing the respiratory rate and depth. **Hyperventilation** refers to very deep, rapid respirations; **hypoventilation** refers to very shallow respirations.

Respiratory rhythm refers to the regularity of the expirations and the inspirations. Normally, respirations are evenly spaced. Respiratory rhythm can be described as *regular* or *irregular*.

Respiratory quality or character refers to those aspects of breathing that are different from normal, effortless breathing. Two of these are the amount of effort a patient must exert to breathe and the sound of breathing. Usually, breathing does not require noticeable effort; some patients, however, breathe only with decided effort, referred to as *laboured breathing*.

The *sound* of breathing is also significant. Normal breathing is silent, but a number of abnormal sounds such as a wheeze are obvious to the nurse's ear. Many sounds occur as a result of the presence of fluid in the lungs and are most clearly heard with a stethoscope.

Patterns and sounds associated with altered breathing are given in the *Practice Guidelines*. *Procedure 15-5* shows the steps for assessing respirations.

PRACTICE GUIDELINES

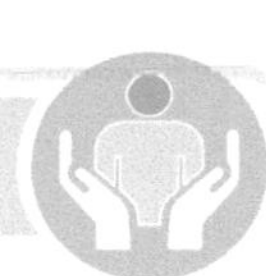

Altered Breathing Patterns and Sounds

Breathing Patterns

Rate

- *Tachypnoea* - quick, shallow breaths
- *Bradypnoea* - abnormally slow breathing
- *Apnoea* - cessation of breathing

Volume

- *Hyperventilation* - overexpansion of the lungs characterised by rapid and deep breaths
- *Hypoventilation* - underexpansion of the lungs, characterised by shallow respirations

Rhythm

- *Cheyne-Stokes breathing* - rhythmic waxing and waning of respirations, from very deep to very shallow breathing and temporary apnoea (nurses may sometimes refer to this when a patient is near to death)

Ease or effort

- *Dyspnoea* - difficult and laboured breathing during which the individual has a persistent, unsatisfied need for air and feels distressed
- *Orthopnoea* - ability to breathe only in upright sitting or standing positions

Breath Sounds

Audible without amplification

- *Stridor* - a shrill, harsh sound heard during inspiration with laryngeal obstruction
- *Stertor* - snoring or sonorous respiration, usually due to a partial obstruction of the upper airway
- *Wheeze* - continuous, high-pitched musical squeak or whistling sound occurring on expiration and sometimes on inspiration when air moves through a narrowed or partially obstructed airway
- *Bubbling* - gurgling sounds heard as air passes through moist secretions in the respiratory tract

Chest movements

- *Intercostal retraction* - indrawing between the ribs
- *Substernal retraction* - indrawing beneath the breastbone
- *Suprasternal retraction* - indrawing above the clavicles

Secretions and coughing

- *Haemoptysis* - the presence of blood in the sputum
- *Productive cough* - a cough accompanied by expectorated secretions
- *Nonproductive cough* - a dry, harsh cough without secretions

PROCEDURE 15-5 Assessing Respirations

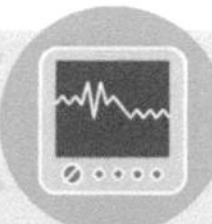

Purposes

- To acquire baseline data against which future measurements can be compared
- To monitor abnormal respirations and respiratory patterns and identify changes
- To assess respirations before the administration of a medication such as morphine (an abnormally slow respiratory rate may warrant withholding the medication)
- To monitor respirations following the administration of a general anaesthetic or any medication that influences respirations
- To monitor patients at risk for respiratory alterations (e.g. those with pyrexia, pain, acute anxiety, chronic obstructive pulmonary disease, respiratory infection, pulmonary oedema or emboli, chest trauma or constriction, brain stem injury)

Assessment

Assess

- Skin and mucous membrane colour (e.g. cyanosis or pallor)
- Position assumed for breathing (e.g. use of **orthopnoeic position**)
- Signs of cerebral anoxia (e.g. irritability, restlessness, drowsiness or loss of consciousness)
- Chest movements (e.g. retractions between the ribs or above or below the sternum)
- Activity tolerance
- Chest pain
- Dyspnoea
- Medications affecting respiratory rate

Planning

Equipment

- Watch with a second hand or indicator

Implementation

Preparation

For a routine assessment of respirations, choose a suitable time to monitor the respirations. A patient who has been exercising will need to rest for a few minutes to permit the accelerated respiratory rate to return to normal.

Performance

1 Follow local policy to ensure that you explain to the patient what you are going to do, why it is necessary and how they can cooperate. Obtain consent and maintain patient privacy and dignity and ensure that the appropriate local infection control procedures are observed.

2 Observe or palpate and count the respiratory rate.
   - The patient's awareness that you are counting the respiratory rate could cause the patient voluntarily to alter the respiratory pattern. If you anticipate this, place a hand against the patient's chest to feel the chest movements with breathing, or place the patient's arm across the chest and observe the chest movements while supposedly taking the radial pulse.
   - Count the respiratory rate for 60 seconds. An inhalation and an exhalation count as one respiration.

3 Observe the depth, rhythm and character of respirations.
   - Observe the respirations for depth by watching the movement of the chest and ensure the patient is unaware you are counting their respirations otherwise they will change the breathing pattern. *During deep respirations a large volume of air is exchanged; during shallow respirations a small volume is exchanged.*
   - Observe the respirations for regular or irregular rhythm. *Normally, respirations are evenly spaced.*
   - Observe the character of respirations - the sound they produce and the effort they require. *Normally, respirations are silent and effortless.*

4 Document the respiratory rate, depth, rhythm and character on the appropriate record.

Evaluation

- Relate respiratory rate to other vital signs, in particular pulse rate, respiratory rhythm and depth to baseline data and health status.
- Report to the medical staff respiratory rate significantly above or below the normal range and any notable change in respirations from previous assessments; irregular respiratory rhythm; inadequate respiratory depth; abnormal character of breathing - orthopnoea, wheezing, stridor or bubbling; and any complaints of dyspnoea.
- Conduct appropriate follow-up such as administering appropriate medications or treatments, positioning the patient to ease breathing, and requesting involvement of other members of the healthcare team such as the physiotherapist.
- Monitor and assess revised treatment.

LIFESPAN CONSIDERATIONS

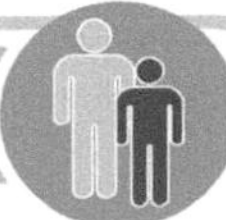

Respirations

Infants

- An infant or child who is crying will have an abnormal respiratory rate and will need quietening before respirations can be accurately assessed.
- If necessary, place your hand gently on the infant's abdomen to feel the rapid rise and fall during respirations.

Children

- Because young children are diaphragmatic breathers, observe the rise and fall of the abdomen.
- If necessary, place your hand gently on the abdomen to feel the rapid rise and fall during respirations.

Mature Adults

- Ask the patient to remain quiet or count respirations after taking the pulse.
- Mature adults experience anatomical and physiological changes that cause the respiratory system to be less efficient. Any changes in rate or type of breathing should be reported immediately.

The effectiveness of respirations is measured in part by the uptake of oxygen from the air into the blood and the release of carbon dioxide from the blood into expired air. The amount of haemoglobin in arterial blood that is saturated with oxygen can be measured indirectly through pulse oximetry. Using a **pulse oximeter** monitor applied to the patient's finger, toe or other site provides a digital readout of both the patient's pulse rate and the oxygen saturation (see *Procedure 15-7* on page 448).

BLOOD PRESSURE

Arterial blood pressure is a measure of the pressure exerted by the blood as it flows through the arteries. Because the blood moves in waves, there are two blood pressure measures: the **systolic pressure**, which is the pressure of the blood as a result of contraction of the ventricles, that is, the pressure of the height of the blood wave; and the **diastolic pressure**, which is the pressure when the ventricles are at rest. Diastolic pressure, then, is the lower pressure, present at all times within the arteries. The difference between the diastolic and the systolic pressures is called the pulse pressure.

Blood pressure is measured in millimetres of mercury (mm Hg) and recorded as a fraction. The systolic pressure is written over the diastolic pressure. The average blood pressure of a healthy adult is 120/80mm Hg, and according to NICE guidelines (NICE, 2006) a systolic rate of less than 140mm Hg and a dyastolic rate of less than 85mm Hg is the norm. A number of conditions are reflected by changes in blood pressure. Because blood pressure can vary considerably among individuals, it is important for the nurse to know a specific patient's baseline blood pressure. For example, a decreased blood pressure following surgery accompanied by a rapid pulse may indicate a haemorrhage.

Determinants of Blood Pressure

Arterial blood pressure is the result of several factors: the pumping action of the heart, the peripheral vascular resistance (the resistance supplied by the blood vessels through which the blood flows), and the blood volume and viscosity.

Pumping Action of the Heart

When the pumping action of the heart is weak, less blood is pumped into arteries (lower cardiac output), and the blood pressure decreases. When the heart's pumping action is strong and the volume of blood pumped into the circulation increases (higher cardiac output), the blood pressure increases.

Peripheral Vascular Resistance

Peripheral resistance can increase blood pressure. The diastolic pressure especially is affected. Some factors that create resistance in the arterial system are the capacity of the arterioles and capillaries, the compliance of the arteries and the viscosity of the blood.

The internal diameter or capacity of the arterioles and the capillaries determines in great part the peripheral resistance to the blood in the body. The smaller the space within a vessel, the greater the resistance. Normally, the arterioles are in a state of partial constriction. Increased vasoconstriction raises the blood pressure, whereas decreased vasoconstriction lowers the blood pressure.

If the elastic and muscular tissues of the arteries are replaced with fibrous tissue, the arteries lose much of their ability to constrict and dilate. This condition, most common in middle-aged and elderly adults, is known as **arteriosclerosis**.

Blood Volume

When the blood volume decreases (e.g. as a result of a haemorrhage or dehydration), the blood pressure decreases because of decreased fluid in the arteries. Conversely, when the volume increases (e.g. as a result of a rapid intravenous infusion), the blood pressure increases because of the greater fluid volume within the circulatory system.

Blood Viscosity

Blood pressure is higher when the blood is highly viscous (thick), that is, when the proportion of red blood cells to the blood plasma is high. This proportion is referred to as the

haematocrit. The viscosity increases markedly when the haematocrit is more than 60% to 65%.

Factors Affecting Blood Pressure

Among the factors influencing blood pressure are age, exercise, stress, race, diet, obesity, sex, medications, diurnal variations and disease processes.

- *Age.* Newborns have a mean systolic pressure of about 75mm Hg. The pressure rises with age, reaching a peak at the onset of puberty, and then tends to decline somewhat. In older people, elasticity of the arteries is decreased – the arteries are more rigid and less yielding to the pressure of the blood. This produces an elevated systolic pressure. Because the walls no longer retract as flexibly with decreased pressure, the diastolic pressure is also high (see Table 15-1 on page 415).
- *Exercise.* Physical activity increases the cardiac output and hence the blood pressure; thus 20–30 minutes of rest following exercise is indicated before the resting blood pressure can be reliably assessed.
- *Stress.* Stimulation of the sympathetic nervous system increases cardiac output and vasoconstriction of the arterioles, thus increasing the blood pressure reading; however, severe pain can decrease blood pressure greatly by inhibiting the vasomotor centre and producing vasodilatation.
- *Race.* According to Holland and Hogg (2010) Asian and African-Caribbean populations have a high number of individuals who are hypertensive.
- *Gender.* After puberty, females usually have lower blood pressures than males of the same age; this difference is thought to be due to hormonal variations. After menopause, women generally have higher blood pressures than before.
- *Medications.* Many medications may increase or decrease the blood pressure.
- *Diet.* Studies have shown that eating too much salt, high intake of caffeine and drinking too much alcohol can increase the blood pressure.
- *Obesity.* Both childhood and adult obesity predispose to hypertension.
- *Diurnal variations.* Pressure is usually lowest early in the morning, when the metabolic rate is lowest, then rises throughout the day and peaks in the late afternoon or early evening.
- *Disease process.* Any condition affecting the cardiac output, blood volume, blood viscosity and/or compliance of the arteries has a direct effect on the blood pressure.

Hypertension

A blood pressure that is persistently above normal is called **hypertension**. It is usually asymptomatic and is often a contributing factor to myocardial infarctions (heart attacks). An elevated blood pressure of unknown cause is called *primary hypertension*. An elevated blood pressure of known cause is called *secondary hypertension*. Hypertension is a widespread health problem. A systolic blood pressure greater than 130 or diastolic greater than 85 requires follow-up (see Table 15.4).

Table 15-4 Recommendations for Follow-up Based on Initial Blood Pressure Measurements for Adults Without Acute End Organ Damage

Initial blood pressure (mmHg)*	SBP mmHg	DBP mmHg	Follow-up recommended
Normal	<120	and <80	Recheck in 2 years
Prehypertension	120-139	or 80-89	Recheck in 1 year**
Stage 1 hypertension	140-159	or 90-99	Confirm within 2 months***
Stage 2 hypertension	≥160	or ≥100	Evaluate or refer to source of care within 1 month. For those with higher pressures (e.g. >180/110 mmHg), evaluate and treat immediately or within 1 week, depending on clinical situation and complications

SBP = systolic blood pressure; DBP = diastolic blood pressure.

* If systolic and diastolic categories are different, follow recommendations for shorter time follow-up (e.g. 160/86 mmHg should be evaluated or referred to source of care within 1 month).

** Modify the scheduling of follow-up according to reliable information about past BP measurements, other cardiovascular risk factors, or target organ disease.

*** Provide advice about lifestyle modifications.

Source: Tables 3 and 4 (pp. 12 and 18), *The Seventh Report of the Joint National Committee on Prevention, Detection, Evaluation, and Treatment of High Blood Pressure*. London: The National Heart, Lung and Blood Institute.

COMMUNITY CARE CONSIDERATIONS

Measuring Blood Pressure in the Community

- Healthcare professionals taking blood pressure measurements need adequate initial training and periodic review of their performance.
- Healthcare providers must ensure that devices for measuring blood pressure are properly validated, maintained and regularly recalibrated according to manufacturers' instructions.
- Where possible, standardise the environment when measuring blood pressure: provide a relaxed, temperate setting, with the patient quiet and seated and with their arm outstretched and supported.
- If the first measurement exceeds 140/90mmHg, if practical, take a second confirmatory reading at the end of the consultation.
- Measure blood pressure on both of the patient's arms with the higher value identifying the reference arm for future measurement.
- In patients with symptoms of postural hypotension (falls or postural dizziness) measure blood pressure while patient is standing. In patients with symptoms or documented postural hypotension (fall in systolic BP when standing of 20mmHg or more) consider referral to a specialist.
- Refer immediately patients with accelerated (malignant) hypertension (BP more than 180/110mmHg with signs of papilloedema and/or retinal haemorrhage) or suspected phaeochromocytoma (possible signs include labile or postural hypotension, headache, palpitations, pallor and diaphoresis).
- To identify hypertension (persistent raised blood pressure, above 140/90mmHg), ask the patient to return for at least two subsequent clinics where blood pressure is assessed from two readings under the best conditions available.
- Measurements should normally be made at monthly intervals. However, patients with more severe hypertension should be re-evaluated more urgently.
- Consider the need for specialist investigation of patients with unusual signs and symptoms, or of those whose management depends critically on the accurate estimation of their blood pressure.

Source: NICE 2006.

The diagnosis of hypertension is made when the average of two or more, diastolic readings on two subsequent visits from the initial assessment is 90mmHg or higher, or when the average of multiple systolic blood pressure readings is higher than 140mmHg (see Table 15-4). Factors associated with hypertension include thickening of the arterial walls, which reduces the size of the arterial lumen, and inelasticity of the arteries as well as such lifestyle factors as cigarette smoking, obesity, heavy alcohol consumption, lack of physical exercise, high blood cholesterol levels and continued exposure to stress. Follow-up care should include lifestyle changes conducive to lowering the blood pressure as well as monitoring the pressure itself.

Hypotension

Hypotension is a blood pressure that is below normal, that is, a systolic reading consistently between 85 and 110mmHg in an adult whose normal pressure is higher than this. **Orthostatic hypotension** is a blood pressure that falls when the patient sits or stands. It is usually the result of peripheral vasodilatation in which blood leaves the central body organs, especially the brain, and moves to the periphery, often causing the person to feel faint. Hypotension can also be caused by analgesics such as morphine sulphate, bleeding, severe burns and dehydration. It is important to monitor hypotensive patients carefully to prevent falls. When assessing for orthostatic hypotension:

- Place the patient in a supine position for 2–3 minutes.
- Record the patient's pulse and blood pressure.
- Assist the patient to slowly sit or stand. Support the patient in case of faintness.
- After one minute in the upright position, recheck the pulse and blood pressure in the same sites as previously.
- Record the results. A rise in pulse of 40 beats per minute or a drop in blood pressure of 30mm Hg indicates abnormal orthostatic vital signs.

Consensus of opinion states that a better result is obtained if a patient is seated for ten minutes to record baseline values which may vary slightly with some nursing practice (Lance *et al.*, 2000).

Assessing Blood Pressure

Blood pressure is generally measured with a mercury sphygmomanometer which includes a *blood pressure cuff*, a *sphygmomanometer* and a *stethoscope*. This method is considered to be reliable and accurate (Dougherty and Lister, 2008).The blood pressure cuff consists of a rubber bag that can be inflated with air. It is called the *bladder* (see Figure 15-24). It is covered with cloth and has two tubes attached to it. One tube connects to a rubber bulb that inflates the bladder. When turned counterclockwise, a small valve on the side of this bulb releases the air in the bladder. When the valve is tightened (turned clockwise), air pumped into the bladder remains there.

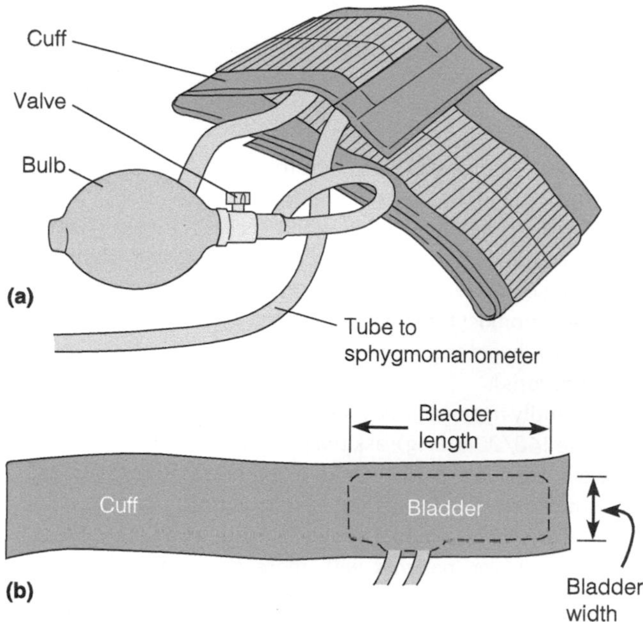

Figure 15-24 (a) A blood pressure cuff and bulb; (b) the bladder inside the cuff.

The other tube is attached to a sphygmomanometer. The sphygmomanometer indicates the pressure of the air within the bladder. There are two types of sphygmomanometers: *aneroid* and *mercury* (see Figure 15-25). The aneroid sphygmomanometer is a calibrated dial with a needle that points to the calibrations.

The mercury sphygmomanometer is a calibrated cylinder filled with mercury. The pressure is indicated at the point to which the rounded curve of the meniscus (the crescent-shaped dome) rises (see Figure 15-26). The blood pressure reading should be made with the eye at the level of the rounded curve in order to be accurate.

CLINICAL ALERT

The mercury sphygmomanometers should be regularly calibrated or they may not record accurate readings. The British Heart Society state that all blood pressure monitors should be tested according to the revised British Heart Society protocol 1993, whether they are used in the clinical area or at home.

The use of *electronic sphygmomanometers* (see Figure 15-27) has become more popular in the clinical environment in the last two decades. They eliminate the need to listen to the sounds of the patient's systolic and diastolic blood pressures through a stethoscope. However, irregular readings are more difficult to identify and the equipment should only be used by staff trained in its use (Beevers *et al.*, 2000). Electronic blood pressure devices should be calibrated periodically to check accuracy in accordance with manufacturer guidelines and local policy. The electronic devices rely on the pulse of the artery to record the blood pressure; therefore accuracy in the positioning of the cuff is essential to record accurately.

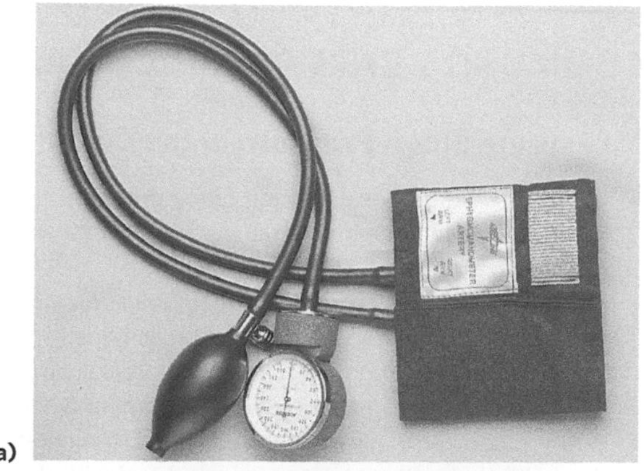

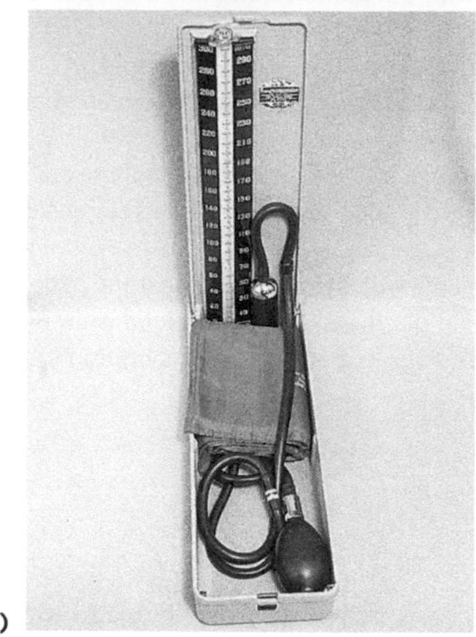

Figure 15-25 Blood pressure equipment: (a) an aneroid manometer and cuff; (b) a mercury manometer and cuff.
Source: Pearson Education Ltd.

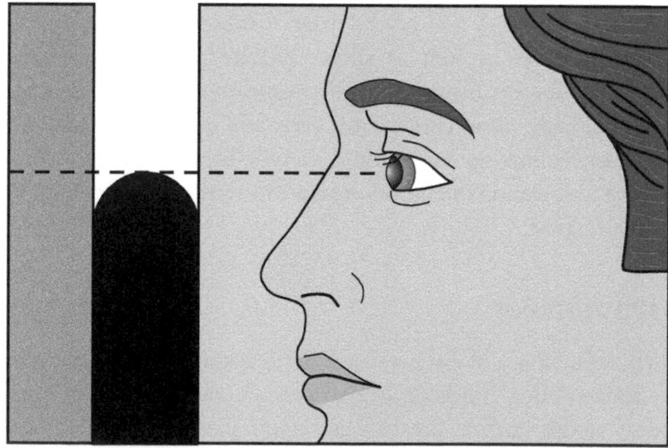

Figure 15-26 To obtain an accurate reading from a mercury manometer, position the meniscus at eye level.

Blood pressure cuffs come in various sizes because the bladder must be the correct width and length for the patient's

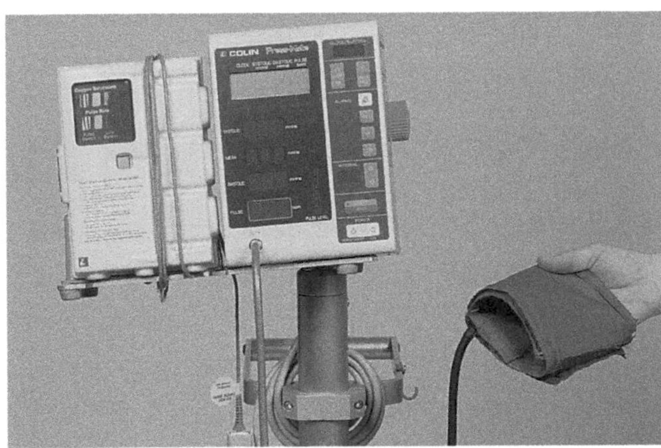

Figure 15-27 Automatic blood pressure monitors register systolic, diastolic and mean blood pressures.

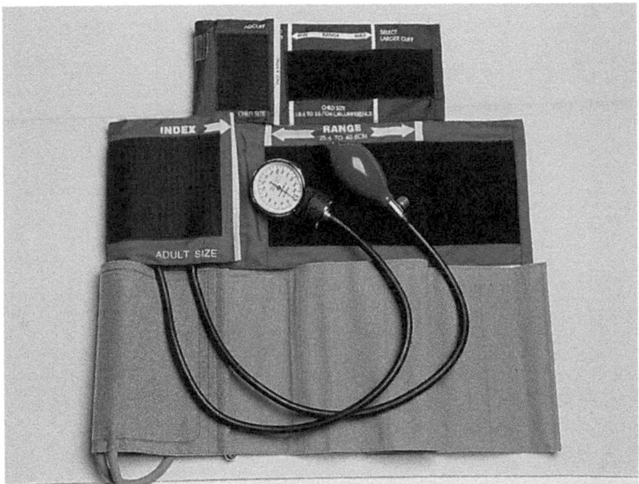

Figure 15-28 Three standard cuff sizes: a small cuff for an infant, small child or frail adult; a normal adult-size cuff; and a large cuff for measuring the blood pressure on the leg or on the arm of an obese adult.

arm (see Figure 15-28). If the bladder is too narrow, the blood pressure reading will be erroneously elevated; if it is too wide, the reading will be erroneously low. The width should be 40% of the circumference, or 20% wider than the diameter of the midpoint of the limb on which it is used. The arm circumference, not the age of the patient, should always be used to determine bladder size. The nurse can also determine whether the width of a blood pressure cuff is appropriate: lay the cuff lengthwise at the midpoint of the upper arm, and hold the outermost side of the bladder edge laterally on the arm. With the other hand, wrap the width of the cuff around the arm, and ensure that the width is 40% of the arm circumference (see Figure 15-29).

The length of the bladder also affects the accuracy of measurement. The bladder should be sufficiently long to cover at least two-thirds of the limb's circumference.

Blood pressure cuffs are made of nondistensible material so that an even pressure is exerted around the limb. Most cuffs are held in place by Velcro. Others have a cloth bandage that is long enough to encircle the limb several times; this type is closed by tucking the end of the bandage into one of the bandage folds.

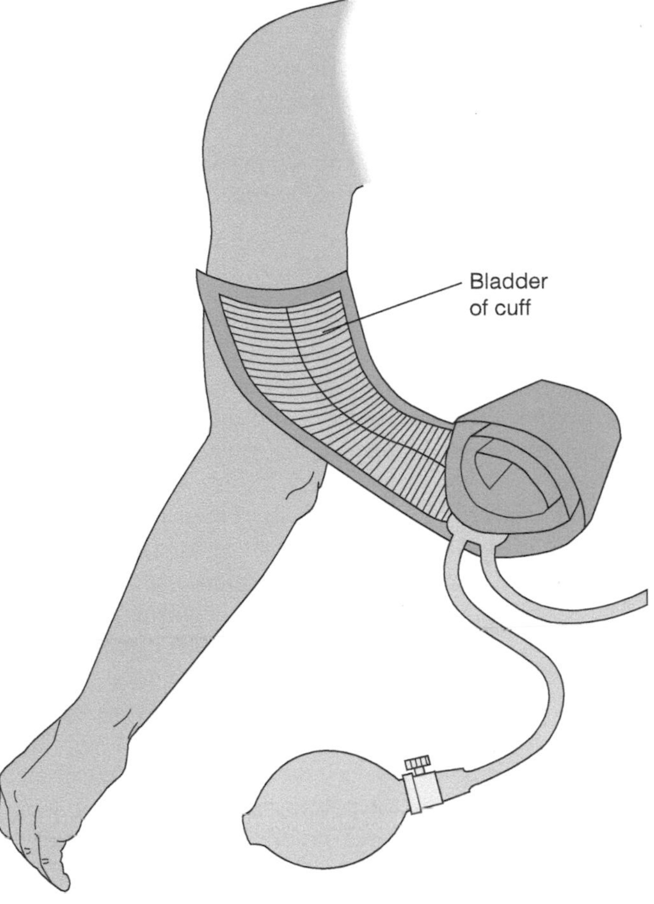

Figure 15-29 Determining that the bladder of a blood pressure cuff is 40% of the arm circumference or 20% wider than the diameter of the mid-point of the limb.

There are an increasing number of individuals who monitor their own blood pressure in the home. According to O'Brien *et al.* (2001), these devices are generally not considered reliable. However, the British Heart Society recommend that patients should be advised to buy carefully and that these monitors need to be tested regularly.

Blood Pressure Sites

The blood pressure is usually assessed in the patient's arm using the brachial artery and a standard stethoscope. Assessing the blood pressure on a patient's thigh is usually indicated in these situations:

- The blood pressure cannot be measured on either arm (e.g. because of burns or other trauma).
- The blood pressure in one thigh is to be compared with the blood pressure in the other thigh.

Blood pressure is not measured on a patient's arm or thigh in the following situations:

- The shoulder, arm or hand (or the hip, knee or ankle) is injured or diseased.
- A cast or bulky bandage is on any part of the limb.
- The patient has had removal of axilla (or hip) lymph nodes on that side.
- The patient has an intravenous infusion in that limb.
- The patient has an arteriovenous fistula (e.g. for renal dialysis) in that limb.

Methods

Blood pressure can be assessed directly or indirectly. *Direct (invasive monitoring) measurement* involves the insertion of a catheter into the brachial, radial or femoral artery. Arterial pressure is represented as wavelike forms displayed on an oscilloscope. With correct placement, this pressure reading is highly accurate.

Two *noninvasive indirect methods* of measuring blood pressure are the *auscultatory* (mercury or aneroid) and *palpatory* methods. The *auscultatory method* is most commonly used in hospitals, clinics and homes. Required equipment is a sphygmomanometer, a cuff and a stethoscope. When carried out correctly, the auscultatory method is relatively accurate.

When taking a blood pressure using a stethoscope, the nurse identifies five phases in the series of sounds called Korotkoff's sounds (see Figure 15-30). First the nurse pumps the cuff up to about 30mmHg above the point where the pulse is no longer felt; that is the point when the blood flow in the artery is stopped. Then the pressure is released slowly (2–3mmHg per sound) while the nurse observes the readings on the manometer and relates them to the sounds heard through the stethoscope. Five phases occur but may not always be audible (see *Practice Guidelines*).

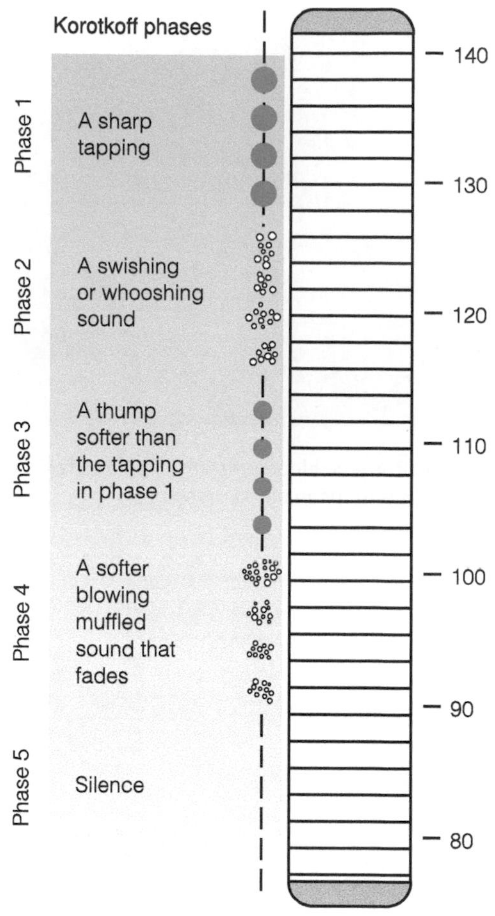

Figure 15-30 Korotkoff's sounds can be differentiated into five phases. In the illustration the blood pressure is 138/90 or 138/102/90.

PRACTICE GUIDELINES

Korotkoff's Sounds

These are the sounds listened for when recording blood pressure manually with a stethoscope and sphygmomanometer.

Phase 1 The pressure level at which the first faint, clear tapping or thumping sounds are heard. These sounds gradually become more intense. To ensure that they are not extraneous sounds, the nurse should identify at least two consecutive tapping sounds. The first tapping sound heard during deflation of the cuff is the systolic blood pressure.

Phase 2 The period during deflation when the sounds have a muffled, whooshing or swishing quality.

Phase 3 The period during which the blood flows freely through an increasingly open artery and the sounds become crisper and more intense and again assume a thumping quality but softer than in phase 1.

Phase 4 The time when the sounds become muffled and have a soft, blowing quality.

Phase 5 The pressure level when the last sound is heard. This is followed by a period of silence. The pressure at which the last sound is heard is the diastolic blood pressure in adults.*

* In clinical areas where the fourth phase is considered the diastolic pressure, three measures are recommended (systolic pressure, diastolic pressure and phase 5). These may be referred to as systolic, first diastolic and second diastolic pressures. The phase 5 (second diastolic pressure) reading may be zero; that is, the muffled sounds are heard even when there is no air pressure in the blood pressure cuff. In some instances, muffled sounds are never heard, in which case a dash is inserted where the reading would normally be recorded (e.g. 190/–/110).

The *palpatory method* is sometimes used when Korotkoff's sounds cannot be heard and electronic equipment to amplify the sounds is not available, or to prevent misdirection from the presence of an auscultatory gap. An auscultatory gap, which occurs particularly in hypertensive patients, is the temporary disappearance of sounds normally heard over the brachial artery when the cuff pressure is high followed by the reappearance of the sounds at a lower level. This temporary disappearance of sound occurs in the latter part of phase 1 and phase 2 and may cover a range of 40 mm Hg. If a palpated estimation of the systolic pressure is not made prior to auscultation, the nurse may begin listening in the middle of this range and underestimate the systolic pressure. In the palpatory method of blood pressure determination, instead of listening for the blood flow sounds, using light to moderate pressure the nurse palpates the pulsations of the artery as the pressure in the cuff is released. The pressure is read from the sphygmomanometer when the first pulsation is felt.

ACTIVITY 15-2

You have been asked by your mentor to record the blood pressure of an obese lady who has just been admitted to your care. You haven't had much experience of recording blood pressures as this is your first ward. Reflect and explore what you need to consider before you approach the patient.

Procedure 15-6 shows the steps in assessing blood pressure.

PROCEDURE 15-6 Assessing Blood Pressure

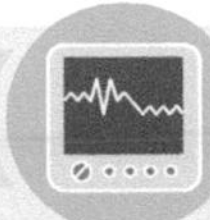

Purposes

- To obtain a baseline measure of arterial blood pressure for subsequent evaluation
- To determine the patient's haemodynamic status (e.g. stroke volume of the heart and blood vessel resistance)
- To identify and monitor changes in blood pressure resulting from a disease process and medical therapy (e.g. presence or history of cardiovascular disease, renal disease, circulatory shock or acute pain; rapid infusion of fluids or blood products)

Assessment

Assess

- Signs and symptoms of hypertension (e.g. headache, ringing in the ears, flushing of face, nosebleeds, fatigue)
- Signs and symptoms of hypotension (e.g. tachycardia, dizziness, mental confusion, restlessness, cool and clammy skin, pale or cyanotic skin)
- Factors affecting blood pressure (e.g. activity, emotional stress, pain and time the patient last smoked or ingested caffeine)

Planning

Equipment

- Stethoscope
- Blood pressure cuff of the appropriate size (approximately covering 80% of the circumference of the upper arm (Petrie *et al.*, 1997)
- Sphygmomanometer

Implementation

Preparation

1 Ensure that the equipment is intact and functioning properly. Check for leaks in the rubber tubing of the sphygmomanometer.

2 Make sure that the patient has not smoked or ingested caffeine within 30 minutes prior to measurement.

Performance

1 Follow local policy to ensure that you explain to the patient what you are going to do, why it is necessary and how they can cooperate. Obtain consent and maintain patient privacy and dignity and ensure that the appropriate local infection control procedures are observed.

2 Position the patient appropriately.
- The adult patient should be sitting unless otherwise specified. Both feet should be flat on the floor *since legs crossed at the knee result in elevated systolic and diastolic blood pressures* (Foster-Fitzpatrick *et al.*, 1999).
- The elbow should be slightly flexed with the palm of the hand facing up and the forearm supported at heart level. Readings in any other position should be specified. The blood pressure is normally similar in sitting, standing and lying positions, but it can vary significantly if patients are not positioned properly. *The blood pressure increases when the arm is below heart level and decreases when the arm is above heart level.*
- Expose the upper arm, and ensure tight or restrictive clothing removed.

3 Ask the patient to rest for 2-3 minutes prior to taking recording.

4 Wrap the deflated cuff evenly around the upper arm. Locate the brachial artery (see Figure 15-15 on page 426). Apply the centre of the bladder directly over the artery. *The bladder inside the cuff must be directly over the artery to be compressed if the reading is to be accurate.*
- For an adult, place the lower border of the cuff approximately 2.5cm (1 inch) above the antecubital space.

5 Position the manometer within 1mm of the patient.

6 If this is the patient's initial examination, perform a preliminary palpatory determination of systolic pressure. The initial estimate tells the nurse the maximal pressure to which the manometer needs to be elevated in subsequent determinations. It also prevents underestimation of the systolic pressure or overestimation of the diastolic pressure should an auscultatory gap occur.
- Palpate the brachial artery with the fingertips.
- Close the valve on the pump by turning the knob clockwise.
- Pump up the cuff until you no longer feel the brachial pulse. At that pressure the blood cannot flow through the artery. Note the pressure on the sphygmomanometer at which pulse is no longer felt. *This gives an estimate of the maximum pressure required to measure the systolic pressure.*
- Release the pressure completely in the cuff, and wait 1-2 minutes before making further measurements. A waiting period gives the blood trapped in the veins time to be released. Otherwise, false high systolic readings will occur.

7 Position the stethoscope appropriately.
- Cleanse the earpieces with alcohol or recommended disinfectant.
- Insert the ear attachments of the stethoscope in your ears so that they tilt slightly forward. *Sounds are heard more clearly when the ear attachments follow the direction of the ear canal.*
- Ensure that the stethoscope hangs freely from the ears to the diaphragm. Rubbing the stethoscope against an object can obliterate the sounds of the blood within an artery.
- Place the bell side of the amplifier of the stethoscope over the brachial pulse. *Because the blood pressure is a low-frequency sound, it is best heard with the bell-shaped diaphragm.* Hold the diaphragm with the thumb and index finger.

8 Auscultate the patient's blood pressure.
- Pump up the cuff until the sphygmomanometer reads 30mm Hg above the point where the brachial pulse disappeared by palpation as in point 6.
- Release the valve on the cuff carefully so that the pressure decreases at the rate of 2-3mmHg per second. *If the rate is faster or slower an error in measurement may occur.*
- As the pressure falls, identify the manometer reading at each of the five phases, if possible.
- Deflate the cuff rapidly and completely.
- Wait 1-2 minutes before making further determinations. *This permits blood trapped in the veins to be released.*
- Repeat the above steps once or twice as necessary to confirm the accuracy of the reading.

9 If this is the patient's initial examination, repeat the procedure on the patient's other arm. There should be a difference of no more than 10mmHg between the arms. The arm found to have the higher pressure should be used for subsequent examinations.

Variation: obtaining a blood pressure by the palpation method

If it is not possible to use a stethoscope to obtain the blood pressure or if the Korotkoff sounds cannot be heard, palpate the radial or brachial pulse site as the cuff pressure is released. The manometer reading at the point where the pulse re-appears represents a blood pressure between what would be auscultated systolic and diastolic values.

Variation: taking a thigh blood pressure

- Help the patient to assume a prone position. If the patient cannot assume this position, measure the blood pressure while the patient is in a supine position with the knee slightly flexed. Slight flexing of the knee will facilitate placing the stethoscope on the popliteal space (see Figure 15-31).
- Expose the thigh, taking care not to expose the patient unduly.
- Locate the popliteal artery (see Figure 15-18 on page 429). Wrap the cuff evenly around the midthigh with the compression bladder over the posterior aspect of the thigh and the bottom edge above the knee. *The bladder must be directly over the posterior popliteal artery if the reading is to be accurate.*

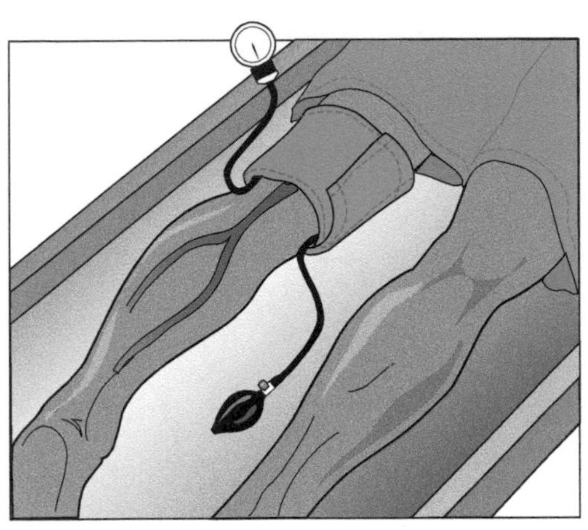

Figure 15-31 Measuring blood pressure in the patient's thigh - location of the popliteal artery and application of the cuff.

- If this is the patient's initial examination, perform a preliminary palpatory determination of systolic pressure by palpating the popliteal artery.
- In adults, the systolic pressure in the popliteal artery is usually 20-30mmHg higher than that in the brachial artery because of use of a larger bladder; the diastolic pressure is usually the same.

Variation: using an electronic blood pressure monitoring device (Figure 15-27). Only use if training on its use has been provided.

- Place the blood pressure cuff on the extremity according to the manufacturer's guidelines.
- Turn on the blood pressure switch.
- If appropriate, set the device for the desired number of minutes between blood pressure determinations.
- When the device has determined the blood pressure reading, note the digital results.

10 Remove the cuff.

11 Wipe the cuff with an approved disinfectant. *Cuffs can become significantly contaminated.* Some clinical areas use disposable blood pressure cuffs. The patient uses it for the length of stay and then it is discarded. This decreases the risk of spreading infection through sharing of cuffs.

12 Document and report pertinent assessment data according to agency policy. Record two pressures in the form '130/80' where '130' is the systolic (phase 1) and '80' is the diastolic (phase 5) pressure. Use the abbreviations *RA* or *RL* for right arm or right leg and *LA* or *LL* for left arm or left leg. Record a difference of greater than 10mmHg between the two arms or legs.

Evaluation

- Relate blood pressure to other vital signs, to baseline data and health status.
- Report any significant change in the patient's blood pressure. Also report these findings:
  - Systolic blood pressure (of an adult) above 140mmHg
  - Diastolic blood pressure (of an adult) above 90mmHg
  - Systolic blood pressure (of an adult) below 100mmHg
- Conduct appropriate follow-up such as administration of medication. If the blood pressure is significantly higher or lower than usual, implement appropriate safety precautions.

CLINICAL ALERT

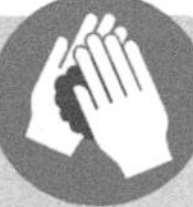

Electronic/automatic blood pressure cuffs can be left in place for many hours. Remove the cuff and check skin condition periodically.

LIFESPAN CONSIDERATIONS

Blood Pressure

Infants

- Use a paediatric stethoscope with small diaphragm.
- The lower edge of the blood pressure cuff can be closer to the antecubital space of an infant.
- Use the palpation method if auscultation with a stethoscope or DUS is unsuccessful.
- Arm and thigh pressures are equivalent in children under one year of age. One quick way to determine the normal systolic blood pressure of a child is to use the following formula:

  Normal systolic BP = 80 + (2 × child's age in years)

Children

- Explain each step of the process and what it will feel like. Demonstrate on a doll.
- Use the palpation technique for children under three years old.
- Cuff bladder *width* should be 40% and *length* should be 80% to 100% of the arm circumference (see Figure 15-32).
- Take the blood pressure prior to other uncomfortable procedures so that the blood pressure is not artificially elevated by the discomfort.
- In children, the diastolic pressure is considered to be the onset of phase 4, where the sounds become muffled.
- In children, the thigh pressure is about 10mm Hg higher than the arm.

Mature Adults

- Skin may be very fragile. Do not allow cuff pressure to remain high any longer than necessary.
- Determine if the patient is taking antihypertensives and, if so, when the last dose was taken.
- Medications that cause vasodilation (antihypertensive medications) along with the loss of baroreceptor efficiency in the elderly place them at increased risk for having orthostatic hypotension. Measuring blood pressure while the patient is in the lying, sitting and standing positions, and noting any changes can determine this.
- If the patient has arm contractures, assess the blood pressure by palpation, with the arm in a relaxed position. If this is not possible, take a thigh blood pressure.

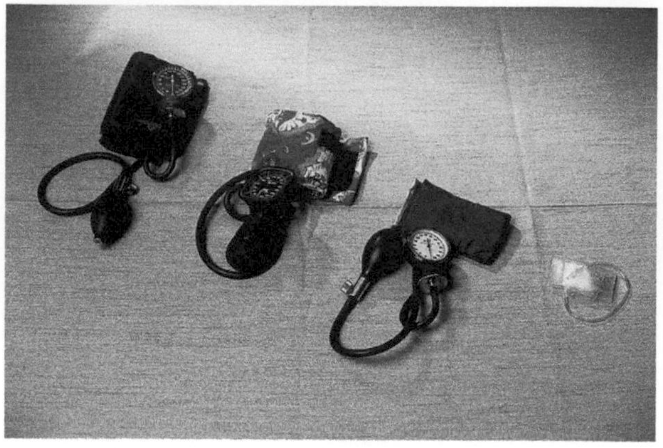

Figure 15-32 Paediatric blood pressure cuffs (with manometers).

Source: Pearson Education Ltd.

Common Errors in Assessing Blood Pressure

The importance of the accuracy of blood pressure assessments cannot be overemphasised. Many judgements about a patient's health are made on the basis of blood pressure. It is an important indicator of the patient's condition and is used extensively as a basis for nursing interventions. Two possible reasons for blood pressure errors are haste on the part of the nurse and subconscious bias. For example, a nurse may be influenced by the patient's previous blood pressure measurements or diagnosis and 'hear' a value consonant with the practitioner's expectations.

According to the British Hypertension Society (2009), errors that occur during the recording of a blood pressure are:

- defective equipment, for example leaking tubing or a faulty valve;
- failure to ensure the mercury column reads 0mm Hg at rest;
- too rapid deflation of the cuff;
- use of an incorrectly sized cuff – if it is too small the BP will be overestimated and if it is too large it will be underestimated;
- the cuff is not at the same level as the heart;
- failure to observe the mercury level properly – the top of the mercury column should be at eye level;
- poor technique, for example failing to notice when the sounds disappear;
- digit preference, for example rounding readings up to the nearest 5mm Hg or 10mm Hg;
- observer bias, for example expecting a young patient's BP to be normal.

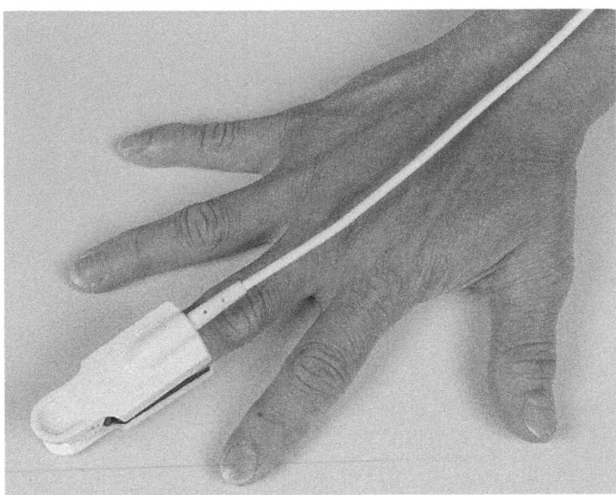

Figure 15-33 Finger tip oximeter sensor (adult).
Source: Jenny Thomas.

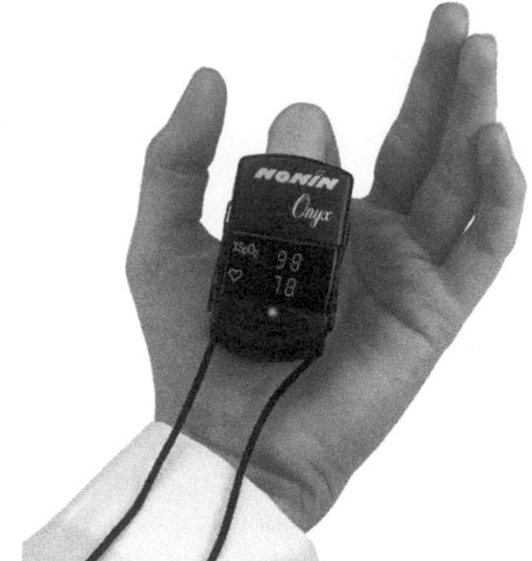

Figure 15-34 Finger tip oximeter sensor (cordless).
Source: Nonin Medical, Inc.

OXYGEN SATURATION

A **pulse oximeter** is a noninvasive device that measures a patient's arterial blood oxygen saturation (SaO_2) by means of a sensor attached to the patient's finger (see Figure 15-33), toe, nose, earlobe or forehead (or around the hand or foot of a neonate). The pulse oximeter can detect hypoxemia (low blood oxygen levels), before clinical signs and symptoms, such as dusky skin colour and dusky nailbeds colour develop.

The pulse oximeter's *sensor* has two parts: (a) two light-emitting diodes (LEDs) – one red the other infrared – that transmit light through nails, tissue, venous blood and arterial blood; and (b) a photodetector placed directly opposite the LEDs (e.g. the other side of the finger, toe or nose). The photodetector measures the amount of red and infrared light absorbed by oxygenated and deoxygenated haemoglobin in arterial blood and reports it as SaO_2. Normal SaO_2 is 95% to 100% and a SaO_2 below 70% is life threatening.

Pulse oximeters with various types of sensors are available. The *oximeter unit* consists of an inlet connection for the sensor cable, a faceplate that indicates (a) the oxygen saturation measurement (expressed as a percentage) and (b) the pulse rate. Cordless units are also available (see Figure 15-34). A preset alarm system signals high and low SaO_2 measurements and a high and low pulse rate. The high and low SaO_2 levels are generally preset at 100% and 85%, respectively, for adults and 95% and 80% for neonates. The high and low pulse rate alarms are usually preset at 140 and 50 BPM for adults. These alarm limits can, however, be changed according to the manufacturer's directions.

Pulse oximeters are now used routinely in hospitals, especially in critical care and acute areas, and in ambulances, with GPs and community nurses. They are used in a number of situations, e.g.

- hypoxaemia – especially in confused elderly patients;
- anasthaesia or sedation;
- prior to or alongside blood gas analysis, e.g. for patients with chronic pulmonary disease;
- to help with the management of oxygen therapy;
- neonates – the acceptable margins are more restrictive in neonates, i.e. 97% to 95%.

Factors Affecting Oxygen Saturation Readings

- *Haemoglobin.* If the haemoglobin is fully saturated with oxygen, the SaO_2 will appear normal even if the total haemoglobin level is low. Thus, the patient could be severely anaemic and have inadequate oxygen to supply the tissues but the pulse oximeter would return a normal value.
- *Circulation.* The oximeter will not return an accurate reading if the area under the sensor has impaired circulation.
- *Activity.* Shivering or excessive movement of the sensor site may interfere with accurate readings.

Procedure 15-7 outlines the steps in measuring oxygen saturation.

PROCEDURE 15-7 Measuring Oxygen Saturation

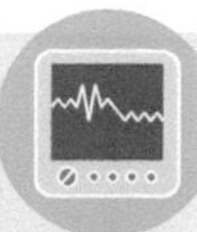

Purposes

- To measure the arterial blood oxygen saturation (SaO_2)
- To detect the presence of hypoemia before visible signs develop

Assessment

Assess

- The best location for a pulse oximeter sensor based on the patient's age and physical condition
- The patient's overall condition including risk factors for development of hypoxemia (e.g. respiratory or cardiac disease) and haemoglobin level
- Vital signs, skin and nail bed colour, and tissue perfusion of extremities as baseline data
- Adhesive allergy

Planning

Many clinical areas have pulse oximeters readily available for use with other vital signs equipment (or even as an integrated part of the electronic blood pressure device).

Equipment

- Nail polish remover as needed
- Alcohol wipe
- Sheet or towel
- Pulse oximeter

Implementation

Preparation

Check that the oximeter equipment is functioning normally and has been calibrated as per manufacturer's specification.

Performance

1 Follow local policy to ensure that you explain to the patient what you are going to do, why it is necessary and how they can cooperate. Obtain consent and maintain patient privacy and dignity and ensure that the appropriate local infection control procedures are observed.

2 Choose a sensor appropriate for the patient's weight, size and desired location. Because weight limits of sensors overlap, a paediatric sensor could be used for a small adult.
- If the patient is allergic to adhesive, use a clip or sensor without adhesive. If using an extremity, assess the proximal pulse and capillary refill at the point closest to the site.
- If the patient has low tissue perfusion due to peripheral vascular disease or therapy using vasoconstrictive medications, use a nasal sensor or a reflectance sensor on the forehead. Avoid using lower extremities that have a compromised circulation and extremities that are used for infusions or other invasive monitoring.

3 Prepare the site.
- Clean the site with an appropriate cleanser before applying the sensor.
- It may be necessary to remove a patient's nail polish/varnish or acrylic nails *since they can interfere with accurate measurements.*

4 Apply the sensor, and connect it to the pulse oximeter.
- Make sure the LED and photodetector are accurately aligned, that is, opposite each other on either side of the finger, toe, nose or earlobe. Many sensors have markings to facilitate correct alignment of the LEDs and photodetector.
- Attach the sensor cable to the connection outlet on the oximeter. Turn on the machine according to the manufacturer's directions. Appropriate connection will be confirmed by an audible beep indicating each arterial pulsation.
- Ensure that the bar of light or waveform on the face of the oximeter fluctuates with each pulsation and reflects the pulse volume or strength.

5 Set and turn on the alarm.
- Check the preset alarm limits for high and low oxygen saturation and high and low pulse rates. Change these alarm limits according to the manufacturer's directions as indicated. Ensure that the audio and visual alarms are on before you leave the patient. A tone will be heard and a number will blink on the faceplate.

6 Ensure patient safety.
- Inspect and/or move or change the location of an adhesive toe or finger sensor every four hours and a spring-tension sensor every two hours.
- Inspect the sensor site tissues for irritation from adhesive sensors.

7 Ensure the accuracy of measurement.
- Minimise motion artefacts by using an adhesive sensor or immobilise the patient's monitoring site. *Movement of the patient's finger or toe may be misinterpreted by the oximeter as arterial pulsations.*

- If indicated, cover the sensor with a sheet or towel to block large amounts of light from external sources (e.g. sunlight or procedure lamps). *Large amounts of outside light may be sensed by the photodetector and alter the SaO_2 value.*

8 Document the oxygen saturation on the appropriate record at designated intervals.

Evaluation

- Compare the oxygen saturation to the patient's previous oxygen saturation level. Relate to pulse rate and other vital signs.
- Conduct appropriate follow-up such as notifying the medical staff, adjusting oxygen therapy or providing breathing treatments.

LIFESPAN CONSIDERATIONS

Pulse Oximetry

Infants

- If an appropriate-sized finger or toe sensor (see Figure 15-35) is not available, consider using an earlobe or forehead sensor.
- The high and low SaO_2 levels are generally preset at 95% and 80% for neonates.
- The high and low pulse rate alarms are usually preset at 200 and 100 for neonates.

Children

- Instruct the child that the sensor does not hurt. Disconnect the probe whenever possible to allow for movement.

Mature Adults

- Use of vasoconstrictive medications, poor circulation or thickened nails may make finger or toe sensors inaccurate.

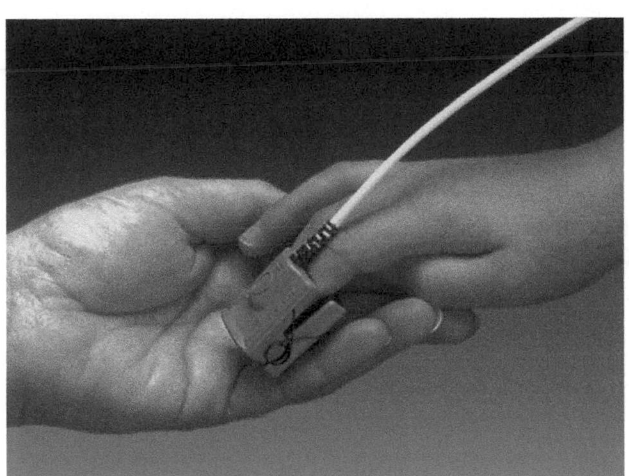

Figure 15-35 Finger tip oximeter sensor (child).

CRITICAL REFLECTION

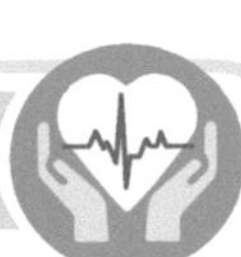

Reading this chapter would have provided you with the information to manage the initial care of Abdullah (the care study on page 415). Using the nursing process diagnose, assess, implement and evaluate Abdullah's care in relation to the symptoms presented in the care study and the vital signs presented. Demonstrate awareness of risk management and effective communication. When reflecting the following points should be considered:

- The disease process.
- Model or theory – Roper, Logan and Tierney or Orem's model.
- Nursing process – assess – diagnose – plan – implement – evaluate.
- Communication: to the patient, non-verbal – skin colour etc., family and members of the multidisciplinary team.
- Communication with the patient – including non-verbal communication, awareness of skin colour, etc.
- Communication with the family and members of the multidisciplinary team.
- Maintaining a safe environment:
  - vital signs – blood pressure, oxygen saturation, respiratory rate, pulse
  - policies/guidelines
  - safe discharge
  - lifespan consideration – interaction with medication.
- Risk assessments:
  - non-compliance
  - falls
  - infection.

CHAPTER HIGHLIGHTS

- Vital signs reflect changes in body function that otherwise might not be observed.
- Body temperature is the balance between heat produced by the body and heat lost from the body.
- Factors affecting body temperature include age, diurnal variations, exercise, hormones, stress and environmental temperatures.
- Hypothermia involves three mechanisms: excessive heat loss, inadequate heat production by body cells and increasing impairment of hypothalamic thermoregulation.
- Body temperature can be measured orally, tympanically, rectally or by axilla. The nurse selects the most appropriate site according to the patient's age and condition.
- Pulse rate and volume reflect the stroke volume output, the compliance of the patient's arteries and the adequacy of blood flow.
- Normally a peripheral pulse reflects the patient's heartbeat, but it may differ from the heartbeat in patients with certain cardiovascular diseases; in these instances, the nurse takes an apical pulse and compares it to the peripheral pulse.
- Many factors may affect a person's pulse rate: age, gender, exercise, presence of fever, certain medications, hypovolaemia, stress (in some situations), position changes and pathology.
- Although the radial pulse is the site most commonly used, eight other sites may be used in certain situations.
- Respirations are normally quiet, effortless and automatic, and are assessed by observing respiratory rate, depth, rhythm, quality and effectiveness.
- Blood pressure reflects cardiac output, peripheral vascular resistance, blood volume and blood viscosity.
- Among the factors influencing blood pressure are age, exercise, stress, race, gender, medications, obesity, diurnal variations and disease processes.
- A blood pressure cuff too large or too small will give false readings.
- During blood pressure measurement, the artery must be held at heart level.
- A pulse oximeter measures the percentage of haemoglobin saturated with oxygen. A normal result is 95% to 100% in adults.
- The importance of recognising and reporting abnormal levels to the appropriate clinician to prevent or reduce deterioration in patient's condition and to maintain patient safety at all times.
- Demonstrate effective communication with the patient at all times, ensure patient is informed and consented to procedure.

ACTIVITY ANSWERS

ACTIVITY 15-1 It is important to consider the patient's general condition and the changes that may have occurred due to his exposure to the changing weather temperatures overnight, some of the points for consideration are as follows:

- lifespan consideration
- hypothermia
- confusion
- disorientation
- safe way of recording temperature
- normal reading
- reporting abnormal readings
- documentation.

ACTIVITY 15-2 Three of the most important aspects to consider are patient dignity, accuracy of reading and recognising one's limitations. However, other points to consider are as follows:

- patient dignity
- wellbeing of the patient
- communication
- consent
- pulse sounds
- position of the cuff
- normal reading
- patient diagnosis
- injury or trauma to the limb going to be used
- reporting abnormal readings
- documentation.

REFERENCES

Beevers, G., Lip, G.Y.H. and O'Brien. E (2000) 'Blood pressure measurement Part 1, Sphygmomanometry: Factors common to all techniques', *British Medical Journal*, 322 (7292), 981–985.

Bindler, R.C. and Ball, J.W. (2003) *Clinical skills manual for pediatric nursing: Caring for children* (3rd edn), Upper Saddle River, NJ: Prentice Hall Health.

British Hypertension Society (2009) *How to measure blood pressure*, Leicester: British Hypertension Society.

Crawford, D., Greene, N. and Wentworth, S. (2005) *Thermometer review: UK market survey*, London: Medicines and Healthcare Products Regulatory Agency. Available at http://bit.ly/a9XYzh (accessed March 2011).

Crawford, D.C., Hicks, B. and Thompson, M.J. (2006) 'Which thermometer? Factors influencing the best choice for intermittent clinical temperature assessment', *Journal of Medical Engineering and Technology*, 30(4), 199–211.

Davie, A. and Amoore, J. (2010) 'Best practice in the measurement of body temperature', *Nursing Standard*, 24(42), 42–49.

Dougherty, L. and Lister, S. (2008) *The Royal Marsden Hospital Manual of Clinical Nursing Procedures* (7th edn), Oxford: Wiley-Blackwell.

Downing, P. (2009) *Fever and the regulation of body temperature*, Springfield, IL: Charles C. Thomas.

Foster-Fitzpatrick, L., Ortiz, A., Sibilano, H., Marcantonio, R. and Braun, L.T. (1999) 'The effects of crossed leg on blood pressure measurement', *Nursing Research*, **48**, 105–108.

Frommelt, T., Ott, C. and Hays, V. (2008) 'Accuracy of different devices to measure temperature', *Medsurg Nursing*, 17(3) 171–174, 176, 182.

Guyton, A.C. (2006) *Textbook of medical physiology* (11th edn), Edinburgh: Elsevier Science.

Holland, K. and Hogg, C. (2010) *Cultural awareness in nursing and health care* (2nd edn), London: Hodder Arnold.

Ladewig, P.W., London, M.L. and Olds, S.B. (1998) *Maternal–newborn nursing care: The nurse, the family, and the community* (4th edn), Menlo Park, CA: Addison Wesley Longman.

Lance, R., Link, M.E., Padua, M., Clavell, L.E., Johnson, G. and Knebel, E. (2000) 'Comparison of different methods of obtaining orthostatic vital signs', *Clinical Nursing Research*, 9, 479–491.

Marieb, E.N. (2010) *Human anatomy and physiology* (8th edn), Menlo Park, London: Benjamin/Cummings.

MHRA (2010) *Mercury in medical devices*, London: Medicines and Healthcare Regulatory Agency.

Muller, P., Van Berkel, L. and de Beaufort, A. (2008) 'Axillary and rectal temperature measurements poorly agree in new born infants', *Neonatology*, 94(1), 31–34.

NICE (2006) *Hypertension – Management of hypertension of adults in primary care, CG 34*, London: NICE.

NICE (2007) *Feverish illness in children – Assessment and initial management in children younger than five years of age, CG 47*, London: NICE.

O'Brien, E., Waeber, B., Parati, G., Staessen, J. and Myers, M.G. (2001) 'Blood pressure measuring devices: Recommendations of the European Society of Hypertension', *British Medical Journal*, 322 (7285), 531–536.

Petrie, J.C., O'Brien, E.T., Litler, W.A. and deSwiet, M. (1997) *British Hypertension Society: Recommendations on blood pressure measurement* (2nd edn), London: British Hypertension Society.

CHAPTER 16
OXYGENATION

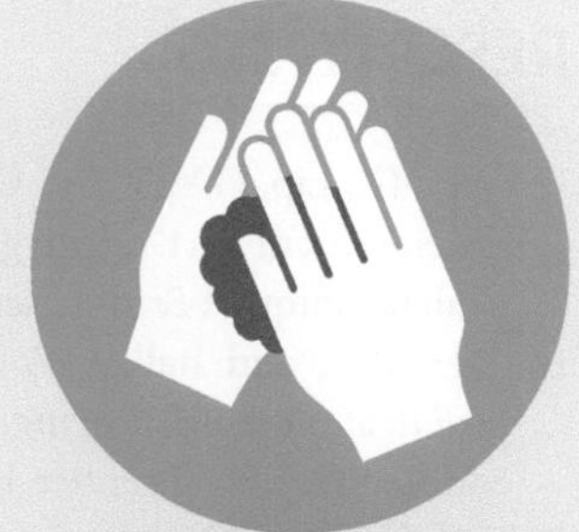

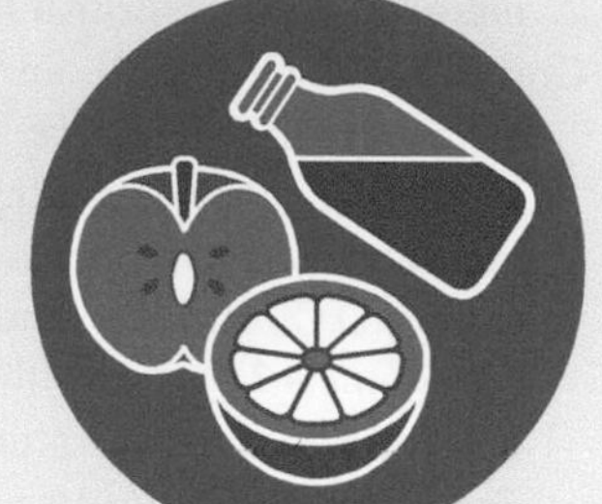

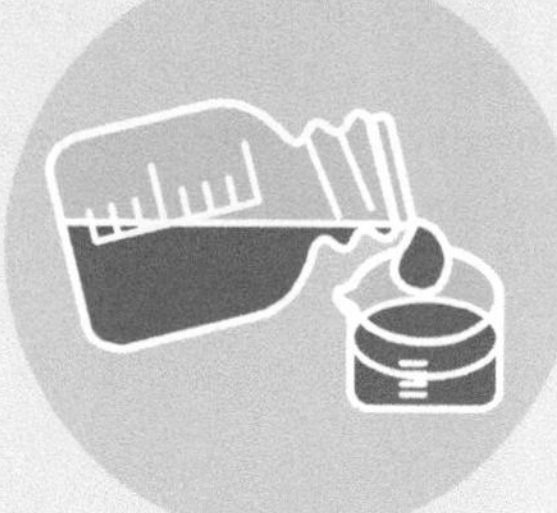

LEARNING OUTCOMES

After completing this chapter, you will be able to:

- Outline the structure and function of the respiratory system.
- Describe the processes of breathing (ventilation) and gas exchange (respiration).
- Explain the role and function of the respiratory system in transporting oxygen and carbon dioxide to and from body tissues.
- Identify factors influencing respiratory function.
- Identify common manifestations of impaired respiratory function.
- Identify and describe nursing measures to promote respiratory function and oxygenation.
- Explain the use of therapeutic measures such as medications, inhalation therapy, oxygen therapy, artificial airways, oropharyngeal suction and chest drainage to promote respiratory function.

After reading this chapter you will be able to discuss the respiratory system, identify common examples of respiratory impairment and describe nursing measures to promote good respiratory function. The chapter relates to **Essential Skills Clusters (NMC, 2010)** 1, 2, 3, 4, 5, 6, 7, 8, 9, 11, 13, 16, as appropriate for each progression point.

Ensure that you really understand this chapter by logging on to your complimentary **MyNursingKit** at **www.pearsoned.co.uk/kozier**. Complete the self-assessment tests to check your progress and utilise further activities to practise and confirm your understanding.

CASE STUDY

Leslie is an 88-year-old gentleman who has smoked all his life. He was recently admitted into hospital following a fall. He was also diagnosed as having had a myocardial infarction (MI), but the doctors were unclear as to whether the fall had caused the MI or whether the MI had caused the fall. During his admission he had some difficulty breathing and was prescribed oxygen therapy. After his admission, Leslie was assessed by the respiratory nurse and Leslie and his family were advised that he would be discharged on continuous oxygen.

On reading this chapter you will be able to discuss the respiratory system, identify possible reasons for the shortness of breath, the implications for Leslie and his family on discharge. You might consider the effects being on continuous oxygen might have on Leslie.

INTRODUCTION

Oxygen, a clear, odourless gas that constitutes approximately 21% of the air we breathe, is necessary for all living cells. The absence of oxygen can lead to death. Although the delivery of oxygen to body tissues is affected at least indirectly by all body systems, the respiratory system is most directly involved in this process. Impaired function of the system can significantly affect our ability to breathe, transport gases and participate in everyday activities.

PHYSIOLOGY OF THE RESPIRATORY SYSTEM

The function of the respiratory system is gas exchange. Oxygen from inspired air diffuses from alveoli in the lungs into the blood in pulmonary capillaries. Carbon dioxide produced during cell metabolism diffuses from the blood into the alveoli and is exhaled. The organs of the respiratory system facilitate this gas exchange and protect the body from foreign matter such as particulates (dust) and pathogens (diseases).

Structure of the Respiratory System

The respiratory system (see Figure 16-1) is divided structurally into the upper respiratory system and the lower respiratory system. The mouth, nose, pharynx and larynx compose the upper respiratory system. The lower respiratory system includes the trachea and lungs, with the bronchi, bronchioles, alveoli, pulmonary capillary network and pleural membranes.

Air enters through the nose, where it is warmed, humidified and filtered. Large particles in the air are trapped by the hairs at the entrance of the nares (nostrils), and smaller particles are filtered and trapped as air changes direction on contact with the nasal turbinates and septum. The sneeze reflex is initiated by irritants in nasal passages. A large volume of air rapidly exits through the nose and mouth during a sneeze, helping to clear nasal passages.

Inspired air passes from the nose through the pharynx. The pharynx is a shared pathway for air and food. It includes both the nasopharynx (upper part) and the oropharynx (lower part), which are richly supplied with lymphoid tissue that traps and destroys pathogens entering with the air.

The larynx is a cartilaginous structure that can be identified externally as the Adam's apple. In addition to its role in providing for speech, the larynx is important for maintaining airway clearance and protecting the lower airways from swallowed food and fluids. During swallowing, the inlet to the larynx (the epiglottis) closes, routing food to the oesophagus. The epiglottis is open during breathing, allowing air to move freely into the lower airways.

Below the larynx, the trachea leads to the right and left main bronchi (primary bronchi) and the conducting airways of the lungs. Within the lungs, the primary bronchi divide repeatedly into smaller and smaller bronchi, ending with the terminal bronchioles. Together these airways are known as the bronchial tree. The trachea and bronchi are lined with mucosal epithelium. These cells produce a thin layer of mucus, that traps pathogens and microscopic particulate matter. These foreign particles are then swept upward towards the larynx and throat by cilia, which are tiny hair-like projections on the epithelial cells. The cough reflex is triggered by irritants in the larynx, trachea or bronchi and occurs when:

- nerve impulses are sent through the vagus nerve (10th cranial) to the medulla;
- a large inspiration of approximately 2.5 l occurs;
- the epiglottis and glottis (vocal cords) close;
- a strong contraction of abdominal and internal intercostal muscles dramatically raises the pressure in the lungs;
- the epiglottis and glottis open suddenly;
- air rushes outward with great velocity;
- mucous and any foreign particles are dislodged from the lower respiratory tract and are propelled up and out.

Until air passes through the terminal bronchioles and enters the respiratory bronchioles and alveoli, no gas exchange occurs. The respiratory zone of the lungs includes the respiratory bronchioles (which have scattered air sacs in their walls); the alveolar ducts and the alveoli (see Figure 16-1). Alveoli have very thin walls, composed of a single layer of epithelial cells covered by a thick mesh of pulmonary capillaries. The alveolar and capillary

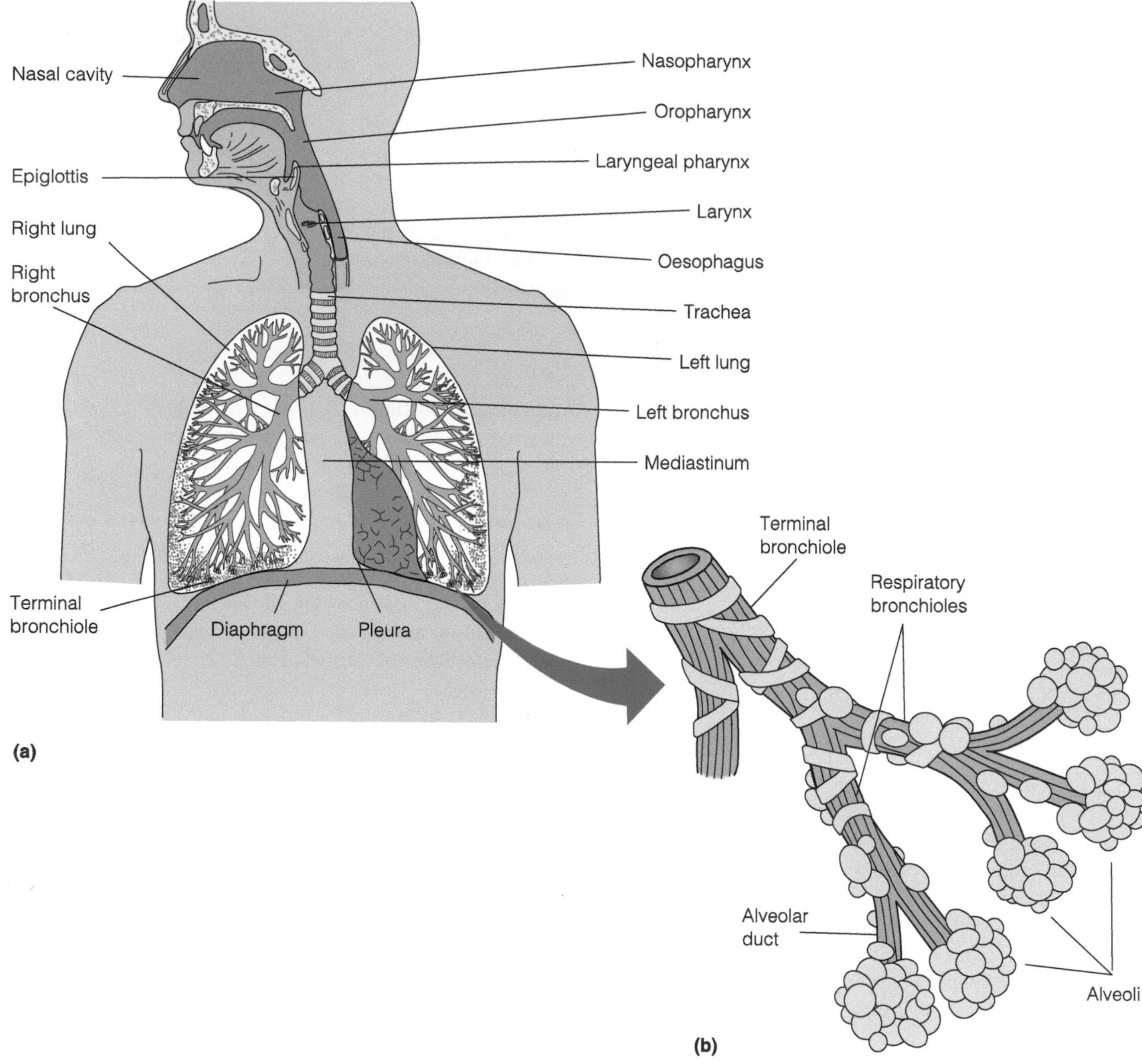

Figure 16-1 (a) Organs of the respiratory tract; (b) Respiratory bronchioles, alveolar ducts and alveoli.

walls form the **respiratory membrane**, where gas exchange occurs between the air on the alveolar side and the blood on the capillary side. The airways move air to and from the alveoli; the right ventricle and pulmonary vascular system transport blood to the capillary side of the membrane.

The outer surface of the lungs is covered by a thin, double layer of tissue known as the pleura. The parietal pleura lines the thorax and surface of the diaphragm. It doubles back to form the visceral pleura, covering the external surface of the lungs. Between these pleural layers is a potential space that contains a small amount of pleural fluid, a serous lubricating solution. This fluid prevents friction during the movements of breathing and serves to keep the layers adherent through its surface tension.

Pulmonary Ventilation

Ventilation of the lungs is accomplished through the act of breathing: inspiration (inhalation) when air flows into the lungs and expiration (exhalation) as air moves out of the lungs. Adequate ventilation depends on several factors:

- clear airways;
- an intact central nervous system and respiratory centre in the medulla oblongata of the brain;
- an intact thoracic cavity capable of expanding and contracting;
- adequate pulmonary compliance and recoil.

A number of mechanisms including ciliary action and the cough reflex work to keep airways open and clear. In some cases, however, these defences may be overwhelmed. The inflammation, oedema and excess mucous production that occur with some types of pneumonia may clog small airways, impairing ventilation of distal alveoli.

The respiratory centres of the medulla and pons in the brain stem control breathing. Severe head injury or drugs that depress the central nervous system (e.g. opiates or barbiturates) can affect the respiratory centres, impairing the drive to breathe.

Expansion and recoil of the lungs occurs passively in response to changes in pressures within the thoracic cavity and the lungs themselves. The intrapleural pressure (pressure in the pleural cavity surrounding the lungs) is always slightly negative in relation to atmospheric pressure. This negative pressure is essential because it creates the suction that holds the visceral pleura and the parietal pleura together as the chest cage expands and contracts. The recoil tendency of the lungs is a major factor in creating this negative pressure. The intrapleural fluid also contributes by causing the pleura to adhere together, much as a film of water can cause two glass slides to adhere together.

The intrapulmonary pressure (pressure within the lungs) always equalises with atmospheric pressure. Inspiration occurs when the diaphragm and intercostal muscles contract, increasing the size of the thoracic cavity. The volume of the lungs increases, decreasing intrapulmonary pressure. Air then rushes into the lungs to equalise this pressure with atmospheric pressure. Conversely, when the diaphragm and intercostal muscles relax, the volume of the lungs decreases, intrapulmonary pressure rises, and air is expelled.

The degree of chest expansion during normal breathing is minimal, requiring little energy expenditure. In adults, approximately 500ml of air is inspired and expired with each breath. This is known as tidal volume. Breathing during strenuous exercise or some types of heart disease requires greater chest expansion and effort. At this time, more than 1,500ml of air may be moved with each breath. Accessory muscles of respiration, including the anterior neck muscles, intercostal muscles and muscles of the abdomen, are employed. Active use of these muscles and noticeable effort in breathing are seen in patients with obstructive pulmonary disease.

Diseases such as muscular dystrophy, or trauma such as spinal cord injury can affect the muscles of respiration, impairing the ability of the thoracic cavity to expand and contract. A penetrating wound or other trauma to the chest wall may allow intrapleural pressure to equalise with the atmosphere, causing the lung to collapse.

Lung compliance, the expansibility or stretchability of lung tissue, plays a significant role in the ease of ventilation. At birth, the fluid-filled lungs are stiff and resistant to expansion, much as a new balloon is difficult to inflate. With each subsequent breath, the alveoli become more compliant and easier to inflate, just as a balloon becomes easier to inflate after several tries. Lung compliance tends to decrease with ageing, making it more difficult to expand alveoli and increasing risk of **atelectasis**, or collapse of a portion of the lung.

In contrast to lung compliance is lung recoil, the continual tendency of the lungs to collapse away from the chest wall. Just as lung compliance is necessary for normal inspiration, lung recoil is necessary for normal expiration. Although elastic fibres in lung tissue contribute to lung recoil, the surface tension of fluid lining the alveoli has the greatest effect on recoil. Fluid molecules tend to draw together, reducing the size of alveoli. **Surfactant**, a **lipoprotein** produced by specialised alveolar cells, acts like a detergent, reducing the surface tension of alveolar fluid. Without surfactant, lung expansion is exceedingly difficult and the lungs collapse. Premature infants whose lungs are not yet capable of producing adequate surfactant develop respiratory distress syndrome.

Alveolar Gas Exchange

After the alveoli are ventilated, the second phase of the respiratory process – the *diffusion* of oxygen from the alveoli and into the pulmonary blood vessels – begins. **Diffusion** is the movement of gases or other particles from an area of greater pressure or concentration to an area of lower pressure or concentration.

Pressure differences in the gases on each side of the respiratory membrane obviously affect diffusion. When the pressure of oxygen is greater in the alveoli than in the blood, oxygen diffuses into the blood. The partial pressure (the pressure exerted by each individual gas in a mixture according to its concentration in the mixture) of oxygen (PO_2) in the alveoli is about 100mm Hg (sometimes referred to as torr (unit of measure) which is the same as millimetres of mercury), whereas the PO_2 in the venous blood of the pulmonary arteries is about 60mm Hg. These pressures rapidly equalise, however, so that the arterial oxygen pressure also reaches about 100mm Hg. By contrast, carbon dioxide in the venous blood entering the pulmonary capillaries has a partial pressure of about 45mm Hg (PCO_2), whereas that in the alveoli has a partial pressure of about 40mm Hg. Therefore, carbon dioxide diffuses from the blood into the alveoli, where it can be eliminated with expired air. When referring to the pressure of oxygen in the arterial blood the abbreviation is PaO_2. When referring to partial pressure in venous blood there is no 'a', that is, PO_2.

Transport of Oxygen and Carbon Dioxide

The third part of the respiratory process involves the transport of respiratory gases. Oxygen needs to be transported from the lungs to the tissues, and carbon dioxide must be transported from the tissues back to the lungs. Normally most of the oxygen (97%) combines loosely with **haemoglobin** (oxygen-carrying red pigment) in the red blood cells and is carried to the tissues as **oxyhaemoglobin** (the compound of oxygen and haemoglobin). The remaining oxygen is dissolved and transported in the fluid of the plasma and cells.

Several factors affect the rate of oxygen transport from the lungs to the tissues:

- cardiac output;
- number of erythrocytes and blood haematocrit;
- exercise.

The **haematocrit** is the percentage of the blood that comprises erythrocytes.

Any pathologic condition that decreases cardiac output (e.g. damage to the heart muscle, blood loss or pooling of blood in the peripheral blood vessels) diminishes the amount of oxygen delivered to the tissues. The heart compensates for inadequate output by increasing its pumping rate; however, with severe damage or blood loss, this compensatory mechanism may not restore adequate blood flow and oxygen to the tissues.

The second factor influencing oxygen transport is the number of erythrocytes (red blood cells, or RBCs) and the haematocrit. In men, the number of circulating erythrocytes normally averages about 5 million per cubic millilitre of blood, and in women, about 4½ million per cubic millilitre. Normally the haematocrit is about 40% to 54% in men and 37% to 48% in women. Excessive increases in the blood haematocrit raise the blood viscosity, reducing the cardiac output and therefore reducing oxygen transport. Excessive reductions in the blood haematocrit, such as anaemia, reduce oxygen transport.

Exercise also has a direct influence on oxygen transport. In well-trained athletes, oxygen transport can be increased up to 20 times the normal rate, due in part to an increased cardiac output and to increased use of oxygen by the cells.

Carbon dioxide, continually produced in the processes of cell metabolism, is transported from the cells to the lungs in three ways. The majority (about 65%) is carried inside the red blood cells as bicarbonate (HCO_3^-) and is an important component of the bicarbonate **buffer** system. A moderate amount of carbon dioxide (30%) combines with haemoglobin as carboxyhaemoglobin for transport. Smaller amounts (5%) are transported in solution in the plasma and as carbonic acid (the compound formed when carbon dioxide combines with water).

RESPIRATORY REGULATION

Respiratory regulation includes both neurological and chemical controls to maintain the correct concentrations of oxygen, carbon dioxide and hydrogen ions in body fluids. The nervous system of the body adjusts the rate of alveolar ventilations to meet the needs of the body so that PO_2 and PCO_2 remain relatively constant. The body's 'respiratory centre' is actually a number of groups of neurons located in the medulla oblongata and pons of the brain.

A chemosensitive centre in the medulla oblongata is highly responsive to increases in blood CO_2 or hydrogen ion concentration. By influencing other respiratory centres, this centre can increase the activity of the inspiratory centre and the rate and depth of respirations. In addition to this direct chemical stimulation of the respiratory centre in the brain, special neural receptors sensitive to decreases in O_2 concentration are located outside the central nervous system in the carotid bodies (just above the bifurcation of the common carotid arteries) and aortic bodies. Decreases in arterial oxygen concentrations stimulate these chemoreceptors, and they in turn stimulate the respiratory centre to increase ventilation. Of the three blood gases (hydrogen, oxygen and carbon dioxide) that can trigger chemoreceptors, increased carbon dioxide concentration normally stimulates respiration most strongly.

However, in patients with certain chronic lung disease such as **emphysema**, oxygen concentrations, not carbon dioxide concentrations, play a major role in regulating respiration. For such patients, decreased oxygen concentrations are the main stimuli for respiration. This is sometimes called the hypoxic drive. Increasing the concentration of oxygen depresses the respiratory rate. Thus, only low concentrations of supplemental oxygen are administered to these patients.

FACTORS AFFECTING RESPIRATORY FUNCTION

Factors that influence oxygenation affect the cardiovascular system as well as the respiratory system. These factors include age, environment, lifestyle, health status, medications and stress.

Age

Developmental factors are important influences on respiratory function. At birth, profound changes occur in the respiratory systems. The fluid-filled lungs drain, the PCO_2 rises and the neonate takes a first breath. The lungs gradually expand with each subsequent breath, reaching full inflation by two weeks of age. Changes of ageing (see Table 16-1) that affect the respiratory system of older adults become especially important if the system is compromised by changes such as infection, physical or emotional stress, surgery, anaesthesia or other procedures. Changes are:

- Chest wall and airways become more rigid and less elastic.
- The amount of exchanged air is decreased.
- The cough reflex and cilia action are decreased.
- Mucous membranes become drier and more fragile.
- Decreases in muscle strength and endurance occur.
- If osteoporosis is present, adequate lung expansion may be compromised.
- A decrease in efficiency of the immune system occurs.

Gastroesophageal reflux disease is more common in older adults and increases the risk of aspiration. The aspiration of stomach contents into the lungs often causes bronchospasm by setting up an inflammatory response.

Table 16-1 Age-related Respiratory Rates

Age	Average range/min
Newborn	30-80
Early Childhood	20-40
Late Childhood	15-25
Adulthood - Male	14-18
Adulthood - Female	16-20

Source: Timby (1989).

LIFESPAN CONSIDERATIONS

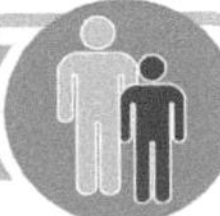

Respiratory Development

Infants

- Respiratory rates are highest and most variable in newborns.
- Infant respiratory rates average about 30 per minute.
- Because of rib cage structure, infants rely almost exclusively on diaphragmatic movement for breathing. This is seen as abdominal breathing, as the abdomen rises and falls with each breath.

Children

- The respiratory rate gradually decreases, averaging around 25 per minute in the pre-school child and reaching the adult rate of 12–18 per minute by late adolescence.
- During infancy and childhood, upper respiratory infections are common and, fortunately, usually not serious. Infants and pre-school children are also at risk for airway obstruction by foreign objects such as coins and small toys. Cystic fibrosis is a congenital disorder that affects the lungs, causing them to become congested with thick, tenacious (sticky) mucus. Asthma is another chronic disease often identified in childhood. The airways of the asthmatic child respond to stimuli such as allergens, exercise or cold air by constricting, becoming oedematous and producing excessive mucus. Airflow is impaired, and the child may wheeze as air moves through narrowed air passages.

Mature Adults

- Mature adults are at increased risk for acute respiratory diseases such as pneumonia and chronic diseases such as emphysema and chronic bronchitis. Chronic obstructive pulmonary disease (COPD) may affect mature adults, particularly after years of exposure to cigarette smoke or industrial pollutants.
- Pneumonia may not present with the usual symptoms of a fever, but will present with atypical symptoms, such as confusion, weakness, loss of appetite, and increase in heart rate and respirations.
- Nursing interventions should be directed towards achieving optimal respiratory effort and gas exchange:
- Always encourage wellness and prevention of disease by reinforcing the need for good nutrition, exercise and immunisations, such as for influenza and pneumonia.
- Increase fluid intake, if not contraindicated by other problems, such as cardiac or renal impairment.
- Correct positioning and frequent changing of positions allow for better lung expansion and air and fluid movement.
- Teach patient to use breathing techniques for better air exchange.
- Pace activities to conserve energy.
- Encourage the patient to eat more frequent, smaller meals to decrease gastric distention, which can cause pressure on the diaphragm.
- Teach patient to avoid extreme hot or cold temperatures that will further tax the respiratory system.
- Explain actions and side-effects of drugs, inhalers and treatments.

Environment

Altitude, heat, cold and air pollution affect oxygenation. The higher the altitude, the lower the PO_2 an individual breathes. As a result, the person at high altitudes has increased respiratory and cardiac rates and increased respiratory depth, which usually become most apparent when the individual exercises.

Healthy people exposed to air pollution, such as smog, often experience stinging of the eyes, headache, dizziness, coughing and choking. People who have a history of existing lung disease and altered respiratory function experience varying degrees of respiratory difficulty in a polluted environment. Some are unable to perform self-care in such an environment.

Lifestyle

Physical exercise or activity increases the rate and depth of respirations and hence the supply of oxygen in the body. Sedentary people, by contrast, lack the alveolar expansion and deep breathing patterns of people with regular activity and are less able to respond effectively to respiratory stressors.

The Department of Health and affiliated organisations are promoting well-being and the healthy person through health promotion and health education, identifying risks and in many instances offering choices to the individual to change their current practice. In the United Kingdom, for example, the government introduced a smoke-free environment in July 2007 stating that this was a huge 'triumph' for Public Health and for Health Protection. The Department of Health was explicit in its view that scientific and medical evidence clearly states that second hand smoking 'causes a range of medical conditions including lung cancer' (Hewitt, 2006).

Within the work place, the government has put in place strategies to identify, prevent and/or reduce risk from external sources. Previous occupations predispose an individual to lung disease, e.g. silicosis was seen in sandstone blasters and potters; asbestosis in asbestos workers; anthracosis in coal miners; and organic dust disease in farmers and agricultural employees who work with mouldy hay. However, due to health and safety measures these are becoming less evident possibly also due to lifestyle changes, e.g. closure of mines. However, according to a study carried out by d'Amato *et al.* (2001), there has been a global increase in respiratory disorders such as asthma and hay fever. While the cause is unknown, they suggest that outdoor air pollution from emissions from vehicles may be the cause. The implication is that maintaining well-being is a local, national and global concern.

Local health boards, trusts and other healthcare organisations are required by government to develop local strategies to reduce risk and promote the well-being of the individual in the community. These local strategies are then discussed and taken forward at a national level (if applicable) to identify, reduce and prevent this type of risk.

Health Status

In the healthy person, the respiratory system can provide sufficient oxygen to meet the body's needs. Diseases of the respiratory system, however, can adversely affect the oxygenation of the blood.

Medications

A variety of medications can decrease the rate and depth of respirations. The most common medications with this effect are analgesics, benzodiazepine sedative-hypnotics and anti-anxiety drugs (e.g. diazepam (Valium), flurazepam, midazolam), barbiturates, and narcotics such as morphine. When administering these, the nurse must carefully monitor respiratory status, especially when the medication is begun or when the dose is increased. Although this is a safety concern, often the importance of the medication outweighs the risk of respiratory depression.

Stress

When stress and stressors are encountered, both psychological and physiological responses can affect oxygenation. Some people may hyperventilate in response to stress. When this occurs, arterial PO_2 rises and PCO_2 falls. The person may experience light-headedness and numbness and tingling of the fingers, toes and around the mouth as a result.

Physiologically, the sympathetic nervous system is stimulated and adrenaline is released. Adrenaline causes the bronchioles to dilate, increasing blood flow and oxygen delivery to active muscles. Although these responses are adaptive in the short term, when stress continues they can be destructive, increasing the risk of cardiovascular disease.

ALTERATIONS IN RESPIRATORY FUNCTION

Respiratory function can be altered by conditions that affect:

- the movement of air into or out of the lungs;
- the diffusion of oxygen and carbon dioxide between the alveoli and the pulmonary capillaries;
- the transport of oxygen and carbon dioxide via the blood to and from the tissue cells.

Three major alterations in respiration are hypoxia, altered breathing patterns and obstructed or partially obstructed airway.

Hypoxia

Hypoxia is a condition of insufficient oxygen anywhere in the body, from the inspired gas to the tissues. It can be related to any of the parts of respiration – ventilation, diffusion of gases or transport of gases by the blood – and can be caused by any condition that alters one or more parts of the process.

Hypoventilation, that is, inadequate alveolar ventilation, can lead to hypoxia. Hypoventilation may occur because of diseases of the respiratory muscles, drugs or anesthesia. With hypoventilation, carbon dioxide often accumulates in the blood, a condition called **hypercarbia (hypercapnia)**.

Hypoxia can also develop when the diffusion of oxygen from alveoli into the arterial blood decreases, as with pulmonary oedema, or it can result from problems in the delivery of oxygen to the tissues (e.g. anaemia, heart failure and embolism). The term **hypoxaemia** refers to reduced oxygen in the blood and is characterised by a low partial pressure of oxygen in arterial blood or low haemoglobin saturation. Clinical signs of hypoxia are:

- rapid pulse;
- rapid, shallow respirations and dyspnoea;
- increased restlessness or light-headedness;
- flaring of the nares;
- substernal or intercostal retractions (sucking in of the chest);
- cyanosis.

Cyanosis (bluish discoloration of the skin, nail beds and mucous membranes, due to reduced haemoglobin-oxygen saturation) may also be present. Cyanosis requires these two conditions: the blood must contain about 5 g or more of unoxygenated haemoglobin per 100 ml of blood, and the surface blood capillaries must be dilated. Factors that interfere with either of these conditions (e.g. severe anaemia or the administration of epinephrine/adrenaline) will eliminate cyanosis as a sign even if the patient is experiencing hypoxia.

Adequate oxygenation is essential for cerebral functioning. The cerebral cortex can tolerate hypoxia for only 3–5 minutes before permanent damage occurs. The face of the acutely hypoxic person usually appears anxious, tired and drawn. The person usually assumes a sitting position, often leaning forward slightly to permit greater expansion of the thoracic cavity.

With chronic hypoxia, the patient often appears fatigued and is lethargic. The patient's fingers and toes may be clubbed as a result of long-term lack of oxygen in the arterial blood supply. With clubbing, the base of the nail becomes swollen and the ends of the fingers and toes increase in size. The angle between the nail and the base of the nail increases to more than 180 degrees.

Altered Breathing Patterns

Breathing patterns refer to the rate, volume, rhythm and relative ease or effort of respiration. Normal respiration (eupnoea) is quiet, rhythmic and effortless. **Tachypnoea** (rapid rate) is seen with fevers, metabolic acidosis, pain and with hypercapnia or hypoxemia. **Bradypnoea** is an abnormally slow respiratory rate, which may be seen in patients who have taken drugs such as morphine, who have **metabolic alkalosis** or who have increased intracranial pressure (e.g. from brain injuries). **Apnoea** is the cessation of breathing.

Hyperventilation, often called *alveolar hyperventilation*, is an increased movement of air into and out of the lungs. During hyperventilation, the rate and depth of respirations increase, and more CO_2 is eliminated than is produced. One particular type of hyperventilation that accompanies **metabolic acidosis** is Kussmaul's breathing, by which the body attempts to compensate (give off excess body acids) by blowing off the carbon dioxide through deep and rapid breathing. This may occur when there is a diabetic ketoacidosis or in severe renal failure. Hyperventilation can also occur in response to stress, as mentioned earlier.

Abnormal respiratory rhythms create an irregular breathing pattern. Two abnormal respiratory rhythms are:

1 **Cheyne-Stokes respirations.** Marked rhythmic waxing and waning of respirations from very deep to very shallow breathing and temporary apnoea; common causes include congestive heart failure, increased intracranial pressure and drug overdose
2 **Biot's (cluster) respirations.** Shallow breaths interrupted by apnoea; may be seen in patients with central nervous system disorders.

Orthopnoea is the inability to breathe except in an upright or standing position. Difficult or uncomfortable breathing is called dyspnoea. The dyspnoeic person often appears anxious and may experience *shortness of breath* (SOB), a feeling of being unable to get enough air (breathlessness). Often the nostrils are flared because of the increased effort of inspiration. The skin may appear dusky; heart rate is increased. Dyspnoea may have many causes, most of which stem from cardiac or respiratory disorders. It is a subjective feeling; that is, dyspnoea may not be directly observed or measured but is reported by the patient. Since treatment is aimed at removing the underlying cause, it is important for the nurse to conduct a thorough history of the onset, duration and precipitating and relieving factors of the patient's dyspnoea.

Obstructed Airway

A completely or partially obstructed airway can occur anywhere along the upper or lower respiratory passageways. An upper airway obstruction – that is, in the nose, pharynx or larynx – can arise because of a foreign object such as food, because the tongue falls back into the oropharynx when a person is unconscious, or when secretions collect in the passageways. In the latter instance, the respirations will sound gurgly or bubbly as the air attempts to pass through the secretions. Lower airway obstruction involves partial or complete occlusion of the passageways in the bronchi and lungs.

Maintaining an open (patient) airway is a nursing intervention, one that often requires immediate action. Partial obstruction of the upper airway passages is indicated by a low-pitched snoring sound during inhalation. Complete obstruction is indicated by extreme inspiratory effort that produces no chest movement. A patient in an effort to obtain air may also exhibit marked sternal and intercostal retractions. Lower airway obstruction is not always as easy to observe. **Stridor**, a harsh, high-pitched sound, may be heard during inspiration. The patient may have altered **arterial blood gas** levels, restlessness, dyspnoea and adventitious breath sounds (abnormal breath sounds).

As previously stated the respiratory system is structurally divided into two sections; the upper respiratory tract and the lower respiratory tract. Altered breathing patterns and respiratory functions may occur for several medical reasons:

- Upper respiratory:
  - Infection: the common cold, pharyngitis (sore throat), tonsillitis
  - Disease: e.g. squamous cell carcinoma
- Lower respiratory:
  - Infection: pneumonia, tuberculosis, bronchitis
  - Neurological disease: spinal cord, motor nerve, infectious disease, muscle wasting disease
  - Chronic obstructive airway disease: bronchiectasis, emphysema, cystic fibrosis, pneumoconiosis
  - Acute obstructive airway disease: bronchiectasis, asthma
  - Traumatic injury: fractured ribs, pleural effusion (empyema), pneumothorax, haemothorax
  - Adult respiratory disease: severe hypoxaemia, loss of lung compliance, secondary disease
  - Industrial disease: asbestosis, silicosis
  - Obesity: obstructive sleep apnoea

ASSESSING OXYGEN STATUS

Nursing assessment of oxygenation status includes a history and review of relevant diagnostic data such as vital signs and oxygen saturation levels.

Patient History

A comprehensive patient history relevant to oxygenation status should include data about current and past respiratory problems; lifestyle; presence of cough, sputum (coughed-up material); pain; medications for breathing; and presence of risk factors for impaired oxygenation status. Examples of interview questions to elicit this information are shown in the *Assessment interview*.

ASSESSMENT INTERVIEW

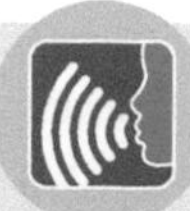

Oxygenation

Current Respiratory Problems

- Have you noticed any changes in your breathing pattern (e.g. shortness of breath, difficulty in breathing, need to be in upright position to breathe, or rapid and shallow breathing)?
- If so, which of your activities might cause these symptom(s) to occur?
- How many pillows do you use to sleep at night?

History of Respiratory Disease

- Have you had colds, allergies, asthma, tuberculosis, bronchitis, pneumonia or emphysema?
- How frequently have these occurred? How long did they last? And how were they treated?
- Have you been exposed to any pollutants?

Lifestyle

- Do you smoke? If so, how much? If not, did you smoke previously, and when did you stop?
- Does any member of your family smoke?
- Is there cigarette smoke or other pollutants (e.g. fumes, dust, coal, asbestos) in your workplace or at home?
- Do you use alcohol? If so, how many drinks (mixed drinks, glasses of wine or beers) do you usually have per day or per week?
- Describe your exercise patterns. How often do you exercise and for how long?
- Do you do any walking? How far are you able to walk? Has this changed?

Presence of Cough

- How often and how much do you cough?
- Is it productive, that is, accompanied by sputum, or nonproductive, that is, dry?
- Does the cough occur during certain activity or at certain times of the day?

Description of Sputum

- Do you produce any sputum?
- When is the sputum produced?
- What is the amount, colour, thickness, odour?
- Is it ever tinged with blood?

Presence of Chest Pain

- Do you experience any pain with breathing or activity?
- Where is the pain located?
- Describe the pain. How does it feel?
- Does it occur when you breathe in or out?
- How long does it last, and how does it affect your breathing?
- Do you experience any other symptoms when the pain occurs (e.g. nausea, shortness of breath or difficulty breathing, light-headedness, palpitations)?
- What activities precede your pain?
- What do you do to relieve the pain?

Presence of Risk Factors

- Do you have a family history of lung cancer, cardiovascular disease (including strokes) or tuberculosis?
- The nurse should also note the patient's weight, activity pattern and dietary assessment. Risk factors include obesity, sedentary lifestyle and diet high in saturated fats.

Medication History

- Have you taken or do you take any over-the-counter or prescription medications for breathing (e.g. bronchodilator, inhalant, narcotic)?
- If so, which ones? And what are the dosages, times taken and results, including side-effects?
- Any known allergies?

Physical Assessment

It is important that while the nurse is taking the patient's history that consideration is given to how this information is gathered, e.g. if the patient is finding it difficult to breathe then this might not be the right time to ask for more than the basic information. The nurse should observe the patient for their current rate, depth rhythm and quality of respirations, taking note of the patient's positioning.

Diagnostic Studies

The doctor may request various diagnostic tests to assess respiratory status, function and oxygenation. Included are sputum specimens, throat cultures, venous and arterial blood specimens, peak flow readings and pulmonary function tests.

Measurement of arterial blood gases is an important diagnostic procedure. Specimens of arterial blood are normally taken by specialty nurses or medical staff. Blood for these tests is taken directly from the radial, brachial or femoral arteries or from central catheters placed in large arteries. Because of the relatively great pressure of the blood in these arteries, it is important to prevent haemorrhaging by applying pressure to the puncture side for about five minutes after removing the needle.

Pulmonary Function Tests

Pulmonary function tests measure lung volume and capacity. Patients undergo pulmonary function tests, which are usually carried out by a respiratory physiologist. The patient breathes into a machine. The tests are painless, but the patient's cooperation is essential. Nurses need to explain the tests to the patient beforehand and help patients to get rest afterward because the tests are often tiring. Table 16-2 describes the measurements taken, and Figure 16-2 shows their relationships and normal adult values.

Table 16-2 Pulmonary Volumes and Capacities

Measurement	Description
Tidal volume (V_T)	Volume inhaled and exhaled during normal quiet breathing
Aspiratory reserve volume (ARV)	Maximum amount of air that can be inhaled over and above a normal breath
Expiratory reserve volume (ERV)	Maximum amount of air that can be exhaled following a normal exhalation
Residual volume (RV)	The amount of air remaining in the lungs after maximal exhalation
Total lung capacity (TLC)	The total volume of the lungs at maximum inaction; calculated by adding the V_T, ARV, ERV and RV
Vital capacity (VC)	Total amount of air that can be exhaled after a maximal inspiration; calculated by adding the V_T, ARV and ERV
Aspiratory capacity	Total amount of air that can be inhaled following normal quiet exhalation; calculated by adding the V_T and ARV
Functional residual capacity (FRC)	The volume left in the lungs after normal exhalation; calculated by adding the ERV and RV
Minute volume (MV)	The total volume or amount of air breathed in 1 minute

Peak Flow Readings

A number of respiratory disorders can alter the mechanical properties of the lungs, which consequently influences airway resistance and lung compliance. Peak expiratory rate (PEF) is a cheap and simple test that measures the maximum expiratory rate in the first 10ml of expiration (see *Procedure 16-1*).

The PEF indicates the presence of airflow obstruction which maybe fixed or variable, as seen in patients with asthma and COPD. When the airways narrow, PEF falls.

Routinely PEF is determined by:

- size of the lungs;
- lung elasticity;
- dimensions and compliance of the central intrathoracic airways;
- strength and speed of contraction of the expiratory muscles.

What is a Peak Flow Reading?

The Peak Expiratory Flow Rate (PEFR) is a measurement of the maximum flow rate, in litres per minute, that can be expelled from the lungs during a forced exhalation. The measurement gives objective information concerning the severity of airway obstruction in patients with symptoms of respiratory distress (Bennett, 2003).

Indications for Peak Flow Recording

Peak flows are recorded for the following reasons:

- serial peak flow readings for management of symptoms of asthma;
- the diagnosis of disease;
- the monitoring of the progression of the disease and its response to treatment;
- to monitor exercise efficiency;
- as a preventative tool.

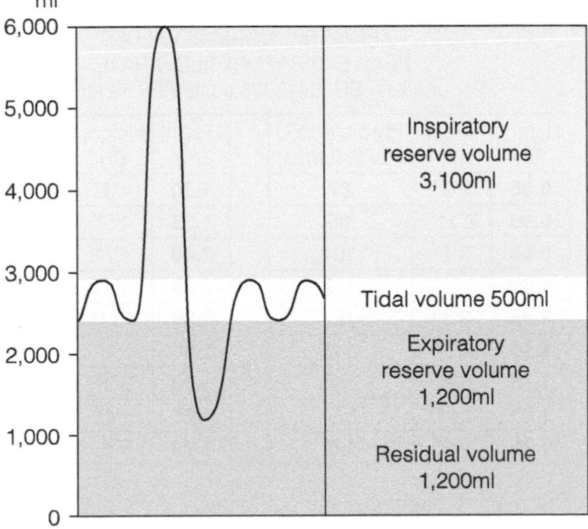

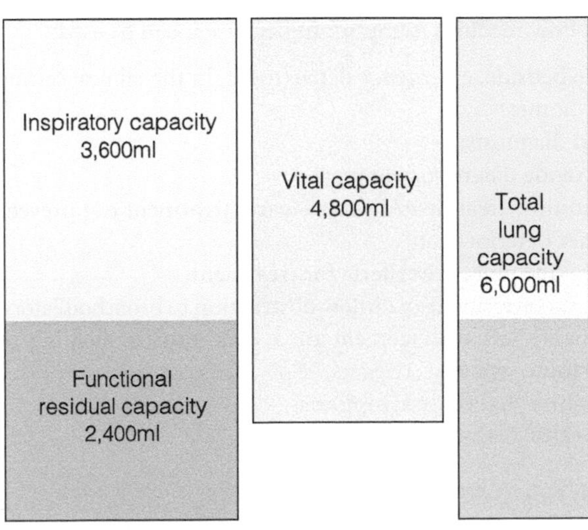

Figure 16-2 The relationship of lung volumes and capacities. Volumes (ml) shown are for an average adult male; female volumes are 20% to 25% smaller.

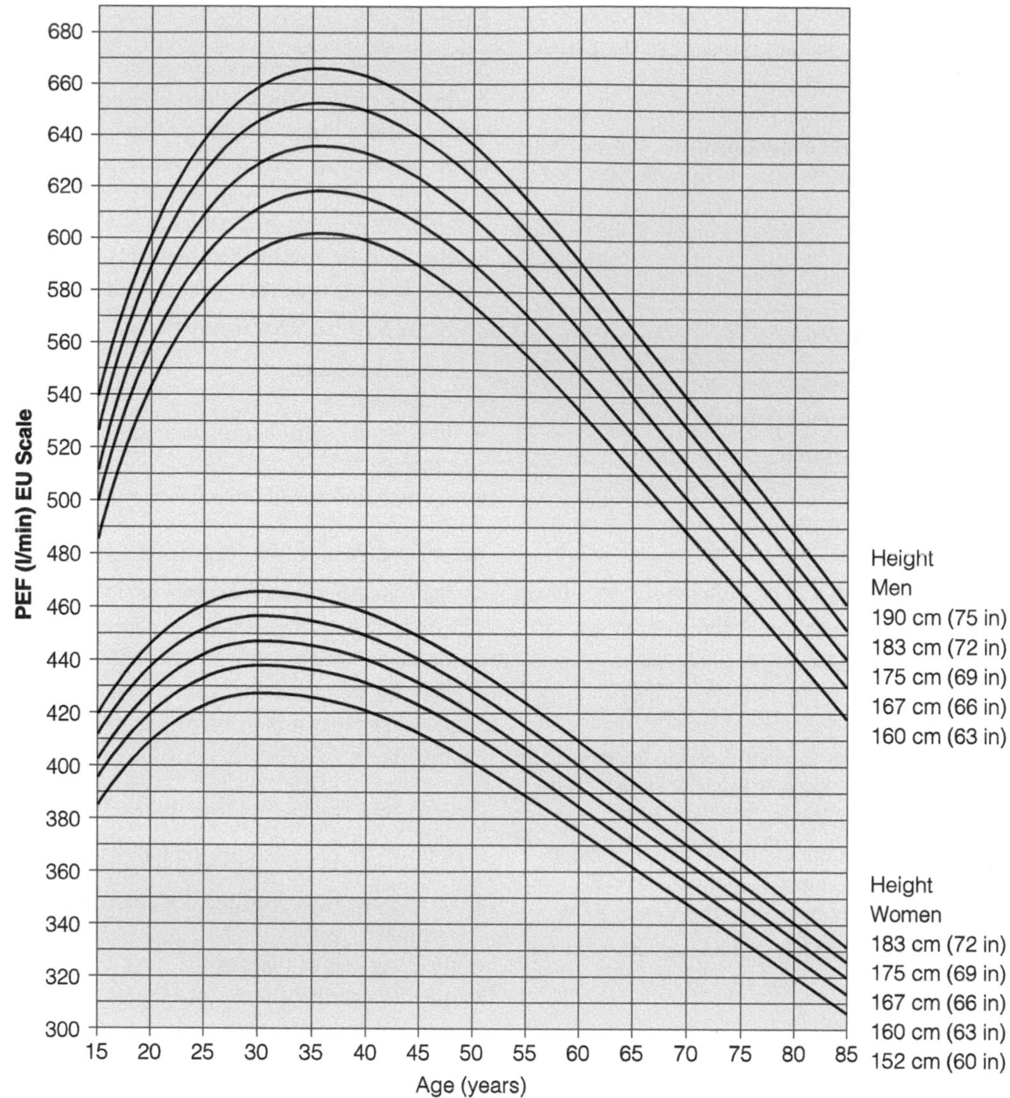

Figure 16-3 Peak expiratory flow rate - normal values.
Source: adapted by Clement Clarke for use with EN13826/EU scale peak flow meters - date of preparation 7 October 2004.

Peak flow readings is important because it can be used:

- at the bedside, emergency department, in the clinical setting or at home;
- to aid diagnosis;
- to provide diagnostic support;
- to monitor treatment/disease – early treatment can prevent further deterioration;
- to provide objective criteria for treatment;
- to assess reversibility of airflow obstruction to bronchodilators;
- to enable self management of a condition by helping to determine specific triggers, e.g. allergens or workplace exposures that cause symptoms;
- for health promotion in general.

Normal Range of Peak Flow Readings

The normal range of peak flow readings can differ depending on age, sex and height of the individual (see Figures 16-3 and 16-4). In an adult the range is normally between 400 and 650 L/min.

PAEDIATRIC NORMAL VALUES
PEAK EXPIRATORY FLOW RATE
For use with EU/EN13826 scale PEF meters only

Height (m)	Height (ft)	Predicted EU PEFR (L/min)	Height (m)	Height (ft)	Predicted EU PEFR (L/min)
0.85	2′9″	87	**1.30**	4′3″	212
0.90	2′11″	95	**1.35**	4′5″	233
0.95	3′1″	104	**1.40**	4′7″	254
1.00	3′3″	115	**1.45**	4′9″	276
1.05	3′5″	127	**1.50**	4′11″	299
1.10	3′7″	141	**1.55**	5′1″	323
1.15	3′9″	157	**1.60**	5′3″	346
1.20	3′11″	174	**1.65**	5′5″	370
1.25	4′1″	192	**1.70**	5′7″	393

Figure 16-4 Paediatric normal values.
Source: adapted by Clement Clarke for use with EU/EN 13826 scale PEF meters only - date of preparation 7 October 2004.

PROCEDURE 16-1 Recording a Peak Flow Measurement

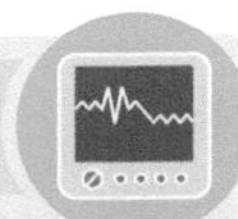

The procedure is effort-dependent and requires training. The manoeuvre should be demonstrated and observed by trained staff.

Purposes

- To record airflow in litres per minute
- To monitor asthma management
- To help diagnosis by monitoring the function of the lung

Assessment

Assess

- The environment to ensure that it is conducive to the patient's well-being
- The patient's position to ensure that it is suitable to record an accurate reading
- Whether the patient is comfortable and able to take the recording
- When the patient received bronchodilators

Planning

Equipment

- Peak flow meter
- Disposable mouthpiece
- Recording chart

Implementation

Preparation

- The patient should be in a standing position or, if unable to stand, then in an upright position (see Figure 16-5).
- Ensure cursor on peak flow meter is set at zero.

Performance

1 Follow local policy to ensure that you explain to the patient what you are going to do, why it is necessary and how they can cooperate. Obtain consent and maintain patient privacy and dignity and ensure that the appropriate local infection control procedures are observed.
2 Attach re-usable/disposable mouthpiece.
3 Ask patient to hold peak flow meter in his/her hand without restricting the cursor.
4 Ask patient to:
   - take a deep breath;
   - hold the breath and seal his/her lips around the mouthpiece, holding the peak flow meter horizontally;
   - blow hard and suddenly, as if blowing out a candle (Bennett, 2003).
5 The measure should be noted and the cursor returned to zero.
6 Repeat this procedure twice more, ensuring the patient is comfortable and not in any distress.
7 The highest of the three attempts to be recorded on the chart.

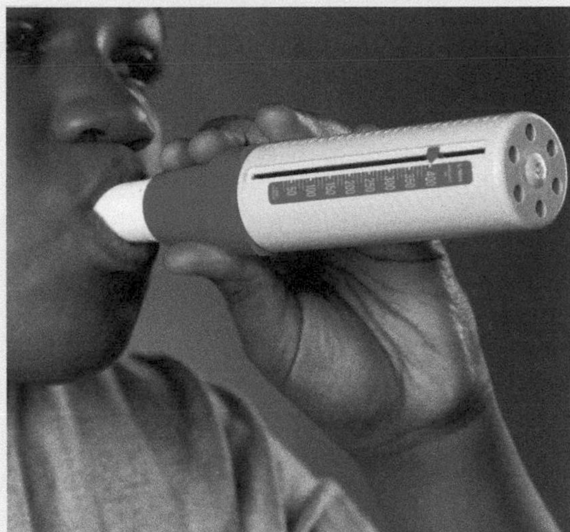

Figure 16-5 Patient sitting when taking peak flow reading.
Source: Science Photo Library Ltd/Coneyl Jay.

8 When inhalers or nebulisers are used, pre- and post-peak flow measurements should be recorded as per hospital policy.
9 Reversibility testing with bronchodilators recording should be taken 15 minutes after short-acting beta two agonist such as salbutamol or 45 minutes after short-acting anti-muscarinic bronchodilators.

Evaluation

- Document the readings.
- Report findings to the doctor.

Other Considerations

- This measurement should not be used in isolation and needs to be evaluated with respiratory symptoms.
- At least two recordings per day are required for monitoring, to obtain an accurate pattern.
- PEF can be reduced in expiratory muscle weakness and poor technique.
- The range limit of different peak flows.
- Suitability for patient.
- The lower range meter for children and the elderly.
- Changing of disposable mouthpieces.
- Trends (PEFR).

Care of Peak Flow Meter

The meter should be kept in its cardboard or plastic box when not in use. Soapy water can be used to wash the mouthpiece, or as per local policy.

PLANNING

The overall goals for a patient with oxygenation problems are to:

- maintain a patent airway;
- improve comfort and ease of breathing;
- maintain or improve pulmonary ventilation and oxygenation;
- improve ability to participate in physical activities;
- prevent risks associated with oxygenation problems such as skin and tissue breakdown, syncope, acid–base imbalances, and feelings of hopelessness and social isolation.

Examples of nursing interventions to facilitate pulmonary ventilation may include ensuring a patent airway, positioning, encouraging deep breathing and coughing, and ensuring adequate hydration. Other nursing interventions helpful to ventilation are suctioning, lung inaction techniques, administration of analgesics before deep breathing and coughing, postural drainage, and percussion and vibration. Nursing strategies to facilitate the diffusion of gases through the alveolar membrane include encouraging coughing, deep breathing and suitable activity. A patient's nursing care plan should also include appropriate dependent nursing interventions such as oxygen therapy, tracheostomy care and maintenance of a chest drain.

IMPLEMENTING

Promoting Oxygenation

Most people in good health give little thought to their respiratory function. Changing position frequently, mobilising and exercising usually maintain adequate ventilation and gas exchange.

When people become ill, however, their respiratory functions may be inhibited for such reasons as pain and immobility. The result of inadequate chest expansion is pooling of respiratory secretions, which ultimately harbour micro-organisms and promote infection. This situation is often compounded by giving opiates for pain, which further depress the rate and depth of respiration.

Interventions by the nurse to maintain the normal respirations of patients include:

- positioning the patient to allow for maximum chest expansion;
- encouraging or providing frequent changes in position;
- encouraging mobilisation;
- implementing measures that promote comfort, such as giving pain medications;
- removing or decreasing any smells that may interfere with the patient's breathing.

The semi-Fowler's or high-Fowler's position allows maximum chest expansion in bed-confined patients, particularly dyspnoeic patients. In these positions the patient is semi-reclining with their knees bent and supported. The nurse should also encourage patients to turn from side to side frequently, so that alternate sides of the chest are permitted maximum expansion. Dyspnoeic patients often sit in bed and lean over their overbed tables (which are raised to a suitable height), usually with a pillow for support. This **orthopnoeic position** is an adaptation of the high-Fowler's position. It has a further advantage in that, unlike in high-Fowler's, the abdominal organs are not pressing on the diaphragm. Also, a patient in the orthopnoeic position can press the lower part of the chest against the table to help in exhaling.

Deep Breathing and Coughing

The nurse can facilitate respiratory functioning by encouraging deep breathing exercises and coughing to remove secretions from the airways. When coughing raises secretions high enough, the patient may either **expectorate** (spit out) or swallow them. Swallowing the secretions is not harmful but does not allow the nurse to view the secretions for documentation purposes or to obtain a specimen for testing.

Breathing exercises are frequently indicated for patients with restricted chest expansion, such as people with COPD or patients recovering from thoracic surgery.

A commonly employed breathing exercise is *abdominal (diaphragmatic)* and pursed-lip breathing. Abdominal breathing permits deep full breaths with little effort. Pursed-lip breathing helps the patient develop control over breathing. The pursed lips create a resistance to the air flowing out of the lungs, thereby prolonging exhalation and preventing airway collapse by maintaining positive airway pressure. The patient purses the lips as if about to whistle and breathes out slowly and gently, tightening the abdominal muscles to exhale more effectively. The patient usually inhales to a count of three and exhales to a count of seven.

Forceful coughing often is less effective than using controlled or huff coughing techniques. Instructions for abdominal (diaphragmatic) and pursed-lip breathing and coughing techniques are provided in *Teaching: patient care.*

Hydration

Adequate hydration maintains the moisture of the respiratory mucous membranes. Normally, respiratory tract secretions are thin and are therefore moved readily by ciliary action. However, when the patient is dehydrated or when the environment has a low humidity, the respiratory secretions can become thick and tenacious. Fluid intake should be as great as the patient can tolerate and disease management allows.

Humidifiers are devices that add water vapour to inspired air. Room humidifiers provide cool mist to room air. Nebulisers are used to deliver humidity and medications. They also are used with oxygen delivery systems to provide moistened air directly to the patient. Their purposes are to prevent mucous membranes from drying and becoming irritated and to loosen secretions for easier expectoration.

Medications

There are a number of different types of medication that can be used for patients with respiratory problems, e.g. bronchodilators, anti-inflammatory drugs, expectorants and cough suppressants. Bronchodilators, including sympathomimetic drugs, beta two agonists, e.g. ventolin, occasionally ephedrine (which are more likely to cause arrhythmias) and theophylline compound bronchodilator preparations reduce bronchospasms by opening tight or congested airways and facilitating ventilation. These drugs may be administered orally or intravenously, but the preferred route is by inhalation to prevent many systemic side-effects.

TEACHING: PATIENT CARE

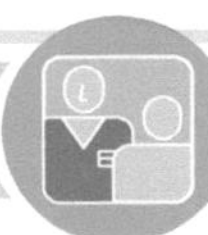

Abdominal (Diaphragmatic) and Pursed-lip Breathing

- Assume a comfortable semi-sitting position in bed or in a chair or a lying position in bed with one pillow.
- Flex your knees to relax the muscles of the abdomen.
- Place one or both hands on your abdomen, just below the ribs.
- Breathe in deeply through the nose, keeping the mouth closed.
- Concentrate on feeling your abdomen rise as far as possible; stay relaxed, and avoid arching your back. If you have difficulty raising your abdomen, take a quick, forceful breath through the nose.
- Then purse your lips as if about to whistle, and breathe out slowly and gently, making a slow 'whooshing' sound without puffing out the cheeks. This pursed-lip breathing creates a resistance to air flowing out of the lungs, increases pressure within the bronchi (main air passages), and minimises collapse of smaller airways, a common problem for people with COPD.
- Concentrate on feeling the abdomen fall or sink, and tighten (contract) the abdominal muscles while breathing out to enhance effective exhalation. Count to seven during exhalation.
- Use this exercise whenever feeling short of breath, and increase gradually to 5–10 minutes four times a day. Regular practice will help you do this type of breathing without conscious effort. The exercise, once learned, can be performed when sitting upright, standing and walking.

Controlled and Huff Coughing

- After using a bronchodilator treatment (if prescribed), inhale deeply and hold your breath for a few seconds.
- Cough twice. The first cough loosens the mucus; the second expels secretions.
- For huff coughing, lean forward and exhale sharply with a 'huff' sound. This technique helps keep your airways open while moving secretions up and out of the lungs.
- Inhale by taking rapid short breaths in succession ('sniffing') to prevent mucus from moving back into smaller airways.
- Rest.
- Try to avoid prolonged episodes of coughing because these may cause fatigue and hypoxia.

Since drugs used to dilate the bronchioles and improve breathing are usually drugs that enhance the sympathetic nervous system, patients must be monitored for side effects of increased heart rate, blood pressure, anxiety and restlessness. This is especially important in older adults, who may also have cardiac problems.

Another class of drugs used is the *anti-inflammatory drugs*, such as glucocorticoids (steroids). They can be given orally, intravenously or by inhaler. They work by decreasing the oedema and inflammation in the airways and allowing a better air exchange. If both bronchodilators and anti-inflammatory drugs are prescribed by inhaler, the patient should be instructed to use the bronchodilator inhaler first and then the anti-inflammatory inhaler. If the bronchioles are dilated first, more tissue is exposed for the anti-inflammatory drugs to act upon.

Expectorants help 'break up' mucus, making it more liquid and easier to expectorate. When frequent or prolonged coughing interrupts sleep, a cough suppressant such as codeine may be prescribed.

Other medications can be used to improve oxygenation by improving cardiovascular function. The *digitalis glycosides* such as digoxin act directly on the heart to improve the strength of contraction and slow the heart rate. *Beta-adrenergic blocking agents* such as propranolol affect the sympathetic nervous system to reduce the workload of the heart. These drugs, however, can negatively affect people with asthma or COPD as they may constrict airways.

Incentive Spirometry

Incentive spirometers (see Figure 16-6), also referred to as *sustained maximal inspiration devices* (SMIs), measure the flow of air inhaled through the mouthpiece and are used to:

- improve pulmonary ventilation;
- counteract the effects of anaesthesia or hypoventilation;
- loosen respiratory secretions;
- facilitate respiratory gaseous exchange;
- expand collapsed alveoli.

They offer an incentive to improve inhalation. When using an SMI, the patient should be assisted into a position, preferably an upright sitting position in bed or a chair, that facilitates maximum ventilation. Studies carried out by Agostini *et al.* (2008) have confirmed that this is still a relatively good measure of recording lung function. *Teaching: patient care* lists instructions for patients in the use of incentive spirometers.

Percussion, Vibration and Postural Drainage

Percussion, vibration and postural drainage (PVD) are frequently performed by physiotherapists; however, in some clinical areas they may be carried out by nursing staff. **Percussion**, sometimes called *clapping*, is forceful striking of the skin with cupped hands. Mechanical percussion cups and vibrators are also available but used less frequently. When the hands are used, the fingers and thumb are held together and flexed slightly to form a cup, as one would to scoop up water. Percussion over congested lung areas can mechanically dislodge tenacious secretions from the bronchial walls. Cupped hands trap the air against the chest. The trapped air sets up vibrations through the chest wall to the secretions.

(a)

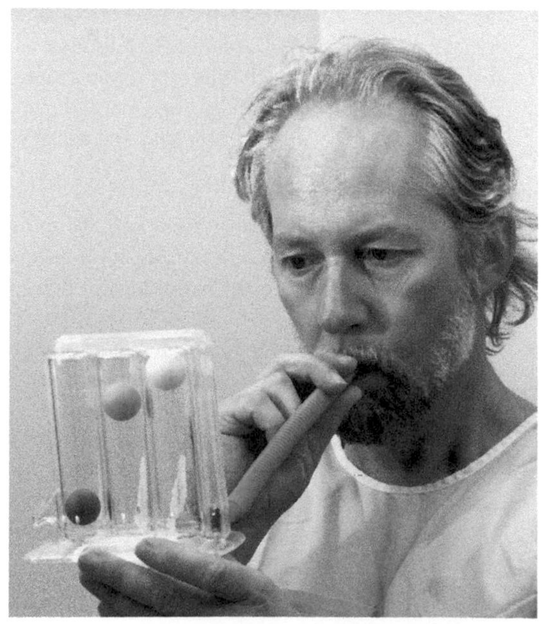

(b)

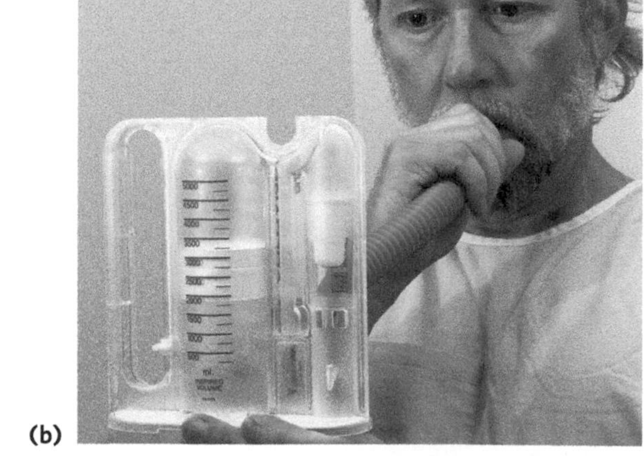

Figure 16-6 (a) Flow-oriented SMI; (b) volume-oriented SMI.

TEACHING: PATIENT CARE

Using an Incentive Spirometer

- Hold or place the spirometer in an upright position. A tilted *flow-oriented* device requires less effort to raise the balls or discs; a *volume-oriented* device will not function correctly unless upright.
- Exhale normally.
- Seal the lips tightly around the mouthpiece.
- Take in a slow, deep breath to elevate the balls or cylinder, and then hold the breath for two seconds initially, increasing to six seconds (optimum), to keep the balls or cylinder elevated if possible.
- For a flow-oriented device, avoid brisk, low-volume breaths that snap the balls to the top of the chamber. Greater lung expansion is achieved with a very slow inspiration than with a brisk, shallow breath, even though it may not elevate the balls or keep them elevated while you hold your breath. Sustained elevation of the balls or cylinder ensures adequate ventilation of the alveoli (lung air sacs).
- If you have difficulty breathing only through the mouth, a nose clip can be used.
- Remove the mouthpiece and exhale normally.
- Cough after the incentive effort. Deep ventilation may loosen secretions, and coughing can facilitate their removal.
- Relax and take several normal breaths before using the spirometer again.
- Repeat the procedure several times and then four or five times hourly. Practice increases inspiratory volume, maintains alveolar ventilation and prevents atelectasis (collapse of the air sacs).
- Clean or dispose of the mouthpiece as directed by the manufacturer and/or hospital or local health board policy.

To percuss a patient's chest, the nurse follows these steps:

1 Cover the area with a towel or gown to reduce discomfort.
2 Ask the patient to breathe slowly and deeply to promote relaxation.
3 Alternately flex and extend the wrists rapidly to slap the chest (see Figure 16-7).
4 Percuss each affected lung segment for 1–2 minutes.

When done correctly, the percussion action should produce a hollow, popping sound. Percussion is avoided over the breasts, sternum, spinal column and kidneys.

Vibration is a series of vigorous quiverings produced by hands that are placed flat against the patient's chest wall. Vibration is used after percussion to increase the turbulence of the exhaled air and thus loosen thick secretions. It is often done alternately with percussion.

To vibrate the patient's chest, the nurse follows these steps:

1 Place hands, palms down, on the chest area to be drained, one hand over the other with the fingers together and extended (see Figure 16-8). Alternatively, the hands may be placed side by side.

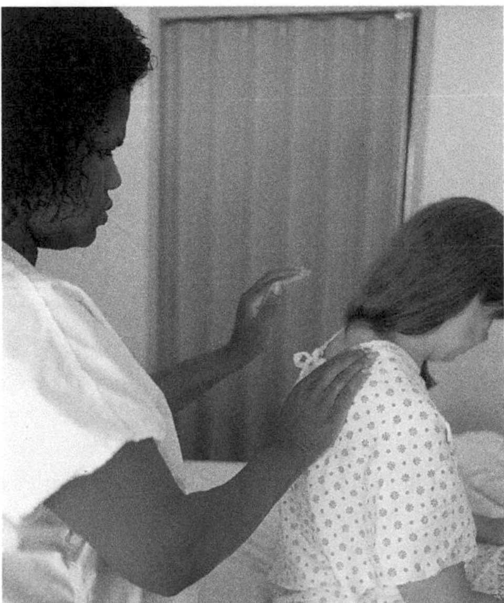

Figure 16-7 Percussing the upper posterior chest.
Source: Pearson Education Ltd.

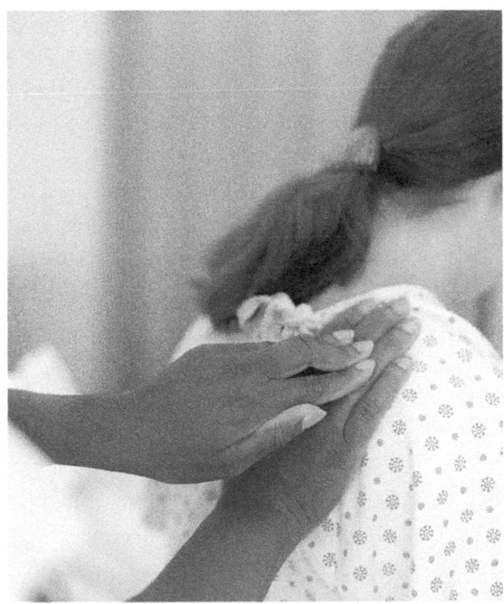

Figure 16-8 Vibrating the upper posterior chest.
Source: Pearson Education Ltd.

2 Ask the patient to inhale deeply and exhale slowly through the nose or pursed lips.
3 During the exhalation, tense all the hand and arm muscles, and using mostly the heel of the hand, vibrate (shake) the hands, moving them downward. Stop the vibrating when the patient inhales.
4 Vibrate during five exhalations over one affected lung segment.
5 After each vibration, encourage the patient to cough and expectorate secretions into the sputum container.

Postural drainage is the drainage by gravity of secretions from various lung segments. Secretions that remain in the lungs or respiratory airways promote bacterial growth and subsequent infection. They also can obstruct the smaller airways and cause atelectasis. Secretions in the major airways, such as the trachea and the right and left main bronchi, are usually coughed into the pharynx, where they can be expectorated, swallowed or effectively removed by suctioning.

A wide variety of positions is necessary to drain all segments of the lungs, but not all positions are required for every patient. Only those positions that drain specific affected areas are used. The lower lobes require drainage most frequently because the upper lobes drain by gravity. Before postural drainage, the patient may be given a bronchodilator medication or nebulisation therapy to loosen secretions. Postural drainage treatments are usually performed two or three times daily, depending on the degree of lung congestion. The best times include before breakfast, before lunch, in the late afternoon, and before bedtime. It is best to avoid hours shortly after meals because postural drainage at these times can be tiring and can induce vomiting.

The nurse needs to evaluate the patient's tolerance of postural drainage by assessing the stability of the vital signs, particularly the pulse and respiratory rates, and by noting signs of intolerance, such as pallor, diaphoresis, dyspnoea and fatigue. Some patients do not react well to certain drainage positions, and the nurse must make appropriate adjustments. For example, some become dyspnoeic in Trendelenburg's position (head of bed tilted lower than the feet), and require only a moderate tilt or a shorter time in that position.

The sequence for PVD is usually as follows: positioning, percussion, vibration and removal of secretions by coughing or suction. Each position is usually assumed for 10–15 minutes, although beginning treatments may start with shorter times and gradually increase.

Following PVD, the nurse should auscultate the patient's lungs, compare the findings to the baseline data, and document the amount, colour and character of expectorated secretions.

Oxygen Therapy

Patients who have difficulty ventilating all areas of their lungs, those whose gas exchange is impaired, or people with heart failure may require oxygen therapy to prevent hypoxia.

Oxygen therapy is a prescribed medication; the prescription should specify the concentration, method of delivery and litre flow per minute. The concentration is of more importance than the litre flow per minute. When administering oxygen is an emergency measure, the nurse may initiate the therapy without a prescription. For patients who have COPD, a low-flow oxygen system is essential.

The following safety precautions are essential during oxygen therapy:

- For home oxygen use or when the facility permits smoking, teach family members to smoke only outside or in provided smoking rooms away from the patient.
- Place cautionary signs reading 'No Smoking: Oxygen in Use' on the oxygen equipment.
- Instruct the patient and visitors about the hazard of smoking with oxygen in use.
- Make sure that electric devices (such as razors, hearing aids, radios, televisions and heating pads) are in good working order to prevent the occurrence of short-circuit sparks.
- Avoid materials that generate static electricity, such as woollen blankets and synthetic fabrics.
- Avoid the use of volatile, flammable materials, such as oils, greases, alcohol and acetone (e.g. nail varnish remover), near patients receiving oxygen.
- Ground electric monitoring equipment, suction machines and portable diagnostic machines.
- Make known the location of fire extinguishers, and make sure personnel are trained in their use.

Although oxygen by itself will not burn or explode, it does facilitate combustion. For example, a bed sheet ordinarily burns slowly when ignited in the atmosphere; however, if saturated with free-flowing oxygen and ignited by a spark, it will burn rapidly and explosively. The greater the concentration of oxygen, the more rapidly fires start and burn, and such fires are difficult to extinguish. Because oxygen is colourless, odourless and tasteless, people are often unaware of its presence.

Oxygen is supplied in several different ways. In hospitals and long-term care facilities, it is usually piped into wall outlets at the patient's bedside, making it readily available for use at all times. Tanks or cylinders of oxygen under pressure are also frequently available for use when wall oxygen either is unavailable or impractical (e.g. for transporting oxygen-dependent patients between clinical areas).

Patients who require oxygen therapy in the home may use small cylinders of oxygen or an oxygen concentrator. Portable oxygen delivery systems are available to increase the patient's independence. Home oxygen therapy services are readily available in communities. These services generally supply the oxygen and delivery devices, training for the patient and family, equipment maintenance and emergency services should a problem occur.

Oxygen administered from a cylinder or wall-outlet system is dry. Dry gases dehydrate the respiratory mucous membranes. Humidifying devices that add water vapour to inspired air are used as an adjunct of oxygen therapy in some patients; particularly for litre flows over 2 L/min (see Figure 16-9). These devices provide 20% to 40% humidity. The oxygen passes through sterile distilled water or tap water and then along a line to the device

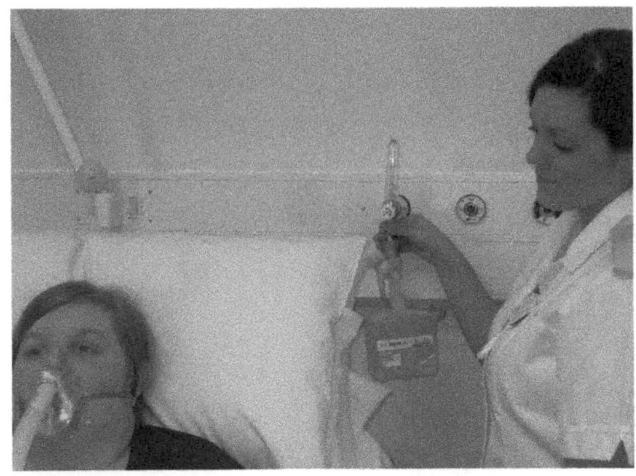
(a)

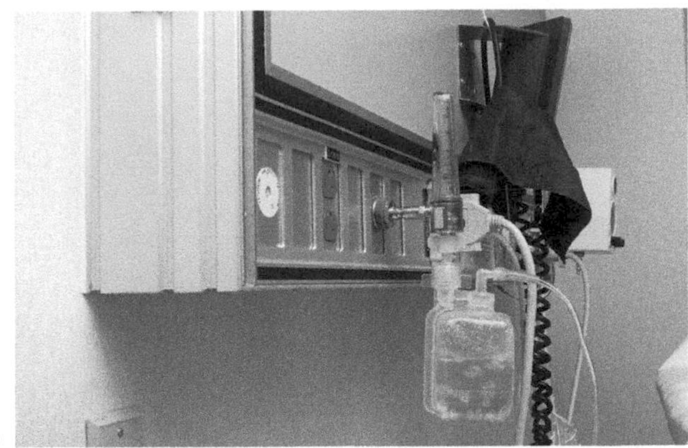
(b)

Figure 16-9 A patient wearing a humidified face mask; (b) humidified oxygen.
Source: (a) © Heulwen Morgan-Samuel; (b) © Shutterstock.com.

through which the moistened oxygen is inhaled (e.g. a nasal cannula, or oxygen mask).

Humidifiers prevent mucous membranes from drying and becoming irritated and loosen secretions for easier expectoration. Oxygen passing through water picks up water vapour before it reaches the patient. The more bubbles created during this process, the more water vapour is produced. Very low litre flows (e.g. 1–2 L/min by nasal cannula) do not require humidification.

Oxygen cylinders need to be handled and stored with caution and strapped securely in wheeled transport devices or stands to prevent possible falls and outlet breakages. They should be placed away from sources of heat.

To use an oxygen wall outlet, the nurse carries out these steps:

1 Attach the flow meter to the wall outlet, exerting firm pressure. The flow meter should be in the off position. (If not already inserted.)
2 Fill the humidifier bottle with distilled or tap water in accordance with local policy. This should be done before coming to the bedside. Some humidifier bottles come prefilled by the manufacturer.
3 Attach the humidifier bottle to the base of the flow meter.
4 Attach the prescribed oxygen tubing and delivery device to the humidifier.
5 Regulate the flow meter to the prescribed level.

Oxygen Delivery Systems

A number of systems are available to deliver oxygen to the patient. The choice of system depends on the patient's oxygen needs, comfort and developmental considerations. With many systems, the oxygen delivered mixes with room air before being inspired. The amount of oxygen delivered is determined by regulating its flow rate (e.g. 2–6 L/min), and precise regulation of the percentage of inspired oxygen, or fraction of inspired oxygen (FiO_2), is not possible. When it is important to regulate the percentage of oxygen received by the patient more precisely, a device such as a Venturi mask may be used.

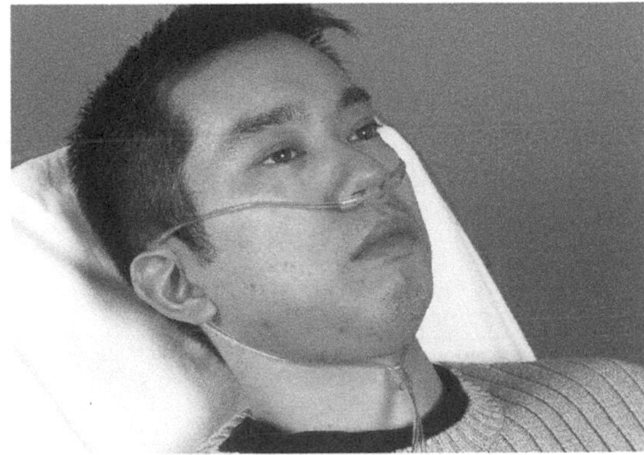

Figure 16-10 A nasal cannula.
Source: Pearson Education Ltd.

Cannula

The nasal cannula (nasal prongs) is the most common inexpensive device used to administer oxygen (see Figure 16-10).

The nasal cannula is easy to apply and does not interfere with the patient's ability to eat or talk. It also is relatively comfortable, permits some freedom of movement, and is well tolerated by the patient. It delivers a relatively low concentration of oxygen (24–45%) at flow rates of 2–6 L/min. Above 6 L/min, the patient tends to swallow air and the FiO_2 is not increased. Also at higher flow rates it causes nasal discomfort for the patient.

Administering oxygen by cannula is detailed in *Procedure 16-2* on page 471.

Face Mask

Face masks that cover the patient's nose and mouth may be used for oxygen inhalation. Exhalation ports on the sides of the mask allow exhaled carbon dioxide to escape. A variety of oxygen masks are available from manufacturers:

- The simple face mask delivers oxygen concentrations from 40–60% at litre flows of 5–8 L/min, respectively (see Figure 16-11).
- The partial rebreather mask delivers oxygen concentrations of 60–90% at litre flows of 6–15 L/min, respectively.

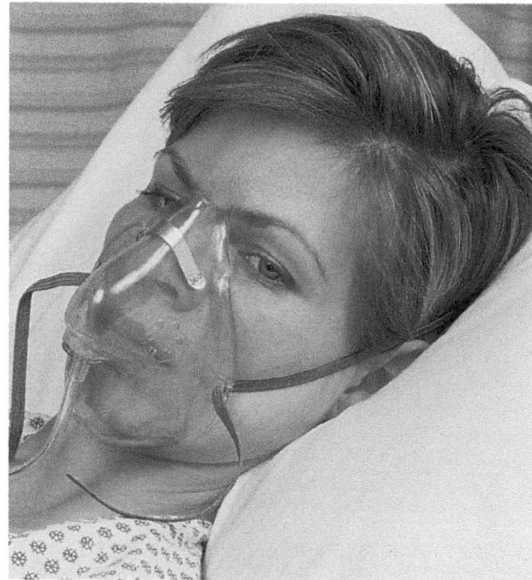

Figure 16-11 A simple face mask.
Source: Elena Dorfmann.

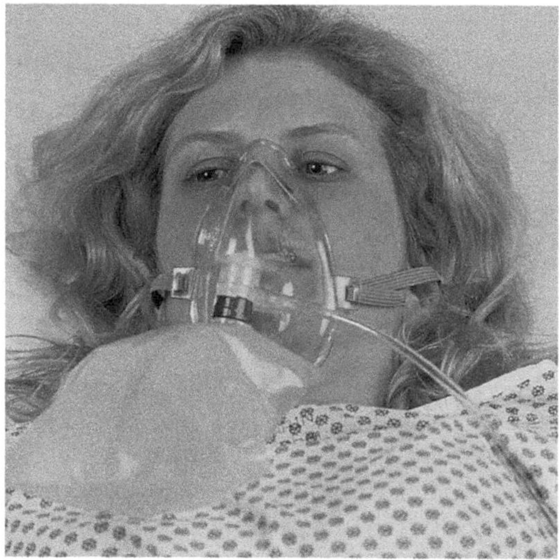

Figure 16-12 A partial rebreather mask.
Source: Jenny Thomas

The oxygen reservoir bag that is attached allows the patient to rebreathe about the first third of the exhaled air in conjunction with oxygen (see Figure 16-12). Thus, it increases the FiO_2 by recycling expired oxygen. The partial rebreather bag must not totally deflate during inspiration to avoid carbon dioxide build up. If this problem occurs, the nurse increases the litre flow of oxygen.

- The nonrebreather mask delivers the highest oxygen concentration possible (95–100%) by means other than intubation or mechanical ventilation, at litre flows of 10–15 L/min. One-way valves on the mask and between the reservoir bag and the mask prevent the room air and the patient's exhaled air from entering the bag so only the oxygen in the bag is inspired (see Figure 16-13). To prevent carbon dioxide build up, the nonrebreather bag must not totally deflate during inspiration. If it does, the nurse can correct this problem by increasing the litre flow of oxygen.

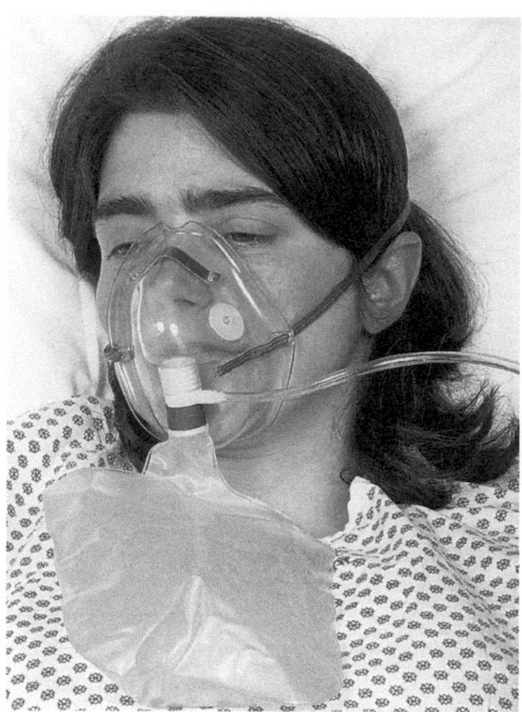

Figure 16-13 A nonrebreather mask.
Source: Jenny Thomas.

- The Venturi mask delivers oxygen concentrations varying from 24–60% or 50% at litre flows of 2–15 L/min (see Table 16-3). The Venturi mask has wide-bore tubing and colour-coded jet adapters that correspond to a precise oxygen concentration and litre flow. For example, a blue adapter delivers a 24% concentration of oxygen at 4 L/min, and a green adapter delivers a 35% concentration of oxygen at 8 L/min.

Initiating oxygen by mask (see Figure 16-14) is much the same as initiating oxygen by cannula, except that the nurse must find a mask of appropriate size. Smaller sizes are available for children and adults with small faces. Administering oxygen by mask or face tent is detailed in *Procedure 16-2.*

Table 16-3 Fixed Performance Oxygen Mask (Venturi-type Masks) Flow Rates

Oxygen flow rate (L/min)	% Oxygen delivered
2	24
6	31
8	35
10	40
15	60

Source: Dougherty and Lister (2008).

CLINICAL ALERT

Oxygen administration in most instances needs to be prescribed!

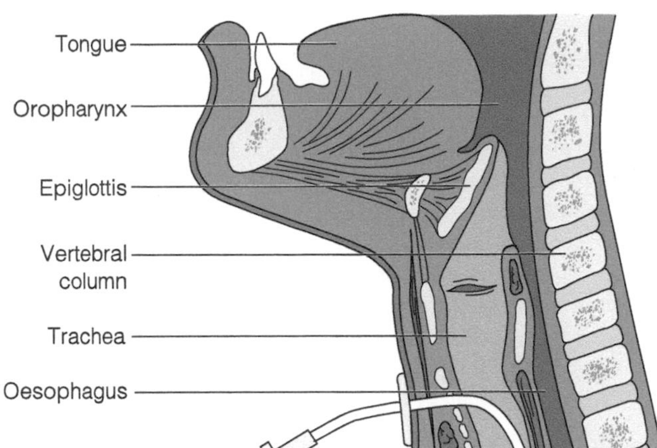

Figure 16-15 A transtracheal oxygen catheter in place.

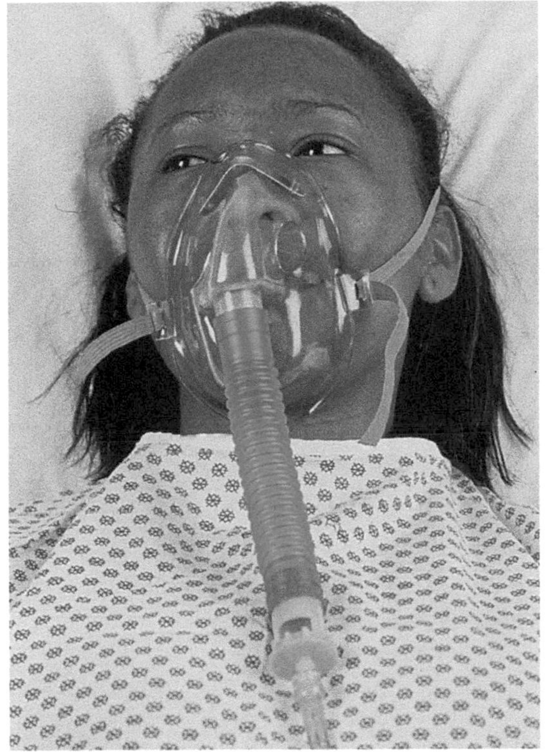

Figure 16-14 A Venturi mask.
Source: Jenny Thomas.

Transtracheal Oxygen Delivery

Transtracheal oxygen delivery may be used for oxygen-dependent patients. Oxygen is delivered through a small, narrow plastic cannula surgically inserted through the skin directly into the trachea (see Figure 16-15). A chain around the neck holds the catheter in place.

With this delivery system, the patient requires less oxygen (0.5–2 l per minute) because all of the flow delivered enters the lungs. The nurse or patient keeps the catheter patent by injecting 1.5ml of normal saline into it, moving a cleaning rod in and out of it, and then injecting another 1.5ml of saline solution. This is done two or three times a day.

Paediatric Oxygen Delivery

A paediatric oxygen tent is often used when poor compliance of cannulae and face masks is noted in a child. A paediatric oxygen tent is a plain clear piece of plastic that is draped over the baby or infant's bed. Oxygen is then administered inside the tent at the required rate.

PROCEDURE 16-2 Administering Oxygen by Cannula, Face Mask or Face Tent

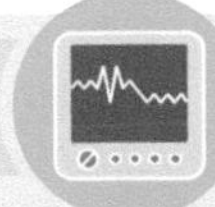

Before administering oxygen, check (a) the prescription for oxygen, including the litre flow rate (L/min) or the percentage of oxygen; (b) the levels of oxygen (PO_2) and carbon dioxide ($PaCO_2$) in the patient's arterial blood (PaO_2 is normally 80-100mmHg; $PaCO_2$ is normally 35-45mmHg); and (c) whether the patient has COPD.

Purposes

Cannula

- To deliver a relatively low concentration of oxygen when only minimal O_2 support is required
- To allow uninterrupted delivery of oxygen while the patient ingests food or fluids

Face Mask/Face Tent

- To provide moderate O_2 support and a higher concentration of oxygen and/or humidity than is provided by cannula

Assessment

Assess

- Skin and mucous membrane colour: Note whether cyanosis is present
- Breathing patterns: Note depth of respirations and presence of tachypnoea, bradypnoea, orthopnoea
- Chest movements: Note whether there are any intercostal, substernal, suprasternal, supraclavicular or tracheal retractions during inspiration or expiration
- Chest wall configuration (e.g. kyphosis)
- Presence of clinical signs of hypoxemia: tachycardia, tachypnoea, restlessness, dyspnoea, cyanosis and confusion. Tachycardia and tachypnoea are often early signs. Confusion is a later sign of severe oxygen deprivation
- Presence of clinical signs of hypercarbia (hypercapnia): restlessness, hypertension, headache, lethargy, tremor
- Presence of clinical signs of oxygen toxicity: tracheal irritation and cough, dyspnoea and decreased pulmonary ventilation

Determine

- Vital signs, especially pulse rate and quality, and respiratory rate, rhythm and depth
- Whether the patient has COPD. A high carbon dioxide level in the blood is the normal stimulus to breathe. However, people with COPD may have a chronically high carbon dioxide level, and their stimulus to breathe is hypoxemia. Low flows of oxygen (2 L/min) stimulate breathing for such persons by maintaining slight hypoxemia. During continuous oxygen administration, arterial blood gas levels of oxygen (PO_2) and carbon dioxide (PCO_2) are measured periodically to monitor hypoxemia
- Results of diagnostic studies
- Haemoglobin, haematocrit, full blood count
- Arterial blood gases
- Pulmonary function tests

Planning

Equipment

Cannula

- Oxygen supply with a flow meter and adapter
- Humidifier with distilled water or tap water according to agency protocol
- Nasal cannula and tubing

Face Mask

- Oxygen supply with a flow meter and adapter
- Humidifier with distilled water or tap water according to local policy
- Face mask of the appropriate size

Face Tent

- Oxygen supply with a flow meter and adaptor
- Humidifier with distilled water
- Face tent of the appropriate size

Implementation

Preparation

Determine the need for oxygen therapy, and verify the prescription for the therapy.

Performance

1. Follow local policy to ensure that you explain to the patient what you are going to do, why it is necessary and how they can cooperate. Obtain consent and maintain patient privacy and dignity and ensure that the appropriate local infection control procedures are observed.
2. Assist the patient to a semi-Fowler's position if possible. This position permits easier chest expansion and hence easier breathing.
3. Explain that oxygen is not dangerous when safety precautions are observed. Inform the patient about the safety precautions connected with oxygen use.
4. Set up the oxygen equipment and the humidifier.
   - Attach the flow meter to the wall outlet or cylinder. The flow meter should be in the off position.
   - If needed, fill the humidifier bottle. (This can be done before coming to the bedside.)
   - Attach the humidifier bottle to the base of the flow meter.
   - Attach the prescribed oxygen tubing and delivery device to the humidifier.
5. Turn on the oxygen at the prescribed rate and ensure proper functioning.
   - Check that the oxygen is flowing freely through the tubing. There should be no kinks in the tubing, and the connections should be airtight. There should be bubbles in the humidifier as the oxygen flows through. You should feel the oxygen at the outlet of the cannula, or mask.
   - Set the oxygen at the flow rate prescribed.
6. Apply the appropriate oxygen delivery device.

Cannula

- Put the cannula over the patient's face, with the outlet prongs fitting into the nares and the elastic band around

the head (see Figure 16-10 on page 469). Some models have a strap to adjust under the chin.
- If the cannula will not stay in place, tape it at the sides of the face.
- Pad the tubing and band over the ears and cheekbones as needed.

Face mask
- Guide the mask towards the patient's face, and apply it from the nose downward.
- Fit the mask to the contours of the patient's face (see Figure 16-11 on page 470). The mask should mould to the face, so that very little oxygen escapes into the eyes or around the cheeks and chin.
- Secure the elastic band around the patient's head so that the mask is comfortable but snug.

7 Assess the patient regularly.
- Assess the patient's vital signs, level of anxiety, colour and ease of respirations, and provide support while the patient adjusts to the device.
- Assess the patient in 15–30 minutes, depending on the patient's condition, and regularly thereafter.
- Assess the patient regularly for clinical signs of hypoxia, tachycardia, confusion, dyspnoea, restlessness and cyanosis. Review arterial blood gas results if they are available.

Face tent
- Position the tent over the child's face.
- Frequent assessment is necessary.
- Vital signs, level of anxiety, colour, and respirations.
- Hypoxia, tachycardia, confusion, dyspnoea, restlessness and cyanosis.

Nasal cannula
- Assess the patient's nares for encrustations and irritation. Apply a *water-soluble* lubricant as required to soothe the mucous membranes.

Face mask or tent
- Inspect the facial skin frequently for dampness or chafing, and dry and treat it as needed.

8 Inspect the equipment on a regular basis.
- Check the litre flow and the level of water in the humidifier in 30 minutes and whenever providing care to the patient.
- Make sure that safety precautions are being followed.

9 Document findings in the patient record using forms or checklists supplemented by narrative notes when appropriate.

Evaluation

- Perform follow-up based on findings that deviated from expected or normal for the patient. Relate findings to previous data if available.
- Report significant deviations from normal to the medical staff.

LIFESPAN CONSIDERATIONS

Oxygen Delivery Equipment

Infants

Oxygen hood
- An oxygen hood is a rigid plastic dome that encloses an infant's head. It provides precise oxygen levels and high humidity.
- The gas should not be allowed to blow directly into the infant's face, and the hood should not rub against the infant's neck, chin or shoulder.

Children

Oxygen tent (see Figure 16-16)
- The tent consists of a rectangular, clear, plastic canopy with outlets that connect to an oxygen or compressed air source and to a humidifier that moisturises the air or oxygen.

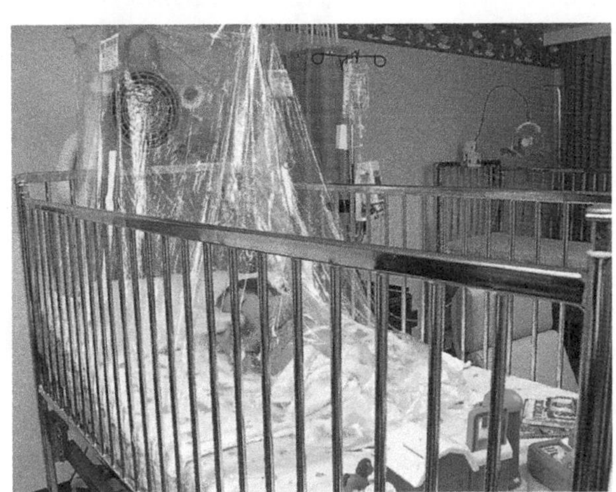

Figure 16-16 Paediatric oxygen tent.
Source: Jenny Thomas.

- Because the enclosed tent becomes very warm, some type of cooling mechanism such as an ice chamber or a refrigeration unit is provided to maintain the temperature at 20–21°C.
- Cover the child with a gown or a cotton blanket. A small towel may be wrapped around the head. *The child needs protection from chilling and from the dampness and condensation in the tent.*
- Flood the tent with oxygen by setting the flow meter at 15 L/min for about five minutes. Then, adjust the flow meter according to orders (e.g. 10–15 L/min). *Flooding the tent quickly increases the oxygen to the desired level.*
- The tent can deliver approximately 30% oxygen.

COMMUNITY CARE CONSIDERATIONS

Community Care Oxygen Equipment

Two major oxygen systems for home care use are available in most communities: cylinders or tanks of compressed gas and oxygen concentrators.

1 Cylinders: These are the system of choice for patients who need oxygen episodically (e.g. on a prn basis). Advantages are that cylinders deliver all litre flows (1–15 L/min). Disadvantages are that some cylinders are heavy and awkward to move, the supply company/community pharmacy must be notified when a refill is needed, and they are costly for the high-use patient (see Figure 16-17).

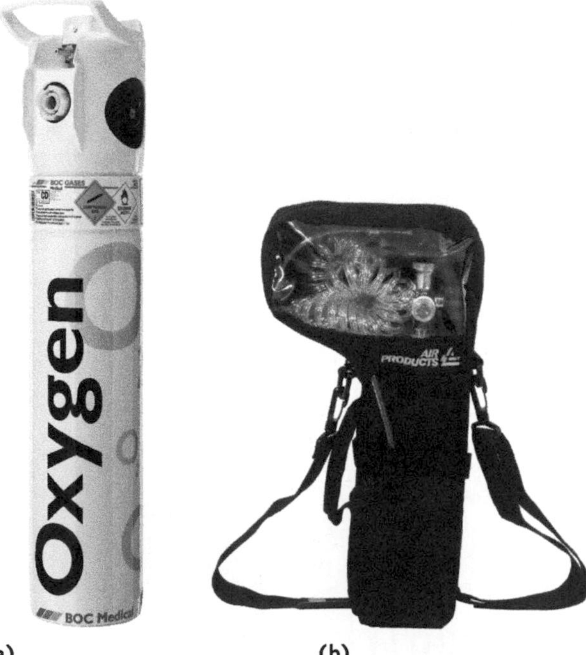

Figure 16-17 Typical oxygen cylinders without (a) and with (b) carrying case.
Source: Air Products and Chemicals 2007, Europe Air Products PLC.

2 Oxygen concentrators: Concentrators are electrically powered systems that manufacture oxygen from room air. At 1 L/min, such a system can deliver a concentration of about 95% oxygen, but the concentration drops when the flow rate increases (e.g. 75% concentration at 4 L/min). Advantages are that they are more attractive in appearance, resembling furniture rather than medical equipment; they eliminate the need for regular delivery of oxygen or refilling of cylinders; because the supply of oxygen is constant, they alleviate the patient's anxiety about running out of oxygen; and they are the most economical system when continuous use is required. Major disadvantages of a concentrator are that it is expensive; lacks real portability; tends to be noisy; is powered by electricity (an emergency backup unit, for example, an oxygen cylinder, must be provided for patients for whom a power failure could be life threatening); and heat produced by the concentrator motor is a problem for those who live in small houses. The oxygen concentrator must also be checked periodically with an O_2 analyser to ensure that it is providing an adequate delivery of oxygen.

Another type of oxygen concentrator is the *oxygen enricher*. It uses a plastic membrane that allows water vapour to pass through with the oxygen, thus eliminating the need for a humidifying device. It is also thought to filter out bacteria present in the air. The enricher provides an O_2 concentration of 40% at all flow rates, it tends to be quieter than the concentrator, there is less chance of combustion (since the gas is only 40% oxygen), it has only two moving parts (thus decreasing the risk of something going wrong), and a nebuliser can be operated off the enricher because of the high flow rate.

The nurse needs to ensure that the patient has an appropriate home oxygen supplier. Services furnished should include:

- a 24-hour emergency service;
- trained personnel to make the initial delivery and instruct the patient in safe, appropriate use of the oxygen and maintenance of the equipment;
- at least monthly follow-up visits to check the equipment and reinstruct the patient as necessary.

Artificial Airways (see also Chapter 25)

Artificial airways are inserted to maintain a patent air passage for a patient whose airway has become or may become obstructed. A patent airway is necessary so that air can flow to and from the lungs. Four of the more common types of airways are oropharyngeal, nasopharyngeal, endotracheal and tracheostomy.

Oropharyngeal and Nasopharyngeal Airways

Oropharyngeal and nasopharyngeal airways are used to keep the upper air passages open when they may become obstructed by secretions or the tongue. These airways are easy to insert and have a low risk of complications. Sizes vary and should be appropriate to the size and age of the patient. For nasopharyngeal airways the device should be well lubricated with water-soluble gel prior to inserting.

Oropharyngeal airways (see Figure 16-18) stimulate the gag reflex and are only used for patients with altered levels of consciousness (e.g. because of general anaesthesia, overdose or head injury) (see Chapter 25 for insertion technique).

Nasopharyngeal airways are tolerated better by alert patients. They are inserted through the nares, terminating in the oropharynx (see Figure 16-19). When caring for a patient with a nasopharyngeal airway, provide frequent oral and nares care, repositioning the airway in the other nostril every 8 hours or as directed to prevent necrosis of the mucosa.

ACTIVITY 16-1

A patient has been admitted to your ward in status asthmaticus (acute asthma attack). Reflect on your care management and discuss what are the key issues to be considered to manage his/her care effectively. Provide a rationale for the decisions you have made.

Endotracheal Tubes

Endotracheal tubes are most commonly inserted for patients who have had general anaesthetics or for those in emergency situations where mechanical ventilation is required. An endotracheal tube is inserted by the practitioner with specialised education through either the mouth or the nose and into the trachea with the guide of a laryngoscope (see Figure 16-20). The tube terminates just superior to the bifurcation of the trachea into the bronchi. The tube may have an air-filled cuff to prevent air leakage around it. Because an endotracheal tube passes through the epiglottis and glottis, the patient is unable to speak while it is in place.

Tracheostomy

Patients who need long-term airway support may have a tracheostomy, a surgical incision in the trachea just below the larynx. A curved tracheostomy tube is inserted to extend through the stoma into the trachea (see Figure 16-21). Tracheostomy tubes may be either plastic or metal and are available in different sizes.

Tracheostomy tubes have an outer cannula that is inserted into the trachea and a flange that rests against the neck and

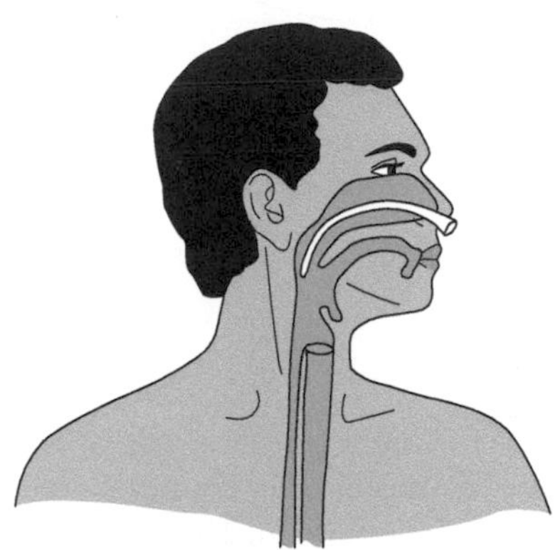

Figure 16-19 A nasopharyngeal airway in place.

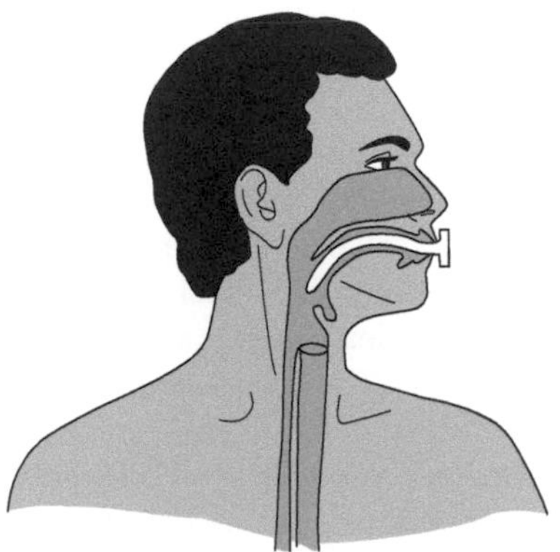

Figure 16-18 An oropharyngeal airway in place.

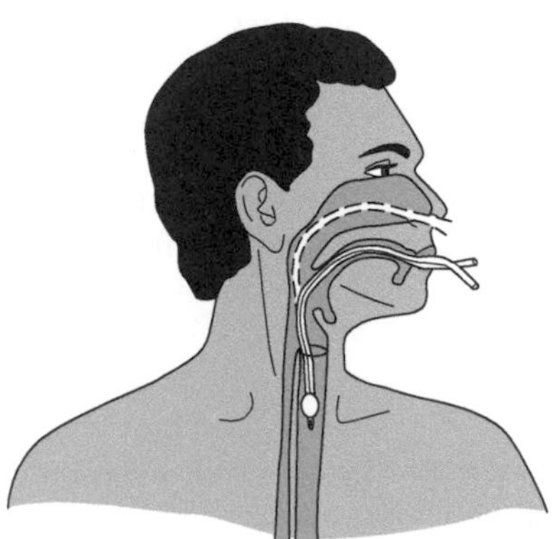

Figure 16-20 An endotracheal tube in place.

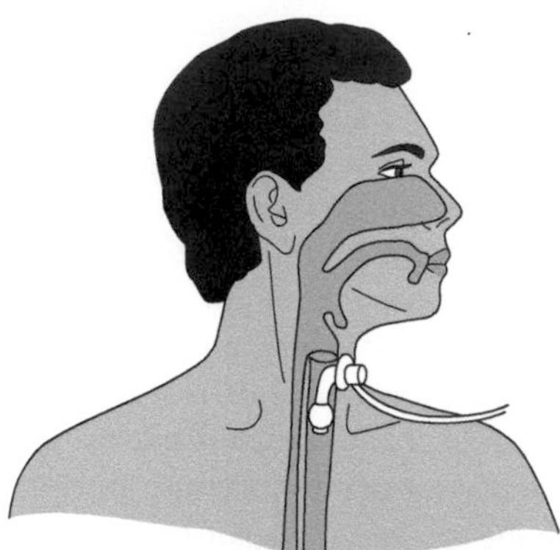

Figure 16-21 A tracheostomy tube in place.

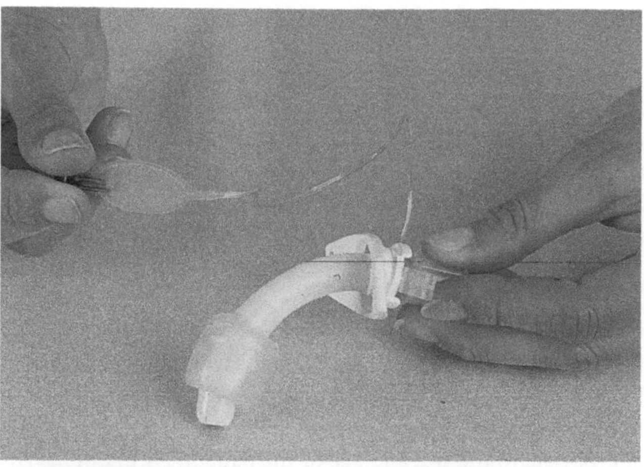

Figure 16-23 A tracheostomy tube with a low pressure cuff.
Source: Smiths Medical International.

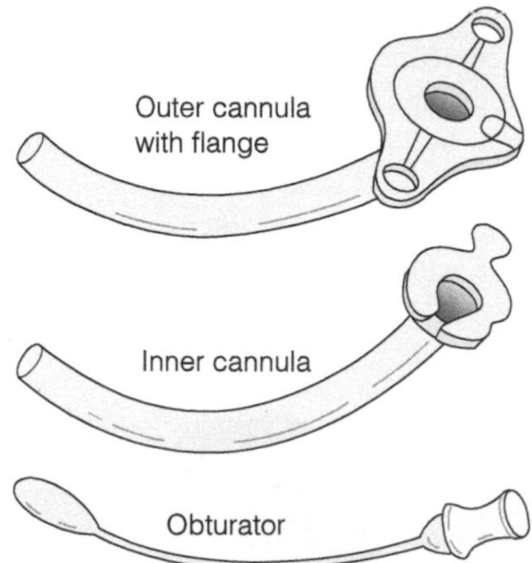

Figure 16-22 Components of a tracheostomy tube.

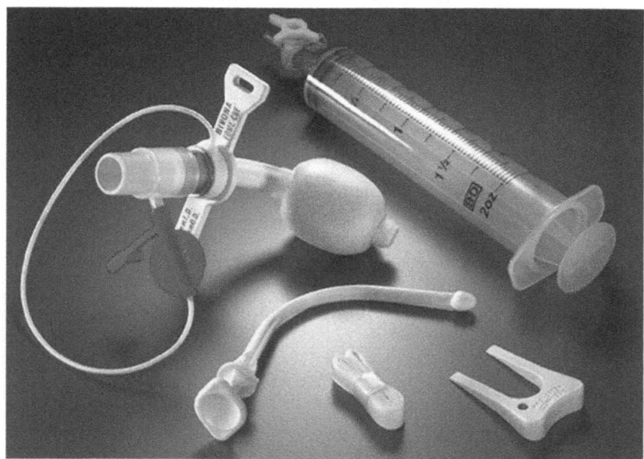

Figure 16-24 A tracheostomy tube with a foam cuff.

allows the tube to be secured in place with tape or ties (see Figure 16-22). All tubes also have an obturator, used to insert the outer cannula and then removed. The obturator is kept at the patient's bedside in case the tube becomes dislodged and needs to be reinserted. Some tracheostomy tubes have an inner cannula that may be removed for periodic cleaning.

Cuffed tracheostomy tubes are surrounded by an inflatable cuff that produces an airtight seal between the tube and the trachea. This seal prevents aspiration of oropharyngeal secretions and air leakage between the tube and the trachea. Cuffed tubes are often used immediately after a tracheostomy and are essential when ventilating a tracheostomy patient with a mechanical **ventilator**. Children do not require cuffed tubes, because their tracheas are resilient enough to seal the air space around the tube.

Low-pressure cuffs (see Figure 16-23) are commonly used to distribute a low, even pressure against the trachea, thus decreasing the risk of tracheal tissue necrosis. They do not need to be deflated periodically to reduce pressure on the tracheal wall. Foam cuffed tracheostomy tubes (see Figure 16-24) do not require injected air; instead, when the port is opened, ambient air enters the balloon, which then conforms to the patient's trachea. Air is removed from the cuff prior to insertion or removal of the tube.

A tracheostomy is normally indicated if the patient is in some respiratory distress. It enables aspiration of tracheobronchial secretions and bypasses upper respiratory tract obstructions. The procedure also aids in weaning patients off ventilator support (Dougherty and Lister, 2008).

The nurse provides tracheostomy care for the patient with a new or recent tracheostomy to maintain patency of the tube and reduce the risk of infection. Initially a tracheostomy may need to be suctioned (see the section on suctioning that follows) and cleaned as often as every one to two hours. After the initial inflammatory response subsides, tracheostomy care may only need to be done once or twice a day, depending on the patient. *Procedure 16-3* describes tracheostomy care.

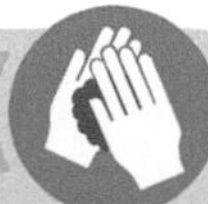

CLINICAL ALERT

'Healthcare professionals and carers who are in contact with tracheostomy patients have to have received training on:
- ***Airway***
- ***Ventilation management of patients with tracheostomy'***

NHS Quality Improvement Scotland (2007) p. 1

When the patient breathes through a tracheostomy, air is no longer filtered and humidified as it is when passing through the upper airways; therefore, special precautions are necessary. Humidity may be provided with a mist collar (see Figure 16-25). Patients with long-term tracheostomies may wear a light scarf or a 4-inch × 4-inch gauze held in place with a cotton tie over the **stoma** to filter air as it enters the tracheostomy.

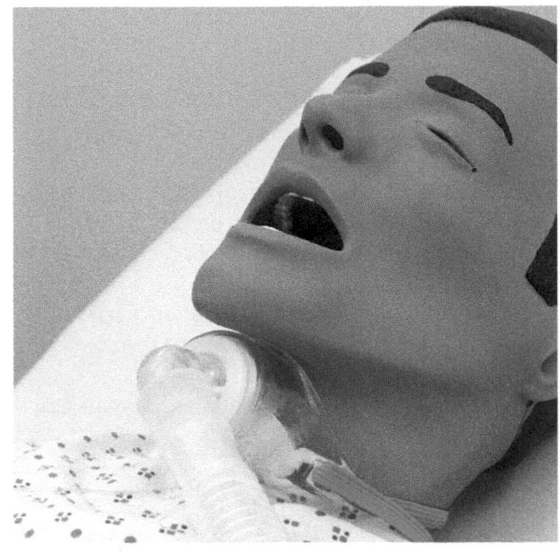

Figure 16-25 A tracheostomy mist collar.

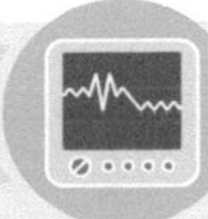

PROCEDURE 16-3 Providing Tracheostomy Care

Purposes

- To maintain airway patency
- To maintain cleanliness and prevent infection at the tracheostomy site to support secretions
- To facilitate healing and prevent skin **excoriation** around the tracheostomy incision
- To promote comfort

Assessment

Determine

- The most appropriate tube for the individual patient
- All patients whenever possible should have a double cannula tracheostomy tube (except for paediatrics or those patients who have a mini tracheostomy)

Assess

- Respiratory status including ease of breathing, rate, rhythm, depth and lung sounds
- Pulse rate
- Character and amount of secretions from tracheostomy site
- Presence of drainage on tracheostomy dressing or ties
- Appearance of incision (note any redness, swelling, purulent discharge or odour)
- Humidifying needs of patient
- Whether the silver tube needs to be changed (recommended every 5–7 days)

Planning

Equipment

- Sterile disposable tracheostomy cleaning kit or supplies including sterile containers, sterile applicators
- Towel or drape to protect bed linens
- Sterile suction catheter kit (suction catheter and sterile container for solution)
- Sterile normal saline
- Warm water
- Sterile gloves (two pairs)
- Clean gloves
- Moisture-proof bag
- Commercially prepared sterile tracheostomy dressing cotton ties
- Clean sterile scissors
- Resuscitation equipment

Implementation

Performance

1 Follow local policy to ensure that you explain to the patient what you are going to do, why it is necessary and how they can cooperate. Obtain consent and maintain patient privacy and dignity and ensure that the appropriate local infection control procedures are observed.

2 Provide for a means of communication, such as eye blinking or raising a finger, to indicate pain or distress.

3 Prepare the patient and the equipment.
- Assist the patient into a position *to promote lung expansion.*
- Open the tracheostomy kit or sterile basins. Pour sterile normal saline into container.
- Establish a sterile field.
- Open other sterile supplies as needed including sterile applicators, suction kit and tracheostomy dressing.

4 Suction the tracheostomy tube.
- Put a clean glove on your non-dominant hand and a sterile glove on your dominant hand (or put on a pair of sterile gloves).
- Suction the full length of the tracheostomy tube to remove secretions and ensure a patent airway (see *Procedure 16-5* on page 485). Suction should only be applied when withdrawing the catheter and should not last for more than 10 seconds.
- Rinse the suction catheter and wrap the catheter around your hand, and peel the glove off so that it turns inside out over the catheter.
- Using the gloved hand, unlock the inner cannula (if present) and remove it by gently pulling it out towards you in line with its curvature. Place the inner cannula in warm water. *This moistens and loosens dried secretions.*
- Remove the soiled tracheostomy dressing. Place the soiled dressing in your gloved hand and peel the glove off so that it turns inside out over the dressing. Discard the glove and the dressing.
- Put on sterile gloves. Keep your dominant hand sterile during the procedure.

5 Clean the inner cannula.
- Remove the inner cannula from the soaking solution.
- Clean the lumen and entire inner cannula thoroughly. Inspect the cannula for cleanliness by holding it at eye level and looking through it into the light.
- Rinse the inner cannula thoroughly in the sterile normal saline.
- After rinsing, gently tap the cannula against the inside edge of the sterile saline container. The inner cannula should be left to air dry as per infection control policy.
- Using sterile technique, suction the outer cannula. *Suctioning removes secretions from the outer cannula.*

6 Replace the inner cannula, securing it in place.
- Insert the inner cannula by grasping the outer **flange** and inserting the cannula in the direction of its curvature.
- Lock the cannula in place by turning the lock (if present) into position to secure the flange of the inner cannula to the outer cannula.

7 Clean the incision site and tube flange with normal saline and apply protective cream around tube flange.
- Observe stoma site for any signs of infection, excoriation, etc.
- Using sterile applicators moistened with normal saline, clean the incision site. Handle the sterile supplies with your dominant hand. Use each applicator only once and then discard. *This avoids contaminating a clean area with a soiled applicator.*

8 Apply a sterile dressing (if necessary).
- Use a commercially prepared tracheostomy dressing only. Cotton lint or gauze fibres can be aspirated by the patient, potentially creating a tracheal abscess.
- Place the dressing under the flange of the tracheostomy tube as shown in Figure 16-26.
- While applying the dressing, ensure that the tracheostomy tube is securely supported. *Excessive movement of the tracheostomy tube irritates the trachea.*

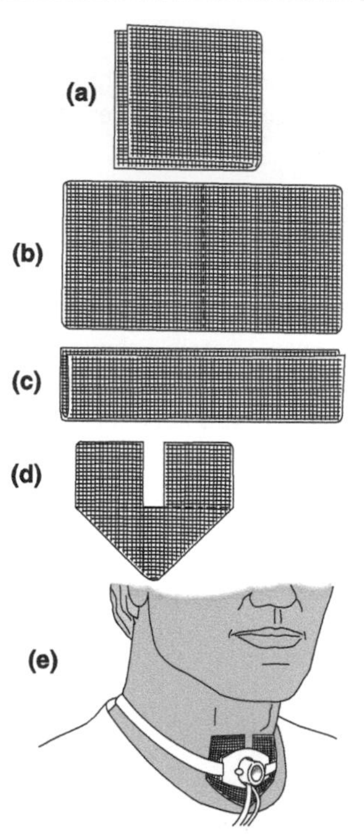

Figure 16-26 (a)-(d) Folding a 4 inch × 4 inch gauze; (e) Placing the tracheostomy dressing wider than the flange of the tracheostomy tube.

9 Change the tracheostomy ties.

Two-strip method

- Cut two unequal strips of twill tape, one approximately 25 cm (10 inch) long and the other about 50 cm (20 inch) long. Cutting one tape longer than the other allows them to be fastened at the side of the neck for easy access and to avoid the pressure of a knot on the skin at the back of the neck.
- Cut a 1 cm (0.5 inch) lengthwise slit approximately 2.5 cm (1 inch) from one end of each strip. To do this, fold the end of the tape back onto itself about 2.5 cm (1 inch), then cut a slit in the middle of the tape from its folded edge.
- Leaving the old ties in place, thread the slit end of one clean tape through the eye of the tracheostomy flange from the bottom side; then thread the long end of the tape through the slit, pulling it tight until it is securely fastened to the flange. *Leaving the old ties in place while securing the clean ties prevents inadvertent dislodging of the tracheostomy tube. Securing tapes in this manner avoids the use of knots, which can come untied or cause pressure and irritation.*
- If old ties are very soiled or it is difficult to thread new ties onto the tracheostomy flange with old ties in place, have an assistant put on a sterile glove and hold the tracheostomy in place while you replace the ties.
- Repeat the process for the second tie.
- Ask the patient to flex the neck. Slip the longer tape under the patient's neck, place one or two finger between the tape and the patient's neck (see Figure 16-27), and tie the tapes together at the side of the neck. *Flexing the neck increases its circumference the way coughing does. Placing two fingers under the ties prevents making the ties too tight, which could interfere with coughing or place pressure on the jugular veins.*

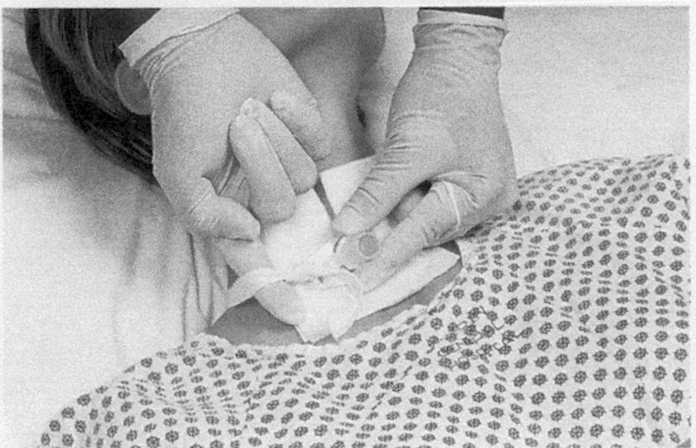

Figure 16-27 Placing a finger underneath the tie tape before tying it.
Source: Elena Dorfmann.

- Tie the ends of the tapes using square knots. Cut off any long ends, leaving approximately 1-2 cm (0.5 inch). *Square knots prevent slippage and loosening. Adequate ends beyond the knot prevent the knot from inadvertently untying.*
- Once the clean ties are secured, remove the soiled ties and discard.

One-strip method

- Cut a length of twill tape 2.5 times the length needed to go around the patient's neck from one tube flange to the other.
- Thread one end of the tape into the slot on one side of the flange.
- Bring both ends of the tape together, take them around the patient's neck, keeping them flat and untwisted.
- Thread the end of the tape next to the patient's neck through the slot from the back to the front.
- Have the patient flex the neck. Tie the loose ends with a square knot at the side of the patient's neck, allowing for slack by placing two fingers under the ties as with the two-strip method. Cut off long ends.

10 Tape and pad the tie knot.

- Place a folded dressing under the tie knot, and apply tape over the knot. *This reduces skin irritation from the knot and prevents confusing the knot with the patient's gown ties.*

11 Check the tightness of the ties.

- Frequently check the tightness of the tracheostomy ties and position of the tracheostomy tube. *Swelling of the neck may cause the ties to become too tight, interfering with coughing and circulation. Ties can loosen in restless patients, allowing the tracheostomy tube to extrude from the stoma.*

12 Document all relevant information.

- Record suctioning, tracheostomy care and the dressing change, noting your assessments.

Variation: using a disposable inner cannula

- Check local policy for frequency of changing inner cannula *because standards vary among clinical areas.*
- Open a new cannula package.
- Using a gloved hand, unlock the current inner cannula (if present) and remove it by gently pulling it out towards you in line with its curvature.
- Check the cannula for amount and type of secretions and discard properly.
- Pick up the new inner cannula touching only the outer locking portion.
- Insert the new inner cannula into the tracheostomy.
- Lock the cannula in place by turning the lock (if present).
- On completion oral hygiene needs of the patient should be met.

Evaluation

- Perform appropriate follow-up such as determining character and amount of secretions, drainage from the tracheostomy, appearance of the tracheostomy incision, pulse rate and respiratory status compared to baseline data, complaints of pain or discomfort at the tracheostomy site.
- Relate findings to previous assessment data if available.
- Report significant deviations from normal to the medical staff.

Suctioning

When patients have difficulty handling their secretions or an airway is in place, suctioning may be necessary to clear air passages. Suctioning is the aspiration of secretions through a catheter connected to a suction machine or wall suction outlet. Even though the upper airways (the oropharynx and nasopharynx) are not sterile, sterile technique is recommended for all suctioning to avoid introducing pathogens into the airways.

Suction catheters may be either open tipped or whistle tipped (see Figure 16-28). The whistle-tipped catheter is less irritating to respiratory tissues, although the open-tipped catheter may be more effective for removing thick mucous plugs. An oral suction tube, or Yankauer device, is used to suction the oral cavity (see Figure 16-29). Most suction catheters have a thumb port on the side to control the suction. The catheter is connected to suction tubing, which in turn is connected to a collection chamber and suction control gauge (see Figure 16-30).

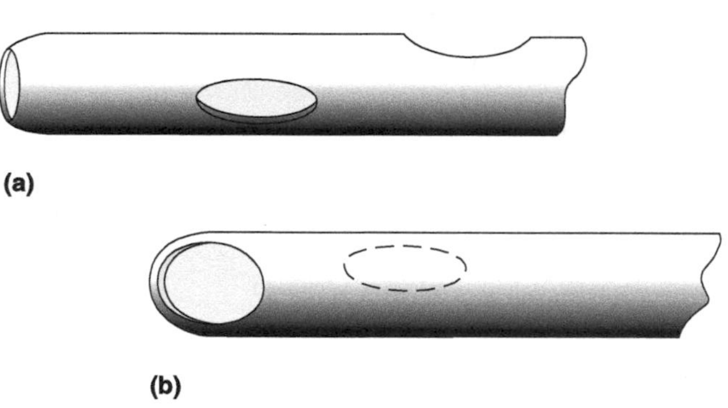

Figure 16-28 Types of suction catheters: (a) open tipped; (b) whistle tipped.

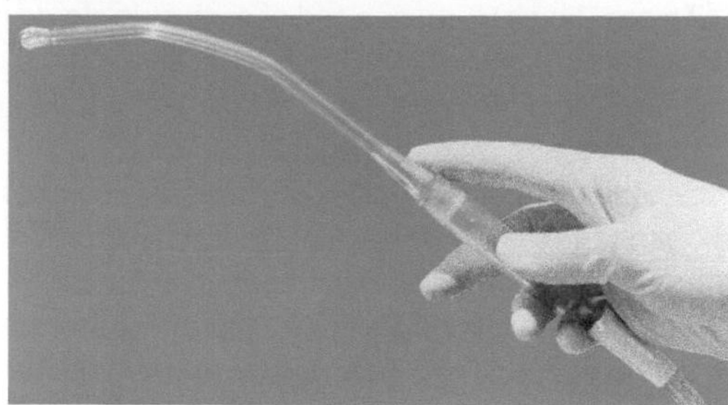

Figure 16-29 Oral (Yankauer) suction tube
Source: Elena Dorfmann.

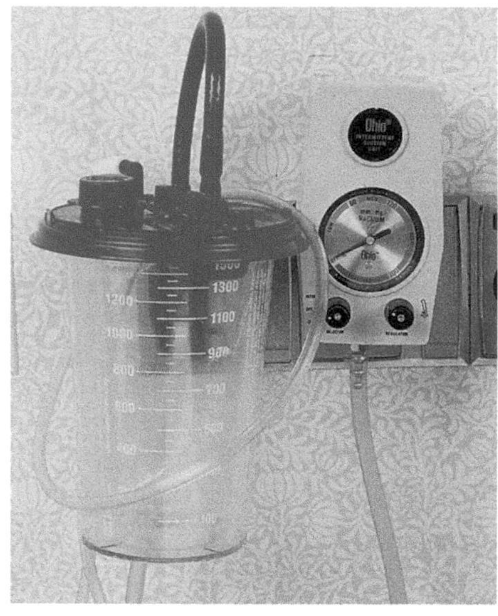

Figure 16-30 A wall suction unit.
Source: Jenny Thomas

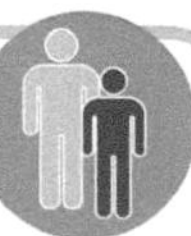

LIFESPAN CONSIDERATIONS

Tracheostomy Care

Infants and Children

- An assistant should *always* be present while tracheostomy care is performed.
- It is good practice to keep a sterile, packaged tracheostomy tube taped to the child's bed so that if the tube dislodges, a new one is available for immediate reintubation.

Mature Adults

- Mature adult skin is more fragile and prone to breakdown. Care of the skin at the tracheostomy stoma is very important.

COMMUNITY CARE CONSIDERATIONS

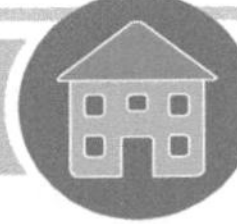

Tracheostomy Care

- Stress the importance of good hand washing technique to the caregiver or patient.
- Tap water may be used for rinsing the inner cannula.
- Teach the caregiver or patient the tracheostomy care procedure and observe a return demonstration.
- Inform the caregiver or patient of the signs and symptoms that may indicate an infection of the stoma site or lower airway.
- Names and telephone numbers of healthcare personnel who can be reached for emergencies or advice must be available to the patient and/or caregiver.

Oropharyngeal or nasopharyngeal suctioning removes secretions from the upper respiratory tract. Endotracheal suctioning is used to remove secretions from the trachea and bronchi. The nurse decides when suctioning is needed by assessing the patient for signs of respiratory distress or evidence that the patient is unable to cough up and expectorate secretions. Dyspnoea, bubbling or rattling breath sounds, poor skin colour (cyanosis), or decreased SaO_2 levels (also called O_2 sats) may indicate the need for suctioning. Good nursing judgement is necessary, because suctioning irritates mucous membranes and can increase secretions if performed too frequently. *Procedure 16-4* outlines oropharyngeal and nasopharyngeal suctioning.

PROCEDURE 16-4 Suctioning Oropharyngeal and Nasopharyngeal Cavities

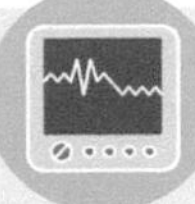

Purposes

- To remove secretions that obstruct the airway
- To facilitate ventilation
- To obtain secretions for diagnostic purposes
- To prevent infection that may result from accumulated secretions

Assessment

Assess

Clinical signs indicating the need for suctioning:

- Restlessness
- Gurgling sounds during respiration
- Adventitious breath sounds when the chest is auscultated
- Change in mental status
- Skin colour
- Rate and pattern of respirations
- Pulse rate and rhythm

Planning

Equipment

- Towel or moisture-resistant pad
- Portable or wall suction machine with tubing and collection receptacle
- Sterile disposable container for fluids
- Sterile normal saline or water
- Sterile gloves
- Goggles or face shield, if appropriate
- Sufficient sterile suction catheter kits (refer to manufacturer's guidelines for appropriate sizes to be used) to complete procedure. If both the oropharynx and the nasopharynx are to be suctioned, one sterile catheter is required for each
- Water-soluble lubricant (for nasopharyngeal suctioning)
- Y-connector
- Sterile gauzes
- Moisture-resistant disposal bag
- Sputum trap, if specimen is to be collected

Implementation

Performance

1 Follow local policy to ensure that you explain to the patient what you are going to do, why it is necessary and how they can cooperate. Obtain consent and maintain patient privacy and dignity and ensure that the appropriate local infection control procedures are observed.

2 Inform the patient that suctioning will relieve breathing difficulty and that the procedure is painless but may be uncomfortable and stimulate the cough, gag or sneeze reflex. *Knowing that the procedure will relieve breathing problems is often reassuring and enlists the patient's cooperation.*

3 Prepare the patient.
- Position a conscious person who has a functional gag reflex in the semi-Fowler's position with the head turned to one side for oral suctioning or with the neck hyperextended for nasal suctioning. *These positions facilitate the insertion of the catheter and help prevent aspiration of secretions.*
- Position an unconscious patient in the lateral position, facing you. *This position allows the tongue to fall forward, so that it will not obstruct the catheter on insertion. The lateral position also facilitates drainage of secretions from the pharynx and prevents the possibility of aspiration.*
- Place the towel or moisture-resistant pad over the pillow or under the chin.

4 Prepare the equipment.
- Set the pressure on the suction gauge in accordance with local policy, and turn on the suction.
- Open the lubricant if performing nasopharyngeal suctioning.
- Open the sterile suction package.

5 Set up container, maintaining asepsis.

6 Pour sterile water or saline into the container.

7 Put on the sterile gloves, or put on a nonsterile glove on the nondominant hand and then a sterile glove on the dominant hand. The sterile gloved hand maintains the sterility of the suction catheter, and the unsterile glove prevents the transmission of the micro-organisms to the nurse.
- With your sterile gloved hand, pick up the catheter and attach it to the suction unit (see Figure 16-31).

8 Make an approximate measure of the depth for the insertion of the catheter and test the equipment.
- Measure the distance between the tip of the patient's nose and the earlobe, or about 13 cm (5 inch) for an adult.
- Mark the position on the tube with the fingers of the sterile gloved hand.
- Test the pressure of the suction and the patency of the catheter by applying your sterile gloved finger or thumb to the port or open branch of the Y-connector (the suction control) to create suction.

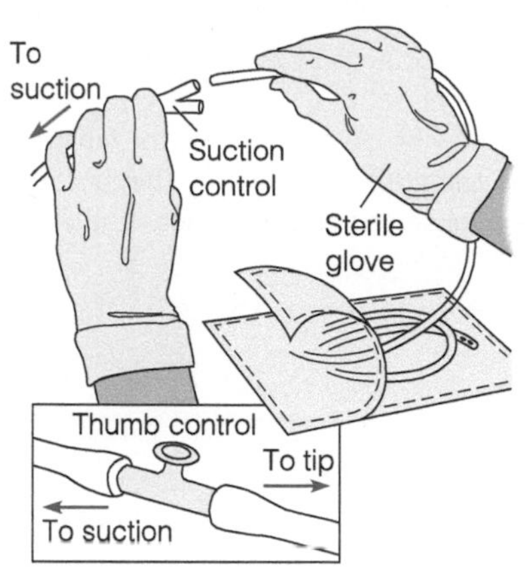

Figure 16-31 Attaching the catheter to the suction unit.

9 Lubricate and introduce the catheter slowly and with care.
- For nasopharyngeal suction, lubricate the catheter tip with sterile water, saline or water-soluble lubricant; for oropharyngeal suction, moisten the tip with sterile water or saline. *This reduces friction and eases insertion.*

For oropharyngeal suction

- Pull the tongue forward, if necessary, using gauze.
- Do not apply suction (that is, leave your finger off the port) during insertion. *Applying suction during insertion causes trauma to the mucous membrane.*
- Advance the catheter about 10–15 cm (4–6 inch) along one side of the mouth into the oropharynx. *Directing the catheter along the side prevents gagging.*

For nasopharyngeal suction

- Without applying suction, insert the catheter the pre-measured or recommended distance into either nostril and advance it along the floor of the nasal cavity. *This avoids the nasal turbinates.*
- Never force the catheter against an obstruction. If one nostril is obstructed, try the other.

10 Perform suctioning.
- Apply your finger to the suction control port to start suction, and gently rotate the catheter. *Gentle rotation of the catheter ensures that all surfaces are reached and prevents trauma to any one area of the respiratory mucosa due to prolonged suction.*
- Apply suction for 5–10 seconds while slowly withdrawing the catheter, then remove your finger from the control and remove the catheter.
- A suction attempt should last only 10 seconds. During this time, the catheter is inserted, the suction applied and discontinued, and the catheter removed.

- It may be necessary during oropharyngeal suctioning to apply suction to secretions that collect in the vestibule of the mouth and beneath the tongue.

11 The catheters should only be used once to reduce the risk of infection.
- Use a clean catheter and repeat the above steps.
- Allow 20- to 30-second intervals between each suction and limit suctioning to five minutes in total. *Applying suction for too long may cause secretions to increase or decrease the patient's oxygen supply.*
- Alternate nares for repeat suctioning.
- Encourage the patient to breathe deeply and to cough between suctions. *Coughing and deep breathing help carry secretions from the trachea and bronchi into the pharynx, where they can be reached with the suction catheter.*

12 Obtain a sputum collection trap (see Figure 16.32).
- Attach the suction catheter to the tubing of the sputum trap.

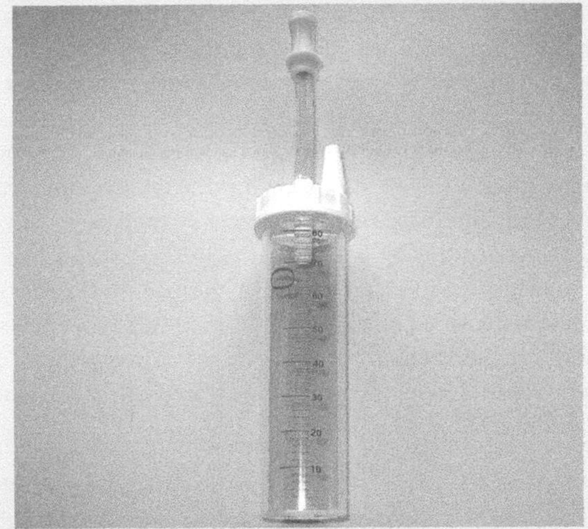

Figure 16-32 A sputum collection trap.
Source: Jenny Thomas.

- Attach the suction tubing to the sputum trap air vent.
- Suction the patient's nasopharynx or oropharynx. The sputum trap will collect the mucus during suctioning.
- Remove the catheter from the patient. Disconnect the sputum trap tubing from the suction catheter. Remove the suction tubing from the trap air vent.
- Connect the tubing of the sputum trap to the air vent. *This retains any micro-organisms in the sputum trap.*
- Connect the suction catheter to the tubing.
- Flush the catheter to remove secretions from the tubing.

13 Promote patient comfort.
- Offer to assist the patient with oral or nasal hygiene.
- Assist the patient to a position that facilitates breathing.

14 Dispose of equipment and ensure availability for the next suction.
- Dispose of the catheter, gloves, water and waste container. Wrap the catheter around your sterile gloved hand and hold the catheter as the glove is removed over it for disposal.
- Rinse the suction tubing as needed by inserting the end of the tubing into the used water container. Empty and rinse the suction collection container as needed or indicated by protocol. Change the suction tubing and container daily.
- Ensure that supplies are available for the next suctioning (suction kit, gloves, water or normal saline).

15 Assess the effectiveness of suctioning.
- Observe skin colour, dyspnoea and level of anxiety.

16 Document relevant data.
- Record the procedure: the amount, consistency, colour and odour of sputum (e.g. foamy, white mucus; thick, green-tinged mucus; or blood-flecked mucus) and the patient's breathing status before and after the procedure.
- If the procedure is carried out frequently (e.g. every hour), it may be appropriate to record only once, at the end of the shift; however, the frequency of the suctioning must be recorded.

Evaluation

- Conduct appropriate follow-up, such as appearance of secretions suctioned; breath sounds; respiratory rate, rhythm and depth; pulse rate and rhythm; and skin colour.
- Compare findings to previous assessment data if available.
- Report significant deviations from normal to the medical staff.

Following **endotracheal intubation** or a tracheostomy, the trachea and surrounding respiratory tissues are irritated and react by producing excessive secretions. Suctioning is necessary to remove these secretions and maintain a patent airway. The frequency of suctioning depends on the patient's health and how recently the intubation was done.

Suctioning is associated with several complications: hypoxemia, trauma to the airway, nosocomial infection and cardiac dysrhythmia, which is related to the hypoxemia. The following techniques are used to minimise or decrease these complications:

- **Hyperinflation**. This involves giving the patient breaths that are 1–1.5 times the tidal volume set on the ventilator through the ventilator circuit or via a manual resuscitation bag valve mask device. Three to five breaths are delivered before and after each pass of the suction catheter.

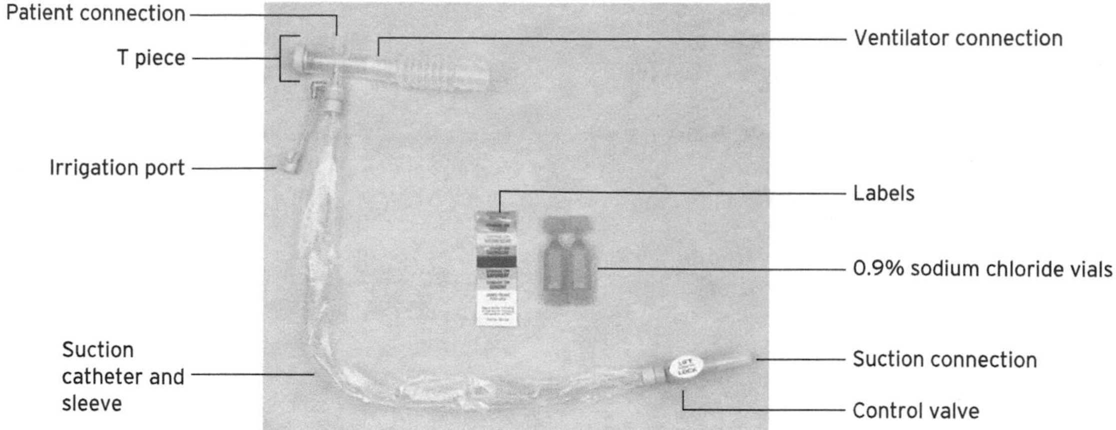

Figure 16-33 A closed airway suction (in-line) system.
Source: Jenny Thomas

- **Hyperoxygenation.** This can be done with a manual resuscitation bag valve mask device or through the ventilator and is performed by increasing the oxygen flow (usually to 100%) before suctioning and between suction attempts.

For tracheostomy and endotracheal suctioning, the diameter of the suction catheter should be about half the inside diameter of the tracheostomy or endotracheal tube so that hypoxia can be prevented. The nurse uses sterile techniques to prevent infection of the respiratory tract (see *Procedure 16-5*). The traditional method of suctioning an endotracheal tube or tracheostomy is sometimes referred to as the *open method.* If a patient is connected to a ventilator, the nurse disconnects the patient from the ventilator, suctions the airway, reconnects the patient to the ventilator, and discards the suction catheter. Drawbacks to the open airway suction system include the nurse needing to wear personal protective equipment (e.g. goggles or face shield, gown) to avoid exposure to the patient's sputum and the potential cost of one-time catheter use, especially if the patient requires frequent suctioning.

With the alternative *closed airway/tracheal suction system (in-line suctioning)* (see Figure 16-33), the suction catheter attaches to the ventilator tubing and the patient does not need to be disconnected from the ventilator. The nurse is not exposed to any secretions because the suction catheter is enclosed in a plastic sheath. The catheter can be reused as many times as necessary until the system is changed. Manufacturers recommend changing closed suction catheter systems on a daily basis. Studies carried out by Rabitsch *et al.* (2004) stated that there was a reduction in infections with the use of closed airway/tracheal systems; however, studies carried out by Siempos *et al.* (2008) concluded that there is no evidence to suggest that closed systems reduce the risk of infection in ventilator-associated pneumonia.

LIFESPAN CONSIDERATIONS

Suctioning

Infants

- A bulb syringe may be used to remove secretions from an infant's nose or mouth. Care needs to be taken to avoid stimulating the gag reflex.

Children

- A catheter is used to remove secretions from an older child's mouth or nose.

COMMUNITY CARE CONSIDERATIONS

Suctioning

- Teach patients and families that the most important aspect of infection control is frequent hand washing.
- The catheter or Yankauer should be flushed by suctioning recently boiled or distilled water to rinse away mucus, followed by the suctioning of air through the device to dry the internal surface and, thus, discourage bacterial growth.

PROCEDURE 16-5 Suctioning a Tracheostomy or Endotracheal Tube

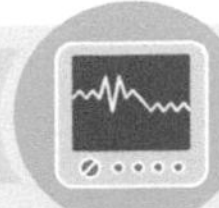

Purposes

- To maintain a patent airway and prevent airway obstructions
- To promote respiratory function (optimal exchange of oxygen and carbon dioxide into and out of the lungs)
- To prevent pneumonia that may result from accumulated secretions

Assessment

Assess the patient for the presence of congestion of the thorax. Note the patient's ability or inability to remove the secretions through coughing.

Planning

Equipment

- Resuscitation bag (bag valve mask device) connected to 100% oxygen
- Sterile towel (optional)
- Equipment for suctioning (see *Procedure 16-4* on page 481)
- Goggles and mask if necessary
- Gown (if necessary)
- Sterile gloves
- Moisture-resistant bag

Implementation

Preparation

Determine if the patient has been suctioned previously and, if so, review the documentation of the procedure. This information can be very helpful in preparing the nurse for both the physiological and psychological impact of suctioning on the patient.

Performance

1 Follow local policy to ensure that you explain to the patient what you are going to do, why it is necessary and how they can cooperate. Obtain consent and maintain patient privacy and dignity and ensure that the appropriate local infection control procedures are observed.

2 Inform the patient that suctioning usually causes some intermittent coughing and that this assists in removing the secretions.

3 Prepare the patient.
   - If not contraindicated because of health, place the patient in the semi-Fowler's position to promote deep breathing, maximum lung expansion and productive coughing. *Deep breathing oxygenates the lungs, counteracts the hypoxic effects of suctioning, and may induce coughing. Coughing helps to loosen and move secretions.*
   - If necessary, provide analgesia before suctioning. Endotracheal suctioning stimulates the cough reflex, which can cause pain for patients who have had thoracic or abdominal surgery or who have experienced traumatic injury. *Pre-medication can increase the patient's comfort during the suctioning procedure.*

4 Prepare the equipment.
   - Attach the resuscitation apparatus to the oxygen source (see Figure 16-34). Adjust the oxygen flow to 100% flush.

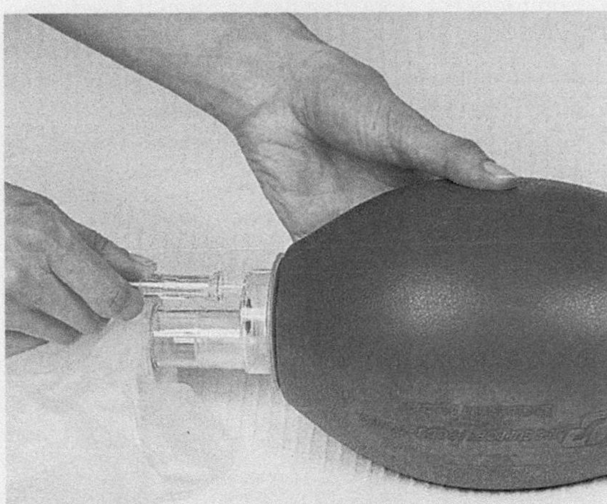

Figure 16-34 Attaching the resuscitation apparatus to the oxygen source.
Source: Jenny Thomas.

   - Open the sterile supplies in readiness for use.
   - Place the sterile towel, if used, across the patient's chest below the tracheostomy.
   - Turn on the suction, and set the pressure in accordance with local policy.

- Put on goggles, mask and gown if necessary.
- Put on sterile gloves. Some clinical policies recommend putting a sterile glove on the dominant hand and an unsterile glove on the nondominant hand to protect the nurse.
- Holding the catheter in the dominant hand and the connector in the nondominant hand, attach the suction catheter to the suction tubing (see Figure 16-29 on page 480).
- Flush and lubricate the catheter.
- Using the dominant hand, place the catheter tip in the sterile saline solution.
- Using the thumb of the nondominant hand, occlude the thumb control and suction a small amount of the sterile solution through the catheter. *This determines that the suction equipment is working properly and lubricates the outside and the lumen of the catheter. Lubrication eases insertion and reduces tissue trauma during insertion. Lubricating the lumen also helps prevent secretions from sticking to the inside of the catheter.*

5 If the patient does not have copious secretions, hyperventilate the lungs with a resuscitation bag before suctioning.

- Summon an assistant, if one is available, for this step.
- Using your nondominant hand, turn on the oxygen to 12-15 L/min.
- If the patient is receiving oxygen, disconnect the oxygen source from the tracheostomy tube using your nondominant hand.
- Attach the resuscitator to the tracheostomy or endotracheal tube (see Figure 16-35).
- Compress the ambu bag device three to five times, as the patient inhales. This is best done by a second person who can use both hands to compress the bag, thus, providing a greater inflation volume.
- Observe the rise and fall of the patient's chest to assess the adequacy of each ventilation.
- Remove the resuscitation device and place it on the bed or the patient's chest with the connector facing up.

Variation - using a ventilator to provide hyperventilation

If the patient is on a ventilator, use the ventilator for hyperventilation and hyperoxygenation. Newer models have a mode that provides 100% oxygen for two minutes and then switches back to the previous oxygen setting as well as a manual breath or sigh button. *The use of ventilator settings provides more consistent delivery of oxygenation and hyperinflation than a resuscitation device.*

6 If the patient has copious secretions, do not hyperventilate with a resuscitator. *Instead*:

- Keep the regular oxygen delivery device on and increase the litre flow or adjust the FiO_2 to 100% for several breaths before suctioning. *Hyperventilating a patient who has copious secretions can force the secretions deeper into the respiratory tract.*

7 Quickly but gently insert the catheter *without* applying any suction.

- With your nondominant thumb off the suction port, quickly but gently insert the catheter into the trachea through the tracheostomy tube (see Figure 16-36). *To prevent tissue trauma and oxygen loss, suction is not applied during insertion of the catheter.*
- Insert the catheter about 12.5 cm for adults, less for children, or until the patient coughs or you feel resistance. *Resistance usually means that the catheter tip has reached the bifurcation of the trachea.* To prevent damaging the mucous membranes at the bifurcation, withdraw the catheter about 1-2 cm (0.4-0.8 inch) before applying suction.

8 Perform suctioning.

- Apply intermittent suction for 5-10 seconds by placing the nondominant thumb over the thumb port. *Suction time is restricted to 10 seconds or less to minimise oxygen loss.*
- Rotate the catheter by rolling it between your thumb and forefinger while slowly withdrawing it. *This prevents tissue trauma by minimising the suction time against any part of the trachea.*

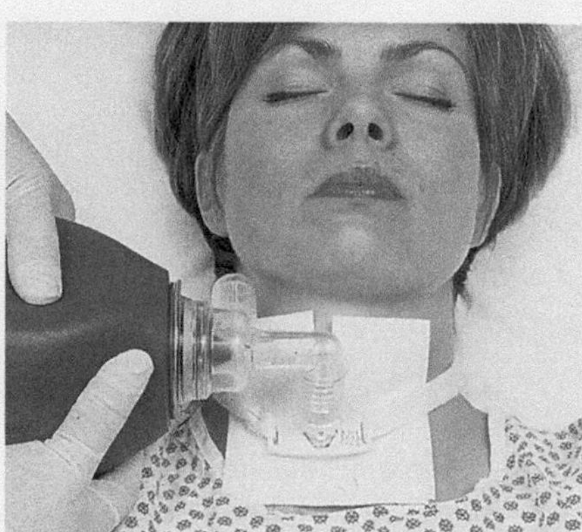

Figure 16-35 Attaching the resuscitator to the tracheostomy.
Source: Jenny Thomas.

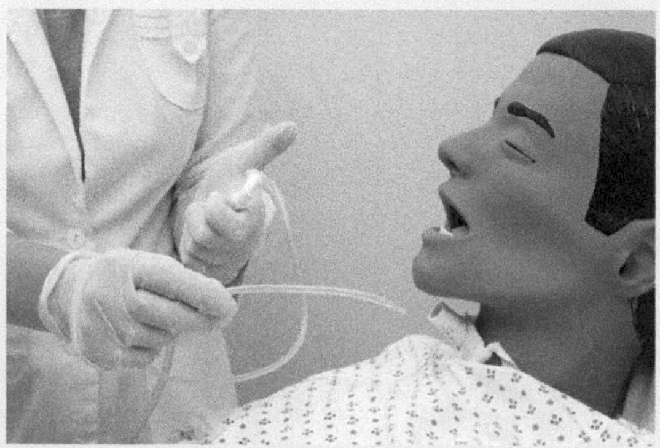

Figure 16-36 Inserting the catheter into the trachea through the tracheostomy tube. *Note*: Suction is not applied while inserting the catheter.
Source: Jenny Thomas.

- Withdraw the catheter completely, and release the suction.
- Hyperventilate the patient.
- Then suction again.

9 Reassess the patient's oxygenation status and repeat suctioning.
- Observe the patient's respirations and skin colour. Check the patient's pulse if necessary, using your nondominant hand.
- Encourage the patient to breathe deeply and to cough between suctions.
- Allow 2-3 minutes between suctions when possible. This provides an opportunity for reoxygenation of the lungs.
- Flush the catheter and repeat suctioning until the air passage is clear and the breathing is relatively effortless and quiet.
- After each suction, pick up the resuscitation bag with your nondominant hand and ventilate the patient with no more than three breaths.

10 Dispose of equipment and ensure availability for the next suction.
- Flush the catheter and suction tubing.
- Turn off the suction and disconnect the catheter from the suction tubing.
- Wrap the catheter around your sterile hand and peel the glove off so that it turns inside out over the catheter.
- Discard the glove and the catheter in the moisture-resistant bag.
- Replenish the sterile fluid and supplies so that the suction is ready for use again. *Patients who require suctioning often require it quickly, so it is essential to leave the equipment at the bedside ready for use.*

11 Provide for patient comfort and safety.
- Assist the patient to a comfortable, safe position that aids breathing. If the person is conscious, a semi-Fowler's position is frequently indicated. If the person is unconscious, Sims' position aids in the drainage of secretions from the mouth.

12 Document relevant data.
- Record the suctioning, including the amount and description of suction returns and any other relevant assessments.

Evaluation

- Perform a follow-up assessment of the patient to determine the effectiveness of the suctioning (e.g. respiratory rate, depth and character; breath sounds; colour of skin and nail beds; character and amount of secretions suctioned; changes in vital signs).
- Relate findings to previous assessment data if available.
- Report significant deviations from normal to the medical staff.

CLINICAL ALERT

If secretions are stubborn then a saline nebuliser (0.9%) should be used 2 hourly (if prescribed).

LIFESPAN CONSIDERATIONS

Suctioning a Tracheostomy or Endotracheal Tube

Infants and Children

- Have an assistant gently support the child to keep the child's hands out of the way. The assistant will need to keep the child's head in the midline position (Bindler and Ball, 2008).

Older Adults

- Older adults often have cardiac and/or pulmonary disease, thus increasing their susceptibility to hypoxemia related to suctioning. Watch closely for signs of hypoxemia. If noted, stop suctioning and hyperoxygenate.
- Do a thorough lung assessment before and after suctioning to determine effectiveness of suctioning and to be aware of any special problems.

COMMUNITY CARE CONSIDERATIONS

Suctioning a Tracheostomy or Endotracheal Tube

- Whenever possible, the patient should be encouraged to clear the airway by coughing.
- Patients may need to learn to suction their secretions if they cannot cough effectively.
- Clean gloves should be used when endotracheal suctioning is performed in the home environment.
- The nurse needs to instruct the caregiver on how to determine the need for suctioning and the correct process of suctioning to avoid potential complications of suctioning.
- Stress the importance of adequate hydration as it thins secretions, which can aid in the removal of secretions by coughing or suctioning.

Chest Tubes and Drainage Systems

If the thin, double-layered pleural membrane is disrupted by lung disease, surgery or trauma, the negative pressure between the pleural layers may be lost. The lung then collapses because it is no longer drawn outward as the diaphragm and intercostal muscles contract during inhalation. When air collects in the pleural space, it is known as a **pneumothorax**. Blood or fluid in the pleural space, a **haemothorax**, places pressure on lung tissue and interferes with lung expansion. Chest tubes may be inserted into the pleural cavity to restore negative pressure and drain collected fluid or blood. Because air rises, chest tubes for pneumothorax are often placed in the upper anterior thorax, whereas chest tubes used to drain fluid generally are placed in the lower lateral chest wall.

When chest tubes are inserted, they must be connected to a sealed drainage system or a one-way valve that allows air and fluid to be removed from the chest cavity but prevents air from entering from the outside. Sterile disposable drainage systems are used to prevent outside air from entering the chest tube. These systems typically have a closed collection chamber for drainage that is connected to a wet or dry seal chamber (see Figure 16-37). With the water-seal system, when the patient inhales, the water prevents air from entering the system from the atmosphere. During exhalation, however, air can exit the chest cavity, bubbling up through the water. Suction can be added to the system to facilitate removing air and secretions from the chest cavity. The drainage system should always be kept below the level of the patient's chest to prevent fluid and drainage from being drawn back into the chest cavity.

A Heimlich valve or comparable system may be used for mobile patients who have a pneumothorax. These valves allow air to escape from the chest cavity, but they close during inhalation to prevent air from entering.

Chest tube insertion and removal require sterile technique and must be done without introducing air or micro-organisms into the pleural cavity.

Nursing responsibilities regarding drainage systems include the following:

- Monitor and maintain the patency and integrity of the drainage system.
- Assess the patient's vital signs, oxygen saturation, cardiovascular status and respiratory status.
- Keep chest tube clamps and a sterile occlusive dressing near the patient. If the tube becomes disconnected from the

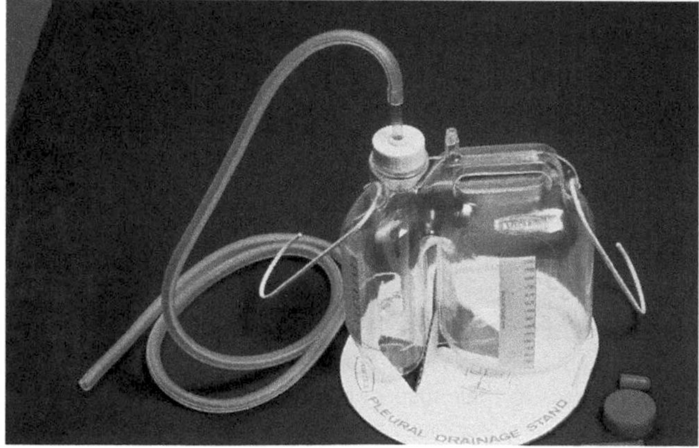

(a)

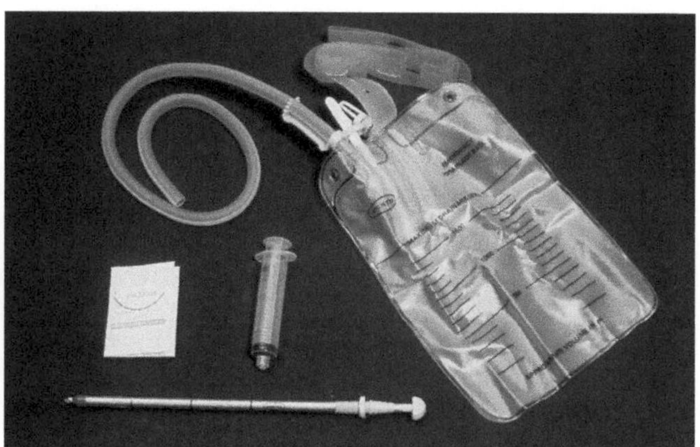

(b)

Figure 16-37 Chest drainage systems.
Source: Wellcome Images, Wellcome Library, London.

collecting system, submerge the end in 5cm of sterile saline or water *to maintain the seal.* If the chest tube is inadvertently pulled out, the wound should be immediately covered with a dry sterile dressing. If you can hear air leaking out of the site, ensure that the dressing is not occlusive. *If the air cannot escape, this would lead to pneumothorax.*

- Use standard precautions and personal protective equipment while manipulating the system and assisting with insertion or removal.
- Observe the dressing site at least every four hours. Inspect the dressing for excessive and abnormal drainage, such as bleeding or foul-smelling discharge. Palpate around the dressing site, and listen for a crackling sound indicative of subcutaneous emphysema. *Subcutaneous emphysema can result from a poor seal at the chest tube insertion site.*
- Determine level of discomfort with and without activity and administer analgesia as required.
- Encourage deep breathing and coughing exercises every two hours (this may be contraindicated in patients who have had a lung removed). Have the patient sit upright to perform the exercises, and splint the chest around the tube insertion site with a pillow or with a hand to minimise discomfort.
- Reposition the patient every two hours. When the patient is lying on the affected side, place rolled towels beside the tubing. Frequent position changes promote drainage, prevent complications and provide comfort. Rolled towels prevent occlusion of the chest tube by the patient's weight.
- Assist the patient with range-of-motion exercises of the affected shoulder three times per day to maintain joint mobility.
- When moving and mobilising the patient:
  - Attach chest drain forceps to the patient's gown/clothing for emergency use.
  - Keep the water-seal unit below chest level and upright.
  - Disconnect the drainage system from the suction apparatus before moving the patient and make sure the air vent is open.

Removal of a chest tube is a brief but quite painful procedure. Administer analgesia before the removal. Remove the dressing around the tube and prepare the dressing that will cover the insertion site. This will be an occlusive dressing if there is no purse-string suture around the insertion site to prevent air from entering the chest. Generally, the medical staff perform the removal but, in some areas, specially trained nurses may be permitted to do so.

EVALUATING

Using the goals and desired outcomes identified in the planning stage of the nursing process, the nurse collects data to evaluate the effectiveness of interventions. If outcomes are not achieved, the nurse and patient need to explore the reasons before modifying the care plan.

CRITICAL REFLECTION

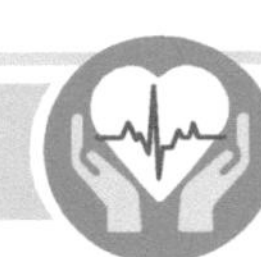

Looking back at the Case Study on page 453, the information provided in this and previous chapters should enable you to apply an appropriate nursing theory or model in order to help you identify the key issues and develop a plan of care that is holistic and individualised for Leslie. Key activities that you may wish to consider are communication, maintaining a safe environment, breathing and discharge planning. By applying the theory to the practice it is important that you provide a rationale for your decisions which will develop your professional understanding of care at the point of delivery. Points to consider:

- Managing and organising care
- Model of nursing - Roper, Logan and Tierney, Orem
- Identify 'problems'
- Follow the nursing process for each problem
- Rationale for making each judgement and decision
- Predisposing factors
- Change of breathing patterns
- Good communication to patient, relatives, multidisciplinary team and providing dignity and respect to the patient
- Change to cognitive thinking and behaviour - health promotion
- Safe practice both in hospital and in the community
- Lifestyle changes and considerations
- Discharge planning

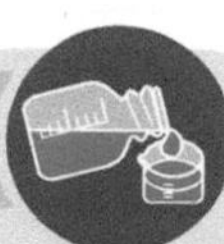

CHAPTER HIGHLIGHTS

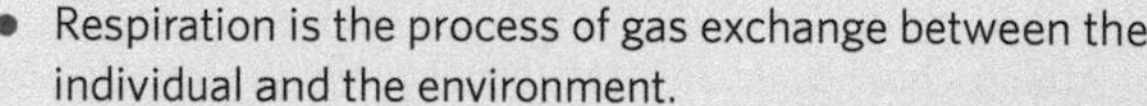

- Respiration is the process of gas exchange between the individual and the environment.
- The respiratory system contributes to effective respiration through pulmonary ventilation (the movement of air between the atmosphere and the lungs) and the diffusion of oxygen and carbon dioxide across the pulmonary membrane.
- Alveoli and the capillaries that surround them form the respiratory membrane, where gas exchange between the lungs and the blood occurs.
- Effective pulmonary ventilation, or breathing, requires clear airways, an intact central nervous system and respiratory centre, an intact thoracic cavity and musculature, and adequate pulmonary compliance (stretch) and recoil.
- Gas exchange occurs by diffusion, as gas molecules move from an area of higher concentration to an area of lower concentration. At the respiratory membrane, oxygen moves from the alveolus into the blood, while carbon dioxide moves from the blood into the alveolus.
- Respiratory rates are normally highest in neonates and infants, gradually slowing to adult ranges.
- Ageing affects the respiratory system: the chest wall becomes more rigid and lungs less elastic.
- Other factors affecting oxygenation include the environment, lifestyle, health status, narcotic analgesics, and stress and coping.
- Hypoxia, insufficient oxygen in the tissues, can result from impaired ventilation (hypoventilation) or diffusion, or from impaired oxygen transportation to the tissues because of anaemia or decreased cardiac output.
- Airway obstruction interferes with ventilation. A low-pitched snoring sound, stridor and abnormal breath sounds may accompany partial airway obstruction. Extreme inspiratory effort with no chest movement indicates complete upper airway obstruction.
- The patient history includes questions about current or past respiratory problems and about lifestyle, presence of symptoms such as cough or shortness of breath, smoking and other risk factors, and medications.
- Nursing interventions to promote oxygenation include promoting healthy breathing and a healthy heart, deep breathing and coughing, and hydration; administering medications; implementing measures to clear secretions (e.g. incentive spirometry, percussion, vibration and postural drainage); initiating and monitoring oxygen therapy; initiating or assisting with procedures to maintain the airway (e.g. artificial airways and suctioning); providing tracheostomy care; and monitoring chest drainage systems.
- The effectiveness of nursing interventions is evaluated by using the goals and desired outcomes identified in the planning stage of the nursing process. If a goal is not met, the nurse asks pertinent questions to assess the reason for not meeting the goal.

ACTIVITY ANSWER

ACTIVITY 16-1 Status asthmaticus is an acute emergency situation and should be treated as a life-threatening illness. The points for consideration are as follows:

- Breathing
- Maintaining a safe environment
- Oxygen therapy
- Delivery
- Position of patient
- Diagnostic tests
- Safety issues with regard to oxygen therapy
- Communication
- Documentation
- Providing the rationale for your clinical decisions and explaining how they enhance the well-being of the patient

REFERENCES

Agostini, P., Calvert, R., Subramanian, H. and Naidu, B. (2008) 'Best evidence topic – thoracic general. Is incentive spirometry effective following thoracic surgery?' *CardioVascular Thoracic Surgery*, 7, 297–300.

Bennett, C. (2003) 'Nursing the breathless patient', *Nursing Standard*, 8 January, 45–51.

Bindler, R.C. and Ball, J.W. (2008) *Clinical skills manual for pediatric nursing: Caring for children* (4th edn), Upper Saddle River, NJ: Prentice Hall Health.

D'Amato, G., Liccardi, G., d'Amato, M. and Cazzola, M. (2001) 'The role of outdoor pollution and climatic changes on the rising trends in respiratory allergy', *Respiratory Medicine*, 95(7), 606–611.

Dougherty, L. and Lister, S. (2008) *The Royal Marsden Hospital manual of clinical nursing procedures* (7th edn), Oxford: Wiley-Blackwell.

Hewitt, P. (2006) 'Date announced for smoking ban in England', available at http://www.direct.gov.uk/en/Nl1/Newsroom/DG_064817 (accessed April 2011).

NHS Quality Improvement Scotland (2007) *Caring for a patient with a tracheostomy*, NHS Quality Improvement Scotland.

Rabitsch, W., Koestler, W., Fiebiger, W., Dileacher, C., Losert, H., Sherif, C., Staudinger, T., Seper, E., Koller, W., Daxböck, F., Schuster, E., Knöbl, P., Bummann, H. and Frass, M. (2004) 'Closed suctioning system reduces cross-contamination between bronchial system and gastric juices', *Anesthesia and Analgesia*, 99(3), 886–892.

Siempos, I., Vardakas, K. and Falagas, M. (2008) 'Closed tracheal suction systems for prevention of ventilator-associated pneumonia', *British Journal of Anaesthesia*, 100(3), 299–306.

Timby, B. (1989) *Clinical nursing procedure*, Philadelphia, PA: Lippincott.

CHAPTER 17

HYGIENE

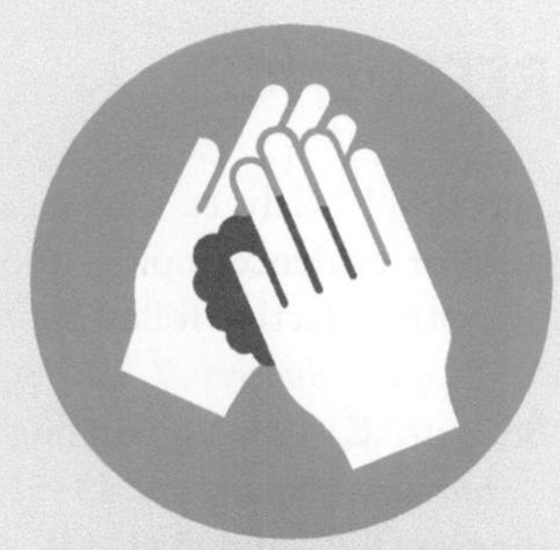

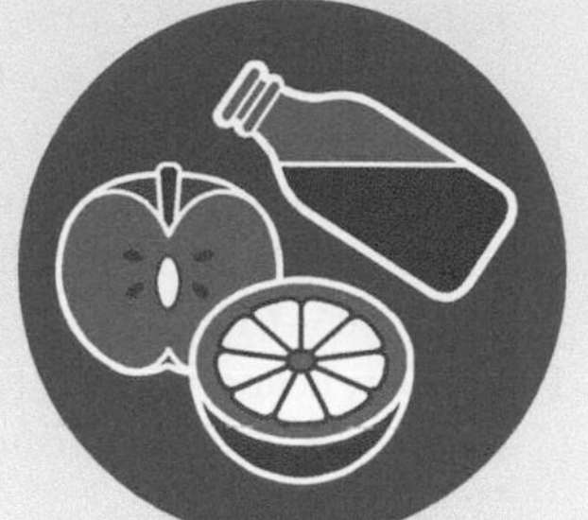

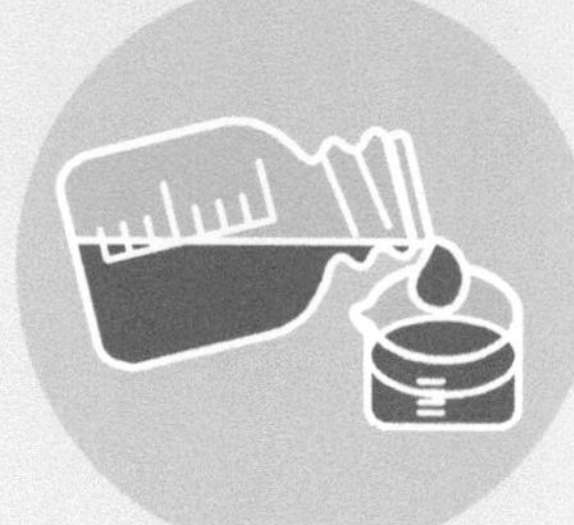

LEARNING OUTCOMES

After completing this chapter, you will be able to:

- Describe hygienic care that nurses provide to patients.
- Identify factors influencing personal hygiene.
- Identify normal and abnormal assessment findings while providing hygiene care.
- Apply the nursing process to common problems related to hygienic care of the skin, feet, nails, mouth, hair, eyes, ears and nose.
- Identify the purposes of bathing.
- Explain specific ways in which nurses help hospitalised patients with hygiene.
- Describe steps for identified hygienic-care procedures.
- Identify steps in removing contact lenses and inserting and removing artificial eyes.
- Describe steps for removing, cleaning and inserting hearing aids.
- Identify safety and comfort measures underlying bed-making procedures.

After reading this chapter you will be able to apply common hygiene techniques to patient care. The chapter relates to **Essential Skills Clusters (NMC, 2010)** 1, 2, 3, 4, 5, 6, 7, 8, 9, 10, as appropriate for each section.

Ensure that you really understand this chapter by logging on to your complimentary **MyNursingKit** at **www.pearsoned.co.uk/kozier**. Complete the self-assessment tests to check your progress and utilise further activities to practise and confirm your understanding.

CASE STUDY

Joseph is an 18-year-old boy who was looking forward to starting university in the Autumn. He is aware that he has been conditionally accepted onto the Sports Science degree, at a university 100 miles away from home.

Joseph is the eldest of three children and is the first member of the family to study at this level. His family are very proud and supportive of him.

Joseph has in the last week confirmed his place on the degree programme and to congratulate him his parents paid for a weekend away where he could enjoy some sporting activities with his friends. Joseph enjoys all types of sport and has played rugby and cricket at county and country level.

Unfortunately, while Joseph was away he was involved in a serious accident with fractures to his C4 and C5. While there is some movement to his limbs, i.e. his fingers and legs, at this point there is very little movement from the waist down. Joseph is used to being totally independent and feels that the future looks very bleak for him. His family are devastated and feel partially responsible and guilty for his injuries as they paid for the holiday.

On reading this chapter, reflect back using an appropriate model, and utilise the nursing process to aid in the collaboration of working out a plan of care for Joseph that meets his personal hygiene needs.

INTRODUCTION

The term 'hygiene' is derived from Hygeia the Greek goddess of health, cleanliness and sanitation. Hygiene is the science of health and its maintenance, and is a level of cleanliness that maintains health and healthy living. The concept of hygiene relates to medicine and both personal and professional practices.

Personal hygiene is the self-care by which people attend to such functions as bathing, toileting, general body hygiene and grooming. According to the Department of Health (2001) 'personal hygiene is the physical act of the cleaning of the body to ensure that the skin, hair and nails are maintained in an optimum condition', and can also include the teeth, oral and nasal cavities, eyes, ears and perineal-genital areas. Personal hygiene is a highly personal matter determined by individual values and practices.

Supporting patients when providing personal hygiene is a very intimate aspect of the nurse's role and needs excellent communication and interpersonal skills in order to maintain patient's dignity and respect during such interventions. Prior to providing any support it is important to assess the patient in relation to culture, religion, preferences and ability in order to gain informed consent, and provide the appropriate care. Patients may require help to wash and change or after urinating or defecating, after vomiting, and whenever they become soiled, for example, from wound drainage or from profuse perspiration. Table 17-1 lists factors that influence hygiene practices.

Table 17-1 Factors Influencing Individual Hygienic Practices

Factor	Variables
Culture	Many people bath or shower once or twice a day, whereas people from some cultures will bathe once a week only. Some cultures consider privacy essential for bathing, whereas others practise communal bathing. Body odour is offensive in some cultures and accepted as normal in others.
Religion	Ceremonial washings are practised by some religions.
Environment	Finances may affect the availability of facilities for bathing. For example, homeless people may not have warm water available; soap, shampoo, shaving equipment and deodorants may be too expensive for people who have limited resources.
Developmental level	Children learn hygiene in the home. Practices vary according to the individual's age; for example, pre-schoolers can carry out most tasks independently with encouragement.
Health and energy	Ill people may not have the motivation or energy to attend to hygiene. Some patients who have neuromuscular impairments/illness may be unable to perform hygienic care.
Personal preferences	Some people prefer a shower to a bath. People share different beliefs about regulating number of baths, etc.

HYGIENIC CARE

Traditionally, personal hygiene care has been provided to patients as they awaken in the morning or after breakfast. However, consideration is now given to patient choice, rest periods and the condition (wellness) of the patient. Early morning washing may not be the preferred choice for the patient, and personal hygiene care should be provided as and when required.

A patient who requires assistance would have their elimination needs provided for, an assisted wash, bath or shower, perineal care, skin pressure areas checked, oral, nail and hair care. Making the patient's bed is part of this care. Personal hygiene and care of the patient's hygiene needs are an ongoing process which should be continually assessed throughout the day and night. Support and care should be offered as necessary. There are a number of aetiologies underlying self-care deficits:

- decreased or lack of motivation;
- weakness or tiredness;
- pain or discomfort;
- perceptual or cognitive impairment;
- inability to perceive body part or **spatial relationship**;
- neuromuscular or musculoskeletal impairment;
- medically imposed restriction;
- therapeutic procedure restraining mobility (e.g. intravenous infusion, cast);
- severe anxiety;
- environmental barriers.

SKIN

The skin is the largest organ of the body. The skin is made up of two layers; the epidermis and the dermis (see Chapter 18). It serves five major functions:

1 It protects underlying tissues from injury by preventing the passage of micro-organisms. The skin and mucous membranes are considered the body's first line of defence.
2 It regulates the body temperature. Cooling of the body occurs through the heat loss processes of evaporation of perspiration, and by radiation and conduction of heat from the body when the blood vessels of the skin are vasodilated. Body heat is conserved through lack of perspiration and vasoconstriction of the blood vessels.
3 It secretes **sebum**, an oily substance that (a) softens and lubricates the hair and skin, (b) prevents the hair from becoming brittle, and (c) decreases water loss from the skin when the external humidity is low. Because fat is a poor conductor of heat, sebum (d) lessens the amount of heat lost from the skin. Sebum also (e) has a bactericidal (bacteria-killing) action.
4 It transmits sensations through nerve receptors, which are sensitive to pain, temperature, touch and pressure.
5 It produces and absorbs vitamin D in conjunction with ultraviolet rays from the sun, which activate a vitamin D precursor present in the skin.

The normal skin of a healthy person has transient and resident micro-organisms that are not usually harmful. In the elderly the skin is thinner and the growth of both the epidermal and dermal cells slow down.

ASSESSING SKIN INTEGRITY

Skin integrity and hygiene practices should be considered and assessed during initial contact with a patient. The assessment should include (a) a nursing health history to determine the patient's skin care practices, self-care abilities and past or current skin problems; (b) physical assessment of the skin; and (c) identification of patients at risk for developing skin impairments.

Personal Hygiene Assessment

Data about the patient's skin care practices enable the nurse to incorporate the patient's needs and preferences as much as possible in the plan of care. The assessment should identify any problems in relation to skin integrity, open wounds, rashes, blemishes, abnormalities of the orifices, the perineal genital area, nails, eyes and nose, and hair conditions.

Assessment of the patient's self-care abilities determines the amount of nursing assistance and the type of bath (e.g. bed, immersion bath or shower) best suited for the patient. Important considerations include the patient's balance (for bath and shower), ability to sit unsupported (in the bath or bed), activity tolerance, coordination, adequate muscle strength, and appropriate joint range of motion, vision, and the patient's preferences. Cognition and motivation are also essential. Patients whose cognitive function is impaired or whose illness alters energy levels and motivation will usually need more assistance. It is important for the nurse to determine the patient's functional level and to maintain and promote as much independence as possible. This also enables the nurse to identify the individual's potential for growth and rehabilitation. There are several models of functional levels of self-care.

The presence of past or current skin problems alerts the nurse to specific nursing interventions or referrals the patient may require. Many skin care conditions have implications for hygienic care. The patient may provide descriptions of these problems during the nursing assessment, or the nurse may observe some during the physical examination that follows. Common skin problems and implications for nursing interventions are shown in Table 17-2. Questions to elicit information about the patient's skin care practices, self-care abilities and skin problems are shown in the *Practice Guidelines*.

Positive responses to any of these require further exploration in terms of duration (When did it start?); frequency (How often have you had this?); description of lesion or rash; any associated signs, such as fever or nausea; aggravating factors (e.g. season of the year, stress, occupation, medication, recent travel, housing, personal contact); alleviating factors (e.g. medications, lotions, home remedies); and any family history of the problem.

Physical Assessment

When assisting with bathing and other hygienic care, the nurse often has the opportunity to collect information about skin discoloration, uniformity of colour, texture, skin elasticity, temperature, intactness and lesions.

Difficulties encountered by the patient in performing bathing activities include the inability to wash the body or body parts, to obtain or get to a water source, and to regulate water temperature or flow. Difficulties in dressing and grooming include inability to obtain, put on, take off, fasten or replace articles of clothing; and to maintain appearance at a satisfactory level. Toileting problems may involve difficulties getting to the toilet or commode or sitting on and rising from it. In addition, the patient may experience problems manipulating clothing for toileting, carrying out proper toilet hygiene, or flushing the

Table 17-2 Common Skin Problems

Problem and appearance	Nursing implications
Abrasion Superficial layers of the skin are scraped or rubbed away. Area is reddened and may have localised bleeding or serous weeping.	• Prone to infection; therefore, wound should be kept clean and dry. • Do not wear rings or jewellery when providing care to avoid causing abrasions to patients (as per hospital policy). • Use appropriate moving and handling techniques (as identified from risk assessment).
Excessive dryness Skin can appear flaky and rough.	• Prone to infection if the skin cracks; therefore, provide alcohol-free lotions to moisturise the skin and prevent cracking. • Use no soap, or use nonirritating soap and limit its use. Rinse skin thoroughly because soap can be irritating and drying. • Encourage increased fluid intake if health permits to prevent dehydration. • Use prescribed **emollient**.
Ammonia dermatitis (nappy rash) Caused by skin bacteria reacting with urea in the urine. The skin becomes reddened and is sore.	• Keep skin dry and clean by applying protective ointments containing zinc oxide to areas at risk (e.g. buttocks and perineum). • If reusable nappy in use boil the infant's nappy or wash them with an antibacterial detergent to prevent infection. Rinse nappy well because detergent is irritating to an infant's skin.
Acne Inflammatory condition with papules and pustules.	• Keep the skin clean to prevent secondary infection. • Treatment varies widely.
Erythema Redness associated with a variety of conditions, such as rashes, exposure to sun, elevated body temperature.	• Wash area carefully to remove excess micro-organisms. • Apply antiseptic spray or lotion to prevent itching, promote healing and prevent skin breakdown.
Hirsutism Excessive hair on a person's body and face, particularly in women.	• Remove unwanted hair by using depilatories, shaving, electrolysis or tweezing. • Enhance patient's self-concept.
Alopecia Hair loss most often in the scalp or beard; however, in some instances it can be hair loss in eyebrows, eye lashes and fine hair all over the body.	• Maintain patient dignity. • Administer sensitizer irritants as prescribed. • Enhance patient self-concept.

PRACTICE GUIDELINES

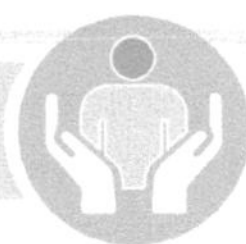

Skin Hygiene

Skin Care Practices

- What are your usual showering or bathing times?
- What cleansing products do you routinely use (e.g. bath oils, powder, facial cleansing creams, body lotions or creams, deodorants, antiperspirants)?
- What facial cosmetic products do you use?
- How and when do you clean makeup applicators? (Applicators should be kept clean, and products used around the eyes in particular should be discarded after four months to prevent bacterial and fungal infections.)
- Are there any cleansing or cosmetic products that you do not use because of the skin problems they create (e.g. skin dryness or allergic reactions)?

Self-Care Abilities

- Do you have any problems managing your hygienic practices (e.g. baths and facial care)? If so, what are these?
- How can the nurses best assist you?

Skin Problems

- Do you have any tendency towards skin dryness, itchiness, rashes, bruising, excessive perspiration or lack of perspiration? Have you had skin or scalp lesions in the past?
- Do you have any allergic tendencies? If so, what?

toilet or emptying the commode. The reasons (aetiologies or related factors) for these problems are varied:

- Deficient knowledge related to:
  - lack of experience with skin condition (acne) and need to prevent secondary infection;
  - new therapeutic regimen to manage skin problems;
  - unfamiliarity with devices available to facilitate sitting on or rising from toilet.
- Change of environment.
- Situational low self-esteem related to:
  - visible skin problem (e.g. acne or alopecia);
  - body odour.
- Post surgery (e.g. stoma, mastectomy or amputation).
- Care provision:
  - lack of experience in providing hygiene care to dependent person.

PLANNING

It is important that the nurse, patient and family/carer (when applicable) discuss each identified problem and agree on the nursing interventions to meet the patient outcomes.

Working in collaboration with the members of the multidisciplinary team, the specific, detailed nursing activities taken by the nurse may include assisting dependent patient with bathing, skin care and perineal care; instructing patients/families about appropriate hygienic practices and alternative methods for dressing; and demonstrating use of assistive equipment and adaptive activities.

Planning to assist a patient with personal hygiene includes consideration of the patient's personal preferences, health and limitations; the best time to give the care; and the equipment, facilities and personnel available. A patient's personal preferences – about when and how to bathe, for example – should be followed as long as they are compatible with the health and the equipment available. Nurses should provide whatever assistance the patient requires, either directly or by delegating this task to other nursing support personnel and taking into consideration the patient's choice.

Planning for Home Care

To provide for continuity of care, it is important that the nurse assesses the patient's and family's abilities for care and the need for referrals and support agency services. One such method of providing this continuity of care and support is by referring the patient, e.g. to the Occupational Therapist, who will normally assess the patient both in the Occupational Therapists' department within a hospital environment (for inpatients) and by an Occupational Therapist for both in and out patients in the patient's normal home environment. The Occupational Therapist will assess the patient on how they manage within their home environment and in collaboration with the patient, relatives and other members of the multidisciplinary team provide the patients with aids and accessories to ensure a safer and supportive environment for the patient.

IMPLEMENTING

The nurse applies the general guidelines for skin care while providing one of the various types of baths available to patients. *Procedure 17-1* on page 499 describes how to bathe an adult or paediatric patient.

General Guidelines for Skin Care

- *An intact, healthy skin is the body's first line of defence.* Nurses need to ensure that all skin care measures prevent injury and irritation. Scratching the skin with jewellery or long, sharp fingernails must be avoided. Harsh rubbing or use of rough towels and washcloths can cause tissue damage, particularly when the skin is irritated or when circulation or sensation is diminished. Bottom bed sheets are kept taut and free from wrinkles to reduce friction and abrasion to the skin. Top bed linens are arranged to prevent undue pressure on the toes. When necessary, bed cradles on footboards are used to keep bedclothes off the feet (see local policies).
- The degree to which the skin protects the underlying tissues from injury depends on the general health of the cells, the amount of subcutaneous tissue and the dryness of the skin. Skin that is poorly nourished and dry is less easily protected and more vulnerable to injury. When the skin is dry, lotions or creams with moisturising agents can be applied, and bathing is limited to once or twice a week because frequent bathing removes the natural oils of the skin and causes dryness.
- *Moisture in contact with the skin for more than a short time can result in increased bacterial growth and irritation.* After a bath, the patient's skin is dried carefully. Particular attention is paid to areas such as the axillae, the groin, beneath the breasts and between the toes, where the potential for irritation is greatest. A non-irritating dusting powder, such as baby talcum, tends to reduce moisture and can be applied to these areas after they are dried. Patients who are incontinent of urine or faeces or who perspire excessively are provided with immediate skin care to prevent skin irritation. This is also the care for patients who are undergoing radiotherapy treatment.
- *Body odours are caused by resident skin bacteria acting on body secretions.* Cleanliness is the best deodorant. Commercial deodorants and antiperspirants can be applied only after the skin is cleaned. Deodorants diminish odours, whereas antiperspirants reduce the amount of perspiration. Neither should be applied immediately after shaving, because of the possibility of skin irritation, nor are they used on skin that is already irritated.
- *Skin sensitivity to irritation and injury varies among individuals and in accordance with their health.* Generally speaking, skin sensitivity is greater in infants, very young children and

Table 17-3 Agents Commonly Used on the Skin

Agent	Action
Soap	Lowers surface tension and thus helps in cleaning. Some soaps contain antibacterial agents, which can change the natural flora of the skin.
Detergent	Used instead of soap for cleaning. Some people who are allergic to soaps may not be allergic to detergents, and vice versa.
Bath oil	Used in bathwater; provides an oily film on the skin that softens and prevents chapping. Oils can make the bath surface slippery, and patients should be instructed about safety measures (e.g. using nonskid bath surface or mat).
Skin cream, lotion	Provides a film on the skin that prevents evaporation and therefore chapping.
Powder	Can be used to absorb water and prevent friction. For example, powder under the breasts can prevent skin irritation. Some powders are antibacterial. However, care is needed as some powders are irritants.
Deodorant	Masks or diminishes body odours.
Antiperspirant	Reduces the amount of perspiration.

older people. A person's nutritional status also affects sensitivity. Emaciated or obese persons tend to experience more skin irritation and injury. The same tendency is seen in individuals with poor dietary habits and insufficient fluid intake. Even in healthy persons, skin sensitivity is highly variable. Some people's skin is sensitive to chemicals in skin care agents and cosmetics. Hypoallergenic cosmetics and soaps or soap substitutes are now available for these people. The nurse needs to ascertain whether the patient has any sensitivity and what agents are appropriate to use.

- Agents used for skin care have selective actions and purposes. Commonly used agents are described in Table 17-3.

Bathing

Bathing removes accumulated oil, perspiration, dead skin cells and some bacteria. The nurse can appreciate the quantity of oil and dead skin cells produced when observing a person after the removal of a cast that has been on for six weeks. The skin is crusty, flaky and dry underneath the cast. Applications of oil over several days are usually necessary to remove the debris.

Excessive bathing, however, can interfere with the intended lubricating effect of the sebum, causing dryness of the skin. This is an important consideration, especially for older adults, who produce less sebum.

In addition to cleaning the skin, bathing also stimulates circulation. A warm or hot bath dilates superficial arterioles, bringing more blood and nourishment to the skin. Vigorous rubbing has the same effect. Rubbing with long smooth strokes from the distal to proximal parts of extremities (from the point farthest from the body to the point closest) is particularly effective in facilitating venous blood flow unless there is some underlying condition (e.g. blood clot) that would preclude this.

Bathing also produces a sense of well-being (Dunn *et al.*, 2002). It is refreshing and relaxing and frequently improves morale, appearance and self-respect. Some people take a morning shower for its refreshing, stimulating effect. Others prefer an evening bath because it is relaxing. These effects are more evident when a person is ill. For example, it is not uncommon for patients who have had a restless or sleepless night to feel relaxed, comfortable and sleepy after a morning bath.

Bathing offers an excellent opportunity for the nurse to assess all patients. The nurse can observe the condition of the patient's skin and physical conditions such as sacral oedema or rashes. While assisting a patient with a bath, the nurse can also assess the patient's psychosocial needs, such as orientation to time and ability to cope with the illness. Learning needs, such as a diabetic patient's need to learn foot care, can also be assessed.

It is important to recognise that care is provided in the community and equipment such as shower seats (Figure 17-1) and hand bars (Figure 17-2) are avariable and discussed in *Community Care Considerations.*

Categories

Two categories of baths are given to patients: personal hygiene and therapeutic. *Personal hygiene/washing baths* are given chiefly for 'cleaning' purposes and include these types:

- *Complete bed bath.* The nurse washes the entire body of a dependent patient in bed.
- *Assisted bedbath.* Patients' confined to bed are able to bathe themselves with help from the nurse for washing the back and perhaps the feet.
- *Partial bath.* Only the parts of the patient's body that might cause discomfort or odour, if neglected, are washed: the face, hands, axillae, perineal area and back.
- *General baths.* General baths are often preferred to bed baths because it is easier to wash and rinse in a bath. The amount of assistance the nurse offers depends on the abilities of the patient. There are specially designed baths for dependent patients.
- Sponge baths are suggested for the newborn because daily general baths are not considered necessary. After the bath, the infant should be immediately dried and wrapped to prevent heat loss. Parents need to be advised that the infant's

COMMUNITY CARE CONSIDERATIONS

Hygiene

Patient and Environment

- *Self-care abilities for hygiene*: Assess the patient's ability to bathe, to manage the temperature of water and flow from taps, to dress and undress, to groom and to use the toilet.
- *Self-care aids required*: Determine if there is a need for a bath/shower seat (see Figure 17-1), a hand shower, a non-skid surface or mat in the bath or shower, hand bars on the sides of the bath (see Figure 17-2), or a raised toilet seat.
- *Facilities:* Check for the presence of laundry facilities and running water.
- *Mechanical barriers:* Note furniture obstructing access to the bathroom and toilet, or a doorway too narrow for a wheelchair.

Family

- *Caregiver availability, skills and responses:* Determine whether individuals are available and able to assist with bathing, dressing, toileting, nail care, hair shampoo, shopping for hygienic or grooming aids, and so on.
- *Education needs:* Assess whether the caregiver needs instruction in how to assist the patient in and out of the bath, on and off the toilet, and so on.
- *Family role changes and coping:* Assess effects of patient's illness on financial status, parenting, spousal roles, sexuality and social roles.

Community

Explore resources that will provide assistance with bathing, laundry and foot care (e.g. home healthcare, podiatrist).

- Consult a social worker as needed to coordinate placement of a patient unable to remain in the home or to identify community resources that will help the patient stay in the home.
- Refer to (a) a physiotherapist for advice and assessment to develop and improve the patient's motor function; (b) a community nurse to provide follow-up for care, teaching and support; and (c) an occupational therapist to assess and develop abilities to perform activities of daily living.

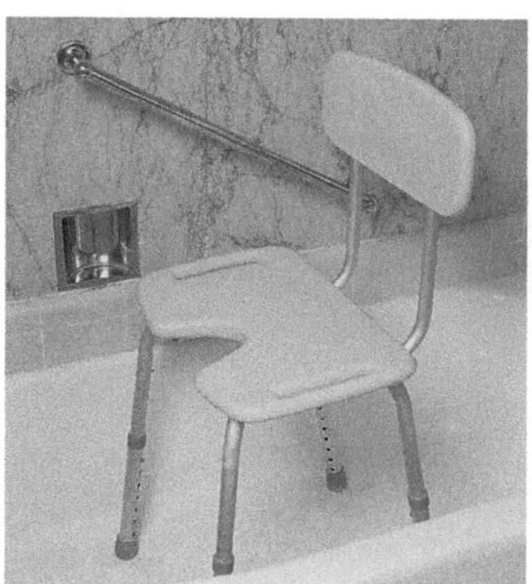

Figure 17-1 Shower seat in the home.

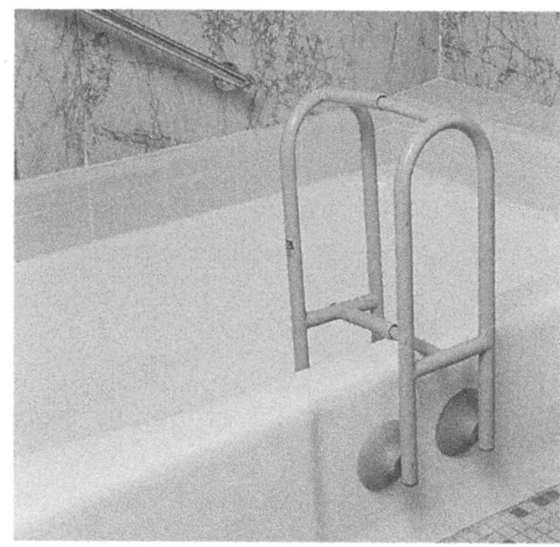

Figure 17-2 Hand bars on the sides of the bath.

ability to regulate body temperature has not yet fully developed. Infants perspire minimally, and shivering starts at a lower temperature than it does in adults; therefore, infants lose more heat before shivering begins. In addition, because the infant's body surface area is very large in relation to body mass, the body loses heat readily.

- *Shower.* Many ambulatory patients are able to use shower facilities and require only minimal assistance from the nurse. Patients in long-term care settings are often given showers with the aid of a shower chair. The wheels on the shower chair allow patients to be transported from their room to the shower. The shower chair also has a commode seat to facilitate cleansing of the patient's perineal area during the shower process (see Figure 17-3).

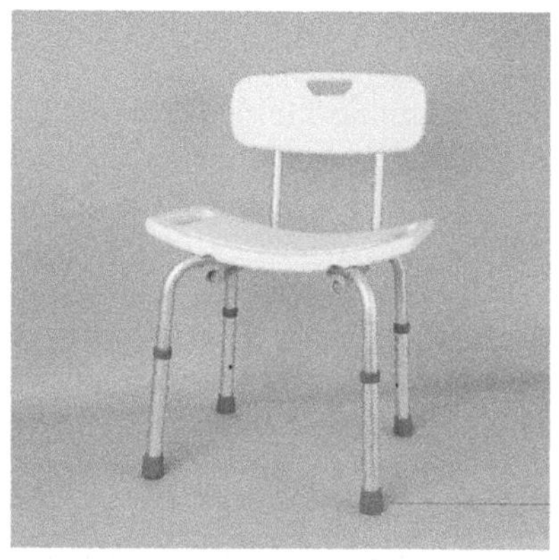

Figure 17-3 A shower chair.
Source: Patterson Medical Ltd.

The water for a bath should feel comfortably warm to the patient. People vary in their sensitivity to heat; generally, the temperature should be 32°C to 42°C. Most patients will verify a suitable temperature. Patients with decreased circulation or cognitive problems will not be able to verify the temperature. Therefore, the nurse must check the water temperature to avoid patient injury with water that is too hot. The water for a bed bath should be changed at least once during procedure (*see Procedure 17-1*) and when it becomes dirty or cold.

Therapeutic baths are given for physical effects, such as to soothe irritated skin or to treat an area (e.g. the perineum). Medications may be placed in the water. A therapeutic bath is generally taken in a bath one-third or one-half full. The patient remains in the bath for a designated time, often 20 to 30 minutes. If the patient's back, chest and arms are to be treated, these areas need to be immersed in the solution. The bath temperature is generally included as part of the treatment. *Procedure 17-1* provides guidelines for bathing patients.

PROCEDURE 17-1 Bathing an Adult or Paediatric Patient

Purposes

- To remove transient micro-organisms, body secretions and excretions, and dead skin cells
- To stimulate circulation to the skin
- To produce a sense of well-being
- To promote relaxation and comfort
- To prevent or eliminate unpleasant body odours
- Stimulate conversation between nurse and patient

Assessment

Assess

- Whether the patient would like a bath and what type of bath
- Condition of the skin (colour, texture and skin integrity, presence of pigmented spots, temperature, lesions, excoriations and abrasions)
- Fatigue
- Presence of pain and need for adjunctive measures (e.g. an analgesic) before the bath
- Movement and range of movement of joints
- Any other aspect of health that may affect the patient's bathing process (e.g. mobility strength, cognition)
- Standard precautions during bathing (e.g. use of gloves, disposal of wipes, etc.)

Planning

Before bathing a patient the nurse must always gain consent from the patient.

- Before bathing a patient, determine:
  - the purpose and type of bath the patient needs;
  - self-care ability of the patient;
  - any movement or positioning precautions specific to the patient;
  - other care the patient may be receiving, such as physiotherapy or x-rays, in order to coordinate all aspects of healthcare and prevent unnecessary fatigue;
  - patient's comfort level with being bathed by someone else;
  - necessary bath equipment (preferred soap, deodorants etc), towels and bed sheets;
  - whether the patient needs hair washed, finger and toe nails cut (as per hospital policy).
- Consider any religious and cultural beliefs.
- Offer the patient urinal, bedpan or commode.

Equipment

- Basin or sink with warm water (check water temperature comfortable for patient requirements) (wash bowl with hot soapy water prior to use).
- Soap and soap dish as per patient choice.
- Towels, washcloth, clean gown or pyjamas or clothes as needed, additional bed linen, if required.
- Gloves, if appropriate (e.g. presence of body fluids or open lesions).
- Personal hygiene articles (e.g. deodorant, powder, lotions).
- Shaving equipment for male patients.
- Hair washing facilities (flannels, preferably disposables).
- Nail clippers.
- Table for bathing equipment.
- Laundry bag as required.

Caution is needed when bathing patients who are receiving intravenous therapy or have multiple connections to equipment. Easy-to-remove gowns that have Velcro or snap fasteners along the sleeves may be used. If a special gown is not available, the nurse needs to pay special attention when changing the patient's gown after the bath (or whenever the gown becomes soiled). General guidelines are provided in the *Practice Guidelines* on page 503. These guidelines do not apply if the patient has an intravenous infusion pump or controller. In this situation, either use a special gown or do not put the sleeve of a gown over the patient's involved arm.

Implementation

Preparation

Before bathing a patient, consider:

- Condition of the skin (colour, texture and elasticity, presence of pigmented spots, temperature, lesions, excoriations and abrasions)
- Fatigue
- Presence of pain and need for adjunctive measures (e.g. an analgesic) before the bath.
- Range of motion of the joints.
- Any other aspect of health that may affect the patient's bathing process (e.g. mobility, strength, cognition).
- Need for use of clean gloves during the bath.

Performance

1 Follow local policy to ensure that you explain to the patient what you are going to do, why it is necessary and how they can cooperate. Obtain consent and maintain patient privacy and dignity and ensure that the appropriate local infection control procedures are observed.

2 Prepare the patient and the environment.
   - Invite a family member or significant other to participate if desired.
   - Close windows and doors to ensure the room is a comfortable temperature. *Air currents increase loss of heat from the body by convection.*
   - Offer the patient a bedpan or urinal or ask whether the patient wishes to use the toilet or commode. Warm water and activity can stimulate the need to void. The patient will be more comfortable after **voiding**, and voiding before cleaning the perineum is advisable.
   - Encourage the patient to perform as much personal self-care as possible. *This promotes independence, exercise and self-esteem.*
   - During the bath, assess each area of the skin carefully.

For a bed bath

3 Prepare the bed and position the patient appropriately.
   - Position the bed at a comfortable working height. Lower the side rail on the side close to you *(if in use)*. Keep the other side rail up. Assist the patient to move near you. This avoids undue reaching and straining and promotes good body mechanics.
   - Place a towel over the top sheet. Remove the top sheet from under the towel by starting at patient's shoulders and moving linen down towards the patient's feet (see Figure 17-4). Ask the patient to grasp and hold the top of the towel while pulling linen to the foot of the bed. *The towel provides comfort, warmth and privacy. Note*: If the bed linen is to be reused, place it over the bedside chair. If it is to be changed, place it in the linen skip.
   - Remove patient's gown/clothing while keeping the patient covered with the towel.

4 Wash the face. Begin the bath at the cleanest area and work downward towards the feet.
   - Place towel under patient's head.
   - Wash the patient's eyes with water only and dry them well (see Figure 17-5). Use a separate corner of the washcloth for each eye. *Using separate corners prevents transmitting micro-organisms from one eye to the other.* Wipe from the inner to the outer canthus. *This prevents secretions from entering the nasolacrimal ducts.*
   - Ask whether the patient wants soap used on the face. Soap has a drying effect, and the face, which is exposed to the air more than other body parts, tends to be drier.
   - Wash, rinse and dry the patient's face, ears and neck.
   - Remove the towel from under the patient's head.

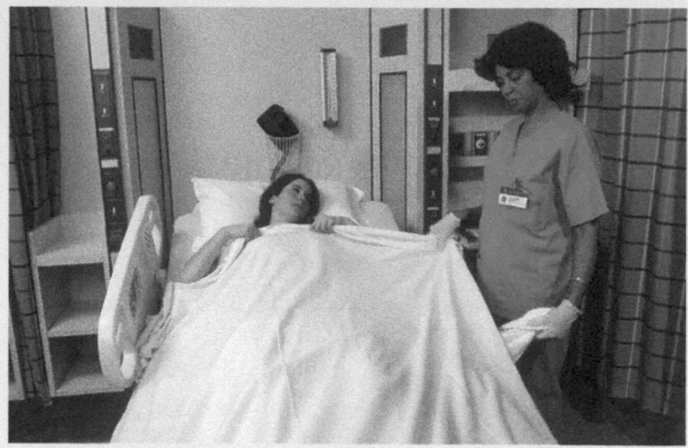

Figure 17-4 Remove top sheet from under the bath towel.
Source: Pearson Education Ltd.

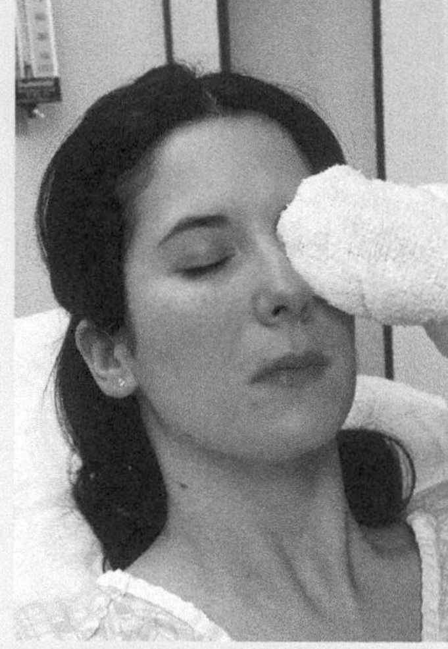

Figure 17-5 Using a separate corner of the washcloth for each eye, wipe from the inner to the outer canthus
Source: Pearson Education Ltd.

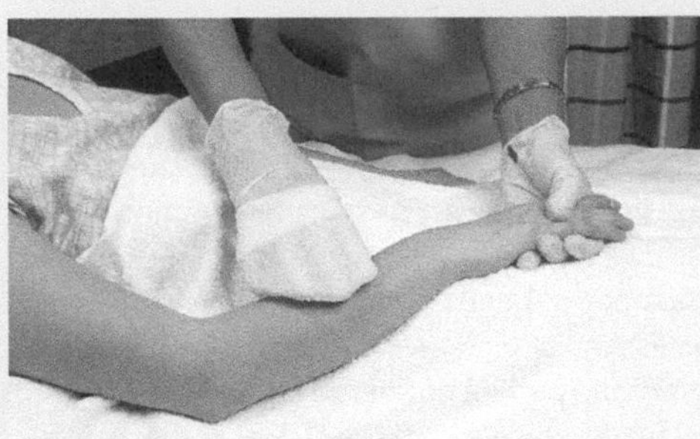

Figure 17-6 Washing the far arm using long, firm strokes from wrist to shoulder area.

5 Wash the arms and hands. (Omit the arms for a partial bath.)
- Place a towel lengthwise under the arm away from you. *It protects the bed from becoming wet.*
- Wash, rinse and dry the arm by elevating the patient's arm and supporting the patient's wrist and elbow (Figure 17-6). Use long, firm strokes from wrist to shoulder, including the axillary area. *Firm strokes from distal to proximal areas promote circulation by increasing venous blood return.*
- (Optional) Place a towel on the bed and put a washbasin on it. Place the patient's hands in the basin. *Many patients enjoy immersing their hands in the basin and washing themselves. Soaking loosens dirt under the nails.* Assist the patient as needed to wash, rinse and dry the hands, paying particular attention to the spaces between the fingers.
- Repeat for hand and arm nearest you. Exercise caution if an intravenous infusion is present, and check its flow after moving the arm.

6 Wash the chest and abdomen. (Particular care is needed under a woman's breast as this area may require bathing if this area is irritated or if the patient has significant perspiration under the breast.)
- Place bath towel lengthwise over chest. Fold bath blanket down to the patient's pubic area. *Keeps the patient warm while preventing unnecessary exposure of the chest.*
- Lift the bath towel off the chest, and bathe the chest and abdomen using long, firm strokes (Figure 17-7). Give special attention to the skin under the breasts and any other skin folds particularly if the patient is overweight. Rinse and dry well.
- Replace the towel when the areas have been dried.
- Change the water now. Raise side rails when refilling basin. *This ensures the safety of the patient.*

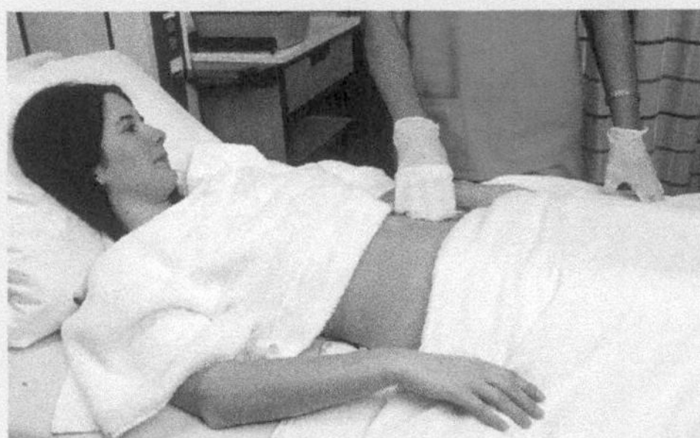

Figure 17-7 Washing the chest and abdomen.
Source: all images on this page © Pearson Education Ltd.

7 Wash the legs and feet.
- Expose the leg farthest from you by folding the towel towards the other leg being careful to keep the perineum covered. *Covering the perineum promotes privacy and maintains the patient's dignity.*
- Lift leg and place the bath towel lengthwise under the leg. Wash, rinse and dry the leg using long, smooth, firm strokes from the ankle to the knee to the thigh (Figure 17-8). *Washing from the distal to proximal areas promotes circulation by stimulating venous blood flow.*
- Reverse the coverings and repeat for the other leg.
- Wash the feet by placing them in the basin of water (Figure 17-9).
- Dry each foot. Pay particular attention to the spaces between the toes. If you prefer, wash one foot after that leg before washing the other leg.
- Obtain fresh, warm bathwater now or when necessary. *Water may become dirty or cold.* Because surface skin cells are removed with washing, the bathwater from dark-skinned patients may be dark; however, this does not mean the patient is dirty. Raise side rails when refilling basin. *This ensures the safety of the patient.*

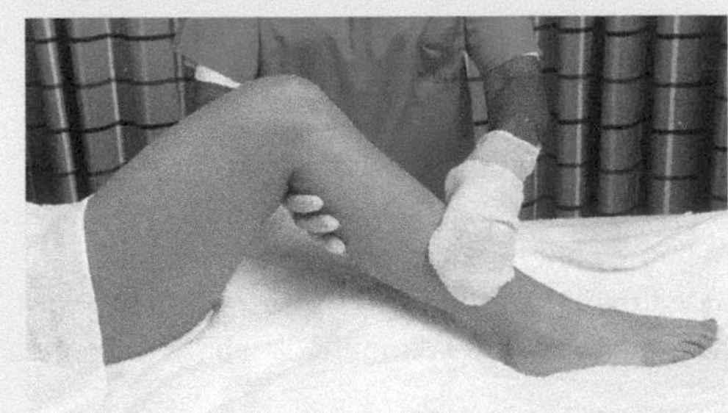

Figure 17-8 Washing far leg.

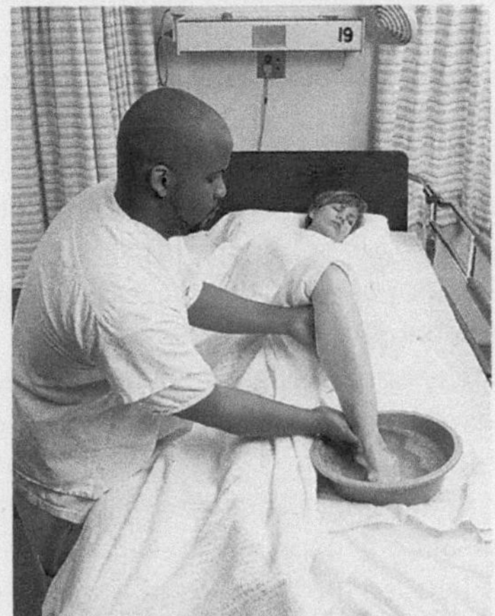

Figure 17-9 Soaking a foot in a basin.

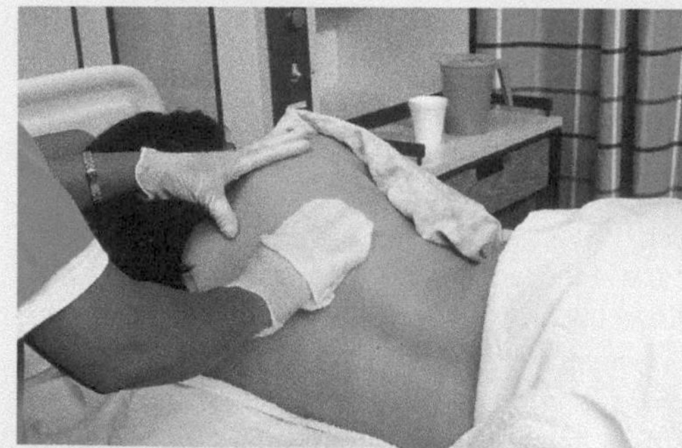

Figure 17-10 Washing the back.

8 Wash the back and then the perineum.
- Assist the patient into a prone or side-lying position facing away from you. Place the bath towel lengthwise alongside the back and buttocks while keeping the patient covered with the towel as much as possible. *This provides warmth and undue exposure.*
- Wash and dry the patient's back, moving from the shoulders to the buttocks, and upper thighs, paying attention to the **gluteal folds** (Figure 17-10).
- Assist the patient to the supine position and determine whether the patient can wash the perineal area independently. If the patient cannot do so, cover the patient as shown in *Procedure 17-2* and wash the area.

9 Assist the patient with grooming aids such as powder, lotion or deodorant.
- Use powder sparingly. Release as little as possible into the atmosphere. This will avoid irritation of the respiratory tract by powder inhalation. Excessive powder can cause caking, which leads to skin irritation.
- Help the patient put on fresh clothing.
- Assist the patient to care for hair, mouth and nails. Some people prefer or need mouth care prior to their bath.

For a general bath or shower

10 Prepare the patient and the bath.
- Fill the bath about one-third to one-half full of water, put cold water in before hot. *Sufficient water is needed to cover the perineal area.*
- Cover all intravenous catheters or wound dressings with plastic coverings, and instruct the patient to prevent wetting these areas if possible.
- Put a rubber bath mat or towel on the floor of the bath if safety strips are not on the bath floor. *These prevent slippage of the patient during the bath or shower.*

11 Assist the patient into the shower or bath.
- Assist the patient taking a standing shower with the initial adjustment of the water temperature and water flow pressure, as needed. Some patients need a chair to sit on in the shower because of weakness. Hot water can cause elderly people to feel faint.
- If the patient requires considerable assistance with an immersion bath, a hydraulic chair/hoist/lift may be required (see Variation below).
- Explain how the patient can signal for help; leave the patient for 2-5 minutes. For safety reasons, do not leave a patient with decreased cognition or patients who may be at risk (e.g. history of seizures, syncope).

12 Assist the patient with washing and getting out of the bath.
- Wash the patient's back, lower legs and feet, if necessary.
- Assist the patient out of the bath. If the patient is unsteady, place a bath towel over the patient's shoulders and drain the water before the patient attempts to get out of it. *Draining the water first lessens the likelihood of a fall. The towel prevents chilling.*

13 Dry the patient, and assist with follow-up care.
- Follow step 9.
- Assist the patient back to his or her room.
- Remember to clean the bath and dispose of the dirty linen as per hospital or local policy.

14 Document in patient's notes:
- Type of bath given (i.e. complete, partial, or self-help).
- Skin assessment, such as excoriation, erythema, exudates, rashes, drainage or skin breakdown.
- Nursing interventions related to skin integrity.
- Ability of the patient to assist or cooperate with bathing.
- Patient response to bathing.
- Educational needs regarding hygiene.
- Information or teaching shared with the patient or their family.

Variation: bathing using a hydraulic bath chair

A hydraulic lift, often used in long-term care or rehabilitation settings, can facilitate the transfer of a patient who is unable to mobilise to the bathroom.

- Bring the patient to the bathroom in a wheelchair or shower chair.
- Fill the bath and check the water temperature with a bath thermometer *to avoid thermal injury to the patient.*

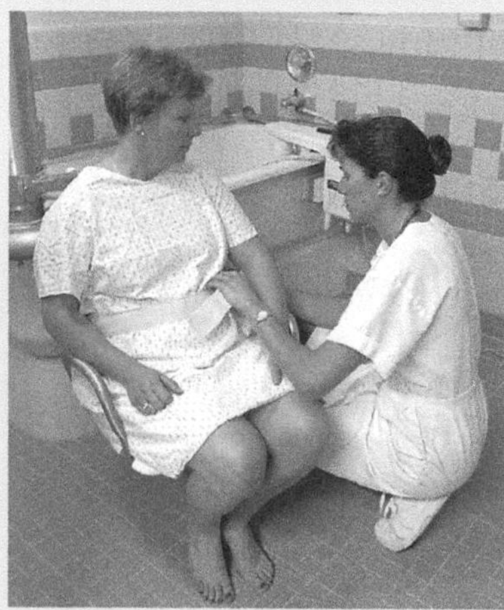

Figure 17-11 Secure the seat belt before moving the patient in a hydraulic bath chair.

- Lower the hydraulic chair lift to its lowest point, outside the bath.
- Transfer the patient to the chair lift and secure the seat belt (Figure 17-11).
- Raise the chair lift above the bath.
- Support the patient's legs as the chair is moved over the bath *to avoid injury to the legs.*
- Position the patient's legs down into the water and slowly lower the chair lift into the bath.
- Assist in bathing the patient, if appropriate.
- Reverse the procedure when taking the patient out of the bath.
- Dry the patient and transfer or transport them back to their room.

Evaluation

- Note the patient's tolerance of the procedure (e.g. respiratory rate and effort, pulse rate, behaviours, statements regarding comfort).
- Conduct appropriate follow up, such as:
  - condition and integrity of skin (dryness, skin elasticity, redness, lesions, and so on);
  - patient strength;
  - percentage of bath done without assistance;
  - relate to careplan for prior assessment, if available.

PRACTICE GUIDELINES

Changing a Hospital Gown for a Patient with an Intravenous Infusion

The intravenous infusion should be stopped and/or capped as per hospital policy.

- If the venflon is stopped only:
  - Slip the gown completely off the arm without the infusion and onto the tubing connected to the arm with the infusion.
  - Holding the container above the patient's arm, slide the sleeve up over the container to remove the used gown.
  - Place the clean gown sleeve for the arm with the infusion over the container as if it were an extension of the patient's arm, from the inside of the gown to the sleeve cuff.
  - Rehang the container. Slide the gown carefully over the tubing towards the patient's hand.
  - Guide the patient's arm and tubing into the sleeve, taking care not to pull on the tubing.
  - Assist the patient to put the other arm into the second sleeve of the gown and fasten as usual.
  - Check the rate of flow of the infusion to make sure it is correct before leaving the bedside.
- If the infusion is capped, care of the venflon site is necessary:
  - Ensure aseptic technique is maintained during 'capping' of venflon.
  - Maintain universal precautions.
  - Observe for any irritation, leakage, swelling, etc.
  - Ensure that venflon is secure.
  - Change gown with care.
  - Ensure that, if infusion is attached to electrical pump, rate, time and volume are as prescribed.

COMMUNITY CARE CONSIDERATIONS

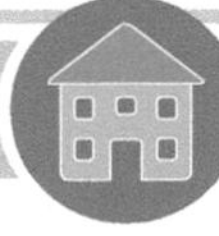

Hygiene at home

Suggest that the patient or family do the following:

- Referral to occupational therapist for assessment.
- Advise re providing a bath seat that fits in the bath or shower.
- Install a hand shower for use with a bath seat and shampooing.
- Use a nonskid surface on the bath or shower.
- Install hand bars on both sides of the bath, shower and toilet to facilitate transfers in, out and onto either the bath, shower or toilet seat.
- Carefully monitor the temperature of the bathwater.
- Apply lotion and oil *after* a bath, not during, because these solutions can make a bath surface slippery.

LIFESPAN CONSIDERATIONS

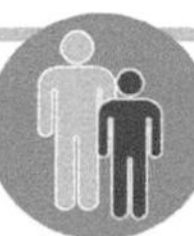

Bathing

Infants

- Sponge baths are suggested for the newborn because daily general baths are not considered necessary (every 3 days). However, once the baby is one month old it is advised to bath them more frequently. After the bath, the infant should be immediately dried and wrapped. Parents need to be advised that the infant's ability to regulate body temperature has not yet fully developed and newborns' bodies lose heat readily.

Children

- Encourage a child's participation appropriate for developmental level.
- Closely supervise children when bathing. Do not leave them unattended.

Adolescents

- Assist adolescents if they need help to choose appropriate creams and emulsifiers. Secretions from newly active sweat glands react with bacteria on the skin, causing a pungent odour.

Mature Adults

- Changes of ageing can decrease the protective function of the skin in older people. These changes include fragile skin, less oil and moisture and a decrease in elasticity.
- To minimise skin dryness in mature adults, avoid excessive use of soap. The ideal time to moisturise the skin is immediately after bathing.
- Avoid powder because it causes moisture loss and is a hazardous inhalant.
- Protect older people and children from injury related to hot water burns.
- Mature patients may prefer to have a general bath on a weekly basis which is their custom at home. Patient preference should be considered.

Long-Term Care Setting

From a historical perspective, the bath has always been a part of nursing care and considered a component of the 'art' of nursing. In today's nursing world, however, the bath or assisted personal body care is often delegated to nonprofessionals or newly qualified nurses as it is a nursing activity that is perceived as unproblematic with few professional challenges (Lomborg and Kirkevold, 2005).

In spite of the previously listed therapeutic values associated with bathing, the choice of bathing procedure often depends on the amount of time available to the nurse or support worker and the patient's self-care ability. Nursing authors (Rader *et al.*, 1996; Hektor and Touhy, 1997; Skewes, 1997; Brawley, 2002) challenge nurses to switch from a task-centred approach to an individualised and aesthetic approach to bathing, especially for the older person in a long-term care setting.

The bath routine (e.g. day, time and number/week) for patients in healthcare settings is often determined by time, resources available and policy, such that the bath becomes routine and depersonalised versus therapeutic, satisfying and person focused. An individualised approach focusing on therapeutic and comforting outcomes of bathing is especially important for patients with dementia.

Providing personal hygiene creates the highest level of stress to any patient and, according to Dunn *et al.* (2002) is often an ongoing challenge in patients with dementia. Being sensitive to the rhythm of their behaviour and looking for cues can often offset problems related to this. Patients with dementia, whether they are at home or in a healthcare facility, often have certain times of the day when they are more agitated – these are times to avoid doing things that will increase their fear and agitation. It is sometimes helpful to wait a while (e.g. half an hour or so) and then try giving the bath because they may forget that they were protesting and be willing to participate. Clark (2006) states that dependency on intimate care is humiliating and some individuals, e.g. those with learning disabilities, are reliant on this intimate care on a daily basis.

Perineal-Genital Care

Perineal-genital care is also referred to as *perineal care* or *pericare.* Perineal care as part of the bed bath is embarrassing for many patients. Nurses also may find it embarrassing initially, particularly with patients of the opposite sex. Most patients who require a bed bath from the nurse are able to clean their own genital areas with minimal assistance. The nurse may need to hand a moistened washcloth and soap to the patient, rinse the washcloth and provide a towel. Extra care is needed with this area especially to patients who are prone to infections. Dougherty and Lister (2008) state that extra vigilance is required from both the nurse and patient following treatment therapies, such as for example radiotherapy, or for fistulae, diarrhea, constipation and urinary tract infections in order to prevent complications due to poor hygiene. According to Ersser *et al.* (2005) there is a strong link between incontinence and skin integrity.

Because some patients are unfamiliar with terminology for the genitals and perineum, it may be difficult for nurses to explain what is expected. Most patients, however, understand what is meant if the nurse simply says, 'I'll give you a washcloth to finish your bath.' Older patients may be familiar with the term *private parts*. Whatever expression the nurse uses, it needs to be one that the patient understands and one that the nurse finds comfortable to use.

The nurse needs to provide perineal care efficiently and matter-of-factly. Nurses should wear gloves while providing this care for the comfort of the patient and to protect themselves from infection. *Procedure 17-2* explains how to provide perineal-genital care.

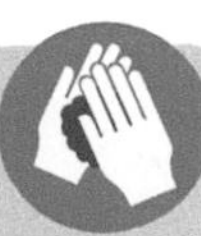

CLINICAL ALERT

Always wash or wipe from 'clean to dirty'. For a female, cleanse perineal area from front to back. For a male, cleanse the urinary meatus by moving in a circular motion from centre of urethral opening around the glans. Provide a sanitary towel to a female patient who is menstruating, and care is needed with disposal of soiled sanitary towels to prevent blood-borne diseases.

PROCEDURE 17-2 Providing Perineal-Genital Care

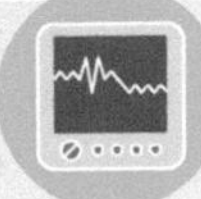

Purposes

- To remove normal perineal secretions and odours
- To promote patient comfort

Assessment

Assess for the presence of:

- Irritation, excoriation, inflammation, swelling
- Excessive discharge
- Odour, pain or discomfort
- Urinary or faecal incontinence
- Recent rectal or perineal surgery
- Indwelling catheter

Determine

- Perineal-genital hygiene practices
- Self-care abilities

Planning

Equipment

Perineal-genital care provided in conjunction with the bed bath:

- Bath towel
- Clean gloves
- Wash basin/bowl with tempered water
- Soap
- Washcloth (preferably disposable)

Special perineal-genital care:

- Bath towel
- Clean gloves
- Cotton wipes
- Solution bottle, or container filled with warm water or a prescribed solution
- Bedpan to receive rinse water
- Soiled linen bag
- Perineal/incontinence sheet or pad

Implementation

Preparation

- Determine whether the patient is experiencing any discomfort in the perineal-genital area.
- Obtain and prepare the necessary equipment and supplies.

Performance

1 Follow local policy to ensure that you explain to the patient what you are going to do, why it is necessary and how they can cooperate. Obtain consent and maintain patient privacy and dignity and ensure that the appropriate local infection control procedures are observed.

2 Prepare the patient (being particularly sensitive to any embarrassment felt by the patient):
   - Fold the top bed linen to the foot of the bed and fold the gown up to expose the genital area.
   - Place a towel under the patient's hips. *The towel prevents the bed from becoming soiled.*

3 Position and drape the patient and clean the upper inner thighs (*see* Figure 17-12).

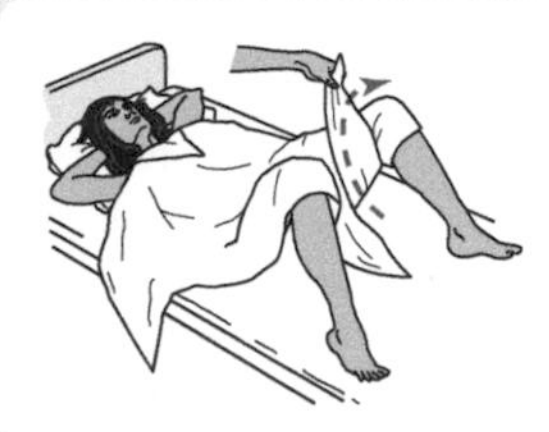

Figure 17-12 Draping the patient for perineal-genital care.

For females

- Position the female in a back-lying position with the knees flexed and spread well apart.
- Cover her body and legs with the towel. Drape the legs by tucking the bottom corners of the towel under the inner sides of the legs (Figure 17-12). *Minimum exposure lessens embarrassment and helps to provide warmth.* Bring the middle portion of the base of the blanket up over the pubic area.
- Put on gloves, wash and dry the upper inner thighs.

For males

- Position the male patient in a supine position with knees slightly flexed and hips slightly externally rotated.
- Put on gloves, wash and dry the upper inner thighs.

4 Inspect the perineal area.
- Note particular areas of inflammation, excoriation or swelling, especially between the labia in females and the scrotal folds in males.
- Also note excessive discharge or secretions from the orifices and the presence of odours.
- Wash and dry the perineal-genital area.

For females

- Clean the labia majora. Then spread the labia to wash the folds between the labia majora and the labia minora (Figure 17-13). *Secretions that tend to collect around the labia minora facilitate bacterial growth.*
- Use separate quarters of the washcloth for each stroke, and wipe from the pubis to the rectum. For menstruating women and patients with indwelling catheters, use clean wipes, or gauze. Take a clean wipe/gauze for each stroke. *Using separate quarters of the washcloth or new gauzes prevents the transmission of micro-organisms from one area to the other. Wipe from the area of least contamination (the pubis) to that of greatest (the rectum).*
- Rinse the area well. Dry the perineum thoroughly, paying particular attention to the folds between the labia. *Moisture supports the growth of many micro-organisms.*

For males

- Wash and dry the penis, using firm strokes. *Handling the penis firmly may prevent an erection.*
- If the patient is uncircumcised, retract the prepuce (foreskin) to expose the glans penis (the tip of the penis) for cleaning. Replace the foreskin after cleaning the glans penis (Figure 17-14). *Retracting the foreskin is necessary to remove the smegma that collects under the foreskin and facilitates bacterial growth. Replacing the foreskin prevents constriction of the penis, which may cause oedema.*
- Wash and dry the scrotum. The posterior folds of the scrotum may need to be cleaned when the buttocks are cleaned (see step 6). *The scrotum tends to be more soiled than the penis because of its proximity to the rectum; thus it is usually cleaned after the penis.*

5 Inspect perineal orifices for intactness.
- Inspect particularly around the urethra in patients with indwelling catheters. *A catheter may cause excoriation around the urethra.*

6 Clean between the buttocks.
- Assist the patient to turn onto the side facing away from you.
- Pay particular attention to the anal area and posterior folds of the scrotum in males. Clean the anus with clean wipes before washing it, if necessary.
- Dry the area well.
- For post child delivery or menstruating females, apply a perineal pad as needed from front to back. *This prevents contamination of the vagina and urethra from the anal area.*

7 Document any unusual findings such as redness, excoriation, skin breakdown, discharge or drainage and any localised areas of tenderness.

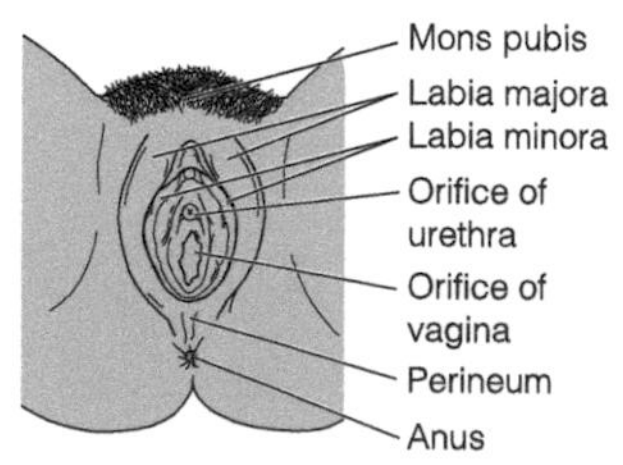

Figure 17-13 Female genitals.

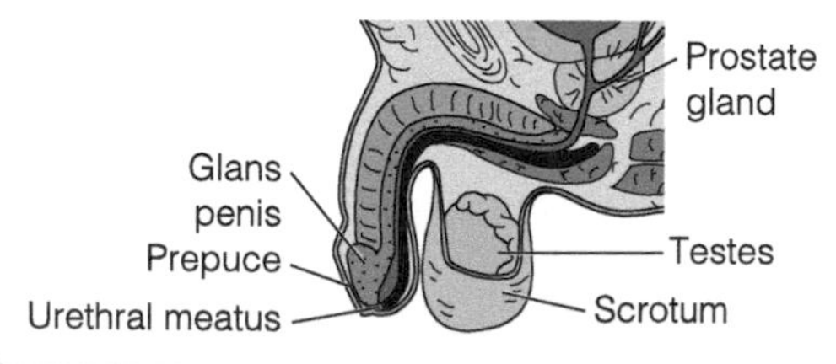

Figure 17-14 Male genitals.

Evaluation

- Relate current assessments to previous assessments.
- Conduct appropriate follow-up such as prescribed ointment for excoriation.
- Report any abnormalities to the doctor.
- Advise patients about dry skin, skin rashes and acne (see *Teaching: Patient Care*).

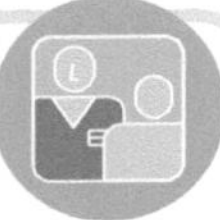

TEACHING: PATIENT CARE

Skin Problems and Care

Dry Skin

- Use cleansing creams to clean the skin rather than soap or detergent, which cause drying and, in some cases, allergic reactions.
- Use bath oils, but take precautions to prevent falls caused by slippery bath surfaces.
- Thoroughly rinse soap or detergent, if used, from the skin.
- Bathe less frequently when environmental temperature and humidity are low.
- Increase fluid intake.
- Humidify the air with a humidifier or by keeping a bucket, bowl or sink full of water.
- Use moisturising or emollient creams that contain lanolin, petroleum jelly or cocoa butter to retain skin moisture.

Skin Rashes

- Keep the area clean by washing it with a mild soap. Rinse the skin well, and pat it dry.
- To relieve itching, try a tepid bath or soak. Some over-the-counter preparations, e.g. E45 cream or Calamine lotion, may help but should be used with full knowledge of the product.
- Avoid scratching the rash to prevent inflammation, infection and further skin lesions.
- Choose clothing carefully. Too much can cause perspiration and aggravate a rash.

Acne

- Wash the face frequently with appropriate soap or detergent and hot water to remove oil and dirt.
- Avoid using oily creams, which aggravate the condition.
- Avoid using cosmetics that block the ducts of the sebaceous glands and the hair follicles.
- Never squeeze or pick at the lesions. This increases the potential for infection and scarring.

EVALUATING

Using data collected during care, the nurse judges whether desired outcomes have been achieved. If the outcomes are not achieved, the nurse explores reasons why. For example:

- Did the nurse overestimate the patient's functional abilities (physical, mental, emotional) for self-care?
- Were provided instructions not clear to all involved?
- Were appropriate aids or supplies not available to the patient?
- Did the patient's condition change?
- Were required analgesics provided before hygienic care?
- What currently prescribed medications and therapies could affect the patient's abilities or tissue integrity?
- Is the patient's fluid and food intake adequate or appropriate to maintain skin and mucous membrane moisture and integrity?

FEET

The feet are essential for ambulation and merit attention even when people are confined to bed. Each foot contains 26 bones, 107 ligaments and 19 muscles, and contain more than a quarter of all the bones in your body. The skin covering the feet has more than 7000 nerve endings. The feet have more sweat glands than anywhere else on the body (125,000 per foot) and daily produce an eggcup's worth of sweat. These structures function together for both standing and walking.

Developmental Variations

At birth, a baby's foot is relatively unformed. The arches are supported by fatty pads and do not take their full shape until five to six years of age. During childhood, the bones and small muscles of the feet are easily damaged by tight, binding socks and ill-fitting shoes. For normal development, it is important that the arches be supported and that the bony structure and the feet grow with no external restrictions. Feet are not fully grown until about age 20. Healthy feet remain relatively unchanged during life. However, the elderly often require special attention for their feet. For example, reduced blood supply and accompanying arteriosclerosis can make a foot prone to ulcers and infection following trauma.

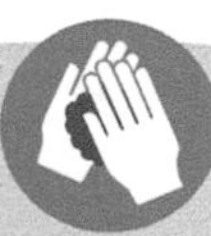

CLINICAL ALERT

Patients with diabetes are at high risk for lower extremity amputations (LEA). Routine foot assessment and patient education in proper foot care can significantly reduce the risk for LEA.

ASSESSING FEET

Assessment of the patient's feet includes identifying patients at risk for foot problems.

Nursing Health History

The nurse determines the patient's history of (a) normal nail and foot care practices, (b) type of footwear worn, (c) self-care abilities, (d) presence of risk factors for foot problems, (e) any foot discomfort and (f) any perceived problems with foot mobility. To elicit such data, the nurse may ask the patient the questions provided in the *Assessment Interview*.

Physical Assessment

Each foot and toe is inspected for shape, size and presence of lesions and is palpated to assess areas of tenderness, oedema and circulatory status. Normally, the toes are straight and flat. Table 17-4 lists physical assessment methods for the feet. Common foot problems include calluses, corns, unpleasant odours, **plantar warts**, fissures between the toes and fungal infections such as athlete's foot.

A callus is a thickened portion of epidermis, a mass of keratotic material. Most calluses are painless and flat and are found on the bottom or side of the foot over a bony prominence. Calluses are usually caused by pressure from shoes. They can be softened by soaking the foot in warm water with Epsom salts, and abraded with pumice stones or similar abrasives. Creams will help to keep the skin soft and prevent the formation of calluses.

ASSESSMENT INTERVIEW

Foot Hygiene

Foot Care Practices

- How often do you wash your feet and cut your toenails?
- What hygiene products do you usually use on your feet (e.g. soap, foot powder or deodorant, lotion or cream)?
- What type of shoes and socks do you wear?
- How often do you change your socks or put on clean socks?
- Do you ever go barefoot? If so, when, where and how often?

Self-Care Abilities

- Do you have any problems managing your foot care? If so, what are these?
- How can the nurses' best help you?

Foot Problems and Risk Factors

- Do you have any problems with foot odour?
- Do you have any foot discomfort? If so, where? When does this occur? What do you do to relieve the discomfort? Does this discomfort affect how you walk?
- Have you noticed any problems with foot mobility (e.g. joint stiffness)?
- Do you have diabetes, any circulatory problems with feet (e.g. swelling, changes in skin colour, arthritis) or any instances of prolonged exposure to chemicals or water?

Table 17-4 Assessment of the Feet

Method	Normal findings	Deviations from normal
Inspect all skin surfaces, particularly between the toes, for cleanliness, odour, dryness, inflammation, swelling, abrasions or other lesions.	Intact skin Absence of swelling or inflammation	Excessive dryness Areas of inflammation or swelling (e.g. corns, calluses) Fissures Scaling and cracking of skin (e.g. athlete's foot) Plantar warts
Palpate anterior and posterior surfaces of ankles and feet for oedema.	No swelling	Swelling or pitting oedema
Palpate dorsalis pedis pulse on dorsal surface of foot.	Strong, regular pulses in both feet	Weak or absent pulses
Compare skin temperature of both feet.	Warm skin temperature	Cool skin temperature in one or both feet

A corn is a keratosis caused by friction and pressure from a shoe. It commonly occurs on the fourth or fifth toe, usually on a bony prominence such as a joint. Corns are usually conical (circular and raised). The base is the surface of the corn and the apex is in deeper tissues, sometimes even attached to bone. Corns are generally removed surgically. They are prevented from reforming by relieving the pressure on the area (i.e. wearing comfortable shoes), and massaging the tissue to promote circulation. The use of oval corn pads should be avoided because they increase pressure and decrease circulation.

Unpleasant odours occur as a result of perspiration and its interaction with micro-organisms. Regular and frequent washing of the feet and wearing clean hosiery help to minimise odour. Foot powders and deodorants also help to prevent this problem.

Plantar warts appear on the sole of the foot. These warts are caused by the virus papovavirus hominis. They are moderately contagious. The warts are frequently painful and often make walking difficult. Curettage of the warts may be performed, freeze them with solid carbon dioxide several times, or apply salicylic acid.

Fissures, or deep grooves, frequently occur between the toes as a result of dryness and cracking of the skin. The treatment of choice is good foot hygiene and application of an antiseptic to prevent infection. Often a small piece of gauze is inserted between the toes in applying the antiseptic and left in place to assist healing by allowing air to reach the area.

CLINICAL ALERT

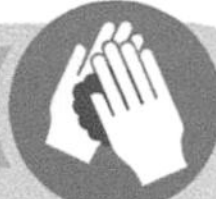

Patients with diabetes often have extremely dry skin. Tell them to use a nonperfumed lotion and to avoid putting lotion between the toes. Advise them not to soak their feet in water because it is drying to the skin.

Athlete's foot, or tinea pedis (ringworm of the foot), is caused by a fungus. The symptoms are scaling and cracking of the skin, particularly between the toes. Sometimes small blisters form, containing a thin fluid. In severe cases, the lesions may also appear on other parts of the body, particularly the hands. Treatments usually involve the application of commercial antifungal ointments or powders. Prevention is important. Common preventive measures are keeping the feet well ventilated, drying the feet well after bathing, wearing clean socks or stockings, and not going barefoot in public showers.

An ingrown toe nail, the growing inward of the nail into the soft tissues around it, most often results from improper nail trimming. Pressure applied to the area causes localised pain. Treatment involves frequent, hot antiseptic soaks and surgical removal of the portion of nail embedded in the skin. Preventing recurrence involves appropriate instruction and adherence to proper nail-trimming techniques.

Identifying Patients at Risk

Because of reduced peripheral circulation to the feet, patients with diabetes or peripheral vascular disease are particularly prone to infection if skin breakage occurs. Many foot problems can be prevented by teaching the patient simple foot care guidelines (see *Teaching: Patient Care* on page 510).

PLANNING

Planning involves (a) identifying nursing interventions that will help the patient maintain or restore healthy foot care practices and (b) establishing desired outcomes for each patient. Interventions may include teaching the patient about correct nail and foot care, proper footwear, wearing the correct size and ways to prevent potential foot problems (e.g. infection, injury and decreased circulation). For patients with self-care difficulties, e.g. visual impairment, limited mobility and/or hand co-ordination, the nurse plans a schedule for soaking the patient's feet and assisting with regular cleaning and trimming of nails (if not contraindicated). Foot and nail care is often provided during the patient's bath but may be provided at any time in the day to accommodate the patient's preference or schedule. The frequency of foot care is determined by the nurse and patient and is based on objective assessment data and the patient's specific problems. For some patients feet may need to be bathed daily; for those whose feet perspire excessively, bathing more than once a day may be necessary.

IMPLEMENTING

Procedure 17-3 describes how to provide foot care. See also the discussion of nails. During these procedures, the nurse has the opportunity to teach the patient appropriate methods for foot care, that is, methods designed to prevent tissue injury and infection (see *Teaching: Patient Care* on page 510).

EVALUATING

Examples of desired outcomes for foot hygiene include the patient being able to:

- participate in self-care (foot hygiene) to optimal level of capacity (specify);
- describe hygienic and other interventions (e.g. proper footwear) to maintain skin integrity, prevent infection and maintain peripheral tissue perfusion;
- demonstrate optimal foot hygiene, as evidenced by:
  - intact, smooth, soft, hydrated and warm skin;
  - intact cuticles and skin surrounding nails;
  - correct foot care and nail care practices.

TEACHING: PATIENT CARE

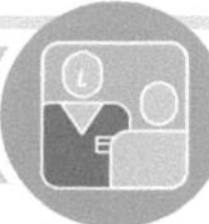

Foot Care

- Feet should be washed daily every day in warm soapy water (prolonged soaking may destroy the natural oils).
- Feet should be dried thoroughly, especially between the toes.
- Advise patients to cut toenails after a bath when the toe nails are softer. Toe nails should be trimmed regularly, using proper nail clippers. Toe nails should be cut straight across, not too short, and not down at the corners as this can lead to in-growing nails. Toe nails can be filed if easier for the patient.
- Any minor cuts or abrasions should be covered with a clean dry dressing, and blisters should be left to dry out on their own. If they burst, a clean dry dressing should be applied. Professional treatment should be sought if they do not heal quickly. Wounds/ulcers should be assessed and treated as a matter of urgency within 24 hours, especially if there is redness or swelling around the area.
- To maintain healthy feet corns and hard skin should be managed by using a foot file, emery board or pumice stone.
- Moisturising cream should be applied to dry skin except for between the toes.
- Prompt treatment for burns, cuts and breaks in the skin, and for any usual changes in colour or temperature. This is particularly important for diabetics.
- Feet should be kept warm and exercised (see below) daily to improve circulation:
  - sitting with feet up for 10 minutes after a long day helps circulation;
  - to refresh feet, massage gently with a foot roller;
  - calf stretches help to keep feet supple and keep a good range of movement;
  - circling feet ten times in each direction, keeping the leg as still as possible;
  - straighten toes and wriggle them around;
  - raise, point, then curl toes for five seconds each, repeated ten times;
  - circle the alphabet with the foot.

Source: Society of Chiropodists and Podiatrists (2011) **http://www.scpod.org/footcare/healthy-feet**.

PROCEDURE 17-3 Providing Foot Care

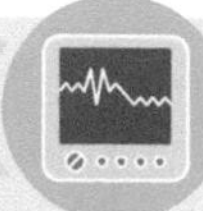

Purposes

- To maintain the skin integrity of the feet
- To prevent foot infections
- To prevent foot odours
- To assess or monitor foot problems

Assessment

Determine

- History of any problems with foot odour, foot discomfort, foot mobility, circulatory problems (e.g. swelling, changes in skin colour and/or temperature, and pain), structural problems (e.g. bunion, hammer toe or overlapping digits)
- Usual foot care practices (e.g. frequency of washing feet and cutting nails, foot hygiene products used, how often socks are changed, whether the patient ever goes barefoot, whether the patient sees a podiatrist)

Assess

- Skin surfaces for cleanliness, odour, dryness and intactness
- Each foot and toe for shape, size, presence of lesions (e.g. corn, callus, wart or rash), and areas of tenderness, ankle oedema
- Skin temperatures of the two feet to assess circulatory status and the dorsalis pedis pulses
- Self-care abilities (e.g. any problems managing foot care)

Planning

Equipment

- Washbowl containing warm water
- Pillow
- Moisture-resistant disposable pad
- Towels
- Soap
- Washcloth
- Toenail cleaning and trimming equipment
- Foot powder or cream

Implementation

Performance

1 Follow local policy to ensure that you explain to the patient what you are going to do, why it is necessary and how they can cooperate. Obtain consent and maintain patient privacy and dignity and ensure that the appropriate local infection control procedures are observed.

2 Prepare the equipment and the patient.
- Fill the washbowl with warm water. *Warm water promotes circulation, comforts and refreshes.*
- Assist the ambulatory patient to a sitting position in a chair, or the bed patient to a supine or semi-Fowler's position.
- Place a pillow under the bed patient's knees. This provides support and prevents muscle fatigue.
- Place the washbowl on the moisture-resistant pad at the foot of the bed for a bed patient or on the floor in front of the chair for an ambulatory patient.
- For a bed patient, pad the rim of the washbowl with a towel. *The towel prevents undue pressure on the skin.*

3 Wash the foot and soak it.
- Place one of the patient's feet in the bowl and wash it with soap, paying particular attention to the interdigital areas. Prolonged soaking is generally not recommended for diabetic patients or individuals with peripheral vascular disease. *Prolonged soaking may remove natural skin oils, thus drying the skin and making it more susceptible to cracking and injury.*
- Rinse the foot well to remove soap. Soap irritates the skin if not properly removed.
- Rub callused areas of the foot with the washcloth. *This helps remove dead skin layers.*
- If the nails are brittle or thick and require trimming, replace the water and allow the foot to soak for a few minutes. *Soaking softens the nails and loosens debris under them.*
- Clean the nails as required. This removes excess debris that harbours micro-organisms.
- Remove the foot from the basin and place it on the towel.

4 Dry the foot thoroughly and apply cream or foot powder.
- Blot the foot gently with the towel to dry it thoroughly, particularly between the toes. *Harsh rubbing can damage the skin. Thorough drying reduces the risk of infection.*
- Apply cream. *This lubricates dry skin.*

or
- Apply a foot powder containing a non-irritating deodorant if the feet tend to perspire excessively. *Foot powders have greater absorbent properties than regular bath powders; some also contain menthol, which makes the feet feel cool.*

5 Trim the nails of the first foot while the second foot is soaking (as per local policy).

6 Document any foot problems observed.
- Foot care is not generally recorded unless problems are noted.
- Record any signs of inflammation, infection, breaks in the skin, corns, troublesome calluses, bunions and pressure areas. This is of particular importance for patients with peripheral vascular disease and diabetes.

Evaluation

- Inspect nails and skin after the soak.
- Compare to prior assessment data.

ACTIVITY 17-1

Fred Bassett is an 82-year-old gentleman who lives alone. He has been a smoker for 60 years and has poor lower limb circulation. He visits the luncheon club once a week but needs the help of a carer as he has poor eyesight and mobility. His carer noticed that he was limping and, on questioning, she was advised that Fred had cut his toenails the previous evening and that, while he was unsure, he thought that he had cut too low and that his toenail bed had bled. Consider the care and reflect on the advice and support that a nurse would give Fred.

NAILS

Nails are normally present at birth. They continue to grow throughout life and change very little until people are elderly. At that time, the nails tend to be tougher, more brittle and in some cases thicker. The nails of an older person normally grow less quickly than those of a younger person and may be ridged and grooved.

ASSESSING NAILS

During the nursing assessment, the nurse explores the patient's usual nail care practices, self-care abilities and any problems associated with them (see the *Assessment Interview*). Physical assessment involves inspection of the nails (e.g. nail shape and texture, nail bed colour and tissues surrounding the nails).

ASSESSMENT INTERVIEW

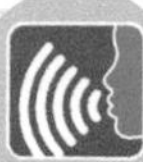

Nail Hygiene

- What are your usual nail care practices?
- Do you have any problems managing your nail care? If so, what are these?
- Have you had any problems associated with your nails (e.g. inflammation of the tissue surrounding the nail, injury, prolonged exposure to water or chemicals, circulatory problems)?

PLANNING

The nurse identifies measures that will assist the patient to develop or maintain healthy nail care practices. A schedule of nail care needs to be established.

IMPLEMENTING

To provide nail care, the nurse needs a nail cutter or sharp scissors, a nail file, hand lotion or mineral oil to lubricate any dry tissue around the nails, and a bowl of water to soak the nails if they are particularly thick or hard.

One hand or foot is soaked, if needed, and dried; then the nail is cut or filed straight across beyond the end of the finger or toe. Avoid trimming or digging into nails at the lateral corners. This predisposes the patient to ingrown fingernails. Patients who have diabetes or circulatory problems should have their nails filed rather than cut; inadvertent injury to tissues can occur if scissors are used. After the initial cut or filing, the nail is filed to round the corners, and the nurse cleans under the nail. The nurse then gently pushes back the cuticle, taking care not to injure it. The next finger or toe is cared for in the same manner. Any abnormalities, such as an infected cuticle or inflammation of the tissue around the nail, are recorded and reported.

EVALUATING

Examples of desired outcomes for nail hygiene include the patient being able to:

- demonstrate healthy nail care practices, as shown by:
  - clean, short nails with smooth edges;
  - intact cuticles and hydrated surrounding skin;
- describe factors contributing to the nail problem;
- describe preventive interventions for the specific nail problem;
- demonstrate nail care as instructed.

In addition, the patient should have pink nail beds and quick return of nail bed colour after capillary refill test.

MOUTH

The mouth is at the entrance or beginning of the alimentary canal. The mouth consists of:

- the oral cavity (*Cavumoris proprium*)
- the epidermal lining of the oral cavity
- gums and teeth
- the tongue.

The mouth has three main functions:

- ingestion
- communication
- breathing.

The Oral Cavity

The oral cavity is secured by the lips and cheeks, and the gums and teeth. The oral cavity is lined with a mucous membrane (the oral mucosa) consisting of a stratified squamous epithelium. Nerve endings supply the oral mucosa. The main functions of the oral cavity are chewing and talking.

Both the salivary glands and tonsils are associated accessory organs to the mouth.

The Epidermal Lining of the Oral Cavity

The entire oral cavity is lined by a stratified squamous epithelium. Stratified epithelium is normally two layered and is found in areas where there is daily 'wear and tear' on the body such as the mouth where there is a need for rapid replication to meet these demands. The functions of epithelial cells are: secretion, selective absorption, protection, sensation and transcellular transport.

Gums and Teeth

The soft tissue lining the mouth is known as **gingiva** (gums). Healthy gums are pink in colour and their function is to form a seal around teeth. Each tooth has three parts: the crown, the root and the pulp cavity (see Figure 17-15). The crown is the

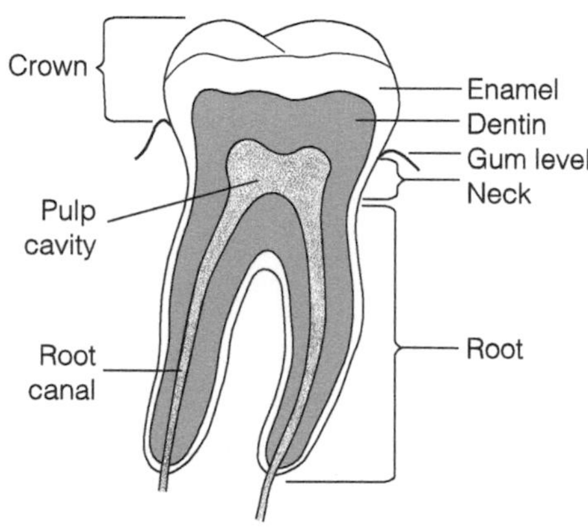

Figure 17-15 The anatomic parts of a tooth.

exposed part of the tooth, which is outside the gum. It is covered with a hard substance called enamel. The ivory-coloured internal part of the crown below the enamel is the dentin. The root of a tooth is embedded in the jaw and covered by a bony tissue called cementum. The pulp cavity in the centre of the tooth contains the blood vessels and nerves.

Developmental Variations (Teeth)

Teeth usually appear five to eight months after birth. Baby-bottle syndrome may result in decay of all of the upper teeth and the lower posterior teeth (Pillitteri, 2003: 824). This syndrome occurs when an infant is put to bed with a bottle of sugar water, formula, milk or fruit juice. The carbohydrates in the solutions causes demineralisation of the tooth enamel, which leads to tooth decay.

By the time children are two years old, they usually have all 20 of their temporary deciduous teeth (see Figure 17-16). At about age six or seven, children start losing their deciduous teeth, and these are gradually replaced by the 32 permanent teeth (see Figure 17-17). By age 25, most people have all of their permanent teeth.

The incidence of periodontal disease increases during pregnancy because the rise in female hormones affects gingival tissue and increases its reaction to bacterial plaque. Many pregnant women experience more bleeding from the gingival sulcus during brushing and increased redness and swelling of the gingiva (the gum).

Some older adults may have few permanent teeth left, and some have dentures. Loss of teeth occurs mainly because of **periodontal disease** (gum disease) rather than **dental caries** (cavities); however, caries are also common in middle-aged adults.

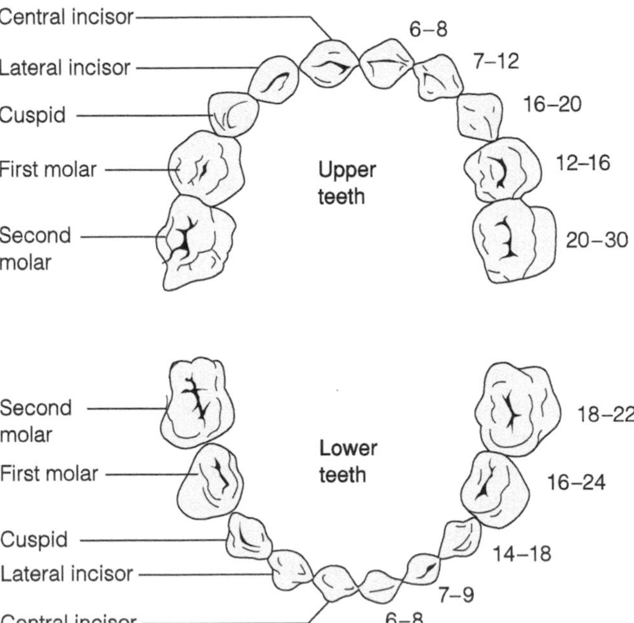

Figure 17-16 Temporary teeth and their times of eruption (stated in months).

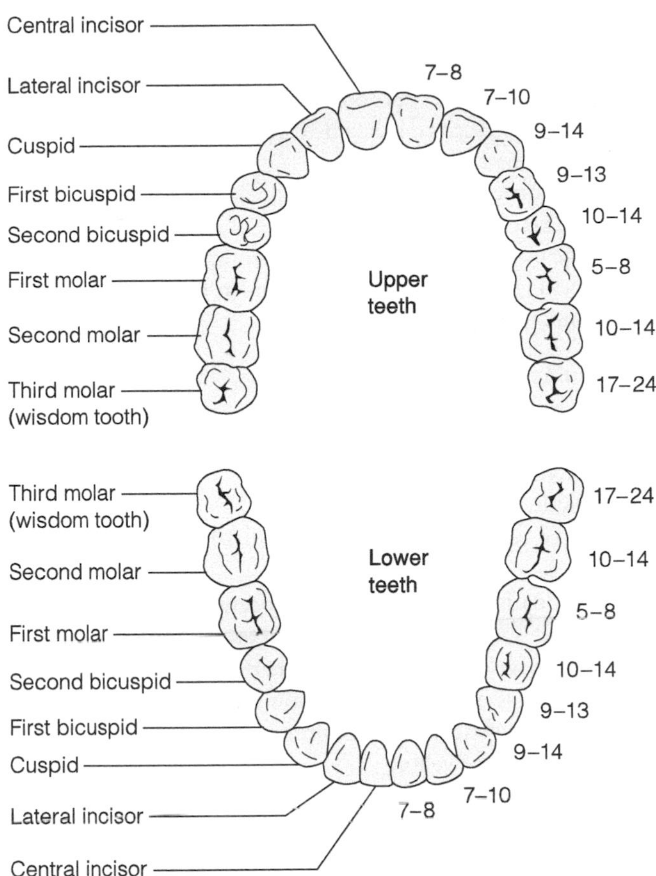

Figure 17-17 Permanent teeth and their times of eruption (stated in years).

Some receding of the gums and a brownish pigmentation of the gums occur with age. Because saliva production decreases with age, dryness of the oral mucosa is a common finding in older people.

Tongue

The skeletal muscle forming the major part of the floor of the mouth cavity is commonly known as the tongue. The skeletal muscle, unlike other muscles, e.g. cardiac muscles, is able to be readily controlled. The tongue has special sensory endings for taste and is known as the primary organ for taste. The tongue works with the other features in the mouth to articulate food around in the mouth cavity (when eating or drinking) and serves as a 'teeth cleaner'. The other main function of the tongue is the manipulation of the mouth to create speech.

Promoting Oral Health Through the Lifespan

A major role of the nurse in promoting oral health is to teach patients about specific oral hygienic measures.

Infants and Toddlers

Most dentists recommend that dental hygiene should begin when the first tooth erupts and be practised after each feeding. Cleaning can be accomplished by using a wet washcloth or small gauze moistened with water.

Dental caries occur frequently during the toddler period, often as a result of the excessive intake of sweets or a prolonged use of the bottle during naps and at bedtime. The nurse should give parents the following instructions to promote and maintain dental health:

- Beginning at about 18 months of age, brush the child's teeth with a soft toothbrush. Use only a toothbrush moistened with water at first and introduce toothpaste later. Use one that contains fluoride.
- Schedule an initial dental visit for the child at about two or three years of age, as soon as all 20 primary teeth have erupted.
- Some dentists recommend an inspection type of visit when the child is about 18 months old to provide an early pleasant introduction to the dental examination.
- Seek professional dental attention for any problems such as discolouring of the teeth, chipping, or signs of infection such as redness and swelling.

Pre-School and School-Age Children

Because deciduous teeth guide the entrance of permanent teeth, dental care is essential to keep these teeth in good repair. Abnormally placed or lost deciduous teeth can cause misalignment of permanent teeth. Fluoride remains important at this stage to prevent dental caries. Pre-schoolers need to be taught to brush their teeth after eating and to limit their intake of refined sugars. Parental supervision may be needed to ensure the completion of these self-care activities. Regular dental checkups are required during these years when permanent teeth appear.

Adolescents and Adults

Proper diet and tooth and mouth care should be evaluated and reinforced to adolescents and adults. Specific measures to prevent tooth decay and periodontal disease are listed in *Procedure 17-4* on page 516.

Oral Mouth Care

Identifying Patients at Risk

Certain patients are prone to oral problems because of lack of knowledge or the inability to maintain oral hygiene. Among these are seriously ill, confused, comatose, depressed and dehydrated patients. In addition, people with nasogastric tubes or receiving oxygen are likely to develop dry oral mucous membranes, especially if they breathe through their mouths. Patients who have had oral or jaw surgery must have meticulous oral hygiene care to prevent the development of infections.

Healthy-appearing individuals, too, may be at risk. High-risk variables such as inadequate nutrition, lack of money for dental care, excessive intake of refined sugars and family history of periodontal disease also need to be identified. Some older people may also be at risk, for example, those who choose salty and enamel-eroding sugary foods because of a decline in their number of taste buds. The decreased saliva production in older adults, which produces a dry mouth and thinning of the oral mucosa, is another factor.

A dry mouth can be aggravated by poor fluid intake, heavy smoking, alcohol use, high salt intake, anxiety and many medications. Medications that can cause dryness of the mouth include diuretics; laxatives, if used excessively; and tranquillisers, such as chlorpromazine and diazepam. Some chemotherapeutic agents used to treat cancer also cause oral dryness and lesions. A common side-effect of the anticonvulsant drug phenytoin is gingival hyperplasia. Optimal oral hygiene (e.g. brushing with a soft toothbrush and flossing) is needed.

Patients who are receiving or have received radiation treatments to the head and neck may have permanent damage to salivary glands. This results in a very dry mouth and can often be treated by providing a thick liquid called *artificial saliva*. Some patients prefer to just sip on liquids to moisten their mouth. Radiation can also cause damage to teeth and jaw structure, with actual damage occurring years after the radiation.

Other common risk factors (Department of Health, 2005) are:

- diets high in sugary foods and drinks, including 'hidden' added sugars in foods that would not be expected to contain sugars;
- inappropriate infant feeding practices;
- poor oral hygiene;
- dry mouth (xerostomia);
- smoking/use of tobacco and other carcinogenic substances;
- excessive alcohol consumption.

Common Problems of the Mouth

Dental caries (cavities) and periodontal disease are the two problems that most frequently affect the teeth. Both problems are commonly associated with plaque and tartar deposits. Plaque is an *invisible* soft film that adheres to the enamel surface of teeth; it consists of bacteria, molecules of saliva and remnants of epithelial cells and leukocytes. When plaque is unchecked, tartar (dental calculus) is formed. **Tartar** is a visible, hard deposit of plaque and dead bacteria that forms at the gum lines. Tartar build-up can alter the fibres that attach the teeth to the gum and eventually disrupt bone tissue. Periodontal disease is characterised by gingivitis (red, swollen gingiva), bleeding, receding gum lines and the formation of pockets between the teeth and gums. In advanced periodontal disease (pyorrhea), the teeth are loose and pus is evident when the gums are pressed. Table 17-5 lists additional problems of the mouth.

Table 17-5 Common Problems of the Mouth

Problem	Description	Nursing implications
Halitosis	Bad breath	Teach or provide regular oral hygiene
Glossitis	Inflammation of the tongue	As above
Gingivitis	Inflammation of the gums	As above
Periodontal disease	Gums appear spongy and bleeding	As above
Reddened or excoriated mucosa		Check for ill-fitting dentures
Excessive dryness of the buccal mucosa		Increase fluid intake as health permits
Cheilosis	Cracking of lips	Lubricate lips, use antimicrobial ointment to prevent infection as prescribed
Dental caries	Teeth have darkened areas, may be painful	Advise patient to see a dentist
Sordes	Accumulation of foul matter (food, micro-organisms and epithelial elements) in the mouth	Teach or provide regular cleaning
Stomatitis	Inflammation of the oral mucosa	Teach or provide regular cleaning
Parotitis	Inflammation of the parotid salivary glands	Teach or provide regular oral hygiene

ASSESSING THE MOUTH

Assessment of the patient's mouth and hygiene practices includes (a) a nursing history to provide a baseline, (b) physical assessment of the mouth and (c) identification of patients at risk for developing oral problems.

Nursing Health History

During the nursing health history, the nurse obtains data about the patient's oral hygiene practices, including dental visits, self-care abilities and past or current mouth problems. Data about the patient's oral hygiene help the nurse determine learning needs and incorporate the patient's needs and preferences in the plan of care. Assessment of the patient's self-care abilities determines the amount and type of nursing assistance to provide. Patients whose hand coordination is impaired, whose cognitive function is impaired, whose illness alters energy levels and motivation, or whose therapy imposes restrictions on activities will need assistance from the nurse. Information about past or current problems alerts the nurse to specific interventions required or referrals that may be necessary. Questions to elicit this information are shown in the *Assessment Interview*.

From the information gathered during the assessment, the medical history of the patient and the physical examination carried out, the care needs of the patient can be planned.

ASSESSMENT INTERVIEW

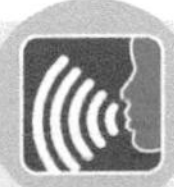

Oral Hygiene

Oral Hygiene Practices

- What are your usual mouth care and/or denture care practices?
- What oral hygiene products do you routinely use (e.g. mouth-wash, type of toothpaste, dental floss, denture cleaner)?
- When was your last dental examination, and how often do you see your dentist?

Self-Care Abilities

- Do you have any problems managing your mouth care?

Past or Current Mouth Problems

- Have you had or do you have any problems such as bleeding, swollen or reddened gums, ulcerations, lumps or tooth pain?

PLANNING

In planning care, the nurse and, if appropriate, the patient and/or family set outcomes for identified problem or self-care deficit. The nurse then performs nursing interventions and activities to achieve the patient outcomes.

During the planning phase, the nurse also identifies interventions that will help the patient achieve these goals. Specific, detailed nursing activities taken by the nurse may include the following:

- Monitor regularly for dryness of the oral mucosa.
- Monitor for signs and symptoms of glossitis (inflammation of the tongue) and stomatitis (inflammation of the mouth).
- Assist dependent patients with oral care.
- Provide special oral hygiene for patients who are debilitated, unconscious or have lesions of the mucous membranes or other oral tissues.
- Teach patients about good oral hygiene practices and other measures to prevent tooth decay.
- Reinforce oral hygiene regimen as part of discharge teaching.

IMPLEMENTING

Good oral hygiene (see *Procedure 17-4*) includes daily stimulation of the gums, mechanical brushing and flossing of the teeth, and flushing of the mouth. The nurse is often in a position to help people maintain oral hygiene by helping or teaching them to clean the teeth and oral cavity, by inspecting whether patients (especially children) have done so, or by actually providing mouth care to patients who are ill or incapacitated. The nurse can also be instrumental in identifying problems that require the intervention of a dentist or oral surgeon and arranging a referral.

PROCEDURE 17-4 Mouth Care

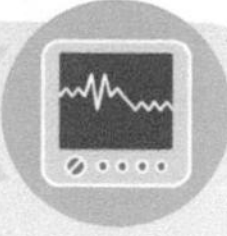

Purposes

- To maintain cleanliness within the oral cavity, in order to reduce the risk of infection, discomfort and pain, thus promoting the patient's ability to take diet and nutrients to ensure their well-being
- To ensure teeth/dentures are kept clean and plaque free to reduce the possibility of ulcers or gum disease

Assessment

Assess

- Whether the patient is in pain or any discomfort
- Whether the patient requires analgesia prior to the procedure
- The patient's normal oral hygiene practice.
- Any dentures or part dentures; if so, it is important to assess whether they fit properly
- Difficulty with swallowing
- Dysphagia
- Medical treatment that may have side-effects, e.g. prone to bleeding gums, etc.
- Patient feeling nauseous

Planning

Equipment

- Clean tray
- Plastic cups
- Mouthwash or clean solutions
- Appropriate equipment for cleaning
- Clean receiver or bowl
- Paper tissues
- Wooden spatula
- Small-headed, soft toothbrush
- Toothpaste
- Disposable gloves
- Denture pot
- Small torch

Implementation

Performance

1 Follow local policy to ensure that you explain to the patient what you are going to do, why it is necessary and how they can cooperate. Obtain consent and maintain patient privacy and dignity and ensure that the appropriate local infection control procedures are observed.

2 Ensure that the patient is pain free and in a comfortable position (normally semi-recumbant position).

3 Put on disposable gloves.

4 Prepare the solutions required. *Solutions must always be prepared immediately before use to maximise their efficacy and minimise the risk of microbial contamination.*

5 Remove the patient's dentures if the patient is unable to do this (see Figure 17-18).
   - Using a tissue or piece of gauze, grasp the upper plate of the front teeth with the thumb and second finger and move the denture up and down slightly. Lower and remove the upper plate and place in denture pot.

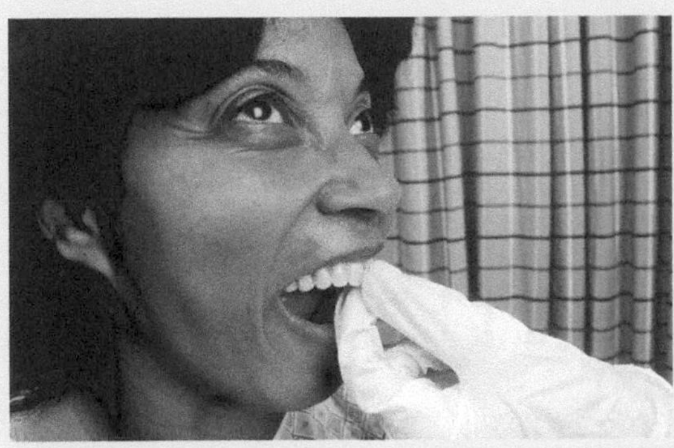

Figure 17-18 Removing the top dentures by first breaking the suction.

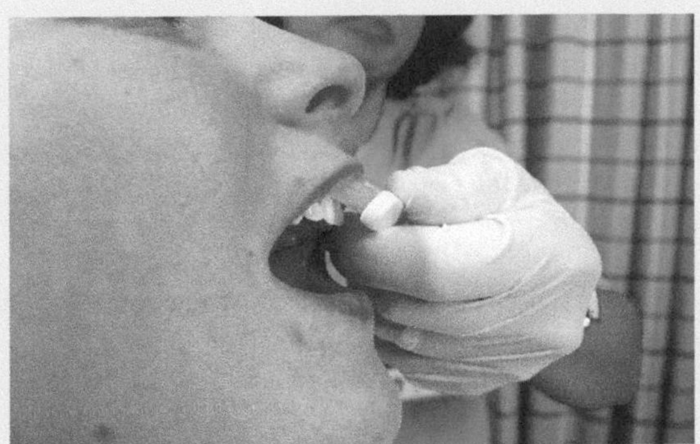

Figure 17-19 The sulcular technique: place the bristles at a 45-degree angle with the tips of the outer bristles under the gingival margins.

Removal of dentures is necessary for cleaning of underlying tissues. A tissue or ***topical*** *swab provides a firmer grip of the dentures and prevents contact with the patient's saliva. The slight movement breaks the suction that secures the plate.*

- Lift the lower plate, turning it so that one side is lower than the other, remove and place in denture pot. *Lifting the lower plate at an angle helps removal of the denture without stretching the lips.*
- Remove a partial denture by exerting equal pressure on the border of each side of the denture. *Holding the clasps could result in damage or breakage.*

6 Inspect the inside of the mouth with the aid of a torch and spatula. *The mouth is examined for changes in condition with respect to moisture, cleanliness, infected or bleeding areas, ulcers, etc.*

7 Clean the patient's natural teeth.

- Using a soft toothbrush and toothpaste (see Figure 17-19) (or foam swab if the gingival is damaged) (see Figure 17-20), brush the patient's natural teeth, gums and tongue, *to remove adherent materials from the teeth, tongue and gum surfaces. Brushing stimulates gingival tissues to maintain tone and prevent circulatory stasis.*
- Hold the brush against the teeth with the bristles at a 45° angle. The tips of the outer bristles should rest against and penetrate under the gingival sulcus to the crowns of the teeth. Repeat until all teeth surfaces have been cleaned. *Brushing loosens and removes debris trapped on and between teeth and gums, reducing the growth medium for pathogenic organisms and minimising the risk of plaque formation and dental caries. Foam swabs are ineffective for this.*
- Clean the biting surfaces by moving the toothbrush back and forth over them in short strokes. Provide a beaker of water or give a mouthwash to the patient.
- Encourage patient to rinse the mouth vigorously then void contents into a receiver. Paper tissues should be to hand. *Rinsing removes loosened debris and toothpaste and makes the mouth taste fresher. The glycerine content of toothpaste will have a drying effect if left in the mouth.*

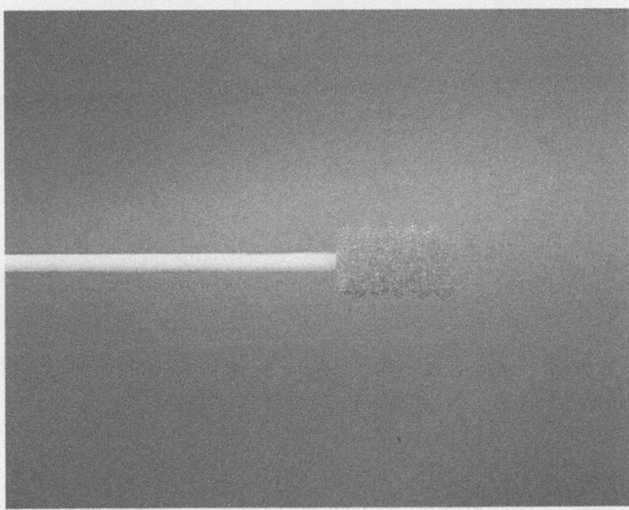

Figure 17-20 Example of foam swab used to clean mouth of a dependent patient.

- If the patient is immunosuppressed, do not allow to rinse directly into a sink. *Reservoirs of stagnant water may harbour Pseudomonas bacteria.*
- If the patient is unable to rinse and void, use a rinsed toothbrush to clean the teeth and moistened foam swabs to wipe the gums and oral mucosa. Foam swabs should be used with a rotating action so that most of the surface is utilised. *To remove debris as effectively as possible.*
- Apply artificial saliva to the tongue if appropriate and/or suitable lubricant to dry lips. *To increase the patient's feeling of comfort and well-being and prevent further tissue damage.*

8 Clean the patient's dentures on all surfaces with a denture brush or toothbrush. Hold dentures over a sink of water in case they are dropped (Clay, 2000; Curzio and McCowan, 2000). Check the dentures for cracks, sharp edges and missing teeth (Curzio and McCowan, 2000). Rinse them

well and return them to the patient. *Cleaning dentures removes accumulated food debris which could be broken down by salivary enzymes to products which irritate and cause inflammation of the adjacent mucosal tissue. Some commercial denture cleaners may have an abrasive effect on the denture surface. This then attracts plaque and encourages bacterial growth.*

9 Dentures should be removed at night and placed in a suitable cleaning solution (Sweeney *et al.* 1995; Clay, 2000).

10 Dentures should be soaked in diluted antifungal for 4-6 hours daily if oral *Candida* species are present. *Soaking in diluted antifungal reduces the risk of re-infecting the mouth with infected dentures.*

11 Floss teeth (unless contraindicated, e.g. clotting abnormality) once in 24 hours using lightly waxed floss (Clay, 2000). To floss upper teeth, use your thumb and index finger to stretch the floss and wrap one end of floss around the third finger of each hand. Move the floss up and down between the teeth from the tops of the crowns to the gum and along the gum lines wherever possible. To floss the lower teeth, use the index fingers to stretch the floss. *Flossing helps to remove debris between teeth.*

12 Discard remaining mouthwash solutions. *To prevent the risk of contamination.*

13 Clean and thoroughly dry the toothbrush. *To reduce the risk of cross-infection.*

14 Wash hands with soap and water or alcohol hand rub and dry with paper towel.

15 Dispose of the equipment appropriately and document any abnormal findings.

Source: Dougherty and Lister, 2008.

Evaluation

- Make sure that the patient remains pain free and comfortable.
- Conduct any follow-up indicated during your care of the patient.

CLINICAL ALERT

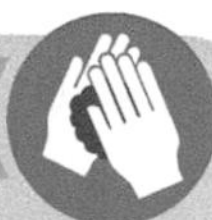

Long-term use of lemon-glycerine swabs can lead to further dryness of the mucosa and changes in tooth enamel. Mineral oil is contraindicated because aspiration of it can initiate an infection (lipid pneumonia).

EVALUATING

Using data collected during care – status of oral mucosa, lips, tongue, teeth, and so on – the nurse judges whether desired outcomes have been achieved.

If outcomes are not achieved, the nurse and patient need to explore the reasons before modifying the care plan. Examples of questions to consider are as follows:

- Did the nurse overestimate the patient's functional abilities?
- Is the patient's hand coordination or cognitive function impaired?
- Did the patient's condition change?
- Has there been a change in the patient's energy level and/or motivation?

ACTIVITY 17-2

Michael is a 69-year-old gentleman who lives with his wife at home. Michael was a chief executive of an organisation and prided himself on his appearance; he is well known and highly thought of locally. During his admission you notice that he has a rather unkempt appearance and it is evident that he has lost weight. From the initial assessment, Michael's wife informs you that during his rugby days Michael lost his two front teeth and has had a bridge which was fitted many years ago. Michael has been admitted into your care as he is very forgetful due to his dementia, and loss of weight. His wife informs you that Michael will often say that he has eaten a large meal when in fact he hasn't eaten anything at all. During Michael's admission you note that, even when he is sat at the table for lunch, Michael appears reluctant to eat. From reading the above section, reflect on the information and explore what you could do to help raise the awareness of any oral problems that Michael may have.

HAIR

Hair is divided into two components: the shaft and the root. The shaft is what is visible to the eye above the skin surface and the root is hidden underneath the skin. Hair growth is cyclical and has both a growing and a resting phase.

The appearance of the hair often reflects a person's feelings, self-concept and socio-cultural well-being. Becoming familiar with hair care needs and practices that may be different than our own is an important aspect of providing competent nursing care to all patients. People who feel ill may not groom their hair as before. A dirty scalp and hair are itchy, uncomfortable and can have an odour. The hair may also reflect state of health (e.g. excessive coarseness and dryness may be associated with endocrine disorders such as hypothyroidism).

Each person has a particular way of caring for hair. Many dark-skinned people need to oil their hair daily because it tends to be dry. Oil prevents the hair from breaking and the scalp from drying. A wide-toothed comb is usually used because finer combs pull and break the hair. Some people brush their hair vigorously before retiring; others comb their hair frequently.

Developmental Variations

Newborns may have lanugo (the fine hair on the body of the foetus, also referred to as *down* or *woolly hair*) over their shoulders, back and sacrum. This generally disappears, and the hair distribution on the eyebrows, head and eyelashes of young children subsequently becomes noticeable. Some newborns have hair on their scalps; others are free of hair at birth but grow hair over the scalp during the first year of life.

Pubic hair usually appears in early puberty followed in about six months by the growth of axillary hair. Boys develop facial hair in later puberty.

In adolescence, the sebaceous glands increase in activity as a result of increased hormone levels. As a result, hair follicle openings enlarge to accommodate the increased amount of sebum, which can make the adolescent's hair more oily.

In older adults, the hair is generally thinner, grows more slowly and loses its colour as a result of ageing tissues and diminishing circulation. Men often lose their scalp hair and may become completely bald. This phenomenon may occur even when a man is relatively young. The older person's hair also tends to be drier than normal. With age, axillary and pubic hair becomes finer and scanter, in contrast to the eyebrows, which become bristly and coarse. Many women develop hair on their faces, which may be a concern to them and impact on their self-esteem and self-image.

ASSESSING HAIR

Assessment of the patient's hair, hair care practices and potential problems includes a nursing health history and physical assessment.

Nursing Health History

During the patient history/assessment the nurse elicits data about usual hair care, self-care abilities, history of hair or scalp problems, and conditions known to affect the hair. Chemotherapeutic agents and radiation of the head may cause alopecia (hair loss). Hypothyroidism may cause the hair to be thin, dry and/or brittle. Use of some hair dyes and curling or straightening preparations can cause the hair to become dry and brittle. Examples of questions to ask to gain information are shown in the *Assessment Interview*.

ASSESSMENT INTERVIEW

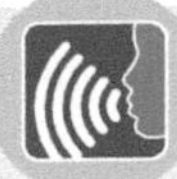

Hair Care

Hair Care Practices

- What is your normal hair care practice?
- What hair care products do you routinely use (e.g. hair gel or wax, hair spray, lubricant, shampoo, conditioners, hair dye, curling or straightening preparations)?

Self-Care Abilities

- Do you have any problems managing your hair?

Past or Current Hair Problems

- Have you had any of the following conditions or therapies: recent chemotherapy, hypothyroidism, radiation of the head, unexplained loss of hair, and growth of excessive body hair?

Physical Assessment

Problems identified may include dandruff, hair loss, **pediculosis**, scabies and hirsutism.

Dandruff

Often accompanied by itching, **dandruff (seborrhea)** appears as a diffuse scaling of the scalp. In severe cases it involves the auditory canals and the eyebrows. Dandruff can usually be treated effectively with a commercial shampoo. In severe or persistent cases, the patient may need specialist prescribed shampoo.

Hair Loss

Hair loss and growth are continual processes. Some permanent thinning of hair normally occurs with ageing. Baldness, common in men, is thought to be a hereditary problem for which there is no known remedy other than the wearing of a hairpiece or a costly surgical hair transplant, in which hair is taken from the back or the sides of the scalp and surgically moved to the hairless area. Although some medications are being developed, their long-term outcomes are unknown.

Pediculosis (Lice)

Lice are parasitic insects that infest mammals. Infestation with lice is called **pediculosis**. Hundreds of varieties of lice infest humans. Three common kinds are *Pediculus capitis* (the head louse), *Pediculus corporis* (the body louse) and *Pediculus pubis* (the crab louse).

Pediculus capitis is found on the scalp and tends to stay hidden in the hairs; similarly, *Pediculus pubis* stays in pubic hair. *Pediculus corporis* tends to cling to clothing, so that when a patient undresses, the lice may not be in evidence on the body; these lice suck blood from the person and lay their eggs on the clothing. The nurse can suspect their presence in the clothing if (a) the person habitually scratches, (b) there are scratches on the skin and (c) there are haemorrhagic spots on the skin where the lice have sucked blood.

Head and pubic lice lay their eggs on the hairs; the eggs look like oval particles, similar to dandruff, clinging to the hair. Bites and pustular eruptions may also be noticed at the hair lines and behind the ears.

Lice are very small, greyish white and difficult to see. The crab louse in the pubic area has red legs. Lice may be contracted from infested clothes and direct contact with an infested person.

The treatment often includes topical pediculicides. Another treatment, occlusive agents, is used by some. The idea is that an oily substance, such as olive oil, smothers the lice and they die.

Removal of nits (eggs) after applying the treatment is not necessary to prevent spread but most people remove them for aesthetic reasons (Frankowski and Weiner, 2002). Fine-toothed 'nit' combs are available. Transmission is from head-to-head contact and it is suggested that the hair care items and bedding of the person who has the lice infestation be washed with hot water.

Scabies

Scabies is a contagious skin infestation by the itch mite. The characteristic lesion is the burrow produced by the female mite as it penetrates into the upper layers of the skin. Burrows are short, wavy, brown or black, threadlike lesions most commonly observed between the webs of the fingers and the folds of the wrists and elbows. The mites cause intense itching that is more pronounced at night because the increased warmth of the skin has a stimulating effect on the parasites. Secondary lesions caused by scratching include vesicles, papules, pustules, excoriations and crusts. Treatment involves thorough cleansing of the body with soap and water to remove scales and debris from crusts, and then an application of a scabicide lotion. All bed linens and clothing should be washed in very hot or boiling water.

Hirsutism

The growth of excessive body hair is called hirsutism. The acceptance of body hair in the axillae and on the legs is largely dictated by culture. Well-groomed women, as depicted in magazines, have no hair on their legs or under their axillae. Equally important to be aware of is that currently many men now partially or fully remove unseemly hair from their body. Excessive facial hair on a woman is thought unattractive in most Western and Asian cultures. For example, some Japanese brides follow the custom of shaving their faces the day before the wedding.

The cause of excessive body hair is not always known. Older women may have some on their faces, and women in menopause may also experience the growth of facial hair. Excessive body hair may be due to the action of the endocrine system. Heredity is also thought to influence the pattern of hair distribution.

PLANNING

In planning care, the nurse and, if appropriate, the patient and/or family set outcomes for each identified nursing problem. The nurse then performs nursing interventions and activities to achieve the patient outcomes.

The specific, detailed nursing activities undertaken by the nurse to assist the patient should take into account the patient's personal preferences, health and energy resources as well as the time, equipment and personnel available. Often, patients like to receive hair care after a bath, before receiving visitors, and before retiring.

IMPLEMENTING

Hair needs to be brushed or combed daily and washed (see *Procedure 17-5*) as needed, to keep it clean. Nurses may need to provide hair care for patients who cannot meet their own self-care needs.

Brushing and Combing Hair

To be healthy, hair needs to be brushed daily. Brushing has three major functions: it stimulates the circulation of blood in the scalp; it distributes the oil along the hair shaft; and it helps to arrange the hair.

Long hair may present a problem for patients confined to bed because it may become matted. It should be combed and brushed at least once a day to prevent this. A brush with stiff bristles provides the best stimulation to blood circulation in the scalp. The bristles should not be so sharp that they injure the patient's scalp, however. A comb with dull, even teeth is advisable. A comb with sharp teeth might injure the scalp; combs that are too fine can pull and break the hair. Some patients are pleased to have their hair tied neatly in place. It is also important to note that dark-skinned people often have thicker, drier, curlier hair than light-skinned people. Very curly hair may stand out from the scalp. Although the shafts of curly or kinky hair look strong and wiry, they have less strength than straight hair shafts and can break easily.

PROCEDURE 17-5 Providing Hair Care for Patients

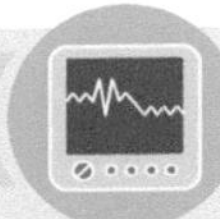

Purposes

- To increase the patient's sense of well-being
- To assess or monitor hair or scalp problems (e.g. matted hair or dandruff)

Assessment

Determine

- History of the following conditions or therapies: recent chemotherapy, hypothyroidism, radiation of the head, unexplained hair loss and growth of excessive body hair
- Usual hair care practices and routinely used hair care products (e.g. hair spray, shampoo, conditioners, hair oil preparation, hair dye, curling or straightening preparations)
- Whether wetting the hair will make it difficult to comb. Kinky hair is easier to comb when wet, however, it is very difficult to comb when it dries (Jackson, 1998: 102)

Assess

- Condition of the hair and scalp. Is the hair straight, curly, kinky? Is the hair matted or tangled? Is the scalp dry?
- Evenness of hair growth over the scalp, in particular, any patchy loss of hair; hair texture, oiliness, thickness or thinness; presence of lesions, infections or infestations on the scalp; presence of hirsutism
- Self-care abilities (e.g. any problems managing hair care)

Planning

Equipment

- Clean brush and comb
- A wide-toothed comb is usually used for many people, especially those who have curly or a thick headset of hair. Finer combs pull the hair into knots and may also break the hair
- Towel
- Hair oil preparation, if appropriate

Implementation

Performance

1 Follow local policy to ensure that you explain to the patient what you are going to do, why it is necessary and how they can cooperate. Obtain consent and maintain patient privacy and dignity and ensure that the appropriate local infection control procedures are observed.

2 Position and prepare the patient appropriately.
   - Assist the patient who can sit to move to a chair. *Hair is more easily brushed and combed when the individual is in a sitting position.* If health permits, assist a patient confined to a bed to a sitting position by raising the head of the bed. Otherwise, assist the patient to alternate side-lying positions, and do one side of the head at a time.
   - If the patient remains in bed, place a clean towel over the pillow and the patient's shoulders. Place it over the sitting patient's shoulders. *The towel collects any removed hair, dirt and scaly material.*
   - Remove any pins or ribbons in the hair.

3 Remove any mats or tangles gradually.
   - Mats can usually be pulled apart with fingers or worked out with repeated brushings.
   - If the hair is very tangled, rub alcohol or an oil, such as mineral oil, on the strands to help loosen the tangles.
   - Comb out tangles in a small section of hair towards the ends. Stablilise the hair with one hand and comb towards the ends of the hair with the other hand. *This avoids scalp trauma.*

4 Brush and comb the hair.
   - For short hair, brush and comb one side at a time. Divide long hair into two sections by parting it down the middle from the front to the back. If the hair is very thick, divide each section into front and back subsections or into several layers.

5 Arrange the hair as neatly and attractively as possible, according to the individual's desires.
   - Braiding long hair helps prevent tangles.

6 Document assessments and special nursing interventions. Daily combing and brushing of the hair are not normally recorded.

Evaluation

- Conduct ongoing assessments for problems such as dandruff, alopecia, pediculosis, scalp lesions or excessive dryness or matting.
- Evaluate effectiveness of medication (e.g. for treating pediculosis), if appropriate.

CLINICAL ALERT

Checking all types of hair is essential as all types of hair could be infested with lice.

Shampooing the Hair

Hair should be washed as often as needed to keep it clean. There are several ways to shampoo patients' hair, depending on their health, strength and age. The patient who is well enough to take a shower can shampoo while in the shower. The patient who is unable to shower may be given a shampoo while sitting on a chair in front of a sink. The back-lying patient who can move to a stretcher can be given a shampoo on a stretcher wheeled to a sink. The patient who must remain in bed can be given a shampoo with water brought to the bedside.

Inflatable hair wash trays or a bowl or large jug can be used as a receptacle for the shampoo water. If possible, the receptacle should be large enough to hold all shampoo water so that it does not have to be emptied during the shampoo.

Water used for the shampoo should be warm enough for an adult or child and be comfortable and not injure the scalp. Dry shampoos are also available. They will remove some of the dirt, odour and oil. Their main disadvantage is that they dry the hair and scalp.

How often a person needs a shampoo is highly individual, depending largely on the person's activities and the amount of **sebum** secreted by the scalp. Oily hair tends to look stringy and dirty, and it feels unclean to the person. *Procedure 17-6* explains how to provide a shampoo for a patient confined to bed.

PROCEDURE 17-6 Shampooing the Hair of a Patient Confined to Bed

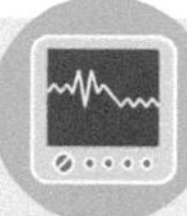

Purposes

- To clean the hair and increase the patient's sense of well-being

Assessment

Determine

- Any routinely used shampoo products

Assess

- Any scalp problems
- Activity tolerance of the patient

Planning

Equipment

- Comb and brush
- Plastic sheet or pad
- Two bath towels
- Shampoo basin
- Washcloth or pad
- Inflatable hair wash tray or receptacle for the shampoo water
- Cotton balls (optional)
- Jug of water
- Liquid or cream shampoo
- Any treatments
- Hair dryer if required

Implementation

Preparation

- Determine the type of shampoo to be used (e.g. medicated shampoo).
- Determine the best time of day for the shampoo. Discuss this with the patient. A person who must remain in bed may find the shampoo tiring. Choose a time when the patient is rested and can rest after the procedure.

Performance

1 Follow local policy to ensure that you explain to the patient what you are going to do, why it is necessary and how they can cooperate. Obtain consent and maintain patient privacy and dignity and ensure that the appropriate local infection control procedures are observed.

2 Position and prepare the patient appropriately.
- Assist the patient to the side of the bed from which you will work.
- Remove all hair accessories, i.e. hair grips, etc. from the hair.

3 Arrange the equipment.
- Put the plastic sheet or pad on the bed under the head. *The plastic keeps the bedding dry.*
- Remove the pillow from under the individual's head, and place it under the shoulders unless there is some underlying condition (e.g. neck surgery, arthritis of the neck). *This hyperextends the neck.*
- Tuck a towel around the patient's shoulders. *This keeps the shoulders dry.*
- Place the inflatable hair wash tray or basin under the head (see Figure 17-21), putting a folded washcloth or pad where the patient's neck rests on the edge of the basin. If the patient is on a stretcher, the neck can rest on the edge of the sink with the washcloth as padding. *Padding supports the muscles of the neck and prevents undue strain and discomfort.*
- Fanfold the top bedding down to the waist, and cover the upper part of the patient with a towel. The folded bedding will stay dry, and the towel, which can be discarded after the shampoo, will keep the patient warm.
- Place the receiving receptacle on a table or chair at the bedside. Put the spout of the inflatable hair wash tray in over the receptacle.

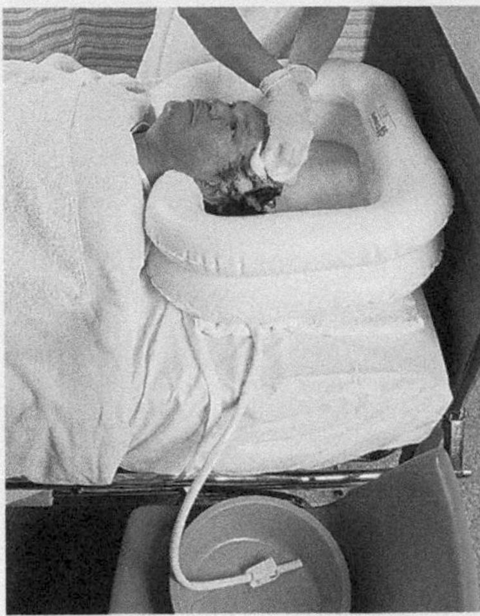

Figure 17-21 Shampooing the hair of a patient confined to bed. Note the shampoo basin and the receptacle below.
Source: Jenny Thomas.

4 Protect the patient's eyes and ears.
- Place a damp washcloth over the patient's eyes. The washcloth protects the eyes from soapy water. A damp washcloth will not slip.
- Place cotton balls in the patient's ears if indicated. *These keep water from collecting in the ear canals.*

5 Shampoo the hair.
- Wet the hair thoroughly with the water.
- Apply shampoo to the scalp. Make a good lather with the shampoo while massaging the scalp with the pads of your fingertips. Massage all areas of the scalp systematically, for example, starting at the front and working towards the back of the head. *Massaging stimulates the blood circulation in the scalp. The pads of the fingers are used so that the fingernails will not scratch the scalp.*
- Rinse the hair briefly, and apply shampoo again.
- Make a good lather and massage the scalp as before.
- Rinse the hair thoroughly this time to remove all shampoo. Shampoo remaining in the hair may dry and irritate the hair and scalp.
- Squeeze as much water as possible out of the hair with your hands.

6 Dry the hair thoroughly.
- Rub the patient's hair with a heavy towel.
- Dry the hair with the dryer. Set the temperature at the setting that is most comfortable for the patient.
- Rotate the position of the hairdryer to prevent burning the patient's scalp.

7 Ensure patient comfort.
- Assist the person confined to bed to a comfortable position.
- Arrange the hair using a clean brush and comb.

8 Document all relevant information following the procedure.

Evaluation

- Conduct ongoing assessments such as any scalp problems or intolerance to the procedure. Report any problems noted to the nurse in charge.

LIFESPAN CONSIDERATIONS

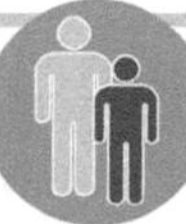

Hair Care

Infants

- Shampoo an infant's hair daily to prevent seborrhea.

Children

- Monitor school-age children for head lice (pediculosis).

Mature Adults

- Ensure adequate warmth for mature adults when shampooing their hair, because they are susceptible to chilling.

Facial Hair - Beard and Moustache Care

Beards and moustaches also require daily care. The most important aspect of the care is to keep them clean. Food particles tend to collect in beards and moustaches, and they need washing and combing periodically. Patients may also wish a beard or moustache trim to maintain a well-groomed appearance.

Male patients often shave or are shaved after a bath/shower (see *Practice Guidelines*).

PRACTICE GUIDELINES

Using a Safety Razor to Shave Facial Hair

Equipment

- Towel
- Safety razor
- Basin of warm water.
- Wipes
- Kidney shaped bowl (to periodically rinse the razor)
- Soap or shaving foam
- Aftershave or face cream
- Disposable sharps box (for razor)

Preparation

- Check with hospital policy to ensure that safety razors may be used. In some areas only personal electric razors may be used.
- Ask the patient which method of shaving they prefer, i.e. wet or dry shave. This is a means of establishing consent.
- Wear gloves in case facial nicks occur and you come in contact with blood.
- Apply shaving cream or soap and water to soften the bristles and make the skin more pliable.
- Hold the skin taut, particularly around creases, to prevent cutting the skin.
- Hold the razor so that the blade is at a 45-degree angle to the skin, and shave in short, firm strokes in the direction of hair growth (see Figure 17-22).
- After shaving the entire area, wipe the patient's face with a wet washcloth to remove any remaining shaving cream and hair.

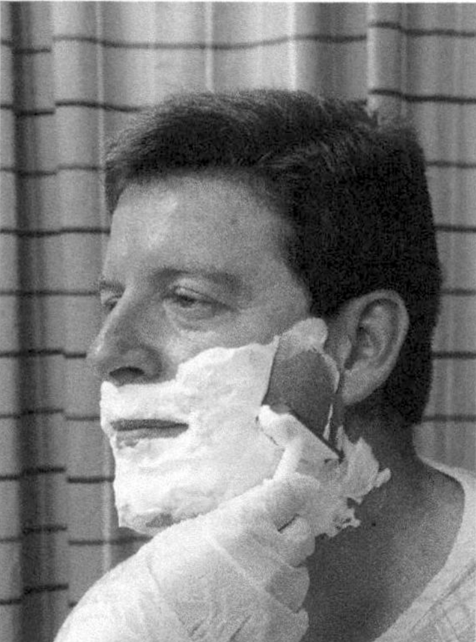

Figure 17-22 Shaving in the direction of hair growth.
Source: Jenny Thomas.

- Dry the face well, then apply aftershave lotion or powder as the patient prefers.
- To prevent irritating the skin, pat on the lotion with the fingers and avoid rubbing the face.
- Clear away both the wash bowl and the kidney dish.
- Dispose or store the razor as per hospital policy.

EVALUATING

Using data collected during care, the nurse judges whether desired outcomes have been achieved. Examples of patient outcomes that are measurable or observable include the patient being able to:

- perform hair grooming with assistance (specify);
- exhibit clean, well-groomed, resilient hair with a healthy sheen;
- reduce or get rid of scalp lesions or infestations;
- describe factors, interventions and preventive measures for specific hair problem (e.g. dandruff).

EYES

Normally eyes require no special hygiene, because lacrimal fluid continually washes the eyes, and the eyelids and lashes prevent the entrance of foreign particles. Special interventions are needed, however, for unconscious patients and for patients recovering from eye surgery or having eye injuries, irritations or infections. In unconscious patients, the blink reflex may be absent, and excessive drainage may accumulate along eyelid margins. In patients with eye trauma or eye infections, excessive discharge or drainage is common. Excessive secretions on the lashes need to be removed before they dry on the lashes as crusts. Individuals who wear eyeglasses, contact lenses or an artificial eye also may require instruction from and care by the nurse.

ASSESSING EYES

Assessment of the patient's eyes includes a nursing health assessment and physical assessment.

Nursing Health History

During the initial assessment the nurse will gather information about the patient's eyeglasses or contact lenses, recent examination by an ophthalmologist, and any history of eye problems and related treatments. Questions to elicit these data are shown in the *Assessment Interview*.

Physical Assessment

In physical assessment, all external eye structures are inspected for signs of inflammation, excessive drainage, encrustations or other obvious abnormalities.

PLANNING

In planning care, the nurse identifies nursing activities that will assist the individual to maintain the integrity of the eye structures or a prosthesis in order to prevent eye injury and infection.

IMPLEMENTING

Nursing activities may include teaching individuals about how to insert, clean and remove contact lenses or a prosthesis, and ways to protect the eyes from injury and strain.

ASSESSMENT INTERVIEW

Eyes

For Patients Who Wear Eyeglasses

- When do you use your glasses?
- Do you wear glasses because of long- or short-sighted problems?
- What is your vision like with and without the glasses?

For Patients Who Wear Contact Lenses

- How often do you wear lenses? Daily? On special occasions?
- How long do you wear your lenses in a given day, including sleep time?
- Do you have any problems with the lenses (e.g. cleaning, insertion, removal, damage)?
- Do you carry an emergency identification label to alert others to remove the lenses and ensure appropriate care in an emergency? (If not, advise the patient to acquire one.)
- What are your insertion and removal procedures?
- What are your cleaning and storage procedures?
- Have you had any problems with either or both eyes or eyelids, such as excessive tearing, burning, redness, sensitivity to light, swelling or feelings of dryness? Describe them.
- Are you using any eyedrops or ointments? (These medications can combine chemically with soft lenses and cause lens damage and eye irritation.)

For All Patients

- When did you last have your eyesight tested?
- Are you currently taking any eye medication? If so, provide name, dosage and frequency.
- Do you have any of the following eye problems: difficulty reading or seeing objects, blurring of vision, tearing, spots or floaters, photophobia (sensitivity to light), burning, itching, pain, double vision, flashing lights or halos around lights?

Eye Care

Dried secretions that have accumulated on the lashes need to be softened and wiped away. Soften dried secretions by placing a sterile gauze moistened with sterile water or normal saline over the lid margins. Wipe the loosened secretions from the inner canthus of the eye to the outer canthus to prevent the particles and fluid from draining into the lacrimal sac and nasolacrimal duct.

If the patient is unconscious and lacks a blink reflex or cannot close the eyelids completely, drying and irritation of the cornea must be prevented. When a comatose patient's corneal reflex is impaired, eye care is essential to keep moist the areas of the cornea that are exposed to air. Lubricating eye drops may be prescribed. Suggestions for providing eye care for the comatose patient are given in the *Practice Guidelines*.

PRACTICE GUIDELINES

Eye Care for the Comatose Patient

- Administer moist compresses to cover the eyes every two to four hours.
- Clean the eyes with saline solution and gauze swabs. Wipe from the inner to outer canthus. This prevents debris from being washed into the nasolacrimal duct.
- Use new gauze for each wipe. This prevents extending infection in one eye to the other eye.
- Instill ophthalmic ointment or artificial tears into the lower lids as ordered. This keeps the eyes moist.
- If the patient's corneal reflex is absent, keep the eyes moist with artificial tears and protect the eye with a protective shield.
- Monitor the eyes for redness, exudate or ulceration.

Eyeglass Care

It is essential that the nurse exercise caution when cleaning eyeglasses to prevent breaking or scratching the lenses. Glass lenses can be cleaned with warm water and dried with a soft tissue that will not scratch the lenses. Plastic lenses are easily scratched and may require special cleaning solutions and drying tissues. When not being worn, all glasses should be placed in an appropriately labelled case and stored at the patient's bedside locker.

Contact Lens Care

Contact lenses, thin curved discs of hard or soft plastic, fit on the cornea of the eye directly over the pupil. They float on the tear layer of the eye. For some people, contact lenses offer several advantages over eyeglasses: (a) they cannot be seen and thus have cosmetic value; (b) they are highly effective in correcting some astigmatisms; (c) they are safer than glasses for some physical activities; (d) they do not fog, as eyeglasses do; and (e) they provide better vision in many cases.

Contact lenses may be either hard or soft or a compromise between the two types – gas-permeable lenses. *Hard contact lenses* are made of a rigid, unwettable, airtight plastic that does not absorb water or saline solutions. They usually cannot be worn for more than 12–14 hours and are rarely recommended for first-time wearers.

Soft contact lenses cover the entire cornea. Being more pliable and soft, they mould to the eye for a firmer fit. The duration of extended wear varies by brand from 1–30 days or more. Eye specialists recommend that long-wear brands be removed and cleaned at least once a week. These lenses require scrupulous care and handling.

Gas-permeable lenses are rigid enough to provide clear vision but are more flexible than the traditional hard lens. They permit oxygen to reach the cornea, thus providing greater comfort, and will not cause serious damage to the eye if left in place for several days.

Most patients normally care for their own contact lenses. In general, each lens manufacturer provides detailed cleaning instructions. Depending on the type of lens and cleaning method used, warm tap water, normal saline, or special rinsing or soaking solutions may be used.

All users should care appropriately for their contact lenses and have a special container to store their lenses. Some contain a solution so that the lenses are stored wet; in others, the lenses are dry. Each lens container has a slot or cup with a label indicating whether it is for the right or left lens. It is essential that the correct lens be stored in the appropriate slot so that it will be placed in the correct eye.

Removing Contact Lenses

Hard contact lenses must be positioned directly over the cornea for proper removal. If the lens is displaced, the nurse asks the patient to look straight ahead, and gently exerts pressure on the upper and lower lids to move the lens back onto the cornea. Figure 17-23 shows the steps needed to remove a hard lens. To avoid lens mixups, the nurse places the first lens in its designated cup in the storage base before removing the second lens (see Figure 17-24).

Removal of soft lenses varies in two ways. First, have the patient look forward. Retract the lower lid with one hand. Using the pad of the index finger of the other hand, move the lens down to the inferior part of the sclera. This reduces the risk of damage to the cornea. Second, remove the lens by gently

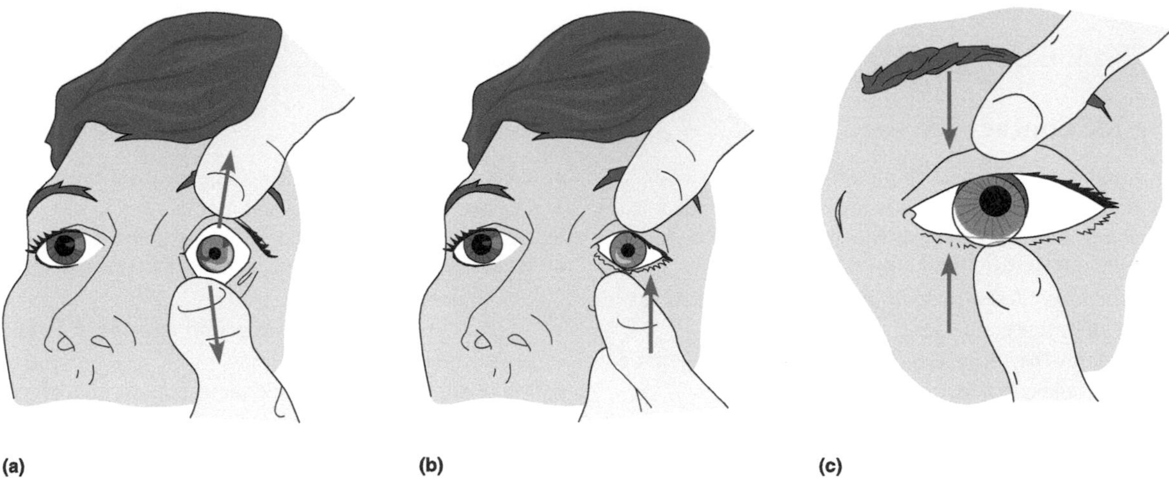

Figure 17-23 Removing hard contact lenses.

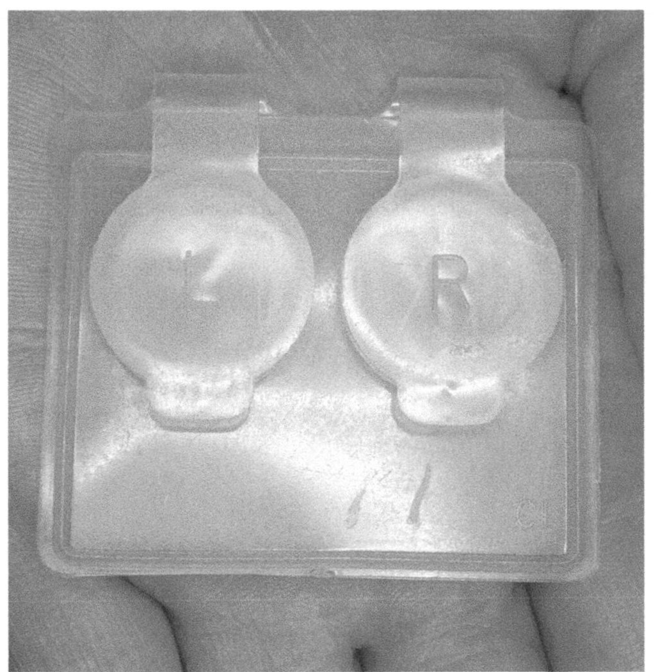

Figure 17-24 Storing lenses. Place the first lens in its designated cup in the storage case before removing the second lens. This avoids mixing up two potentially different lenses.
Source: David Parker/Science Photo Library Ltd.

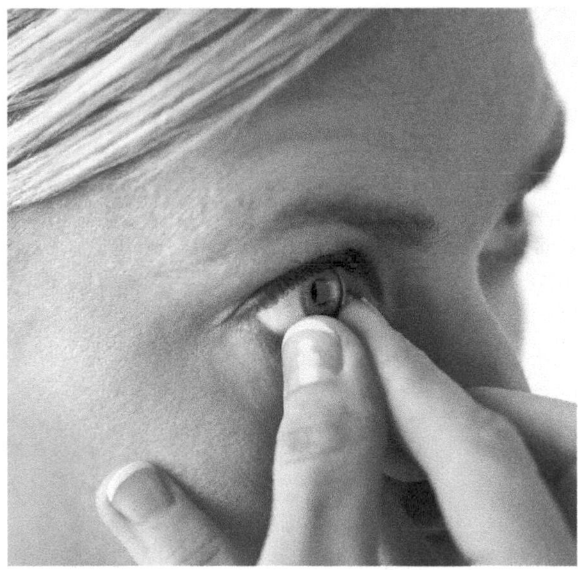

Figure 17-25 Removing a soft lens by pinching it between the pads of the thumb and index finger.
Source: Fotolia.com./Corbis.

pinching the lens between the pads of the thumb and index finger. Pinching causes the lens to double up, so that air enters underneath the lens, overcoming the suction and allowing removal. Use the pads of the fingers to prevent scratching the eye or the lens with the fingernails. Figure 17-25 shows an individual removing her own contact lens using the method described. Please note that a nurse should wear gloves.

Inserting Contact Lenses

Seriously ill patients whose contact lenses have been removed will not need them reinserted until they become more active in their care and require the lenses to see properly. Contact lenses need to be lubricated in a sterile, nonirritating wetting solution (usually a saline solution) before they are inserted. The wetting solution helps the lens glide over the cornea, thus reducing the risk of injury. Most patients, when well, will reinsert the lenses independently.

Instructions for caring for contact lenses are given in the *Practice Guidelines*.

PRACTICE GUIDELINES

Caring for Contact Lenses

- Wash and dry hands prior to handling the lenses.
- Rub, rinse and store the lenses in the recommended solution before and after each use (except single-use lenses, which should be discarded after each wear).
- Clean the lens case with solution, wipe with a clean tissue then air-dry after each use.
- Always apply the same lens first to avoid mixing them up.
- Check the lens is not inside out before applying.
- Handle carefully to avoid damaging the lens.
- Apply the lenses before putting on make-up or creams, etc.
- Remove lenses then remove make-up (if appropriate).
- Keep eyes closed when using hairspray or other aerosols.
- Replace the lens case at least monthly.
- Discard lenses and solutions that are past their expiry date.
- Wear only the lenses specified by the contact lens practitioner.
- Stick strictly to the recommended wearing schedule and replacement frequency.
- Make sure there is an adequate supply of replacement lenses or a spare pair.
- Have an up-to-date pair of spectacles for when the lenses need to be removed.

Source: British Contact Lens Association, 2010.

Artificial Eyes

Artificial eyes are usually made of glass or plastic. Some are permanently implanted; others are removed regularly for cleaning. Most individuals who wear a removable artificial eye follow their own care regimen. Even for an unconscious patient, daily removal and cleaning are not necessary.

There are several types of prosthesis (National Artificial Eye Service, 2011):

- *Conformer* – an acrylic resin prosthesis fitted post operatively to retain the socket shape and support lids.
- *Half sphere* – an acrylic resin prosthesis manufactured using preformed moulds and cut to fit the patient's socket.
- *Special half sphere* – as for 'half sphere' but the iris and sclera are hand-painted to the patient's requirements.
- *Mould eye* – an acrylic resin prosthesis approximating to the unique shape obtained from an impression or the patient's socket. The iris and sclera are hand-painted to match patient's requirements.
- *Cosmetic shell* – an acrylic resin prosthesis approximating to the unique shape obtained from an impression taken over the patient's blind eye. The iris and sclera are hand-painted to the patient's requirements.

CLINICAL ALERT

An implant is not an ocular prosthesis.

To remove an artificial eye, the nurse puts on clean gloves and retracts the patient's lower eyelid down over the infraorbital bone while exerting slight pressure below the eyelid to overcome the suction (see Figure 17-26). An alternate method is to compress a small rubber bulb and apply the tip directly to the eye. As the nurse gradually releases the finger pressure on the bulb, the suction of the bulb counteracts the suction holding the eye in the socket and draws the eye out of the socket.

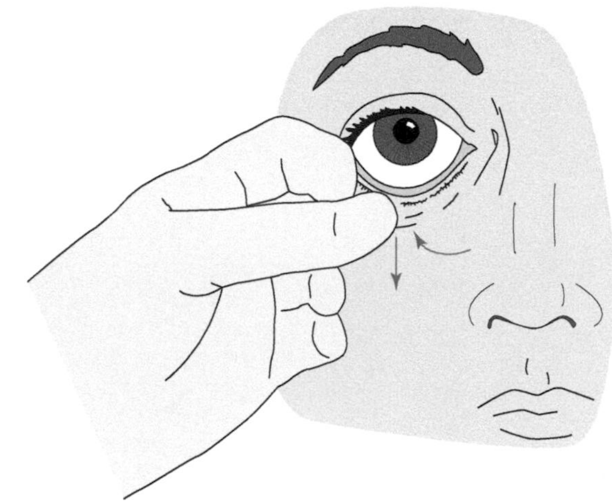

Figure 17-26 Removing an artificial eye by retracting the lower eyelid and exerting slight pressure below the eyelid.

The eye is cleaned with warm normal saline and placed in a container filled with water or saline solution. The socket and tissues around the eye are usually cleaned with cotton wipes and normal saline. To reinsert the eye, the nurse uses the thumb and index finger of one hand to retract the eyelids, exerting pressure on the supraorbital and infraorbital bones. Holding the eye between the thumb and index finger of the other hand, the nurse slips the eye gently into the socket (see Figure 17-27).

General Eye Care

Many individuals may need to learn specific information about care of the eyes. Some examples follow.

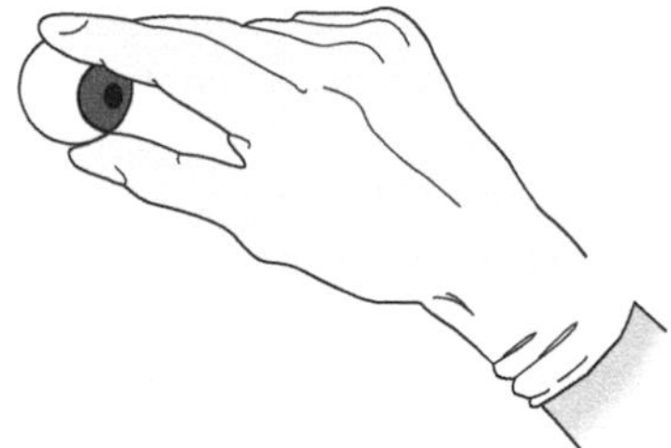

Figure 17-27 Holding an artificial eye between the thumb and index finger for insertion.

- Avoid home remedies for eye problems. Eye irritations or injuries at any age should be treated medically and immediately.
- If dirt or dust gets into the eyes, clean them copiously with clean, tepid water as an emergency treatment.
- Take measures to guard against eyestrain and to protect vision, such as maintaining adequate lighting for reading and obtaining shatterproof lenses for glasses.
- Schedule regular eye examinations, particularly after age 40, to detect problems such as **cataracts** and **glaucoma**.

EVALUATING

Using data collected during care, the nurse judges whether desired outcomes have been achieved. Examples of desired outcomes to evaluate the effectiveness of nursing interventions follow:

- conjunctive and sclera free of inflammation;
- eyelids free of secretions;
- no tearing;
- no eye discomfort;
- demonstrates appropriate methods of caring for contact lenses;
- describes interventions to prevent eye injury and infection.

EARS

Normally ears require minimal hygiene. Individuals who have excessive cerumen (earwax) and dependent patients who have hearing aids may require assistance from the nurse. Hearing aids are usually removed before surgery.

Cleaning the Ears

The auricles of the ear are cleaned during the bed bath. The nurse or patient must remove excessive cerumen that is visible or that causes discomfort or hearing difficulty. Visible cerumen may be loosened and removed by retracting the auricle up and back. If this measure is ineffective, irrigation is necessary. Patients need to be advised never to use keys, toothpicks or cotton-tipped applicators to remove cerumen. Keys and toothpicks can injure the ear canal and rupture the tympanic membrane; cotton-tipped applicators can cause wax to become impacted within the canal.

Care of Hearing Aids

A hearing aid is a battery-powered, sound-amplifying device used by persons with hearing impairments. It consists of a microphone that picks up sound and converts it to electric energy, an amplifier that magnifies the electric energy electronically, a receiver that converts the amplified energy back to sound energy, and an earmould that directs the sound into the ear. There are several types of hearing aids:

- *Behind-the-ear (BTE, or postaural) aid.* This is the most widely used type because it fits snugly behind the ear. The hearing aid case, which holds the microphone, amplifier and receiver, is attached to the earmould by a plastic tube (see Figure 17-28).
- *In-the-ear aid (ITE, or intra-aural).* This one-piece aid has all its components housed in the earmould (see Figure 17-29).
- *In-the-canal (ITC) aid.* This is the most compact and least visible aid, fitting completely inside the ear canal. In addition to having cosmetic appeal, the ITC does not interfere with telephone use or the wearing of eyeglasses. However, it is not

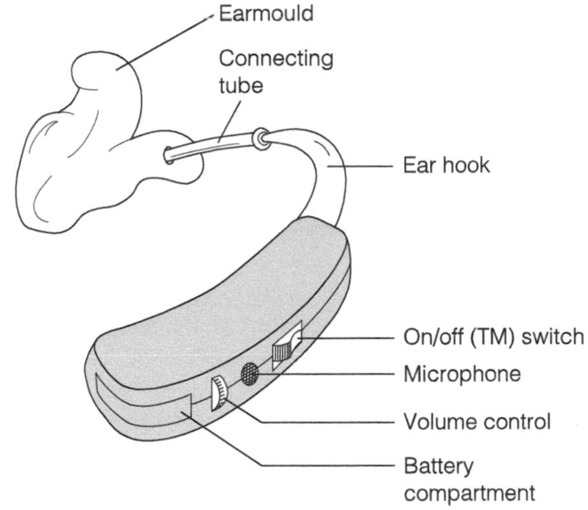

Figure 17-28 A behind-the-ear hearing aid.

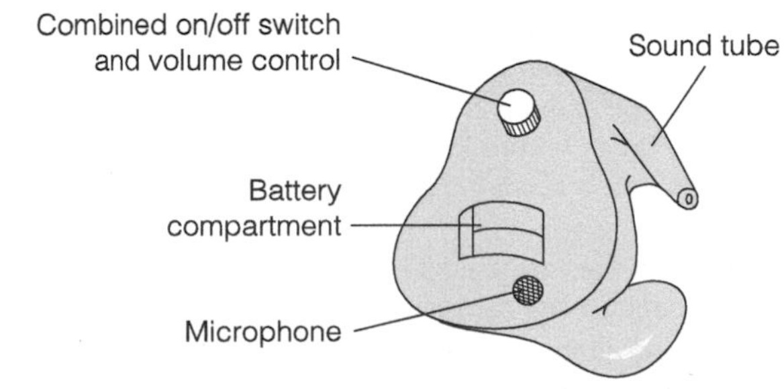

Figure 17-29 An in-the-ear hearing aid.

suitable for individuals with progressive hearing loss; it requires adequate ear canal diameter and length for a good fit; and it tends to plug with cerumen more than other aids.

- *Eyeglasses aid.* This is similar to the behind-the-ear aid, but the components are housed in the temple of the eyeglasses. A hearing aid can be in one or both temples of the glasses.
- *Body hearing aid.* This pocket-sized aid, used for more severe hearing losses, clips onto an undergarment, shirt pocket or harness carrier supplied by the manufacturer. The case, containing the microphone and amplifier, is connected by a cord to the receiver, which snaps into the earpiece.

For correct functioning, hearing aids require appropriate handling during insertion and removal, regular cleaning of the earmould, and replacement of dead batteries. With proper care, hearing aids generally last 5–10 years. Earmoulds generally need readjustment every 2–3 years. *Procedure 17-7* describes how to remove, clean and insert a hearing aid.

PROCEDURE 17-7 Removing, Cleaning and Inserting a Hearing Aid

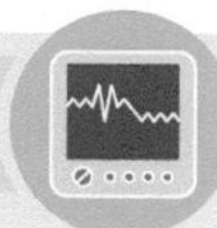

Purpose

- To maintain proper hearing aid function

Assessment

- Determine if the individual has experienced any problems with the hearing aid and hearing aid practices.
- Assess for the presence of inflammation, excessive wax, drainage or discomfort in the external ear.

Planning

Equipment

- Individual's hearing aid
- Soap, water and towels or a damp cloth
- New battery (if needed)

Implementation

Performance

1 Follow local policy to ensure that you explain to the patient what you are going to do, why it is necessary and how they can cooperate. Obtain consent and maintain patient privacy and dignity and ensure that the appropriate local infection control procedures are observed.

2 Remove the hearing aid.
- Turn the hearing aid off and lower the volume. The on/off switch may be labelled 'O' (off), 'M' (microphone), 'T' (telephone) or 'TM' (telephone/microphone). *The batteries continue to run if the hearing aid is not turned off.*
- Remove the earmould by rotating it slightly forward and pulling it outward.
- If the hearing aid is not to be used for several days, remove the battery. *Removal prevents corrosion of the hearing aid from battery leakage.*
- Store the hearing aid in a safe place and label with individual's name. Avoid exposure to heat and moisture. *Proper storage prevents loss or damage.*

3 Clean the earmould.
- Detach the earmould if possible.
- Disconnect the earmould from the receiver of a body hearing aid or from the hearing aid case of behind-the-ear and eyeglass hearing aids where the tubing meets the hook of the case. Do not remove the earmould if it is glued or secured by a small metal ring. *Removal facilitates cleaning and prevents inadvertent damage to the other parts.*
- If the earmould is detachable, soak it in a mild soapy solution. Rinse and dry it well. Do not use isopropyl alcohol. *Alcohol can damage the hearing aid.*
- If the earmould is not detachable or is for an in-the-ear aid, wipe the earmould with a damp cloth.
- Check that the earmould opening is patent. Blow any excess moisture through the opening or remove debris (e.g. earwax) with a pipe cleaner or toothpick.
- Reattach the earmould if it was detached from the rest of the hearing aid.

4 Insert the hearing aid.
- Determine from the patient if the earmould is for the left or the right ear.
- Check that the battery is inserted in the hearing aid. Turn off the hearing aid, and make sure the volume is turned all the way down. *A volume that is too loud is distressing.*
- Inspect the earmould to identify the ear canal portion. Some earmoulds are fitted for only the ear canal and

concha; others are fitted for all the contours of the ear. The canal portion, common to all, can be used as a guide for correct insertion.
- Line up the parts of the earmould with the corresponding parts of the patient's ear.
- Rotate the earmould slightly forward, and insert the ear canal portion.
- Gently press the earmould into the ear while rotating it backward.
- Check that the earmould fits snugly by asking the patient if it feels secure and comfortable.
- Adjust the other components of a behind-the-ear or body hearing aid.
- Turn the hearing aid on and adjust the volume according to the individual's needs.

5 Correct problems associated with improper functioning.
- If the sound is weak or there is no sound:
  (a) Ensure that the volume is turned high enough.
  (b) Ensure that the earmould opening is not clogged.
  (c) Check the battery by turning the hearing aid on, turning up the volume, cupping your hand over the earmould, and listening. A constant whistling sound indicates the battery is functioning. If necessary, replace the battery. Be sure that the negative (–) and positive (+) signs on the battery match those where indicated on the hearing aid.
  (d) Ensure that the ear canal is not blocked with wax, which can obstruct sound waves.
- If the individual reports a whistling sound or squeal after insertion:
  (a) Turn the volume down.
  (b) Ensure that the earmould is properly attached to the receiver.
  (c) Reinsert the earmould.

6 Document pertinent data.
- The removal and the insertion of a hearing aid are not normally recorded.
- Report and record any problems the patient has with the hearing aid.

Evaluation

- Speak to the patient in a normal conversational tone and observe patient behaviours.
- Compare the patient's hearing ability to previous assessments.

NOSE

Nurses usually need not provide special care for the nose, because patients can ordinarily clear nasal secretions by blowing gently into a soft tissue. When the external nares are encrusted with dried secretions, they should be cleaned with a cotton-tipped applicator or moistened with saline or water. The applicator should not be inserted beyond the length of the cotton tip; inserting it further may cause injury to the mucosa.

SUPPORTING A HYGIENIC ENVIRONMENT

When patient's personal hygiene needs have been met it is important to complete the procedure by changing/making the patient's bed. Because people are usually confined to bed when ill, often for long periods, the bed becomes an important element in the patient's life. A place that is clean, safe and comfortable contributes to the individual's ability to rest and sleep and to a sense of well-being. Basic furniture in a healthcare environment includes the bed, bedside table, overbed table, one or more chairs and a storage space for clothing. Most bed units also have a call light, light fixtures, electric outlets and hygienic equipment in the bedside table. Two types of equipment often installed in an acute care facility are a suction outlet for several kinds of suction and an oxygen outlet for most oxygen equipment.

Hospital Beds

The frame of a hospital bed is divided into three sections. This permits the head and the foot to be elevated separately. Many hospital beds have electric motors to operate the movable joints. The motor is activated by pressing a button or moving a small lever, located either at the side of the bed or on a small panel separate from the bed but attached to it by a cable, which the patient can readily use. Common bed positions are shown in Table 17-6.

Mattresses

Mattresses are usually covered with a water-repellent material that resists soiling and can be cleaned easily as per local policy. Many special mattresses are also used in hospitals to relieve pressure on the body's bony prominences, such as the heels. They are particularly helpful for individuals confined to bed for a long time, and should be used following an appropriate risk assessment such as the Waterlow Scale or Pressure Sore Prediction Score.

Side Rails/Cot Sides

Side rails, or safety sides, have been used on both hospital beds and trolleys. They are of various shapes and sizes and are usually

Table 17-6 Commonly Used Bed Positions

Flat Head of bed Foot of bed	Mattress is completely horizontal.	Patient sleeping in a variety of bed positions, such as back-lying, side-lying and prone (face down) To maintain spinal alignment for clients with spinal injuries To assist patients to move and turn in bed Bed-making by nurse
Fowler's position	Semi-sitting position in which head of bed is raised to angle of at least 45°. Knees may be flexed or horizontal.	Convenient for eating, reading, visiting, watching TV Relief from lying positions To promote lung expansion for client with respiratory problem
Semi-Fowler's position	Head of bed is raised only to 30° angle.	To assist a patient to a sitting position on the edge of the bed
Trendelenburg's position	Head of bed is lowered and the foot raised in a straight incline.	Relief from lying position To promote lung expansion
Reverse Trendelenburg's position	Head of bed raised and the foot lowered. Straight tilt in direction opposite to Trendelenburg's position.	To promote venous circulation in certain clients To provide postural drainage of basal lung lobes To promote stomach emptying and prevent oesophageal reflex in client with hiatus hernia

made of metal. A bed can have two full-length side rails or four half- or quarter-length side rails (also called split rails). Devices to raise and lower side rails differ. Often one or two knobs are pulled to release the side and permit it to be moved. When side rails are being used, it is important that the nurse never leaves the bedside while the rail is lowered. Some side rails have two positions: up and down. Others have three: high, intermediate and low.

For decades, the use of side rails has been routine practice with the rationale that the side rails serve as a safe and effective means of preventing patients from falling out of bed. However, research has identified that in many instances when patients are restricted they are exposed to different injuries from e.g. climbing over cot sides. Several studies have shown that raised side rails do not deter older patients from getting out of bed unassisted and have led to more serious falls, injuries and even death (Talerico, 2003; Wagner *et al.*, 2007). It is therefore imperative that an appropriate risk assessment is undertaken prior to using cot sides. The use of cot sides should only be used as per local and national policies. Alternatives to side rails do exist and can include low-height bed, mats placed at the side of the bed, motion sensors and bed alarms.

Bed Cradles

A bed cradle is a device designed to keep the top bedclothes off the feet, legs and even abdomen of a patient. The bedclothes are arranged over the device and may be pinned in place. There are several types of bed cradles. One of the most common is a curved metal rod that fits over the bed. Part of the cradle fits under the mattress, and small metal brackets press down on each side of the mattress to keep the cradle in place. The frame of some cradles extends over half of the width of the bed, above one leg. The use of bed cradles is controversial and an appropriate risk assessment should be undertaken before their use and local and national policies adhered to.

Intravenous Stands

Intravenous stands usually made of metal, support intravenous (IV) infusion containers while fluid is being administered to a patient. These rods were traditionally freestanding on the floor beside the bed. Now, intravenous stands are often attached to the hospital beds and attached to an electric power point, making moving patients when making beds more difficult.

MAKING BEDS

Nurses need to be able to prepare hospital beds in different ways for specific purposes. Indeed it is evident from clinical observation that even within one hospital bed-making differs from clinical area to clinical area.

In most instances, beds are made after the patient receives certain care and when beds are unoccupied. At times, however, nurses need to make an occupied bed or prepare a bed for a patient who is having surgery (an anaesthetic, post-operative or surgical bed). Regardless of what type of bed equipment is available, whether the bed is occupied or unoccupied, or the purpose for which the bed is being prepared, certain *Practice Guidelines* pertain to all bed-making.

PRACTICE GUIDELINES

Bed-Making

- It is good practice to make beds with a colleague, as it is better use of resources and time management. Wash hands thoroughly after handling a patient's bed linen. Linens and equipment that have been soiled with secretions and excretions harbour micro-organisms that can be transmitted to others directly or by the nurse's hands or uniform.
- Hold soiled linen away from uniform.
- Linen for one patient is never (even momentarily) placed on another patient's bed.
- Place soiled linen directly in a portable linen skip or tucked into a pillow case at the end of the bed before it is gathered up for disposal.
- Do not shake soiled linen in the air because shaking can disseminate secretions and excretions and the micro-organisms they contain.
- When stripping and making a bed, conserve time and energy by stripping and making up one side as much as possible before working on the other side.
- To avoid unnecessary trips to the linen supply area, gather all linen before starting to strip a bed.

Unoccupied Bed

An unoccupied bed can be either closed or open. Generally the top covers of an open bed are folded back (thus the term *open bed*) to make it easier for a patient to get in. Open and closed beds are made the same way, except that the top sheet, blanket and bedspread of a *closed bed* are drawn up to the top of the bed and under the pillows.

Beds are often changed after bed baths. The linen can be collected before the bath. The linen is not usually changed unless it is soiled. Unfitted sheets, blankets and bedspreads are mitred at the corners of the bed. The purpose of mitring is to secure the bedclothes while the bed is occupied. Figure 17-30 shows how to mitre the corner of a bed. *Procedure 17-8* explains how to change an unoccupied bed.

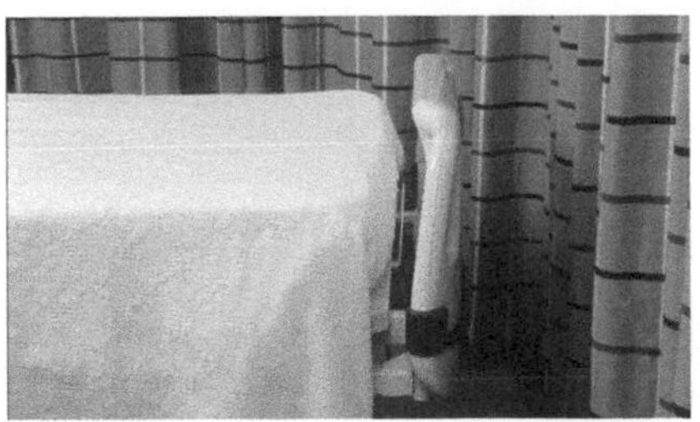

(a)

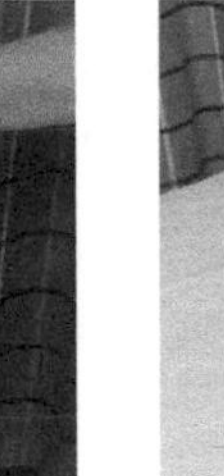

(b)

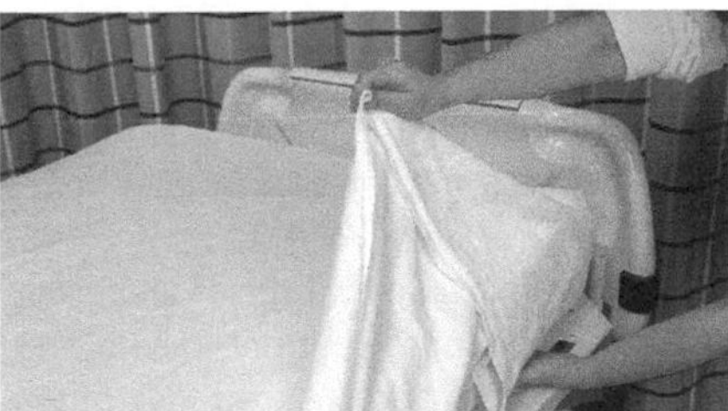

(c)

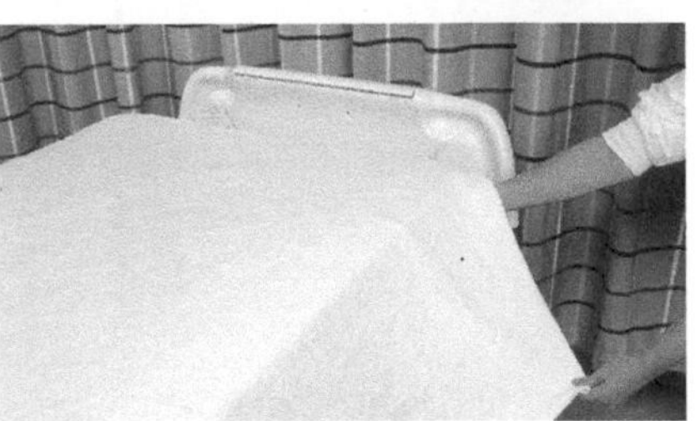

(d)

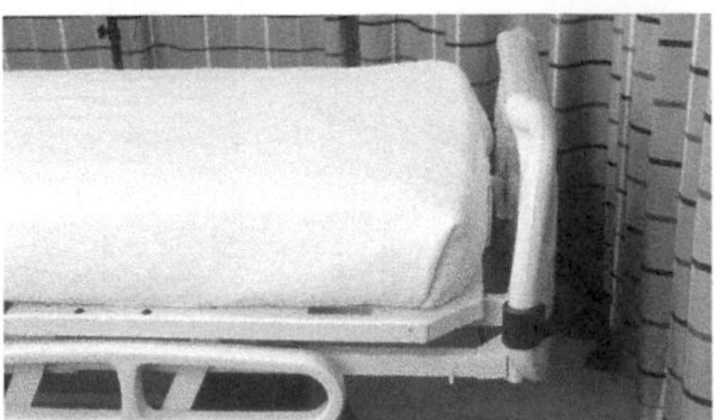

(e)

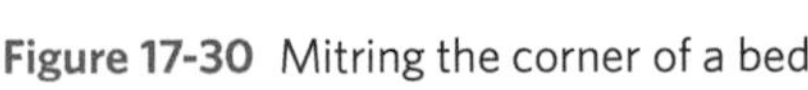

Figure 17-30 Mitring the corner of a bed.
Source: Pearson Education Ltd.

PROCEDURE 17-8 Changing an Unoccupied Bed

Purposes

- To promote the individual's comfort
- To provide a clean neat environment for the patient
- To provide a smooth, wrinkle-free bed foundation, thus minimising sources of skin irritation

Assessment

- Assess the patient's health status to determine that the person can safely get out of bed
- Note all the tubes and equipment connected to the patient because this may influence the need for additional linens or waterproof pads

Planning

Equipment

- One pair of sheets
- Cloth drawsheet (optional)
- One blanket
- One bedspread
- Waterproof drawsheet or waterproof pads (optional)
- Pillowcase(s) for the head pillow(s)
- Plastic laundry bag or portable linen basket/skip, if available

Implementation

Preparation

Determine what linens the patient may already have in the room *to avoid stockpiling of unnecessary extra linens.*

Performance

1 Follow local policy to ensure that you explain to the patient what you are going to do, why it is necessary and how they can cooperate. Obtain consent and maintain patient privacy and dignity and ensure that the appropriate local infection control procedures are observed.
2 Place the fresh linen on the patient's chair or overbed table; do not use another patient's bed. This prevents cross-contamination (the movement of micro-organisms from one patient to another) via soiled linen.
3 Assess and assist the patient out of bed (as per moving and handling policy).
   - Make sure that this is an appropriate and convenient time for the patient to be out of bed.
   - Assess and ensure safety of any infusions or any drainage tubes attached to the patient or the bed linen.
   - Assist the patient to a comfortable chair.
4 Raise the bed to a comfortable working height.
5 Strip the bed.
   - Check bed linens for any items belonging to the patient and detach the call bell or any drainage tubes from the bed linen.
   - Loosen all bedding systematically, starting at the head of the bed on the far side and moving around the bed up to the head of the bed on the near side. *Moving around the bed systematically prevents stretching and reaching and possible muscle strain.*
   - Remove the pillowcases, if soiled, and place the pillows on the bedside chair near the foot of the bed.
   - Fold reusable linens, such as the bedspread and top sheet on the bed, into fourths. First, fold the linen in half by bringing the top edge even with the bottom edge, and then grasp it at the centre of the middle fold and bottom edges (see Figure 17-31). *Folding linens saves time and energy when reapplying the linens on the bed.*
   - Remove the waterproof pad and discard it if soiled.

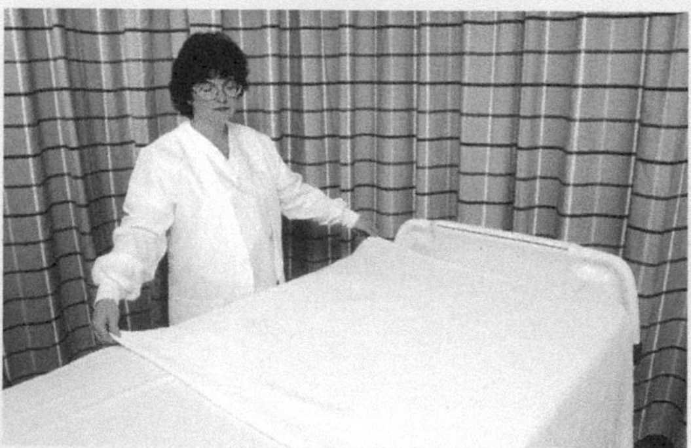

Figure 17-31 Fold reusable linens into fourths when removing them from the bed.
Source: Pearson Education Ltd.

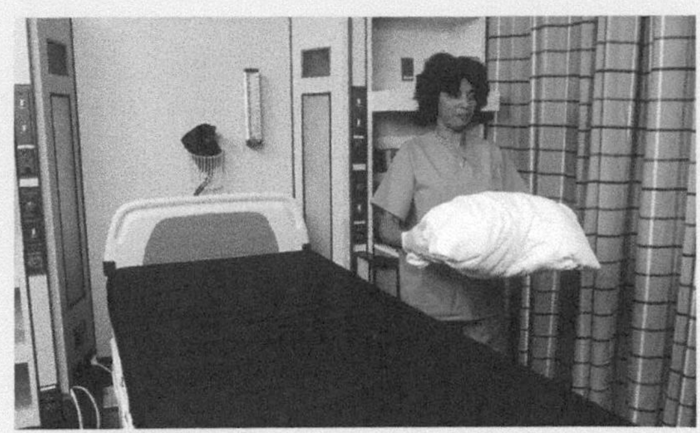

Figure 17-32 Roll soiled linen inside bottom sheet and hold away from body.

- Roll all soiled linen inside the bottom sheet, hold it away from your uniform, and place it directly in the linen hamper (see Figure 17-32). *These actions are essential to prevent the transmission of micro-organisms to the nurse and others.*
- Grasp the mattress securely, using the lugs if present, and move the mattress up to the head of the bed.

6 Apply the bottom sheet and drawsheet.

- Place the folded bottom sheet with its centre fold on the centre of the bed. Make sure the sheet is hem side down for a smooth foundation. Spread the sheet out over the mattress, and allow a sufficient amount of sheet at the top to tuck under the mattress (see Figure 17-33). *The top of the sheet needs to be well tucked under to remain securely in place, especially when the head of the bed is elevated.* Place the sheet along the edge of the mattress at the foot of the bed and do not tuck it in (unless it is a contour or fitted sheet).
- Mitre the sheet at the top corner on the near side (Figure 17-30, earlier) and tuck the sheet under the mattress, working from the head of the bed to the foot.
- If a waterproof drawsheet is used, place it over the bottom sheet so that the centre fold is at the centreline of the bed and the top and bottom edges extend from the middle of the patient's back to the area of the midthigh or knee. Fanfold the uppermost half of the folded drawsheet at the centre or far edge of the bed and tuck in the near edge (see Figure 17-34).

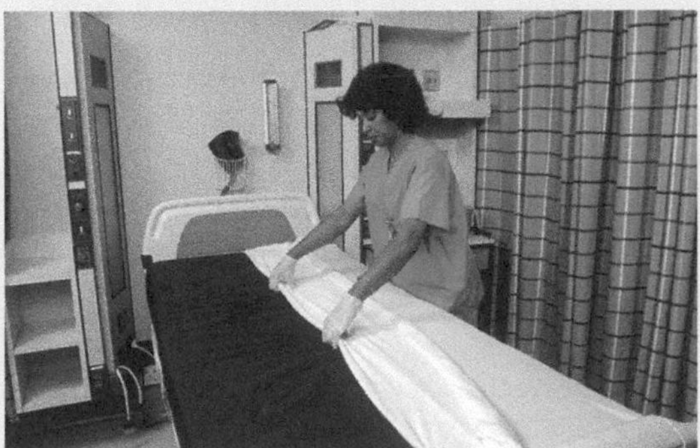

Figure 17-33 Placing bottom sheet on bed.

Source: all images on this page © Pearson Education Ltd.

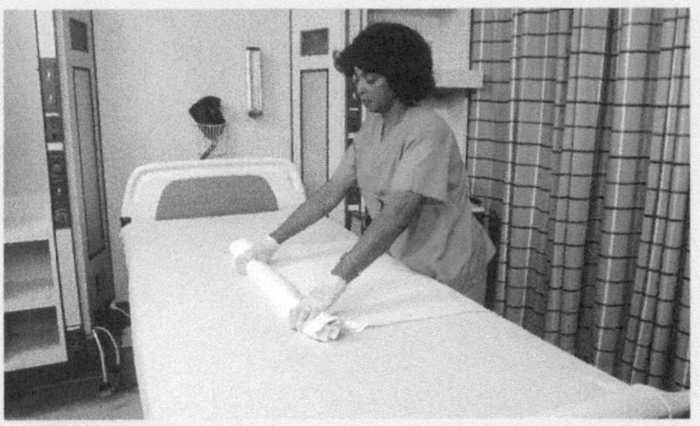

Figure 17-34 Placing drawsheet on bed.

- Lay the cloth drawsheet over the waterproof sheet in the same manner.
- *Optional:* Before moving to the other side of the bed, place the top linens on the bed hemside up, unfold them, tuck them in and mitre the bottom corners. *Completing one entire side of the bed at a time saves time and energy.*

7 Move to the other side and secure the bottom linens.

- Tuck in the bottom sheet under the head of the mattress, pull the sheet firmly and mitre the corner of the sheet.
- Pull the remainder of the sheet firmly so that there are no wrinkles. Wrinkles can cause discomfort for the patient. Tuck the sheet in at the side.
- Complete this same process for the drawsheet(s).

8 Apply or complete the top sheet, blanket and spread.

- Place the top sheet, hemside up, on the bed so that its centre fold is at the centre of the bed and the top edge is even with the top edge of the mattress.
- Unfold the sheet over the bed.
- *Optional:* Make a vertical or a horizontal toe pleat in the sheet to provide additional room for the patient's feet.
  a) *Vertical toe pleat:* Make a fold in the sheet 5–10cm perpendicular to the foot of the bed (see Figure 17-35).
  b) Horizontal toe pleat: Make a fold in the sheet 5–10cm across the bed near the foot (see Figure 17-36).

  Loosening the top covers around the feet after the patient is in bed is another way to provide additional space.
- Follow the same procedure for the blanket and the spread, but place the top edges about 15cm from the head of the bed to allow a cuff of sheet to be folded over them.
- Tuck in the sheet, blanket and spread at the foot of the bed, and mitre the corner, using all three layers of linen. Leave the sides of the top sheet, blanket and spread hanging freely unless toe pleats where provided.

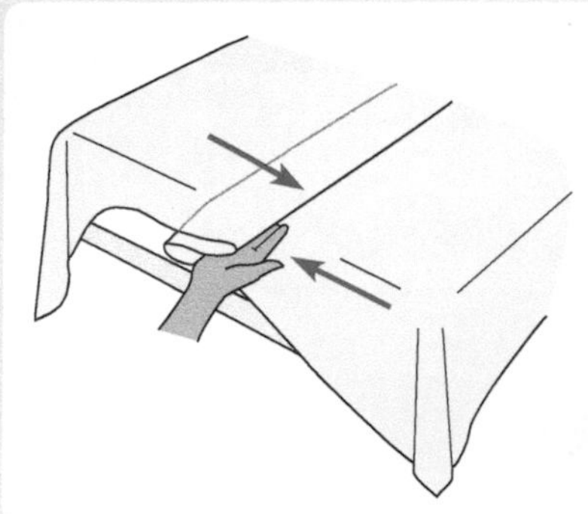

Figure 17-35 A vertical toe pleat.

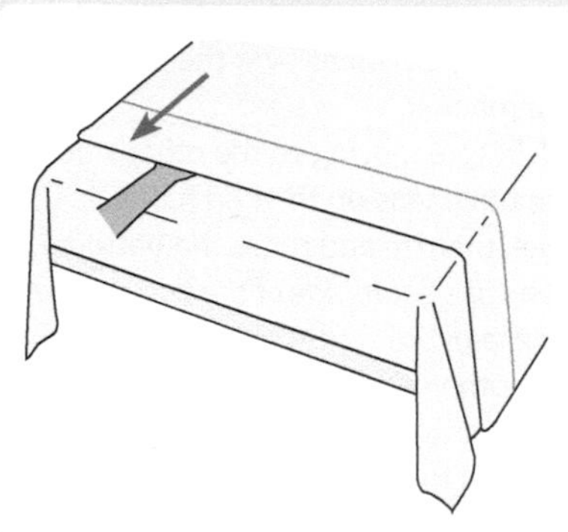

Figure 17-36 A horizontal toe pleat.

- Fold the top of the top sheet down over the spread, providing a cuff (see Figure 17-37). *The cuff of sheet makes it easier for the patient to pull the covers up.*
- Move to the other side of the bed and secure the top bedding in the same manner.

9 Put clean pillowcases on the pillows as required.
- Grasp the closed end of the pillowcase at the centre with one hand.

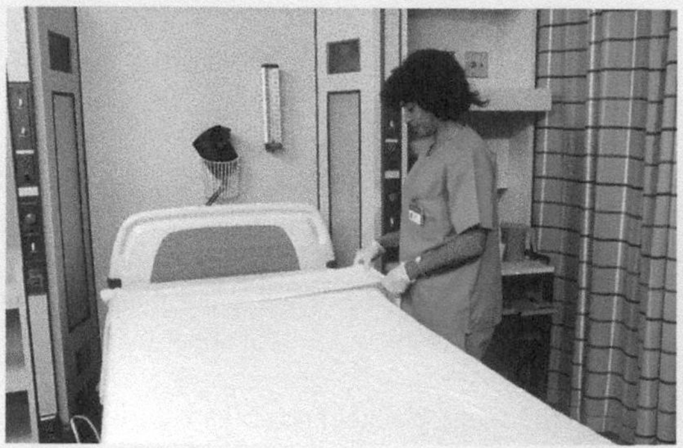

Figure 17-37 Making a cuff of the top linens.

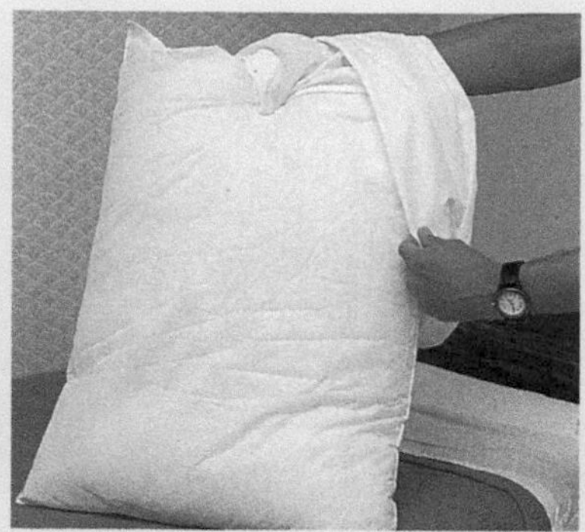

Figure 17-38 Method for putting a clean pillowcase on a pillow.

- Gather up the sides of the pillowcase and place them over the hand grasping the case. Then grasp the centre of one short side of the pillow through the pillowcase (see Figure 17-38).
- With the free hand, pull the pillowcase over the pillow.
- Adjust the pillowcase so that the pillow fits into the corners of the case and the seams are straight. *A smoothly fitting pillowcase is more comfortable than a wrinkled one.*
- Place the pillows appropriately at the head of the bed.

10 Provide for patient comfort and safety.
- Attach the signal cord so that the patient can conveniently use it. Some cords have clamps that attach to the sheet or pillowcase.
- If the bed is currently being used by a patient, either fold back the top covers at one side or fanfold them down to the centre of the bed. *This makes it easier for the patient to get into the bed.*
- Place the bedside table and the overbed table so that they are available to the patient.
- Leave the bed in the high position if the patient is returning by trolley or place in the low position if the patient is returning to bed after being out of bed.

Variation 1: surgical bed

While the patient is in the operating theatre, the patient's bed is prepared for the post-operative phase. In some clinical areas, the patient is brought back to the ward on a trolley and transferred to the bed in the room. In others, the patient's bed is brought to the operating department and the patient is transferred there. In the latter situation, the bed needs to be made with clean linens as soon as the patient goes to theatre so that it can be taken to the operating department when needed.

- Strip the bed.
- Place and leave the pillows on the bedside chair. *Pillows are left on a chair to facilitate transferring the patient into the bed.*
- Apply the bottom linens as for an unoccupied bed.

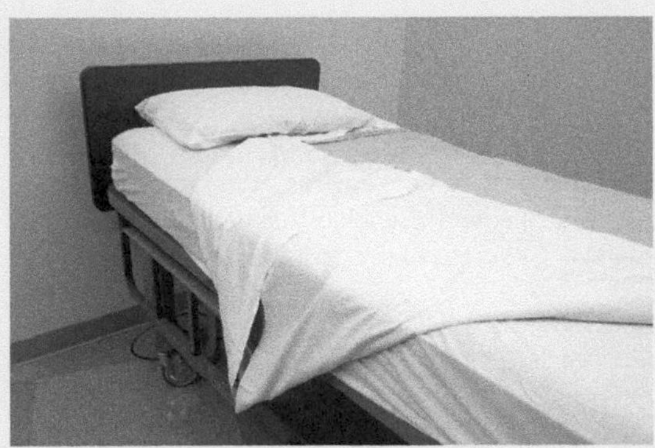

Figure 17-39 Fold up the two outer corners of the top linens forming a triangle.

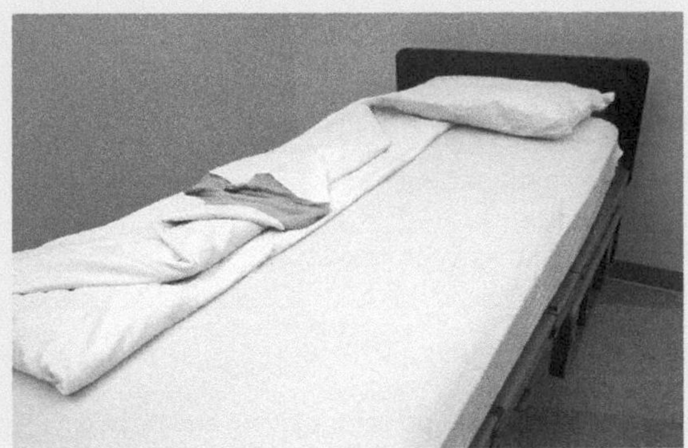

Figure 17-40 Surgical bed. The linens are horizontally fanfolded to the other side of the bed to facilitate transfer of the patient into the bed.

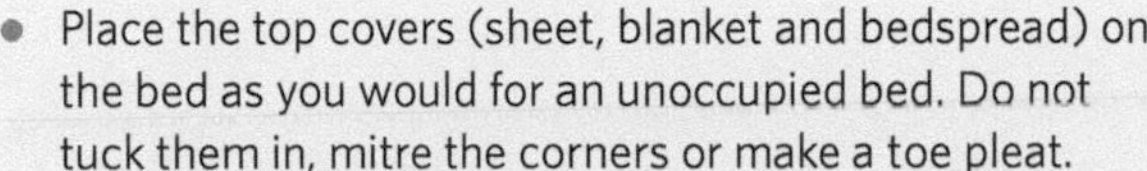

- Place the top covers (sheet, blanket and bedspread) on the bed as you would for an unoccupied bed. Do not tuck them in, mitre the corners or make a toe pleat.
- Make a cuff at the top of the bed as you would for an unoccupied bed. Fold the top linens up from the bottom.
- On the side of the bed where the patient will be transferred, fold up the two outer corners of the top linens so they meet in the middle of the bed forming a triangle (see Figure 17-39).
- Pick up the apex of the triangle and fanfold the top linens lengthwise to the other side of the bed *to facilitate the patient's transfer into the bed* (see Figure 17-40).
- Leave the bed in high position with the side rails down. *The high position facilitates the transfer of the patient.*
- Lock the wheels of the bed if the bed is not to be moved. *Locking the wheels keeps the bed from rolling when the patient is transferred from the trolley to the bed.*

Variation 2: duvet bed

Many organisations for various reasons have changed their bed linen to follow current day preferences in the home. While these changes are noted in the more traditional healthcare environment, there is a higher prevalence of duvets when caring for children and young adults, in the mental health environment and indeed in patient's homes.

Changing the bottom sheet remains as noted above and the changing of a duvet cover mimics that of changing a pillow.

Evaluation

- Make sure the call light is accessible to the patient.
- Relate patient parameters of activity (e.g. pulse and respirations) to previous assessment data particularly if the patient has been on bedrest for an extended period of time or it is the first time that the patient is getting out of bed after surgery.

Changing an Occupied Bed

Some patients may be too weak to get out of bed. Either the nature of their illness may contraindicate their sitting out of bed, or they may be restricted in bed by the presence of traction or other therapies. When changing an occupied bed (see *Procedure 17-9*), the nurse works quickly and disturbs the patient as little as possible to conserve the patient's energy, using the following guidelines:

- Maintain the patient in good body alignment. Never move or position a patient in a manner that is contraindicated by the patient's health. Obtain help to ensure safety.
- Move the patient gently and smoothly. Rough handling can cause the patient discomfort and abrade the skin.
- Explain what you plan to do throughout the procedure before you do it. Use terms that the patient can understand.
- Use the bed-making time, like the bed bath time, to assess and meet the patient's needs.

PROCEDURE 17-9 Changing an Occupied Bed

Purposes

- To conserve the patient's energy and maintain current healthy status
- To promote patient comfort
- To provide a clean, neat environment for the patient
- To provide a smooth, wrinkle-free bed foundation, thus minimising sources of skin irritation

Assessment

- Note specific precautions for moving and positioning the patient
- Determine presence of incontinence or excessive drainage from other sources indicating the need for protective waterproof pads
- Assess skin condition and need for special mattress, footboard or heel protectors
- Assess whether you will need assistance with the procedure and seek help (if so) before you begin.

Planning

Equipment

- Two flat sheets
- Cloth drawsheet (optional)
- One blanket
- One bedspread
- Waterproof drawsheet or waterproof pads (optional)
- Pillowcase(s) for the head pillow(s)
- Plastic laundry bag or portable linen basket /skip, if available

Implementation

Performance

1 Follow local policy to ensure that you explain to the patient what you are going to do, why it is necessary and how they can cooperate. Obtain consent and maintain patient privacy and dignity and ensure that the appropriate local infection control procedures are observed.

2 Remove the top bedding.
   - Remove any equipment attached to the bed linen, such as a call bell.
   - Loosen all the top linen at the foot of the bed and remove the spread and the blanket.
   - Leave the top sheet over the patient (the top sheet can remain over the patient if it is being changed and if it will provide sufficient warmth).

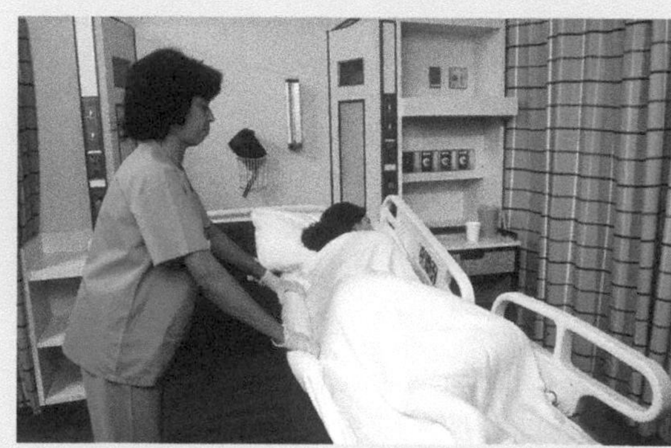

Figure 17-41 Moving soiled linen as close to the patient as possible.
Source: Pearson Education Ltd.

3 Change the bottom sheet and drawsheet.
   - Assist the patient to turn on the side facing away from the side where the clean linen is.
   - If applicable raise the side rail nearest the patient. *This protects the patient from falling.* If there is no side rail, have another nurse support the patient at the edge of the bed.
   - Loosen the foundation of the linen on the side of the bed near the linen supply.
   - Fanfold the drawsheet and the bottom sheet at the centre of the bed (see Figure 17-41), as close to the patient as possible. *Doing this leaves the near half of the bed free to be changed.*
   - Place the new bottom sheet on the bed, and vertically fanfold the half to be used on the far side of the bed as close to the patient as possible (see Figure 17-42). Tuck the sheet under the near half of the bed and mitre the corner if a contour sheet is not being used.
   - Place the clean drawsheet on the bed with the centre fold at the centre of the bed. Fanfold the uppermost half vertically at the centre of the bed and tuck the near side edge under the side of the mattress (Figure 17-43).
   - Assist the patient to roll over towards you onto the clean side of the bed. The patient rolls over the fanfolded linen at the centre of the bed.

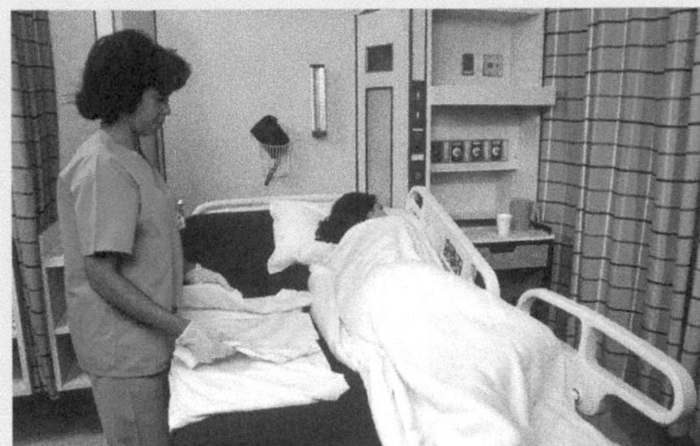

Figure 17-42 Placing new bottom sheet on half of the bed.
Source: Pearson Education Ltd.

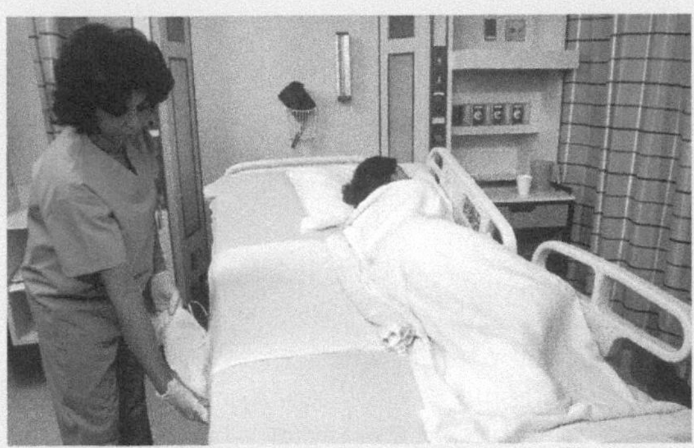

Figure 17-43 Placing clean drawsheet on the bed.
Source: Pearson Education Ltd.

- Move the pillows to the clean side for the patient's use. Raise the side rail before leaving the side of the bed.
- Move to the other side of the bed and lower the side rail.
- Remove the used linen and place it in the portable skip.
- Unfold the fanfolded bottom sheet from the centre of the bed.
- Facing the side of the bed, use both hands to pull the bottom sheet so that it is smooth and tuck the excess under the side of the mattress.
- Unfold the drawsheet fanfolded at the centre of the bed and pull it tightly with both hands. Pull the sheet in three sections: (a) face the side of the bed to pull the middle section, (b) face the far top corner to pull the bottom section and (c) face the far bottom corner to pull the top section.
- Tuck the excess drawsheet under the side of the mattress.

4 Reposition the patient in the centre of the bed.
   - Reposition the pillows at the centre of the bed.
   - Assist the patient to the centre of the bed. Determine what position the patient requires or prefers and assist the patient to that position.

5 Apply or complete the top bedding.
   - Spread the top sheet over the patient and either ask the patient to hold the top edge of the sheet or tuck it under the shoulders.
   - Complete the top of the bed.

6 Ensure continued safety of the patient.
   - Raise the side rails. Place the bed in the low position before leaving the bedside.
   - Attach the signal cord to the bed linen within the patient's reach.
   - Put items used by the patient within easy reach.

Evaluation

- Conduct appropriate follow-up, such as determining patient's comfort and safety, patency of all drainage tubes and patient's access to call light to summon help when needed.

CRITICAL REFLECTION

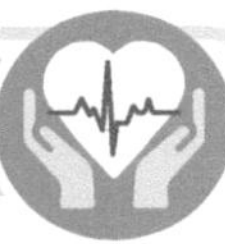

There have been several opportunities within the chapter to reflect on some of the personal hygiene practices discussed within the chapter. The case study on page 493 highlights the difficulties of maintaining these standards when accidents happen that are life changing and impede on the individual's ability to maintain their own standards. Personal hygiene encompasses all areas that affect the individual in your care and, upon reflecting on this chapter and your experience in clinical practice, you should consider the issues raised within the chapter, explore, discuss and reflect on how your practice has changed in light of the information gained and how this would improve patient care, especially in relation to Joseph and his family. Points to consider are:

- Managing and organising care
- Caring and empathy
- Respect and dignity
- Physiological, psychological and psychosocial
- Communication
- Breathing
- Eating and drinking
- Personal hygiene
- Sleeping
- Sexuality
- Mobility
- Work and play
- Family support

CHAPTER HIGHLIGHTS

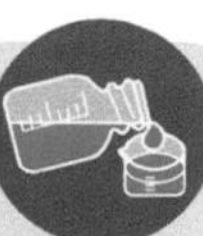

- Patients' hygienic practices are influenced by numerous factors including culture, religion, environment, developmental level, health and energy and personal preferences.
- The major functions of the skin are to: protect underlying tissues; help regulate body temperature; secrete sebum; transmit sensations through nerve receptors for sensory perception; and produce and absorb vitamin D in conjunction with ultraviolet rays from the sun.
- When planning hygiene care, the nurse must take the patient's preferences into consideration.
- Nurses provide perineal-genital care for patients who are unable to do so for themselves.
- Nurses can often teach patients how to prevent foot problems.
- Oral hygiene should include daily dental flossing and mechanical brushing of the teeth.
- Regular dental checkups and fluoride supplements are recommended to maintain healthy teeth.
- Nurses provide special oral care to patients who are unconscious or debilitated.
- Hair care includes daily combing and brushing and regular shampooing.
- Nurses may need to assist dependent patients with their artificial eyes, eyeglasses and contact lenses.
- Patients with a hearing aid may require nursing assistance with the device.
- Changing bed linens is a part of maintaining hygiene.
- It is important to keep beds clean and comfortable for patients.

ACTIVITY ANSWERS

ACTIVITY 17-1 Fred is an elderly gentleman who lives alone and is obviously at risk. There are several aspects of care for consideration relating to the cutting of Fred's toe nails and to his general well-being. On reflection, you should consider the following issues when exploring issues related to Fred's holistic care:

- Maintaining a safe environment
- Communication
- Multidisciplinary team referrals
- Infection control
- Home care support
- Health promotion

ACTIVITY 17-2 It is evident from the initial assessment of Michael that he is a respected member of the community with good social skills. It is evident, however, that both physical and psychological issues are affecting his ability to maintain his general well-being. It is evident that his dementia and possibly mouthcare issues are affecting his weight, diet any intake, etc. On reflection, it is important to recognise these issues and provide the rationale as to why, for example, ill-fitting dentures may affect his general health. Points to consider when reflecting are:

- Patient dignity
- Eating and drinking
- Personal hygiene
- Communication
- Mouth assessment
- Patient autonomy
- Psychological assessment
- Psychosocial assessment
- Self-esteem

REFERENCES

Brawley, E.C. (2002) 'Bathing environments: How to improve the bathing experience', *Alzheimer's Care Quarterly*, 3(1), 38–41.

British Contact Lens Association (2010) *The does and don'ts of contact lens wear*, London: British Contact Lens Association.

Clark, J. (2006) 'Intimate care: Theory, research and practice', *Learning Disability Practice*, 9(10), 12–17.

Clay, M. (2000) 'Oral health in older people', *Nursing Older People*, 12(7): 21–5.

Department of Health (2001) *Essence of Care*, London: Department of Health.

Department of Health (2005) *Choosing better oral healthcare – an oral health plan for England*, London: Department of Health.

Dougherty, L. and Lister, S. (2008) *The Royal Marsden Hospital manual of clinical nursing procedures* (7th edn), Oxford: Wiley-Blackwell.

Dunn J.C., Thiru-Chelvam, B., and Beck, C.H.M. (2002) 'Interdisciplinary care. Bathing: pleasure or pain?' *Journal of Gerontological Nursing*, 28(11), 6–13.

Ersser, S.J., Getliffe, K., Voegeli, D. and Regan, S. (2005) 'A critical review of the inter-relationship between skin vulnerability and urinary incontinence and related nursing intervention', *International Journal of Nursing Studies*, 42(7), 823–835.

Frankowski, B.L. and Weiner, L.B. (2002) 'Head lice', *Pediatrics*, 110(3), 638–643.

Hektor, L.M. and Touhy, T.A. (1997) 'The history of the bath: From art to task?' *Journal of Gerontological Nursing*, 23(5), 7–15.

Jackson, F. (1998) 'The ABC's of black hair and skin care', *The ABNF Journal*, 9(5), 100–104.

Lomborg, K. and Kirkevold, M. (2005) 'Curtailing: Handling the complexity of body care in people hospitalized with severe COPD', *Scandinavian Journal of Caring*, 19(2), 148–156.

National Artifical Eye Service (2011) *Definitions – types of ocular prostheses*, available at http://www.bfwh.nhs.uk/aes/definitions.htm (accessed April 2011).

NMC (2010) *Standards for pre-registration nursing education*, London: NMC.

Pillitteri, A. (2003) *Maternal and child health nursing: Care of the child bearing and child-rearing family* (4th edn), Philadelphia, PA: Lippincott Williams and Wilkins.

Rader, J., Lavelle, M., Hoeffer, B. and McKenzie, D. (1996) 'Maintaining cleanliness: An individualised approach', *Journal of Gerontological Nursing*, 22(3), 31–38.

Skewes, S. (1997) 'Bathing: It's a tough job!', *Journal of Gerontological Nursing*, 23(5), 45–49.

Society of Chiropodists and Podiatrists (2011) *Healthy feet*, available at http://www.scpod.org/footcare/healthy-feet/ (accessed April 2011).

Sweeney, M.P., Shaw, A., Yip, B. and Baqq, J. (1995) 'Oral health in elderly patients', *British Journal of Nursing*, 4(20): 1204–8.

Talerico, K.A. (2003) 'A new revolution in healthcare: Mental healthcare of older people is vital', *Journal of Psychosocial Nursing and Mental Health Services*, 41(5), 12–15.

Wagner, L.M., Capezuti, E., Brush, B., Boltz, M., Renz, S. and Talerico, K.A. (2007) 'Description of an advanced practice nursing consultative model to reduce restrictive siderail use in nursing homes', *Research in Nursing and Health*, 30(2), 131–140.

CHAPTER 18

SKIN INTEGRITY AND WOUND CARE

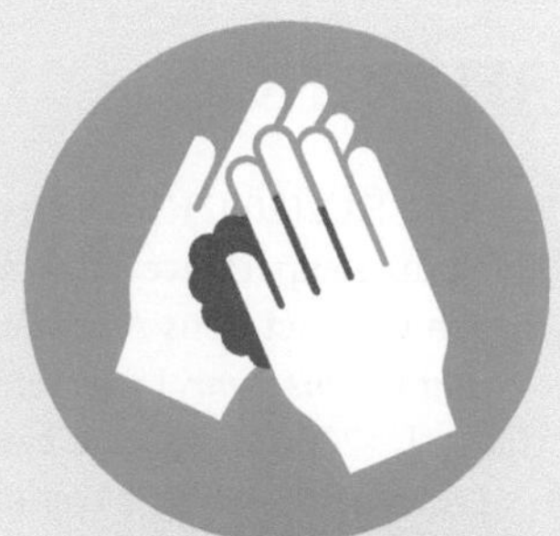

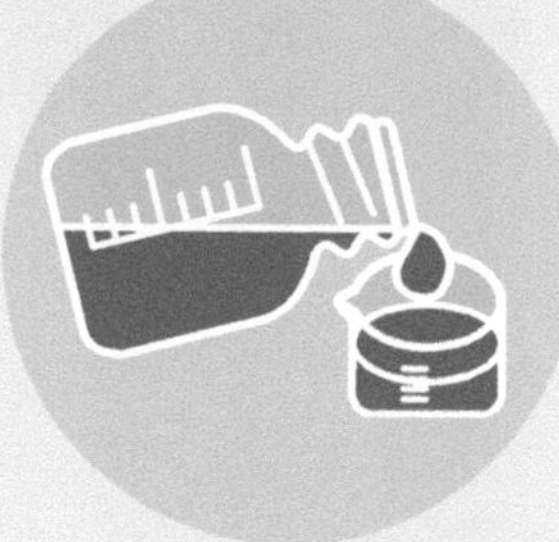

LEARNING OUTCOMES

After completing this chapter, you will be able to:

- Discuss the structure and functions of the skin.
- Describe factors affecting skin integrity.
- Describe the aetiology of pressure ulcers.
- Identify patients at risk for pressure ulcer formation and describe the four stages of pressure ulcer development.
- Discuss measures to prevent pressure ulcer formation.
- Discuss assessment information required when assessing a patient with a wound.
- Differentiate primary and secondary wound healing.
- Describe the three phases of wound healing.
- Identify the main complications of and factors that affect wound healing.
- Describe nursing strategies to treat pressure ulcers, promote wound healing and prevent complications of wound healing.
- Identify purposes of commonly used wound dressing materials and binders.

After reading this chapter you will be able to consider the factors that lead to the development of pressure ulcers and develop skills appropriate for patient wound care. The chapter relates to **Essential Skills Clusters (NMC, 2010) 1–22, 24–27, 34–36, 38–42**, as appropriate for each progression point.

Ensure that you really understand this chapter by logging on to your complimentary **MyNursingKit** at **www.pearsoned.co.uk/kozier**. Complete the self-assessment tests to check your progress and utilise further activities to practise and confirm your understanding.

CASE STUDY

Charles is a 32-year-old man who has a moderate learning disability together with **hydrocephalus**, **spastic diplegia**, **epilepsy** and is visually impaired. He currently lives at home with his aging parents, who have support from social services to care for Charles. Charles is unable to walk, normally using a customised wheelchair to get around. Over recent weeks Charles has lost approximately 10 kilograms in weight, his **Body Mass Index (BMI)** is now 19. He occasionally suffers urinary incontinence, has a poor appetite and has become withdrawn, choosing to sit in front of the television for long periods. He has developed a small grade 1 **pressure ulcer** on his coccyx.

This chapter will help you to consider the factors that have lead to the development of the pressure ulcer as well as the pressure area care required by Charles.

INTRODUCTION

Maintaining patients' skin integrity and promoting wound healing are some of the most important goals of nursing practice. Impaired skin integrity is not a frequent problem for most healthy people but is a threat to older people; to patients with restricted mobility, chronic illnesses or trauma; and to those undergoing invasive procedures. To protect the skin and manage wounds effectively, the nurse must understand the factors affecting skin integrity, the physiology of wound healing and specific measures that promote optimal skin conditions.

THE SKIN

The skin is the largest organ in the body, accounting for approximately 16% of a person's body weight (BBC, 2010). It covers the entire body and varies in thickness from 0.5 millimetres on the eyelids to 4 millimetres on the palms of an adult's hand (BBC, 2010).

Skin is made up of two main layers; the outer epidermis and the inner dermis (see Figure 18-1). The **epidermis** (outer layer of the skin) is made up of flat, scale-like squamous cells, under which are found the basal cells. The deepest part of the epidermis also contains **melanocytes**. These cells produce melanin, which gives the skin its colour. While the **dermis**, or inner layer of skin, contains blood and lymph vessels, hair follicles, nerve endings and glands.

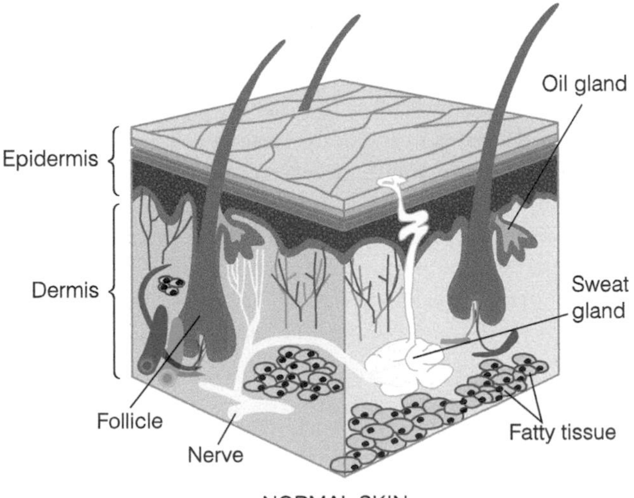

Figure 18-1 Structure of the skin.

Skin has five important functions in maintaining health and protecting the individual from injury (see Table 18-1).

Table 18-1 Functions of the Skin

Function	Action
Barrier	The skin acts as a physical barrier and first line defence against the external environment, preventing micro-organisms and other substances from entering the body (Voegeli, 2008).
Sensation	Nerve endings within the skin provide the body with information about the external environment. It provides the sense of touch and sensation.
Regulator	The skin regulates body temperature even under extreme external temperatures. The production (evaporation) of sweat in the skin cools the body, while the erection of hair follicles traps a layer of air which insulates the body from the cold.
Excretion	Waste products in solution (sweat) are excreted through the skin. Water is lost continuously through the skin as insensible sweating. More pronounced water loss through sweating occurs as part of temperature regulation.
Synthesiser	The skin has the ability to synthesise the use of vitamin D in the presence of sunlight and ultra violet radiation. Vitamin D is essential in the absorption of calcium and phosphates.

SKIN INTEGRITY

Maintaining skin integrity is a fundamental goal in nursing practice (Gardiner *et al.*, 2008). It is the nurse's role to prevent, restore and, where possible, heal skin breakages. The skin is a physical barrier to the external environment and, as such, its integrity is vital to the health of the patient. However, skin appearance and integrity can be affected by a number of intrinsic and extrinsic factors. These factors must be taken into account to prevent or manage skin breakdown:

- age
- skin type
- nutrition
- hydration
- peripheral circulation
- oedema
- reduced mobility
- trauma
- faecal/urinary incontinence
- drying or desiccation of skin
- fever/infection
- immunosuppression
- reduced sensation
- medications
- underlying diseases such as diabetes
- stress/mental health
- metabolic state.

PRESSURE ULCERS

Pressure ulcers, otherwise known as pressure sores, bedsores and decubitus ulcers, are areas of localised tissue damage believed to be caused by a combination of pressure, shear and friction (European Pressure Ulcer Advisory Panel (EPUAP), 2010).

Pressure ulcers are a problem in primary, acute and long-term care settings. Although inextricably linked with the aging adult, pressure ulcers can develop in all age groups. Vanderwee *et al.* (2007) found that 20% of patients in European acute care settings will develop a pressure ulcer, whilst the prevalence of pressure ulcers amongst hospitalised children has been estimated to be between 0.47% and 13.1% (Willock *et al.*, 2009).

Pressure ulcers place an immense strain on the NHS, costing approximately £2.64 billion per annum (Posnett and Franks, 2007). However, the true extent of the problem is difficult to measure as currently there are no standardised means of measuring incidence and prevalence of pressure ulcers across the UK (Riordan and Voegeli, 2009).

Aetiology of Pressure Ulcers

Pressure ulcers are due to localised **ischaemia**, a deficiency in the blood supply to the tissue. The tissue is caught between two hard surfaces, usually the surface of the bed and the bony skeleton. When blood cannot reach the tissue, the cells are deprived of oxygen and nutrients, the waste products of metabolism accumulate in the cells and the tissue consequently dies. Prolonged, unrelieved pressure also damages the small blood vessels.

After the skin has been compressed, it appears pale, as if the blood had been squeezed out of it. When pressure is relieved, the skin takes on a bright red flush, called **reactive hyperaemia**, which is the body's mechanism for preventing pressure ulcers. The flush is due to **vasodilation**, a process in which extra blood floods to the area to compensate for the preceding period of impeded blood flow.

Two other factors frequently act in conjunction with pressure to produce pressure ulcers: friction and shearing force. Friction is force acting parallel to the skin surface. For example, sheets rubbing against skin create friction. Friction can abrade the skin, that is, remove the superficial layers, making it more prone to breakdown.

Shearing force is a parallel force that twists and stretches tissues in opposite directions and causes tissue ischaemia by moving vessels laterally and impeding the flow of blood. This can be best illustrated by observing a patient sitting up in bed. The body will tend to slide downwards towards the foot of the bed. This downward movement is transmitted to the sacral bone and the deep tissues. At the same time, the skin over the sacrum tends not to move because of the adherence between the skin and the bed sheets. The skin and superficial tissues are thus relatively unmoving in relation to the bed surface, whereas the deeper tissues are firmly attached to the skeleton and move downward. This causes a shearing force in the area where the deeper tissues and the superficial tissues meet.

ACTIVITY 18-1

Reflect on a patient you have recently cared for. What actual or potential risk factors were evident that could have led to the development of a pressure ulcer?

Risk Factors

Several factors contribute to the formation of pressure ulcers: immobility and inactivity, inadequate nutrition, faecal and urinary incontinence, decreased mental capacity, diminished sensation, excessive body heat, ageing and the presence of certain chronic conditions.

Immobility

Normally people move when they experience discomfort due to pressure on an area of the body. Healthy people rarely exceed their tolerance to pressure. However, paralysis, extreme weakness, pain or any cause of decreased activity can hinder a person's ability to change positions independently and relieve the pressure, even if the person can perceive the pressure. According to Baumgarten *et al.* (2010) immobility is consistently a determining factor in the development of pressure ulcers.

Inadequate Nutrition

According to Riordan and Voegeli (2009) adequate nutrition is needed to maintain skin integrity. Prolonged inadequate nutrition causes weight loss, muscle atrophy and the loss of subcutaneous tissue. These three reduce the amount of padding between the skin and the bones, thus increasing the risk of pressure ulcer development. More specifically, inadequate intake of protein, carbohydrates, fluids and vitamin C contributes to pressure ulcer formation.

Hypoproteinemia (abnormally low protein content in the blood), due either to inadequate intake or abnormal loss, predisposes the patient to dependent **oedema**. Oedema (the presence of excess fluid in the tissues) makes skin more prone to injury by decreasing its elasticity, resilience and vitality. Oedema increases the distance between the capillaries and the cells, thereby slowing the diffusion of oxygen to the tissue cells and of metabolites away from the cells.

Faecal and Urinary Incontinence

Moisture from incontinence promotes skin **maceration** (tissue softened by prolonged wetting or soaking) and makes the epidermis more easily eroded and susceptible to injury. Digestive enzymes in faeces also contribute to skin **excoriation** (area of loss of the superficial layers of the skin). Any accumulation of secretions or excretions is irritating to the skin, harbours microorganisms, and makes an individual prone to skin breakdown and infection. Ersser *et al.* (2005) recognise that incontinence is a major causative factor in pressure ulcer development and state that maintaining skin integrity for a patient with incontinence is challenging for healthcare professionals.

Decreased Mental Capacity

Individuals with a reduced level of awareness, for example, those who are unconscious or heavily sedated, are at risk for pressure ulcers because they are less able to recognise and respond to pain associated with prolonged pressure (Bours *et al.*, 2001).

Diminished Sensation

Paralysis, stroke or other neurological disease may cause loss of sensation in a body area. Loss of sensation reduces a person's ability to respond to injurious heat and cold and to feel the tingling ('pins and needles') that signals loss of circulation. Keller *et al.* (2002) suggest that this is a particular problem with intensive care patients as they have reduced sensation due to analgesics and sedation and are unable to feel the painful stimuli of pressure so do not feel the need to or cannot change position to relieve the pressure.

Excessive Body Heat

Body heat is another factor in the development of pressure ulcers. An elevated body temperature increases the metabolic rate, thus increasing the cells' need for oxygen. This increased need is particularly severe in the cells of an area under pressure, which are already oxygen deficient. Severe infections with accompanying elevated body temperatures may affect the body's ability to deal with the effects of tissue compression.

Age

The ageing process brings about several changes in the skin and its supporting structures, making the older person more prone to impaired skin integrity. These changes include the following:

- loss of lean body mass;
- generalised thinning of the epidermis;
- decreased strength and elasticity of the skin due to changes in the collagen fibres of the dermis;
- increased dryness due to a decrease in the amount of oil produced by the sebaceous glands;
- diminished pain perception due to a reduction in the number of cutaneous end organs responsible for the sensation of pressure and light touch.

Older people are at increased risk of developing pressure ulcers as their skin is thinner and the layers of fat and muscle are less dense (NHS Choices, 2010). Therefore, the age of the individual should be taken into account when measuring a patient's risk of developing pressure ulcers.

Chronic Health Conditions

Certain chronic conditions such as diabetes and cardiovascular disease are risk factors for skin breakdown and delayed healing. These conditions compromise oxygen delivery to tissues by poor perfusion and thus cause poor and delayed healing and increase risk of pressure sores. Margolis *et al.* (2003) suggest that the presence of a medical condition such as diabetes increases the patient's likelihood of developing pressure ulcers and state that identification of these medical conditions should override identification of other risk factors such as incontinence and immobility.

Other Factors

Other factors contributing to the formation of pressure ulcers are poor lifting techniques (RCN, 2001), incorrect positioning, repeated injections in the same area, hard support surfaces, and incorrect application of pressure-relieving devices.

Assessment of Skin Integrity

Ongoing assessment is the key to preventing skin breakdown and the development of pressure ulcers. The initial assessment of the patient should include a physical examination of the skin as well as obtaining information about the patient's skin condition from the patient, their notes or from a family member. The nurse should establish if the patient has any skin diseases, previous bruising, tendency to bruising, any skin lesions or unusual healing of wounds. Information on assessing pressure sites is given in the *Practice Guidelines*.

Physical examination of the skin will allow the nurse to gain information about the patient's skin colour, skin turgor (elasticity), presence of oedema (swelling) and the characteristics of any wounds that may be present. In adults, particular attention should be paid to skin condition in areas most likely to break down: in skin folds such as under the breasts, in areas that are frequently moist such as the perineum, and in areas that receive extensive pressure such as the coccyx and trochanters (hips) (see Figure 18-2). Children under the age of two have larger heads, less hair and less occipital subcutaneous tissue than older children and adults; therefore, particular attention should be paid to the occiput (back of the head) as well as the ears, heels and sacrum (Great Ormond Street Hospital for Children NHS Trust, 2003).

PRACTICE GUIDELINES

Assessing Common Pressure Sites

- Be sure the lighting is good, preferably natural or fluorescent.
- The room should not be too hot or too cold. Heat can cause the skin to flush; cold can cause the skin to blanch or become cyanotic.
- Inspect pressure areas (see Figure 18-2) for any whitish or reddened spots; discoloration can be caused by impaired blood circulation to the area.
- Inspect pressure areas for abrasions and excoriations. An abrasion can occur when skin rubs against a sheet (e.g. when the patient is pulled). Excoriations can occur when the skin has prolonged contact with body secretions or excretions or with dampness in skin folds.
- Palpate the surface temperature of the skin over the pressure areas (warm your hands first). Normally, the temperature is the same as that of the surrounding skin. Increased temperature is abnormal and may be due to inflammation or blood trapped in the area.
- Palpate over bony prominences and dependent body areas for the presence of oedema, which feels spongy.

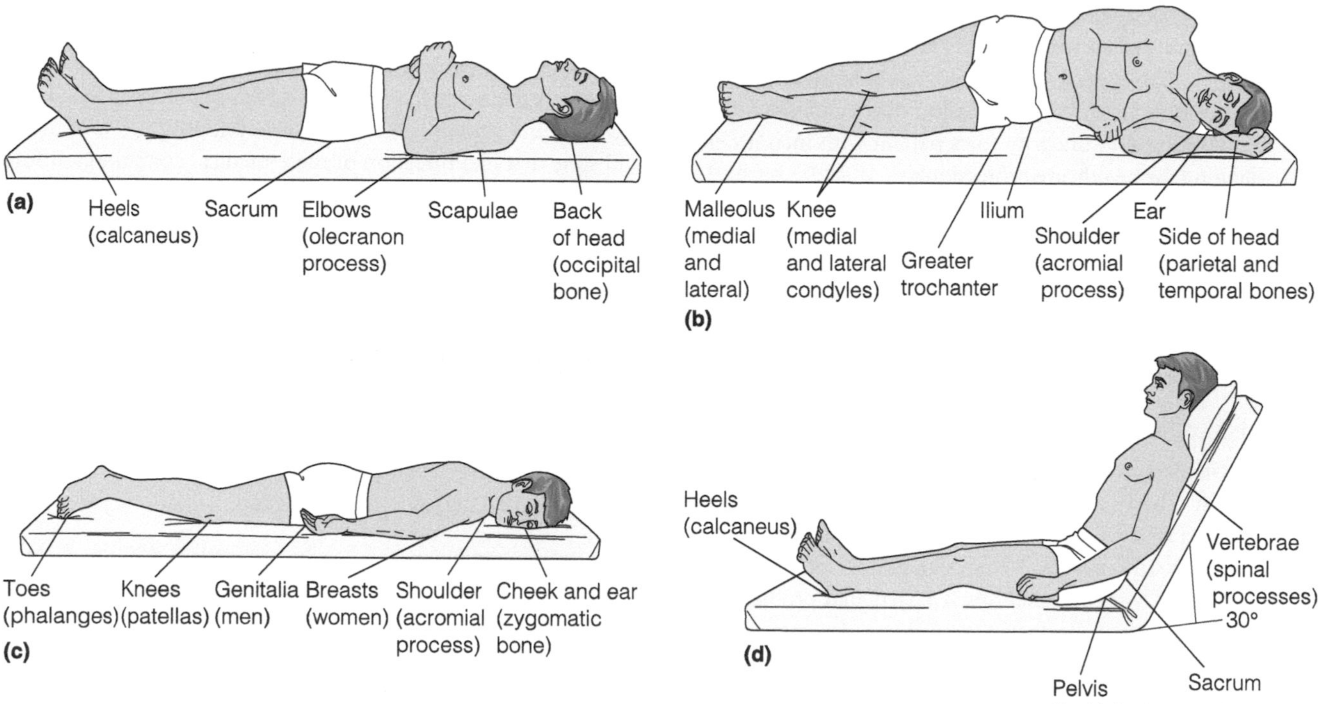

Figure 18-2 Body pressure areas: in (a) supine position; (b) lateral position; (c) prone position; (d) Fowler's position.

Risk Assessment Tools

Risk assessment tools aid the identification of people vulnerable to pressure ulcer development, guiding the selection of nursing interventions needed (NICE, 2005) and should be completed within 6 hours of admission (NICE, 2003). Schoonhoven *et al.* (2005) note that there are approximately 40 risk assessment tools available to nurses in the UK. However, they go on to state that only the Waterlow, Norton and Braden scales have been subject to any form of scrutiny. With so many risk assessment tools available, this can cause confusion and inconsistencies in care, particularly when patients are transferred from one ward or hospital to another.

Waterlow (Waterlow, 1997), The Knoll Scale (see Figure 18-3), Norton (see Table 18-2) and Braden (see Figure 18-4) are numerical scales that include the risk factors attributed to the development of pressure ulcers. Although simple to use, there is little evidence that these tools reduce the incidence of pressure ulcers (Pancorbo-Hidalgo *et al.*, 2006). The Royal College of Nursing (RCN) in conjunction with the National Institute for Health and Clinical Excellence (NICE, 2005) suggest that these tools should be used as an adjunct to the assessment process and should not replace clinical judgement.

Preventing Pressure Ulcers

To reduce the likelihood of pressure ulcer development in all patients, the nurse needs to employ a variety of preventive measures. Patients and their families should be involved in any

Modified Knoll Risk Assessment Scale

Directions: Use the following tool to assess the patient for risk of skin breakdown. Record the scores and total on the appropriate sheets.

General Health Status

0 Good - Injury limited to one area, free of major health problems
1 Fair - Major surgery, major health problems are controlled
2 Poor - Chronic/serious health problem, predisposing disease
3 Moribund - Prognosis poor predicted, stay in the acute care area >1 month. Death expected within 3 months

Mental Status

0 Alert - Aware of time and place, communicates properly
1 Lethargic - Responds only with stimulation (eg. verbal, noise). Sleeps for long periods, sleeps most of the day and night
2 Semicomatose/confused - Responds appropriately to painful stimulus only, does not cooperate in the relief of pressure
3 Comatose - Does not respond appropriately to pain, under paralysing agents

Activity

0 Ambulatory - Walks freely without help
1 Needs help - Needs assistance to walk/get out of bed, gets out of bed by standing and pivoting
4 Chairfast - Cannot ambulate, confined to chair/wheelchair, total lift out of bed
6 Bedfast - Cannot sit in chair, remains constantly in bed

Mobility

0 Full - Can move all extremities at will
1 Limited - Cannot voluntarily move all extremities, cast on arm/leg, pain with joint movement
4 Very limited - Moves extremities only with assistance, severe pain with joint movement, paralysis of upper/lower extremities, turning frame/eg. RotoRest* bed (KCI, San Antonio, Tex)
6 Immobile - Never voluntarily changes position, contractures prevent movement, paralysis of all extremities

Incontinence

0 None - Has control of bladder/bowels, Foley/condom in place
1 Occasional - Loses bladder control at times, Foley/condom intermittently in place, loses control of bowels but no diarrhea, ostomy/fistula with drainage protection
4 Usually - No control of bladder without Foley/condom, diarrhea less than every 4 hours, ostomy/drainage with intermittent protective drainage system
6 Total - No control of bladder without Foley/condom, diarrhea more than every 4 hours, ostomy/drainage without protective drainage system

Nutritional Intake

0 Good - Serum albumin normal (3.5-5), weight gain in the absence of edema, no obesity/underweight
1 Fair - Serum albumin between 3.0-3.5, no peripheral edema, overweight/underweight, constant weight
2 Poor - Serum albumin between 2.5-3.0, losing weight slowly, in the absence of edema/dialysis, obese
3 None - Serum albumin less than 2.5, losing weight rapidly, in the absence of edema/dialysis, increased weight with edema

Fluid Intake

0 Good - Good skin turgor, skin warm and resilient, intake and output equal with no peripheral edema
1 Fair - Skin dry and flaccid, output is greater than intake
2 Poor - Lips parched and mouth dry, cracked and flaking skin, edema to dependent areas
3 None - Generalised edema of body, weeping of fluid from the skin

Predisposing Disease

0 Absent - Has no vascular disease, immune suppression, neuropathies, diabetes, anemias, paralysis, hypoxia, no contributing dermal ulcer formation
1 Slight - Controlled diabetes, anemia, incipient vascular disease, incipient skin disease
2 Moderate - Brittle diabetic, sepsis but no shock, immune suppression with no infections, PO2 between 60 and 80, advanced vascular disease as manifested by absent pulses, or poor capillary refill, frequent unhealed areas of skin
3 Severe - Uncontrolled diabetes/anemia, PO2 <60, shock, paralysis, immune suppression with infection, well advanced vascular disease as manifested by lack of sensation, unhealed areas of the skin, edema of the arides and feet, necrotic toes of fingers, evidence of stasis ulcers.

Figure 18-3 The Knoll Scale

Source: The Knoll scale of liability to pressure sores, *Guide to the practice of nursing*, St Louis: Mosby, pp. 83-86 (McFarlane, S. and Castledine, G., 1977), Copyright Elsevier 1977.

Table 18-2 Norton's Pressure Area Risk Assessment Form (Scoring System)

A. General physical condition		B. Mental state		C. Activity		D. Mobility		E. Incontinence	
Good	4	Alert	4	Ambulatory	4	Full	4	Absent	4
Fair	3	Apathetic	3	Walks with help	3	Slightly limited	3	Occasional	3
Poor	2	Confused	2	Chairbound	2	Very limited	2	Usually urinary	2
Very bad	1	Stuporous	1	Bedfast	1	Immobile	1	Double	1

Source: *An Investigation of Geriatric Nursing Problems in Hospitals*, by D. Norton, R. McLaren and A.N. Exton-Smith, 1975, Edinburgh, UK: Churchill Livingstone. Reprinted with permission.

measures employed to maintain skin integrity and prevent the development of pressure ulcers.

Providing Nutrition

Inadequate intake of calories, protein, vitamins and iron is believed to be a risk factor for pressure ulcer development; therefore, nutritional supplements should be considered for nutritionally compromised patients. Patients at risk of developing pressure ulcers require a diet rich in protein, carbohydrates, lipids, vitamins A and C and minerals, such as iron, zinc and copper (Anderson, 2005). Patient weight should be monitored regularly to help assess their nutritional status. Blood tests should be performed to monitor lymphocyte (white cell) count, protein (especially albumin) and haemoglobin.

Maintaining Skin Hygiene

When bathing the patient, the nurse should minimise the force and friction applied to the skin, using mild cleansing agents that minimise irritation and dryness and that do not disrupt the skin's 'natural barriers' (Voegeli, 2008). Also, avoid using hot water, which increases skin dryness and irritation. The patient's skin should be kept clean and dry and free of irritation and maceration by urine, faeces, sweat, incomplete drying after a bath, soap or alcohol. Apply skin protection if indicated.

BRADEN SCALE FOR PREDICTING PRESSURE SORE RISK

Patient's Name ______________________ Evaluator's Name ______________________

					Date of Assessment			
SENSORY PERCEPTION Ability to respond meaningfully to pressure-related discomfort	**1. Completely Limited:** Unresponsive (does not moan, flinch or grasp) to painful stimuli, due to diminished level of consciousness or sedation, OR limited ability to feel pain over most of body surface.	**2. Very Limited:** Responds only to painful stimuli. Cannot communicate discomfort except by moaning or restlessness, OR has a sensory impairment which limits the ability to feel pain or discomfort over 1/2 of body.	**3. Slightly Limited:** Responds to verbal commands but cannot always communicate discomfort or need to be turned, OR has some sensory impairment which limits ability to feel pain or discomfort in 1 or 2 extremities.	**4. No Impairment:** Responds to verbal commands. Has no sensory deficit which would limit ability to feel or voice pain or discomfort.				
MOISTURE Degree to which skin is exposed to moisture	**1. Constantly Moist:** Skin is kept moist almost constantly by perspiration, urine, etc. Dampness is detected every time patient is moved or turned.	**2. Moist:** Skin is often but not always moist. Linen must be changed at least once a shift.	**3. Occasionally Moist:** Skin is occasionally moist, requiring an extra linen change approximately once a day.	**4. Rarely Moist:** Skin is usually dry; linen requires changing only at routine intervals.				
ACTIVITY Degree of physical activity	**1. Bedfast:** Confined to bed.	**2. Chairfast:** Ability to walk severely limited or nonexistent. Cannot bear own weight and/or must be assisted into chair or wheelchair.	**3. Walks Occasionally:** Walks occasionally during day but for very short distances, with or without assistance. Spends majority of each shift in bed or chair.	**4. Walks Frequently:** Walks outside the room at least twice a day and inside room at least once every 2 hours during waking hours.				
MOBILITY Ability to change and control body position	**1. Completely Immobile:** Does not make even slight changes in body or extremity position without assistance.	**2. Very Limited:** Makes occasional slight changes in body or extremity position but unable to make frequent or significant changes independently.	**3. Slightly Limited:** Makes frequent though slight changes in body or extremity position independently.	**4. No Limitations:** Makes major and frequent changes in position without assistance.				
NUTRITION Usual food intake pattern	**1. Very Poor:** Never eats a complete meal. Rarely eats more than 1/3 of any food offered. Eats 2 servings or less of protein (meat or dairy products) per day. Takes fluids poorly. Does not take a liquid dietary supplement, OR is NPO and/or maintained on clear liquids or IVs for more than 5 days.	**2. Probably Inadequate:** Rarely eats a complete meal and generally eats only about 1/2 of any food offered. Protein intake includes only 3 servings of meat or dairy products per day. Occasionally will take a dietary supplement, OR receives less than optimum amount of liquid diet or tube feeding.	**3. Adequate:** Eats over half of most meals. Eats a total of 4 servings of protein (meat, dairy products) each day. Occasionally will refuse a meal, but will usually take a supplement if offered, OR is on a tube feeding or TPN regimen, which probably meets most of nutritional needs.	**4. Excellent:** Eats most of every meal. Never refuses a meal. Usually eats a total of 4 or more servings of meat and dairy products. Occasionally eats between meals. Does not require supplementation.				
FRICTION AND SHEAR	**1. Problem:** Requires moderate to maximum assistance in moving. Complete lifting without sliding against sheets is impossible. Frequently slides down in bed or chair, requiring frequent repositioning with maximum assistance. Spasticity, contractures or agitation leads to almost constant friction.	**2. Potential Problem:** Moves feebly or requires minimum assistance. During a move skin probably slides to some extent against sheets, chair, restraints or other devices. Maintains relatively good position in chair or bed most of the time but occasionally slides down.	**3. No Apparent Problem:** Moves in bed and in chair independently and has sufficient muscle strength to lift up completely during move. Maintains good position in bed or chair at all times.					
				Total Score				

Figure 18-4 Braden Scale for predicting pressure sore risk.

Source: 'Clinical Practice Guideline, Pressure Ulcers in Adults: Prediction and Prevention,' by U.S. Department of Health and Human Services, PPPPUA Pub no. 92-0047, pp. 16-17, 1992, Rockville, MD: Public Health Service.

Moisture or skin barriers are very effective in preventing moisture or drainage from collecting on the skin.

Avoiding Skin Trauma

Providing the patient with a smooth, firm and wrinkle-free foundation on which to sit or lie helps prevent skin trauma. To prevent injury due to friction and shearing forces, patients must be positioned, transferred and turned correctly (see Chapter 13).

Frequent shifts in position, even if only slight, effectively change pressure points. The patient should shift weight every 15–30 minutes and, whenever possible, exercise or ambulate to stimulate blood circulation.

Providing Pressure-Relieving Equipment

Capillary closing pressure is estimated to be between 12mmHg and 32mmHg in healthy adults and children. Therefore, for circulation to remain uncompromised, pressure on the bony prominences should remain below capillary pressure for as much time as possible through a combination of turning, positioning and use of pressure-relieving surfaces.

There are a number of devices available to relieve pressure. Decisions regarding which device to use should be based on a holistic assessment of the individual and should include the level of risk, comfort and general health state (NICE, 2005). All patients assessed as at risk of developing pressure ulcers should be nursed on high specification foam mattresses with pressure-relieving properties and consideration should be given to using an alternating pressure system (NICE, 2005). The RCN (2001) strongly advise that synthetic sheepskins should not be used as pressure-relieving aids, although there is some evidence from Australia that genuine sheepskins may have some pressure-relieving properties (NICE, 2003; Jolley *et al.*, 2004). Table 18-3 lists selected mechanical devices for reducing pressure on body parts.

Table 18-3 Mechanical Devices for Reducing Pressure on Body Parts

Device	Description/comments
Gel or viscoelastic filled pads	Polyvinyl, silicone or Silastic pads filled with a gelatinous substance similar to fat
Pillows and wedges (foam, gel, air, fluid)	Can raise a body part (e.g. heels) off the bed or surface
Foam mattress	Foam moulds to the body
Alternating pressure mattress	Composed of a number of cells in which the pressure alternately increases and decreases; uses a pump (see Figure 18-5)
Air fluidised bed (high-air-loss bed)	Forced temperature-controlled air is circulated around millions of tiny silicone-coated beads, producing a fluid-like movement. Provides uniform support to body contours. Decreases skin maceration by its drying effect. Moisture from the patient penetrates the bed sheet and soaks the beads. Air flow forces the beads away from the patient and rapidly dries the sheet (see Figure 18-6)
Static low-air-loss (LAL) bed	Consists of many air-filled cushions divided into four or five sections. Separate controls permit each section to be inflated to a different level of firmness; thus pressure can be reduced on bony prominences but increased under other body areas for support (see Figure 18-7)
Active or second-generation LAL bed	Like the static LAL bed, but in addition gently pulsates or rotates from side to side, thus stimulating capillary blood flow and facilitating movement of pulmonary secretions

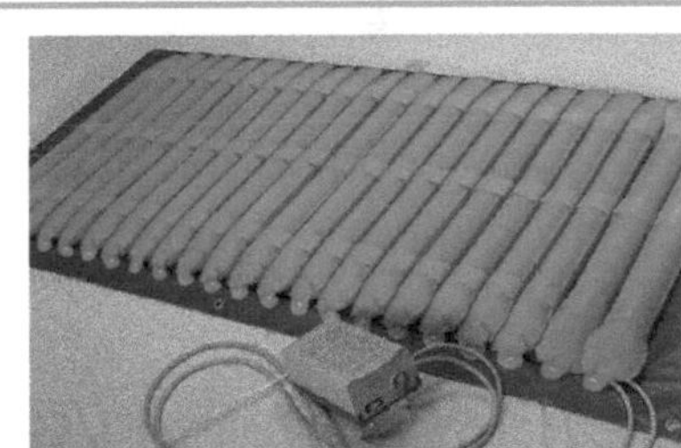

Figure 18-5 Alternating pressure (EASE).
Source: EASE.

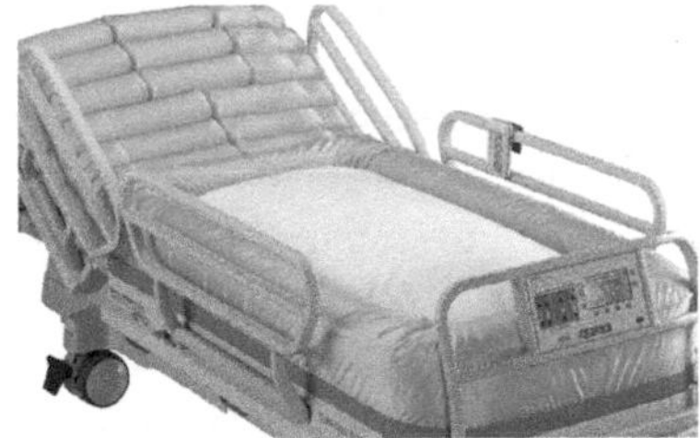

Figure 18-6 Air-fluidised bed (Clinitron).
Source: Hill-Rom Services Inc.

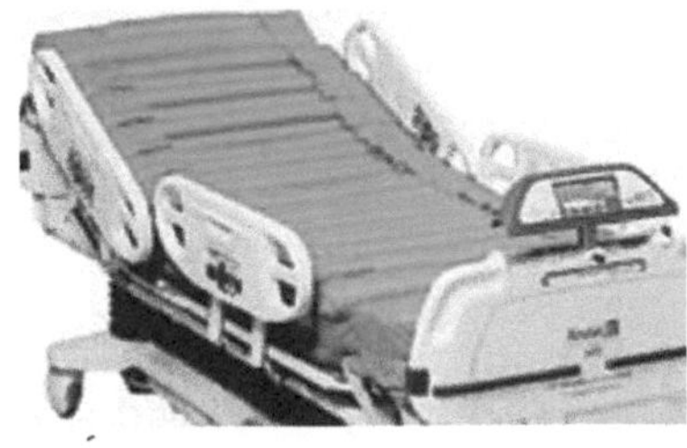

Figure 18-7 Low-air-loss bed. (Therapulse®)
Source: KCI Licensing Inc.

The Limits of Pressure Ulcer Prevention

According to the National Patient Safety Agency (NPSA, 2009) over 14,000 pressure ulcer incidents are reported to the Reporting and Learning System (RLS). Although many of these can be prevented, not all pressure ulcers can be avoided. A study by Hagisawa and Barbehel (1999) found that even when 'best current practice' was used to prevent the incidence of pressure ulcers, between 4.4% and 5.1% of patients still developed a pressure ulcer. It is therefore important that the nurse not only knows how to prevent pressure ulcers but also how to assess and treat them.

ACTIVITY 18-2

Reflect on a patient you have cared for who has a pressure ulcer. How did you prevent the pressure ulcer from deteriorating further?

RESEARCH NOTE

Effects of Education and Experience on Nurses' Value of Ulcer Prevention

Using a qualitative research report, Samuriwo (2010) used the data from semi-structured interviews of 16 nurses in one NHS trust and university to determine the value that nurses place on pressure ulcer prevention. The findings of the study showed how the participants underwent a transition from placing low value on pressure ulcer prevention to high value based on their experience of caring for patients with pressure ulcers rather than the education they receive on pressure ulcer prevention. Caring for patients with pressure ulcers allowed the nurses to re-evaluate the care that they delivered.

Source: Samuriwo, R. (2010) Effects of education and experience on nurses' value of ulcer prevention, *British Journal of Nursing*, 19(20 supplement), S8–S18.

ASSESSMENT OF THE PATIENT WITH A WOUND

Nurses play a vital role in the management of wounds. In order to manage a wound effectively, the patient should be fully assessed. Wound assessment should be done in conjunction with a holistic assessment of the patient. Wound assessment is shown in the *Practice Guidelines* on page 551.

Assess the Patient

During the assessment process, the nurse is responsible for taking an accurate history, examining the patient and documenting and communicating these findings to appropriate healthcare professionals. A holistic assessment of the patient is the key to understanding possible factors that could affect wound healing. This assessment should consider the following factors:

- Nutritional status
- Age
- Associated illness/immunity
  - Diabetes
  - Cardiovascular disease
  - Depression
- Medications
  - Steroids
  - Non-steroidal anti-inflammatory medications, e.g. aspirin
  - Chemotherapy
- Allergies

When caring for an older adult some of these factors may be more problematic. It is vitally important therefore that special consideration is given to the aging process when holistically assessing the older patient's ability to heal (see *Practice Guidelines*).

PRACTICE GUIDELINES

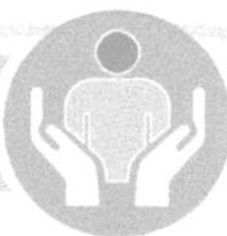

Factors Inhibiting Wound Healing in Older Adults

- Vascular changes associated with ageing, such as atherosclerosis and atrophy of capillaries in the skin, can impair blood flow to the wound.
- Collagen tissue is less flexible, which increases the risk of damage from pressure, friction and shearing.
- Scar tissue is less elastic.
- Changes in the immune system may reduce the formation of the antibodies and monocytes necessary for wound healing.
- Nutritional deficiencies may reduce the numbers of red blood cells and leukocytes, thus impeding the delivery of oxygen and the inflammatory response essential for wound healing. Oxygen is needed for the synthesis of collagen and the formation of new epithelial cells.
- Having diabetes or cardiovascular disease increases the risk of delayed healing due to impaired oxygen delivery to these tissues.
- Cell renewal is slower, leading to delayed healing.

Assess the Wound

Accurate assessment of the wound is crucial to its management. Assessment of the patient and wound is an ongoing process that can be aided by photographing the site. This acts as a visual record of the progress, particularly of chronic wounds, although it is important to note that nurses may have to seek consent from the patient before taking the photographs.

Assessment of the wound should begin with the wound history. Establishing the history of the wound can help with determining the aetiology of the wound. The nurse should consider the following:

- How long has the patient had the wound?
- What caused or may have caused the wound?
- Does the patient have a history of previous wounds?
- If the patient has a history of wounds, how have these wounds healed in the past?
- Have any previous diagnostic tests been performed?

Once the history of the wound has been established, the wound itself needs to be examined and accurately documented (see *Practice Guidelines*).

PRACTICE GUIDELINES

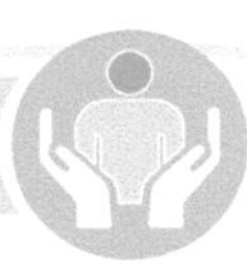

Wound Assessment

Wound assessment should include:

- Location of wound
- Dimensions of the wound
- Extent of tissue loss
- Characteristics of the wound base
- Wound drainage/exudates
- Condition of surrounding skin
- Signs of infection
- The presence of any foreign material
- Pain associated with the wound

COMMUNITY CARE CONSIDERATIONS

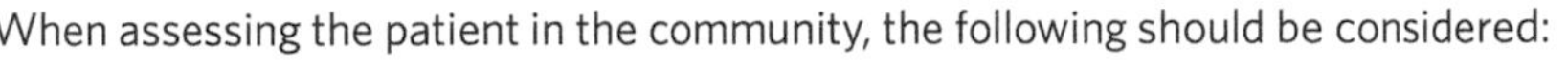

When assessing the patient in the community, the following should be considered:

- The patient's current level of knowledge/understanding.
- Their ability to change position, ambulate and transfer using appropriate assistive devices.
- The patient's home environment such as bathroom facilities.
- The patient's nutritional status.
- Family or carer's willingness to assist in actions to promote wound healing and prevent skin breakdown.
- The patient's social status such as financial status, employment, family roles.
- The need for respite carers.
- Community/social resources such as meals on wheels, financial assistance.

Classification of Wounds

There are a number of wound classification methods available to nurses; by aetiology, location, type of injury or presenting symptoms, wound depth and tissue loss or clinical appearance of the wound.

General wounds are classified as being:

- **Superficial** – where there is only loss of the epidermis.
- **Partial thickness** – confined to the dermis and epidermis.
- **Full thickness** – involving the dermis, epidermis, subcutaneous tissue and possibly muscle and bone.

Classification of Pressure Ulcers

In collaboration, the European Pressure Ulcer Advisory Panel (EPUAP) and the National Pressure Ulcer Advisory Panel (NPUAP) have developed a classification system for pressure ulcers (EPUAP and NPUAP, 2009). They recognise four categories of injury associated with pressure ulcers as shown in Figure 18-8. It is important to note that pressure ulcers do not necessarily progress or deteriorate from one category to another.

Wound Location and Dimensions

The exact location and dimensions of the wound should be assessed and accurately documented. Consistency in terminology and measurement style is key in the written communication of wound area. Skeletal charts can be used to diagrammatically communicate the location of the wound (see Figure 18-9).

Pressure ulcers are generally found over bony prominences, but may also be found in an area where localised high pressure or shear forces is applied. It is important to accurately identify the bony prominence. For instance, the coccyx bone is at the tip of the spinal bones, whereas the sacrum is the triangular-shaped bone superior to the coccyx. The sacral site is a common site of pressure ulcers and occurs in individuals who are recumbent in

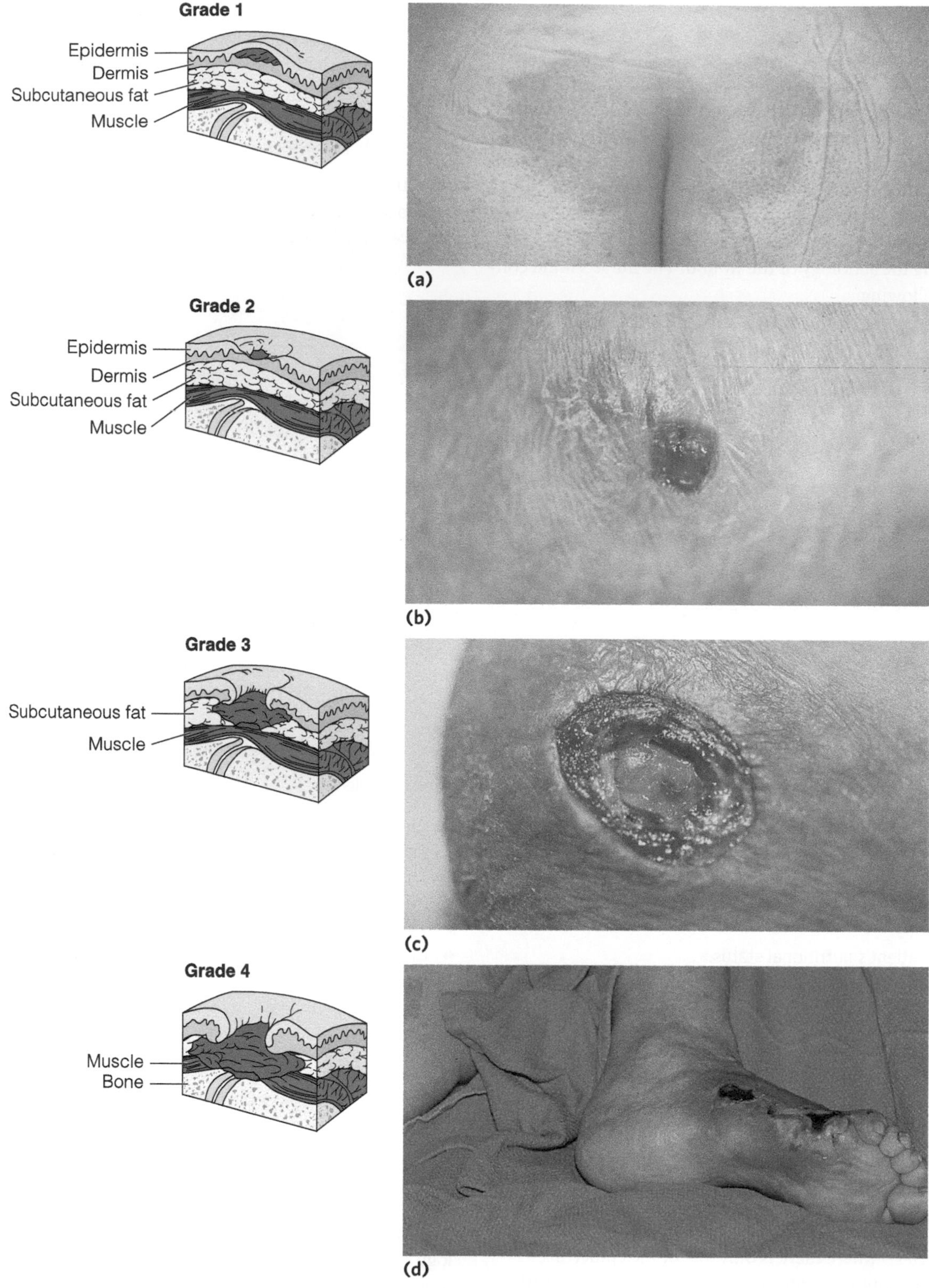

Figure 18-8 Four grades of pressure ulcers. (a) grade 1: nonblanchable erythema signalling potential ulceration; (b) grade 2: partial-thickness skin loss (abrasion, blister or shallow crater) involving the epidermis and possibly the dermis; (c) grade 3: full-thickness skin loss involving damage or necrosis of subcutaneous tissue that may extend down to, but not through, underlying fascia. The ulcer presents clinically as a deep crater with or without undermining of adjacent tissue; (d) grade 4: full-thickness skin loss with tissue necrosis or damage to muscle, bone or supporting structures, such as a tendon or joint capsule. Undermining and sinus tracts may also be present.

Source: Line Art From 'Clinical Practice Guideline, Pressure Ulcers in Adults: Prediction and Prevention,' by U.S. Department of Health and Human Services, PPPPUA, Pub. no. 92-0047, 1992, Rockville, MD: Public Health Service. EPUAP (2003) Classification system.

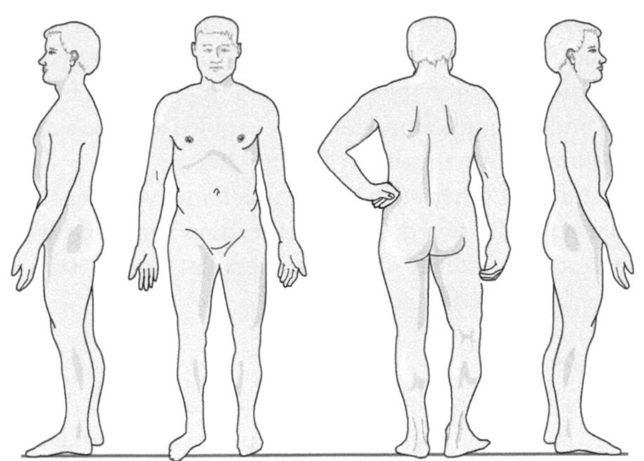

Description of Pressure Ulcers and Classification

Stage I: Characterised by erythema that does not resolve within minutes of pressure relief. Skin remains intact.

Stage II: Partial thickness loss of skin involving the epidermis or dermis – may involve both. The ulcer is superficial and may present as a blister, abrasion or shallow crater. Free of eschar.

Stage III: Full thickness loss which goes through the dermis to the subcutaneous tissue but does not extend through the underlying fascia. Appears as a crater and may include undermining.

Stage IV: Full thickness skin loss with extensive damage through the subcutaneous tissue to the fascia and may involve muscle layers, joint and/or bone.

1 cm 2 cm 3 cm 4 cm 5 cm

- IDENTIFY LOCATION OF ALL PRESSURE ULCERS ABOVE BY NUMBERING (1, 2, 3): IF MORE THAN 3, USE ADDITIONAL SHEET.
- COMPLETE CHART BELOW FOR SITE #1, USE REVERSE SIDE FOR SITES 2 & 3.

Patient Admitted On: ______________________

Date Sheet Initiated: ______________________

Pressure relief methods in use:

❑ Low Airloss Bed

❑ Low Airloss Mattress Overlay

❑ Turning Q2h when pt. supine and Q1h if HOB↑

❑ Pressure Reducing Mattress Overlay

❑ Other ______________________

Date MD notified of ulcer: ______________________

DOCUMENT WEEKLY AND P.R.N. SIGNIFICANT CHANGE IN ULCER'S APPEARANCE

SITE #1: LOCATION		DESCRIBE TREATMENT:			FREQUENCY:
DATE / TIME					
DIMENSIONS: (in. cm.) LENGTH					
WIDTH					
DEPTH					
ODOUR (None or Foul)					
DESCRIBE DRAINAGE (Purulent, Serous, Serosanguinous) and AMOUNT (Scant, Moderate, Copious)					
STAGE (See Above)					
COMMENTARY: i.e.: Describe tissue surrounding ulcer: is there undermining? % necrotic vs % granular, etc.					
NURSE					

Figure 18-9 Wound/skin documentation sheet.

bed and in individuals who sit in a reclined position either in a chair or wheelchair. Coccyx ulcers occur in individuals who sit upright in a chair.

Lower leg wounds may occur over a bony prominence or in soft tissue between bones. Lower leg wounds may be identified in relation to body side: **anterior**, **posterior**, **lateral** or **medial**. Pedal wounds are generally identified by foot position: for instance, **plantar**, **dorsal**, lateral or medial aspect of the foot. Pedal wounds may also be identified by bone location: for instance, **metatarsal**, **phalange** (1st through 5th digit), calcaneus (heel) or **mallelous** (ankle).

Wounds, such as incisions, may present over the trunk of the body or a limb. In this case, the body location is identified as the anatomical position: abdominal, groin, calf, chest etc.

The dimensions of the wound should be assessed regularly to provide a means of measuring the amount of tissue lost and assessing the progress or deterioration of the wound. The dimensions of the wound, including length, width, depth (if measurable depth is present), surface area and volume (where appropriate), should be recorded. A number of techniques exist to measure wounds (Fette, 2006).

The simplest and cheapest means of measuring a wound is to calculate the wound surface area by measuring the wound's length and width with a tape measure or ruler. The volume of a wound can be measured using the Kundin gauge (Kundin, 1989) (see Figure 18-10). However, both these methods become problematic if the wound is not linear in shape.

Another widely used and relatively inexpensive two-dimensional wound measurement tool is wound tracing. The wound measurements are recorded by tracing the outline of the wound onto sterile transparent film (Yenidunya and Demirseren, 2004). Although there are limitations to this method of measuring wounds (Fette, 2006), the tracings can be easily stored in the patient's records or entered into electronic database (Yenidunya and Demirseren 2004).

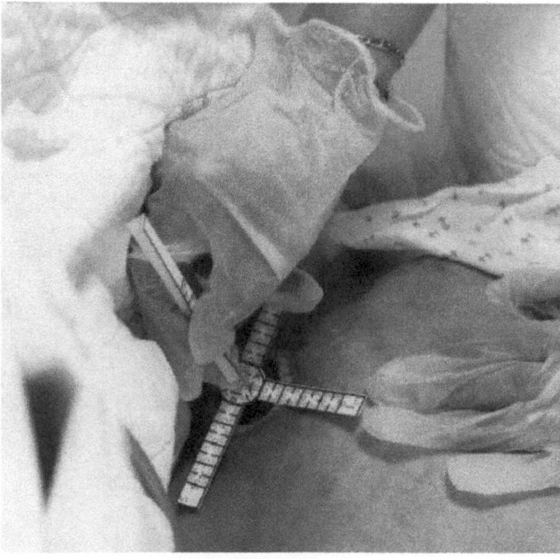

Figure 18-10 Kundin ruler.

Source: Kundin, J.I. (1989) 'A new way to size up a wound', *American Journal of Nursing*, 89(2): 206–207.

Measurement of the wound should also include tunnels, sinus tracts or cavities. These can be measured by gently inserting a sterile probe into the wound margins at varying intervals. Cotton buds or applicators should be avoided as these can leave cotton fibres within the sinus (Butcher, 2002).

A number of other methods are used; however, they tend to be more expensive or require specialist equipment and training, for instance, moulding, scaled photography, planimetrics and computerised stereophotogrammetry.

Wound bed

The characteristic of the wound bed guides clinical decision-making in determining the most appropriate treatment and dressing. Evaluation of the progress of the wound can be made based on the tissue type and amount (see Table 18-4). As the characteristics of the wound change, treatment choices are reviewed and renewed as necessary.

Wound Drainage

Exudate is material, such as fluid and cells, which has escaped from blood vessels during the inflammatory process and is deposited in tissue or on tissue surfaces. The nature and amount of exudate vary according to the tissue involved, the intensity and duration of the inflammation, and the presence of microorganisms.

There are three major types of exudate: serous, purulent and sanguineous (haemorrhagic). A **serous exudate** consists chiefly of serum (the clear portion of the blood) derived from blood and the serous membranes of the body. It looks watery and has few cells. An example is the fluid in a blister from a burn.

A **purulent exudate** is thicker than serous exudate because of the presence of **pus**, which consists of leukocytes, liquefied dead tissue debris and dead and living bacteria. Purulent exudates

Table 18-4 Wound Bed Tissue Types

Tissue Type	Description
Eschar	Necrotic tissue, which appears black and leathery with varying degrees of adherence to the wound margin and wound bed.
Slough	Necrotic tissue, which is in the process of liquefying and separating from the wound bed. The colour of slough tissue may vary from yellow, tan, grey or brown tones. The tissue generally has a gelatinous or stringy consistency.
Granulation	Occurs during the proliferative phase of healing. Healthy granulation tissue appears red. Pale granulation tissue can indicate poor circulation while deep red granulation tissue may indicate infection.
Epithelial	Occurs in the proliferative phase of wound healing. Epithelial tissue migrates across a clean healthy wound bed. Once the wound bed is covered with epithelial tissue, the tissue differentiates and matures forming epidermal tissue.

vary in colour, some acquiring tinges of blue, green or yellow. The colour may depend on the causative organism.

Haemorrhagic exudate consists of large amounts of red blood cells, indicating damage to capillaries that is severe enough to allow the escape of red blood cells from plasma. This type of exudate is frequently seen in open wounds.

CLINICAL ALERT

A bright haemorrhagic exudate indicates fresh bleeding, whereas dark sanguineous exudate denotes older bleeding.

Mixed types of exudates are often observed. A *haemoserous* (consisting of clear and blood-tinged drainage) exudate is commonly seen in surgical incisions.

Laboratory Tests

Laboratory tests can often support the nurse's clinical assessment of the wound's progress in healing. A decreased white cell (leucocyte) count can delay healing and increase the possibility of infection. A haemoglobin level below normal range indicates poor oxygen delivery to the tissues. Blood coagulation studies are also significant. Prolonged coagulation times can result in excessive blood loss and prolonged clot absorption. Hypercoagulability can lead to intravascular clotting. Intra-arterial clotting can result in a deficient blood supply to the wound area. Serum protein analysis provides an indication of the body's nutritional reserves for rebuilding cells. Wound cultures can either confirm or rule out the presence of infection. Sensitivity studies are helpful in the selection of appropriate antibiotic therapy. The nurse obtains a wound culture whenever an infection is suspected.

Procedure 18-1 provides guidelines to obtain a specimen of wound drainage.

PROCEDURE 18-1 Collecting a Wound Swab for Culture and Sensitivity

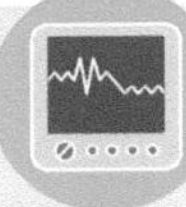

Purposes

- To identify the micro-organisms potentially causing an infection and the antibiotics to which they are sensitive.

Assessment

Assess

- For signs of infection in the wound, e.g. pain, inflammation (remember this can be a normal part of the healing process), exudates (type, volume, colour, odour)
- For systemic signs of infection such as fever, chills or elevated white blood cell count (WBC).

Wound swabs should only be taken if clinically indicated. The nurse should use their clinical judgement when assessing for infection before doing a wound swab. This is important as almost all wounds are colonised with micro-organisms, therefore a wound swab will almost always show micro-organisms. However, colonisation with micro-organisms poses very little risk to the patient, whereas infection causes localised problems, such as malodorous exudate and pain, and systemic problems such as fever. Colonisation with micro-organisms requires no treatment, whereas infection requires the use of antibiotics. Over prescribing antibiotics leads to resistant bacteria such as multi-resistant staphylococcus aureus (MRSA).

Planning

Before collecting the specimen, ensure collection of equipment and that an appropriate microbiology form is completed. Remember when collecting wound specimens the wound should not be cleansed prior to collection.

Equipment

- Clean gloves
- Sterile gloves
- Sterile dressing set
- Normal saline (for cleansing after collection of the specimen)
- Culture tube with swab
- Appropriate sterile wound dressing
- Completed microbiology form

Implementation

Preparation

If appropriate, administer analgesia 30 minutes before the procedure if the patient is complaining of pain at the wound site.

Performance

1. Follow local policy to ensure that you explain to the patient what you are going to do, why it is necessary and how they can cooperate. Obtain consent and maintain patient privacy and dignity and ensure that the appropriate local infection control procedures are observed.
2. Remove any dressings that cover the wound. *To allow access to wound.*
3. Put on clean/sterile gloves according to local policy. *To prevent cross-contamination.*
4. Observe any drainage on the dressing, note amount, colour and type of exudates. *To assess appropriateness of swabbing.*
5. Discard the dressing in the clinical waste bin. *To prevent cross-contamination.*
6. Remove your gloves and dispose of them properly. *To prevent cross-contamination.*
7. Wash hands again and open the sterile dressing set using aseptic technique.
8. Assess the wound.
9. Put on sterile gloves.
10. Obtain the specimen by rotating the swab back and forth over the wound. Then return the swab to the culture tube, taking care not to touch the top or the outside of the tube. *This ensures adequate collection of wound exudate.*
11. Cleanse the wound if appropriate, *in order to remove foreign material/excessive exudate.*
12. Dress the wound with an appropriate dressing, *in order to prevent contamination/maintain moist wound bed/prevent wound from cooling.*
13. Arrange for the specimen to be transported to the laboratory immediately. Be sure to include the completed form.
14. Document all relevant information.

Evaluation

- Compare findings of wound assessment and drainage to previous assessments to determine any changes.
- Report the culture results to the doctor or nurse practitioner.
- Conduct appropriate follow-up such as administering medications as ordered.

Wound Margins

Examination of the wound margins or edges can provide clues as to the aetiology of the wound and to the progress of healing. The wound margin can be attached to the wound bed, detached from the wound bed (undermining) or rolled under. A rolled edge can indicate that the wound is too dry and would require a moist wound dressing. The wound margins should also be checked for oedema, colour and any signs of **erythema** or **maceration**.

Periwound or Surrounding Skin

The skin surrounding a wound can provide the nurse with invaluable information about the condition of the wound. Erythema and warmth could indicate inflammation and infection, while interruptions in the integrity of the surrounding skin such as pustules could indicate allergic reaction to dressings. The nurse should examine and palpate the surrounding skin to establish if there are any signs of induration, eczema, maceration or desiccation.

Wound Pain

The duration, intensity and causation of wound should be monitored regularly. Pain may be persistent or occur during wound treatments, such as wound cleansing, dressing changes or debridement. Pain may be an indication of additional tissue trauma, infection or bone involvement. Pain should be assessed according to local policy. Chapter 24 considers some of the pain assessment tools available to nurses.

Wound Healing

An assessment should consider the wound's phase of healing. Acute, uncomplicated wounds tend to progress through a predictable series of events that result in the wound healing. In contrast, chronic or complex wounds usually fail to proceed through these events in an orderly fashion leading to an extended healing time or even leading to a non-healing wound.

For living organisms, the ability to repair tissue that has been damaged is imperative to survival. Regardless of the severity of the injury, there are two mechanisms for the repair of tissue: regeneration (renewal of tissues) or connective tissue repair (replacement of the damaged tissue with a scar). Humans have limited ability to regenerate new tissue, but tend to heal by connective tissue repair.

Healing can be considered in terms of *types of healing* and *phases of healing.*

Types of Wound Healing

There are two types of healing, influenced by the amount of tissue loss. **Primary intention** healing occurs where the tissue surfaces have been approximated (closed) and there is minimal or no tissue loss; it is characterised by the formation of minimal granulation tissue and scarring. An example of wound healing by primary intention is a closed surgical incision.

A wound that is extensive and involves considerable tissue loss, and in which the edges cannot or should not be approximated, heals by **secondary intention** healing. An example of wound healing by secondary intention is a pressure ulcer. Secondary intention healing differs from primary intention healing in three ways: (a) the repair time is longer, (b) the scarring is greater and (c) the susceptibility to infection is greater.

Phases of Wound Healing

Wound healing can be broken down into three stages: inflammatory, proliferative and maturation or remodelling.

Inflammatory Phase

The *inflammatory phase* is initiated immediately after injury and lasts three to six days. Two major processes occur during this phase: haemostasis and phagocytosis.

Haemostasis (the cessation of bleeding) results from vasoconstriction of the larger blood vessels in the affected area, retraction (drawing back) of injured blood vessels, the deposition of **fibrin** (connective tissue) and the formation of blood clots in the area. The blood clots, formed from blood platelets, provide a matrix of fibrin that becomes the framework for cell repair. A scab also forms on the surface of the wound. Consisting of clots and dead and dying tissue, this scab serves to aid haemostasis and inhibit contamination of the wound by micro-organisms. Below the scab, epithelial cells migrate into the wound from the edges. The epithelial cells serve as a barrier between the body and the environment, preventing the entry of micro-organisms.

The inflammatory phase also involves vascular and cellular responses intended to remove any foreign substances and dead and dying tissues. The blood supply to the wound increases, bringing with it oxygen and nutrients needed in the healing process. The area appears reddened and oedematous as a result.

During cell migration, leukocytes (specifically, neutrophils) move into the interstitial space. These are replaced about 24 hours after injury by macrophages, which arise from the blood monocytes. These macrophages engulf micro-organisms and cellular debris by a process known as **phagocytosis**. The macrophages also secrete an angiogenesis factor (AGF), which stimulates the formation of epithelial buds at the end of injured blood vessels. The microcirculatory network that results sustains the healing process and the wound during its life. This inflammatory response is essential to healing, and measures that impair inflammation, such as steroid medications, can place the healing process at risk.

Proliferative Phase

The *proliferative phase*, the second phase in healing, extends from day three or four to about day 21 post-injury. Fibroblasts (connective tissue cells), which migrate into the wound starting about 24 hours after injury, begin to synthesise collagen. **Collagen** is a whitish protein substance that adds tensile strength to the wound. As the amount of collagen increases, so does the strength of the wound; thus, the chance that the wound will open progressively decreases. If the wound is sutured, a raised 'healing ridge' appears under the intact suture line. In a wound that is not sutured, the new collagen is often visible.

Capillaries grow across the wound, increasing the blood supply. Fibroblasts move from the bloodstream into the wound, depositing fibrin. As the capillary network develops, the tissue becomes a translucent red colour. This tissue, called **granulation tissue**, is fragile and bleeds easily.

When the skin edges of a wound are not sutured, the area must be filled in with granulation tissue. When the granulation tissue matures, marginal epithelial cells migrate to it, proliferating over this connective tissue base to fill the wound. If the wound does not close by **epithelialisation**, the area becomes covered with dried plasma proteins and dead cells. This is called **eschar**. Initially, wounds healing by secondary intention seep blood-tinged (serosanguineous) drainage. Later, if they are not covered by epithelial cells, they become covered with thick, grey, fibrinous tissue that is eventually converted into dense scar tissue.

Maturation Phase

The *maturation phase* begins about day 21 and can extend one or two years after the injury. Fibroblasts continue to synthesise collagen. The collagen fibres themselves, which were initially laid in a haphazard fashion, reorganise into a more orderly structure. During maturation, the wound is remodelled and contracted. The scar becomes stronger, but the repaired area is never as strong as the original tissue. In some individuals, particularly dark-skinned persons, an abnormal amount of collagen is laid down. This can result in a hypertrophic scar, or **keloid**.

Complications of Wound Healing

Several untoward events can occur to interfere with the healing of a wound. These include excessive bleeding, infection and **dehiscence**.

Haemorrhage

Some escape of blood from a wound is normal. **Haemorrhage** (massive bleeding), however, is abnormal. It may be caused by a dislodged clot, a slipped stitch or erosion of a blood vessel, for example.

Internal haemorrhage may be detected by swelling or distention in the area of the wound and, possibly, by the presence of blood in a surgical drain. Some patients will have a **haematoma**, a localised collection of blood underneath the skin that may appear as a reddish blue swelling (bruise). A large haematoma may be dangerous in that it places pressure on blood vessels and can thus obstruct blood flow.

The risk of haemorrhage is greatest during the first 48 hours after surgery. Haemorrhage is an emergency; the nurse should apply pressure dressings to the area and monitor the patient's vital signs. Medical advice should be sought immediately as the patient may need to be taken to theatre for surgical intervention.

Infection

Colonisation is the presence of micro-organisms without illness or reaction. Most if not all wounds are contaminated as the skin is surrounded by micro-organisms. These micro-organisms compete with the new cells in the wound for oxygen and nutrition and as a result can delay wound healing. If these micro-organisms multiply excessively or invade tissues, infection can result. If a wound and surrounding tissues become infected there are generally a few tell-tale signs including:

- pain;
- change in the colour of the wound bed;
- malodorous (offensive smelling) exudate;
- heat;
- swelling.

If infection is suspected the nurse should swab the wound and send it for culture and sensitivity. This test will identify the micro-organism and suggest a drug that the micro-organism is sensitive to. Severe infection causes fever and elevated white blood cell count. Patients who are immunosuppressed are especially susceptible to wound infections.

A wound can be infected with micro-organisms at the time of injury, during surgery or post-operatively. Wounds that occur as a result of injury (e.g. bullet and knife wounds) are most likely to be contaminated at the time of injury. Surgery involving the intestines can also result in infection from the micro-organisms inside the intestine.

Dehiscence

Dehiscence is the partial or total rupturing of a sutured wound. Dehiscence usually involves an abdominal wound in which the layers below the skin also separate. A number of factors, including obesity, poor nutrition, multiple trauma, failure of suturing, excessive coughing, vomiting and dehydration, heighten a patient's risk of wound dehiscence. Wound infection can be the cause of the wound dehiscing (Tobon *et al.*, 2003).

Dehiscence may be preceded by sudden straining, such as coughing or sneezing. It is not unusual for a patient to feel that 'something has given away'. When dehiscence occurs, the wound should be quickly supported by large sterile dressings, the patient should be placed in a bed in a position that puts as little pressure on the wound as possible. The surgeon must be notified because immediate surgical repair of the area may be necessary.

MANAGEMENT OF THE PATIENT WITH A WOUND

Management of the patient with wounds tends to lie within the nursing domain. It is therefore the nurse's responsibility to encourage wound healing where possible. The plan of care for a patient with a wound should address causative factors or factors that could impede the healing process and treat the wound with appropriate dressings and interventions.

There are three major areas in which nurses can help patients develop optimal conditions for healing pressure ulcers: obtaining sufficient nutrition and fluids, preventing wound infections and proper positioning.

Nutrition and Fluids

Patients should be assisted to take in at least 2,500 ml of fluids a day unless conditions contraindicate this amount. Although there is no evidence that excessive doses of vitamins or minerals enhance wound healing, adequate amounts are extremely important. The nurse should ensure that patients receive sufficient protein, vitamins C, A, B_1 and B_5 and zinc (Anderson, 2005).

Preventing Infection

There are two main aspects to controlling wound infection: preventing micro-organisms from entering the wound and preventing the transmission of blood borne pathogens to or from the patient to others. Although most wounds are contaminated with micro-organisms, particularly chronic wounds such as pressure ulcers, the nurse must use an aseptic technique in order to minimise the introduction of further micro-organisms into the wound. *Procedure 18-2* explains how to perform an aseptic technique for wound care.

Cleaning Wounds

Wound cleaning involves the removal of debris (i.e. foreign materials, excess slough, necrotic tissue and excess exudate). It is important to point out that exudate should only be removed if it is excessive as it is believed to contain growth factors and nutrients vital to wound healing (White and Cutting, 2006). In order to make a decision about whether to cleanse a wound, the nurse must fully assess the wound.

The choices of cleaning agent and method depend largely on local policy; however, antiseptics and disinfectants are not recommended as they have been found to be inactivated by body fluid, can damage healing tissue and can lead to systemic toxicity (Khan and Naqvi, 2006). Although normal saline (0.9% saline) is favoured as wound cleansing solution in hospitals, tap water, which is easily accessible, efficient and cost effective, is commonly used in the community setting (Fernandez *et al.*, 2007). Normal saline is an isotonic solution that is purported to be less likely to interfere with the normal healing process (Fernandez et *al.*, 2007).

Nurses are guided by evidence-based practice and local policy when deciding whether to cleanse a wound and what cleanser to use. Recommended guidelines for cleaning wounds are shown in the *Practice Guidelines.*

Cleansing Technique

The most common means of cleansing a wound is by swabbing (or scrubbing) and irrigation (see *Procedure 18-3*); however, showering and bathing are acceptable options for some individual patients (Atiyeh *et al.*, 2009). Cleansing a wound with cotton wool or gauze is not recommended as they can leave fibres behind which can lead to infection (Dowsett *et al.*, 2004). It is also believed that the pressure exerted on the wound during swabbing can be detrimental to the wound (Oliver, 1997).

The technique of choice for cleansing a wound is irrigation (Atiyeh *et al.*, 2009); however, there are problems associated with this technique. Too much irrigation pressure and new tissue is damaged while too little pressure does not remove debris (Davies *et al.*, 2005).

PRACTICE GUIDELINES

Cleaning Wounds

- Use solutions such as isotonic saline or tap water to clean or irrigate wounds (Fernandez *et al.*, 2007).
- When possible, warm the solution to body temperature before use. *This prevents lowering the wound temperature, which slows the healing process.*
- If a wound is grossly contaminated by foreign material, bacteria, slough or necrotic tissue, clean the wound at every dressing change. *Foreign bodies and devitalised tissue act as a focus for infection and can delay healing.*
- If a wound is clean, has little exudate, and reveals healthy granulation tissue, avoid cleaning. *Unnecessary cleaning can delay wound healing by traumatising newly produced, delicate tissues, reducing the surface temperature of the wound, and removing exudate which itself may have bactericidal properties.*
- Use gauze squares. Avoid using cotton balls and other products that shed fibres onto the wound surface. *The fibres become embedded in granulation tissue and can act as foci for infection. They may also stimulate 'foreign body' reactions, prolonging the inflammatory phase of healing and delaying the healing process.*
- Clean superficial noninfected wounds by irrigating them with normal saline. *The hydraulic pressure of an irrigating stream of fluid dislodges contaminating debris and reduces bacterial colonisation.*
- *To retain wound moisture*, avoid drying a wound after cleaning it.
- Clean from the wound in an outward direction *to avoid transferring organisms from the surrounding skin into the wound.*

PROCEDURE 18-2 Aseptic Technique for Wound Care

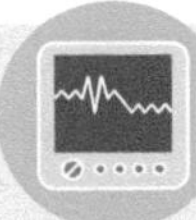

Purposes

- To remove a soiled dressing
- To clean the area (if necessary)
- To apply a new sterile dressing

Assessment

Assess

- The patient's care plan and notes to determine previous appearance, size of the wound and dressing choice
- If the patient is experiencing any pain
- The most appropriate position for the patient

Planning

Equipment

- Clean trolley or appropriate surface for equipment
- Sterile dressing pack
- Sterile syringe for irrigation
- Cleansing solution (normal saline)
- New dressing or other equipment needed for the procedure
- Clinical waste bag
- Sterile gloves and clean gloves
- Apron
- Alcohol gel

Implementation

Performance

1. Follow local policy to ensure that you explain to the patient what you are going to do, why it is necessary and how they can cooperate. Obtain consent and maintain patient privacy and dignity and ensure that the appropriate local infection control procedures are observed.
2. Position the patient as required.
3. Remove soiled gloves. *To prevent contamination.*
4. Prepare the trolley to create a 'sterile field'. *To provide a clean area to work.*
5. Open the sterile dressing pack onto the sterile field without touching the contents. *To prevent contamination of the equipment.*
6. Open other packs onto sterile field. *To prevent contamination.*

→

7 Pour cleansing solution into the gallipot or other sterile container. *To have solution in a sterile container.*
8 Put on sterile gloves being careful to only touch the wrist sections. *To prevent contamination.*
9 Cleanse the wound (if necessary) either by irrigation using the syringe or with a gauze swab. *To remove visible foreign material.*
10 Apply a new dressing using gloved hands. *To prevent contamination of the wound.*
11 Place used or opened disposable equipment. *To avoid contaminating the environment.*
12 Wash hands using handwash followed by alcohol gel. *To prevent cross-contamination.*
13 Reposition the patient. *To promote patient comfort.*
14 Discuss the outcomes with the patient and document findings in the patient's notes. *To inform the patient and other healthcare professionals.*

Evaluation

- Relate findings from dressing change to previous assessment information.
- Report any significant changes to doctor or nurse specialist.

Positioning

To promote wound healing, patients must be positioned to keep pressure off the wound. Changes of position and transfers can be accomplished without shear or friction damage. In addition to proper positioning, the patient should be assisted to be as mobile as possible because activity enhances circulation. If the patient cannot move independently, range-of-motion exercises and regular repositioning should be implemented.

PROCEDURE 18-3 Irrigating a Wound

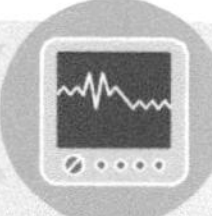

Purposes

- To clean the area
- To apply heat and hasten the healing process

Assessment

Assess

- The patient's care plan and notes to determine previous appearance and size of the wound
- The character of the exudate
- Presence of pain and the time of the last pain medication
- Clinical signs of systemic infection
- Allergies to the wound irrigation agent or tape

Planning

- Before irrigating a wound, determine (a) the type of irrigating solution to be used, (b) the frequency of irrigations and (c) the temperature of the solution.
- If possible, schedule the irrigation at a time convenient for the patient. Some irrigations require only a few minutes and others can take much longer.

Equipment

- Sterile dressing equipment and dressing materials
- Sterile syringes (e.g. a 30 to 60ml syringe)
- Sterile gallipot for the irrigating solution
- Clinical waste bag
- Receiver for the irrigation returns
- Irrigating solution warmed to body temperature
- Sterile gloves and clean gloves
- Moisture-proof sterile drape

Implementation

Preparation

Check that the irrigating fluid is at the proper temperature.

Performance

1 Follow local policy to ensure that you explain to the patient what you are going to do, why it is necessary and how they can cooperate. Obtain consent and maintain patient privacy and dignity and ensure that the appropriate local infection control procedures are observed.
2 Position the patient as required. *To improve access to the site, ensure the irrigating solution will flow by gravity from the upper end of the wound to the lower end and improve patient comfort.*
3 Place the waterproof drape over the patient and the bed. *To prevent cross-contamination and improve patient comfort.*
4 Put on clean gloves and remove and discard the old dressing. *To prevent contamination and allow the wound to be assessed.*
5 Assess the wound and drainage. *To ensure treatment is appropriate.*
6 Remove and discard clean gloves and wash hands. *To prevent cross contamination.*
7 Open the sterile dressing pack and supplies onto a clean trolley. *To prevent contamination of equipment.*
8 Pour the cleansing solution into the gallipot. *To have solution in a sterile container.*
9 Position the receiver below the wound to receive the irrigating fluid.
10 Irrigate the wound:
- Instil a steady stream of irrigating solution into the wound. Make sure all areas of the wound are irrigated.

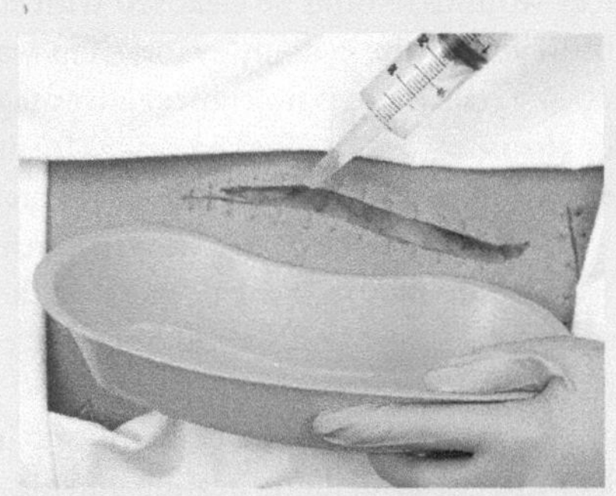

Figure 18-11 Irrigating a wound.

- Use a syringe with a catheter tip to flush the wound (Figure 18-11).
- Continue irrigating until the solution becomes clear (no exudate is present).

11 Dry the area around the wound. *Moisture left on the skin promotes the growth of micro-organisms and can cause skin irritation and breakdown.*
12 Assess the wound.
13 Using aseptic technique, apply a dressing to the wound based on the amount of drainage expected (see Tables 18-5 and 18-6). *To prevent contamination of the wound.*
14 Discuss the outcomes with the patient and document the findings of the procedure. *To inform the patient and other healthcare professionals.*

Evaluation

- Relate findings from dressing change to previous assessment information.
- Report any significant changes to doctor or nurse specialist.

Treating Pressure Ulcers

Pressure ulcers are a challenge for nurses because of the number of variables involved (e.g. risk factors, types of ulcers and degrees of impairment) and the numerous treatment/dressings available. Existing and potential infections are the most serious complications of pressure ulcers. In treating pressure ulcers, nurses should follow the local trust's policies and national guidelines. Prompt treatment can prevent further tissue damage and pain and facilitate wound healing. See Table 18-5 regarding dressings for pressure ulcers.

Pressure ulcer treatment usually combines effective wound care with pressure-reducing techniques and holistic management of the patient such as maintaining adequate nutritional intake.

Table 18-5 Dressings for Pressure Ulcers

Dressing	Mechanism of action	Grade 1	Grade 2	Grade 3	Grade 4
Transparent barrier	Retains wound moisture, allows gas exchange, does not stick to wound surface	✓	✓		
Hydrocolloid	Occlusive, repels moisture and dirt, maintains moist wound environment	✓		✓	
Hydrogel	Maintains moist wound environment		✓	✓	✓
Alginate	Maintains moist wound environment, absorbs exudate			✓	✓

Note: Some dressings may be used on other pressure ulcer grades. See Figure 18-8 on page 552 for European Pressure Ulcer Advisory Panel Pressure Ulcer Grading and Classification.

Pressure ulcer wounds should be cleansed with sterile saline in hospitals; however, in the patient's home tap water can be used as research suggests there is no clinical advantage for using sterile saline for chronic wounds (Joanna Briggs Institute, 2008). It is acceptable for some individuals to cleanse the area by means of showering particularly for large or awkward areas. Minimal mechanical force should be used when cleansing the wound as this will delay healing. The wound should only be cleansed with antiseptics if clinically indicated.

Tissue that is non-viable should be removed in order to reduce the risk of infection, facilitate healing and aid assessment of the wound. The removal of non-viable tissue can be achieved by a number of techniques including surgery, autolysis (breakdown of the dead tissue by self-produced enzymes), enzymatic (use of topical ointments to promote debridement (removal of dead tissue)) and larval (maggot) therapy.

Surgical removal of non-viable tissue can range from the use of scissors or scalpel at the bedside to full surgery. The use of hydrocolloids and hydrogels dressings aid the autolysis of non-viable tissue by providing a moist environment.

Dressing Wounds

Dressings are applied for the following purposes:

- to protect the wound from mechanical injury;
- to protect the wound from microbial contamination;
- to provide or maintain a moist environment;
- to provide thermal insulation;
- to absorb drainage or debride a wound or both;
- to prevent haemorrhage (when applied as a pressure dressing or with elastic bandages);
- to splint or immobilise the wound site and thereby facilitate healing and prevent injury.

Types of Dressing

Various dressing materials are available to cover wounds. The type of dressing used depends on (a) the location, size and type of the wound; (b) the amount of exudate; (c) whether the wound requires debridement or is infected; and (d) such considerations as frequency of dressing change, ease or difficulty of dressing application and cost. Table 18-6 describes these materials.

Table 18-6 Selected Types of Wound Dressings

Dressing	Description	Purpose	Examples
Transparent adhesive films/ wound barriers	Adhesive plastic, semi-permeable, nonabsorbent dressings allow exchange of oxygen between the atmosphere and wound bed. They are impermeable to bacteria and water.	To provide protection against contamination and friction; to maintain a clean moist surface that facilitates cellular migration; to provide insulation by preventing fluid evaporation; and to facilitate wound assessment. For procedure for applying this dressing see *Procedure 18-4*.	Op-Site, Tegaderm, Bioclusive
Impregnated nonadherent dressings	Woven or nonwoven cotton or synthetic materials are impregnated with petrolatum, saline, zinc-saline, antimicrobials or other agents. Require secondary dressings to secure them in place, retain moisture and provide wound protection.	To cover, soothe and protect partial- and full-thickness wounds without exudates.	Adaptic, Carrasyn, Xeroform
Hydrocolloids	Waterproof adhesive wafers, pastes or powders. Wafers, designed to be worn for up to seven days, consist of two layers. The inner adhesive layer has particles that absorb exudate and form a hydrated gel over the wound; the outer film provides a seal.	To absorb exudate; to produce a moist environment that facilitates healing but does not cause maceration of surrounding skin; to protect the wound from bacterial contamination, foreign debris and urine or faeces; and to prevent shearing. For procedure for applying this dressing see *Procedure 18-5*.	DuoDerm, Comfeel, Tegasorb, Granuflex
Hydrogels	Glycerin or water-based non-adhesive jellylike sheets, granules or gels are oxygen permeable, unless covered by a plastic film. May require secondary occlusive dressing.	To liquefy necrotic tissue or slough, rehydrate the wound bed and fill in dead space.	Aquasorb, Elasto-Gel, Vigilon
Polyurethane foams	Nonadherent hydrocolloid dressings; these need to have their edges taped down or sealed. Require secondary dressings to obtain an occlusive environment. Surrounding skin must be protected to prevent maceration.	To absorb light to moderate amounts of exudate; to debride wounds.	Lyofoam, Allevyn
Exudate absorbers (alginates)	Nonadherent dressings of powder, beads or granules, ropes, sheets or paste conform to the wound surface and absorb up to 20 times their weight in exudate; require a secondary dressing.	To provide a moist wound surface by interacting with exudate to form a gelatinous mass; to absorb exudate; to eliminate dead space or pack wounds; and to support debridement.	Sorbsan, Kaltostat

PROCEDURE 18-4 Applying a Transparent Wound Barrier

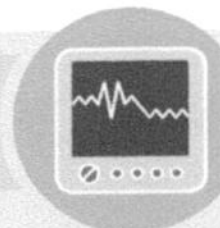

Purposes

- To provide a moist wound environment and promote wound healing
- To protect the wound from trauma and infectious agents
- To facilitate assessment of wound healing

Assessment

Assess

- Appearance and size of the wound or at-risk skin area
- Amount and character of exudate
- For complaints of discomfort or pain
- For signs of infection such as fever, chills or elevated WBC count

Planning

Equipment

- Clean gloves
- Sterile gloves (optional)
- Hair scissors or clippers
- Alcohol or acetone to remove adhesive from old dressing
- Clinical waste bag
- Saline and gauze or syringe for wound irrigation
- Wound barrier dressing
- Scissors

Implementation

Preparation

Review patient's notes regarding frequency and type of dressing change. Ensure where possible that the dressing is done at a time that is convenient for the patient (e.g. not at visiting time).

Performance

1 Follow local policy to ensure that you explain to the patient what you are going to do, why it is necessary and how they can cooperate. Obtain consent and maintain patient privacy and dignity and ensure that the appropriate local infection control procedures are observed.

2 Position the patient as required. *To improve access to the site and patient comfort.*

3 Wash hands, apply clean gloves and remove the existing dressing. *To assess appropriateness of new dressing.*

4 Remove soiled gloves and wash hands. *To prevent cross-contamination.*

5 Put on clean or sterile gloves in accordance with local policy. *To prevent cross-contamination.*

6 Clean the wound if indicated. *To remove visible debris/ foreign material or excess exudate.*

7 Dry the surrounding skin with dry gauze. *To prevent maceration of surrounding skin.*

8 Assess the wound. *To help determine progression of the wound.*

9 Remove part of the paper backing on the dressing (see Figure 18-12). *To help with the application of the dressing.*

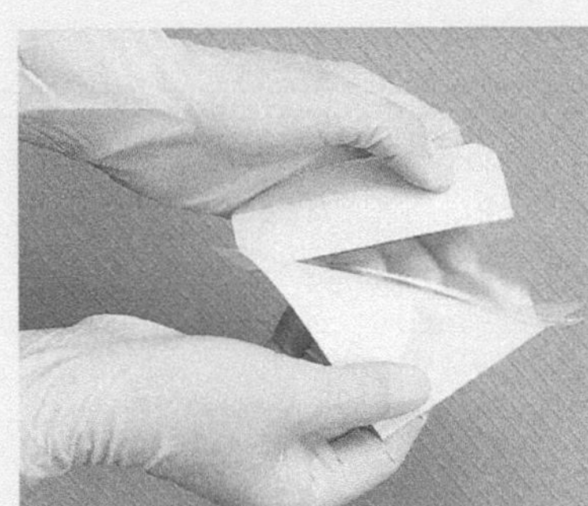

Figure 18-12 A transparent wound dressing.
Source: Jenny Thomas.

10 Apply the dressing at one edge of the wound site, allowing at least 2.5cm (1 inch) coverage of the skin surrounding the wound. *To ensure the wound is adequately covered.*

11 Gently lay or press the barrier over the wound. Keep it free of wrinkles, but avoid stretching it too tightly. *A stretched dressing restricts mobility.*

12 Remove and dispose of gloves appropriately. *To prevent cross-contamination.*

13 Assess the wound at least daily. *To ensure any changes are recorded and assess the necessity for changing dressing.*

14 Discuss the outcomes with the patient and document the findings in the patient's notes (see Figure 18-9 on page 553). *To inform the patient and other healthcare professionals.*

Evaluation

- Perform follow-up based on findings that deviate from expected or normal for the patient.
- Relate findings to previous assessment information if available.
- Report significant deviations from normal to the doctor.

PROCEDURE 18-5 Applying a Hydrocolloid Dressing

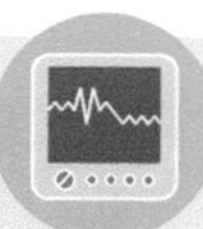

Purposes

- To maintain a moist wound surface and promote healing
- To prevent the entrance of micro-organisms into the wound
- To minimise wound discomfort
- To promote autolysis of necrotic material by white blood cells
- To decrease the frequency of dressing changes

Assessment

Assess

- Appearance and size of the wound or at-risk skin area
- Amount and character of exudate
- For complaints of discomfort
- For signs of infection such as fever, chills or elevated WBC count

Planning

If possible, review the patient notes to note details regarding previous hydrocolloid dressing changes.

Equipment

- Clean gloves
- Sterile gloves (optional)
- Dressing set including scissors
- Clinical waste bag
- Sterile gauze and saline (if required)
- Hydrocolloid dressing at least 3-4cm (1.5 inch) larger than wound on all four sides

Implementation

Preparation

- Review the care plan for information regarding frequency and type of dressing change.
- Change the dressing if it leaks, is dislodged or develops an odour. Otherwise, it may remain in place up to one week.
- If possible, schedule the dressing change at a time convenient for the patient. Some dressing changes require only a few minutes and others can take much longer.

Performance

1 Follow local policy to ensure that you explain to the patient what you are going to do, why it is necessary and how they can cooperate. Obtain consent and maintain patient privacy and dignity and ensure that the appropriate local infection control procedures are observed.

2 Position the patient as required. *To improve access to the site and patient comfort.*

3 Wash hands, apply clean gloves and remove the existing dressing. *To assess appropriateness of new dressing.*

4 Remove soiled gloves and wash hands. *To prevent cross-contamination.*

5 Put on clean or sterile gloves in accordance with local policy. *To prevent cross-contamination.*

6 Clean the wound if indicated. *To remove visible debris/ foreign material or excess exudates.*

7 Leave the residue that is difficult to remove on the skin. It will wear off in time. *Attempts to remove residue can irritate the surrounding skin.*

8 Dry the surrounding skin with dry gauze. *To prevent maceration of surrounding skin.*

9 Assess the wound. *To help determine progression of the wound.*

10 Apply the dressing. Follow the manufacturer's instructions.

11 Hold the dressing in place for about one minute with your hand. *The warmth helps the dressing conform and adhere.*

12 Remove and dispose of gloves appropriately. *To prevent cross-contamination.*

13 Assess the wound at least daily. *To ensure any changes are recorded and assess the necessity for changing dressing.*

14 Discuss the outcomes with the patient and document the findings in the patient's notes. *To inform the patient and other healthcare professionals.*

Evaluation

- Perform follow-up based on findings that deviate from expected or normal for the patient.
- Relate findings to previous assessment information if available.
- Report significant deviations from normal to the doctor or specialist wound care nurse.

Supporting and Immobilising Wounds

Bandages and binders serve various purposes:

- supporting a wound (e.g. a fractured bone);
- immobilising a wound (e.g. a strained shoulder);
- applying pressure (e.g. elastic bandages on the lower extremities to improve venous blood flow);
- securing a dressing (e.g. for an extensive abdominal surgical wound).

There are several types of bandages and binders and several ways in which they are applied. When correctly applied, they promote healing, provide comfort and can prevent injury (see the *Practice Guidelines*).

Bandages

A bandage is a strip of cloth used to wrap some part of the body. Bandages are available in various widths, most commonly 1.5–7.5cm, and are usually supplied in rolls for easy application to a body part.

PRACTICE GUIDELINES

Bandaging

- Whenever possible, bandage the part in its normal position, with the joint slightly flexed *to avoid putting strain on the ligaments and the muscles of the joint.*
- Pad between skin surfaces and over bony prominences *to prevent friction from the bandage and consequent abrasion of the skin.*
- Always bandage body parts by working from the distal to the proximal end *to aid the return flow of venous blood.*
- Bandage with even pressure *to prevent interference with blood circulation.*
- Whenever possible, leave the end of the body part (e.g. the toe) exposed *so that you will be able to determine the adequacy of the blood circulation to the extremity.*
- Cover dressings with bandages at least 5cm beyond the edges of the dressing *to prevent the dressing and wound from becoming contaminated.*
- Face the patient when applying a bandage *to maintain uniform tension and the appropriate direction of the bandage.*

Many types of materials are used for bandages. Gauze is one of the most commonly used, because it is light and porous and readily moulds to the body. It is also relatively inexpensive, so it is generally discarded when soiled. Gauze is used to retain dressings on wounds and to bandage the fingers, hands, toes and feet. It supports dressings and at the same time permits air to circulate, while elastic conforming bandages are applied to provide pressure to an area.

The width of the bandage used depends on the size of the body part to be bandaged. For example, a 2.5cm (1 inch) bandage is used for a finger, a 5cm bandage for an arm, and a 7.5cm or 10cm bandage for a leg. Padding (e.g. abdominal pads and gauze squares) is frequently used to cover bony prominences (e.g. the elbow) or to separate skin surfaces (e.g. the fingers).

Before applying a bandage, the nurse needs to know its purpose and to assess the area requiring support (see the *Practice Guidelines*). When bandages are used to secure dressings, the nurse wears gloves to prevent contact with body fluids.

PRACTICE GUIDELINES

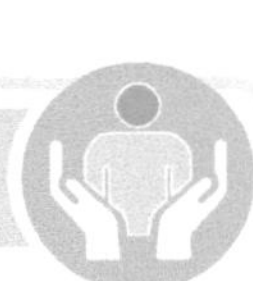

Assessing before Applying Bandages or Binders

- Inspect and palpate the area for swelling.
- Inspect for the presence of and status of wounds (open wounds will require a dressing before a bandage or binder is applied).
- Note the presence of drainage (amount, colour, odour, viscosity).
- Inspect and palpate for adequacy of circulation (skin temperature, colour and sensation). *Pale or cyanotic skin, cool temperature, tingling and numbness can indicate impaired circulation.*
- Ask the patient about any pain experienced (location, intensity, onset, quality).
- Assess the ability of the patient to reapply the bandage or binder when needed.
- Assess the capabilities of the patient regarding activities of daily living (e.g. to eat, dress, comb hair, bathe) and assess the assistance required during the convalescence period.

Basic Turns for Roller Bandages

Applying bandages to various parts of the body involves one or more of five basic bandaging turns.

1 *Circular* turns are used to anchor bandages and to terminate them. Circular turns usually are not applied directly over a wound because of the discomfort the bandage would cause.
2 *Spiral* turns are used to bandage parts of the body that are fairly uniform in circumference, for example, the upper arm or upper leg.
3 *Spiral reverse* turns are used to bandage cylindrical parts of the body that are not uniform in circumference, for example, the lower leg or forearm.
4 *Recurrent* turns are used to cover distal parts of the body, for example, the end of a finger, the skull or the stump of an amputation.
5 *Figure-eight* turns are used to bandage an elbow, knee or ankle, because they permit some movement after application.

Circular Turns

- Hold the bandage in your dominant hand, keeping the roll uppermost, and unroll the bandage about 8cm. This length of unrolled bandage allows good control for placement and tension.
- Apply the end of the bandage to the part of the body to be bandaged. Hold the end down with the thumb of the other hand (see Figure 18-13).
- Encircle the body part a few times or as often as needed, making sure that each layer overlaps one-half to two-thirds of the previous layer. This provides even support to the area.
- The bandage should be firm, but not too tight. Ask the patient if the bandage feels comfortable. A tight bandage can interfere with blood circulation, whereas a loose bandage does not provide adequate protection.
- Secure the end of the bandage with tape or a safety pin over an uninjured area. Pins can cause discomfort when situated over an injured area.

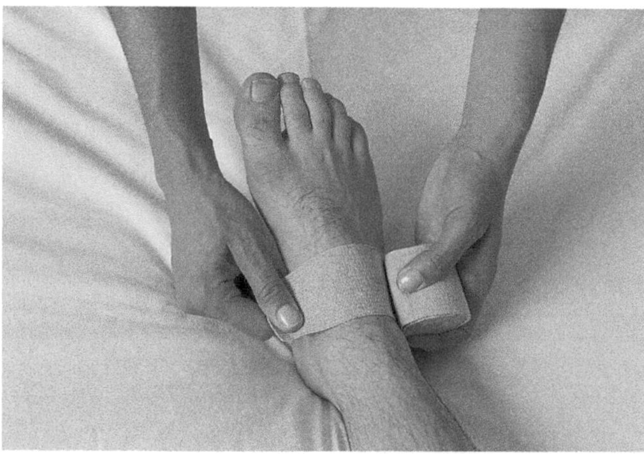

Figure 18-13 Starting a bandage with two circular turns.
Source: Elena Dorfmann.

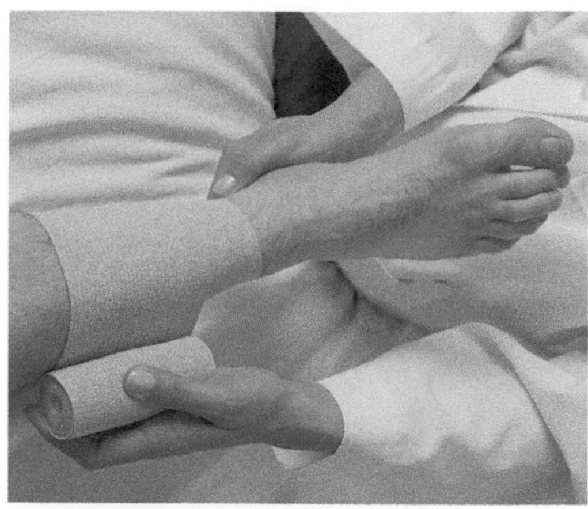

Figure 18-14 Applying spiral turns.
Source: Elena Dorfmann.

Spiral Turns

- Make two circular turns. Two circular turns anchor the bandage.
- Continue spiral turns at about a 30-degree angle, each turn overlapping the preceding one by two-thirds the width of the bandage (see Figure 18-14).
- Terminate the bandage with two circular turns and secure the end as described for circular turns.

Spiral Reverse Turns

- Anchor the bandage with two circular turns, and bring the bandage upward at about a 30-degree angle.
- Place the thumb of your free hand on the upper edge of the bandage (see Figure 18-15(a)). The thumb will hold the bandage while it is folded on itself.
- Unroll the bandage about 15cm, and then turn your hand so that the bandage falls over itself (see Figure 18-15(b)).
- Continue the bandage around the limb, overlapping each previous turn by two-thirds the width of the bandage. Make each bandage turn at the same position on the limb so that the turns of the bandage will be aligned (see Figure 18-15(c)).
- Terminate the bandage with two circular turns, and secure the end as described for circular turns.

Recurrent Turns

- Anchor the bandage with two circular turns.
- Fold the bandage back on itself, and bring it centrally over the distal end to be bandaged (see Figure 18-16).
- Holding it with the other hand, bring the bandage back over the end to the right of the centre bandage but overlapping it by two-thirds the width of the bandage.
- Bring the bandage back on the left side, also overlapping the first turn by two-thirds the width of the bandage.
- Continue this pattern of alternating right and left until the area is covered. Overlap the preceding turn by two-thirds the bandage width each time.
- Terminate the bandage with two circular turns (see Figure 18-17). Secure the end appropriately.

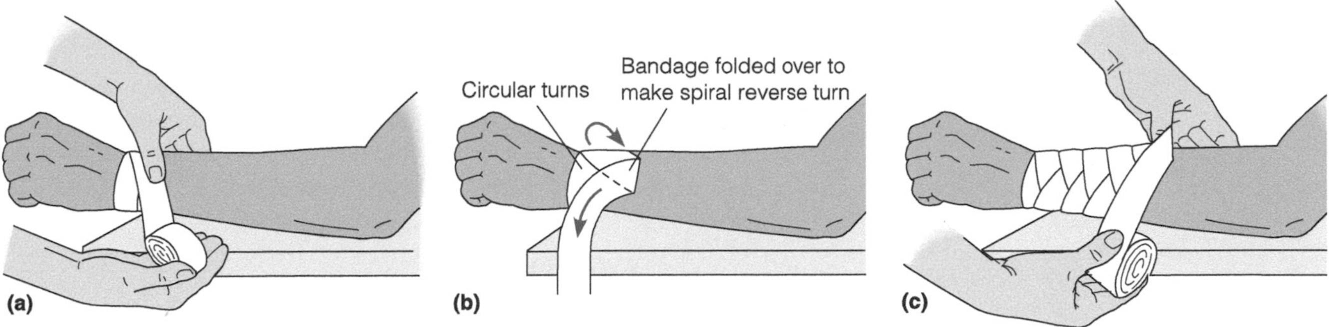

Figure 18-15 Applying spiral reverse turns.

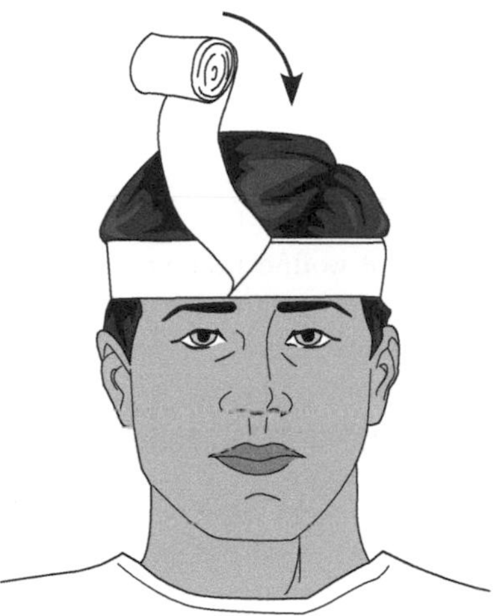

Figure 18-16 Starting a recurrent bandage.

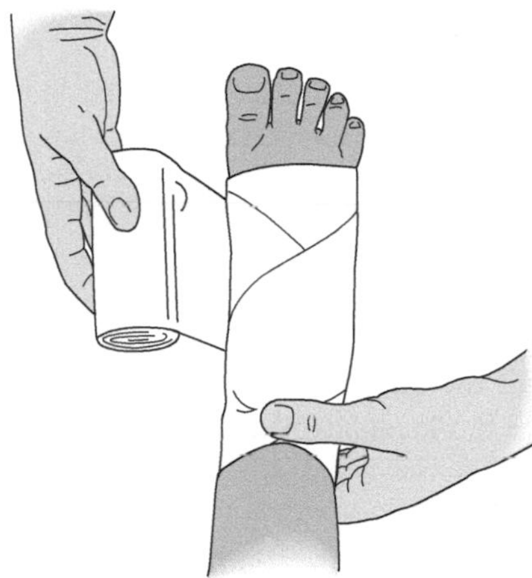

Figure 18-18 Applying a figure-eight bandage.

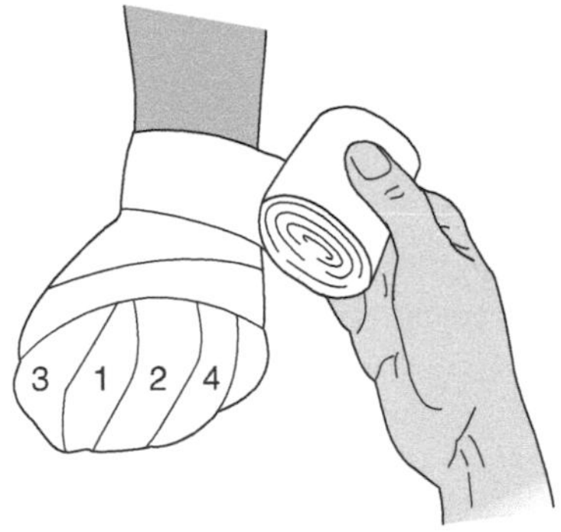

Figure 18-17 Completing a recurrent bandage.

Figure-Eight Turns

- Anchor the bandage with two circular turns.
- Carry the bandage above the joint, around it and then below it, making a figure-eight (see Figure 18-18).
- Continue above and below the joint, overlapping the previous turn by two-thirds the width of the bandage.
- Terminate the bandage above the joint with two circular turns and then secure the end appropriately.

Tubular Support and Retention Bandages

Tubular retention bandages are made out of a gauze material and are used to retain dressings. They are particularly useful when dressing awkward areas such as the trunk of the body. Tubular support bandages are elasticated and when applied in a double layer can support strains and sprains of limbs.

Binders

A binder is a type of bandage designed for a specific body part, for example, the triangular binder (sling) fits the arm. Binders are used to support large areas of the body, such as the abdomen, arm or chest.

Triangular Arm Sling

- Ask the patient to flex the elbow to an 80-degree angle or less, depending on the purpose. The thumb should be facing upward or inward towards the body. *An 80-degree angle is sufficient to support the forearm, to prevent swelling of the hand, and to relieve pressure on the shoulder joint (e.g. to support the paralysed arm of a stroke patient whose shoulder might otherwise become dislocated).* A more acute angle is preferred if there is swelling of the hand (see how to apply a sling for maximum hand elevation, below).

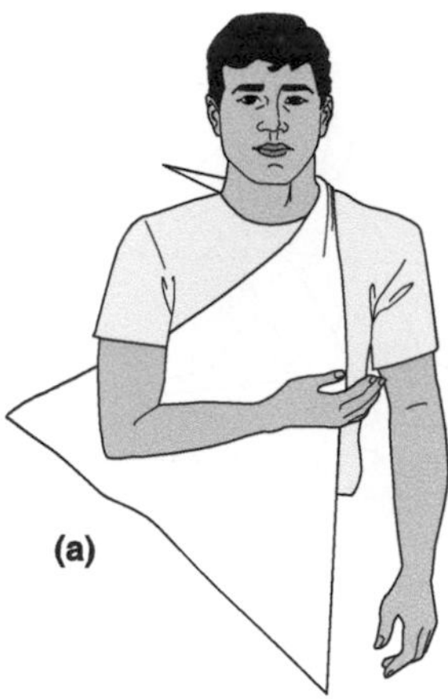

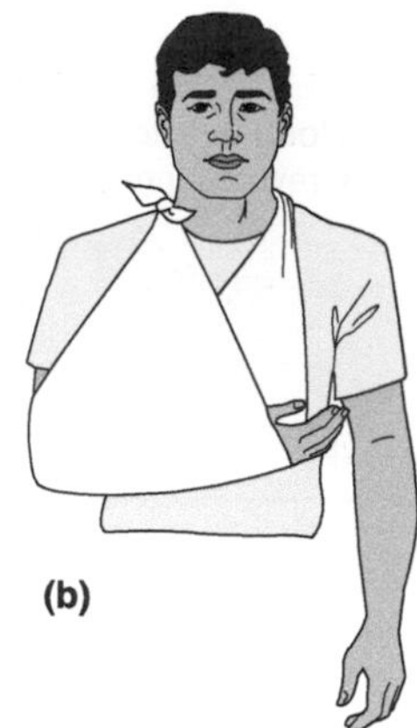

Figure 18-19 Large arm sling.

- Place one end of the unfolded triangular binder over the shoulder of the uninjured side so that the binder falls down the front of the chest of the patient with the point of the triangle (apex) under the elbow of the injured side.
- Take the upper corner and carry it around the neck until it hangs over the shoulder on the injured side.
- Bring the lower corner of the binder up over the arm to the shoulder of the injured side. Using a square knot, secure this corner to the upper corner at the side of the neck on the injured side (see Figure 18-19(a)). *A square knot will not slip. Tying the knot at the side of the neck prevents pressure on the bony prominences of the vertebral column at the back of the neck.*
- Make sure the wrist is supported, to maintain alignment.
- Fold the sling neatly at the elbow and secure it with safety pins or tape. It may be folded and fastened at the front (see Figure 18-19(b)).
- Remove the sling periodically to inspect the skin for indications of irritation, especially around the site of the knot.

It is important to note that once the dressing or bandage is applied, circulation beyond that dressing bandage should be checked. The nurse must note the colour of the skin, temperature, any sensation of 'pins and needles' or numbness.

EVALUATING

Evaluation of the care provided as measured against the desired outcomes should be undertaken as usual. Ongoing assessment judges whether patient outcomes have been achieved. In particular, the nurse assesses skin integrity (particularly over bony prominences), nutritional and fluid intake, and signs of healing. If outcomes are not achieved, the nurse should explore the reasons why and consider other interventions to achieve the desired outcomes.

Wound management is one of the most challenging and varied roles within nursing. Effective wound management requires knowledge of wound healing, assessment and dressings. Generally wound management is not a role that can be delegated to nursing assistants as it requires a level of expertise to make rational decisions and evaluate previous treatment.

Key to wound management is accurate documentation. Assessment of the whole person is vital in understanding the underlying factors that could affect wound healing. This along with assessment of the wound should provide the nurse with the information to establish effective treatment. It is important to note that no dressing will ever heal a wound – the wound is healed from the inside out – and for some patients their wounds will never heal as their underlying condition is not conducive with healing.

CRITICAL REFLECTION

Let us revisit the case study on page 543. Now that you have read this chapter, reflect on how you would begin to assess Charles. What extrinsic and intrinsic factors could affect wound healing for Charles? How would you promote wound healing and what type of dressing would you choose?

CHAPTER HIGHLIGHTS

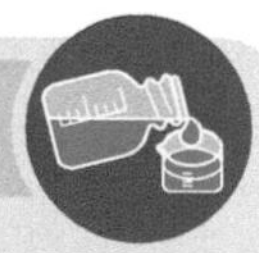

- Maintaining skin integrity is an important function of the nurse.
- A pressure ulcer is any lesion caused by unrelieved pressure that results in damage to underlying tissues. Pressure ulcers usually occur over bony prominences.
- Two other factors that act in conjunction with pressure to produce a pressure ulcer are friction and shearing forces.
- Several factors increase the risk for the development of pressure ulcers: immobility and inactivity, inadequate nutrition, faecal and urinary incontinence, decreased mental status, diminished sensation, excessive body heat and advanced age.
- There are four grades of pressure ulcer development, which vary according to the degree of tissue damage.
- Several risk assessment tools are available to identify patients at risk for pressure ulcer development. They include scoring systems to evaluate a person's degree of risk.

- Meticulous skin examination of common pressure ulcer sites by the nurse is an important ongoing assessment activity for patients at risk.
- Nursing interventions to prevent the formation of pressure ulcers include conducting ongoing assessment of risk factors and skin status, providing skin care to maintain skin integrity, ensuring adequate nutrition, implementing measures to avoid skin trauma, providing supportive devices and patient education.
- When a pressure ulcer is present, the nurse describes the ulcer in terms of location, size, depth, stage, colour, status of wound margins and surrounding skin, and specific signs of infection, if present.
- Wound assessment is an ongoing process to evaluate healing. The nurse assesses wounds by visual inspection, palpation and the sense of smell. Essential information acquired from the assessment of wounds include wound appearance, size, drainage, swelling and pain.
- There are two types of wound healing, which are distinguished by the amount of tissue loss: primary intention healing and secondary intention healing.
- The wound-healing process has three phases: inflammatory, proliferative and maturation.
- Major types of wound exudate are serous, purulent and haemorrhagic. Exudate can be a combination of two or three of these types.
- Laboratory tests that may be used to assess the progress of wound healing include leukocyte count, haemoglobin, blood coagulation studies, serum protein analysis and wound cultures. Nurses are usually responsible for obtaining specimens of wound drainage for culture.
- The main complications of wound healing are haemorrhage, infection and dehiscence, each of which is identifiable by specific clinical signs and symptoms.
- Factors affecting wound healing include developmental stage, nutritional status, lifestyle, medications and the presence of infection.
- Treatment for pressure ulcers varies according to the stage of the ulcer and local policy.
- Major nursing responsibilities related to wound care include assisting the patient in obtaining sufficient nutrition and fluids, preventing wound infections and proper positioning.
- Wound care may involve cleaning wounds, changing dressings, irrigating and applying bandages and binders.
- Various dressing materials are available to protect wounds, absorb exudate and keep the wound bed moist, thus facilitating healing.
- Synthetic dressings have been developed for use with specific types of wounds. These include transparent adhesive films, hydrocolloids, hydrogels, polyurethane foams and exudate absorbers. The nurse must be aware of the specific purposes of each and their indications for use.
- The type of dressing used depends on (a) location, size and type of the wound; (b) amount of exudate; (c) whether or not the wound requires debridement, is infected or has sinus tracts; and (d) such considerations as frequency of dressing change, ease or difficulty of dressing applications and cost.

ACTIVITY ANSWERS

ACTIVITY 18-1 Depending on your patient, one or more of the following factors may lead to your patient developing a pressure ulcer:

- age
- skin type
- nutrition
- hydration
- peripheral circulation
- oedema
- reduced mobility
- trauma
- faecal/urinary incontinence
- drying or desiccation of skin
- fever/infection
- immunosuppression
- reduced sensation
- medications
- underlying diseases such as diabetes
- stress/mental health
- metabolic state

ACTIVITY 18-2 Although your patient may already have developed a pressure ulcer, there are a number of interventions that could prevent this wound from deteriorating and also prevent the development of further pressure ulcers. Interventions could include:

- Encouraging food intake
- Providing supplemental drinks
- Ensuring skin hygiene is maintained
- Avoiding skin trauma by using appropriate manual handling techniques
- Providing pressure relieving equipment (if it has not already been provided)

REFERENCES

Anderson, B. (2005) 'Nutrition and wound healing: The necessity of assessment', *British Journal of Nursing*, 14(19 Suppl.), S30, S32, S34, S36, S38.

Atiyeh, B.S., Dibo, S.A. and Hayek, S.N. (2009) 'Wound cleansing, topical antiseptics and wound healing', *International Wound Journal*, 6, 420–430.

Baumgarten, M., Margolis, D., Orwig, D., Hawkes, W., Rich, S., Langenberg, P., Shardell, M., Palmer, M.H., McArdle, P., Sterling, R., Jones, P.S. and Magaziner, J. (2010) 'Use of pressure-redistributing support surfaces among elderly hip fracture patients across the continuum of care: Adherence to pressure ulcer prevention guidelines', *The Gerontologist*, 50(2), 253–262.

BBC (2010) *Organs – Skin*, London: BBC, available from http://www.bbc.co.uk/science/humanbody/body/factfiles/skin/skin.shtml (accessed March 2011).

Bours, G.J.J.W., De Laat, E., Halfens, R.J.G. and Lubbers, M. (2001) 'Prevalence, risk factors and prevention of pressure ulcers in Dutch intensive care units – results of a cross-sectional survey', *Intensive Care Medicine*, 27, 1599–1605.

Butcher, M. (2002) 'Wound care: Managing wound sinuses', *Nursing Times*, 98(2), 63–65.

Davies, C.E., Turton, G., Woolfrey, G., Elley, R. and Taylor, M. (2005) 'Exploring debridement options for chronic venous leg ulcers', *British Journal of Nursing*, 14(7), 393–397.

Dowsett, C., Edwards-Jones, V. and Davies, S. (2004) 'Infection control for wound bed preparation', *British Journal of Community Nursing*, 9(9 Supp), 12–17.

Ersser, S.J., Getliffe, K., Voegeli, D. and Regan, S. (2005) 'A critical review of the inter-relationship between skin vulnerability and urinary incontinence and related nursing intervention', *International Journal of Nursing Studies*, 42(7), 823–835.

European Pressure Ulcer Advisory Panel (EPUAP) (2010) *Pressure ulcer classification. Differentiation between pressure ulcers and moist lesions*, available at http://www.epuap.org/review6_3/page6.html (accessed March 2011).

EPUAP and NPUAP (2009) *Pressure ulcer treatment quick reference guide*, available at http://www.epuap.org/guidelines/Final_Quick_Treatment.pdf (accessed March 2011).

Fernandez, R.T., Griffiths, R. and Ussia, C. (2007) 'Water for wound cleansing', *International Journal of Evidence-based Healthcare*, 5(3), 305–323.

Fette, A.M. (2006) 'A clinimetric analysis of wound measurement tools', *World Wide Wounds*, available at http://www.worldwidewounds.com/2006/january/Fette/Clinimetric-Analysis-Wound-Measurement-Tools.html (accessed March 2011).

Gardiner, L., Lampshire, S., Biggins, A., McMurray, A., Noake, N., van Zyl, M., Vickery, J., Woodage, T., Lodge, J. and Edgar, M. (2008) 'Evidence-based best practice in maintaining skin integrity', *Wound Practice and Research*, 16(2), 5–15.

Great Ormond Street Hospital for Children NHS Trust (2003) *Pressure ulcer prevention and management*, available at http://www.ich.ucl.ac.uk/clinical_information/clinical_guidelines/copy%20of%20cpg_guideline_00005 (accessed March 2011).

Hagisawa, S. and Barbenel, J. (1999) 'The limits of pressure sore prevention', *Journal of the Royal Society of Medicine*, 92, 576–578.

Joanna Briggs Institute (2008) 'Solutions, techniques and pressure in wound cleansing', *Nursing Standard*, 22(27), 35–39.

Jolley, D.J., Wright, R., McGowan, S., Hickey, M.B., Campbell, D.A., Sinclair, R.D. and Montgomery, K.C. (2004) 'Preventing pressure ulcers with the Australian Medical Sheepskin: An open-label randomized controlled trial', *The Medical Journal of Australia*, 180, 324–327.

Keller, B.P.J.A., Wille, J., van Ramshorst, B. and van der Werken, C. (2002) 'Pressure ulcers in intensive care patients: A review of risks and prevention', *Intensive Care Medicine*, 28, 1379–1388.

Khan, M.N. and Naqvi, A.H. (2006) 'Antiseptics, iodine, povidone iodine and traumatic wound cleansing', *Journal of Tissue Viability*, 16(4), 6–10.

Kundin, J.I. (1989) 'A new way to size up a wound', *American Journal of Nursing*, 89(2), 206–207.

Margolis, D.J., Knauss, J., Bilker, W. and Baumgarten, M. (2003) 'Medical conditions as risk factors for pressure ulcers in an outpatient setting', *Age and Ageing*, 32, 259–264.

NHS Choices (2010) *Pressure ulcers – causes*, available at http://www.nhs.uk/Conditions/Pressure-ulcers/Pages/Causes.aspx (accessed March 2011).

NICE (2003) *Pressure ulcer prevention: Pressure ulcer risk assessment and prevention, including the use of pressure-relieving devices (beds, mattresses and overlays) for the prevention of pressure ulcers in primary and secondary care*, CG 7, London: NICE.

NICE (2005) *Pressure ulcers: The management of pressure ulcers in primary and secondary care*, CG 29, London: NICE.

NMC (2007) *Essential skills clusters for pre-registration nursing programmes*, London: NMC.

NMC (2010) *Standards for pre-registration nursing education*, London: NMC.

Norton, D., McLaren, R. and Exton-Smith, A.N. (1975) *An investigation of geriatric nursing problems in hospital*, Edinburgh: Churchill Livingstone.

NPSA (2009) *Pressure ulcers: An analysis of RLS data*, available at http://www.npsa.nhs.uk/EasySiteWeb/GatewayLink.aspx?alId=29229 (accessed March 2011).

Oliver, L. (1997) 'Wound cleansing', *Nursing Standard*, 11(20), 47–56.

Pancorbo-Hidalgo, P.I., Garcia-Fernandez, F.P., Lopez-Medina, I.M. and Alvarez-Nieto, C. (2006) 'Risk assessment scales for pressure ulcer prevention: A systematic review', *Journal of Advanced Nursing*, 54(1), 94–110.

Posnett, J. and Franks, P.J. (2007) 'The costs of skin breakdown and ulceration in the UK', in Pownall, M. (ed.) *Skin breakdown: The silent epidemic*. Hull: Smith and Nephew, 6–12.

Riordan, J. and Voegeli, D. (2009) 'Prevention and treatment of pressure ulcers', *British Journal of Nursing*, 18(20), S20–S27.

RCN (2001) *Clinical practice guidelines: Pressure ulcer risk assessment and prevention*, London: RCN.

Samuriwo, R. (2010) 'Effects of education and experience on nurses' value of ulcer prevention', *British Journal of Nursing*, 19(20 supplement), S8–S18.

Schoonhoven, L., Grobber, D.E., Bousema, M.T. and Buskins, E. (2005) 'Predicting pressure ulcers: Cases missed using a new clinical prediction rule', *Journal of Advanced Nursing*, 49(1), 16–22.

Tobon, A., Arango, M., Fernandez, D. and Restrepo, A. (2003) 'Mucormycosis (zygomycosis) in a heart-kidney transplant recipient. Recovery after posaconazole therapy', *Clinical Infectious Diseases*, 36, 1488–1491.

Vanderwee, K., Clark, M., Dealey, C. *et al.* (2007) 'Pressure ulcer prevalence in Europe: A pilot study', *Journal of Evaluation in Clinical Practice*, 13(2), 227–235.

Voegeli, D. (2008) 'Care or harm: Exploring essential components in skin care regimens', *British Journal of Nursing*, 17(1), 24–30.

Waterlow, J. (1997) 'Practical use of the Waterlow tool in the community', *British Journal of Community Nursing*, 2(2), 83–86.

White, R. and Cutting, K.F. (2006) 'Modern exudates management: A review of wound treatments', *World Wide Wounds*, available at http://www.worldwidewounds.com/2006/september/White/Modern-Exudate-Mgt.html (accessed March 2011).

Willock, J., Baharestani, M.M. and Anthony, D. (2009) 'The development of the Glamorgan paediatric pressure ulcer risk assessment scale', *Journal of Wound Care*, 18(1), 17–21.

Yenidunya, M.O. and Demirseren, M.E. (2004) 'A useful method for pre-operative planning with a plastic sheet', *Plastic and Reconstructive Surgery*, 114(1), 271–272.

CHAPTER 19
NUTRITION

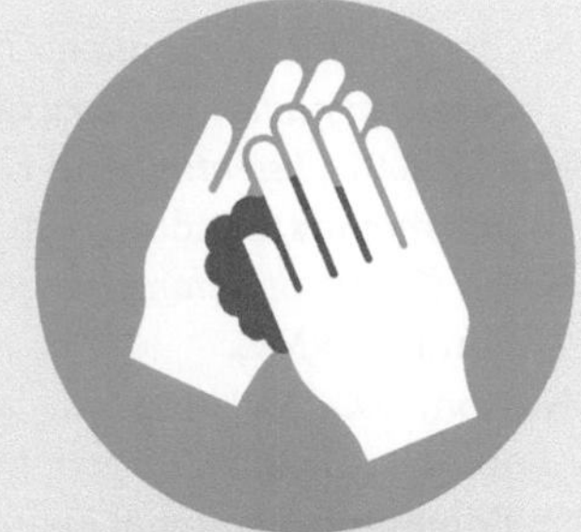

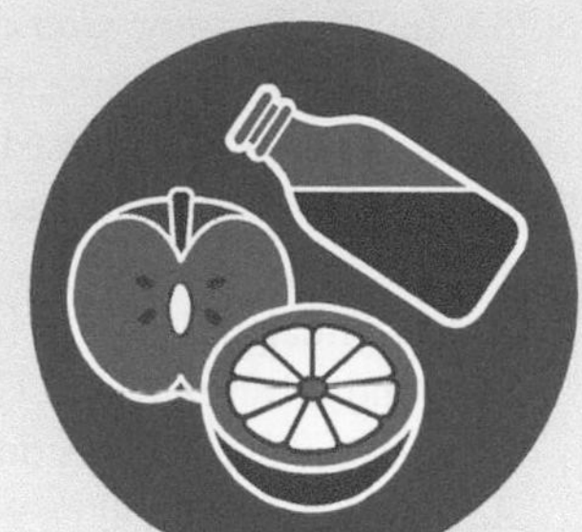

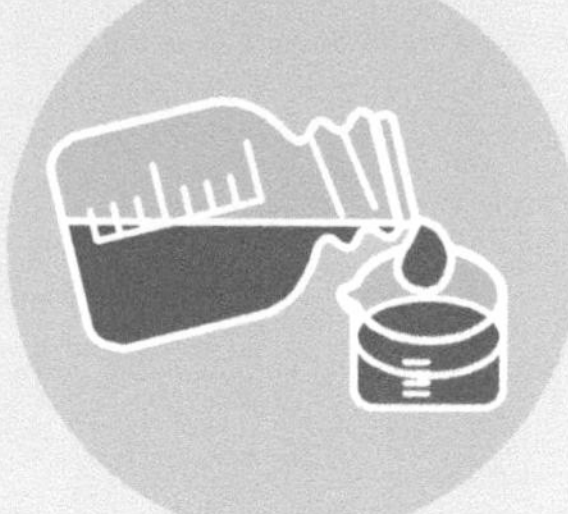

LEARNING OUTCOMES

After completing this chapter, you will be able to:

- Identify essential nutrients and dietary sources of each.
- Explain essential aspects of energy balance.
- Discuss body weight and the body mass index.
- Identify factors influencing nutrition.
- Identify developmental nutritional considerations.
- Discuss essential components and purposes of nutritional screening and nutritional assessment.
- Identify risk factors for and clinical signs of malnutrition.
- Describe nursing interventions to promote optimal nutrition.
- Discuss nursing interventions to treat patients with nutritional problems.
- Assess, plan, implement and evaluate nursing care for a patient that is unable to maintain his or her nutritional needs.

After reading this chapter you will be able to reflect on the nursing role in providing healthcare and promoting well-being. It relates to **Essential Skills Clusters (NMC, 2010)** 1, 2, 3, 4, 5, 6, 7, 8, 9, 10, 28, 29, 30, 31, 32, as appropriate for each progression point.

Ensure that you really understand this chapter by logging on to your complimentary **MyNursingKit** at **www.pearsoned.co.uk/kozier**. Complete the self-assessment tests to check your progress and utilise further activities to practise and confirm your understanding.

CASE STUDY

William is a 78-year-old gentleman who lives at home with his wife. They are both active social people who enjoy outdoor activities such as rambling, camping and watching sport such as rugby. On retiring William and his wife have spent two or three holidays a year abroad when they were not looking after their grandchildren and now their great grandchildren. William was admitted to your care following a cerebrovascular accident which left him with a left-sided weakness and dysphagia. Since admission he is reluctant to acknowledge his weakness and would prefer not to eat than embarrass himself by admitting he has difficulties in feeding himself. This has been going on for a few days and his nutritional needs are not being met.

INTRODUCTION

Nutrition is the interaction between the components that are found in what we eat and how they affect the body. According to Dudek (2006) the body's need for food and nutrition is on the same level of Maslow's Hierarchy of Needs as its need for oxygen to breathe. Individuals require essential nutrients in food for the growth, maintenance of body functions and body tissues. While water is essential for survival, research has classified two types of nutrients essential to our diet in order to maintain health and well-being. There are:

- **Macronutrients** – carbohydrates, proteins fats/lipids.
- **Micronutrients** – vitamins, minerals.

Webb (2008) states that a deficiency in any micronutrients could lead ultimately to a deficiency disease.

MACRONUTRIENTS

Carbohydrates

Carbohydrates are considered one of the most important sources of stored energy (Mann and Truswell 2007). The basic components of carbohydrates are carbon, hydrogen and oxygen which are then subdivided into two basic kinds: simple carbohydrates (sugars) and complex carbohydrates (starch).

Sugars are the simplest of all carbohydrates; they are water soluble and are produced naturally by both plants and animals. Sugars (building blocks) may be **monosaccharides**, e.g. glucose, fructose and galactose. Glucose is the major carbohydrate in blood and closely monitored for in people with diabetes in order to manage the diabetes effectively. **Disaccharides** are made up of two monosaccharides, e.g. glucose and fructose, bound together (sucrose) through a dehydration reaction. There is no real practical difference between these two types of sugars and it certainly does not mean that a monosaccharide is easier to digest that a disaccharide.

Starches are the insoluble, nonsweet forms of carbohydrate. They are **polysaccharides**; that is, they are composed of branched chains of dozens, sometimes hundreds, of monosaccharide molecules. Like sugars, nearly all starches exist naturally in plants, such as grains, legumes and potatoes.

Proteins

Proteins contain carbon, hydrogen, oxygen and nitrogen bound together by covalent bonds (Seeley *et al.*, 2011). Proteins act as a form of transport regulating body processes. Complete proteins are made up of **amino acids** which are further broken down into essential or nonessential amino acids. Complete proteins contain all nine essential amino acids which are found in meat, fish, poultry, eggs, milk and milk products. Incomplete proteins lack some amino acids but are usually derived from vegetables.

- Essential amino acids cannot be manufactured in the body and therefore must be ingested in the diet. For example arginine, which has a role in the immune system, and leucine, which is necessary for tissue growth and maintenance, can only be derived from food.
- Nonessential amino acids can be manufactured by the body. The body extracts amino acids from the diet and develops new ones from the carbon-hydrates and nitrogens. Nonessential amino acids include glycine, alanine, aspartic acid, glutamic acid, proline, hydroxyproline, cystine, tyrosine and serine.

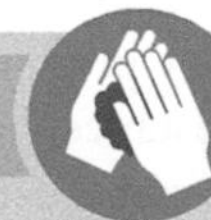

CLINICAL ALERT

A balanced diet is necessary in order to maintain health and well-being. Eating too much protein (meat) may cause health problems such as high cholesterol and gout, while too little protein may affect the immune system and possibly cause anaemia.

Lipids/Fats

Lipids are organic molecules composed mainly of carbon, hydrogen and oxygen, with some lipids presenting with small amounts of, for example, phosphorous and nitrogen. They are a group of compounds that dissolve in solvents such as alcohol or acetate but are normally insoluble in water. Lipids regulate physiological processes, form plasma membranes and provide protection and insulation to the body.

Fats are a type of lipid which, when ingested, break down, store and release energy for use when needed. Fats are a group of lipids known as triglycerides. Triglycerides are found in food such as meat, dairy products and cooking oils. There are three major lipids commonly referred to as fats: (1) triglycerides (fats and oils), (2) phospholipids (lecithin) and (3) sterols (cholesterol).

Triglycerides

Triglycerides account for 98% of the lipids in food (Dudek, 2006). Triglycerides consist of two different components, i.e. glycerol and three fatty acids. Glycerol attaches itself to three fatty acids and a triglyceride molecule is formed. Fatty acids are differentiated by the length and degree of saturation of their carbon chains.

Fatty acids are the basic structural units of all fats and can be saturated or unsaturated:

- Saturated fatty acids are mainly sourced from beef, pork, whole milk, cheese, butter, eggs, coconut oil and palm oil.
- Unsaturated fatty acids can be divided into three groups:
  - Monounsaturated fatty acids are found in olive oil and peanut oils. Monounsaturated fats are liquid at room temperature and semi-solid when refrigerated.
  - Polyunsaturated fatty acids are found in corn, fish oils and sunflowers, nuts and leafy green vegetables. Omega 3 fatty acids have been found to lower the risk of heart attacks.
  - Trans-fats are either monounsaturated or polyunsaturated fats and only occur in small amounts in dairy products and meat.

Phospholipids

Phospholipids are both fat and water soluble. This factor enables phospholipids to act as emulsifiers (a chemical agent which stops liquid and solid parts separating). Thus they keep blood and other body fluids suspended in fats.

Sterols

Cholesterol is the main sterol and is found only in eggs, meat, dairy products, fish and poultry. Cholesterol is a fat-like waxy substance that is both produced by the body and found in foods of animal origin. It is an important steroid as other steroid molecules copy from it, e.g. bile salts which increase fat absorption in the intestines.

MICRONUTRIENTS

Micronutrient is a term commonly known for the vitamins, essential minerals and trace elements (Webb, 2008) which are found in small amounts in food.

Vitamins

A vitamin is an organic compound that cannot be manufactured by the body and is needed in small quantities to catalyse metabolic processes. Thus, when vitamins are lacking in the diet, metabolic deficits result. Vitamins are generally classified as follows:

- Water-soluble vitamins include C and the B-complex vitamins: B_1 (thiamine), B_2 (riboflavin), B_3 (niacin or nicotinic acid), B_6 (pyridoxine), B_9 (folic acid), B_{12} (cobalamin), pantothenic acid and biotin. The body cannot store water-soluble vitamins; thus, people must get a daily supply in the diet. Water-soluble vitamins can be affected by food processing, storage and preparation.
- Fat-soluble vitamins include A, D, E and K. The body can store these vitamins, although there is a limit to the amounts of vitamin E and K the body can store. Therefore, a daily supply of fat-soluble vitamins is not absolutely necessary. Vitamin content is highest in fresh foods that are consumed as soon as possible after harvest.

Minerals

Minerals are inorganic compounds such as sodium, calcium and iron which are found in organic compounds. There are two categories of minerals:

1. Macro-minerals are those that people require daily in amounts over 100mg. They include calcium, phosphorus, sodium, potassium, magnesium, chloride and sulphur.
2. Microminerals are those that people require daily in amounts less than 100mg. They include iron, zinc, manganese, iodine, fluoride, copper, cobalt, chromium and selenium.

CLINICAL ALERT

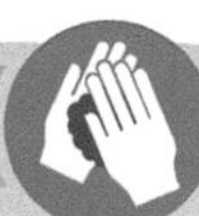

There are at least 15 minerals that are essential to the body, but only in trace amounts. One of these is fluoride which is sourced from tea and sea food. In the UK fluoride is sold as a medicine. Infants up to 6 months should not be given fluoride supplements at all (The British Dental Association as cited in Webb, 2008).

Common problems associated with the lack of mineral nutrients are iron deficiency resulting in anaemia, and osteoporosis resulting from loss of bone calcium.

ENERGY BALANCE

Energy balance is the relationship between the energy derived from food and the energy used by the body. The body obtains energy in the form of calories from carbohydrates, protein and fat. The body uses energy for voluntary activities such as walking and talking and for involuntary activities such as breathing and secreting enzymes. A person's energy balance is determined by comparing their energy intake with energy output.

Energy Intake

The amount of energy that nutrients or foods supply to the body is their caloric value. A **calorie** (c, cal and kcal) is a unit of heat energy. A calorie is the amount of heat required to raise the temperature of 1g of water 1°C and one kilo-calorie (kcal) is the amount needed to raise 1kg of water by 1°C. The energy liberated from the metabolism of food has been determined to be:

- 4 calories/gram of carbohydrates;
- 4 calories/gram of protein;
- 9 calories/gram of fat.

Energy Output

Metabolism refers to all biochemical and physiological processes by which the body grows and maintains itself. Metabolic rate is normally expressed in terms of the rate of heat liberated during these chemical reactions. The basal metabolic rate (BMR) is the rate at which the body metabolises food to maintain the energy requirements of a person who is awake and at rest. The energy in food maintains the basal metabolic rate of the body and provides energy for activities such as running and walking.

BODY WEIGHT

Maintaining a healthy body weight requires a balance between the expenditure of energy and the intake of nutrients. Generally, when energy requirements of an individual equate with the daily calorie intake, the body weight remains stable.

The **body mass index (BMI)** has been used since the 1960s to assess obesity in adults and more recently in children (Cole *et al.*, 2007). Many countries now make use of centile charts to record BMI, and in 1995 the WHO expert committee approved the use of BMI slimness in young adults (WHO, 1995). More recently, the WHO introduced growth standards for children (WHO, 2006a). Thomas and Bishop (2007) suggest that a child's BMI should be recorded against an age-related centile chart.

For people older than 18 years, the BMI is an indicator of changes in body fat stores and whether a person's weight is appropriate for height, and may provide a useful estimate of malnutrition. To calculate the BMI:

- Measure the person's height in metres, e.g. 1.5m
- Measure the weight in kilograms, e.g. 60kg
- Calculate the BMI using the following formula

$$\text{BMI} = \frac{\text{Weight in kilograms}}{(\text{Height in metres})^2}$$

- or

$$\frac{60 \text{ kilograms}}{1.5 \times 1.5\ (\text{metres})^2} = 26.6$$

The WHO revised their BMI classifications in 2006, as shown in Table 19-1.

According to Walters (1998) a BMI of less than 16 in adults suggests that the individual is malnourished, 16–19 is underweight, 20–25 is normal, 26–30 is overweight. With a BMI between 31 and 40, the individual is moderately obese and above 40 is morbidly obese. The WHO introduced global child growth standards in 2006 for infants up to 5 years of age. They are used as a tool in public health, medicine and by governmental and health organisations for monitoring the well-being of children and for detecting children or populations not growing properly or under- or overweight and who may require specific medical or public health responses (Vesel *et al.*, 2010).

Table 19.1 International Classification of Adult Underweight, Overweight and Obesity According to BMI.

Classification	BMI(kg/m²)	
	Principal cut-off points	**Additional cut-off points**
Underweight	<18.50	<18.50
Severe thinness	<16.00	<16.00
Moderate thinness	16.00-16.99	16.00-16.99
Mild thinness	17.00-18.49	17.00-18.49
Normal range	18.50-24.99	18.50-22.99 23.00-24.99
Overweight	≥25.00	≥25.00
Pre-obese	25.00-29.99	25.00-27.49 27.50-29.99
Obese	≥30.00	≥30.00
Obese class I	30.00-34-99	30.00-32.49 32.50-34.99
Obese class II	35.00-39.99	35.00-37.49 37.50-39.99
Obese class III	≥40.00	≥40.00

Source: WHO (2006b).

FACTORS AFFECTING NUTRITION

Although the nutritional content of food is an important consideration when planning a diet, an individual's food preferences and habits are often a major factor affecting actual food intake. Eating habits are influenced by developmental considerations, gender, ethnicity and culture, beliefs about food, personal preferences, religious practices, lifestyle, medications and therapy, health, alcohol consumption, advertising and psychological factors.

Gender

Nutrient requirements are different for men and women because of body composition and reproductive functions. The larger muscle mass of men translates into a greater need for calories and proteins. Also, prior to the menopause, women require more iron than men due to menstruation, and pregnant and breast feeding women need a higher calorie and fluid intake.

Ethnicity and Culture

Food is a part of our culture and ethnicity often determines food preferences. Children learn about food at a young age and our beliefs and choices are developed at this early stage. Babies for example may be weaned much later in developing countries than here in the UK. This is common practice where malnutrition is more common (Holland and Hogg, 2010). Jews for example do not eat pork or pork products while Hindus don't eat beef or beef products. Traditional foods (e.g. rice for Asians, and pasta for Italians) can be eaten as long as there is variety in the diet to ensure that all the macronutrients (e.g. protein, fat and carbohydrate) and micronutrients, vitamins and minerals are consumed.

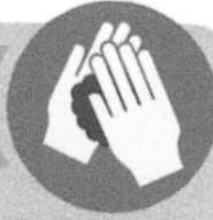

CLINICAL ALERT

We live in a multicultural society and, as with all nationalities, traditional food does not always please everyone. With travelling becoming more prominent and easier, individuals now have more awareness of other food choices. Assumptions should not be made in relation to patient choice in the clinical area. Good communication and assessment should gain this information.

Beliefs about Food

Beliefs about effects of foods on health and well-being can affect food choices. Many people acquire their beliefs about food from television, magazines and other media.

Personal Preferences

People develop likes and dislikes based on associations with a typical food. Individual likes and dislikes can also be related to familiarity. Preferences in the tastes, smells, flavours (blends of taste and smell), temperatures, colours, shapes, textures and sizes of food influence a person's food choices.

It is important to note that some people choose not to eat meat or meat products (vegetarians), and this can be for a variety of reasons. While there are eight or more classifications of vegetarians within the UK, vegans and lacto-vegans are the more frequently used terms. While not an entirely accurate definition, vegans use only plant foods while lacto-vegetarians don't eat meat or fish. Consideration of these preferences should be taken into account when meals are provided.

Religious Practices

Religious practice also affects diet. Some Roman Catholics avoid meat on certain days, and some Protestant faiths prohibit meat, tea, coffee or alcohol. Both Orthodox Judaism and Islam prohibit pork. Orthodox Jews observe kosher customs, eating certain foods only if they are inspected by a rabbi and prepared according to dietary laws. The nurse must be sensitive to such religious dietary practices.

Lifestyle

Certain lifestyles are linked to food-related behaviours. People who are always in a hurry probably buy convenience grocery items or eat restaurant meals. Culture changes are evident with more people spending less time at home (working, leisure, travelling) and having less time to prepare the 'complete' meal 'from scratch'. Individual differences also influence lifestyle patterns (e.g. cooking skills, concern about health). Some people work at different times, such as evening or night shifts. They might need to adapt their eating habits to this and also make changes in their medication schedules if they are related to food intake.

What, how much and how often a person eats are frequently affected by socioeconomic status. For example, people with limited income, including some older people, may not be able to afford meat and fresh vegetables. In contrast, people with higher incomes may purchase more proteins and fats and fewer complex carbohydrates.

Medications and Therapy

The effects of drugs on nutrition vary considerably. They may alter appetite, disturb taste perception or interfere with nutrient absorption or excretion. Nurses need to be aware of the nutritional effects of specific drugs when evaluating a patient for nutritional problems.

Health

An individual's health status greatly affects eating habits and nutritional status. Lack of teeth, ill-fitting teeth or a sore mouth make chewing food difficult. Difficulty swallowing (dysphagia) due to a painfully inflamed throat or a stricture of the oesophagus can prevent a person from obtaining adequate nourishment. Disease processes and surgery of the gastro-intestinal tract can affect digestion, absorption, metabolism and excretion of essential nutrients. Gastrointestinal and other diseases also create anorexia (loss of appetite), nausea, vomiting and diarrhoea, all of which can adversely affect a person's appetite and nutritional status.

Alcohol Consumption

Excessive alcohol use contributes to nutritional deficiencies in a number of ways. Alcohol may replace food in a person's diet and it can depress the appetite. Excessive alcohol can have a toxic effect on the intestinal mucosa, thereby decreasing the absorption of nutrients. The need for vitamin B increases, because it is used in alcohol metabolism. Alcohol can impair the storage of nutrients and increase nutrient catabolism (break down or metabolism) and excretion.

The Media

Television, magazines and advertising boards are just a few examples of how individuals can be influenced on what they eat or do not eat. There is pressure on individuals to 'conform' to what 'looks good' from peers, relatives, friends and society. Since the early 1960s some teenagers have emulated professional models, etc. and have restricted their eating in order to become the popular size 6 or 8. Many created health problems for themselves. Currently, internationally there is much publicity regarding obesity. There is a significant increase in children, adolescents and adults being overweight and the media is used to try and advise and educate the public on a healthy diet alongside healthcare professionals.

Psychological Factors

Although some people overeat when stressed, depressed or lonely, others eat very little under the same conditions. Anorexia and weight loss can indicate severe stress or depression. Anorexia nervosa and bulimia are severe psychophysiological conditions seen most frequently in female adolescents, probably as a result of puberty and the unhealthy images of thin models in the media.

Lifespan Requirements

Nutritional requirements change throughout the lifecycle. While Table 19-2 sourced from the Public Health Action Team (PHAST) (2010) demonstrates the requirements of individuals at different stages of their lives, it is important to recognise that these may vary from person to person.

Table 19-2 Changing Nutritional Requirements Among Different Age Groups

Infants	First 4-6 months of life (period of rapid growth and development) - breast milk (or infant formula) contains all the nutrients required.
	Between 6 and 12 months - requirements for iron, protein, thiamin, niacin, vitamin B6, vitamin B12, magnesium, zinc, sodium and chloride increase.
	Department of Health advice recommends exclusive breastfeeding until 6 months of age with weaning introduced at 6 months.
1-3 years	Energy requirements increase (children are active and growing rapidly). Protein requirements increase slightly. Vitamins requirements increase (except vitamin D). Mineral requirements decrease for calcium, phosphorus and iron and increase for the remaining minerals (except for zinc).
4-6 years	Requirements for energy, protein, all the vitamins and minerals increase except C and D and iron.
7-10 years	Requirements for energy, protein, all vitamins and minerals increase except thiamin, vitamin C and A.
11-14 years	Requirements for energy continue to increase and protein requirements increase by approximately 50%.
	By the age of 11, the vitamin and mineral requirements for boys and girls start to differ.
	Boys: increased requirement for all the vitamins and minerals.
	Girls: no change in the requirement for thiamin, niacin, vitamin B6, but there is an increased requirement for all the minerals. Girls have a much higher iron requirement than boys (once menstruation starts).
15-18 years	***Boys***: requirements for energy and protein continue to increase as do the requirements for a number of vitamins and minerals (thiamin, riboflavin, niacin, vitamins B6, B12, C and A, magnesium, potassium, zinc, copper, selenium and iodine). Calcium requirements remain high as skeletal development is rapid.
	Girls: requirements for energy, protein, thiamin, niacin, vitamins B6, B12 and C, phosphorus, magnesium, potassium, copper, selenium and iodine all increase.
	Boys and girls have the same requirement for vitamin B12, folate, vitamin C, magnesium, sodium, potassium, chloride and copper. Girls have a higher requirement than boys for iron (due to menstrual losses) but a lower requirement for zinc and calcium.
19-50 years	Requirements for energy, calcium and phosphorus are lower for both men and women than adolescents and a reduced requirement in women for magnesium, and in men for iron. The requirements for protein and most of the vitamins and minerals remain virtually unchanged in comparison to adolescents (except for selenium in men which increases slightly).
Pregnancy	Increased requirements for some nutrients. Women intending to become pregnant and for the first 12 weeks of pregnancy are advised to take supplements of folic acid. Additional energy and thiamin are required only during the last three months of pregnancy. Mineral requirements do not increase.
Lactation	Increased requirement for energy, protein, all the vitamins (except B6), calcium, phosphorus, magnesium, zinc, copper and selenium.
50+ years	Energy requirements decrease gradually after the age of 50 in women and age 60 in men as people typically become less active and the basal metabolic rate is reduced. Protein requirements decrease for men, but continue to increase slightly in women. The requirements for vitamins and minerals remain virtually unchanged for both men and women.
	After the menopause, women's requirement for iron is reduced to the same level as that for men.
	After the age of 65 there is a reduction in energy needs but vitamins and minerals requirements remain unchanged. This means that the nutrient density of the diet is even more important.

Source: PHAST (2010) Public Health Action Support Team CIC (registered in England and Wales).

It is important to understand that activity, rest and illness would have an effect on these requirements. Many formulae have been developed to assess nutritional energy requirements.

ALTERED NUTRITION

Malnutrition is commonly defined as the lack of necessary or appropriate food substances but, in practice, includes both undernutrition and overnutrition. Overnutrition refers to a caloric intake in excess of daily energy requirements, resulting in storage of energy in the form of adipose tissue. As the amount of stored fat increases, the individual becomes overweight or obese.

Undernutrition refers to an intake of nutrients insufficient to meet daily energy requirements because of inadequate food intake or improper digestion and absorption of food. An inadequate food intake may be caused by the inability to acquire and prepare food, inadequate knowledge about essential nutrients and a balanced diet, discomfort during or after eating, dysphagia, anorexia (loss of appetite), nausea or vomiting, and so on. Improper digestion and absorption of nutrients may be caused by an inadequate production of hormones or enzymes or by medical conditions resulting in inflammation or obstruction of the gastrointestinal tract.

Inadequate nutrition is associated with marked weight loss, generalised weakness, altered functional abilities, delayed wound healing, and increased susceptibility to infection, immunosuppression, impaired pulmonary function and prolonged length of hospitalisation. In response to undernutrition, carbohydrate reserves, stored as liver and muscle glycogen, are mobilised. However, these reserves can only meet energy requirements for a short time (e.g. 24 hours) and then body protein is mobilised which results in depletion of protein reserves (muscle mass).

Protein energy malnutrition (PEM), once associated with the manifestation of malnutrition seen in starving children of third world countries, is now recognised as a significant problem of patients with long-term deficiencies in caloric intake (e.g. those with cancer and chronic disease). Characteristics of PEM are depressed visceral proteins (proteins that are in blood, e.g. albumin), weight loss and visible muscle and fat wasting.

HEALTHY DIET

Nationally there are numerous guidelines to help individuals, healthcare professionals and carers to advise and meet the daily essential nutrient requirements. Indeed, all food packages now inform customers of the contents within each item sold. There are strategies in place initiated by local government to educate and inform young children of eating 'healthy' and incentives (free milk, breakfast clubs, etc.) in some schools to support these strategies.

External factors such as financial stress, work commitments etc. can influence the individual's well-being, and it is essential that care and time is denoted to dietary/nutritional requirements.

An accurate assessment, both physical and psychological, is necessary before any decisions can be made regarding nutritional requirements, as this will enable a nurse to make an informed decision. It is important to consider age, health condition and mobility of the patient when considering the amount, content of food, etc.

Fundamental to the ability of the nurse to make a valid judgement is an awareness of the components of a healthy diet (as discussed throughout the chapter). Figure 19.1 illustrates an 'eatwell plate' as designed by the Food Standards Agency.

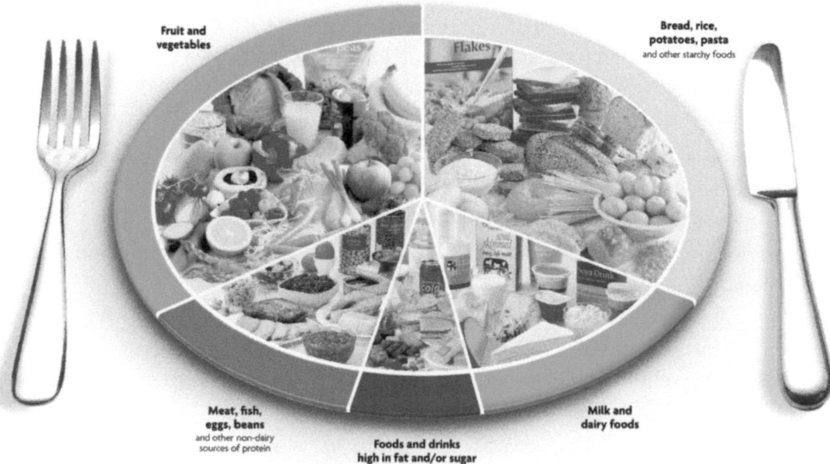
The eatwell plate
Use the eatwell plate to help you get the balance right. It shows how much of what you eat should come from each food group.
Fruit and vegetables
Bread, rice, potatoes, pasta and other starchy foods
Meat, fish, eggs, beans and other non-dairy sources of protein
Foods and drinks high in fat and/or sugar
Milk and dairy foods

Figure 19-1 The eatwell plate.
Source: Department of Health in association with the Welsh Government, the Scottish Government and the Food Standards Agency in Northern Ireland © Crown copyright.

ASSESSING NUTRITION

The purpose of a nutritional assessment is to identify patients at risk of malnutrition and those with poor nutritional status. In most healthcare environments, the responsibility for nutritional assessment and support is shared by the doctor, the dietician and the nurse. Generally, nurses perform a nutritional screen. A comprehensive nutritional assessment is often performed by a nutritionist or a dietician. In 2003 The British Association of Parental and Enteral Nutrition (BAPEN) published a nutritional screening tool (the Malnutrition Universal Screening Tool – MUST) based on BMI, unintentional weight loss and the effect of illness on the nutritional status of a patient. This screening tool has been widely used and local Trusts and Health Boards have indeed implemented and revised the tool for their own use. The MUST tool was reviewed and minor changes were made to it in 2008 (BAPEN, 2008) (see Figure 19-2).

ACTIVITY 19-1

A 20-year-old fully active young lady enjoys sport of all types and competes at county levels in tennis, hockey and swimming. She has asked you to prepare her a nutritional diet to meet her needs. On reflection, can you provide her with an appropriate meal and provide the rationale as to why some foods have been included or excluded.

Nutritional Screening

The Royal College of Nursing (RCN, 2006) state that every nurse has a responsibility to identify whether an individual is at risk of malnutrition. Malnutrition refers to both under nutrition an overnutrition. The RCN (2006, p. 1) defines malnutrition as:

- Undernutrition is the result of a deficiency of energy and/or nutrients.
- Overnutrition is the result of an excess nutrients e.g., obesity.

Before the introduction of any nutritional support or supplements, it is important that an initial screening or assessment is undertaken. Indeed, most Trusts or Health Boards include a risk assessment form within the initial assessment in order to identify risk within the first meeting.

According to Thomas and Bishop (2007) a nutritional assessment can be undertaken by taking a diet history, and a 24-hour recall can provide information in relation to frequency, habits, preferences meal patterns, etc. Dougherty and Lister (2008) argue that a diet history should be accompanied by a percentage weight loss. A nutritional screening should be undertaken during this initial assessment using a model such as Roper, Logan and Tierney's Activities of Living (Roper *et al.*, 2000). The nurse would look for variables to determine whether the patient is at risk of nutritional problems. Some of the issues that a nurse can identify from the initial assessment are noted below:

- unintentional weight loss;
- skin integrity;
- poor or decreased appetite;
- current diet;
- height and weight history;
- present illness or diagnosis;
- cognitive or physical impairments that make it difficult for the patient to understand;
- age;
- clinical observation of hair, nails mucous membrane;
- elimination (excessive).

However, it is important to realise that blood tests provide significant information regarding an individual's nutritional status. It is also important to identify risk factors that can indicate whether a patient is at risk, and these are summarised below:

- chewing or swallowing difficulties (including ill-fitting dentures, dental caries and missing teeth);
- inadequate food budget;
- inadequate food intake;
- inadequate food preparation facilities;
- inadequate food storage facilities;
- living and eating alone;
- physical disabilities;
- alcohol or substance abuse;
- conditions that cause increased metabolism such as burns or trauma;
- chronic illness: end-stage renal disease, liver disease, HIV, pulmonary disease (COPD), cancer;
- fluid and electrolyte imbalance;
- gastrointestinal problems: anorexia, dysphagia (inability to swallow), nausea, vomiting, diarrhoea, constipation;
- neurological or cognitive impairment;
- oral and gastrointestinal surgery.

Patient History

The importance of obtaining accurate past and current history regarding the health and well-being of the patient has been frequently discussed throughout this chapter. By utilising a model such as that of Roper, Logan and Tierney, any concerns regarding eating and drinking should have been highlighted. Information can also be gathered from direct or indirect observation (see Table 19-3), biochemistry (lab results) (see later in chapter) current and previous health history (patient notes) and body measurements – anthropometric measurements.

Anthropometric Measurements

While anthropometric measurements are not often used in the acute sector on a daily basis, they do provide important

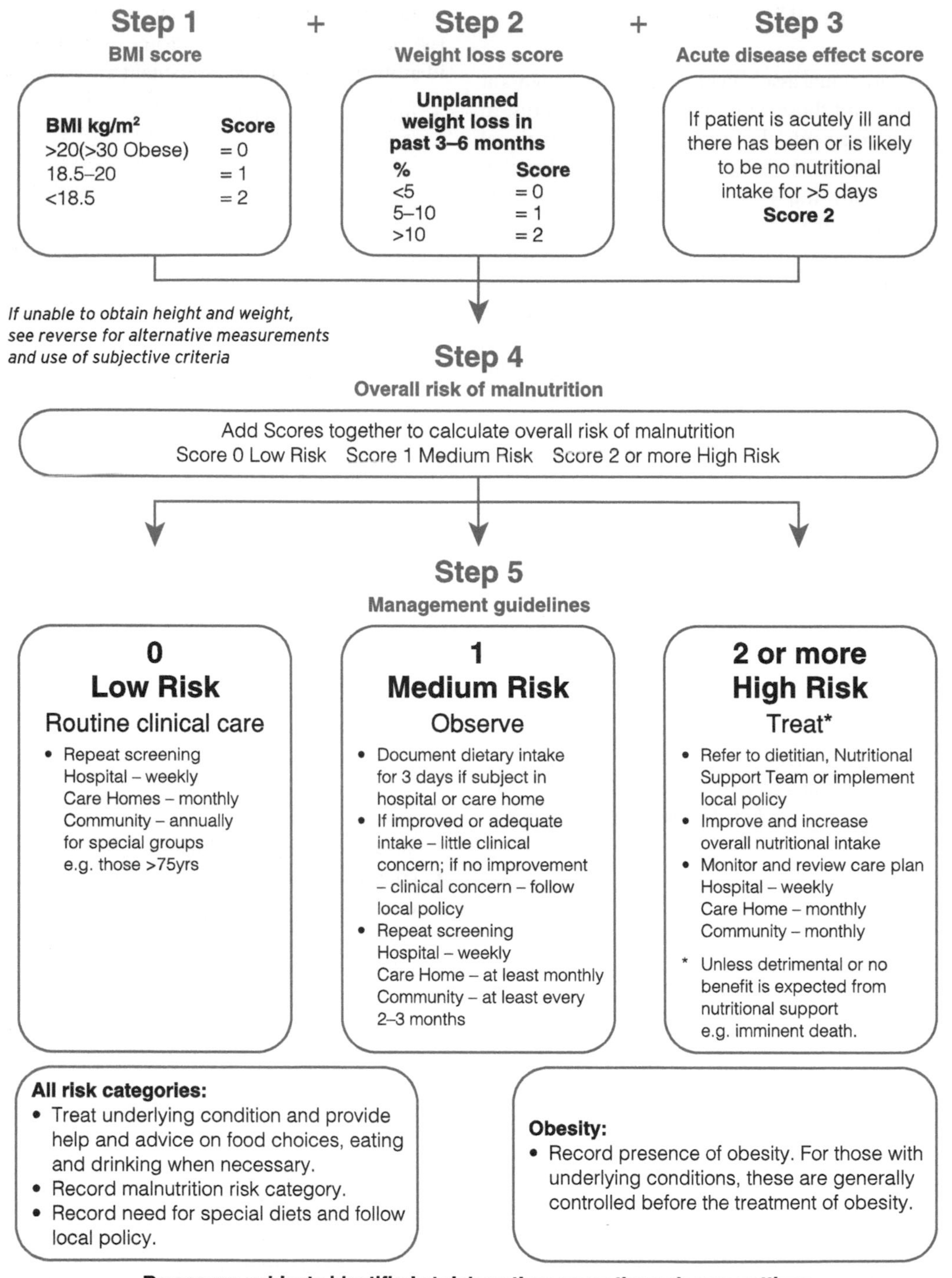

Step 1
BMI score
+
Step 2
Weight loss score
+
Step 3
Acute disease effect score
BMI kg/m² Score
>20(>30 Obese) = 0
18.5–20 = 1
<18.5 = 2
Unplanned weight loss in past 3–6 months
% Score
<5 = 0
5–10 = 1
>10 = 2
If patient is acutely ill and there has been or is likely to be no nutritional intake for >5 days
Score 2
If unable to obtain height and weight, see reverse for alternative measurements and use of subjective criteria
Step 4
Overall risk of malnutrition
Add Scores together to calculate overall risk of malnutrition
Score 0 Low Risk Score 1 Medium Risk Score 2 or more High Risk
Step 5
Management guidelines
0
Low Risk
Routine clinical care
• Repeat screening
Hospital – weekly
Care Homes – monthly
Community – annually
for special groups
e.g. those >75yrs
1
Medium Risk
Observe
• Document dietary intake for 3 days if subject in hospital or care home
• If improved or adequate intake – little clinical concern; if no improvement – clinical concern – follow local policy
• Repeat screening
Hospital – weekly
Care Home – at least monthly
Community – at least every 2–3 months
2 or more
High Risk
Treat*
• Refer to dietitian, Nutritional Support Team or implement local policy
• Improve and increase overall nutritional intake
• Monitor and review care plan
Hospital – weekly
Care Home – monthly
Community – monthly
* Unless detrimental or no benefit is expected from nutritional support e.g. imminent death.
All risk categories:
• Treat underlying condition and provide help and advice on food choices, eating and drinking when necessary.
• Record malnutrition risk category.
• Record need for special diets and follow local policy.
Obesity:
• Record presence of obesity. For those with underlying conditions, these are generally controlled before the treatment of obesity.
Re-assess subjects identified at risk as they move through care settings
See The 'MUST' Explanatory Booklet for further details and The 'MUST' Report for supporting evidence.

Figure 19-2 The Malnutrition Universal Screening Tool flowchart.

Source: The 'MUST' Report-nutritional screening of adults: a multi-disciplinary responsibility. Development and use of the 'Malnutrition Universal Screening Tool' (MUST) for Adults, Editor: Professor Marinos Elia, BAPEN.

information if there is significant weight loss. Anthropometric measurements are not invasive and a skinfold measurement aims to determine fat stores. The most common site for skinfold measurement is the triceps (the area at the back of the upper arm) skinfold. The midarm circumference (MAC) is also used to measure fat muscle and skeleton. All these are undertaken by expert practitioners and not carried out routinely.

Changes in anthropometric measurements often occur slowly and reflect chronic rather than acute changes in nutritional status. They are, therefore, used to monitor the patient's

Table 19-3 Clinical Signs of Malnutrition

Area of examination	Signs associated with malnutrition
General appearance	Apathetic, listless, looks tired, easily fatigued
Weight	Overweight or underweight
Skin	Dry, flaky or scaly; pale or pigmented; presence of petechiae (bruising); lack of subcutaneous fat
Nails	Brittle, pale ridged or spoon shaped
Hair	Dry, dull, sparse, loss of colour, brittle
Eyes	Pale or red conjunctiva, dryness, soft cornea, dull cornea
Lips	Swollen, red cracks at side of mouth, vertical fissures
Tongue	Swollen, beefy red or magenta coloured; smooth appearance; decrease or increase in size
Gums	Spongy, swollen, inflamed; bleed easily
Muscles	Underdeveloped, flaccid, wasted, soft
Gastrointestinal system	Anorexia, indigestion, diarrhoea, constipation, enlarged liver
Nervous system	Decreased reflexes, sensory loss, burning and tingling of hands and feet, mental confusion or irritability

progress for months to years rather than days to weeks. Ideally, initial and subsequent measurements need to be taken by the same healthcare professional to ensure similar measurements, and measurements obtained need to be interpreted with caution. Fluctuations in hydration status that often occur during illness can influence the accuracy of results. In addition, normal standards often do not account for normal changes in body composition such as those that occur with ageing.

Laboratory Data

Laboratory tests provide objective data to the nutritional assessments but, because many factors can influence these tests, no single test specifically predicts nutritional risk or measures the presence or degree of a nutritional problem. The tests most commonly used are serum proteins, urinary urea nitrogen and creatinine, and total lymphocyte count.

Serum Proteins

Serum protein levels provide an estimate of protein stores. Tests commonly include haemoglobin, albumin and transferrin. For example, a low haemoglobin level may be evidence of iron deficiency anaemia. It is important to recognise that other causes for iron deficiency anaemia may be pathological such as gastrointestinal cancer.

Albumin is a protein which is made in the liver that accounts for more than 50% of the total serum proteins and is one of the key proteins measured to assess nutritional status. An abnormal serum albumin blood result would indicate liver or kidney disease, malnutrition, inflammation or low protein diet. High volumes of intravenous fluids may affect these results.

Transferrin is a trace protein in the blood that binds and transfers iron from the intestine to the bloodstream onto the liver spleen and bone marrow. Transferrin has a shorter half life than albumin and is more likely to respond quicker to protein deficiency in the body. Transferrin levels below normal indicate protein loss, iron deficiency anaemia, pregnancy, hepatitis and liver dysfunction.

Prealbumin, also referred to as thyroxine-binding albumin and transthyretin, has the shortest half life and therefore identifies protein deficiencies fastest. Cost implications restrict the frequency of testing in the UK.

Urinary Tests

Measurements of urinary urea, nitrogen and creatinine are often used to determine the protein nutritional status of an individual. **Urea** is the end product of amino acid metabolism which is eventually excreted via the kidneys.

Blood urea nitrogen (BUN) is a blood test that measures the urea level in the blood. A rise in the level would indicate dehydration. Nitrogen is an element of amino acid and thus a protein. It is necessary for growth and development. A low level of nitrogen in the blood test could indicate malnutrition.

Creatinine is a breakdown of creatine which helps to supply energy to the muscle in the body. Creatinine is the end product of the creatine produced when energy is released during skeletal muscle metabolism. The greater the muscle mass, the greater the excretion of creatinine, which is excreted from the bloodstream through the kidneys. As skeletal muscle atrophies during malnutrition, creatinine excretion decreases. Urinary creatinine is also influenced by protein intake, exercise, age, renal function and thyroid function.

Total Lymphocyte Count

Certain nutrient deficiencies and forms of PEM can depress the immune system. The total number of lymphocytes decreases as protein depletion occurs.

PLANNING

Following the assessment and during the planning of care it is essential that there is involvement from the appropriate member/s of the multidisciplinary team and the patient and/or relatives/carers. Collaboration ensures the effective management of the patient during this period of care whether at home or in the community. Working as part of a team ensures that the patient receives optimum care through current knowledge and practice.

Major goals for patients with or at risk for nutritional problems include:

- maintain or restore optimal nutritional status;
- promote healthy nutritional practices;
- prevent complications associated with malnutrition;
- decrease weight;
- regain specified weight;
- maintain or improve skin integrity.

Planning the care will take into consideration the patient's own needs and the ability or support that is necessary to ensure that the care is delivered. The care planned for the patient should be realistic, measurable and achievable. The decisions made should reflect current management and long-term management at home (discharge planning).

IMPLEMENTING

Nursing interventions to promote optimal nutrition for patients are often provided in collaboration with the multidisciplinary team. The nurse is accountable and responsible in ensuring that the plan of care is carried out in the practice area. This can either be undertaken by him/herself or by delegating to other members of staff. Documentation is important to ensure that the plan of care is implemented at all times. Special diets should be ordered, equipment should be made available and nutrition provided as agreed between the multidisciplinary team. Fluid and diet intake should be recorded as per hospital policy and any issues should be referred to the appropriate member of staff. Recording the fluid and dietary intake will provide the nurse with the information required to reassess the effectiveness of the support provided.

Assisting with Special Diets

Some patients require changes to their diet. This may be due to a disease process such as diabetes mellitus. It could be to increase or decrease weight, to restore nutritional deficits or to allow an organ to rest and promote healing. Diets can be modified in a number of ways including: change in texture, change in amount of calories in food, specific nutrients, seasonings and consistency.

It is important to include the patient in any decisions made regarding diet alterations as they are more likely to concord with the treatment if their needs and wishes have been considered.

Stimulating an Appetite

Physical illness, unfamiliar or unpalatable food, environmental and psychological factors, and physical discomfort or pain may depress the appetites of many patients. A short-term decrease in food intake usually is not a problem for adults; over time, however, it leads to weight loss, decreased strength and stamina, and other nutritional problems. A decreased food intake is often accompanied by a decrease in fluid intake, which may cause fluid and electrolyte problems. Stimulating a person's appetite requires the nurse to determine the reason for the lack of appetite and then deal with the problem. Some interventions for improving the patient's appetite are summarised in the *Practice Guidelines*.

PRACTICE GUIDELINES

Improving Appetite

- Provide familiar food that the person likes. Often the relatives of patients are pleased to bring food from home but may need some guidance about special diet requirements.
- Smaller portions may encourage the patient to attempt some food, especially when they have a poor appetite.
- Avoid unpleasant or uncomfortable treatments immediately before or after a meal.
- Provide a tidy, clean environment that is free of unpleasant sights and odours. A soiled dressing, a used bedpan, an uncovered irrigation set or even used dishes can negatively affect the appetite.
- Encourage or provide oral hygiene before mealtime. This improves the patient's ability to taste.
- Relieve illness symptoms that depress appetite before mealtime; for example, give an analgesic for pain or an antipyretic for a fever or allow rest for fatigue.
- Reduce psychological stress. A lack of understanding of therapy, the anticipation of an operation and fear of the unknown can cause anorexia. Often, the nurse can help by discussing feelings with the patient, giving information and assistance, and allaying fears.

Assisting Patients with Eating

Most patients can manage to eat food on their own; however, illness, accident trauma, etc. may make this difficult for patients. Helping patients to eat can be both an intrusive and embarrassing process. Patients, e.g. who have a left-sided weakness following a cerebrovascular accident (stroke), very often find it difficult to accept this weakness, and indeed often ignore the affected side. It is important for a nurse to understand how to help a patient previously able to eat independently feels when finding themselves in a position of needing assistance with eating. Some patients feel resentful at this loss of autonomy. Advice on providing patient meals is given in the *Practice Guidelines*.

PRACTICE GUIDELINES

Providing Patient Meals

- Offer the patient help with hand washing and oral hygiene before a meal.
- Most people sit during a meal; if the patient's condition permits, assist them into a comfortable position in bed or in a chair, whichever is appropriate.
- Ensure that the correct meal is served to the patient; this is particularly important for patients on specific diets such as those with diabetes.
- If the patient is blind, it is useful to identify the placement of food as you would describe the time on a clock (see Figure 19-3). For instance, the nurse might say, 'The potatoes are at eight o'clock, the chicken at 12 o'clock and the green beans at 4 o'clock'.
- Following mealtime observe how much and what the patient has eaten and the amount of fluid taken. Record fluid intake and quantity of food eaten as required.
- If the patient is on a special diet or is having problems eating, record the amount of food eaten and any pain, fatigue or nausea experienced.

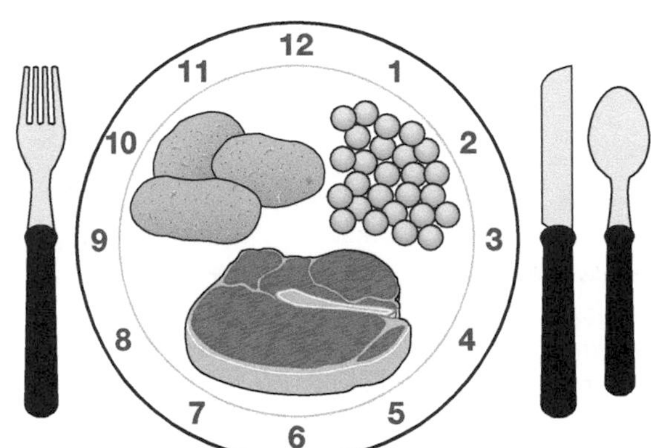

Figure 19-3 For a patient who is blind, the nurse can use the clock system to describe the location of food on the plate.
Source: adapted from Queensland Blind Association Inc.

- If the patient is not eating, document this so that changes can be made, such as rescheduling the meals, providing smaller, more frequent meals or obtaining special self-feeding aids.

Assisting patients with their meals can be time-consuming and often there is more than one patient who needs help. It is important that a nurse does not 'rush' this process and ensures that the patient feels relaxed and not hurried during this time. Whenever possible it is important that the patient feeds him or herself with minimal assistance. Specialised equipment (see Figures 19-4 and 19-5) can be provided by the occupational therapy department. It is therefore important that early referrals are made to the occupational therapist in order to facilitate these.

Figure 19-4 Left to right: glass holder, cup with hole for nose, two-handled cup holder.
Source: Pearson Education Ltd.

Patients with disabilities, e.g. blindness (some of whom normally manage on their own), are not now in their 'safe' environment and find it difficult to adjust. Care is needed and providing them with simple advice on where the plate is in relation to themselves and what the food is and where it is placed on the plate would provide them with greater independence (see Figure 19-3).

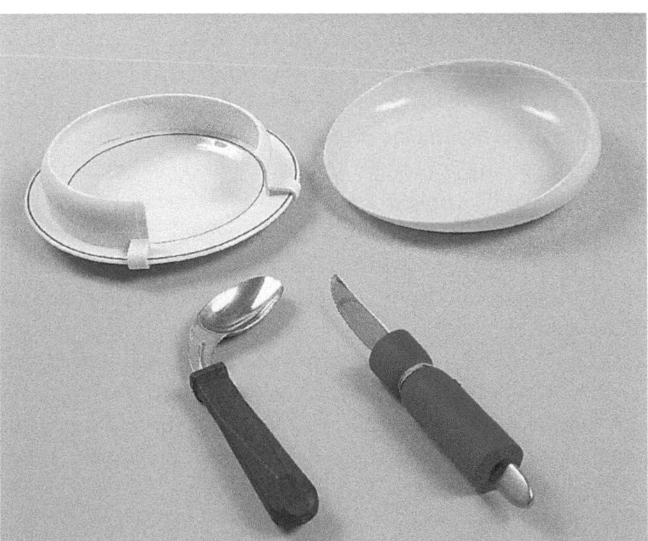

Figure 19-5 Dinner plate with guard attached and lipped plate facilitates scooping; wide-handled spoon and knife facilitate grip.
Source: Pearson Education Ltd.

When feeding a patient, ask in which order the patient would like to eat the food. If the patient cannot see, tell the patient which food is being given. Always allow ample time for the patient to chew and swallow the food before offering more. Also, provide fluids as requested or, if the patient is unable to communicate, offer fluids after every three or four mouthfuls of solid food.

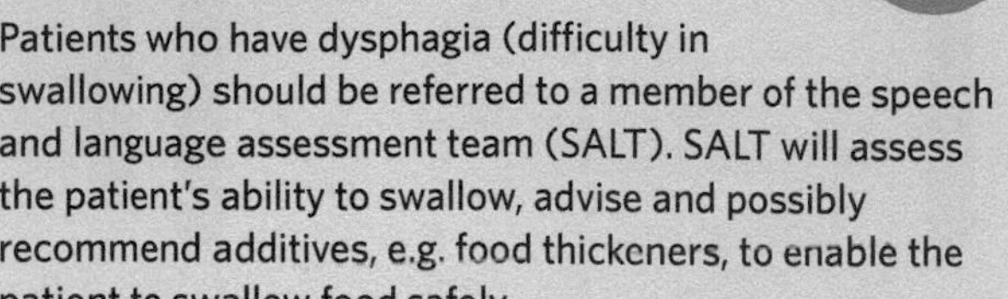

CLINICAL ALERT

Patients who have dysphagia (difficulty in swallowing) should be referred to a member of the speech and language assessment team (SALT). SALT will assess the patient's ability to swallow, advise and possibly recommend additives, e.g. food thickeners, to enable the patient to swallow food safely.

Poor appetite can be compensated by food supplements and it is important to offer these before offering a more invasive procedure such as enteral support.

Enteral Nutrition

Some patients may need an alternative means of ensuring adequate nutrition. Enteral nutrition (through the gastrointestinal system) is one alternative feeding method either for short- or long-term use. There are several types of feeding tubes, e.g. nasogastric/nasoduodenal, **gastrostomy** and **jejunostomy**.

A nasogastric/nasoduodenal (NG) tube (enteral tube) is the most common tube used (see Figure 19-6). It can be inserted at the patient's bed and sedation of the patient is not often required. However, consent must be gained. NG tubes are available in a number of different sizes and designs, the choice of which should be based on the patient's needs. The most commonly used are the wide or large bore tube (>12 Fr) (see Figure 19-6(a)) and the fine-bore tube (≤12 Fr) (see Figure 19-6(b)). Fine bore tubes are the more comfortable choice for the patients as they stay in situ for longer and are less likely to develop complications. An NG tube is inserted through one of the nostrils, down the nasopharynx, and into the alimentary tract. The accuracy of positioning should be checked as per hospital or health board policy by checking the pH of the gastric content and/or by X-ray prior to use.

Nasogastric tubes are used for patients who have intact gag and cough reflexes, who have adequate gastric emptying, and who require short-term feedings. It is important to note that in some trusts nurses are not allowed to insert nasogastric tubes without further training. *Procedure 19-1* provides guidelines for inserting a nasogastric tube. *Procedure 19-2* outlines the steps for removing a nasogastric tube.

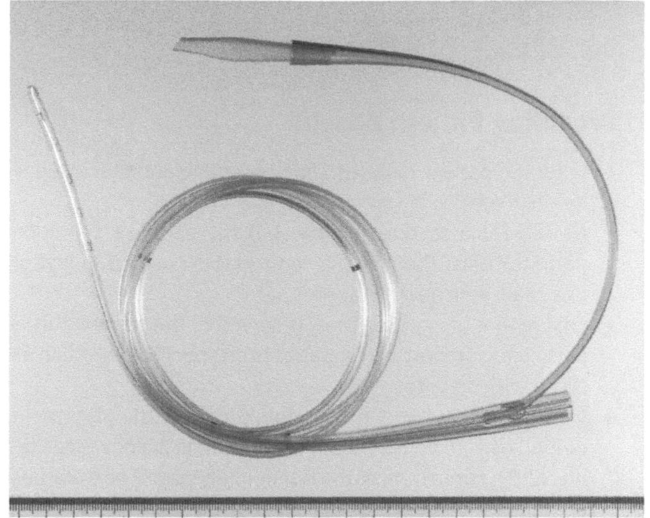

(a)

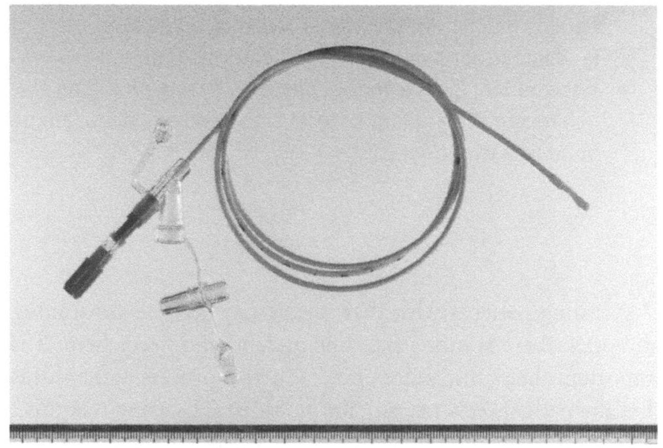

(b)

Figure 19-6 (a) Wide bore nasogastric tube. (b) Fine bore nasogastric tube with stylet and Y-Port connector for administration of medication.

Source: (a) http://www.yuyumedical.com/medidis1.asp. (b) http://www.silmag.com/Imagenes/Productos/394_c.jpg.

CLINICAL ALERT

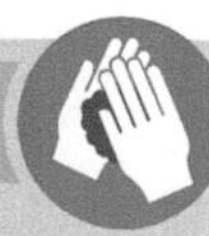

A nasogastric tube should only be inserted by an appropriately qualified or experienced healthcare professional.

PROCEDURE 19-1 Inserting a Nasogastric Tube

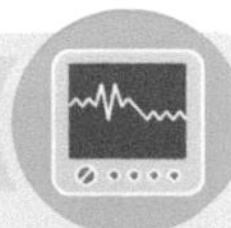

Purposes

- To administer tube feedings and medications to patients unable to eat by mouth or swallow a sufficient diet
- To establish a means for suctioning stomach contents to prevent gastric distention, nausea and vomiting

Assessment

- Check patency of nostrils and intactness of nasal tissues. Check for history of nasal surgery or deviated septum.
- Determine presence of gag reflex.
- Assess mental status or ability to cooperate with procedure.

Planning

Before inserting a nasogastric tube, determine the size of tube to be inserted.

Equipment

- Clinically clean tray
- Large- or small-bore tube (enteral tube)
- Guidewire or stylet for small-bore tube
- Nonallergenic adhesive tape
- Adhesive patch if available
- Clean gloves
- Water-soluble lubricant
- Tissues
- Glass of water
- 10ml catheter tip syringe
- Sterile receiver
- pH indicator strips
- Stethoscope
- Disposable pad or towel
- Free drainage bag if required.
- Spigot

Implementation

Preparation

- Assist the patient to a semi-upright position in the bed or chair if their condition permits. It is often easier to swallow in this position and gravity helps the passage of the tube.
- Place a towel or disposable pad across the chest.

Performance

1 Follow local policy to ensure that you explain to the patient what you are going to do, why it is necessary and how they can cooperate. Obtain consent and maintain patient privacy and dignity and ensure that the appropriate local infection control procedures are observed. The passage of a gastric tube is not painful, but it is unpleasant because the gag reflex is activated during insertion.

2 Arrange with the patient some form of signalling as a form of communication if he/she wishes to stop the procedure at any time.

3 Follow manufacturer's instruction to prepare the tube.

4 Assess the patient's nostrils.
   - Ask the patient to hyperextend the head and, using a flashlight, observe the intactness of the tissues of the nostrils, including any irritations or abrasions.
   - Examine the nostrils for any obstructions or deformities by asking the patient to breathe through one nostril while occluding the other.
   - Select the nostril that has the greater airflow.

5 Determine how far to insert the tube.
   - Use the tube to mark off the distance from the tip of the patient's nose to the tip of the earlobe and then from the tip of the earlobe to the tip of the xiphoid (see Figure 19-7). *This length approximates the distance from the nostril to the stomach. This distance varies among individuals.*
   - Note this length on the tubes graduated marks.

6 Insert the tube.
   - Put on gloves.
   - Lubricate the tip of the tube well with water-soluble lubricant or water to ease insertion. A water-soluble lubricant dissolves if the tube accidentally enters the lungs. An oil-based lubricant, such as petroleum jelly, will not dissolve and could cause respiratory complications if it enters the lungs.
   - Insert the tube, with its natural curve towards the patient, into the selected nostril. Ask the patient to

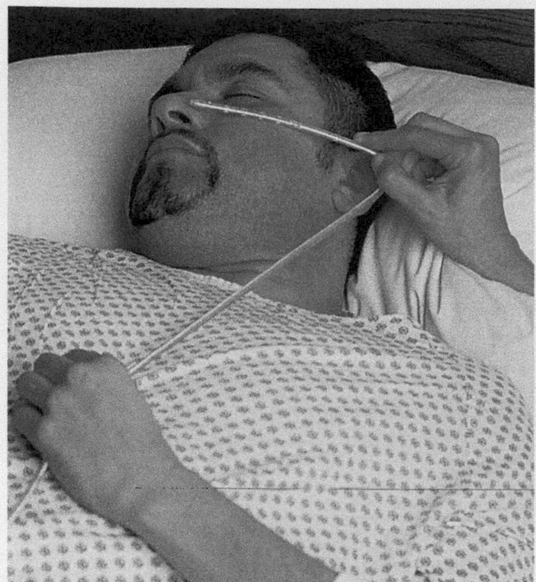

Figure 19-7 Measuring the appropriate length to insert a nasogastric tube.
Source: Pearson Education Ltd.

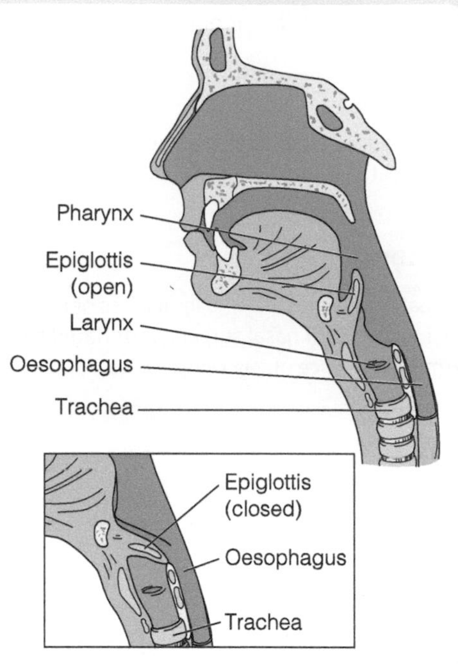

Figure 19-8 Swallowing closes the epiglottis.

hyperextend the neck, and gently advance the tube towards the nasopharynx. *Hyperextension of the neck reduces the curvature of the nasopharyngeal junction.*

- Direct the tube along the floor of the nostril and towards the ear on that side.
- Slight pressure is sometimes required to pass the tube into the nasopharynx and some patients' eyes may water at this point. *Tears are a natural body response.* Provide the patient with tissues as needed.
- If the tube meets resistance, withdraw it, relubricate it and insert it in the other nostril. *The tube should never be forced against resistance because of the danger of injury.*
- Once the tube reaches the oropharynx (throat), the patient will feel the tube in the throat and may gag and retch. Ask the patient to tilt the head forward, and encourage the patient to drink and swallow. *Tilting the head forward facilitates passage of the tube into the posterior pharynx and oesophagus rather than into the larynx; swallowing moves the epiglottis over the opening to the larynx* (see Figure 19-8).
- If the patient gags, stop passing the tube momentarily. Have the patient rest, take a few breaths and take sips of water to calm the gag reflex.
- In cooperation with the patient, pass the tube 5–10cm with each swallow, until the indicated length is inserted.
- If the patient continues to gag and the tube does not advance with each swallow, withdraw it slightly, and inspect the throat by looking through the mouth. *The tube may be coiled in the throat.* If so, withdraw it until it is straight, and try again to insert it.

7 Ascertain correct placement of the tube according to local policy.
   - Aspirate stomach contents, and check the pH, which should be acidic.
   - In some areas introducing 5ml of air into the stomach and using a stethoscope over the epigastrium is used to listen to sounds.
   - Depending on local policy the position of the tube can be checked by x-ray. However, this should not be routinely performed. It is important when using a small-bore tube that the guidewire is left in place when x-ray is performed.
   - If the signs do not indicate placement in the stomach, advance the tube 5cm, and repeat the tests.

8 Secure the tube by taping it to the bridge of the patient's nose.
   - If the patient has oily skin, wipe the nose first with alcohol.
   - Cut 7.5cm of tape, and split it lengthwise at one end, leaving a 2.5cm tab at the end.
   - Place the tape over the bridge of the patient's nose, and bring the split ends either under and around the tubing or under the tubing and back up over the nose (see Figure 19-9). *Taping in this manner prevents the tube from pressing against and irritating the edge of the nostril. An adhesive patch can sometimes be placed over the tube and secure it to the patient's cheek.*

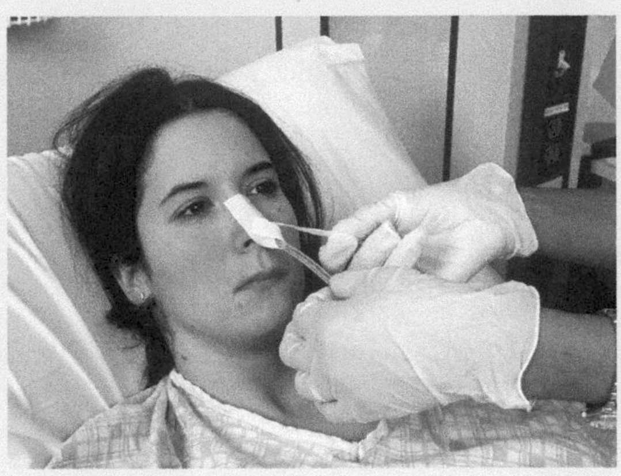

Figure 19-9 Taping a nasogastric tube to the bridge of the nose.
Source: Pearson Education Ltd.

9 Attach the tube to the feeding apparatus or free drainage as required as ordered, or clamp the end of the tubing.
10 Document relevant information: the insertion of the tube, the means by which correct placement was determined and patient responses (e.g. discomfort or abdominal distention).
11 Establish a plan for providing daily nasogastric tube care.
   - Inspect the nostril for discharge and irritation.
   - Clean the nostril and tube.
   - Apply water-soluble lubricant to the nostril if it appears dry or encrusted.
   - Change the adhesive tape as required.
   - Give frequent mouth care as the patient may breathe through the mouth.

Evaluation

There may be an immediate response from the patient if the tube is wrongly situated. These may be signs of respiratory problems, e.g. shortness of breath, coughing, cyanosed patient, etc. The patient may become agitated. Repositioning or removal of the tube is essential if this occurs. If the patient does not show any of these symptoms then, as per hospital policy aspiration, insertion of air bubble and/or confirmation by x-ray can be sought.

PROCEDURE 19-2 Removing a Nasogastric Tube

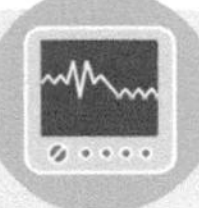

Purpose

To safely remove the nasogastric tube and restore the patient's normal eating pattern

Assessment

Assess

- For the presence of bowel sounds.
- For the absence of nausea or vomiting when tube is clamped.

Planning

Equipment

- Disposable pad
- Tissues
- Clean gloves
- 50ml syringe (optional)
- Clinical waste bag
- Washing bowl
- Towel
- Soap and wipes

Implementation

Preparation

- Confirm that both medical and nursing staff agree that the patient's condition is stable and it is safe to remove the nasogastric tube.
- Assist the patient to a sitting position if condition permits.
- Place the disposable pad across the patient's chest to collect any spillage of mucous and gastric secretions from the tube.
- Provide tissues to the patient to wipe the nose and mouth after tube removal.

Performance

1 Follow local policy to ensure that you explain to the patient what you are going to do, why it is necessary and how they can cooperate. Obtain consent and maintain patient privacy and dignity and ensure that the appropriate local infection control procedures are observed. Explain that the procedure will cause no discomfort.
2 Detach the tube.
   - Disconnect the nasogastric tube from the feeding apparatus.
   - Remove the adhesive tape securing the tube to the nose.
3 Remove the nasogastric tube.
   - Put on disposable gloves.
   - Ask the patient to take a deep breath and to hold it. *This closes the glottis, thereby preventing accidental aspiration of any gastric contents.*
   - Pinch the tube with the gloved hand. *Pinching the tube prevents any contents inside the tube from draining into the patient's throat.*
   - Quickly and smoothly withdraw the tube.
   - Place the tube in the clinical waste bag. *Placing the tube immediately into the bag prevents the transference of micro-organisms from the tube to other articles or people.*
   - Observe the intactness of the tube.
4 Ensure patient comfort.
   - Provide mouth care if desired.
   - Assist the patient as required to blow the nose. Excessive secretions may have accumulated in the nasal passages.
5 Dispose of the equipment appropriately.
6 Offer to assist the patient in washing face and nose, especially where the adhesive tape and patch were attached to the skin.
7 Document all relevant information.
   - Record the removal of the tube, the amount and appearance of any drainage and any relevant assessments of the patient.

Evaluation

- Perform a follow-up examination, such as presence of bowel sounds, absence of nausea or vomiting when tube is removed, and intactness of tissues of the nostrils.

Gastrostomy and **jejunostomy** devices are used for long-term nutritional support, generally more than 6–8 weeks. Conventional tubes are placed surgically or by laparoscopy through the abdominal wall into the stomach (gastrostomy) or into the jejunum (jejunostomy).

A **percutaneous** endoscopic gastrostomy (PEG) (see Figure 19-10) or percutaneous endoscopic jejunostomy (PEJ) (see Figure 19-11) is created by using an endoscope to visualise the inside of the stomach, making a puncture through the skin and subcutaneous tissues of the abdomen into the stomach, and inserting the PEG or PEJ catheter through the puncture. The catheter has internal and external bumpers and an inflatable retention balloon to maintain placement. Once the opening has healed, replacement tubes can be inserted without the use of **endoscopy**. These procedures are invasive and would require some form of sedation.

Guidelines for care of a PEG are given in *Procedure 19-3*.

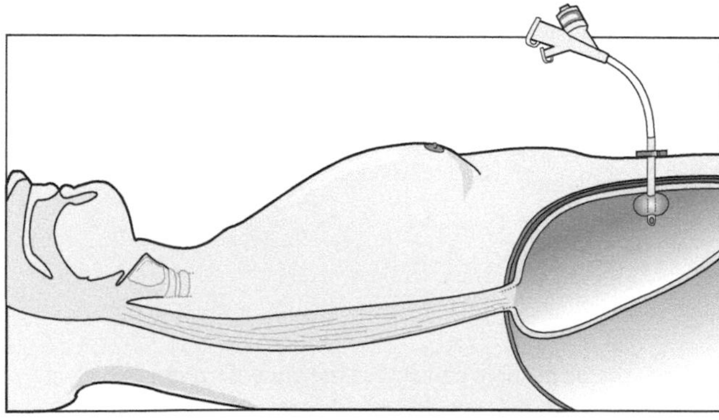

Figure 19-10 Percutaneous endoscopic gastrostomy (PEG) tube.

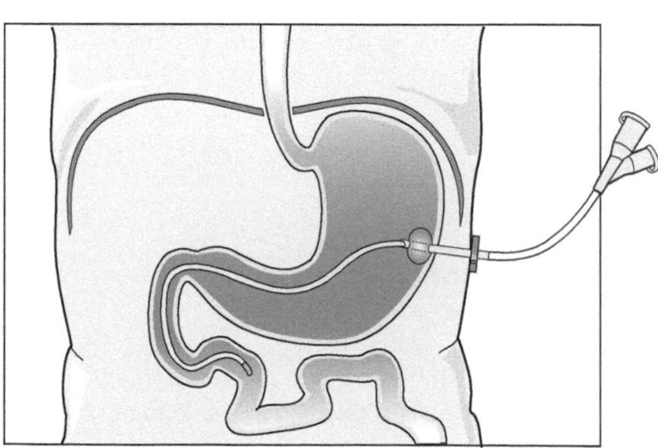

Figure 19-11 Percutaneous endoscopic jejunostomy (PEJ) tube.

PROCEDURE 19-3 Care of Percutaneous Endoscopic Gastrostomy Tube (PEG)

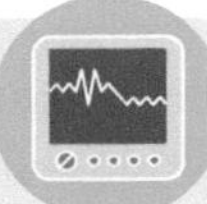

Purposes

- For the patient to maintain adequate nutritional intake
- For the patient to receive medication as prescribed

Assessment

Assess

- When the PEG tube was inserted (recommended 36-48 hours post-insertion)
- Patency of tube
- Patient's knowledge of PEG tube

Planning

Equipment

- Sterile procedure pack
- Sterile saline to clean area
- Sterile gloves

Implementation

Performance

1 Follow local policy to ensure that you explain to the patient what you are going to do, why it is necessary and how they can cooperate. Obtain consent and maintain patient privacy and dignity and ensure that the appropriate local infection control procedures are observed.
2 Prepare area (aseptic especially if first removal of dressing following insertion).
3 Turn off any pumps that are attached to the tube.
4 Wash hands and maintain all infection control procedures.
5 Remove the dressing and observe site for signs of infection or any abnormal discharge from the site.
6 Clean the stoma site with normal saline, using sterile wipes.
7 Rotate the gastrostomy tube 360°.
8 Push the external fixation gently against the abdomen.
9 If the tube is removed from the fixation device then ensure that it is reattached.
10 Do not replace the dressing, unless there is discharge from the stoma site.
11 Reattach any pumps and recommence as prescribed.
12 Dispose of all soiled wipes, etc. appropriately.
13 Document all relevant information.

Evaluation

Check and clean daily and observe area for any discharge, irritation or excoriation. Check for any leakage and patency of infusion.

Enteral Feeds

The frequency of feedings and amounts to be administered are usually prescribed by the doctor or dietician. Liquid feeding mixtures are available commercially or may be prepared by the dietary department in accordance with the patient's individual needs. A standard formula will provide the patient with the required nutrients as assessed and calculated by the dietician.

Enteral feedings can be given intermittently or continuously. Intermittent feedings are the administration of 300–500ml of enteral formula several times per day. The stomach is the preferred site for these feedings, which are usually administered over at least 30 minutes. Bolus intermittent feedings are those that use a syringe to deliver the formula into the stomach. Because the formula is delivered rapidly by this method, it is not usually recommended but may be used in long-term situations if the patient tolerates them. These feedings must be given only into the stomach; the patient must be monitored closely for distention and aspiration.

Continuous feedings are generally administered over a 24-hour period using an infusion pump that guarantees a constant flow rate (see Figure 19-12). Continuous feedings are essential when feedings are administered in the small bowel. They are also used when smaller bore gastric tubes are in place or when gravity flour is insufficient to instill the feeding.

Cyclic feedings are continuous feedings that are administered in less than 24 hours (e.g. 12–16 hours). These feedings, often administered at night and referred to as nocturnal feedings, allow the patient to attempt to eat regular meals through the day. Because nocturnal feedings may use higher nutrient densities and higher infusion rates than the standard continuous feeding, particular attention needs to be given to monitoring fluid status and circulating volume overload.

Procedure 19-4 provides the essential steps involved in administering a tube feeding, and *Procedure 19-5* indicates the steps involved in administering a gastrostomy or jejunostomy tube feeding.

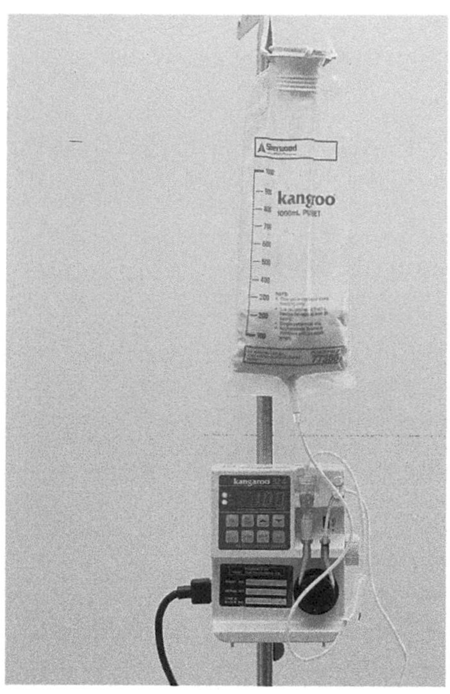

Figure 19-12 An enteric feeding pump.
Source: Pearson Education Ltd.

PROCEDURE 19-4 Administering Food and/or Drugs via an Enteral Feeding Tube

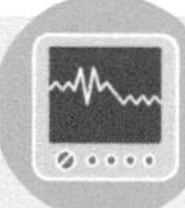

Purposes

- To restore or maintain nutritional and hydration status
- To ensure that the patient receives prescribed medication

Assessment

Assess

- For any clinical signs of malnutrition or dehydration.
- Check for allergies to any food in the feeding.
- For the presence of bowel sounds.
- Note any problems that suggest lack of tolerance of previous feedings (e.g. delayed gastric emptying, abdominal distention, constipation or dehydration).
- Assess whether the patient's condition has changed and the need for the medication remains.
- Ensure that the 6 R's are applied (see Chapter 23).

Planning

Before commencing a nasogastric feed, determine the type, amount and frequency of feedings and tolerance of previous feedings.

Equipment

- Correct amount of feeding solution
- Receiver
- Clean gloves
- pH test strip
- Water (at room temperature)
- Feeding pump as required
- 50ml catheter tipped syringe
- Mortar and pestle or tablet crusher if oral solutions are not available and the medication is necessary.
- Check is absorbable from point of delivery.

Implementation

Preparation

- Assist the patient to sit in the Fowler's position (sitting up) in a bed or a chair, the normal position for eating. However, if the patient cannot sit up they should be placed with their head tilted upwards at a 30–40 degree angle. *These positions enhance the gravitational flow of the solution and prevent aspiration of fluid into the lungs.*
- Check whether the patient can take **buccal**, **transdermal**, **topical**, rectal or subcutaneous medication. Gain consent both for the nutrients and the medication. Ensure that the patient is aware of both administrations.

Performance

1 Follow local policy to ensure that you explain to the patient what you are going to do, why it is necessary and how they can cooperate. Obtain consent and maintain patient privacy and dignity and ensure that the appropriate local infection control procedures are observed. Inform the patient that the feeding should not cause any discomfort but may cause a feeling of fullness.

2 Assess tube placement.
  - Check graduations on the nasogastric tube.
  - Ensure that there are no signs that the tube has been dislodged, such as coughing, gagging and retching.

3 Assess residual feeding contents.
  - Aspirate all stomach contents and measure the amount before administering the feeding. *This is done to evaluate absorption of the last feeding; that is, whether undigested formula from a previous feeding remains.*
  - If 100ml (or more than half the last feeding) is withdrawn, check with the nurse in charge or refer to local policy before proceeding.
  - Re-instil the gastric contents into the stomach if this is the local policy. *Removal of the contents could disturb the patient's electrolyte balance.*
  - If the patient is on a continuous feeding regimen, check the gastric residual every 4–6 hours or according to local protocol.

4 Administer the feeding.
  - Before administering feeding: check the expiration date of the feeding; and warm the feeding to room temperature. *An excessively cold feeding may cause cramps.*
  - Remove the screw-on cap from the container and attach the administration set with the drip chamber and tubing (see Figure 19-13).
  - Close the clamp on the tubing.
  - Hang the container on an intravenous pole about 30cm above the tube's insertion point into the patient. *At this height, the formula should run at a safe rate into the stomach or intestine.*
  - Squeeze the drip chamber to fill it to one-third to one-half of its capacity.
  - Open the tubing clamp, run the formula through the tubing, and reclamp the tube. *The formula will displace the air in the tubing, thus preventing the instillation of excess air.*
  - Attach the feeding set tubing to the feeding tube and regulate the drip rate to deliver the feeding over the desired length of time.

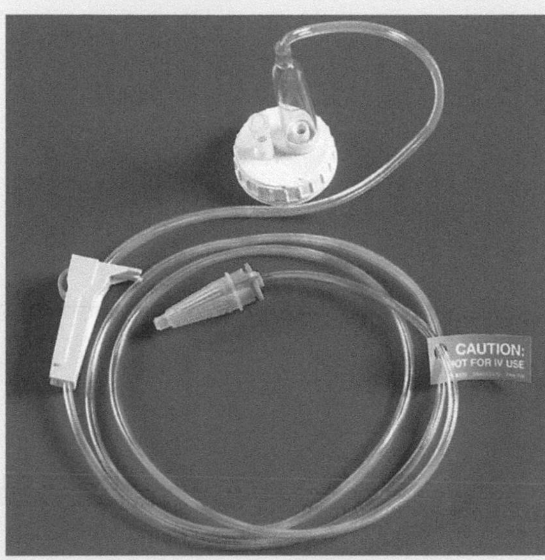

Figure 19-13 Feeding set tubing with drip chamber.
Source: Ross Products Division, Abbott Laboratories.

5 Rinse the feeding tube immediately before all of the formula has run through the tubing.
  - The amount of water will be guided by the patient's condition and any contraindications, i.e. fluid restrictions. *Water flushes the lumen of the tube, preventing future blockage by sticky formula.*

6 Ensure patient comfort and safety.
  - Ask the patient to remain sitting upright in sitting position or in a slightly elevated right lateral position for at least 30 minutes. *These positions facilitate digestion and movement of the feeding from the stomach along the alimentary tract, and prevent the potential aspiration of the feeding into the lungs.*
  - Check local policy on the frequency of changing the nasogastric tube and the use of smaller lumen tubes if a large-bore tube is in place. *These measures prevent irritation and erosion of the pharyngeal and oesophageal mucous membranes.*

7 Dispose of equipment appropriately.
  - Change the equipment every 24 hours or according to local policy.

8 Document all relevant information.
  - Document the amount of gastric contents aspirated, the amount and kind of feed given, duration of the feeding and assessments of the patient.
  - Record the volume of the feeding and water administered on the patient's intake and output record.

9 Monitor the patient for possible problems.
   - Carefully assess patient's receiving tube feedings for problems.
   - To prevent dehydration, give the patient supplemental water in addition to the prescribed tube feeding as ordered.

When drugs are being administered:

- Stop the enteral feed and flush the tube with between 30 and 50ml of water. (If there is a contraindication between the drug and the food discontinue the feed for up to 2 hours as advised by pharmacy.)
- Each medication should be given separately and should be diluted appropriately, i.e. thick liquids should be diluted in equal amounts of water and tablets in 10-15ml of water.
- Medication should never be added directly to the enteral feeding tube.
- If tablets are crushed, the container should be washed with water and this should be used as a flush between drugs.
- The tube should be flushed with 10ml of water between each medication.
- The tube should be flushed with between 30 and 50ml of water before recommencing feeds.
- Fluid restrictions should be discussed with pharmacist prior to administering of drugs.

Evaluation

- Perform a follow-up examination of the following:
  - tolerance of feeding;
  - regurgitation and feelings of fullness after feedings;
  - weight gain or loss;
  - faecal elimination pattern (e.g. diarrhoea, flatulence, constipation);
  - skin elasticity;
  - urine output;
  - glucose tolerance;
- Relate findings to previous assessment data if available. Report significant changes.

PROCEDURE 19-5 Administering a Gastrostomy or Jejunostomy Feeding

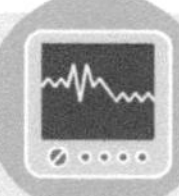

Purposes

See *Procedure 19-4*.

Assessment

See *Procedure 19-4*.

Planning

Before commencing a gastrostomy or jejunostomy feeding, determine the type and amount of feeding to be instilled, frequency of feedings and any pertinent information about previous feedings (e.g. the positioning which the patient best tolerates the feeding).

Equipment

- Pump
- Appropriate giving set
- 50ml syringe
- Sterile water
- Cap
- Supplement

Implementation

Preparation

See *Procedure 19-4*.

Performance

1 Follow local policy to ensure that you explain to the patient what you are going to do, why it is necessary and how they can cooperate. Obtain consent and maintain patient privacy and dignity and ensure that the appropriate local infection control procedures are observed.

2 Assess and prepare the patient. See *Procedure 19-4*.

3 Check the patency of a tube.
   - Administer 50ml of sterile water via the tube.
   - If the water does not flow freely, notify the nurse in charge and/or physician.

4 Check for residual formula, if required by local policy.
   - Attach the syringe to the end of the feeding tube, and withdraw and measure the stomach or jejunal contents.
   - For continuous feedings, check the residual every 4-6 hours and hold feedings according to local policy. The doctor and/or dietician should be notified if a large residual persists.

5 Administer the feeding.
   See point 4 of *Procedure 19-4*.

6 Ensure patient comfort and safety.
   - After the feeding, ask the patient to remain in the sitting position or head is elevated at 30-40 degrees for at least 30 minutes. *This minimises the risk of aspiration.*
   - Assess status of peristomal skin. Gastric or jejunal drainage contains digestive enzymes that can irritate the skin. Document any redness and broken skin areas.
   - Check orders about cleaning the peristomal skin, applying a skin protectant and applying appropriate dressings. Generally, the peristomal skin is washed with mild soap and water at least once daily.
   - Observe for common complications of enteral feedings: aspiration, hyperglycemia, abdominal distention, diarrhoea and faecal impaction. Report findings to the doctor and/or dietician. Often, a change in formula or rate of administration can correct problems.
   - When appropriate, teach the patient how to administer feedings and when to notify the nurse concerning problems.

Variation: percutaneous endoscopic gastrostomy (PEG)

A PEG is kept in place with a short crosspiece or bolster near the skin level at the stoma.

- Clean the stoma daily with soap and water using a cotton swab or small piece of gauze in a circular motion.
- Rotate the external fixation device 360° and clean the skin under it.
- After cleaning, allow the skin to air dry.
- Report any signs of redness, pain, soreness, swelling or drainage to the nurse.
- Do not apply a dressing over the PEG. A dressing and tape may result in skin excoriation and breakdown.

7 Document all assessments and interventions.

Evaluation

See *Procedure 19-4*.

Before administering a tube feed, the nurse must determine any food allergies which the patient may have and assess tolerance to previous feedings. Table 19-4 lists essential assessments to conduct before administering tube feedings. The nurse must also check the expiration date on a commercially prepared formula or the preparation date and time of locally prepared solution, discarding any formula that has passed the expiration date or solution more than 24 hours old.

Parenteral Nutrition

Parenteral nutrition (PN), also referred to as total parenteral nutrition (TPN), is provided when the gastrointestinal tract is non-functional because of an interruption in its continuity or because its absorptive capacity is impaired. Parenteral nutrition is administered intravenously such as through a **central venous catheter** into the superior vena cava.

Table 19-4 Assessing Patients Receiving Tube Feedings

Assessments	Rationale
Allergies to any food in the feeding	Common allergenic foods include milk, sugar, water, eggs and vegetable oil.
Bowel sounds before each feeding or, for continuous feedings, every 4-8 hours	To determine intestinal activity.
Correct placement of tube, before feedings	To prevent aspiration of feedings.
Presence of regurgitation and feelings of fullness after feedings	May indicate delayed gastric emptying, need to decrease quantity or rate of the feeding, or high fat content of the formula.
Abdominal distention, at least daily Measure abdominal girth at the umbilicus	Abdominal distention may indicate intolerance to a previous feeding.
Nausea, vomiting, diarrhoea, constipation or flatulence	The lack of bulk in liquid feedings may cause constipation. The presence of hypertonic or concentrated ingredients may cause diarrhoea and flatulence.
Urine for sugar and acetone	Hyperglycaemia may occur if the sugar content is too high.
Haematocrit	Increases as a result of dehydration.

Parenteral feedings are solutions of dextrose, water, fat, proteins, electrolytes, vitamins and trace elements; they provide all needed calories. Because TPN solutions are hypertonic (highly concentrated in comparison to the **solute** concentration of blood), they are injected only into high-flow central veins, where they are diluted by the patient's blood.

TPN is a means of giving nutrition and fluid to patients such as those with severe malnutrition, severe burns, bowel disease disorders (e.g. ulcerative colitis or enteric fistula), acute renal failure, hepatic failure, metastatic cancer or major surgeries where nothing may be taken by mouth for more than five days.

TPN is not risk free. Infection control is of utmost importance during TPN therapy. The nurse must always observe surgical aseptic technique when changing solutions, tubing, dressings and filters. Patients are at increased risk of fluid, electrolyte and glucose imbalances, and require frequent evaluation and modification of the TPN mixture.

Enteral or parenteral feedings may be continued beyond hospital care in the patient's home or may be initiated in the home.

CRITICAL REFLECTION

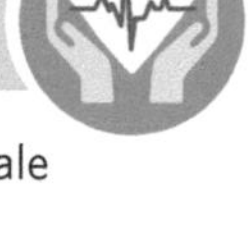

Look back at the Case Study on page 573. Following the knowledge gained from reading this and previous chapters, can you reflect and consider how effective communication, working with the multidisciplinary team, organising care effectively and collaborating with William and his wife can improve the current management of care for William. Points to consider:

- Good communication and provide the rationale.
- Factors of good assessment and provide rationale for decisions made.
- Early referrals to appropriate members of the multidisciplinary team identifying the appropriate members and provide explanation as to why.
- Note the support offered in relation to cutlery, diet and positioning when eating.
- Evaluation and provide rationale.

CHAPTER HIGHLIGHTS

- Although people are bombarded with information about what to eat and what not to eat, each person is responsible for selecting foods that provide essential nutrients. Nurses assist people to evaluate the information they receive about nutrients.
- Essential nutrients are grouped into six categories: water, carbohydrates, fats, proteins, vitamins and minerals.
- Nutrients serve three basic purposes: forming body structures (such as bones and blood), providing energy, and helping to regulate the body's biochemical reactions.
- Energy balance is the relationship between the energy derived from food and the energy used by the body.
- The amount of energy that nutrients or foods supply to the body is their caloric value.
- A person's state of energy balance can be determined by comparing caloric intake with caloric expenditure.
- Body mass index (BMI) or percentage body fat are indicators of changes in body fat stores, whether a person's weight is appropriate for height, and may provide a useful estimate of nutrition.
- Factors influencing a person's nutrition include development, gender, ethnicity and culture, beliefs about foods, personal preferences, religious practices, lifestyle, medications and medical therapy, health status, alcohol abuse, advertising, and psychological factors such as stress, isolation and depression.
- A well-balanced diet includes a healthy balance of the different food groups and fluid. The tilted plate can show the patient the correct portions of the different food groups. The vegetarian tilted plate can be used for all types of vegetarians.
- Both inadequate and excessive intakes of nutrients result in malnutrition. The effects of malnutrition can be general or specific, depending on which nutrients and what level of deficiency or excess are involved.
- Some of the long-range effects of certain nutrient excesses are among the many factors involved in certain diseases, such as coronary artery disease and cancer.
- Assessment of nutritional status may involve all or some of the following: patient history, nutritional screening, physical examination, calculation of the percentage of weight loss, a dietary history, anthropometric measurements and laboratory tests.
- Major goals for patients with or at risk for nutritional problems include the following: maintain or restore optimal nutritional status, decrease or regain specified weight, promote healthy nutritional practices and prevent complications associated with malnutrition.
- Assisting and supporting patients with therapeutic diets is a function shared by the nurse and the dietician. The nurse reinforces the dietician's instructions, assists the patient to make beneficial changes and evaluates the patient's response to planned changes.
- Because many hospitalised patients have poor appetites, a major responsibility of the nurse is to provide nursing interventions that stimulate their appetites.

- Whenever possible, the nurse should help incapacitated patients to feed themselves; a number of self-feeding aids help patients who have difficulty handling regular utensils.
- Enteral feedings, administered through nasogastric, nasointestinal, gastrostomy or jejunostomy tubes, are provided when the patient is unable to ingest foods or the upper gastrointestinal tract is impaired.
- A nasogastric or nasointestinal tube is used to provide enteral nutrition for short-term use (less than six weeks) while a gastrostomy or jejunostomy tube can be used to supply nutrients via the enteral route for long-term use.
- Parenteral nutrition (PN), provided when the gastrointestinal tract is nonfunctional (e.g. absorptive capacity impaired), is given intravenously into a large central vein (e.g. the superior vena cava).

ACTIVITY ANSWERS

ACTIVITY 19-1 Competitors digest and absorb nutrients at a different speed and have different needs compared to other individuals in order to maintain a good activity level. In order to develop a nutritional meal for a 20-year-old athlete there are several key issues that need to be considered. Some of these points are as follows:

- Physical activity level
- Note body mass
- Identify any cultural or other beliefs
- Carbohydrates
- Protein
- Fats

On reflection, please discuss the rationale for your decision making process.

REFERENCES

BAPEN (2008) *The Malnutrition Universal Screening Tool flowchart*, available at http://www.bapen.org.uk/must-tool.htm (accessed March 2011).

Cole, T., Flegal, K., Nicholls, D. and Jackson, A. (2007) 'Body mass index cut offs to define thinness in children and adolescents: International survey', *British Medical Journal*, 335, 194

Dougherty, L. and Lister, S. (2008) *The Royal Marsden Hospital manual of clinical nursing procedures* (7th edn), Oxford: Wiley-Blackwell.

Dudek, S.G. (2006) *Nutrition essentials for nursing practice* (5th edn), Philadelphia, PA: Lippincott.

Holland, K. and Hogg, C. (2010) *Cultural awareness in nursing and health* care (2nd edition), London: Hodder Arnold.

Mann, J. and Truswell, S. (2007) *Essentials of human nutrition* (3rd edn). Oxford: Oxford: University Press.

NMC (2010) *Standards for pre-registration nursing education*, London: NMC.

PHAST (2010) *Dietary Reference Values (DRVs), current dietary goals, recommendations, guidelines and the evidence for them*, London: Department of Health.

RCN (2006) *Malnutrition*, London: RCN.

Roper, N., Logan, W.W. and Tierney, A.J. (2000) *The Roper–Logan–Tierney model of nursing: Based on activities of living*, Oxford: Churchill Livingstone.

Seeley, R., VanPutte, C., Regan, J. and Russo, A. (2011) *Anatomy and physiology* (9th edn), New York: McGraw Hill.

Thomas, B. and Bishop, J. (2007) *Manual of dietetic practice* (4th edn), Oxford: Blackwell Science.

Vesel, L., Bahl, R., Martines, J., Penny, M., Bhandari, N., Kirkwood, B.R. and the WHO Immunization-linked Vitamin A Supplementation Study Group (2010) 'Use of new World Health Organization child growth standards to assess how infant malnutrition relates to breastfeeding and mortality', *Bulletin of the World Health Organization*, 88, 39–48.

Viner, R. and Booy, R. (2005) 'Epidemiology of health and illness', *British Medical Journal*, 330, 411–414.

Walters, E. (1998) 'Know how: Nutritional assessment', *Nursing Times*, 94(8), 68–69.

Webb, G. (2008) *Nutrition: A health promotion approach* (3rd edn), London: Hodder.

WHO (1995) *Physical status: The use and interpretation of anthropometry. Report of a WHO Expert Committee*, WHO Technical Report Series 854, Geneva: World Health Organization.

WHO (2006a) *The WHO child growth standards*, Geneva: World Health Organization, available at http://www.who.int/childgrowth/en/ (accessed March 2011).

WHO (2006b) *BMI Classification*, Geneva: World Health Organization, available at http://apps.who.int/bmi/index.jsp?introPage=intro_3.html (accessed March 2011).

FURTHER RESOURCES

The WHO Child Growth Standards: http://www.who.int/childgrowth/en/index.html

CHAPTER 20
HYDRATION

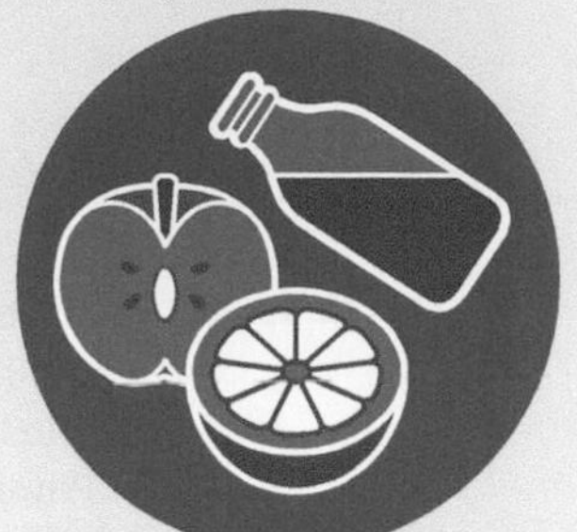

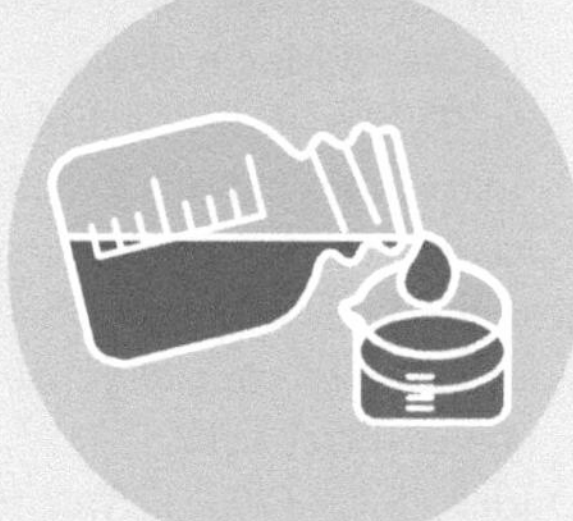

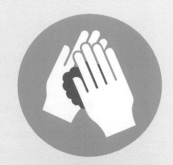

LEARNING OUTCOMES

After completing this chapter, you will be able to:

- Identify factors influencing hydration, electrolyte and acid-base balance.
- Identify developmental hydration considerations.
- Identify risk factors for and clinical signs of dehydration.
- Describe nursing interventions to alter fluid, electrolyte or acid-base imbalances.
- Teach patients measures to maintain fluid and electrolyte balance.
- Implement measures to correct imbalances of fluids and electrolytes or acids and bases such as enteral or parenteral replacements.
- Evaluate the effect of nursing interventions on the patient's fluid, electrolyte or acid-base balance.

This chapter will help you explore the importance of hydration and understand how to identify those at risk of problems associated with hydration and the management of the patient with altered hydration status. It relates to **Essential Skills Clusters (NMC, 2010) 27, 30 and 32**, as appropriate for each progression point.

Ensure that you really understand this chapter by logging on to your complimentary **MyNursingKit** at **www.pearsoned.co.uk/kozier**. Complete the self-assessment tests to check your progress and utilise further activities to practise and confirm your understanding.

CASE STUDY

Thomas Creal, a 75-year-old man, is admitted to a medical ward after collapsing at home. In accident and emergency (A&E) he is diagnosed with a left-sided stroke which has resulted in a profound right-side weakness and dysphagia (difficulty with swallowing).

Thomas has a past medical history of Type II diabetes, coronary heart disease and hypertension. His current medication includes furosemide, captopril, aspirin, clopidogrel and atenolol.

INTRODUCTION

Humans have basic need for fluid to maintain normal functioning of the body. Fluid intake must match fluid output in order to maintain homeostasis. Maintaining adequate fluid balance is essential to maintain health across the lifespan. The role of the nurse is to identify individuals at risk of dehydration or overhydration and manage patients with identified problems associated with hydration.

BODY FLUIDS AND ELECTROLYTES

In good health, fluids, **electrolytes**, acids and bases are finely balanced, a condition known as physiological homoeostasis (stability). This balance depends on a number of physiological processes that regulate fluid intake and output, and the movement of water and the substances dissolved in it between the body compartments.

Almost every illness has the potential to threaten this balance. Even in daily living, excessive temperatures or vigorous activity can disturb the balance if adequate water and salt intake is not maintained. Medical and nursing interventions used to treat the patient, such as use of diuretics (medications used to make the patient urinate more) or aspiration of a nasogastric tube (see Chapter 19) can also affect this balance.

Body Fluids

Survival is said to be based on the rule of three; humans can survive three minutes without oxygen, three days without water and three weeks without food. Water is fundamental for survival and vital as it is:

- a medium for metabolic reactions within cells;
- a transporter for nutrients, waste products and other substances;
- a lubricant;
- an insulator and shock absorber;
- a means of regulating and maintaining body temperature.

Water makes up 50–80% of the human body depending on age (Stockslager *et al.*, 2007) (see Table 20-1), and without regular intake of water many bodily functions would be affected. Age, sex and body fat affect total body water. For example, infants have the highest proportion of water, accounting for 70–80% of their body weight, but the proportion of body water decreases with ageing. In people older than 60, it decreases to approximately 50%.

Table 20-1 Total Body Water as a Percentage of Total Body Weight According to Age and Gender

Age and gender	Total body water as percentage of body weight
Preterm infant	80
Newborn to 6 months	74
6 months to 1 year	60
1 year to 12 years	60
12 years to 18 years (Male)	59
12 years to 18 years (Female)	56
19 years to 50 years (Male)	59
19 years to 50 years (Female)	50
51+ years (Male)	56
51+ years (Female)	47

On average an adult needs to drink between 2.0 and 3.0 litres of fluid a day in order to function efficiently (Stockslager *et al.*, 2007). At least 60% of this should come from fluids, the rest will come from food and metabolism. Children, however, need differing amounts of fluid according to their body weight (see *Practice Guidelines*).

Approximately 9l of fluid passes through an adult's gastrointestinal (GI) tract every day but 7.7l are reabsorbed in the small intestine. Hydration status can be assessed by checking the patient's urine output. An adult should pass 0.5 millilitres of urine for every kilogram of body weight every hour: for example, an adult weighing 70kg should pass 35ml of urine every hour. However, it is important to note that an individual's urine output may be reduced if their insensible losses are increased, e.g. if the person is sweating profusely or has a pyrexia (high temperature).

PRACTICE GUIDELINES

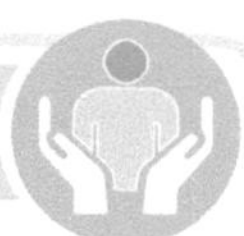

Fluid Requirements for Children

Body weight	Fluid requirements
1-10kg	100ml/kg
11-20kg	1000ml plus 50ml/kg over 10kg
< 20kg	1500ml
> 20kg	1500ml plus 20ml/kg over 20kg

Source: Hogston, R. and Simpson, P.M. (eds) (1999) *Foundations of Nursing Practice*; 4th edition, Basingstoke: Palgrave Macmillan.

Distribution of Body Fluids

The body's fluid is divided into two major compartments: intracellular (inside the cells) and extracellular (outside the cells). Intracellular fluid is found within the cells of the body and constitutes approximately two-thirds of the total body fluid in adults. Extracellular fluid is found outside the cells and accounts for about one-third of total body fluid.

The extracellular fluids comprise:

- Intravascular fluid or **plasma**, which is found within the vascular system (arteries, capillaries and veins).
- Interstitial fluid which surrounds the cells.
- **Lymph** which carries lymphocytes and is transported through the lymphatic system. Lymph forms part of the body's immune system.
- Transcellular fluid includes cerebrospinal, pericardial, pancreatic, pleural, intraocular, biliary, peritoneal and synovial fluids (see Figure 20-1). The transcellular fluid is often termed the 'third space' (see later in the chapter).

Intracellular fluid is vital to normal cell functioning. It contains **solutes** such as oxygen, electrolytes and glucose, and it provides a medium in which metabolic processes of the cell take place.

Although extracellular fluid is in the smaller of the two compartments, it is vital to the transport system of the body. Extracellular fluid carries nutrients to and waste products away from the cells. For example, plasma carries oxygen from the lungs to the capillaries of the vascular system. From there, the oxygen moves across the capillary membranes into the interstitial spaces and then across the cellular membranes into the cells. The opposite route is taken for waste products, such as carbon dioxide going from the cells to the lungs. Interstitial fluid transports wastes from the cells by way of the lymph system as well as directly into the blood plasma through capillaries.

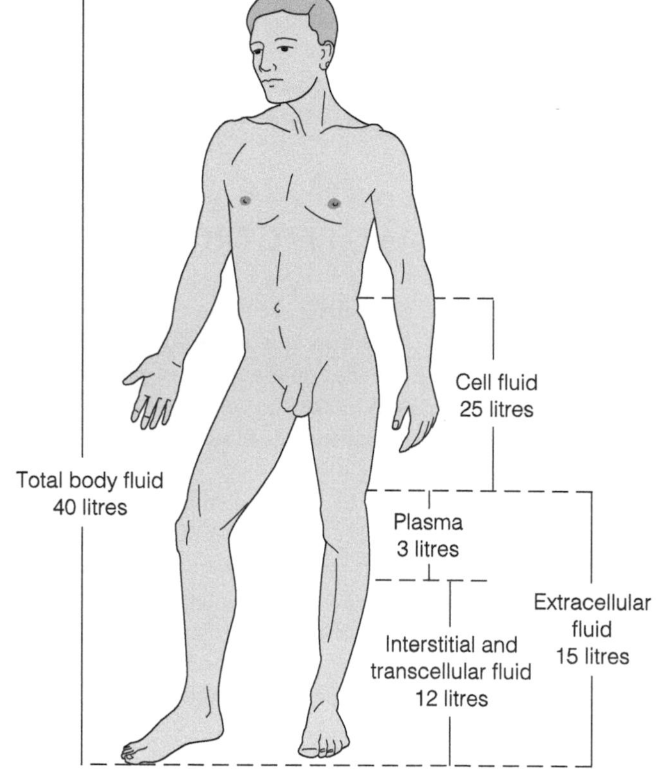

Figure 20-1 Total body fluid represents 40 litres in an adult male weighing 70kg.

Composition of Body Fluids

Extracellular and intracellular fluids contain oxygen from the lungs, dissolved nutrients from the GI tract, excretory products of metabolism such as carbon dioxide, and electrolytes such as sodium (Na^+).

Electrolytes are charged ions that when dissolved in water can conduct electricity. They form as a result of a salt breaking up in water, for example the salt sodium chloride breaks up into one ion of sodium (Na^+) and one ion of chloride (Cl^-). The composition of fluids varies from one body compartment to another.

- Extracellular fluid has ↑ sodium, chloride and bicarbonate and ↓ potassium, calcium and magnesium, and interstitial fluid also contains ↑ protein.

- Intracellular fluid has ↑ potassium, magnesium, phosphate and sulphate and ↓ sodium, chloride and bicarbonate.
- Intravascular fluid (plasma) contains ↑ protein (albumin).
- Interstitial fluid has ↓ protein (albumin).

Maintaining a balance of fluid volumes and electrolyte compositions in the fluid compartments of the body is essential to health. Normal and unusual fluid and electrolyte losses must be replaced if homoeostasis is to be maintained.

Other body fluids such as gastric and intestinal secretions also contain electrolytes. This is of particular concern when these fluids are lost from the body (e.g. in severe vomiting or diarrhoea or when gastric suction removes the gastric secretions). Fluid and electrolyte imbalances can result from excessive losses through these routes.

Movement of Body Fluids and Electrolytes

The body fluid compartments are separated from one another by cell membranes and the capillary membranes. These membranes allow substances across them at different rates and are described as **selectively permeable**. They almost act like a sieve. Small particles such as electrolytes, oxygen and carbon dioxide easily move across these membranes, but larger molecules like glucose and proteins have more difficulty moving between fluid compartments.

Solutes, which are substances dissolved in liquid such as electrolytes, oxygen and protein, and water, move across these membranes by a number of different methods: osmosis, diffusion, filtration and active transport.

Osmosis

Osmosis is the movement of water across cell membranes, from the less concentrated solution to the more concentrated solution (Figure 20-2). In other words, water moves towards the higher concentration of solute in an attempt to equalise the concentrations.

For example, a marathon runner loses a significant amount of water through perspiration, increasing the concentration of solutes in the plasma because of water loss. This higher solute concentration draws water from the interstitial space and cells into the vascular compartment to equalise the concentration of solutes in all fluid compartments. Osmosis is an important mechanism for maintaining homoeostasis and fluid balance.

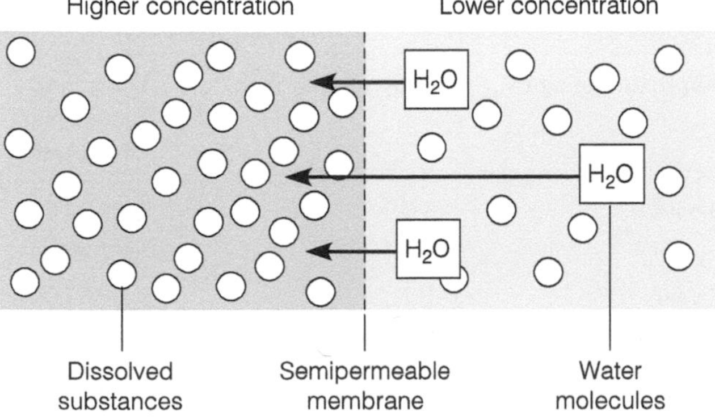

Figure 20-2 Osmosis: water molecules move from the less concentrated area to the more concentrated area in an attempt to equalise the concentration of the solutions on two sides of a membrane.

The concentration of solutes in body fluids is usually expressed as the **osmolality (tonicity)** and is reported as milliosmols per kilogram (mOsm/kg). Sodium is the best determinant of plasma osmolality (concentration of solutes in the blood) otherwise known as *serum osmolality*, while potassium, glucose and urea are primary contributors to the osmolality of intracellular fluid. Serum osmolality can be checked easily by taking a blood sample from a vein in the arm. However, intracellular osmolality is far more difficult to test.

It is important that the nurse understands osmolality (tonicity), particularly when giving patients intravenous fluids (fluids straight into the vein). Most intravenous fluids administered are termed as **isotonic** solutions, which means they have the same osmolality as body fluids, for example 0.9% sodium chloride is an isotonic solution. Other fluids that are administered are **hypertonic** solutions which have a higher osmolality than body fluids, such as 3% sodium chloride, and **hypotonic** solutions which have a lower osmolality than body fluids, such as 0.45% sodium chloride.

Infusing a hypertonic intravenous solution such as 3% sodium chloride will draw fluid out of red blood cells (RBCs), causing them to shrink. On the other hand, a hypotonic solution administered intravenously will cause the RBCs to swell as water is drawn into the cells.

Diffusion

Diffusion is spontaneous intermingling (spreading) of particles. Diffusion can be demonstrated by adding high coloured solution (squash) to a clear fluid (water); the squash intermingles with the water until the final solution is a mixture of the squash and water. The process of diffusion occurs even when two substances are separated by a thin membrane. In the body, diffusion of water, electrolytes and other substances occurs through the capillary membranes.

The rate of diffusion of substances varies according to (a) the size of the molecules, (b) the concentration of the solution and (c) the temperature of the solution. Larger molecules move less quickly than smaller ones because they require more energy to move about. With diffusion, the molecules move from a solution of higher concentration to a solution of lower concentration (see Figure 20-3). Increases in temperature increase the rate of motion of molecules and therefore the rate of diffusion.

Filtration

Filtration is a process whereby fluid and solutes move together across a membrane from one compartment to another. The movement is from an area of higher pressure to one of lower pressure. An example of filtration is the movement of fluid and nutrients from the capillaries of the arterioles to the interstitial fluid around the cells.

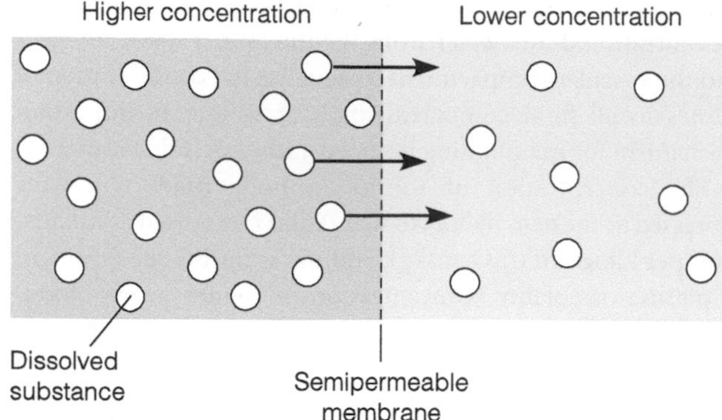

Figure 20-3 Diffusion: the movement of molecules through a semipermeable membrane from an area of higher concentration to an area of lower concentration.

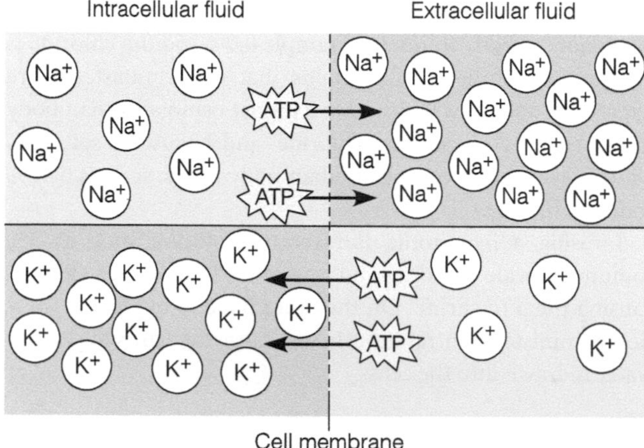

Figure 20-4 An example of active transport. Energy ATP is used to move sodium molecules and potassium molecules across a semipermeable membrane against sodium's and potassium's concentration gradients (i.e. from areas of lesser concentration to areas of greater concentration).

Active Transport

Substances can move across cell membranes from a less concentrated solution to a more concentrated one by **active transport** (see Figure 20-4). This process differs from diffusion and osmosis in that energy is required for it to take place. In active transport, a substance combines with a carrier on the outside surface of the cell membrane, and they move to the inside surface of the cell membrane. Once inside, they separate, and the substance is released to the inside of the cell.

Regulating Body Fluids

In a healthy person, fluid intake and fluid loss are balanced; however, illness can upset this balance so that the body has too little or too much fluid.

Fluid Intake

Fluid intake comes from a number of sources:

- fluids such as water, squash, pop and coffee;
- food such as fruit, vegetables;
- metabolism.

A moderately active adult requires approximately 2.5l of fluid each day. However the average adult normally drinks about 1.5l of fluid each day which is insufficient to maintain health. The outstanding fluid comes from food and the metabolism of food. The water content of food is relatively large and accounts for approximately 750ml of fluid each day, while the metabolism of food, the physical and chemical processes used to breakdown the food, makes up the remaining fluid volume required (see Table 20-2).

The body's thirst mechanism is the main regulator of fluid intake. The thirst centre is located in the hypothalamus of the brain and is stimulated by volume of fluid in the vascular system and angiotensin (a hormone released in response to decreased blood flow to the kidneys). For example, a long-distance runner loses significant amounts of water through perspiration and rapid breathing during a race, increasing the concentration of solutes of body fluids. This stimulates the thirst centre causing the runner to experience the sensation of thirst and the desire to drink to replace lost fluids.

Thirst, however, is not a reliable indicator of hydration status as the body is already dehydrated before the thirst mechanism is stimulated. It is also important to note that the thirst mechanism can be affected by a number of factors including the patient's age. In particular, reduced thirst has been noted in older adults (Royal College of Nursing (RCN), 2007).

ACTIVITY 20-1

Calculate the fluid intake requirements for a child who weighs 32kg.

Table 20-2 Average Daily Fluid Requirements by Age and Weight

Approximate age	Body weight (kg)	Daily fluid requirement (ml/24 hr)
3 days	3.0	250-300
1 year	9.5	1,150-1,300
2 years	11.8	1,350-1,500
6 years	20.0	1,800-2,000
10 years	28.7	2,000-2,500
14 years	45.0	2,200-2,700
18 years (adult)	54.0	2,200-2,700

Source: *Nelson Textbook of Pediatrics* (p. 107), by R.E. Behrman, 1992, Philadelphia: Saunders. Adapted with permission.

Table 20-3 Average Daily Fluid Output for an Adult

Route	Amount (ml)
Urine	1,400–1,500
Insensible losses	
Lungs	350–400
Skin	350–400
Sweat	100
Faeces	100–200
Total	2,300–2,600

Fluid Output

Fluid losses from the body counterbalance the adult's 2.5l average daily intake of fluid, as shown in Table 20-3. There are three main routes of fluid output:

1 urine;
2 insensible loss through the skin as perspiration and through the lungs as water vapour in the expired air;
3 loss through the intestines in faeces.

Urine

Urine formed by the kidneys and excreted from the urinary bladder is the major avenue of fluid output. Normal urine output for an adult is 1,400–1,500ml per 24 hours, or at least 0.5ml per kilogram per hour. In healthy people, urine output may vary noticeably from day to day. Urine volume automatically increases as fluid intake increases. If fluid loss through perspiration is large, however, urine volume decreases to maintain fluid balance in the body.

Insensible losses

Insensible fluid loss occurs through the skin, in the form of perspiration and lungs, as water vapour. It is not noticeable and therefore cannot be measured. Insensible losses can increase and decrease according to the climate, activity and any skin losses such as a burn or abrasion.

Faeces

Partly digested food or chime contains water and electrolytes. Approximately 1.5l of chime enters the large intestine in an adult; however, only 100ml is reabsorbed.

Maintaining Homoeostasis

The volume and composition of body fluids is regulated by a number of body systems including the kidneys, the endocrine system, the cardiovascular system, the lungs and the GI system.

Kidneys

The kidneys are the primary regulator of body fluids and electrolyte balance. The kidneys adjust the amount of water reabsorbed from the plasma (extracellular fluid) and therefore regulate how much fluid is excreted as urine. Approximately 1.5l of urine is excreted daily by the average adult. The kidneys also select which and how much electrolytes are excreted.

Antidiuretic hormone (ADH)

Antidiuretic hormone regulates water excretion from the kidney. When serum osmolality rises (plasma electrolytes increase), ADH is produced and causes the kidneys to reabsorb more water back into the plasma. This results in urine output falling. Conversely, if serum osmolality decreases (plasma electrolytes decrease), ADH is suppressed and the urine output increases.

Rennin-angiotensin-aldosterone system

Specialised receptors in the kidneys respond to changes in renal perfusion (the amount of blood passing through the kidneys for filtration) and initiate the rennin-angiotensin-aldosterone system. If blood flow to the kidney decreases, rennin, an enzyme, is released. Rennin causes the conversion of angiotensinogen to angiotensin I, which is then converted to angiotensin II by angiotensin-converting enzyme. Angiotensin II acts directly on the kidneys to promote sodium and water retention. In addition, it stimulates the release of aldosterone from the adrenal cortex. Aldosterone also promotes sodium retention in the distal kidneys. The net effect of the rennin-angiotensin-aldosterone system is to restore blood volume (and renal perfusion) by sodium and water retention.

Regulating Electrolytes

Electrolytes are present in all body fluids and fluid compartments. Just as maintaining the fluid balance is vital to normal body function, so is maintaining electrolyte balance. Although the concentration of specific electrolytes differs between fluid compartments, a balance of cations (positively charged ions) and anions (negatively charged ions) always exists. Electrolytes are important for:

- maintaining fluid balance;
- contributing to acid–base regulation;
- facilitating enzyme reactions;
- transmitting neuromuscular reactions.

Most electrolytes enter the body through dietary intake and are excreted in the urine. Some electrolytes, such as sodium and chloride, are not stored by the body and must be consumed daily to maintain normal levels. Potassium and calcium, on the other hand, are stored in the cells and bone, respectively. The regulatory mechanisms and functions of the major electrolytes are summarised in Table 20-4.

Sodium (Na^+)

Sodium is the most abundant electrolyte in extracellular fluid. Sodium's main function is to control and regulate water balance. Sodium is found in many foods, such as bacon, ham, processed cheese and table salt.

Potassium (K^+)

Potassium is the major electrolyte in intracellular fluids, with only a small amount found in plasma and interstitial fluid.

Table 20-4 Regulation and Functions of Electrolytes

Electrolyte	Regulation	Function
Sodium (Na^+)	Reabsorbed or excreted by kidneys	Regulating extracellular fluid volume Maintaining blood volume Transmitting nerve impulses and contracting muscles
Potassium (K^+)	Excreted or conserved by the kidneys Renal excretion and conservation Movement into cells from plasm by insulin Movement out of cells when cells are damaged or if there is acidosis (see later in chapter)	Maintaining intracellular osmolality Transmitting nerve and other electrical impulses Regulating cardiac impulse transmission and muscle contraction Skeletal and smooth muscle function Regulating acid-base balance
Calcium (Ca^{2+})	Redistribution between bones and extracellular fluid Parathyroid hormone and calcitriol increase serum Ca^{2+} levels; calcitonin decreases serum levels	Forming bones and teeth Transmitting nerve impulses Regulating muscle contractions Maintaining cardiac pacemaker (automaticity) Blood clotting Activating enzymes such as pancreatic lipase and phospholipase
Magnesium (Mg^{2+})	Conservation and excretion by kidneys Intestinal absorption increased by vitamin D and parathyroid hormone	Intracellular metabolism Operating sodium-potassium pump Relaxing muscle contractions Transmitting nerve impulses Regulating cardiac function
Chloride (Cl^-)	Excreted and reabsorbed along with sodium in the kidneys Aldosterone increases chloride reabsorption with sodium	HCl production Regulating extra-cellular fluid balance and vascular volume Regulating acid-base balance Buffer in oxygen-carbon dioxide exchange in RBCs
Phosphate (PO_4^-)	Excretion and reabsorption by the kidneys Parathyroid hormone decreases serum levels by increasing renal excretion Reciprocal relationship with calcium: increasing serum calcium levels decrease phosphate levels; decreasing serum calcium increases phosphate	Forming bones and teeth Metabolising carbohydrate, protein and fat Cellular metabolism; producing ATP and DNA Muscle, nerve and RBC function Regulating acid-base balance Regulating calcium levels
Bicarbonate (HCO_3^-)	Excretion and reabsorption by the kidneys Regeneration by kidneys	Major body buffer involved in acid-base regulation

Potassium is important in maintaining intracellular water balance, and it is a vital electrolyte for skeletal, cardiac and smooth muscle activity. It is involved in maintaining **acid-base balance** as well. Potassium is found in a range of foods:

- Vegetables
  - Avocado
  - Raw carrot
  - Baked potato
  - Raw tomato
  - Spinach
- Meats and fish
  - Beef
  - Cod
  - Pork
  - Veal
- Fruits
  - Dried fruits (e.g. raisins and dates)
  - Banana
  - Apricot
  - Cantaloupe melon
  - Orange
- Beverages
  - Milk
  - Orange juice
  - Apricot nectar

Calcium (Ca^{2+})

The vast majority of calcium in the body is in the skeletal system, with a relatively small amount in extracellular fluid. Calcium is important in the development of bones, regulating muscle contraction and relaxation and cardiac function. Extracellular calcium is regulated by the parathyroid hormone, calcitonin and calcitriol (derived from vitamin D). When extracellular calcium falls the parathyroid hormone and calcitriol cause calcium to be released from the bones and when there is a rise in extracellular calcium calcitonin stimulates the deposition of calcium in bones.

With ageing, more calcium is excreted by the kidneys causing osteoporosis (brittle bones) increasing the risk of fractures of the bones. Milk and milk products are the richest sources of calcium, with other foods such as dark green leafy vegetables and canned salmon containing smaller amounts.

Magnesium (Mg^{2+})

Magnesium is primarily found in the skeleton and in intracellular fluid. It is important for intracellular metabolism, being particularly involved in the production and use of ATP (adenosine triphosphate) which gives the cells energy. Magnesium also is necessary for protein and deoxyribonucleic acid (DNA) synthesis within the cells. Extracellular magnesium is involved in neuromuscular and cardiac function. Maintaining and ensuring adequate magnesium levels is an important part of care of patients with heart problems. Cereal grains, nuts, dried fruit, legumes and green leafy vegetables are good sources of magnesium in the diet, as are dairy products, meat and fish.

Chloride (Cl^-)

Chloride is found in extracellular fluid and is regulated by the kidneys. Chloride is a major component of gastric juice as hydrochloric acid (HCl) and is involved in regulating acid–base balance. Chloride is found in the same foods as sodium.

Phosphate (PO_4^-)

Phosphate is found in intracellular fluid, extracellular fluid, bone, muscle and nerve tissue. Phosphate is involved in many chemical actions of the cell; it is essential for functioning of muscles, nerves and red blood cells. It is also involved in the metabolism of protein, fat and carbohydrate. Phosphate is absorbed from the intestine and is found in many foods such as meat, fish, poultry, milk products and legumes.

Bicarbonate (HCO_3^-)

Bicarbonate is present in both intracellular and extracellular fluids. Its primary function is regulating acid–base balance. Extracellular bicarbonate levels are regulated by the kidneys. Bicarbonate is excreted when too much is present; if more is needed, the kidneys both regenerate and reabsorb bicarbonate. Unlike other electrolytes that must be consumed in the diet, adequate amounts of bicarbonate are produced through metabolic processes to meet the body's needs.

ACID–BASE BALANCE

An important part of regulating the chemical balance or homoeostasis of body fluids is regulating their acidity or alkalinity. An **acid** is a substance that releases hydrogen ions (H^+) in solution while **bases** or *alkalis* have a low hydrogen ion concentration and can accept hydrogen ions in solution. The relative acidity or alkalinity of a solution is measured as **pH**. The pH reflects the hydrogen ion concentration of the solution: the higher the hydrogen ion concentration (and the more acidic the solution), the lower the pH. Water has a pH of 7 and is neutral; that is, it is neither acidic in nature nor is it alkaline; solutions with a pH lower than 7 are acidic; those with a pH higher than 7 are alkaline.

Regulation of Acid–Base Balance

Body fluids are maintained within a narrow range that is slightly alkaline. The normal pH of arterial blood is between 7.35 and 7.45 (Figure 20-5). Acids are continually produced during metabolism. Several body systems, including buffers, the respiratory system and the renal system, are actively involved in maintaining the narrow pH range necessary for optimal function.

Buffers

Buffers prevent excessive changes in pH by removing or releasing hydrogen ions. If excess hydrogen ion is present in body fluids, buffers bind with the hydrogen ion, minimising the change in pH. When body fluids become too alkaline, buffers can release hydrogen ion, again minimising the change in pH. The action of a buffer is immediate, but limited in its capacity to maintain or restore normal acid–base balance.

The major buffer system in extracellular fluids is the bicarbonate (HCO_3^-) and carbonic acid (H_2CO_3) system. So when an acid, for example hydrochloric acid, is added it will cause a condition called acidosis. This acid combines with the bicarbonate which prevents the pH from dropping too much. When a base (alkali), for example sodium hydroxide, is added it combines with carbonic acid which prevents the pH from rising too much. If a strong acid is added to extracellular fluid the bicarbonate is used up quickly to try to neutralise the acid. This causes a drop in the pH and causes a condition known as **acidosis**. If a strong base is added to extracellular fluid carbonic acid is depleted quickly causing the pH to rise causing a condition known as **alkalosis**.

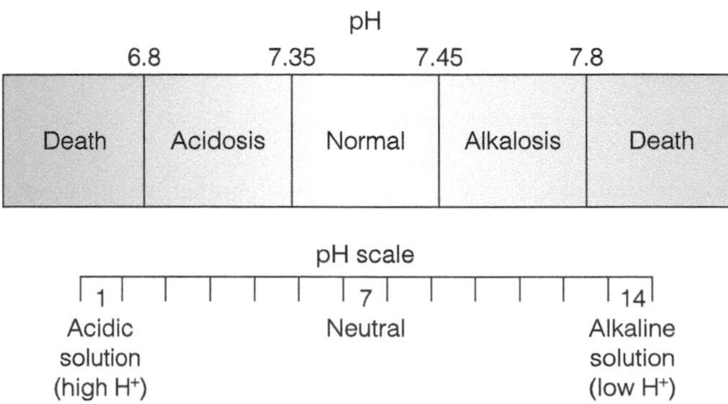

Figure 20-5 Body fluids are normally slightly alkaline, a pH between 7.35 and 7.45.

Respiratory Regulation

The lungs help regulate acid–base balance by eliminating or retaining carbon dioxide (CO_2) which is a potential acid. When carbon dioxide combines with water, carbonic acid is formed. Working together with the bicarbonate–carbonic acid buffer system, the lungs regulate acid–base balance and pH by altering the rate and depth of respirations. The response of the respiratory system to changes in pH is rapid, occurring within minutes.

When carbon dioxide and carbonic acid rises in the blood, the respiratory centre of the brain is stimulated; this increases the rate and depth of respirations. Carbon dioxide is exhaled, and carbonic acid levels fall. By contrast, when bicarbonate levels are excessive, the rate and depth of respirations are reduced. This causes carbon dioxide to be retained, carbonic acid levels to rise and the excess bicarbonate to be neutralised.

Carbon dioxide levels in the blood are measured as the PCO_2, or partial pressure of the dissolved gas in the blood. PCO_2 refers to the pressure of carbon dioxide in venous blood. $PaCO_2$ refers to the pressure of carbon dioxide in arterial blood. The normal $PaCO_2$ is 35–45mmHg.

Renal Regulation

Although buffers and the respiratory system can compensate for changes in pH, the kidneys are the ultimate long-term regulator of acid–base balance. They are slower to respond to changes, requiring hours to days to correct imbalances, but their response is more permanent and selective than that of the other systems.

The kidneys maintain acid–base balance by selectively excreting or conserving bicarbonate and hydrogen ions. When excess hydrogen ion is present and the pH falls (acidosis), the kidneys reabsorb and regenerate bicarbonate and excrete hydrogen ion. In the case of alkalosis and a high pH, excess bicarbonate is excreted and hydrogen ion is retained. The normal serum bicarbonate level is 22–26mmol/l.

FACTORS AFFECTING BODY FLUID, ELECTROLYTES AND ACID-BASE BALANCE

The ability of the body to adjust fluids, electrolytes and acid–base balance is influenced by age, gender and body size, environmental temperature and lifestyle.

Age

Infants and growing children have a much higher metabolic rate than adults which increases fluid loss. Infants lose more fluid through the kidneys because immature kidneys are less able to conserve water than adult kidneys. In addition, infants respirations are more rapid and the body surface area is proportionately greater than that of adults, increasing insensible fluid losses. This rapid turnover of fluid and an increase in losses, such as fever, associated with illness can create critical fluid imbalances in children far more rapidly than in adults.

In older people, the normal ageing process may affect fluid balance. The thirst response often is blunted (RCN, 2007). This, added to the fact that the kidneys are less able to conserve water, increases the risk of dehydration.

Gender and Body Size

Total body water also is affected by gender and body size (see Table 20-1 on page 597). Because fat cells contain little or no water and lean tissue has a high water content, people with a higher percentage of body fat have less body fluid. Women have proportionately more body fat and less body water than men.

Environmental Temperature

People with an illness and those participating in strenuous activity are at risk of fluid and electrolyte imbalances when the environmental temperature is high. Fluid losses through sweating are increased in hot environments as the body attempts to dissipate heat. These losses are even greater in people who have not been acclimatised to the environment.

Both salt and water are lost through sweating. When only water is replaced, salt depletion is a risk. The person who is salt depleted may experience fatigue, weakness, headache and GI symptoms such as anorexia (loss of appetite) and nausea. If water is not replaced, body temperature rises, and the person is at risk for heat exhaustion or heatstroke.

Drinking adequate amounts of cool liquids, particularly during strenuous activity, reduces the risk of adverse effects from heat. Balanced electrolyte solutions and carbohydrate–electrolyte solutions such as sports drinks are recommended because they replace both water and electrolytes lost through sweat.

Lifestyle

Other factors such as diet, exercise and stress affect fluid, electrolyte and acid–base balance.

The intake of fluids and electrolytes is affected by the diet. For example, people with anorexia nervosa or bulimia are at risk of severe fluid and electrolyte imbalances because of inadequate intake, induced vomiting and use of diuretics and laxatives.

Stress can increase production of ADH, which decreases urine production. The overall response of the body to stress is to increase the blood volume.

Other lifestyle factors can also affect fluid, electrolyte and acid–base balance. Heavy alcohol consumption affects electrolyte balance, increasing the risk of low calcium, magnesium and phosphate levels. The risk of acidosis associated with breakdown of fat tissue also is greater in the person who drinks large amounts of alcohol.

ACTIVITY 20-2

What factors could affect a patient's body fluid, electrolyte and acid-base balance?

DISTURBANCES IN FLUID VOLUME, ELECTROLYTE AND ACID-BASE BALANCES

Hypovolaemia

Hypovolaemia or decreased blood volume occurs when the body loses both water and electrolytes. Hypovolaemia generally occurs as a result of (a) abnormal losses through the skin, GI tract or kidney; (b) decreased intake of fluid; (c) bleeding; or (d) movement of fluid into a third space. See the section on third space syndrome that follows.

For the risk factors and clinical signs related to hypovolaemia, see Table 20-5.

Third Space Syndrome

Third space syndrome is caused by movement of fluid from the vascular space (plasma) into an area where it is not readily accessible as extracellular fluid. This fluid remains in the body but is essentially unavailable for use. The fluid may be found in the bowel, in the interstitial space as oedema, in inflamed tissue, or in potential spaces such as the peritoneal or pleural cavities.

Oedema

Oedema is excess interstitial fluid caused by increased water and sodium content. Oedema typically is most apparent in areas where the tissue pressure is low, such as around the eyes.

Oedema can be caused by several different mechanisms.

- Pressure building within the capillaries pushes fluid into the tissues. This is principally found in the feet, ankles and sacrum and is mainly due to gravity.
- Low levels of protein in the plasma as a result of malnutrition can also cause oedema because fluid is not drawn out of the tissues into the capillaries.

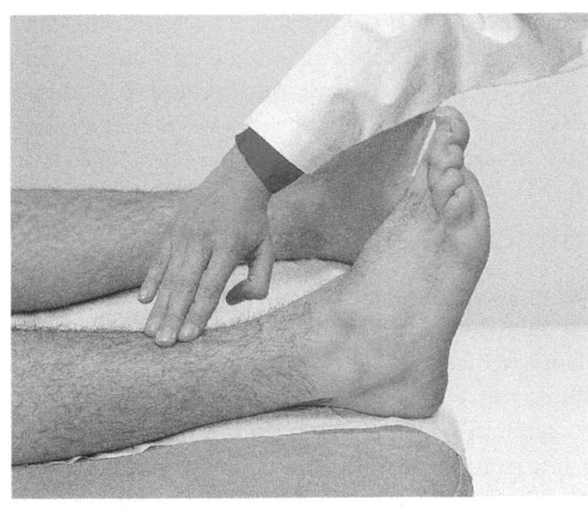

Figure 20-6 Evaluation of oedema. Palpate for oedema over the tibia as shown here and behind the medial malleolus, and over the dorsum of each foot.

- Tissue trauma and some disorders such as allergic reactions cause the capillaries to become more permeable, allowing fluid to escape into interstitial tissues.
- Obstructed lymph flow impairs the movement of fluid from interstitial tissues back into the vascular compartment, resulting in oedema.

Pitting oedema is oedema that leaves a small depression or pit after finger pressure is applied to the swollen area. The pit is caused by movement of fluid to adjacent tissue, away from the point of pressure (see Figure 20-6). Within 10 to 30 seconds the pit normally disappears.

Dehydration

Dehydration occurs when water is lost from the body without significant loss of electrolytes. Because water is lost while electrolytes, particularly sodium, are retained, the serum osmolality (concentration of sodium in the blood) increases. Water is

Table 20-5 Hypervolaemia

Risk factors	Clinical manifestations	Nursing interventions
Excess intake of sodium-containing intravenous fluids. Excess ingestion of sodium in diet or medications (e.g. sodium bicarbonate antacids such as Alka-Seltzer or hypertonic enema solutions such as Fleet's). Impaired fluid balance regulation related to: • heart failure • renal failure • cirrhosis of the liver.	Weight gain. Fluid intake greater than output. Moist mucous membranes. Full, bounding pulse; tachycardia. Increased blood pressure and central venous pressure. Distended neck and peripheral veins; slow vein emptying. Moist crackles in lungs; dyspnoea, shortness of breath. Mental confusion.	Assess for clinical manifestations of hypervolaemia. Monitor weight and vital signs. Assess for oedema. Assess breath sounds. Monitor fluid intake and output. Monitor laboratory findings. Place in Fowler's position. Administer diuretics as ordered. Restrict fluid intake as indicated. Restrict dietary sodium as ordered. Implement measures to prevent skin breakdown.

drawn into the vascular compartment from the interstitial space and cells, resulting in cells becoming dehydrated. Older adults are at particular risk for dehydration because of decreased thirst sensation (RCN, 2007). This type of water deficit also can affect patients who are hyperventilating or have prolonged fever.

Overhydration

Overhydration, also known as *water intoxication*, occurs when water is gained in excess of electrolytes, resulting in low serum osmolality (concentration of sodium in the blood). Water is drawn into the cells, causing them to swell. In the brain this can lead to cerebral oedema and impaired neurological function. Water intoxication often occurs when both fluid and electrolytes are lost, for example, through excessive sweating, but only water is replaced. It can also result from the syndrome of inappropriate antidiuretic hormone (SIADH), a disorder that can occur with some malignant tumours, AIDS, head injury or administration of certain drugs such as barbiturates or anaesthetics.

Electrolyte Imbalances

The most common and most significant electrolyte imbalances involve sodium, potassium, calcium, magnesium, chloride and phosphate.

Sodium

Sodium (Na^+), the most abundant electrolyte in the extracellular fluid, is found in most body secretions, for example, saliva, gastric and intestinal secretions, bile and pancreatic fluid. Therefore, continuous excretion of any of these fluids, such as vomiting, can result in a sodium deficit.

Hyponatraemia is a sodium deficit, or serum sodium level of less than 135mmol/l. As a result, water is drawn out of the vascular compartment into interstitial tissues and the cells (see Figure 20-7(a)), causing the clinical manifestations associated with this disorder.

Hypernatraemia is excess sodium, or a serum sodium of greater than 145mmol/l. As a result, fluid moves out of the cells into the extracellular fluid (see Figure 20-7(b)) and the cells become dehydrated.

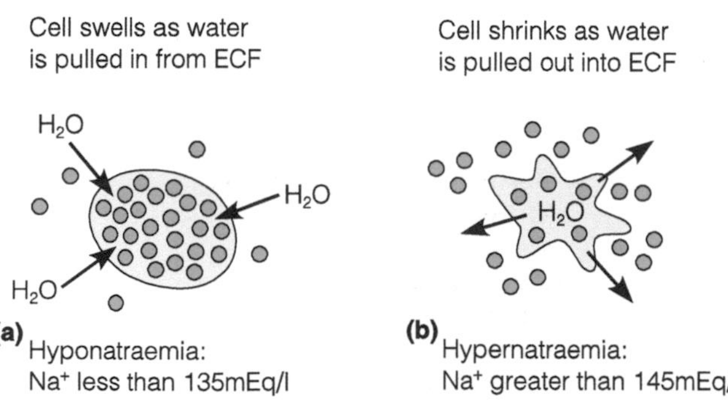

Figure 20-7 The extracellular sodium level affects cell size. (a) In hyponatraemia, cells swell; (b) in hypernatraemia, cells shrink in size.

Table 20-6 lists risk factors and clinical signs for hyponatraemia and hypernatraemia.

Potassium

Although the amount of potassium (K^+) in extracellular fluid is small, it is vital to normal neuromuscular and cardiac function. Potassium is usually excreted by the kidneys. However, the kidneys do not regulate potassium excretion as effectively as they do sodium excretion. Therefore, an acute potassium deficiency can develop rapidly. Of the body's secretions, the GI secretions are high in potassium.

Hypokalaemia is a potassium deficit or a serum potassium level of less than 3.5mmol/l. Gastrointestinal losses of potassium through vomiting and gastric suction are common causes of hypokalaemia, as are the use of potassium-wasting diuretics, such as thiazide diuretics or loop diuretics (e.g. frusemide).

Hyperkalaemia is a potassium excess or a serum potassium level greater than 5.0mmol/l, is less common than hypokalaemia and rarely occurs in patients with normal renal (kidney) function. It is, however, more dangerous than hypokalaemia, and can lead to cardiac arrest. Table 20-6 lists risk factors and clinical signs for hypokalaemia and hyperkalaemia.

CLINICAL ALERT

Potassium may be given intravenously for severe hypokalemia. It must always be diluted appropriately and never given in a bolus. Potassium that is to be given IV should be mixed in the pharmacy and double checked prior to administration by two nurses. The usual concentration of IV potassium is 20–40mmol/l.

Calcium

Regulating levels of calcium (Ca^{2+}) in the body is more complex than the other major electrolytes so calcium balance can be affected by many factors. Imbalances of this electrolyte are relatively common.

Hypocalcaemia is a calcium deficit, or a total serum calcium level of less than 8.5mg/dl. Severe depletion of calcium can cause muscle spasms and paresthesias (abnormal sensation such as pins and needles) and can lead to convulsions. Low serum magnesium levels (hypomagnesaemia) and chronic alcoholism also increase the risk of hypocalcaemia.

Hypercalcaemia, or serum calcium levels greater than 10.5mg/dl, most often occurs when calcium is mobilised from the bony skeleton. This may be due to malignancy or prolonged immobilisation.

The risk factors and clinical manifestations related to calcium imbalances are found in Table 20-6.

Magnesium

Magnesium (Mg^{2+}) imbalances are relatively common in hospitalised patients, although they may be unrecognised.

Table 20-6 Electrolyte Imbalances

Risk factors	Clinical manifestations	Nursing interventions
Hyponatraemia		
Loss of sodium • Gastrointestinal fluid loss • Sweating • Use of diuretics *Gain of water* • Hypotonic tube feedings • Drinking water • Excess intravenous infusion of dextrose in water administration *Syndrome of inappropriate ADH (SIADH)* • Head injury • AIDS • Malignant tumours	Lethargy, confusion, apprehension Muscle twitching Abdominal cramps Anorexia, nausea, vomiting Headache Seizures, coma *Laboratory findings:* Serum sodium below 135mmol/l Serum osmolality below 280mOsm/kg	Assess clinical manifestations. Monitor fluid intake and output. Monitor laboratory data (e.g. serum sodium). Assess patient closely if administering hypertonic saline solutions. Encourage food and fluid high in sodium if permitted (e.g. table salt, bacon, ham, processed cheese). Limit water intake as indicated.
Hypernatraemia		
Loss of fluids • Insensible water loss (hyperventilation or fever) • Diarrhoea *Water deprivation* Excess salt intake: • Parenteral administration of saline solutions • Hypertonic tube feedings without adequate water • Excessive use of table salt Conditions such as: • Diabetes insipidus • Heat stroke	Thirst Dry, sticky mucous membranes Tongue red, dry, swollen Weakness Postural hypotension, dyspnoea Severe hypernatraemia: • Fatigue, restlessness • Decreasing level of consciousness • Disorientation • Convulsions *Laboratory findings:* Serum sodium above 145mmol/l Serum osmolality above 300mOsm/kg	Monitor fluid intake and output. Monitor behaviour changes (e.g. restlessness, disorientation). Monitor laboratory findings (e.g. serum sodium). Encourage fluids as ordered. Monitor diet as ordered (e.g. restrict intake of salt and foods high in sodium).
Hypokalaemia		
Loss of potassium • Vomiting and gastric suction • Diarrhoea • Heavy perspiration Use of potassium-wasting drugs (e.g. diuretics) Poor intake of potassium (as with debilitated patients, alcoholics, anorexia nervosa) Hyperaldosteronism	Muscle weakness, leg cramps Fatigue, lethargy Anorexia, nausea, vomiting Decreased bowel sounds, decreased bowel motility Cardiac dysrhythmias Depressed deep-tendon reflexes *Laboratory findings:* Serum potassium below 3.5mmol/l Arterial blood gases (ABGs) may show alkalosis T wave flattening and ST segment depression on ECG	Monitor heart rate and rhythm. Monitor patients receiving digitalis (e.g. digoxin) closely, because hypokalemia increases risk of digitalis toxicity. Administer oral potassium as ordered with food or fluid to prevent gastric irritation. Administer IV potassium solutions at a rate no faster than 10-20mmol/h; never administer undiluted potassium intravenously. For patients receiving IV potassium, monitor for pain and inflammation at the injection site. Teach patient about potassium-rich foods. Teach patients how to prevent excessive loss of potassium (e.g. through abuse of diuretics and laxatives).
Hyperkalaemia		
Decreased potassium excretion • Renal failure • Hypoaldosteronism • Potassium-conserving diuretics *High potassium intake* • Excessive use of K+ containing salt substitutes • Excessive or rapid IV infusion of potassium Potassium shift out of the tissue cells into the plasma (e.g. infections, burns, acidosis)	Gastrointestinal hyperactivity, diarrhoea Irritability, apathy, confusion Cardiac dysrhythmias or arrest Muscle weakness, areflexia (absence of reflexes) Paresthesias and numbness in extremities *Laboratory findings:* Serum potassium above 5.0mmol/l Peaked T wave, widened QRS on ECG	Closely monitor cardiac status and ECG. Administer diuretics and other medications such as glucose and insulin as ordered. Hold potassium supplements and K^+ conserving diuretics. Monitor serum K^+ levels carefully; a rapid drop may occur as potassium shifts into the cells. Teach patients to avoid foods high in potassium and salt substitutes.

→

Table 20-6 *(continued)*

Risk factors	Clinical manifestations	Nursing interventions
Hypocalcaemia		
Surgical removal of the parathyroid glands Conditions such as • Hypoparathyroidism • Acute pancreatitis • Hyperphosphataemia • Thyroid carcinoma *Inadequate vitamin D intake* • Malabsorption • Hypomagnesaemia • Alkalosis • Sepsis • Alcohol abuse	Numbness, tingling of the extremities and around the mouth Muscle tremors, cramps; if severe can progress to tetany and convulsions Cardiac dysrhythmias; decreased cardiac output Confusion, anxiety, possible psychoses *Laboratory findings:* Serum calcium less than 8.5mg/dL or 4.5mmol/l (total)	Closely monitor respiratory and cardiovascular status. Take precautions to protect a confused patient. Administer oral or parenteral calcium supplements as ordered. When administering intravenously, closely monitor cardiac status and ECG during infusion. Teach patients at high risk for osteoporosis about • Dietary sources rich in calcium • Recommendation for 1,000–1,500mg of calcium per day • Calcium supplements • Regular exercise • Oestrogen replacement therapy for postmenopausal women.
Hypercalcaemia		
Prolonged immobilisation Conditions such as • Hyperparathyroidism • Malignancy of the bone • Paget's disease	Lethargy, weakness Depressed deep-tendon reflexes Anorexia, nausea, vomiting Constipation Polyuria, hypercalciuria Flank pain secondary to urinary calculi Dysrhythmias, possible heart block *Laboratory findings:* Serum calcium greater than 10.5mg/dL or 5.5mmol/l (total)	Increase patient movement and exercise. Encourage oral fluids as permitted to maintain a dilute urine. Teach patients to limit intake of food and fluid high in calcium. Encourage ingestion of fibre to prevent constipation. Protect a confused patient; monitor for pathologic fractures in patients with long-term hypercalcemia. Encourage intake of acid-ash fluids (e.g. prune or cranberry juice) to counteract deposits of calcium salts in the urine.
Hypomagnesaemia		
Excessive loss from the GI tract (e.g. from nasogastric suction, diarrhoea, fistula drainage) Long-term use of certain drugs (e.g. diuretics, aminoglycoside antibiotics) Conditions such as • Chronic alcoholism • Pancreatitis • Burns	Neuromuscular irritability with tremors Increased reflexes, tremors, convulsions Tachycardia, elevated blood pressure, dysrhythmias Disorientation and confusion Vertigo *Laboratory findings:* Serum magnesium below 1.5mmol/l	Assess patients receiving digitalis for digitalis toxicity. Hypomagnesemia increases the risk toxicity. Take protective measures when there is a possibility of seizures. Assess the patient's ability to swallow water prior to initiating oral feeding. Initiate safety measures to prevent injury during seizure activity. Carefully administer magnesium salts as ordered. Encourage patients to eat magnesium-rich foods if permitted (e.g. whole grains, meat, seafood and green leafy vegetables). Refer patients to alcohol treatment programmes as indicated
Hypermagnesaemia		
Abnormal retention of magnesium, as in • Renal failure • Adrenal insufficiency Treatment with magnesium salts	Peripheral vasodilation, flushing Nausea, vomiting Muscle weakness, paralysis Hypotension, bradycardia Depressed deep-tendon reflexes Lethargy, drowsiness Respiratory depression, coma Respiratory and cardiac arrest if hypomagnesaemia is severe *Laboratory findings:* Serum magnesium above 2.5mmol/l Electrocardiogram showing prolonged QT interval; an atrioventricular (AV) block may occur	Monitor vital signs and level of consciousness when patients are at risk. If patellar reflexes are absent, notify the physician. Advise patients who have renal disease to contact their care provider before taking over-the-counter drugs.

Hypomagnesaemia or deficiency in magnesium occurs more frequently than hypermagnesaemia. Chronic alcoholism is the most common cause of hypomagnesaemia. Magnesium deficiency also may aggravate the manifestations of alcohol withdrawal, such as delirium tremens (DTs).

Hypermagnesaemia is present when the serum magnesium level rises. It is due to increased intake or decreased excretion. It is often iatrogenic, that is, a result of overzealous magnesium therapy.

Table 20-6 lists risk factors and manifestations for patients with altered magnesium balance.

Chloride

Because of the relationship between sodium ions and chloride ions (Cl^-), imbalances of chloride commonly occur in conjunction with sodium imbalances.

Hypochloraemia is a decreased serum chloride level and is usually related to excess losses of chloride through the GI tract, kidneys or sweating. Hypochloremic patients are at risk for alkalosis and may experience muscle twitching, tremors or tetany.

Conditions that cause sodium retention also can lead to a high serum chloride level or **hyperchloraemia**. Excess replacement of sodium chloride or potassium chloride is additional risk factors for high serum chloride levels. The manifestations of hyperchloraemia include acidosis, weakness and lethargy, with a risk of dysrhythmias and coma.

Phosphate

The phosphate anion (PO_4^-) is found both in intracellular and extracellular fluid. Phosphate is critical for cellular metabolism because it is a major component of ATP.

Phosphate imbalances are frequently related to therapeutic interventions for other disorders. Glucose and insulin administration and total parenteral nutrition can cause phosphate to shift into the cells from extracellular fluid compartments, leading to **hypophosphataemia**, a low serum phosphate. Alcohol withdrawal, acid–base imbalances and the use of antacids that bind with phosphate in the GI tract are other possible causes of low serum phosphate levels. Manifestations of hypophosphataemia include paresthesias, muscle weakness and pain, mental changes and possible seizures.

Hyperphosphataemia occurs when phosphate shifts out of the cells into extracellular fluids (e.g. due to tissue trauma or chemotherapy for malignant tumours), in renal failure or when excess phosphate is administered or ingested. Infants who are fed cow's milk are at risk for hyperphosphataemia, as are people using phosphate-containing enemas or laxatives. Patients who have high serum phosphate levels may experience numbness and tingling around the mouth and in the fingertips, muscle spasms and tetany.

Acid–Base Imbalances

Acid–base imbalances generally are classified as *respiratory* or *metabolic* by the general or underlying cause of the disorder. Carbonic acid levels are normally regulated by the lungs through the retention or excretion of carbon dioxide, and problems of regulation lead to respiratory acidosis or alkalosis. Bicarbonate and hydrogen ion levels are regulated by the kidneys, and problems of regulation lead to metabolic acidosis or alkalosis. Healthy regulatory systems will attempt to correct acid–base imbalances, a process called compensation.

Respiratory Acidosis

Hypoventilation and carbon dioxide retention cause carbonic acid levels to increase and the pH to fall below 7.35, a condition known as **respiratory acidosis**. Serious lung diseases such as asthma and chronic obstructive pulmonary disease (COPD) are common causes of respiratory acidosis. Central nervous system depression due to anaesthesia or a narcotic overdose can sufficiently slow the respiratory rate so that carbon dioxide is retained. When respiratory acidosis occurs, the kidneys retain bicarbonate to restore the normal carbonic acid to bicarbonate ratio. Recall, however, that the kidneys are relatively slow to respond to changes in acid–base balance, so this compensatory response may require hours to days to restore the normal pH.

Respiratory Alkalosis

When a person hyperventilates, more carbon dioxide than normal is exhaled, carbonic acid levels fall, and the pH rises to greater than 7.45. This condition is termed **respiratory alkalosis**. Psychogenic or anxiety-related hyperventilation is a common cause of respiratory alkalosis. Other causes include fever and respiratory infections. In respiratory alkalosis, the kidneys will excrete bicarbonate to return the pH to within the normal range. Often, however, the cause of the hyperventilation is eliminated and the pH returns to normal before renal compensation occurs.

Metabolic Acidosis

When bicarbonate levels are low in relation to the amount of carbonic acid in the body, the pH falls and **metabolic acidosis** develops. This may develop because of renal failure and the inability of the kidneys to excrete hydrogen ion and produce bicarbonate. It also may occur when too much acid is produced in the body, for example, in diabetic ketoacidosis or starvation when fat tissue is broken down for energy. Metabolic acidosis stimulates the respiratory centre, and the rate and depth of respirations increase. Carbon dioxide is eliminated and carbonic acid levels fall, minimising the change in pH. This respiratory compensation occurs within minutes of the pH imbalance.

Metabolic Alkalosis

In **metabolic alkalosis**, the amount of bicarbonate in the body exceeds normal values. Ingestion of bicarbonate of soda as an antacid is one cause of metabolic alkalosis. Another cause is prolonged vomiting with loss of hydrochloric acid from the stomach. The respiratory centre is depressed in metabolic alkalosis, and respirations slow and become shallower. Carbon dioxide is retained and carbonic acid levels increase, helping balance the excess bicarbonate.

The risk factors and manifestations for acid–base imbalances are listed in Table 20-7.

Table 20-7 Acid-Base Imbalances

Risk factors	Clinical manifestations	Nursing interventions
Respiratory acidosis		
Acute lung conditions that impair alveolar gas exchange (e.g. pneumonia, acute pulmonary oedema, aspiration of foreign body, near-drowning) Chronic lung disease (e.g. asthma, cystic fibrosis or emphysema) Overdose of narcotics or sedatives that depress respiratory rate and depth Brain injury that affects the respiratory centre	Increased pulse and respiratory rates Headache, dizziness Confusion, decreased level of consciousness (LOC) Convulsions Warm, flushed skin **Chronic:** Weakness Headache *Laboratory findings:* Arterial blood pH less than 7.35 $PaCO_2$ above 45mm Hg HCO_3^- normal or slightly elevated in acute; above 26mmol/l in chronic	Frequently assess respiratory status and lung sounds. Monitor airway and ventilation; insert artificial airway and prepare for mechanical ventilation as necessary. Administer pulmonary therapy measures such as inhalation therapy, percussion and postural drainage, bronchodilators and antibiotics as ordered. Monitor fluid intake and output, vital signs and arterial blood gases. Administer narcotic antagonists as indicated. Maintain adequate hydration (2-3l of fluid per day).
Respiratory alkalosis		
Hyperventilation due to • Extreme anxiety • Elevated body temperature • Overventilation with a mechanical ventilator • Hypoxia • Salicylate overdose	Complaints of shortness of breath, chest tightness Light-headedness with circumoral paresthesias and numbness and tingling of the extremities Difficulty concentrating Tremulousness, blurred vision *Laboratory findings (in uncompensated respiratory alkalosis):* Arterial blood pH above 7.45 $PaCO_2$ less than 35mm Hg	Monitor vital signs and ABGs. Assist patient to breathe more slowly. Help patient breathe in a paper bag or apply a rebreather mask (to inhale CO_2).
Metabolic acidosis		
Conditions that increase nonvolatile acids in the blood (e.g. renal impairment, diabetes mellitus, starvation) Conditions that decrease bicarbonate (e.g. prolonged diarrhoea) Excessive infusion of chloride-containing IV fluids (e.g. NaCl)	Kussmaul's respirations (deep, rapid respirations) Lethargy, confusion Headache Weakness Nausea and vomiting *Laboratory findings:* Arterial blood pH below 7.35 Serum bicarbonate less than 22mmol/l $PaCO_2$ less than 38mm Hg with respiratory compensation	Monitor ABG values, intake and output, and LOC. Administer IV sodium bicarbonate carefully if ordered. Treat underlying problem as ordered.
Metabolic alkalosis		
Excessive acid losses due to • Vomiting • Gastric suction Excessive use of potassium-losing diuretics Excessive adrenal corticoid hormones due to • Cushing's syndrome • Hyperaldosteronism Excessive bicarbonate intake from • Antacids • Parenteral $NaHCO_3$	Decreased respiratory rate and depth Dizziness Circumoral paresthesias, numbness and tingling of the extremities Hypertonic muscles, tetany *Laboratory findings:* Arterial blood pH above 7.45 Serum bicarbonate greater than 26mmol/l $PaCO_2$ higher than 45mm Hg with respiratory compensation	Monitor intake and output closely. Monitor vital signs, especially respirations, and LOC. Administer ordered IV fluids carefully. Treat underlying problem.

ASSESSING HYDRATION STATUS

Assessing a patient's fluid, electrolyte and acid–base balance and imbalances is an important nursing function. Components of the assessment include (a) the patient history, (b) physical assessment of the patient, (c) clinical measurements and (d) review of laboratory test results.

Patient History

The patient history is particularly important for identifying patients who are at risk of fluid, electrolyte and acid–base imbalances. The current and past medical history may reveal conditions such as chronic lung disease or diabetes mellitus that can disrupt normal balances. Medications prescribed to treat acute or chronic conditions (e.g. diuretic therapy for hypertension) also may place the risk of fluid, electrolyte and acid base disturbances (see *Practice Guidelines*).

When obtaining the patient history, the nurse needs not only to recognise risk factors but also to elicit data about the patient's food and fluid intake, fluid output, and the presence of signs or symptoms suggestive of altered fluid and electrolyte balance, such as headaches, lethargy and nausea and vomiting.

Physical Assessment

Physical assessment of the patient will usually focus on the skin, oral cavity, heart, lungs, muscles and neurological status. The findings from the physical assessment are used to expand and verify information gained when taking the patient history of the patient. Table 20-8 expands on the physical assessment of the patient. You may also want to refer to Tables 20-6 and 20-7 for possible abnormal findings related to specific imbalances.

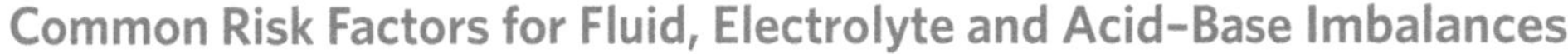

Common Risk Factors for Fluid, Electrolyte and Acid–Base Imbalances

Chronic Diseases and Conditions

- Chronic lung disease (COPD, asthma, cystic fibrosis)
- Heart failure
- Kidney disease
- Diabetes mellitus
- Cushing's syndrome or Addison's disease
- Cancer
- Malnutrition, anorexia nervosa, bulimia
- Ileostomy (an operation that involves bringing the end of the ileum to the surface of the skin and a stoma formed)

Acute Conditions

- Acute gastroenteritis
- Bowel obstruction
- Head injury or decreased level of consciousness
- Trauma such as burns or crush injuries
- Surgery
- Fever, draining wounds, fistulas (an abnormal opening between two organs)

Medications

- Diuretics
- Corticosteroids
- Nonsteroidal anti-inflammatory drugs

Treatments

- Chemotherapy
- IV therapy and total parenteral nutrition
- Nasogastric suction
- Enteral feeding
- Mechanical ventilation

Other Factors

- Age: very old or very young
- Inability to access food and fluids independently

Clinical Measurements

Three simple clinical measurements that can be initiated by the nurse to detect signs of fluid and nutritional problems.

Daily Weights

Daily weight measurements provide a relatively accurate assessment of a patient's fluid status. Significant changes in weight over a short time (e.g. days to a week or two) are indicative of acute fluid changes. Each kilogram (2.2lb) of weight gained or lost is equivalent to 1l of fluid gained or lost. Such fluid gains or losses indicate changes in total body fluid volume rather than in any specific compartment, such as the intravascular compartment. Rapid losses or gains of 5–8% of total body weight indicate moderate to severe fluid volume deficits or excesses.

To obtain accurate weight measurements, the nurse should weigh the patient (a) at the same time each day (e.g. before breakfast), (b) wearing the same or similar clothing, and (c) on the same scale. The type of scale (i.e. standing, bed, chair) should be documented.

Vital Signs

Changes in the vital signs may indicate, or in some cases precede, fluid, electrolyte and acid–base imbalances. For example, elevated body temperature may be a result of dehydration or a cause of increased body fluid losses.

Table 20-8 Focused Physical Assessment for Fluid, Electrolyte or Acid-Base Imbalances

System	Assessment focus	Technique	Possible abnormal findings
Skin	Colour, temperature, moisture	Inspection, palpation	Flushed, warm, very dry Moist or diaphoretic Cool and pale
	Turgor	Gently pinch up a fold of skin over sternum or inner aspect of thigh for adults, on the abdomen or medial thigh for children	Poor turgor: Skin remains tented for several seconds instead of immediately returning to normal position (sign of dehydration)
	Oedema	Inspect for visible swelling around eyes, in fingers and in lower extremities	Skin around eyes is puffy, lids appear swollen; rings are tight; shoes leave impressions on feet (oedema)
		Compress the skin over the dorsum of the foot, around the ankles, over the tibia, in the sacral area	Depression remains (pitting): see scale for describing oedema in Figure 20-6
Mucous membranes	Colour, moisture	Inspection	Mucous membranes dry, dull in appearance; tongue dry and cracked (dehydration)
Eyes	Firmness	Gently palpate eyeball with lid closed	Eyeball feels soft to palpation
Fontanels (soft spot on the top of an infant's head)	Firmness, level	Inspect and gently palpate anterior fontanel	Fontanel bulging, firm Fontanel sunken, soft
Cardiovascular system	Heart rate	Auscultation, cardiac monitor	Tachycardia, bradycardia; irregular; dysrhythmias
	Peripheral pulses	Palpation	Weak and thready; bounding
	Blood pressure	Auscultation of Korotkoff's sounds	Hypotension
	Capillary refill	BP assessment lying and standing	Postural hypotension
	Venous filling	Palpation	Slowed capillary refill
		Inspection of jugular veins and hand veins	Jugular venous distention; flat jugular veins, poor venous refill
Respiratory system	Respiratory rate and pattern	Inspection	Increased or decreased rate and depth of respirations
	Lung sounds	Auscultation	Crackles or moist rales
Neurological	Level of consciousness (LOC)	Observation, stimulation	Decreased LOC, lethargy, stupor or coma
	Orientation, cognition	Questioning	Disoriented, confused; difficulty concentrating
	Motor function	Strength testing	Weakness, decreased motor strength
	Reflexes	Deep-tendon reflex (DTR) testing	Hyperactive or depressed DTRs
	Abnormal reflexes	*Chvostek's sign*: Tap over facial nerve about 2cm anterior to tragus of ear	Facial muscle twitching including eyelids and lips on side of stimulus
		Trousseau's sign: Inflate a blood pressure cuff on the upper arm to 20mmHg greater than the systolic pressure, leave in place for 2–5 minutes	Carpal spasm: contraction of hand and fingers on affected side

Respiratory rate is the clearest indicator that the patient is having some difficulty with fluid, electrolyte and/or acid–base balances. The 'Patient at risk' scoring system, a means of assessing the patient's stability, is currently widely used within the UK as a means of identifying those patients at risk of deterioration. One of the vital signs that this scoring system focuses on is respiratory rate as this is one of the first indicators of potential health problems.

Tachycardia is an early sign of hypovolaemia. Pulse volume will decrease in hypovolaemia and increase in hypervolaemia.

Irregular pulse rates may occur with electrolyte imbalances. Changes in respiratory rate and depth may cause respiratory acid–base imbalances or act as a compensatory mechanism in metabolic acidosis or alkalosis.

Blood pressure, a sensitive measure to detect blood volume changes, may fall significantly with hypovolaemia or increase with hypervolaemia. Postural, or **orthostatic, hypotension** may also occur with hypovolaemia.

To assess for orthostatic hypotension, measure the patient's blood pressure and pulse in a supine position. Allow the patient to remain in that position for 3–5 minutes, leaving the blood pressure cuff on the arm. Stand the patient up and immediately reassess the blood pressure and pulse. A drop of 10–15mmHg in the systolic blood pressure with a corresponding drop in diastolic pressure and an increased pulse rate (by 10 or more beats per minute) is indicative of orthostatic or postural hypotension.

Fluid Intake and Output

The measurement and recording of all fluid intake and output (I and O) during a 24-hour period provides important data about the patient's fluid and electrolyte balance.

The unit used to measure intake and output is the millilitre (ml). Most hospitals have a form for recording fluid balance, usually a bedside record on which the nurse lists all items measured and the quantities per shift (see Figure 20-8). Some agencies have another form for recording the specifics of intravenous

Fluid balance chart

Hospital/Ward: Date:

Hospital number:

Surname:

Forenames:

Date of birth:

Sex:

	Fluid intake			Fluid output				
Time (hrs)	**Oral**	**IV**	**Other (specify route)**	**Urine**	**Vomit**	**Other (specify)**		
01.00								
02.00								
03.00								
04.00								
05.00								
06.00								
07.00								
08.00								
09.00								
10.00								
11.00								
12.00								
13.00								
14.00								
15.00								
16.00								
17.00								
18.00								
19.00								
20.00								
21.00								
22.00								
23.00								
24.00								
TOTAL								

Figure 20-8 Fluid balance chart.

Source: Nicol *et al.* (2000) *Essential Nursing Skills*, Mosby.

fluids, such as the type of solution, additives, time started, amounts absorbed and amounts remaining per shift.

It is important to inform patients, family members and all caregivers that accurate measurements of the patient's fluid intake and output are required, explaining why and emphasising the need to use a bedpan, urinal or commode. Instruct the patient not to put toilet tissue into the container with urine. Patients who wish to be involved in recording fluid intake measurements need to be taught how to compute the values and what foods are considered fluids.

To measure fluid intake, the nurse records on the fluid balance form each fluid item taken (if the patient has not already done so), specifying the time and type of fluid. All of the following fluids need to be recorded:

- Oral fluids.
- Water.
- Milk.
- Juice.
- Soft drinks.
- Coffee or tea.
- Cream.
- Soup.
- Any other beverages including water taken with medications.
- Foods that are or tend to become liquid at room temperature, including ice cream, sherbet, custard and gelatine.
- Do not measure foods that are pureed, because purees are simply solid foods prepared in a different form.
- Tube feedings. Remember to include the water flushes at the end of intermittent feedings or during continuous feedings.
- Parenteral fluids (intravenous fluids). The exact amount of intravenous fluid administered is to be recorded, since some fluid containers may be overfilled. Blood transfusions are included.
- Intravenous medications. Intravenous medications that are prepared with solutions such as normal saline (NS) and are administered as an intermittent or continuous infusion must also be included.
- Catheter or tube irrigants. Fluid used to irrigate urinary catheters, nasogastric tubes and intestinal tubes must be measured and recorded if not immediately withdrawn.

To measure fluid output, measure the following fluids (remember to observe appropriate infection control precautions):

- Urinary output. Following each **voiding**, pour the urine into a measuring container, observe the amount, and record it and the time of voiding on the fluid balance form.
- For patients with retention catheters, empty the drainage bag into a measuring container at the end of the shift (or at prescribed times if output is to be measured more often). Note and record the amount of urine output.
- In intensive care areas, urine output often is measured hourly.
- If the patient is incontinent of urine, estimate and record these outputs. For example, for an incontinent patient the nurse might record 'Incontinent × 3' or 'Drawsheet soaked in 12 inch diameter'. A more accurate estimate of the urine output of infants and incontinent patients may be obtained by first weighing nappies or incontinent pads that are dry, and then subtracting this weight from the weight of the soiled items. Each gram of weight left after subtracting is equal to 1ml of urine. If urine is frequently soiled with faeces, the number of voidings may be recorded rather than the volume of urine.
- Vomitus and liquid faeces. The amount and type of fluid and the time need to be specified.
- Tube drainage, such as gastric or intestinal drainage.
- Wound drainage and draining fistulas. Wound drainage may be recorded by documenting the type and number of dressings or linen saturated with drainage or by measuring the exact amount of drainage collected in a vacuum drainage or gravity drainage system.

Fluid intake and output measurements are totalled at the end of the shift (every 8–12 hours), and the totals are recorded in the patient's permanent record. In intensive care areas, the nurse may record intake and output hourly. Usually the staff member on night shift totals the amounts of input and output recorded for each shift and records the 24-hour total.

To determine whether the fluid output is proportional to fluid intake or whether there are any changes in the patient's fluid status, the nurse (a) compares the total 24-hour fluid output measurement with the total fluid intake measurement and (b) compares both to previous measurements. Urinary output is normally equivalent to the amount of fluids ingested; the usual range is 1.5–2l in 24 hours, or 40–80ml in 1 hour (0.5ml/kg/hour). Patients whose output substantially exceeds intake are at risk for fluid volume deficit. By contrast, patients whose intake substantially exceeds output are at risk for fluid volume excess. In assessing the patient's fluid balance it is important to consider additional factors that may affect intake and output. The patient who is extremely diaphoretic (excess perspiration) or who has rapid, deep respirations has fluid losses that cannot be measured but must be considered in evaluating fluid status.

When there is a significant discrepancy between intake and output or when fluid intake or output is inadequate (e.g. a urine output of less than 500ml in 24 hours or less than 0.5ml per kilogram per hour in an adult), this information should be reported to the charge nurse or doctor immediately.

Laboratory Tests

Laboratory tests provide objective information about the patient's fluid, electrolyte and acid–base balance.

Full Blood Count (FBC)

The full blood count, a basic screening test, includes information about the haematocrit (Hct). The **haematocrit** measures the volume (percentage) of whole blood that is composed of RBC in relation to plasma. Therefore, haematocrit is affected by changes in plasma volume. Normal haematocrit values are 40–54% in men and 37–47% in women. With severe dehydration haematocrit increases and conversely severe overhydration decreases haematocrit.

Osmolality

Serum osmolality is a measure of the solute concentration of the blood and is used primarily to evaluate fluid balance. Normal values are 280–300mOsm/kg. An increase in serum osmolality indicates a fluid volume deficit; a decrease reflects a fluid volume excess.

Serum Electrolytes

Serum electrolyte levels are often routinely ordered for any patient admitted to hospital as a screening test for electrolyte and acid–base imbalances. Serum electrolytes also are routinely assessed for patients at risk in the community, for example, patients who are being treated with a diuretic for hypertension or heart failure. The most commonly ordered serum tests are for sodium, potassium, chloride, magnesium and bicarbonate ions. Normal values of commonly measured electrolytes are shown in the *Practice Guidelines*.

Urine pH

Measurement of urine pH may be obtained by laboratory analysis or by using a dipstick on a fresh urine specimen. Because the kidneys play a critical role in regulating acid–base balance, assessment of urine pH can be useful in determining whether the kidneys are responding appropriately to acid–base imbalances. Normally the pH of the urine is relatively acidic, averaging about 6.0, but a range of 4.6–8.0 is considered normal. In metabolic acidosis, urine pH should decrease as the kidneys excrete hydrogen ions; in metabolic alkalosis, the pH should increase.

PRACTICE GUIDELINES

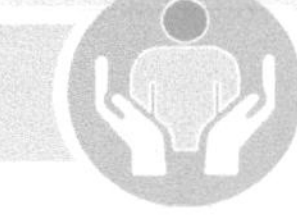

Normal Electrolyte Values for Adults

Venous Blood

Sodium	135-145mmol/l
Potassium	3.5-5.0mmol/l
Chloride	85-105mmol/l
Calcium (total)	4.5-5.5mmol/l or 8.5-10.5mg/dl
Magnesium	1.5-2.5mmol/l or 1.6-2.5mg/dl
Phosphate	1.8-2.6mmol/l (phosphorus)
Serum osmolality	280-300mOsm/kg water

Note: normal laboratory values may vary from Trust to Trust.

Urine Specific Gravity

Specific gravity is an indicator of urine concentration that can be performed quickly and easily by nursing staff. Normal specific gravity ranges from 1.005 to 1.030 (usually 1.010 to 1.025). When the concentration of solutes in the urine is high, the specific gravity rises; in very dilute urine with few solutes, it is abnormally low.

Arterial Blood Gases

Arterial blood gases are performed to evaluate the patient's acid–base balance and oxygenation. Arterial blood is used because it provides a truer reflection of gas exchange in the pulmonary system than venous blood. Blood gases may be drawn by nurses with specialised skills and can be taken by inserting a needle into the artery or by taking blood from a line that has already been inserted into the artery which is commonly found in critical care areas.

Six measurements are commonly used to interpret arterial blood gas tests:

1 pH, a measure of the relative acidity or alkalinity of the blood.
2 PaO_2, the pressure exerted by oxygen dissolved in the plasma of arterial blood; an indirect measure of blood oxygen content.
3 $PaCO_2$, the partial pressure of carbon dioxide in arterial plasma; the respiratory component of acid–base determination.
4 Bicarbonate (HCO_3^-) a measure of the metabolic component of acid–base balance.
5 Base excess (BE), a calculated value of bicarbonate levels, also reflective of the metabolic component of acid–base balance.
6 Oxygen saturation (SaO_2), the percentage of haemoglobin saturated (combined) with oxygen.

Normal ABG values are listed in the *Practice Guidelines* and changes seen in common acid–base imbalances are summarised in Table 20-9. However, please note that although the PaO_2 and SaO_2 are important for assessing respiratory status, they generally do not provide useful information for assessing acid–base balance and so are not included in this table.

When evaluating ABG results to determine acid–base balance, it is important to use a systematic approach such as the one outlined in the *Practice Guidelines*. Nurses need to assess each measurement individually, then look at the interrelationships to determine what type of acid–base imbalance may be present.

Table 20-9 Arterial Blood Gas Values in Common Acid-Base Disorders

Disorder		**ABG values**
Respiratory acidosis	pH	< 7.35
	$PaCO_2$	> 45mmHg (excess CO_2 and carbonic acid)
	HCO_3^-	Normal; > 26mmol/l with renal compensation
Respiratory alkalosis	pH	> 7.45
	$PaCO_2$	< 35mmHg (inadequate CO_2 and carbonic acid)
	HCO_3^-	Normal; < 22mmol/l with renal compensation
Metabolic acidosis	pH	< 7.35
	$PaCO_2$	Normal; < 35mmHg with respiratory compensation
	HCO_3^-	< 22mmol/l
	BE	< −2mmol/l
Metabolic alkalosis	pH	< 7.45
	$PaCO_2$	Normal; > 45mmHg with respiratory compensation
	HCO_3^-	> 26mmol/l (excess bicarbonate)
	BE	> +2mmol/l

PRACTICE GUIDELINES

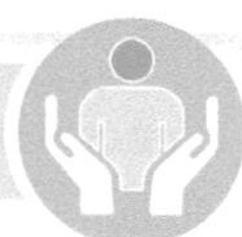

Normal Values of Arterial Blood Gases

pH	7.35–7.45	HCO_3^-	22–26mmol/l
PaO_2	80–100mmHg	Base excess	−2 to +2mmol/l
$PaCO_2$	35–45mmHg	O_2 saturation	95–98%

Note: some normal values will vary according to the kind of test carried out in the laboratory.

PRACTICE GUIDELINES

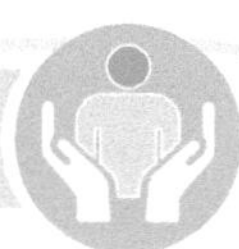

Interpreting ABGs

1 Assess the pH:
- If the pH is less than 7.35, the problem is acidosis
- If the pH is more than 7.45, the problem is alkalosis

2 Look at the $PaCO_2$:
- If the $PaCO_2$ is less than 35mmHg, more carbon dioxide is being exhaled than normal
- If the $PaCO_2$ is greater than 45mmHg, less carbon dioxide is being exhaled than normal

3 Assess the pH and $PaCO_2$ relationship for a possible respiratory problem:
- If the pH is less than 7.35 (acidosis) and the $PaCO_2$ is greater than 45mmHg, retained carbon dioxide is causing respiratory acidosis
- If the pH is greater than 7.45 (alkalosis), and the $PaCO_2$ is less than 35mmHg, lack of carbon dioxide is causing **respiratory alkalosis**

4 Look at the bicarbonate:
- If the HCO_3 is less than 22mmol/l, bicarbonate levels are lower than normal
- If the HCO_3^- is greater than 26mmol/l, bicarbonate levels are higher than normal

5 Assess pH, HCO_3^- and BE values for a possible metabolic problem
- If the pH is less than 7.35 and the bicarbonate is less than 22mmol/l, and the BE is less than −2mmol/l this is **metabolic acidosis**
- If the pH is more than 7.45 (alkalosis) and the bicarbonate is greater than 26mmol/l, and the BE is greater +2mmol/l this is **metabolic alkalosis**

ACTIVITY 20-3

What would you include in an assessment of a patient's fluid, electrolyte and acid-base balances?

COMMUNITY CARE CONSIDERATIONS

Fluid, Electrolyte and Acid-Base Balance

When assessing a patient's fluid, electrolyte and acid-base balance in the community setting the following should be considered:

- The risk factors for imbalances.
- The patient's ability to maintain food and fluid intake such as their mobility, swallow, access to fluids, ability to purchase food and prepare a balanced diet.
- The patient's current knowledge and understanding of their condition and any medications that they may be taking.
- The family or carer's willingness to provide assistance in preventing fluid, electrolyte and imbalances.

PLANNING

Major goals for patients with or at risk for nutritional and hydration problems include:

- Maintain or restore normal fluid balance.
- Maintain or restore normal balance of electrolytes in the intracellular and extracellular compartments.
- Maintain or restore pulmonary ventilation and oxygenation.
- Prevent associated risks (tissue breakdown, decreased cardiac output, confusion, other neurologic signs).

Obviously, goals will vary according to the diagnosis and defining characteristics for each individual. Appropriate preventive and corrective nursing interventions that relate to these must be identified.

IMPLEMENTING

Promoting Wellness

Most people rarely think about their fluid, electrolyte or acid–base balance. They know it is important to drink adequate fluids and consume a balanced diet, but they may not understand the potential effects when this is not done. Nurses can promote patients' health by providing education that will help them maintain fluid and electrolyte balance.

Enteral Fluid and Electrolyte Replacement

Fluids and electrolytes can be provided orally in the hospital and the home if the patient's health permits, that is, if the patient is not vomiting, has not experienced an excessive fluid loss, and has an intact GI tract and gag and swallow reflexes. Patients who are unable to ingest solid foods may be able to ingest fluids.

Modifications to Fluid

Increased fluids are often prescribed for patients with actual or potential fluid volume deficits arising, for example, from mild diarrhoea or mild to moderate fevers. Guidelines for helping patients increase fluid intake are shown in the *Practice Guidelines*.

Restricted fluids may be necessary for patients who have fluid retention (fluid volume excess) as a result of renal failure, congestive heart failure, SIADH or other disease processes. Fluid restrictions vary from 'nothing by mouth' to a precise amount ordered by a doctor. The restriction of fluids can be difficult for some patients, particularly if they are experiencing thirst. Guidelines for helping patients restrict fluid intake are shown in the *Practice Guidelines*.

Dietary Changes

Specific fluid and electrolyte imbalances may require simple dietary changes. For example, patients receiving potassium-depleting diuretics need to be informed about foods with a high potassium content (e.g. bananas, oranges and leafy greens). Some patients with fluid retention need to avoid foods high in sodium. Most healthy patients can benefit from foods rich in calcium.

Oral Electrolyte Supplements

Some patients can benefit from oral supplements of electrolytes, particularly when a medication is prescribed that affects electrolyte balance, when dietary intake is inadequate for a specific electrolyte, or when fluid and electrolyte losses are excessive as a result of, for example, excessive perspiration.

PRACTICE GUIDELINES

Facilitating Fluid Intake

- Explain to the patient the reason for the required intake and the specific amount needed. This provides a rationale for the requirement and promotes concordance.
- Set short-term goals that the patient can realistically meet. Examples include drinking a glass of fluid every hour while awake or a pitcher of water by 12 noon.
- Identify fluids the patient likes and make available a variety of those items, including fruit juices, soft drinks and milk (if allowed). Remember that beverages such as coffee and tea have a diuretic effect, so their consumption should be limited.
- Help patients to select foods that tend to become liquid at room temperature (e.g. ice cream, sherbet, custard), if these are allowed.
- For patients who are confined to bed, supply appropriate cups and glasses to facilitate appropriate fluid intake and keep the fluids within easy reach.
- Make sure fluids are served at the appropriate temperature: hot fluids hot and cold fluids very cold.
- Encourage patients when possible to participate in maintaining the fluid intake record. This assists them to evaluate the achievement of desired outcomes.
- Be alert to any cultural implications of food and fluids. Some cultures may restrict certain foods and fluids and view others as having healing properties.

RESEARCH NOTE

The efficacy of pre-thickened fluid on total fluid and nutrition consumption among extended care residents requiring thickened fluids due to risk of aspiration

The aim of this quantitative study was to assess whether the use of pre-thickened, standardised consistency fluids resulted in an increase in fluid and nutrient intake in patients with dysphagia. The study looked at eleven adult patients who were in a residential facility in Dublin. The patients ranged in age from 51 to 109 years. The researchers used a cross-over study design with patients assigned to two groups over a six-week period. The first group received pre-thickened, standardised consistency fluids while the second group received fluids thickened at the bedside with modified maize starch. Midway through the study the groups were then changed over with the first group receiving bedside thickened fluids and the second group receiving pre-thickened fluids. Over a six-week period data was collected about the patients daily fluid, protein, calorie, vitamin intake and constipation rates. The results showed that patients had significantly higher energy, protein, calcium and vitamin intake when given pre-thickened fluids. The fluids taken in the pre-thickened form were found to have a higher nutritional value, however no difference in constipation rates were noted. The researchers suggest that pre-thickened fluids may offer a beneficial alternative, however they recognise the small sample used in the study and suggest that this may need larger scale study may be worthwhile.

Source: based on McCormick, S.E., Stafford, K.M., Saqib, G., Chronin, D.N. and Power, D. (2008) 'The efficacy of pre-thickened fluid on total fluid and nutrition consumption among extended care residents requiring thickened fluids due to risk of aspiration', *Age and Ageing*, 37, 714-718.

PRACTICE GUIDELINES

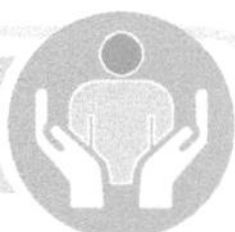

Helping Patients Restrict Fluid Intake

- Explain the reason for the restricted intake and how much and what types of fluids are permitted orally. Many patients need to be informed that ice cubes, gelatin and ice cream, for example, are considered fluid.
- Identify fluids or fluid-like substances the patient likes and make sure that these are provided, unless contraindicated.
- Set short-term goals that make the fluid restriction more tolerable. For example, schedule a specified amount of fluid at one- or two-hourly intervals between meals. Some patients may prefer fluids only between meals if the food provided at mealtime helps relieve thirst.
- Place allowed fluids in small containers.
- Periodically offer the patient ice cubes as an alternative to water, because ice cubes when melted are approximately half of the frozen volume.
- Provide frequent mouth care and rinses to reduce the thirst sensation.
- Instruct the patient to avoid eating salty or sweet foods because these foods tend to produce thirst. Sugarless gum may be an alternative for some patients.
- Encourage the patient when possible to participate in maintaining the fluid intake record.

Parenteral Fluid and Electrolyte Replacement

Intravenous (IV) fluid therapy is essential when patients are unable to take food and fluids orally. It is an efficient and effective method of supplying fluids directly into the intravascular fluid compartment and replacing electrolyte losses. Intravenous fluid therapy is prescribed by a doctor. The nurse is responsible for administering and maintaining the therapy, and also monitoring the patient receiving the therapy.

Intravenous Solutions

Intravenous solutions can be classified as isotonic, hypotonic or hypertonic. Most IV solutions are *isotonic*, having the same concentration of solutes as blood plasma. Isotonic solutions are often used to restore blood volume. *Hypertonic* solutions have a greater concentration of solutes than plasma; *hypotonic* solutions have a lesser concentration of solutes. Table 20-10 provides examples of IV solutions and nursing implications.

Volume expanders or colloids are used to increase the blood volume following severe loss of blood (e.g. from haemorrhage) or loss of plasma (e.g. from severe burns, which draw large amounts of plasma from the bloodstream to the burn site). Examples of expanders are fresh frozen plasma, blood and albumin.

Venepuncture Sites

The site chosen for venepuncture varies with the patient's age, the length of time the infusion is to run, the type of solution used and the condition of veins. For adults, veins in the hand and arm are commonly used; for infants, veins in the scalp and dorsal foot veins are often used. Larger veins are preferred for infusions that need to be given rapidly and for solutions that could be irritating (e.g. certain medications).

The metacarpal, basilic and cephalic veins are commonly used for intermittent or continuous infusions (see Figure 20-9(b)). The ulna and radius act as natural splints at these sites, and the patient has greater freedom of arm movements for activities such as eating. Although the basilic and median cubital veins in the antecubital space are convenient sites for venepuncture, they are usually used for blood sampling, and insertion sites for a peripherally inserted central catheter line (see Figure 20-9(a)).

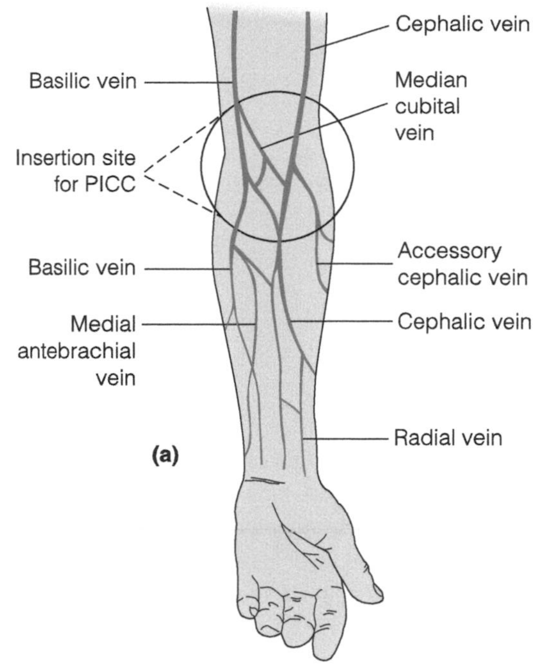

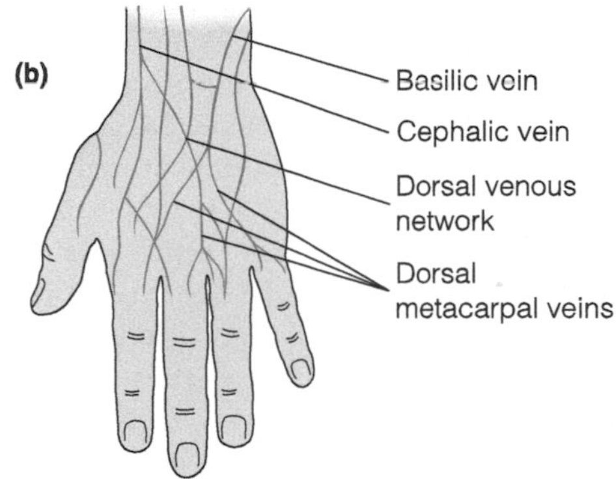

Figure 20-9 Commonly used venepuncture sites of the (a) arm; (b) hand. (a) also shows the site used for a peripherally inserted central catheter (PICC).

Table 20-10 Selected Intravenous Solutions

Type/examples	Comments/Nursing implications
Isotonic solutions 0.9% NaCl (normal saline) Lactated Ringer's (a balanced electrolyte solution) 5% dextrose in water (D5W)	Isotonic solutions such as normal saline and lactated Ringer's initially remain in the vascular compartment, expanding vascular volume. Assess patients carefully for signs of hypervolaemia such as bounding pulse and shortness of breath. D5W is isotonic on initial administration but provides free water when dextrose is metabolised, expanding intracellular and extracellular fluid volumes.
Hypotonic solutions 0.45% NaCl (half normal saline) 0.33% NaCl (one-third normal saline)	Hypotonic solutions are used to provide free water and treat cellular dehydration. These solutions promote waste elimination by the kidneys.
Hypertonic solutions 5% dextrose in normal saline (D5NS) 5% dextrose in 0.45% NaCl (D5 1/2NS) 5% dextrose in lactated Ringer's (D5LR)	Hypertonic solutions draw fluid out of the cells and interstitial compartments into the vascular compartment, expanding vascular volume. Do not administer to patients with kidney or heart disease or patients who are dehydrated. Watch for signs of hypervolaemia.

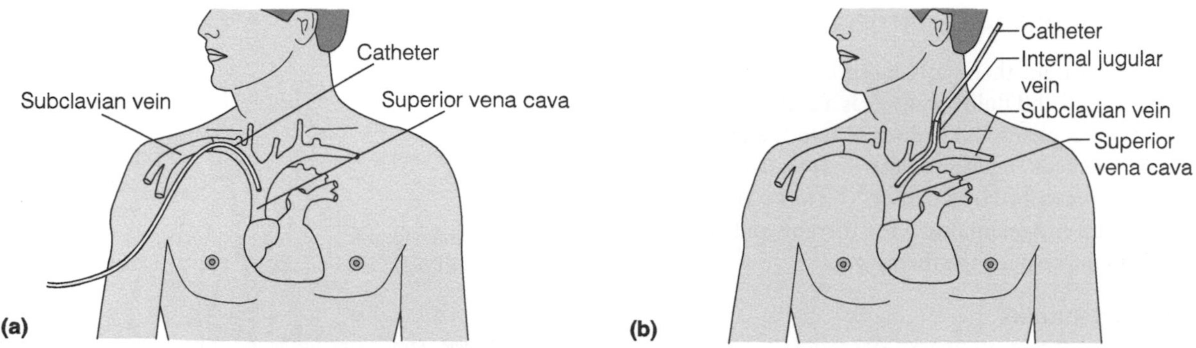

Figure 20-10 Central venous lines with (a) subclavian vein insertion and (b) left jugular insertion.

When long-term IV therapy or parenteral nutrition is anticipated or the patient is receiving IV medications that are damaging to vessels (e.g. chemotherapy), a central venous catheter may be inserted. **Central venous catheters** usually are inserted into the subclavian or jugular vein, with the distal tip of the catheter resting in the superior vena cava just above the right atrium (see Figure 20-10). They may be inserted at the patient's bedside or, for longer-term access, surgically inserted. Subclavian central venous catheters permit freedom of movement for ambulation; however, there is a risk of **pneumothorax** on catheter insertion. Assess the patient closely for manifestations such as shortness of breath, chest pain, cough, hypotension, tachycardia and anxiety after the insertion procedure.

With a peripherally inserted central venous catheter (PICC), the catheter is inserted in the basilic or cephalic vein just above or below the antecubital space of the right arm. The tip of the catheter rests in the superior vena cava. The risk of pneumothorax is eliminated with PICC. These catheters frequently are used for long-term intravenous access when the patient will be managing IV therapy at home.

Implantable venous access devices or ports (see Figure 20-11) are used for patients with chronic illness who require long-term IV therapy (e.g. intermittent medications such as chemotherapy, total parenteral nutrition and frequent blood samples). The device is designed to provide repeated access to the central venous system, avoiding the trauma and complications of multiple venepunctures. Using local anaesthesia, implantable ports are surgically placed into a small subcutaneous pocket, usually on the upper chest. The distal end of the catheter is placed in the subclavian or jugular vein. There are different kinds of implantable venous access devices and they may be tunnelled or nontunnelled.

Special precautions need to be taken with all central lines and venous access ports to ensure asepsis and catheter patency. Nursing care of patients with these devices is outlined in *Practice Guidelines*.

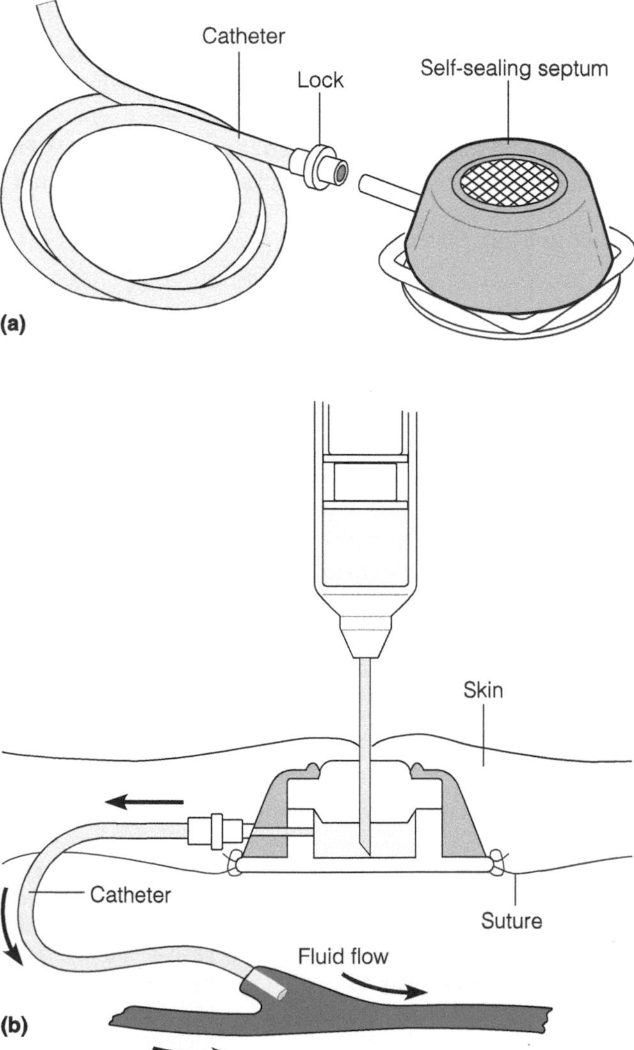

Figure 20-11 An implantable venous access device: (a) components; (b) the device in place.

Intravenous Equipment

Because equipment varies according to the manufacturer, the nurse must become familiar with the equipment used in each particular hospital or care environment and receive appropriate training on the equipment.

Most solutions are currently dispensed in plastic bags (see Figure 20-12). However, glass containers may need to be used if the administered medications are incompatible with plastic, such as albumin infusions. Glass containers require an air vent so that air can enter the bottle and replace the fluid that enters the patient's vein. Air vents usually have filters to prevent contamination from the air that enters the container. Air vents are not required for plastic solution containers, because plastic bags collapse under atmospheric pressure when the solution enters the vein.

Avoid selecting a container whose volume is greater than the volume ordered. For example, if 750ml 5% dextrose has been prescribed, the nurse should use one 500ml container and one 250ml container, which total 750ml. Do not obtain a 1,000ml container with the intention of stopping the solution after 750ml has been administered. Too often, the incorrect amount can be instilled unless an electronic device is used to regulate the volume. If a 1,000ml solution container must be used, remove 250ml before starting the infusion.

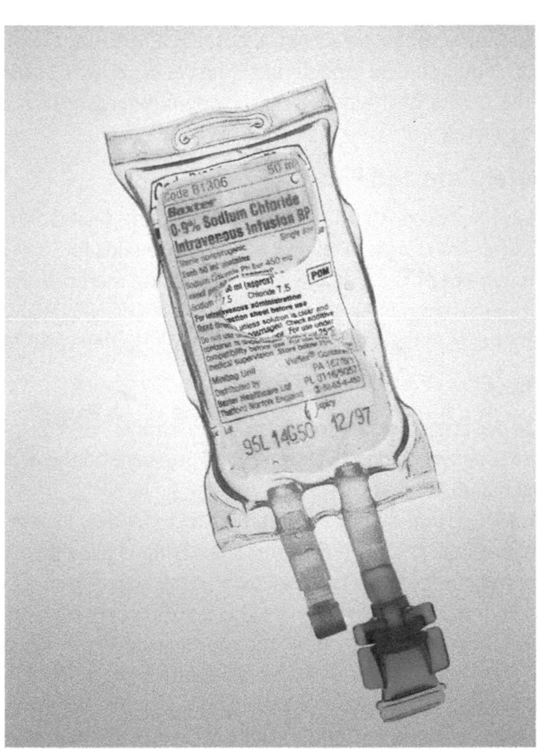

Figure 20-12 A plastic intravenous fluid container.

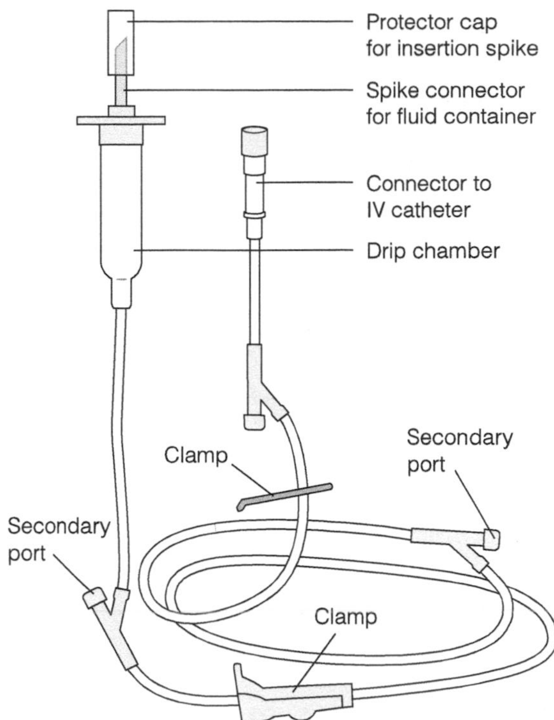

Figure 20-13 A standard IV administration set.

It is essential that the solution be sterile and clear. Cloudiness, evidence that the container has been opened previously or leaks indicate possible contamination. Always check the expiration date on the label. Return any questionable or contaminated solutions to pharmacy.

Infusion sets usually include an insertion spike, a drip chamber, a roller valve, tubing with secondary ports and a protective cap over the needle adapter (see Figure 20-13). The insertion spike is kept sterile and inserted into the solution container when the equipment is set up and ready to start. The drip chamber permits a predictable amount of fluid to be delivered. The roller valve or screw clamp, which compresses the lumen of the tubing, controls the rate of the flow. The protective cap over the needle adapter maintains the sterility of the end of the tubing so that it can be attached to a sterile venous cannula inserted in the patient's vein.

Most infusion sets include one or more injection ports for administering IV medications or secondary infusions. Needleless systems are increasingly used because they reduce the risk of needlestick injury and contamination of the intravenous line. With a needleless system, a blunt cannula is inserted into a special injection port or adapter on the IV tubing to administer medications or secondary infusions (see Figure 20-14). Many infusion sets include an in-line filter to trap air, particulate matter and microbes. A special infusion set may be required if the IV flow rate will be regulated by an infusion pump.

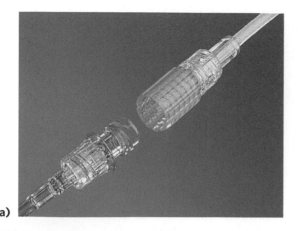

(a)

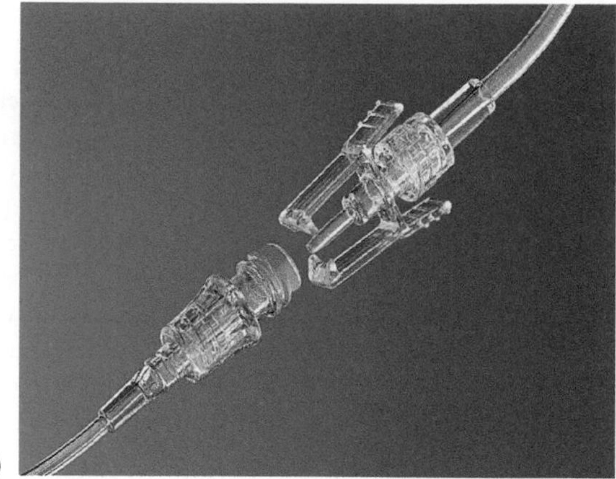

(b)

Figure 20-14 Cannulae used to connect the tubing of additive sets to primary infusions: (a) threaded-lock cannula; (b) lever-lock cannula.

Source: (BD) Becton, Dickinson and Company and courtesy of Baxter Healthcare Corporation. All rights reserved.

PRACTICE GUIDELINES

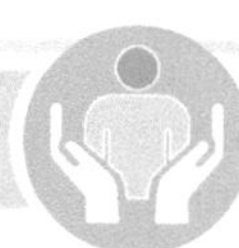

Caring for Patients with a Venous Access Device (VAD)

On Insertion

Document the following information:

- Evidence of informed consent (Nursing and Midwifery Council (NMC), 2008)
- Date and time of insertion of VAD (Department of Health (DH), 2007)
- Reason for insertion of VAD (Pratt *et al.*, 2007)
- Site preparation (Camp Sorrell, 2004)
- Number and location of attempts and the technique used to insert the VAD (Wernstein, 2007)
- Insertion site and vein used (Wernstein, 2007)
- Any bruising or bleeding noted after insertion (Wernstein, 2007)
- Length of catheter (Wernstein, 2007)

Site Care

- Local policies should be adhered.
- Aseptic technique should be used when performing VAD site care. Standard precautions should be adhered to (Dougherty and Watson, 2008).
- Site care should involve observation of the site, the VAD and surrounding tissues. Findings should be documented (DH, 2007).
- Follow local protocol for cleaning solutions and types of dressings. RCN (2010) advise the use of antimicrobial solutions such as Chlorhexadine for cleansing of VAD sites.
- The insertion site should be assessed on a daily basis (Dougherty, 2006).
- Ideally, VAD should be dressed with sterile, transparent, semi-permeable dressings (RCN, 2010) to aid assessment of the insertion site.
- If a gauze dressing is used, this should be changed every day or if the integrity of the dressing is compromised (RCN, 2010). If a transparent, semi-permeable dressing is used this can remain in situ for up to 7 days but should be changed immediately if the integrity of the dressing is compromised (RCN, 2010).
- Before using the port it should be cleaned using a single use antimicrobial swab (in accordance with local policy and manufacturers guidelines) (Pratt *et al.*, 2007), starting at the centre of the port site, moving outwards. Allow the site to air dry.

Catheter Care and Flushing

- Flush the port with normal saline, a heparin flush solution (10 units/ml), or as local protocol recommends for the specific type of port being used. After infusing medications or solutions, again flush the port with saline (RCN, 2010).
- Remember to flush all lumens for multiple-lumen catheters.

Teaching

Provide patients with the following instructions:

- Do not allow anyone to take a blood pressure on the arm in which a PICC line is inserted.
- For a PICC, you do not need to restrict activities, except do not immerse the arm in water. Showering is allowed if the site and catheter are covered by an occlusive dressing.
- For an implanted venous port there are no activity restrictions, but remember that the port or catheter tip can become dislodged. Signs of a dislodged catheter tip include pain in the neck or ear on the affected side, swishing or gurgling sounds, or palpitations. Free movement of the port, swelling or difficulty accessing the port may indicate port dislodgement. Notify the physician should any of these occur or if symptoms of infection develop.

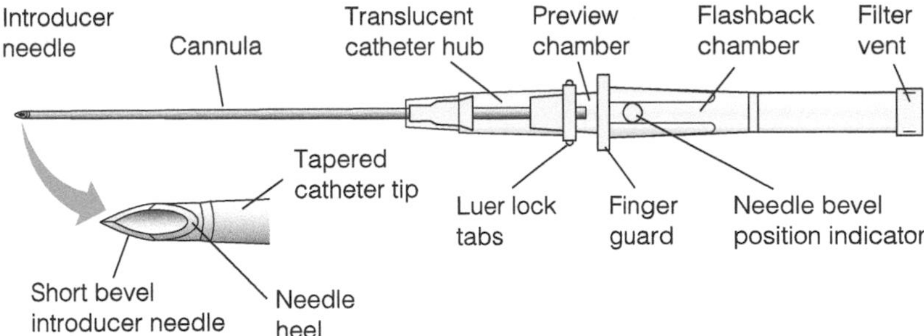

Figure 20-15 An over-the-needle catheter.

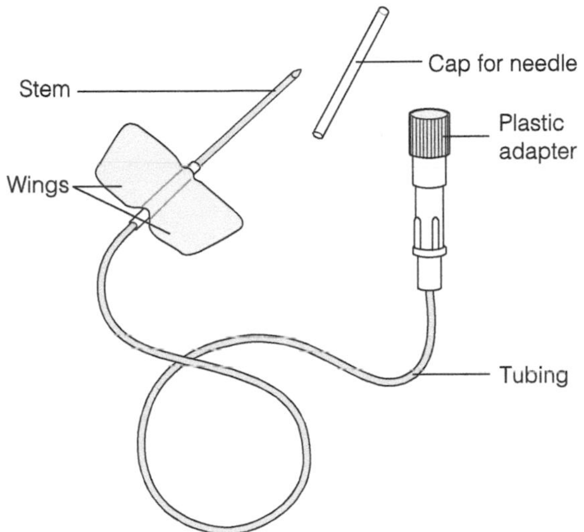

Figure 20-16 Schematic of a butterfly needle with adapter.

Catheters and needles are commonly used for intravenous infusions. Over-the-needle catheters are commonly used for adult patients. The plastic catheter fits over a needle used to pierce the skin and vein wall (see Figure 20-15). Once inserted into the vein, the needle is withdrawn and discarded, leaving the catheter in place. IV catheters allow the patient more mobility and rarely infiltrate, that is, become dislodged from the vein and allow fluid to flow into interstitial spaces.

Butterfly, or wing-tipped, needles with plastic flaps attached to the shaft are sometimes used (see Figure 20-16). The flaps are held tightly together to hold the needle securely during insertion; after insertion, they are flattened against the skin and secured with tape.

IV poles are used to hang the solution container. Some poles are attached to hospital beds; others stand on the floor or hang from the ceiling. The height of most poles is adjustable. The higher the solution container, the greater the force of the solution as it enters the patient and the faster the rate of flow.

Starting an Intravenous Infusion

Although the doctor is responsible for prescribing IV therapy for patients, nurses initiate, monitor and maintain the prescribed IV infusion. This is true not only in hospitals and long-term care facilities but increasingly in community-based settings such as clinics and patients' homes.

Before starting an infusion, the nurse determines the following:

- the type and amount of solution to be infused;
- the exact amount (dose) of any medications to be added to a compatible solution;
- the rate of flow or the time over which the infusion is to be completed.

If solutions are prepared by the pharmacy or another department, the nurse must verify that the solution supplied exactly matches that which the doctor has prescribed. The nurse needs to understand the purpose for the infusion in order to assess the patient effectively.

To start an intravenous infusion, see *Procedure 20-1*.

> **ACTIVITY 20-4**
>
> What interventions would you implement to prevent a patient from becoming dehydrated?

EVALUATING

The goals established in the planning phase are evaluated according to specific desired outcomes. If the outcomes are not achieved, the nurse should explore the reasons.

Management of patients with fluid, electrolyte and acid–base disturbances is a vital role within nursing. It is important to note that all nurses should be able to manage a patient's fluid and electrolyte balance; however, not all nurses are able to administer intravenous fluids or medications without further often formal education. The safe administration of intravenous medications and fluid requires knowledge and experience.

PROCEDURE 20-1 Starting an Intravenous Infusion

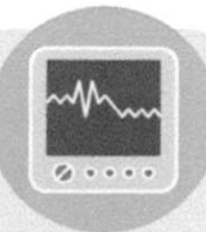

Before preparing the infusion, the nurse first checks the prescription chart. The nurse needs to know the type of solution required, the amount to be administered, the rate of flow of the infusion and any patient allergies.

Purposes

- To supply fluid when patients are unable to take in an adequate volume of fluids by mouth
- To provide salts needed to maintain electrolyte balance
- To provide glucose (dextrose), the main fuel for metabolism
- To provide medications

Assessment

Assess

- Vital signs (pulse, respiratory rate and blood pressure) for baseline data
- Skin turgor
- Allergy to tape or iodine

Planning

Prior to initiating the IV infusion, consider how long the patient is likely to have the IV, what kinds of fluids will be infused, mobility and any physical constraints.

Equipment

- Infusion set
- Container of sterile parenteral solution
- IV pole
- Adhesive or nonallergenic tape
- Clean gloves
- Alcohol swabs
- Electronic infusion device or pump (the nurse decides what device is needed as appropriate to the patient's condition.)

Implementation

Preparation

- Prepare the patient.
- Make sure that the patient's clothing or gown can be removed over the IV apparatus if necessary.

Performance

1 Follow local policy to ensure that you explain to the patient what you are going to do, why it is necessary and how they can cooperate. Obtain consent and maintain patient privacy and dignity and ensure that the appropriate local infection control procedures are observed.

2 Open and prepare the infusion set.
   - Remove tubing from the container and straighten it out.
   - Slide the tubing clamp along the tubing until it is just below the drip chamber to facilitate its access.
   - Close the clamp.
   - Leave the ends of the tubing covered with the plastic caps until the infusion is started. *To maintain the sterility of the ends of the tubing.*

3 After checking that it is the correct solution and the expiry date, spike the solution container.
   - Remove the protective cover from the entry site of the bag.
   - Remove the cap from the spike and insert the spike into the insertion site of the bag or bottle (see Figure 20-17). Follow the manufacturer's instructions.

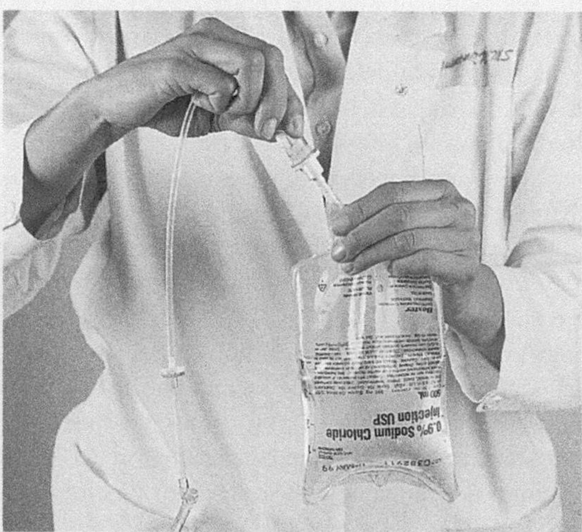

Figure 20-17 Inserting the spike.

4 Apply a medication label to the solution container if a medication is added.

5 Hang the solution container on the pole.
- Adjust the pole so that the container is suspended about 1m (3 feet) above the patient's head. *To enable gravity to overcome venous pressure and facilitate flow of the solution into the vein.*

6 Partially fill the drip chamber with solution. Squeeze the chamber gently until it is half full of solution (see Figure 20-18).

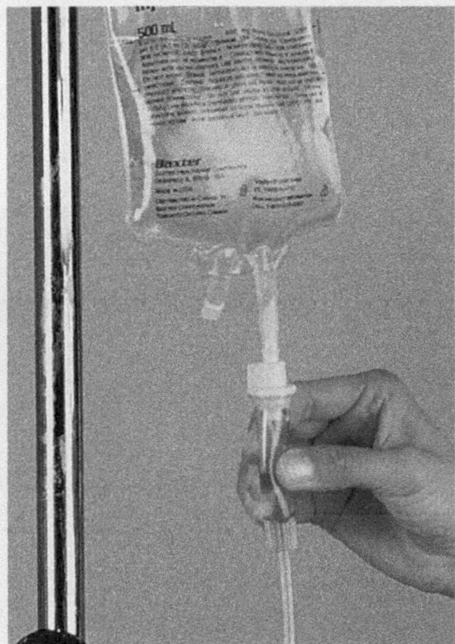

Figure 20-18 Squeezing the drip chamber.

7 Prime the tubing.
- Remove the protective cap and hold the tubing over a container. Maintain the sterility of the end of the tubing and the cap.
- Release the clamp and let the fluid run through the tubing until all bubbles are removed. Tap the tubing if necessary with your fingers to help the bubbles move. *The tubing is primed to prevent the introduction of air into the patient.*
- Air bubbles smaller than 0.5ml usually do not cause problems in peripheral lines.
- Reclamp the tubing and replace the tubing cap, maintaining sterile technique.
- If an infusion control pump, electronic device or controller is being used, follow the manufacturer's directions for inserting the tubing and setting the infusion rate.

8 Clean port of venous catheter with antimicrobial swab and allow to dry.

9 Flush venous access with sodium chloride (please see local policy) to ensure the line is patent.

10 Attach infusion line to venous catheter and commence infusion according to the prescription.

11 Document relevant data, including assessments.
- Record the start of the infusion on the patient's chart.
- Include the date and time of commencement of infusion; amount and type of solution used, including any additives (e.g. kind and amount of medications); fluid batch number; flow rate; and the patient's general response.

Evaluation

- Assess the skin status at the IV site (warm temperature and absence of pain, redness and swelling).
- Assess the status of the dressing.
- Check that the IV flow rate is consistent with that prescribed.
- Assess the patient's ability to perform self-care activities and understanding of any mobility limitations.
- Compare the patient's vital signs to baseline level.

Regulating and Monitoring Intravenous Infusions

Orders for IV infusions may take several forms: '3,000ml over 24 hours'; '1,000ml every 8 hours × 3 bags'; '125ml/h until oral intake is adequate'. The nurse initiating the IV calculates the correct flow rate, regulates the infusion and monitors the patient's responses. Unless an infusion control device is used, the nurse manually regulates the drops per minute of flow using the roller clamp to ensure that the prescribed amount of solution will be infused in the correct timespan. If the flow is incorrect, problems such as hypervolaemia, hypovolaemia or inadequate medication administration can result.

The number of drops delivered per millilitre of solution varies with different brands and types of infusion sets. This rate, called the *drop factor*, generally is printed on the package of the infusion set. Commonly infusion giving sets have drop factors of 10, 12, 15 or 20 drops/ml.

To calculate flow rates, the nurse must know the volume of fluid to be infused and the specific time for the infusion. Two commonly used methods of indicating flow rates are designating the number of millilitres to be administered in 1 hour (ml/hr) and the number of drops to be given in 1 minute (drops/min).

Millilitres per hour

Hourly rates of infusion can be calculated by dividing the total infusion volume by the total infusion time in hours. For example, if 3,000ml is infused in 24 hours, the number of millilitres per hour is

$$\frac{\text{3,000ml (total infusion volume)}}{\text{24 hours (total infusion time)}} = \text{125ml/hr}$$

Nurses need to check infusions at least every hour to ensure that the indicated millilitres per hour have infused and that IV patency is maintained.

Drops per minute

The nurse initiating and monitoring an infusion via a gravity set (not using a pump) must regulate the drops per minute to ensure that the prescribed amount of solution will infuse. Drops per minute are calculated by the following formula:

$$\text{Drops per minute} = \frac{\text{Total infusion volume} \times \text{drop factor}}{\text{Total time of infusion in minutes}}$$

If the requirements are 1,000ml in 8 hours and the drop factor is 20 drops/ml, the drops per minute should be

$$\frac{1{,}000\text{ml} \times 20 \text{ (drops/ml)}}{8 \times 60 \text{ mins (480 mins)}} = 41 \text{ drops/min}$$

Approximating this rate as 40 drops/min, the nurse regulates the drops per minute by tightening or releasing the IV tubing clamp and counting the drops for 1 minute. A number of factors influence flow rate:

- The position of the forearm. Sometimes a change in the position of the patient's arm decreases flow. Bending of the arm can also alter the flow rate.
- The position and patency of the tubing. Tubing can be obstructed by the patient's weight, a kink or a clamp closed too tightly. The flow rate also diminishes when part of the tubing dangles below the puncture site.
- The height of the infusion bag. Elevating the height of the infusion bag a few inches can speed the flow by creating more pressure.
- Possible infiltration or fluid leakage. Swelling, a feeling of coldness and tenderness at the venepuncture site may indicate infiltration.
- Size of the venous catheter, a narrow catheter will slow infusion rates.

Devices to Control Infusions

A number of devices are used to control the rate of an infusion. *Electronic infusion devices* regulate the infusion rate at preset limits. They also have an alarm that is triggered when the solution in the IV bag is low, when there is air in the tubing, or when the tubing is not high enough. The *Dial-A-Flo* in-line device (see Figure 20-19) is a regulator that controls the amount of fluid to be administered. Hospitals may stock the Dial-A-Flo for use in situations where a pump is not required, but prevention of fluid overload is important. It is preset at the volume to be infused and can be attached at the time the infusion is set up or when the tubing is changed. Another variation is a *volume-control set*, which is used if the volume of fluid administered is to be carefully controlled.

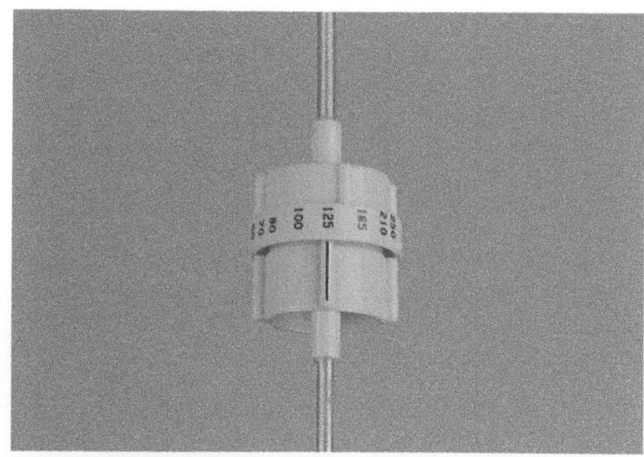

Figure 20-19 The Dial-A-Flo in-line device.

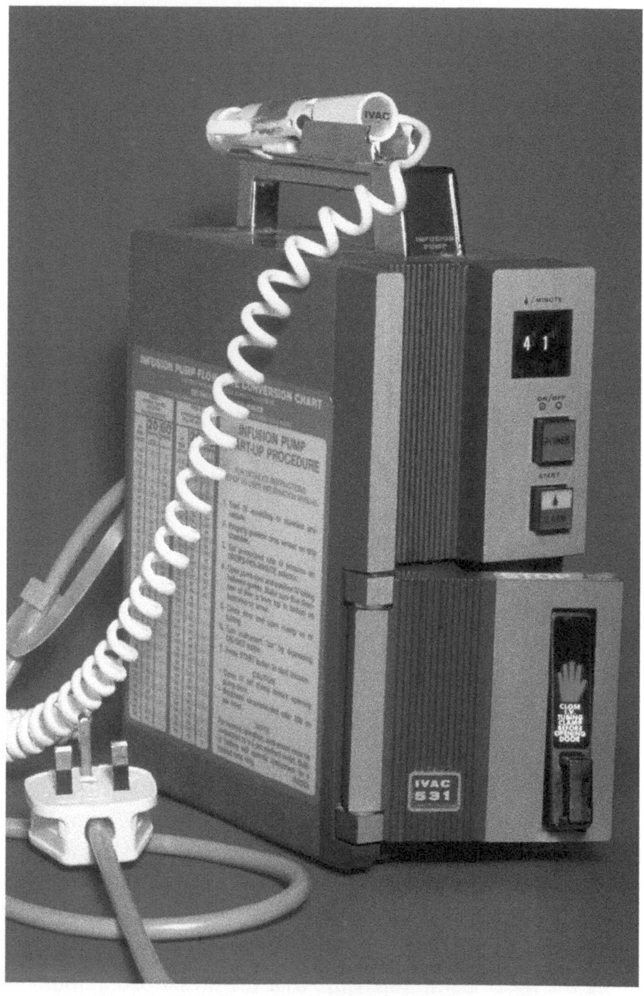

Figure 20-20 Intravenous infusion pump.
Source: **http://www.medcatalog.com/images/medequip2.jpg.**

CLINICAL ALERT

A flow rate control device should be used when administering IV fluid to high risk patient groups (RCN, 2010) including older and paediatric patients. Both of these age groups are especially at risk for complications of fluid overload, which can occur with rapid infusion of IV fluids.

An infusion pump (see Figure 20-20) delivers fluids intravenously by exerting positive pressure on the tubing or on the fluid. In situations where the fluid flow is unrestricted, the pump pressure is comparable to that of gravity flow. However, if restrictions develop (increased venous resistance), the pump can maintain the fluid flow by increasing the pressure applied to the fluid.

Procedure 20-2 outlines the steps involved in monitoring an intravenous infusion.

PROCEDURE 20-2 Monitoring an Intravenous Infusion

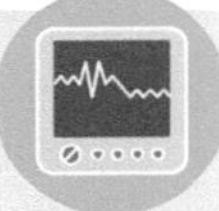

Purposes

- To maintain the prescribed flow rate
- To prevent complications associated with IV therapy

Assessment

Assess

- Appearance of infusion site; patency of system
- Type of fluid being infused and rate of flow
- Response of the patient

Planning

Review the type of equipment needed away from the patient's bedside.

Implementation

Preparation

- Gather the relevant information.
- From the prescription chart, determine the type and sequence of solutions to be infused.
- Determine the rate of flow and infusion regimen.

Performance

1. Follow local policy to ensure that you explain to the patient what you are going to do, why it is necessary and how they can cooperate. Obtain consent and maintain patient privacy and dignity and ensure that the appropriate local infection control procedures are observed.
2. Ensure that the correct solution is being infused.
   - If the solution is incorrect stop the infusion immediately and flush the intravenous catheter to maintain patency of the cannula.
   - Change the solution to the correct one. Document and report the error according to local protocol.
3. Observe the rate of flow every hour.
   - Compare the rate of flow regularly, for example, every hour, against the prescription chart. *Infusions that are infusing incorrectly can be harmful to a patient.*
   - If the rate is too fast, slow it so that the infusion will be completed at the planned time. *Solution administered too quickly may cause a significant increase in circulating blood volume. Hypervolaemia may result in pulmonary oedema and cardiac failure.*
   - Assess the patient for manifestations of hypervolaemia and its complications, including dyspnoea; rapid, laboured breathing; cough; crackles in the lung bases; tachycardia; and bounding pulses.
   - If the rate is too slow adjust the flow to the specified rate in the prescription chart. *Solution that is administered too slowly can supply insufficient fluid, electrolytes or medication for a patient's needs.*

→

4 Inspect the patency of the IV tubing and needle.
- Observe the position of the solution container and readjust height if needed. *If the container is too low, the solution may not flow into the vein because there is insufficient gravitational pressure to overcome the pressure of the blood within the vein.*
- Observe the drip chamber. If it is less than half full, squeeze the chamber to allow the correct amount of fluid to flow in.
- Inspect the tubing for pinches or kinks or obstructions to flow. Arrange the tubing so that it is lightly coiled and under no pressure. Sometimes the tubing becomes caught under the patient's body and the weight blocks the flow.
- Observe the position of the tubing. *The solution may not flow upward into the vein against the force of gravity.*
- If there is leakage, locate the source. If the leak is at the catheter connection, tighten the tubing into the catheter. If the leak cannot be stopped, slow the infusion as much as possible without stopping it, and replace the tubing with a new sterile set. Estimate the amount of solution lost, if it was substantial.

5 Inspect the insertion site for fluid infiltration.
- When an IV needle becomes dislodged from the vein, fluid flows into interstitial tissues, causing swelling. This is known as *infiltration* and is manifested by localised swelling, coolness, pallor and discomfort at the IV site.
- If an infiltration is present, stop the infusion and remove the catheter. Restart the infusion at another site.
- Apply a warm compress to the site of the infiltration. *Warmth promotes comfort and vasodilation, facilitating absorption of the fluid from interstitial tissues.*

6 If infiltration is not evident but the infusion is not flowing, determine whether the needle is dislodged from the vein.
- Use a sterile syringe of saline to withdraw fluid from the port. If blood does not return, discontinue the intravenous solution.

7 Inspect the insertion site for phlebitis (inflammation of a vein).
- Inspect and palpate the site at least every eight hours. Phlebitis can occur as a result of injury to a vein, for example, because of mechanical trauma or chemical irritation. Chemical injury to a vein can occur from intravenous electrolytes (especially potassium and magnesium) and medications. The clinical signs are redness, warmth and swelling at the intravenous site and burning pain along the course of a vein.
- If phlebitis is detected, discontinue the infusion, and apply warm compresses to the venepuncture site.
- Do not use this injured vein for further infusions.

8 Inspect the intravenous site for bleeding.
- Oozing or bleeding into the surrounding tissues can occur while the infusion is freely flowing but is more likely to occur after the needle has been removed from the vein.
- Observation of the venepuncture site is extremely important for patients who bleed readily, such as those receiving anticoagulants.
- Teach the patient ways to maintain the infusion system, for example:
  - Avoid sudden twisting or turning movements of the arm with the needle or catheter.
  - Avoid stretching or placing tension on the tubing.
  - Try to keep the tubing from dangling below the level of the needle.

9 Notify a nurse if:
- The flow rate suddenly changes or the solution stops dripping.
- The solution container is nearly empty.
- There is blood in the IV tubing.
- Discomfort or swelling is experienced at the IV site.

10 Document all relevant information.

Evaluation

- Check that the amount of fluid infused corresponds with to the schedule.
- Check that the IV system is intact.
- Assess the appearance of the IV site (e.g. dry, tissue infiltration, discomfort).
- Compare urinary output to urinary intake.
- Tissue turgor; specific gravity of urine.
- Compare the patient's vital signs and lung sounds to baseline data.

Changing Intravenous Containers, Tubing and Dressings

Intravenous solution containers are changed when only a small amount of fluid remains in the neck of the container and fluid still remains in the drip chamber. However, all IV bags should be changed every 24 hours, regardless of how much solution remains, to minimise the risk of contamination. *Procedure 20-3* provides guidelines for changing an IV solution container, tubing and the IV site dressing.

PROCEDURE 20-3 Changing an Intravenous Container, Tubing and Dressing

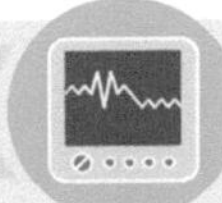

Purposes

- To maintain the flow of required fluids
- To maintain sterility of the IV system and decrease the incidence of phlebitis and infection
- To maintain patency of the IV tubing
- To prevent infection at the IV site

Assessment

Assess

- Presence of fluid infiltration, bleeding or phlebitis at IV site
- Allergy to tape or other substances
- Infusion rate
- Blockages in IV system
- Appearance of the dressing for integrity, moisture and need for change
- The date and the time of the previous dressing change

Planning

Review prescription chart for changes in fluid administration.

Equipment

- Container with the correct type and amount of sterile solution
- Administration set

For the dressing

- Sterile gloves
- Transparent dressing
- Sodium chloride or other solution for cleaning puncture site
- Alcohol swabs
- Tape
- Sterile dressing pack

Implementation

Preparation

- Obtain the correct solution container.
- Read the label of the new container.
- Verify that you have the correct solution, correct patient, correct additives (if any) and correct dose (number of bags or total volume ordered).

Performance

1 Follow local policy to ensure that you explain to the patient what you are going to do, why it is necessary and how they can cooperate. Obtain consent and maintain patient privacy and dignity and ensure that the appropriate local infection control procedures are observed.

2 Set up the intravenous equipment with the new bag of fluid. See *Procedure 20-1* earlier.
- Prime the tubing.

3 Prepare the IV catheter site.
- Open all equipment: swabs, cleansing fluid and dressing. *This facilitates access to supplies after gloves have been put on.*
- Place a towel under the extremity. *This prevents soiling of bed linens.*
- Apply sterile gloves.

4 Remove the soiled dressing and all tape, except the tape holding the catheter or IV needle in place.
- Remove tape and gauze from the old dressing one layer at a time. *This prevents dislodgement of the catheter or needle in case tubing becomes entangled between layers of dressing.*
- Remove adhesive dressings in the direction of the patient's hair growth when possible. *This minimises discomfort when adhesive is removed from the skin.*
- Discard the used dressing materials in the appropriate container.

5 Assess the IV site.
- Inspect the IV site for the presence of infiltration or inflammation. *Inflammation or infiltration necessitates removal of the IV needle or catheter to avoid further trauma to the tissues.*

6 Disconnect the used tubing.
- Place a sterile swab under the hub of the catheter. *This absorbs any leakage that might occur when the tubing is disconnected.*

- Clamp the tubing.
- Holding the hub of the catheter with the nondominant hand, loosen the tubing with the dominant hand, using a twisting, pulling motion. *Holding the catheter firmly but gently maintains its position in the vein.*
- Remove the used IV tubing.
- Place the end of the tubing in the basin or other receptacle.

7 Connect the new tubing, and re-establish the infusion.
- Continue to hold the catheter and grasp the new tubing with the dominant hand.
- Remove the protective tubing cap and, maintaining sterility, insert the tubing end securely into the needle hub. Twist it to secure it.
- Open the clamp to start the solution flowing.

8 Remove the tape securing the needle or catheter.
- When removing this tape and while cleaning the site, stabilise the needle or catheter hub with one hand. *This prevents inadvertent dislodgement of the needle or catheter.*

9 Clean the IV site.
- Use appropriate cleansing fluid such as sodium chloride or chlorhexidine (as per local policy).
- Clean the site, beginning at the catheter or needle and cleaning outward in an 8cm diameter. *Cleaning in this manner prevents contamination of the IV site from bacteria on the peripheral skin areas. Antiseptics reduce the number of micro-organisms present at the site, thus reducing the risk of infection.*

10 Retape the needle or catheter.

11 Apply the dressing.
- Apply a sterile transparent dressing over the site.
- Remove gloves.

12 Secure IV tubing with additional tape as required.

13 Regulate the rate of flow of the solution according to the prescription chart.

14 Document all relevant information.
- Record the change of the solution container, tubing and/or dressing in the appropriate place on the patient's chart. Also record the fluid intake according to local practice. Also record your assessments.

Evaluation

The following should be checked:
- status of the IV site;
- patency of the IV system;
- accuracy of flow.

When an IV infusion is no longer necessary to maintain the patient's fluid intake or to provide a route for medication administration, the infusion is either discontinued and the catheter removed or the catheter is left in place and converted to a saline or heparin lock. Guidelines for discontinuing an IV infusion are outlined in *Procedure 20-4*.

PROCEDURE 20-4 Discontinuing an Intravenous Infusion

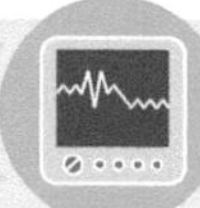

Purpose

To discontinue an intravenous infusion when the therapy is complete or when the IV site needs to be changed.

Assessment

Assess

- Appearance of the venepuncture site
- Any bleeding from the infusion site
- Amount of fluid infused
- Appearance of IV catheter

Planning

Review prescription chart.

Equipment

- Clean gloves
- Gauze swabs
- Small sterile dressing and tape

Implementation

Performance

1. Follow local policy to ensure that you explain to the patient what you are going to do, why it is necessary and how they can cooperate. Obtain consent and maintain patient privacy and dignity and ensure that the appropriate local infection control procedures are observed.
2. Prepare the equipment.
   - Clamp the infusion tubing. *Clamping the tubing prevents the fluid from flowing out of the needle onto the patient or bed.*
   - Loosen the tape at the venepuncture site while holding the needle firmly and applying countertraction to the skin. *Movement of the needle can injure the vein and cause discomfort to the patient. Countertraction prevents pulling the skin and causing discomfort.*
   - Put on clean gloves and hold a sterile gauze above the venepuncture site.
3. Withdraw the needle or catheter from the vein.
   - Withdraw the needle or catheter by pulling it out along the line of the vein. *Pulling it out in line with the vein avoids injury to the vein.*
   - Immediately apply firm pressure to the site, using sterile gauze, for 2–3 minutes. *Pressure helps stop the bleeding and prevents haematoma formation.*
   - Hold the patient's arm or leg above the body if any bleeding persists. *Raising the limb decreases blood flow to the area.*
4. Examine the catheter removed from the patient.
   - Check the catheter to make sure it is intact. *If a piece of tubing remains in the patient's vein it could move centrally (toward the heart or lungs) and cause serious problems.*
   - Report a broken catheter to the nurse in charge or doctor immediately.
5. Cover the venepuncture site.
   - Apply the sterile dressing. *The dressing continues the pressure and covers the open area in the skin, preventing infection.*
6. Discard the IV solution container properly, if infusions are being discontinued, and discard the used supplies appropriately.
7. Document all relevant information.
   - Record the amount of fluid infused on the intake and output record and on the chart, according to local practice. Include the container number, type of solution used, time of discontinuing the infusion and the patient's response.

Evaluation

- Check the appearance of the venepuncture site.
- Compare the patient's pulse with baseline level.
- Assess the patient's respirations, skin colour, oedema, sputum, cough and urine output.
- And how the person feels physically and psychologically.

CRITICAL REFLECTION

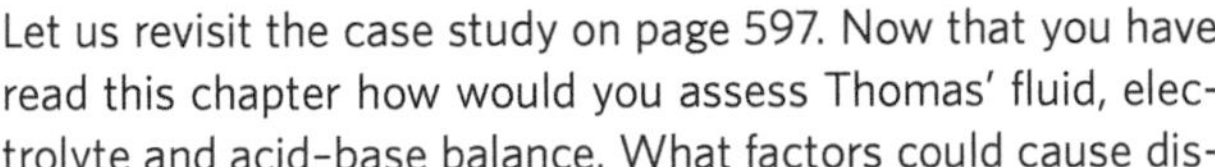

Let us revisit the case study on page 597. Now that you have read this chapter how would you assess Thomas' fluid, electrolyte and acid-base balance. What factors could cause disturbance of Thomas' fluid, electrolyte and acid-base balances? What interventions would you implement in order to prevent further deterioration?

CHAPTER HIGHLIGHTS

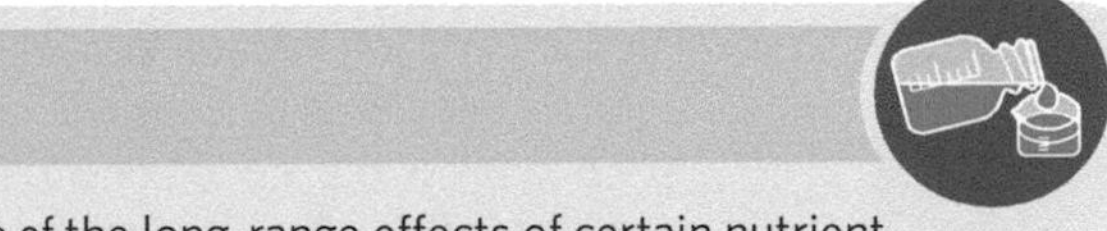

- Factors influencing a person's hydration include development, gender, ethnicity and culture, beliefs about foods, personal preferences, religious practices, lifestyle, medications and medical therapy, health status, alcohol abuse, advertising, and psychological factors such as stress, isolation and depression.
- A balance of fluids, electrolytes, acids and bases in the body is necessary for health and life.
- Some of the long-range effects of certain nutrient excesses are among the many factors involved in certain diseases, such as coronary artery disease and cancer.
- Assessment of hydration status may involve all or some of the following: patient history, nutritional screening, physical examination, calculation of the percentage of weight loss, a dietary history, anthropometric measurements and laboratory tests.

- In healthy adults, measurable fluid intake and output should balance (about 1,500ml per day). The output of urine normally approximates the oral intake of fluids. Water from food and oxidation is balanced by fluid loss through the skin, respiratory process and faeces.
- Fluid imbalances include:
  - hypovolaemia
  - hypervolaemia
  - dehydration, a deficit in water only
  - overhydration, an excess of water only.
- The most common electrolyte imbalances are deficits or excesses in sodium, potassium and calcium.
- The acid-base balance (pH range) of body fluids is maintained within a precise range of 7.35 to 7.45.
- Acid-base balance is regulated by buffers that neutralise excess acids or bases; the lungs, which eliminate or retain carbon dioxide, a potential acid; and the kidneys, which excrete or conserve bicarbonate and hydrogen ions.
- Acid-base imbalance occurs when the normal 20-to-1 ratio of bicarbonate to carbonic acid is upset. Imbalances may be either respiratory or metabolic in origin; either can result in acidosis or alkalosis.
- Fluid, electrolyte and acid-base imbalance is most accurately determined through laboratory examination of blood plasma.
- For patients with fluid retention, fluids may need to be restricted; a schedule and short-term goals that make the fluid restriction more tolerable need to be developed.
- For patients experiencing excessive fluid losses, the administration of fluids and electrolytes intravenously is necessary. Meticulous aseptic technique is required when caring for patients with intravenous infusions.
- Preventing complications such as infiltration, phlebitis, hypervolaemia (circulatory overload), and infection are an important aspect of intravenous therapy.

ACTIVITY ANSWERS

ACTIVITY 20-1 A child weighing 32kg will require 1740ml over a 24-hour period.

ACTIVITY 20-2 The factors that may affect a patient's body fluid, electrolytes and acid-base balance include:
- The patient's age
- The patient's physical condition, e.g. swallowing and mobility difficulties
- The patient's mental condition, e.g. depression
- Medications, e.g. furosemide

ACTIVITY 20-3 When assessing a patient's body fluid, electrolyte and acid-base balance disturbance, the following would need to be considered:
- Full patient history - any problems with urination, defecation, swallowing and his past medical history
- Full physical assessment
- Vital signs - BP, pulse, respiratory rate, consciousness level, oxygen saturations, temperature
- Weight
- ECG - to detect any arrhythmias
- Urine - including amount, colour, odour, specific gravity, dipstick test
- Head to toe assessment - including skin and mucous membranes
- Gut function - bowels sounds, flatus
- Swallowing assessment
- Laboratory tests:
  - full blood count - to check haematocrit, haemoglobin, white cell count
  - urea and electrolytes - to check renal function and detect any electrolyte imbalances

ACTIVITY 20-4 The following interventions could be implemented in order to prevent a patient from becoming dehydrated:
- Site a peripheral intravenous cannula
- Commence the patient on an isotonic intravenous fluid replacement (as prescribed by the doctor)
- Monitor the patient's condition closely:
  - regular vital signs
  - fluid balance
  - electrolytes
  - renal function
  - swallowing
- Longer term - may need to consider enteral fluid via nasogastric tube or percutaneous endoscopic gastrostomy (PEG)

REFERENCES

Behrman, R.E. (1992) *Nelson text book of pediatrics*, Philadelphia, PA: Saunders.

Camp Sorrell, D. (2004) *Access device guidelines, recommendations for nursing practice and education* (2nd edn), Philadelphia PA: Oncology Nursing Society.

Department of Health (DH) (2007) *Saving lives: Reducing infection delivering clean and safe care. Huge impact intervention No.1. Central venous catheter care bundle.* London: DH.

Dougherty, L. (2006) *Central venous access devices. Care and management*, Oxford: Blackwell.

Dougherty, L. and Watson, J. (2008) 'Vascular access devices', in Dougherty, L. and Lister, S. (eds), *The Royal Marsden Hospital manual of clinical nursing procedures* (7th edn), Oxford: Wiley-Blackwell, 724–773.

Hogston, R. and Simpson, P.M. (2002) *Foundations of nursing practice: Making the difference*, Basingstoke: Palgrave Macmillan.

McCormick, S.E., Stafford, K.M., Saqib, G., Chronin, D.N. and Power, D. (2008) 'The efficacy of pre-thickened fluid on total fluid and nutrition consumption among extended care residents requiring thickened fluids due to risk of aspiration', *Age and Ageing*, 37, 714–718.

NMC (2008) *The Code: Standards of conduct, performance and ethics for nurses and midwives*, London: NMC.

NMC (2010) *Standards for pre-registration nursing education*, London: NMC.

Pratt, R.J., Pellowe, C., Wilson, J.A., Loveday, H.P., Harper, P.J., Jones, S.R.L.J., McDougall, C. and Wilcox, M.H. (2007) epic 2: 'National evidence-based guidelines for preventing healthcare-associated infection in NHS hospitals in England', *Journal of Hospital Infection*, 655(Supp), S1–S64.

RCN (2007) *Hospital hydration best practice toolkit: Practical tips for encouraging water consumption*, London: RCN, available at http://www.rcn.org.uk/__data/assets/pdf_file/0003/70383/6-tips.pdf (accessed 29 June 2011).

RCN (2010) *Standards for infusion therapy*, London: RCN.

Stockslager, J.L., Mayer, B.H., Munden, J., Munson, C. and Theodore, R. (2007) *Nutrition made incredibly easy*, London: Lippincott, Williams and Wilkins.

Wernstein, S.M. (2007) *Plumer's principles and practice of infusion therapy* (8th edn), Philadelphia, PA: Lippincott, Williams and Wilkins.

CHAPTER 21
URINARY ELIMINATION

LEARNING OUTCOMES

After completing this chapter, you will be able to:

- Understand the physiology of urination.
- Identify factors that influence urinary elimination.
- Identify common causes of selected urinary problems.
- Describe the assessment of urinary elimination.
- Identify measures that maintain normal elimination patterns.
- Explain the care of patients with indwelling catheters or urinary diversions.

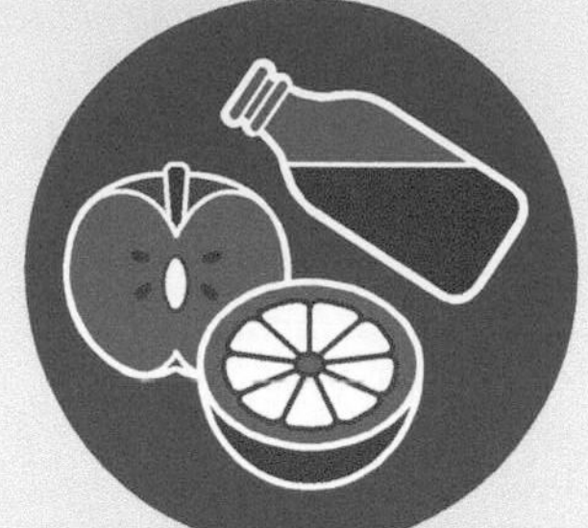

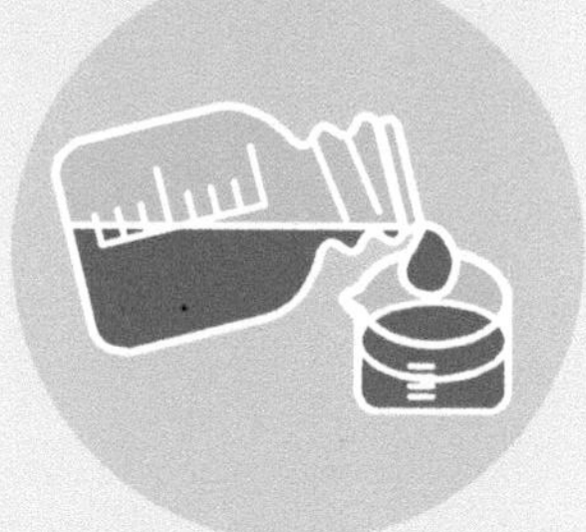

After reading this chapter you will be able to discuss ways in which **continence** can be promoted and understand the process of **urination**. This chapter relates to the **Essential Skills Clusters (NMC, 2010) 1 to 11, 13, 14, 15, 16, 18, 22, 24, 26 and 36**, as appropriate for each progression point.

Ensure that you really understand this chapter by logging on to your complimentary **MyNursingKit** at **www.pearsoned.co.uk/kozier**. Complete the self-assessment tests to check your progress and utilize further activities to practice and confirm your understanding.

CASE STUDY

Sally is a 12-year-old girl who has just returned from theatre after having an appendectomy. She is complaining of pain around the incision site but is able to move with some assistance. Sally tells you that she needs to pass urine.

INTRODUCTION

Urinary elimination is a private, independent function that is usually taken for granted. Control of urinary elimination is usually learnt in infancy (Richardson, 2003); however, problems can exist for both children and adults. It is only when a problem arises that most people become aware of their urinary habits and any associated symptoms. However, nurses are frequently consulted or involved in assisting patients with elimination problems. These problems can be embarrassing to patients and can cause considerable discomfort. Nurses need to have an understanding of the normal physiology of urination and ways in which associated problems can be managed.

PHYSIOLOGY OF URINARY ELIMINATION

Urinary elimination depends on effective functioning of four urinary tract organs: kidneys, **ureters**, bladder and **urethra** (see Figure 21-1).

The paired kidneys are situated on either side of the spinal column, behind the peritoneal cavity. They are the primary regulators of fluid and acid–base balance in the body. The functional units of the kidneys, called **nephrons**, filter the blood and remove metabolic wastes. In the average adult 1,200 ml of blood, or about 21% of the **cardiac output**, passes through the kidneys every minute. Each kidney contains approximately 1 million nephrons. Each nephron has a **glomerulus**, a tuft of capillaries surrounded by Bowman's capsule (see Figure 21-2). The endothelium of glomerular capillaries is porous, allowing fluid and solutes to readily move across this membrane into the capsule. Plasma proteins and blood cells, however, are too large to cross the membrane normally. Glomerular filtrate is similar in composition to plasma, made up of water, electrolytes, glucose, amino acids and metabolic wastes.

From Bowman's capsule the filtrate moves into the tubule of the nephron. In the **proximal** convoluted tubule, most of the water and **electrolytes** are reabsorbed. **Solutes** such as glucose are reabsorbed in the loop of Henle, but in the same area, other substances are secreted into the filtrate, concentrating the urine. In the distal convoluted tubule, additional water and sodium are reabsorbed under the control of hormones such as antidiuretic hormone (ADH) and aldosterone. This controlled reabsorption allows fine regulation of fluid and electrolyte balance in the body. When fluid intake is low or the concentration of solutes in the blood is high, ADH is released from the anterior pituitary,

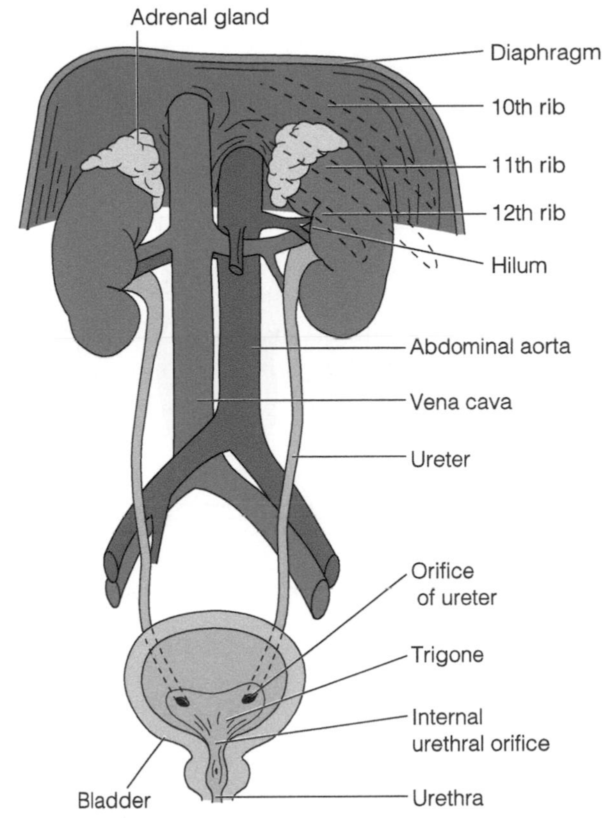

Figure 21-1 Anatomic structures of the urinary tract.

more water is reabsorbed in the distal tubule, and less urine is excreted. By contrast, when fluid intake is high or the blood solute concentration is low, ADH is suppressed. Without ADH, the distal tubule becomes impermeable to water, and more urine is excreted. Aldosterone also affects the tubule. When aldosterone is released from the adrenal cortex, sodium and water are reabsorbed in greater quantities, increasing the blood volume and decreasing urinary output.

Once the urine is formed in the kidneys, it moves through the collecting ducts into the calyces of the renal pelvis and from there into the ureters. The ureters are from 25–30cm long in the adult and about 1.25cm in diameter. The upper end of each ureter is funnel shaped as it enters the kidney. The lower ends of the ureters enter the bladder at the posterior corners of the floor of the bladder (see Figure 21-1). At the junction between the ureter and the bladder, a flaplike fold of mucous membrane acts as a valve to prevent **reflux** (backflow) of urine up the ureters.

The urinary bladder is a hollow, muscular organ that serves as a reservoir for urine and as the organ of excretion. When

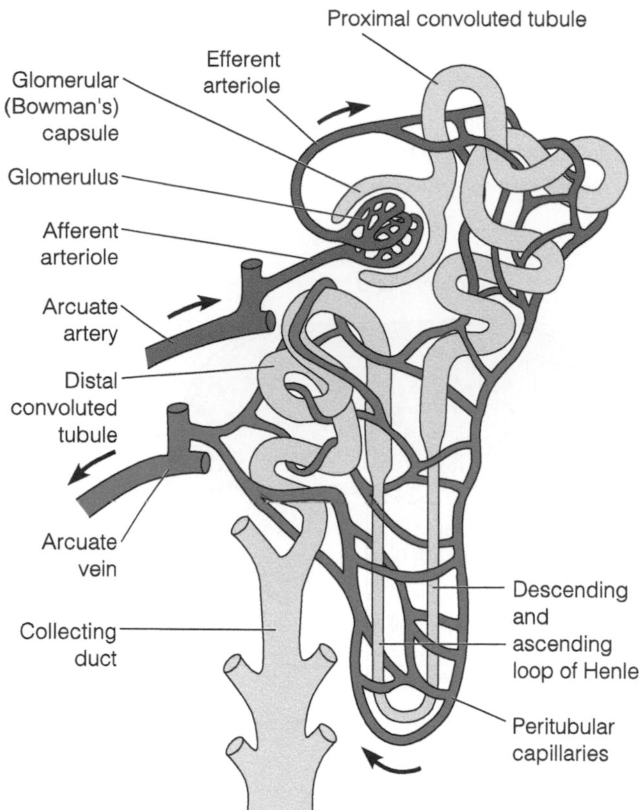

Figure 21-2 The nephrons of the kidney are composed of six parts: the glomerulus, Bowman's capsule, proximal convoluted tubule, loop of Henle, distal convoluted tubule and collecting duct.

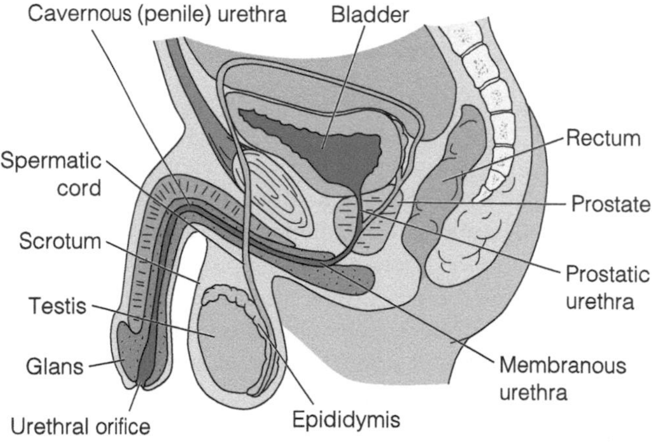

Figure 21-3 The male urogenital system.

empty, it lies behind the symphysis pubis. In men, the bladder lies in front of the rectum and above the prostate gland (see Figure 21-3); in women it lies in front of the uterus and vagina (see Figure 21-4). The wall of the bladder is made up of four layers: (a) an inner mucous layer, (b) a connective tissue layer, (c) three layers of smooth muscle fibres, some of which extend lengthwise, some obliquely, and some more or less circularly, and (d) an outer serous layer. The smooth muscle layers are

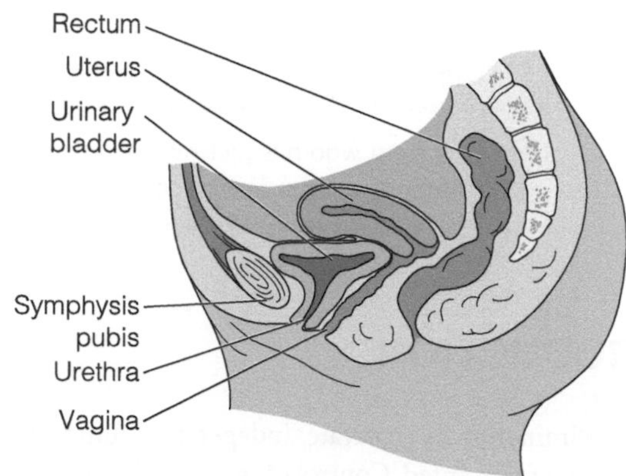

Figure 21-4 The female urogenital system.

collectively called the **detrusor muscle**. The **trigone** at the base of the bladder is a triangular area marked by the ureter openings at the posterior corners and the opening of the urethra at the anterior inferior corner.

The bladder is capable of considerable distention because of rugae (folds) in the mucous membrane lining and because of the elasticity of its walls. When full, the dome of the bladder may extend above the symphysis pubis; in extreme situations, it may extend as high as the umbilicus.

The urethra extends from the bladder to the urinary **meatus** (opening). In the adult woman, the urethra lies directly behind the symphysis pubis, anterior to the vagina, and is about 3.7cm long (see Figure 21-4). The urethra serves only as a passageway for the elimination of urine. The urinary meatus is located between the labia minora, in front of the vagina and below the clitoris. The male urethra is about 20cm long and serves as a passageway for semen as well as urine (see Figure 21-3). The meatus is located at the distal end of the penis.

The internal sphincter muscle situated at the base of the urinary bladder is under involuntary control. The external sphincter muscle is under voluntary control, allowing the individual to choose when urine is eliminated.

In both men and women, the urethra has a mucous membrane lining that is continuous with the bladder and the ureters. Thus, an infection of the urethra can extend through the urinary tract to the kidneys. Women are particularly prone to urinary tract infections because of their short urethra and the proximity of the urinary meatus to the vagina and anus.

URINATION

Micturition, **voiding** and urination all refer to the process of emptying the urinary bladder. Urine collects in the bladder until pressure stimulates special sensory nerve endings in the bladder wall called stretch receptors. This occurs when the adult bladder contains 250–450ml of urine. In children, a considerably smaller volume, 50–200ml, stimulates these nerves.

The stretch receptors transmit impulses to the spinal cord, specifically to the voiding reflex centre located at the level of the second to fourth sacral vertebrae, causing the internal sphincter to relax and stimulating the urge to void. If the time and place are appropriate for urination, the conscious portion of the brain relaxes the external urethral sphincter muscle and urination takes place. If the time and place are inappropriate, the micturition reflex usually subsides until the bladder becomes more filled and the reflex is stimulated again.

Voluntary control of urination is possible only if the nerves supplying the bladder and urethra, the neural tracts of the cord and brain, and the motor area of the cerebrum are all intact. The individual must be able to sense that the bladder is full. Injury to any of these parts of the nervous system – for example, by a cerebral haemorrhage or spinal cord injury above the level of the sacral region – results in intermittent involuntary emptying of the bladder. Older adults whose cognition is impaired may not be aware of the need to urinate or able to respond to this urge by seeking toilet facilities. Likewise, people with severe learning disabilities experience urinary incontinence (Stenson and Danaher, 2005).

Factors Affecting Voiding

Numerous factors affect the volume and characteristics of the urine produced and the manner in which it is excreted. An individual's age can have an effect on the characteristics of urine output. Table 21-1 summarises developmental changes that affect urine output.

Psychosocial factors can also affect a person's ability to pass urine. Urination is a private function that requires privacy, time and normal positioning. If these conditions are not met it can lead to anxiety and muscle tension. As a result, the person is unable to relax abdominal and perineal muscles and the external urethral sphincter and voiding is inhibited.

In order to maintain a normal micturition, the body maintains a balance between the amount of fluid ingested and the amount of fluid eliminated. When the amount of fluid intake increases, the urine output normally increases. Certain fluids, such as alcohol, increase fluid output by inhibiting the production of antidiuretic hormone. By contrast, food and fluids high in sodium can cause fluid retention because water is retained to maintain the normal concentration of electrolytes. Some patients will require careful monitoring of their fluid balance, particularly if they are receiving intravenous fluid, are catheterised or have urination problems (see Chapter 20).

Many medications can also affect micturition, particularly those affecting the autonomic nervous system, interfere with the normal urination process and may cause urinary dysfunction (see *Practice Guidelines*). **Diuretics** (e.g. furosemide) increase urine formation by preventing the reabsorption of water and electrolytes from the tubules of the kidney into the bloodstream. Some medications may also alter the colour of the urine.

Good muscle tone is important to maintain the stretch and contractility of the detrusor muscle so the bladder can fill adequately and empty completely. Patients who require an indwelling catheter for a long period may have poor bladder muscle tone because continuous drainage of urine prevents the bladder from filling and emptying normally. Abdominal muscle contraction also assists in bladder emptying while pelvic muscle tone is a factor in being able to retain urine voluntarily once the urge to urinate is perceived.

Table 21-1 Changes in Urinary Elimination through the Lifespan

Stage	Variations
Foetuses	The foetal kidney begins to excrete urine between the 11th and 12th week of development.
Infants	Ability to concentrate urine is minimal; therefore, urine appears light yellow. Because of neuromuscular immaturity, voluntary urinary control is absent.
Children	Kidney function reaches maturity between the first and second year of life; urine is concentrated effectively and appears a normal amber colour. Between 20 and 24 months of age, the child starts to recognise bladder fullness and is able to hold urine beyond the urge to void. At approximately 2½ to 3 years of age, the child can perceive bladder fullness, hold urine after the urge to void, and communicate the need to urinate. Full urinary control usually occurs at age 4 or 5 years; daytime control is usually achieved by age 3 years. The kidneys grow in proportion to overall body growth.
Adults	The kidneys reach maximum size between 35 and 40 years of age. After 50 years, the kidneys begin to diminish in size and function. Most shrinkage occurs in the cortex of the kidney as individual nephrons are lost.
Older adults	An estimated 30% of nephrons are lost by age 80. Renal blood flow decreases because of vascular changes and a decrease in cardiac output. The ability to concentrate urine declines. Bladder muscle tone diminishes, causing increased frequency of urination and nocturia (awakening to urinate at night). Diminished bladder muscle tone and contractibility may lead to residual urine in the bladder after voiding, increasing the risk of bacterial growth and infection. Urinary incontinence may occur due to mobility problems or neurological impairments.

PRACTICE GUIDELINES

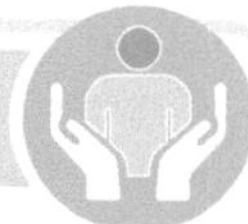

Medications that may Affect Urinary Function

Drug	Side Effect
Anticholinergic and antispasmodics (e.g. atropine)	Retention
Antidepressant and antipsychotics (e.g. phenothiazines)	Sedation and retention
Antihistamine preparations (pseudoephedrine (Actifed and Sudafed))	Retention
Antihypertensives (e.g. hydralazine)	Retention
Antiparkinsonism drugs (e.g. levodopa)	Retention
Beta-adrenergic blockers (e.g. propranolol)	Retention
Opioids	Sedation and retention
Diuretics	Frequency and urgency
Caffeine	Frequency and urgency
Alcohol	Sedation and frequency
Alpha-adrenergic blockers (e.g. terazoscin)	Stress incontinence

Some diseases and pathologies can affect the formation and excretion of urine. Diseases of the kidneys may affect the ability of the nephrons to produce urine. Abnormal amounts of protein or blood cells may be present in the urine, or the kidneys may virtually stop producing urine altogether, a condition known as renal failure. Heart and circulatory disorders such as heart failure, shock or hypertension can affect blood flow to the kidneys, interfering with urine production. If abnormal amounts of fluid are lost through another route (e.g. vomiting or high fever), water is retained by the kidneys and urinary output falls.

Processes that interfere with the flow of urine from the kidneys to the urethra affect urinary excretion. A urinary stone (calculus) may obstruct a ureter, blocking urine flow from the kidney to the bladder. Hypertrophy of the prostate gland, a common condition affecting older men, may obstruct the urethra, impairing urination and bladder emptying.

Some surgical and diagnostic procedures can affect the passage of urine and the urine itself. The urethra may swell following a **cystoscopy**, and surgical procedures on any part of the urinary tract may result in some post-operative bleeding; as a result, the urine may be red or pink tinged for a time.

Also, spinal anaesthetics can affect the passage of urine because they decrease the patient's awareness of the need to void. Surgery on structures adjacent to the urinary tract (e.g. the uterus) can also affect voiding because of swelling in the lower abdomen.

Urinary Elimination Problems

Although people's patterns of elimination are highly individual, most adults urinate about five times a day; however, children may urinate more often. Table 21-2 shows the average urinary output per day at different ages.

Table 21-2 Average Daily Urine Output by Age

Age	Amount (ml)
1 to 2 days	15-60
3 to 10 days	100-300
10 days to 2 months	250-450
2 months to 1 year	400-500
1 to 3 years	500-600
3 to 5 years	600-700
5 to 8 years	700-1,000
8 to 14 years	800-1,400
14 years through adulthood	1,500
Older adulthood	1,500 or less

There are a number of problems associated with the urinary system. **Polyuria** (or **diuresis**) is the production of abnormally large amounts of urine by the kidneys and is associated with excessive fluid intake, diabetes mellitus and chronic nephritis.

Oliguria and **anuria** are terms used to describe decreased urinary output. Oliguria is low urine output, usually less than 500ml a day or 30ml an hour, and is associated with poor fluid intake or impaired blood flow to the kidneys, while anuria refers to a lack of urine production.

Urinary frequency means urinating at frequent intervals, that is, more often than usual. An increased intake of fluid causes some increase in the frequency of voiding. Conditions such as urinary tract infection, stress and pregnancy can cause frequent voiding of small quantities (50–100ml) of urine.

Nocturia, on the other hand, is a term used to describe the need to urinate two or more times a night.

Urgency is the feeling that the person must urinate. There may or may not be a great deal of urine in the bladder, but the person feels a need to urinate immediately. It is common in young children who have poor external sphincter control.

Dysuria means voiding that is either painful or difficult. It can accompany a stricture (decrease in calibre) of the urethra, urinary infections and injury to the bladder and urethra. Often patients will say they have to push to void or that burning accompanies or follows voiding. Often, urinary hesitancy (a delay and difficulty in initiating voiding) is associated with dysuria.

Enuresis is involuntary urination in children beyond the age when voluntary bladder control is normally acquired, usually four or five years of age. **Nocturnal enuresis** is often irregular in occurrence and affects boys more often than girls. **Diurnal** (daytime) **enuresis** may be persistent and pathologic in origin. It affects women and girls more frequently.

Urinary incontinence, or involuntary urination, is a symptom, not a disease. It can have a significant impact on the patient's life, creating physical problems such as skin breakdown and possibly leading to psychosocial problems such as embarrassment, isolation and social withdrawal. Although incontinence is sometimes common in older adults, it is not a normal consequence of ageing and can often be treated. All patients should be asked about their voiding patterns. If incontinence is described, a thorough history and assessment is indicated. Treatment may include surgery, medication or behavioural therapies.

Urinary retention refers to accumulated urine in the bladder which becomes over distended. Overdistention (overstretching) of the bladder causes poor contractility of the detrusor muscle, further impairing urination. Common causes of urinary retention include prostatic hypertrophy (enlargement), surgery and some medications.

Neurogenic bladder refers to an impairment of the neurological function interfering with the normal mechanisms of urine elimination. The patient with a neurogenic bladder does not perceive bladder fullness and is unable to control the urinary sphincters. The bladder may become flaccid and distended or spastic, with frequent involuntary urination.

A number of factors can be associated with altered urinary elimination (see Table 21-3).

Table 21-3 Selected Factors Associated with Altered Urinary Elimination

Pattern	Selected associated factors
Polyuria	Ingestion of fluids containing caffeine or alcohol Prescribed diuretic Presence of thirst, dehydration and weight loss History of diabetes mellitus, diabetes insipidus or kidney disease
Oliguria, anuria	Decrease in fluid intake Signs of dehydration Presence of hypotension, shock or heart failure History of kidney disease Signs of renal failure such as elevated blood urea nitrogen (BUN) and serum creatinine, oedema, hypertension
Frequency or nocturia	Pregnancy Increase in fluid intake Urinary tract infection
Urgency	Presence of psychological stress Urinary tract infection
Dysuria	Urinary tract inflammation, infection or injury Hesitancy, haematuria, pyuria (pus in the urine) and frequency
Enuresis	Family history of enuresis Difficult access to toilet facilities Home stresses
Incontinence	Bladder inflammation or other disease Difficulties in independent toileting (mobility impairment) Leakage when coughing, laughing, sneezing Cognitive impairment
Retention	Distended bladder on palpation and percussion Associated signs, such as pubic discomfort, restlessness, frequency and small urine volume Recent anaesthesia Recent perineal surgery Presence of perineal swelling Medications prescribed Lack of privacy or other factors inhibiting micturition

Managing Urinary Elimination

Managing urinary elimination is a key role within nursing. Nurses need to be sensitive, empathetic and use effective communication skills to manage elimination problems (Baillie and Arrowsmith, 2009). As indicated on the following pages, assessment is vital to effective management of patients with urinary problems and the nurse needs to have knowledge of normal physiology as well as altered physiology and associated problems in order to implement effective interventions.

ASSESSING URINARY FUNCTION

A complete assessment of a patient's urinary function includes the following:

- patient history;
- physical assessment of the genitourinary system, hydration status and examination of the urine;
- relating the data obtained to the results of any diagnostic tests and procedures.

Patient History

The nurse determines the patient's normal voiding pattern and frequency, appearance of the urine and any recent changes, any past or current problems with urination, the presence of an **ostomy** and factors influencing the elimination pattern.

Physical Assessment

Complete physical assessment of the urinary tract usually includes percussion of the kidneys to detect areas of tenderness, palpation and percussion of the bladder, and if indicated examination of the urethral meatus for swelling, discharge or inflammation.

Problems with urination affect the excretion of waste products from the body; therefore, it is important that the nurse assess the patient's skin for colour, texture and tissue turgor as well as the presence of oedema. If incontinence, dribbling or dysuria is noted in the history, the skin of the perineum should be inspected for irritation because contact with urine can excoriate the skin and can lead to the development of pressure ulcers (see Chapter 18).

Assessing Urine

Normal urine consists of 96% water and 4% solutes. Organic solutes include urea, ammonia, creatinine and uric acid. Urea is the chief organic solute. Inorganic solutes include sodium, chloride, potassium, sulphate, magnesium and phosphorus. Sodium chloride is the most abundant inorganic salt.

Urinalysis is an important diagnostic test used to assess patients for conditions such as urinary tract infections and renal calculi (kidney stones). Urine should be collected midstream or from a catheter using sterile equipment (Dougherty and Lister, 2004). This poses problems when collecting from children who are not toilet-trained or from adults who may suffer urinary incontinence. Although the application of a urine bag is the chosen method for collecting urine in these circumstances, this method is often uncomfortable (Farrell *et al.* 2002). Indeed, a study by Liaw *et al.* (2000) of three methods of collecting urine at home found that parents preferred pads to collection bags and the clean catch method. However, Farrell *et al.* (2002) stated that there were significant concerns over the reliability of results from this method of collection. Macfarlane *et al.* (1999) therefore suggest that the clean catch method, although time-consuming and messy, is the best means of collecting urine from non-toilet-trained infants.

Whatever method of collection is used it important that the sample be tested immediately as any delay may result in unreliable results (Simerville *et al.*, 2005). The urine can be tested in a laboratory and/or using reagent strips (dipsticks). The reagent strips can be used to detect a number substances (see *Practice Guidelines*). Reagent strips cannot be used to definitively diagnose disease process but act only as an indicator in conjunction with clinical history and other diagnostic tests (Wells, 2007). However, if used according to manufacturer's guidelines these strips are relatively accurate.

PRACTICE GUIDELINES

Urinalysis Reagent Strips

Glucose	Glucosuria is often indicative but never diagnostic of Diabetes mellitus
Protein	Can indicate renal disease in hypertensive or diabetic patients
Blood	Haematuria is usually found when there is urinary tract infection or urological cancer
Urobilinogen	Normally found in urine but raised levels can indicate hepatic disease
Bilirubin	Indicative of obstructive jaundice
Nitrites	Usually indicative of urinary tract infections
Leucocytes	Usually indicative of urinary tract infections
Ketones	Produced from anaerobic metabolism. Can indicate dehydration or starvation but is particularly serious if found in a diabetic patient
pH	pH of urine is usually between 4.5 and 8.0 and reflects the acid-base balance
Specific gravity	Normally urine specific gravity varies within the range of 1.002-1.035

(Adapted from Wells, 2007)

Table 21-4 Characteristics of Normal and Abnormal Urine

Characteristic	Normal	Abnormal	Nursing considerations
Amount in 24 hours (adult)	1,200-1,500ml	Under 1,200ml A large amount over intake	Urinary output normally is approximately equal to fluid intake. Output of less than 30ml/hr may indicate decreased blood flow to the kidneys and should be immediately reported.
Colour, clarity	Straw, amber Transparent	Dark amber Cloudy Dark orange Red or dark brown Mucous plugs, viscid, thick	Concentrated urine is darker in colour. Dilute urine may appear almost clear or very pale yellow. Some foods and drugs may colour urine. Red blood cells in the urine (haematuria) may be evident as pink, bright red or rusty brown urine. Menstrual bleeding can also colour urine but should not be confused with haematuria. White blood cells, bacteria, pus or contaminants such as prostatic fluid, sperm or vaginal drainage may cause cloudy urine.
Odour	Faint aromatic	Offensive	Some foods (e.g. asparagus) cause a musty odour; infected urine can have a fetid odour; urine high in glucose has a sweet odour.
Sterility	No micro-organisms present	Micro-organisms present	Urine specimens may be contaminated by bacteria from the perineum during collection.
pH	4.5-8	Over 8 Under 4.5	Freshly voided urine is normally somewhat acidic. Alkaline urine may indicate a state of alkalosis, urinary tract infection or a diet high in fruits and vegetables. More acidic urine (low pH) is found in starvation, diarrhoea or with a diet high in protein foods or cranberries.
Specific gravity	1.010-1.025	Over 1.025 Under 1.010	Concentrated urine has a higher specific gravity; diluted urine has a lower specific gravity.
Glucose	Not present	Present	Glucose in the urine indicates high blood glucose levels (> 180mg/dl) and may be indicative of undiagnosed or uncontrolled diabetes mellitus.
Ketone bodies (acetone)	Not present	Present	Ketones, the end product of the breakdown of fatty acids, are not normally present in the urine. They may be present in the urine of patients who have uncontrolled diabetes mellitus, are in a state of starvation or who have ingested excessive amounts of aspirin.
Blood	Not present	Occult (microscopic) Bright red	Blood may be present in the urine of patients who have urinary tract infection, kidney disease or bleeding from the urinary tract.

Another important diagnostic test used to assess patients' urinary function is a 24-hour urine collection. This test looks for sodium, creatinine and protein (Schrier, 2009) and involves collecting urine from the patient over a 24-hour period. Descriptions of other tests related to urinary functions, such as collecting urine specimens, measuring specific gravity and visualisation procedures, are given in Chapter 11.

Characteristics of normal and abnormal urine are shown in Table 21-4.

ACTIVITY 21-1

Reflect on a patient you have recently cared for who needed to pass urine. What did you need to assess in order to choose the appropriate intervention for the patient? What options were available to you?

Measuring Urinary Output

Normally, the kidneys produce urine at a rate of approximately 0.5ml per kg of body weight and is affected by many factors, including fluid intake, body fluid losses through other routes such as perspiration, and the cardiovascular and renal status of the individual. Urine outputs below 0.5ml per kg of body weight may indicate low blood volume or kidney malfunction and must be reported.

In order to measure urine output, the following procedure should be followed. Standard precautions should be implemented as urine can carry a number of infections. Once the patient has passed urine into a clean urinal, bedpan or commode the nurse should pour the urine into a measuring jug or if appropriate weigh the urine by weighing the container plus the urine, then weighing the container without the urine and subtract the two weights to determine the volume of urine: 1 gram = 1 millilitre. Once the volume of urine has been established, this information should be recorded on a fluid balance chart which is usually kept at the bedside. The fluid intake and output are then calculated at the end of each shift and at the end of 24 hours.

When measuring urine output from a patient with an indwelling urinary catheter, a similar procedure can be carried out. However, it is important that the spout of the catheter bag does not come into contact with the container used to collect the urine, as there is a high risk of infection (Pratt *et al.*, 2007).

Measuring Residual Urine

After passing urine, there is normally very little **residual urine** (urine remaining in the bladder following the voiding) present. However, if there is obstruction in the urethra (e.g. enlarged prostate gland) or loss of bladder muscle tone, the bladder may not empty fully. Residual urine is measured to assess the amount of retained urine after voiding and determine the need for interventions (e.g. medications to promote detrusor muscle contraction).

Measuring residual urine can be achieved by either using a bladder scanner or by catheterising the patient immediately after voiding. Catheterisation, however, is avoided if at all possible as it carries an increased risk of infection. Interpretation of the results is important as large volumes of residual urine can be indicative of significant urinary problems and may be the cause of recurring urinary tract infections (Docherty and McCallum, 2009).

PLANNING

The goals established will vary according to the diagnosis and defining characteristics. Examples of overall goals for patients with urinary elimination problems may include the following:

- maintain or restore a normal voiding pattern;
- regain normal urine output;
- prevent associated risks such as infection, skin breakdown, fluid and electrolyte imbalance, and lowered self-esteem;
- perform toilet activities independently with or without assistive devices.

Appropriate preventive and corrective nursing interventions that relate to these must be identified. Specific nursing activities associated with each of these interventions can be selected to meet the patient's individual needs.

IMPLEMENTING

Maintaining Normal Urinary Elimination

Most interventions to maintain normal urinary elimination are independent nursing functions. These include promoting adequate fluid intake, maintaining normal voiding habits and assisting with toileting.

Promoting Fluid Intake

Increasing fluid intake increases urine production, which in turn stimulates the micturition reflex. A normal daily intake averaging 1,500ml of measurable fluids is adequate for most adult patients.

Many patients have increased fluid requirements, necessitating a higher daily fluid intake. For example, patients who are perspiring excessively (have diaphoresis) or who are experiencing abnormal fluid losses through vomiting, gastric suction, diarrhoea or wound drainage require fluid to replace these losses in addition to their normal daily intake requirements.

Patients who are at risk of urinary tract infection or urinary calculi (stones) should consume 2,000–3,000ml of fluid daily. Dilute urine and frequent urination reduce the risk of urinary tract infection as well as stone formation.

Increased fluid intake may be contraindicated for some patients such as people with kidney failure or heart failure. For these patients, a fluid restriction may be necessary to prevent fluid overload and oedema.

Maintaining Normal Voiding Habits

The hospital environment and medications can interfere with the patient's normal voiding habits. As far as possible, it is the nurse's responsibility to maintain and encourage these normal voiding habits (see *Practice Guidelines*).

Assisting with Toileting

Patients who are ill are often weak and may require assistance with toileting. In order to maintain privacy and dignity, patients should be assisted to the bathroom where possible and the nurse should remain with them if there is a risk of falling. Patients who have difficulty with walking can be helped using wheelchairs or stand aids (see Chapter 13). Only if the patient is unable to go to the bathroom should a commode or bedpan be offered.

Preventing Urinary Tract Infections

Infections of the urinary tract are very common. Most women will have at least one urinary tract infection in their lives; however, it is more unusual in men as they have longer urethras. Most urinary tract infections (UTI) are caused by bacteria common to the intestinal environment (e.g. *Escherichia coli*). These gastrointestinal bacteria can colonise the perineal area and move into the urethra, especially when there is urethral trauma, irritation or manipulation.

For women who have experienced a UTI, nurses need to provide instructions about ways to prevent a recurrence. NHS Choices (2008) suggests a number of ways to prevent recurrence of infection:

- Drink plenty of water to flush bacteria out of the system.
- Drink cranberry juice daily. Patients who are taking warfarin should be told to avoid drinking cranberry juice as it can interfere with the metabolism of the drug (Suvarna *et al.*, 2003).

PRACTICE GUIDELINES

Maintaining Normal Voiding Habits

Positioning

- Assist the patient to a normal position for voiding: standing for male patients; for female patients, squatting or leaning slightly forward when sitting. These positions enhance movement of urine through the tract by gravity.
- If the patient is unable to ambulate to the bathroom, use a bedside commode for females and a urinal for males standing at the bedside.
- If necessary, encourage the patient to push over the pubic area with the hands or to lean forward to increase intra-abdominal pressure and external pressure on the bladder.

Relaxation

- Provide privacy for the patient. Many people cannot void in the presence of another person.
- Allow the patient sufficient time to void.
- Suggest the patient read or listen to music.
- Provide sensory stimuli that may help the patient relax. Pour warm water over the perineum of a female or have the patient sit in a warm bath to promote muscle relaxation. Applying a hot water bottle to the lower abdomen of both men and women may also foster muscle relaxation.
- Turn on running water within hearing distance of the patient to stimulate the voiding reflex and to mask the sound of voiding for people who find this embarrassing.
- Provide ordered analgesics and emotional support to relieve physical and emotional discomfort to decrease muscle tension.

Timing

- Assist patients who have the urge to void immediately. Delays only increase the difficulty in starting to void, and the desire to void may pass.
- Offer toileting assistance to the patient at usual times of voiding, for example, on awakening, before or after meals and at bedtime.

For Bed-confined Patients

- Warm the bedpan. A cold bedpan may prompt contraction of the perineal muscles and inhibit voiding.
- Elevate the head of the patient's bed to Fowler's position, place a small pillow or rolled towel at the small of the back to increase physical support and comfort, and have the patient flex the hips and knees. This position simulates the normal voiding position as closely as possible.

- Go to the toilet as the need arises, never hold on to the urine.
- Girls and women should always wipe the perineal area from front to back following urination or defecation in order to prevent introduction of gastrointestinal bacteria into the urethra.
- Practice good hygiene, wash genitalia daily.
- Empty the bladder after sex.
- Avoid nylon and other types of synthetic underwear, as these can help promote the growth of bacteria. Loose fitting cotton underwear should be worn instead.

ACTIVITY 21-2

A patient informs you that it burns when she passes urine. What would you need to do?

Managing Urinary Incontinence

It is important to remember that urinary incontinence is not a normal part of ageing and often is treatable. Independent nursing interventions for patients with urinary incontinence (UI) include (a) a behaviour-oriented continence training programme that may consist of bladder training, habit training, prompted voiding, pelvic muscle exercises and positive reinforcement; (b) meticulous skin care; and (c) for males, application of an external drainage device (condom-type catheter device).

Promoting Continence

Promoting continence requires the involvement of the patient, the patient's family and the multidisciplinary team, in order for an individualised programme to be designed. The programme may include the following:

- Education of the patient and their family.
- Bladder training, involves the patient postponing voiding, resisting the sensation of urgency and voiding according to a timetable rather than according to the urge to void. Over the course of the programme, the patient will be required to lengthen the intervals between urination with the ultimate goal of bladder stabilisation and diminished urgency. This form of training may be used for patients who have bladder instability and urge incontinence.
- Habit training, also referred to as timed voiding or scheduled toileting, attempts to keep patients dry by having them void at regular intervals. With habit training, there is no attempt to motivate the patient to delay voiding if the urge occurs.

- Prompted voiding supplements habit training by encouraging the patient to try to use the toilet (prompting) and reminding the patient when to void.

Pelvic Floor Exercises

Pelvic floor exercises strengthen pelvic floor muscles in women and can reduce episodes of incontinence. The patient can identify perineal muscles by stopping urination mid-stream or by tightening the anal sphincter as if to hold a bowel movement.

Pelvic floor exercises can be performed anytime, anywhere, sitting or standing – even when voiding. Specific patient instructions for performing pelvic floor exercises are summarised in *Teaching: Patient Care.*

TEACHING: PATIENT CARE

Pelvic Floor Exercises

- First, sit or stand with the legs apart.
- Pull your rectum, urethra and vagina up inside, and hold for a count of 3-5 seconds. The pull should be felt at the cleft of your buttocks.
- Initially perform each contraction 10 times, five times daily.
- Develop a schedule that will help remind you to do these exercises.
- Try to start and stop your stream of urine.
- To control episodes of stress incontinence squeeze the pelvic floor muscles when doing any activity that increases intra-abdominal pressure, such as coughing, laughing, sneezing or lifting.

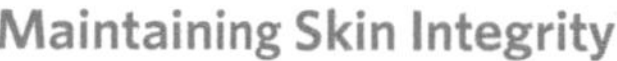

Maintaining Skin Integrity

Skin that is continually moist becomes macerated (softened). Urine that accumulates on the skin is converted to ammonia, which is very irritating to the skin. Because both skin irritation and maceration predispose the patient to skin breakdown and ulceration, the incontinent person requires meticulous skin care. To maintain skin integrity, the nurse washes the patient's perineal area with soap and water after episodes of incontinence, rinses it thoroughly, dries it gently and thoroughly, and provides clean, dry clothing or bed linen. If the skin is irritated, the nurse applies barrier creams such as zinc oxide ointment to protect it from contact with urine. If it is necessary to pad the patient's clothes for protection, the nurse should use products that absorb wetness and leave a dry surface in contact with the skin.

Specially designed incontinence sheets are double layered, quilted and have a waterproof backing on the underside. The design of the sheet allows fluid (i.e. urine) to pass through the upper quilted layer and be absorbed, leaving the quilted surface dry to the touch. This absorbent sheet helps maintain skin integrity; it does not stick to the skin when wet and reduces odour.

Applying External Urinary Drainage Devices (Penile Sheath)

The application of a penile sheath or external catheter connected to a urinary drainage system is commonly prescribed for incontinent males. Use of a penile sheaths is preferable to insertion of an indwelling catheter because the risk of urinary tract infection is minimal. *Procedure 21-1* on page 650 describes how to apply and remove a penile sheath.

Managing Urinary Retention

Interventions that assist the patient to maintain a normal voiding pattern, discussed earlier, also apply when dealing with urinary retention. Patients who have a flaccid bladder (weak, soft and lax bladder muscles) may use manual pressure on the bladder to promote bladder emptying. This is known as Credé's manoeuvre or Credé's method, which is normally only used for patients who have lost and are not expected to regain voluntary bladder control. When all measures fail to initiate voiding, urinary catheterisation may be necessary to empty the bladder completely. An indwelling Foley catheter may be inserted until the underlying cause is treated. Alternatively, intermittent catheterisation (every 3–4 hours) may be performed because the risk of urinary tract infection may be less than with an indwelling catheter.

Urinary Catheterisation

Urinary catheterisation is the introduction of a catheter through the urethra into the urinary bladder. This is usually performed only when absolutely necessary, because the danger exists of introducing micro-organisms into the bladder. Patients who are immunocompromised are at the greatest risk. Once an infection is introduced into the bladder, it can ascend the ureters and eventually involve the kidneys. The hazard of infection remains after the catheter is in place because normal defence mechanisms such as intermittent flushing of micro-organisms from the urethra through voiding are bypassed. Therefore urinary catheters have to be inserted under strict asepsis.

Another hazard is trauma, particularly in the male patient, whose urethra is longer and more tortuous. It is important to insert a catheter along the normal contour of the urethra. Damage to the urethra can occur if the catheter is forced through strictures or at an incorrect angle. In males, the urethra is normally curved, but it can be straightened by elevating the penis to a position perpendicular to the body.

Catheters are commonly made of rubber or plastics although they may be made from latex, silicone or polyvinyl chloride (PVC). They are sized by the diameter of the lumen using the French (Fr) scale: the larger the number, the larger the lumen. Some catheters are designed for intermittent catheterisation whereby the tube is inserted, the bladder drained and the tube is removed. Others, indwelling catheters, are designed to remain within the bladder.

There are two basic types of catheters available for intermittent catheterisation, uncoated and coated PVC Nelaton. They both come in various sizes from 10–14 Charrier (ch) and come in female or male lengths. The uncoated catheter requires separate lubrication in order to enter the urethra easily and prevent discomfort and can be reused while the coated catheters are single use only and do not require separate lubrication to be inserted.

The indwelling, or Foley, catheter is a double-lumen catheter. The larger lumen drains urine from the bladder. A second, smaller lumen is used to inflate a balloon near the tip of the catheter to hold the catheter in place within the bladder (see Figure 21-5). Patients who require continuous or intermittent bladder irrigation may have a three-way Foley catheter (see Figure 21-6). The three-way catheter has a third lumen through which sterile irrigating fluid can flow into the bladder. The fluid then exits the bladder through the drainage lumen, along with the urine.

The balloons of indwelling catheters are various sizes; paediatric catheters hold 2.5–5ml while adult catheters hold 10–50ml depending on the manufacturer. The *Practice Guidelines* provides guidance on catheter selection.

Indwelling catheters are connected via tubing to a gravity drainage system. This system consists of a drainage tube and a collecting bag for the urine and depends on the force of gravity to drain urine from the bladder to the collecting bag. *Procedure 21-2* (see page 651) describes catheterisation of females and males, using straight and retention catheters.

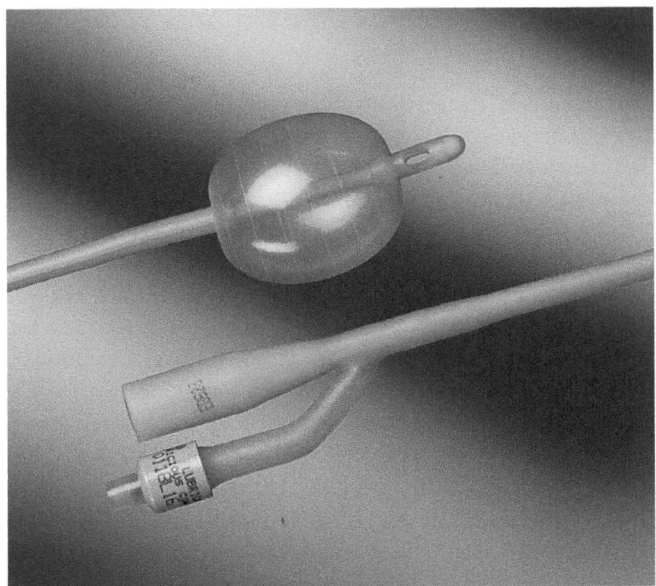

Figure 21-5 A retention (Foley) catheter with the balloon inflated.
Source: courtesy of C.R. Bard Inc.

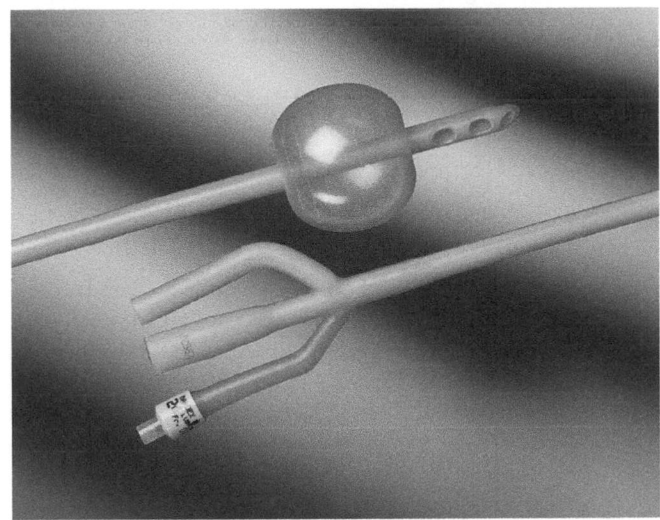

Figure 21-6 A three-way Foley catheter.
Source: courtesy of C.R. Bard Inc.

ACTIVITY 21-3

Urinary catheterisation is a procedure that should only be used when all other options have been considered. Think of three reasons why you would not routinely catheterise a patient.

Nursing Interventions for Patients with Indwelling Catheters

Nursing care of the patient with an indwelling catheter and continuous drainage is largely directed towards preventing infection of the urinary tract and encouraging urinary flow through the drainage system.

The patient with an indwelling catheter should drink up to 3,000ml per day if permitted. Large amounts of fluid ensure a large urine output, which keeps the bladder flushed out and decreases the likelihood of urinary stasis and subsequent infection. Large volumes of urine also minimise the risk of sediment or other particles obstructing the drainage tubing.

Acidifying the urine of patients with an indwelling catheter may reduce the risk of urinary tract infection and calculus formation. Foods such as eggs, cheese, meat and poultry, whole grains, cranberries, plums, prunes and tomatoes tend to increase the acidity of urine. Conversely, most fruits and vegetables, legumes and milk and milk products result in alkaline urine.

No special cleaning other than routine hygienic care is necessary for patients with retention catheters, nor is special meatal care recommended. Local policy regarding catheter care should be adhered to.

Routine changing of catheter and tubing is not recommended. A collection of sediment in the catheter or tubing or impaired urine drainage are indicators for changing the catheter and drainage system. When this occurs, the catheter and drainage system are removed and discarded, and a new sterile catheter is inserted and attached to a new drainage system.

Guidelines to prevent catheter-associated urinary tract infections are given in the *Practice Guidelines*. Ongoing assessment of patients with indwelling catheters is a high priority. The nurse should:

- Ensure that there are no obstructions in the drainage. Check that there are no kinks in the tubing, the patient is not lying on the tubing, and the tubing is not clogged with mucus or blood.
- Check that there is no tension on the catheter or tubing.
- Ensure that gravity drainage is maintained. Make sure there are no loops in the tubing below its entry to the drainage receptacle and that the drainage receptacle is below the level of the patient's bladder.
- Ensure that the drainage system is well sealed and that there are no leaks at the connection sites.
- Observe the flow of the urine as indicated by the patient's condition, and note colour, odour and any abnormal constituents. If sediment is present, check the catheter more frequently to ascertain whether it is plugged.

PRACTICE GUIDELINES

Selecting an Appropriate Urinary Catheter

- Select the type of material in accordance with the estimated length of the catheterisation period.
- Use polyvinyl chlorine or plastic catheters for short periods only (e.g. one week or less), because they are inflexible.
- Use plain latex catheters for periods of 2-3 weeks. Latex may be used for patients with no known latex allergy. However, because of these allergies, latex is being phased out of healthcare products.
- Use polytetrafluorothylene (PTFE) for up to four weeks.
- Use silicone elastomer catheters for long-term use (e.g. 2-3 months) because they create less encrustation at the urethral meatus. However, they are expensive.
- Use hydrogel catheters for periods of up to 12 weeks.
- Use polymer hydromer for up to 12 weeks.
- Use pure silicone catheters for patients who have latex allergies. There can be left in place for up to 12 weeks.
- Determine appropriate catheter length by the patient's gender. For adult female patients, use a 22cm catheter; for adult male patients, a 40cm catheter.
- Determine appropriate catheter size by the size of the urethral canal. Use sizes such as #8 or #10 for children, #14 or #16 for adults. Men frequently require a larger size than women, for example, #18.

Removing Indwelling Catheters

Indwelling catheters are removed when clinically indicated. If the catheter has been in place for a short time (e.g. a few days), the patient usually has little difficulty regaining normal urinary elimination patterns. Swelling of the urethra, however, may initially interfere with voiding, so the nurse should regularly assess the patient for urinary retention until voiding is re-established.

Patients who have had an indwelling catheter for a prolonged period may require bladder retraining to regain bladder muscle tone. With an indwelling catheter in place, the bladder muscle does not stretch and contract regularly as it does when the bladder fills and empties by voiding. A few days before removal, the catheter may be clamped for specified periods of time (e.g. 2–4 hours), then released to allow the bladder to empty. This allows the bladder to distend and stimulates its musculature. Check local policy regarding bladder training procedures.

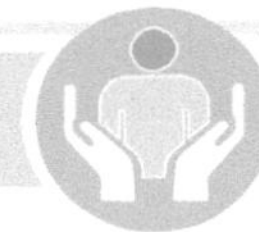

PRACTICE GUIDELINES

Preventing Catheter-Associated Urinary Infections

- Have an established infection control programme.
- Catheterise patients only when necessary, by using aseptic technique and sterile equipment.
- Do not disconnect the catheter and drainage tubing unless absolutely necessary.
- Remove the catheter as soon as possible.
- Follow and reinforce good hand-washing technique.
- Provide routine perineal hygiene.
- Prevent contamination of the catheter with faeces in the incontinent patient.

To remove a retention catheter, the nurse follows these steps:

- Obtain a receptacle for the catheter (e.g. a disposable basin); a clean, disposable towel; clean gloves; and a sterile syringe to deflate the balloon. The syringe should be large enough to withdraw all the solution in the catheter balloon. The size of the balloon is indicated on the label at the end of the catheter.
- Ask the patient to assume a supine position as for a catheterisation.
- Put on clean gloves and place the towel between the legs of the female patient or over the thighs of the male.
- Insert the syringe into the injection port of the catheter, and withdraw the fluid from the balloon.
- Do not pull the catheter while the balloon is inflated; doing so may injure the urethra.
- After all of the fluid is withdrawn from the balloon, gently withdraw the catheter and place it in the waste receptacle.
- It may be necessary, if clinically indicated, to send the tip of the catheter to the pathology laboratory. The tip should be removed using a sterile scissors and placed in an appropriate sterile container which is labelled with the patient's details.
- Dry the perineal area with a towel.
- Remove gloves.
- Measure the urine in the drainage bag, and record the removal of the catheter. Include in the recording (a) the time the catheter was removed; (b) the amount, colour and clarity of the urine; (c) the intactness of the catheter; and (d) instructions given to the patient.
- Following removal of the catheter, determine the time of the first voiding and the amount voided during the first eight hours. Compare this output to the patient's intake.

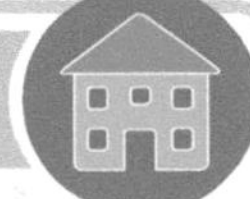

COMMUNITY CARE CONSIDERATIONS

Issues for People Living with Long-Term Urinary Catheters in the Community

- Urinary tract infections
- Leakage
- Discomfort
- Interference in daily life
- Need to seek urgent medical care

Source: based on O'Donahue *et al.* (2010).

Clean Intermittent Self-Catheterisation

Clean intermittent self-catheterisation (CISC) is performed by many patients who have some form of neurogenic bladder dysfunction, such as that caused by spinal cord injury. Clean or medical aseptic technique is used. Intermittent self-catheterisation:

- enables the patient to retain independence and gain control of the bladder;
- reduces incidence of urinary tract infection;
- protects the upper urinary tract from reflux;
- allows normal sexual relations without incontinence;
- reduces the use of aids and appliances;
- frees the patient from embarrassing dribbling.

The procedure for self-catheterisation is similar to that used by the nurse to catheterise a patient. Essential steps are outlined in the *Teaching: Patient Care*. Because the procedure requires physical and mental preparation, patient assessment is important. The patient should have:

- sufficient manual dexterity to manipulate a catheter;
- sufficient mental ability;
- motivation and acceptance of the procedure;
- for women, reasonable agility to access the urethra;
- bladder capacity greater than 100ml.

Before teaching CISC, the nurse should establish the patient's voiding patterns, the volume voided, fluid intake and residual amounts. CISC is easier for males to learn because of the visibility of the urinary meatus. Females need to learn initially with the aid of a mirror but eventually should perform the procedure by using only the sense of touch (as described in *Teaching: Patient Care*).

TEACHING: PATIENT CARE

Clean Intermittent Self-Catheterisation

- Catheterise as often as needed. At first, catheterisation may be necessary every 2–3 hours, increasing to 4–6 hours.
- Attempt to void before catheterisation; insert the catheter to remove residual urine if unable to void or if amount voided is insufficient (e.g. less than 100ml).
- Assemble all needed supplies ahead of time. Good lighting is essential, especially for women.
- If a woman, remove a tampon before catheterising. *A tampon can inhibit catheterisation.*
- Wash your hands.
- Clean the urinary meatus with either a flannel or soapy washcloth, and then rinse with a wet washcloth. Women should clean the area from front to back.
- Assume a position that is comfortable and that facilitates passage of the catheter, such as a semi-reclining position in bed or sitting on a chair or the toilet. Men may prefer to stand over the toilet; women may prefer to stand with one foot on the side of the bathtub.
- Apply lubricant to the catheter tip (2.5cm) for women; (5–15cm) for men.
- Insert the catheter until urine flows through.

(a) If a woman, locate the **meatus** using a mirror or other aid, or use the 'touch' technique as follows:
  - Place the index finger of the nondominant hand on the clitoris.
  - Place the third and fourth fingers at the vagina.
  - Locate the meatus between the index and third fingers.
  - Direct the catheter through the meatus and then upward and forward.

(b) If a man, hold the penis with a slight upward tension at a 60- to 90-degree angle to insert the catheter. Return the penis to its natural position when urine starts to flow.
  - Hold the catheter in place until all urine is drained.
  - Withdraw the catheter slowly to ensure complete drainage of urine.
  - Wash the catheter with soap and water; store in a clean container. Replace the catheter when it becomes difficult to clean, or too soft or hard to insert easily.
  - The patient should be told to inform their general practitioner if their urine becomes cloudy or contains sediment; if there is bleeding, difficulty or pain when passing the catheter; or if the patient has a fever.
  - Drink at least 2,000–2,500ml of fluid a day to ensure adequate bladder filling and flushing.

Urinary Diversions

A urinary diversion is the surgical rerouting of urine from the kidneys to a site other than the bladder. Urinary diversions are usually created when the bladder must be removed, for example, because of cancer or trauma. The most common urinary diversion is the ileal conduit or ileal loop (see Figure 21-7). In this procedure, a segment of the ileum is removed and the intestinal ends are reattached. One end of the portion removed is closed with sutures to create a pouch, and the other end is brought out through the abdominal wall to create a stoma. The ureters are implanted into the ileal pouch and urine drains continuously.

When caring for patients with a urinary diversion, the nurse must accurately assess intake and output, note any changes in urine colour, odour or clarity (mucous shreds are commonly seen in the urine of patients with an ileal diversion), and frequently assess the condition of the stoma and surrounding skin. Patients who must wear a urine collection appliance are at risk for impaired skin integrity because of irritation by urine. Well-fitting appliances are vital. The nurse should consult with a stoma nurse and continence nurse to identify the most appropriate appliance for the patient's needs.

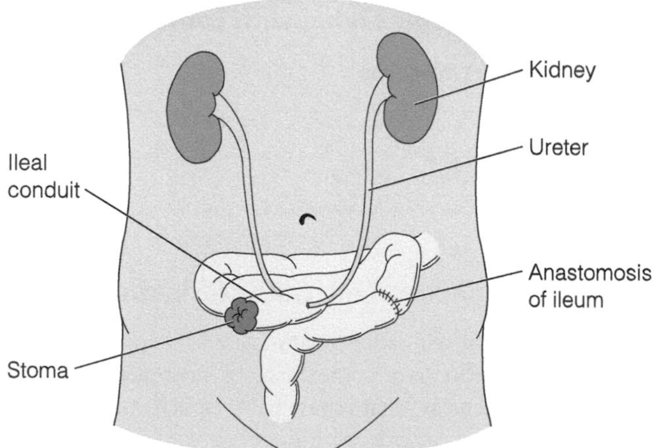

Figure 21-7 An ileal conduit.

Patients with urinary diversions may experience problems with their body image and sexuality and may require assistance in coping with these changes and managing the stoma. Most patients are able to resume their normal activities and lifestyle.

Suprapubic Catheter Care

A suprapubic catheter is inserted through the abdominal wall above the symphysis pubis into the urinary bladder (see Figure 21-8). It is inserted using local anaesthesia or during bladder or vaginal surgery. The catheter may be secured in place with sutures if a retention balloon is not used. The suprapubic catheter may be placed for temporary bladder drainage until the patient is able to resume normal voiding or may be a permanent device.

Care of patients with a suprapubic catheter includes regular assessments of the patient's urine, fluid intake and comfort; maintenance of a patent drainage system; skin care around the insertion site; and periodic clamping of the catheter preparatory to removing it if it is not a permanent appliance. If the catheter is temporary, orders generally include leaving the catheter open to drainage for 48–72 hours, then clamping the catheter for three- to four-hour periods during the day until the patient can void satisfactory amounts. Satisfactory voiding is determined by measuring the patient's residual urine after voiding.

Care of the catheter insertion site involves sterile technique. Dressings around the newly placed suprapubic catheter are changed whenever they are soiled with drainage to prevent bacterial growth around the insertion site and reduce the potential for infection. For catheters that have been in place for an extended period, no dressing may be needed and the healed insertion tract enables removal and replacement of the catheter as needed. The nurse assesses the insertion area at regular intervals. Any redness or discharge at the skin around the insertion site must be reported.

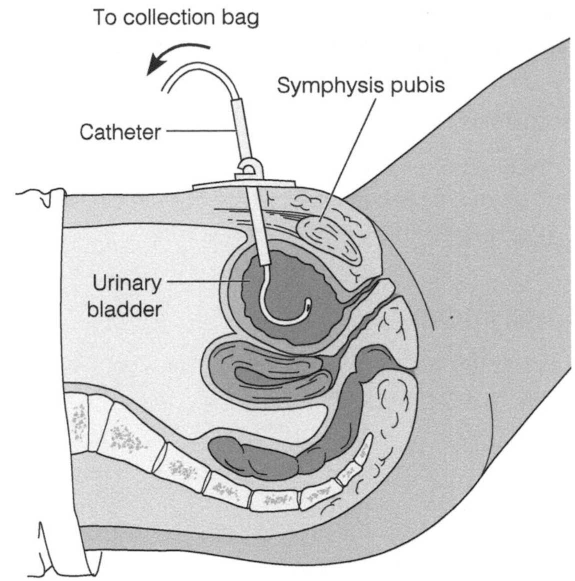

Figure 21-8 A suprapubic catheter in place.

RESEARCH NOTE

RCT of Urethral versus Suprapubic Catheterisation

This randomised controlled trial aimed to compare the use of intermittent urethral catheterisation with indwelling suprapubic catheterisation in women undergoing surgery for urodynamic stress incontinence or uterovaginal prolapsed. Seventy-two women participated in the study and were put into two groups. Group one had bladder drainage using a suprapubic catheter and group two was catheterised intermittently post-operatively. The results showed that intermittent catheterisation following urogynaecological surgery was associated with a more rapid return to normal micturation and a shorter hospital stay. No difference was noted in the rate of urinary tract infections between the two groups.

Source: based on Dixon, L., Dolan, L.M., Brown, K. and Hilton, P. (2010) 'RCT of urethral versus suprapubic catheterisation', *British Journal of Nursing* (Continence Care Supplement), 19(18), S7–S13.

EVALUATING

Using the overall goals and desired outcomes identified in the planning stage, the nurse collects data to evaluate the effectiveness of nursing activities. If the desired outcomes are not achieved, explore the reasons before modifying the care plan.

PROCEDURE 21-1 Applying a Penile Sheath

Purposes

- To collect urine and control urinary incontinence
- To permit the patient physical activity without fear of embarrassment because of leaking urine
- To prevent skin irritation as a result of urine incontinence

Assessment

- Review the patient record to determine a pattern to voiding and other pertinent data.
- Apply clean gloves and examine the patient's penis for swelling or excoriation that would contraindicate use of the condom catheter.

Planning

Determine if the patient has had an external catheter previously and any difficulties with it. Perform any procedures that are best completed without the catheter in place, for example, weighing the patient would be easier without the tubing and bag. Ensure that the correct size of external catheter is ordered.

Equipment

- Leg drainage bag with tubing or urinary drainage bag with tubing
- Penile sheath with adhesive
- Clean gloves
- Basin of warm water and soap
- Washcloth and towel
- Elastic tape or Velcro strap

Implementation

Preparation

- Assemble the leg drainage bag or urinary drainage bag for attachment to the condom sheath.
- Roll the condom outward onto itself to facilitate easier application (see Figure 21-9). On some models, an inner flap will be exposed. This flap is applied around the urinary meatus to prevent the reflux of urine.
- Position the patient in either a supine or a sitting position.

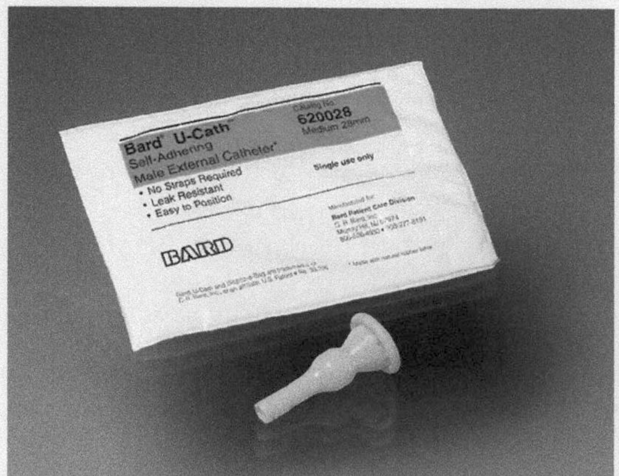

Figure 21-9 Before application, roll the condom outward onto itself.

Source: courtesy of C.R. Bard Inc.

Performance

1. Explain to the procedure to the patient. *To gain consent and reduce anxiety.*
2. Wash hands, apply clean gloves and observe appropriate infection control procedures. *To prevent cross-contamination.*
3. Provide for patient privacy. *To maintain patient dignity and reduce anxiety.*
4. Drape the patient appropriately with the bath blanket, exposing only the penis. *To maintain patient dignity and reduce anxiety.*
5. Clean the genital area and dry it thoroughly. *This minimises skin irritation and excoriation after the sheath is applied.*
6. Apply and secure the condom. Roll the sheath smoothly over the penis, leaving 2.5cm between the end of the penis and the rubber or plastic connecting tube (see Figure 21-10). *This space prevents irritation of the tip of the penis and provides for full drainage of urine.*
   - Secure the sheath firmly, but not too tightly, to the penis. *To ensure blood supply to the penis.*
   - Make sure that the tip of the penis is not touching the sheath and that the sheath is not twisted. *A twisted sheath could obstruct the flow of urine.*
   - Attach the urinary drainage system to the sheath. *To prevent leakage.*
   - Remove the gloves and wash your hands.

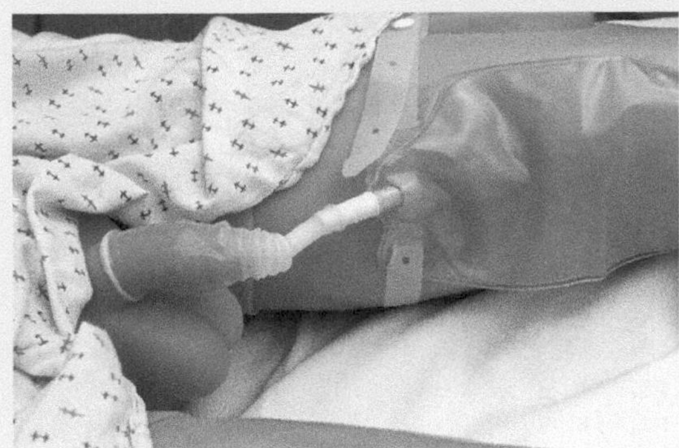

Figure 21-10 The condom rolled over the penis.

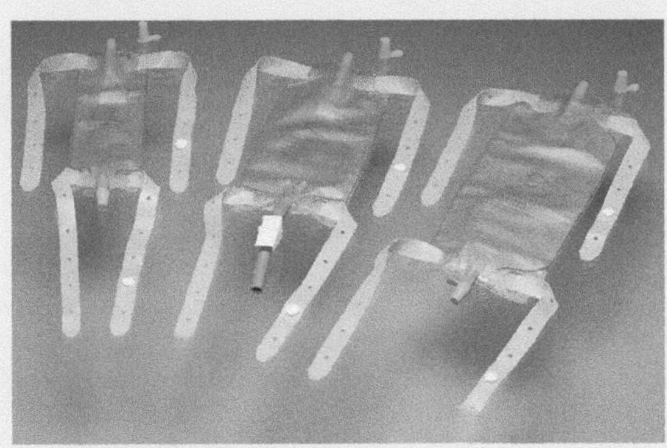

Figure 21-11 Urinary drainage leg bags.
Source: courtesy of C.R. Bard Inc.

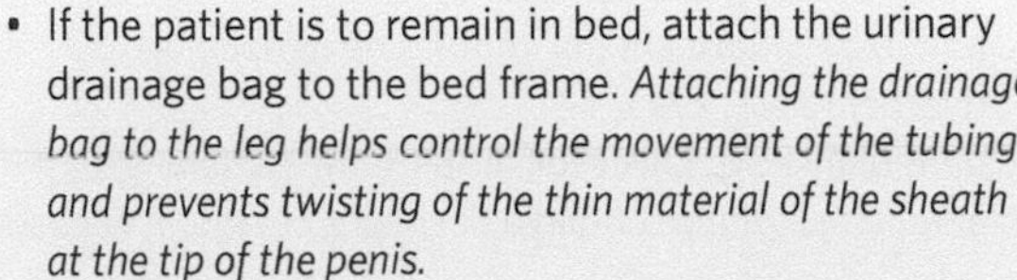

- If the patient is to remain in bed, attach the urinary drainage bag to the bed frame. *Attaching the drainage bag to the leg helps control the movement of the tubing and prevents twisting of the thin material of the sheath at the tip of the penis.*
- If the patient is ambulatory, attach the bag to the patient's leg (see Figure 21-11).

7 The patient should be taught to keep the drainage bag below the level of the sheath and to avoid loops or kinks in the tubing. *To facilitate drainage of urine.*

8 Inspect the penis 30 minutes following the sheath application, and check urine flow.

9 Assess the penis for swelling and discoloration. *This may indicate that the sheath is too tight.*

10 Change the sheath daily and provide skin care. *To prevent infection.*

11 To remove sheath - apply clean gloves and roll the sheath off and wash the penis with water, rinse and dry thoroughly. Reapply a new sheath as necessary.

12 Discuss the outcomes with the patient and document findings in the patient's notes. *To inform the patient and other healthcare professionals.*

Evaluation

- Regularly review the patient, particularly if there are any signs of swelling or discoloration or if there is reduced urine output.
- If necessary report any findings to the doctor or senior nurse.

PROCEDURE 21-2 Performing Urinary Catheterisation

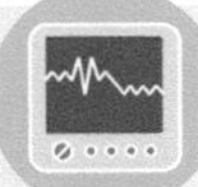

Purposes

- To relieve discomfort due to bladder distention or to provide gradual decompression of a distended bladder
- To assess the amount of residual urine if the bladder empties incompletely
- To empty the bladder completely prior to surgery
- To facilitate accurate measurement of urinary output for critically ill patients whose output needs to be monitored hourly
- To provide for intermittent or continuous bladder drainage and irrigation
- To prevent urine from contacting an incision after perineal surgery
- To manage incontinence when other measures have failed

Assessment

- Determine the most appropriate method of catheterisation based on the purpose and any criteria specified in the order such as total amount of urine to be removed or size of catheter to be used.

- Assess the patient's overall condition. Determine if the patient is able to cooperate during the procedure and if the patient can be positioned supine with head relatively flat.
- Determine when the patient last voided or was last catheterised.
- Palpate the bladder to check for fullness or distension.

Planning

Allow adequate time to perform the catheterisation. Although the entire procedure can require as little as 15 minutes, several sources of difficulty could result in a much longer time. If possible, it should not be performed just prior to or after the patient eats.

Equipment

- Sterile catheter of appropriate size. (An extra catheter should also be at hand.)
- Catheterisation kit (see Figure 21-12) or individual sterile items:
  - foil bowl
  - cotton wool balls
  - gauze swabs
  - forceps
  - cardboard tray
  - small gallipot
  - paper towels
  - paper sheet
  - sterile gloves
  - cleansing fluid as in local policy
- For an indwelling catheter:
  - syringe and sterile water to fill balloon
  - collection bag and tubing
  - antiseptic, lubricant gel containing lignocaine hydrochloride 2%
  - bath blanket or sheet for draping the patient
  - adequate lighting (obtain a flashlight or lamp if necessary).

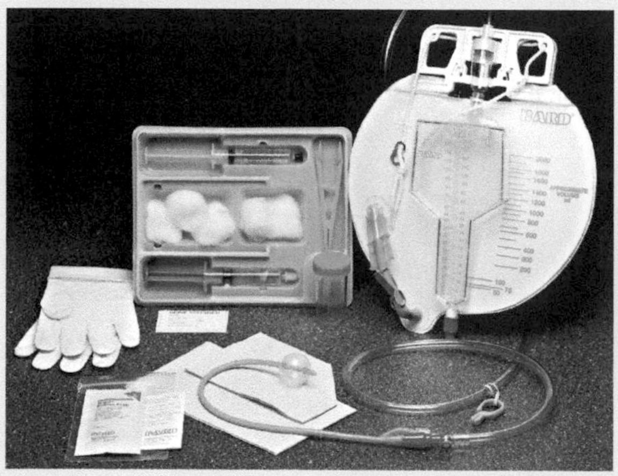

(a)

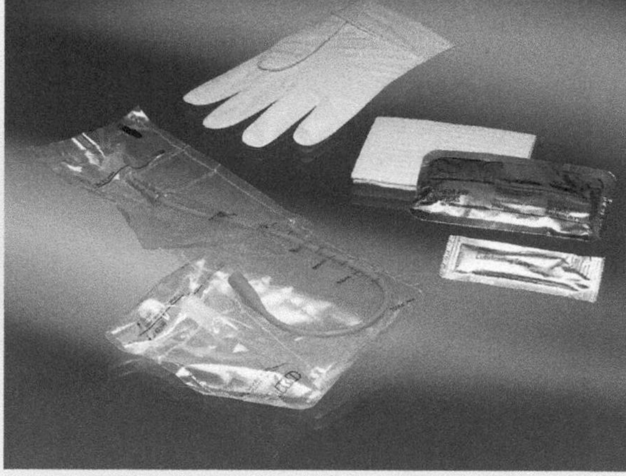

(b)

Figure 21-12 Catheter insertion kits: (a) indwelling; (b) straight. (Courtesy of C.R. Bard Inc.)

Implementation

Preparation

- If using a catheterisation kit check the expiry date.

Performance

1. Follow local policy to ensure that you explain to the patient what you are going to do, why it is necessary and how they can cooperate. Obtain consent and maintain patient privacy and dignity and ensure that the appropriate local infection control procedures are observed.
2. Position the patient appropriately:
   - **Female**: supine with knees flexed and externally rotated.
   - **Male**: supine, legs slightly abducted. *To provide easy access and comfort for the patient.*
3. Make sure there is adequate lighting.
4. Wash hands and dry hands and observe appropriate infection control procedures. *To prevent cross-contamination.*
5. Prepare a sterile field and equipment using an aseptic technique. *To prevent cross-contamination.*
6. If using a collecting bag and it is not contained within the catheterisation kit, open the drainage package and place the end of the tubing within reach. *Since one hand is needed to hold the cathether once it is in place, open the package while two hands are still available.*
7. Repeat handwashing, then dry hands and put on sterile gloves. *To prevent cross-contamination.*

8 Arrange sterile towels to cover the surrounding area and fill the syringe with the sterile water and attach to the indwelling catheter inflation hub and test the balloon. *If the balloon malfunctions, it is important to replace it prior to use.*

9 Cleanse the meatus. *To prevent cross-contamination.*
Note: The nondominant hand is considered contaminated once it touches the patient's skin.
- **Women**: Use your nondominant hand to spread the labia. Using the forceps moisten a cotton ball/gauze with solution (see local policy for type of solution) and wipe one side of the labia majora in an anteroposterior direction (see Figure 21-13).
  Use a new cotton ball/gauze for the opposite side. Repeat process for labia minora. Then finally cleanse the meatus.
- **Men**: Use your nondominant hand to grasp the penis just below the glans. If necessary, retract the foreskin. Hold the penis firmly upright, with slight tension. *Lifting the penis in this manner helps straighten the urethra.* Using the forceps moisten a cotton ball/gauze with solution (see local policy for type of solution) and wipe the centre of the meatus in a circular motion around the glans. Repeat three more times.

10 Insert local anaesthetic gel into the urethral meatus according to manufacturer's instructions. *The local anaesthetic will act both as a lubricant and numb the area.*

11 Wait 3–4 minutes for the anaesthetic gel to take effect.

12 Wash and dry hands and put on a new pair of sterile gloves. *To prevent cross-contamination.*

13 Place the collecting tray on paper towel close to the patient. *To collect urine once the catheter has been inserted.*

14 Open the catheter on the sterile field so that it is ready to use.

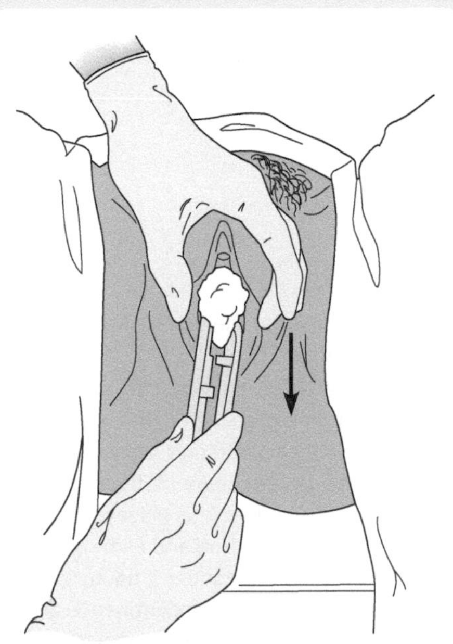

Figure 21-13 When cleaning the urinary meatus, move the swab downward.

15 Insert the catheter.
- Grasp the catheter firmly 4–6cm from the tip. Ask the patient to take a slow deep breath and insert the catheter as the patient exhales. Slight resistance is expected as the catheter passes through the sphincters. If necessary, twist the catheter or hold pressure on the catheter until the sphincter relaxes.
- Advance the catheter 4cm further after the urine begins to flow through it. *To be sure the catheter is fully in the bladder.*
- If the catheter accidentally contacts the labia or slips into the vagina, it is considered contaminated and a new, sterile catheter must be used. The contaminated catheter may be left in the vagina until the new catheter is inserted to help avoid mistaking the vaginal opening for the urethral meatus. For an indwelling catheter, inflate the retention balloon with the designated volume.
- Pull gently on the catheter until resistance is felt to ensure that the balloon has inflated and to place it in the trigone of the bladder (see Figure 21-14(a) and (b)).

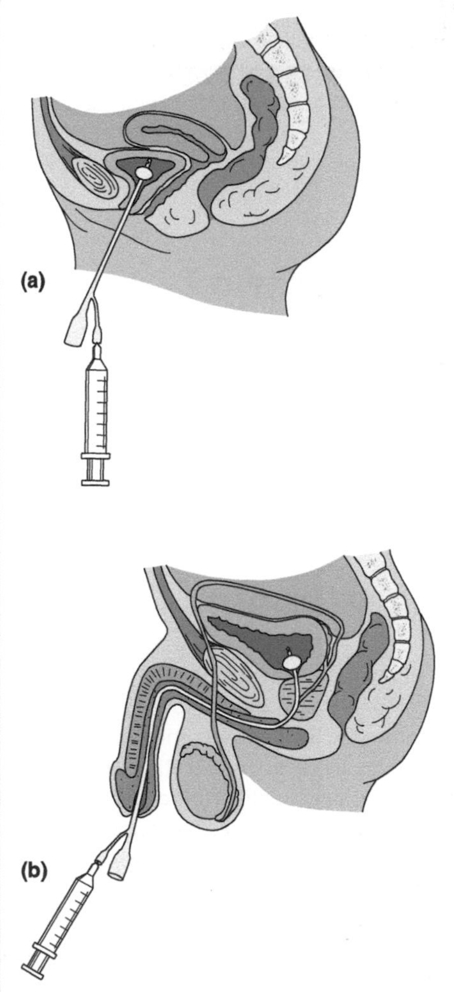

Figure 21-14 Placement of retention catheter and inflated balloon in (a) female patient; and (b) male patient.

16 For intermittent catheterisation, when the urine flow stops remove the catheter. For an indwelling catheter, secure the collecting tubing to the bed linens and hang the bag below the level of the bladder. No tubing should fall below the top of the bag (see Figure 21-15). *To prevent pulling on the catheter and aid drainage of urine.*

17 Wipe the perineal area of any remaining antiseptic or lubricant. Replace the foreskin if retracted earlier. Return the patient to a comfortable position. *To provide comfort for the patient.*

18 Discard all used supplies appropriately and wash your hands.

19 Document the catheterisation procedure including catheter size and results in the patient's notes. *To inform other healthcare professionals.*

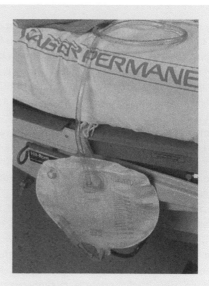

Figure 21-15 Correct position for urine drainage bag and tubing.

Evaluation

- Perform a detailed follow-up based on findings that deviated from expected or normal for the patient. Relate findings to previous assessment data if available.
- Teach the patient how to care for the indwelling catheter, to drink more fluids, and other appropriate instructions.

CRITICAL REFLECTION

Let us revisit the case study on page 635. Now that you have read this chapter reflect on the process of urination and the impact incontinence can have on the individual. How would you assess a patient with urinary incontinence? What interventions would you implement to promote continence?

CHAPTER HIGHLIGHTS

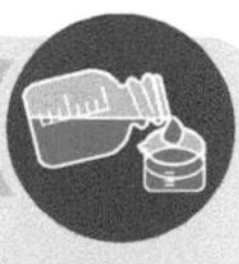

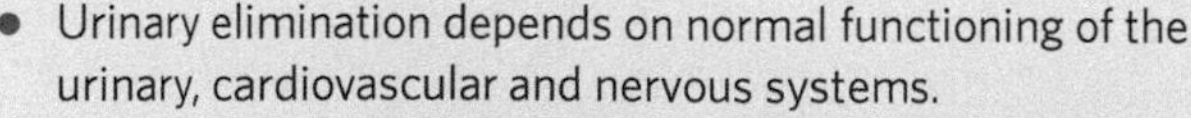

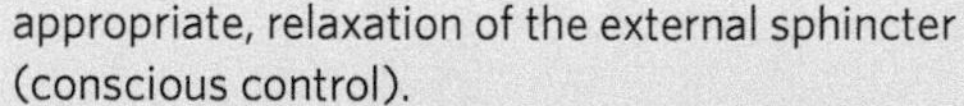

- Urinary elimination depends on normal functioning of the urinary, cardiovascular and nervous systems.
- Urine is formed in the nephron, the functional unit of the kidney, through a process of filtration, reabsorption and secretion. Hormones such as antidiuretic hormone (ADH) and aldosterone affect the reabsorption of sodium and water, thus affecting the amount of urine formed.
- The normal process of urination is stimulated when sufficient urine collects in the bladder to stimulate stretch receptors. Impulses from stretch receptors are transmitted to the spinal cord and the brain, causing relaxation of the internal sphincter (unconscious control) and, if appropriate, relaxation of the external sphincter (conscious control).
- In the adult, urination generally occurs after 250–450ml of urine has collected in the bladder.
- Many factors influence a person's urinary elimination, including growth and development, fluid intake, stress, activity, medications and various diseases.
- Alterations in urine production and elimination include polyuria, oliguria, anuria, frequency, nocturia, urgency, dysuria, enuresis, haematuria, incontinence and retention. Each may have various influencing and associated factors that need to be identified.

- Assessment of a patient's urinary function includes (a) patient history that identifies voiding patterns, recent changes, past and current problems with urination, and factors influencing the elimination pattern; (b) a physical assessment of the genitourinary system; (c) inspection of the urine for amount, colour, clarity and odour; and, if indicated; (d) testing of urine for specific gravity, pH and the presence of glucose, ketone bodies, protein and occult blood.
- Incontinence can be physically and emotionally distressing to patients because it is considered socially unacceptable.
- Bladder training can often reduce episodes of incontinence.
- Patients with urinary retention not only experience discomfort but also are at risk of urinary tract infection.
- The most common cause of urinary tract infection is invasive procedures such as catheterisation and cystoscopic examination. Women in particular are prone to ascending urinary tract infections because of their short urethras.
- Goals for the patient with problems with urinary elimination include maintaining or restoring normal elimination patterns and preventing associated risks such as skin breakdown.
- Nursing interventions related to urinary elimination are generally directed towards facilitating the normal functioning of the urinary system or towards assisting the patient with particular problems.
- Interventions include (a) assisting the patient to maintain an appropriate fluid intake, (b) assisting the patient to maintain normal voiding patterns, (c) monitoring the patient's daily fluid intake and output, and (d) maintaining cleanliness of the genital area.
- Urinary catheterisation is frequently required for patients with urinary retention but is only performed when all other measures to facilitate voiding fail. Sterile technique is essential to prevent ascending urinary infections.
- Care of patients with indwelling catheters is directed towards preventing infection of the urinary tract and encouraging urinary flow through the drainage system.
- Patients with urinary retention may be taught to perform clean intermittent self-catheterisation to enhance their independence, reduce the risk of infection and eliminate incontinence.
- When the urinary bladder is removed, a urinary diversion is formed to allow urine to be eliminated from the body. The ileal conduit or ileal loop is the most common diversion and requires that the patient wear a urine collection device continually over the stoma.

ACTIVITY ANSWERS

ACTIVITY 21-1 You would need to assess the patient's mobility, pain levels and vital signs. If the patient is stable and is able to mobilise they should be encouraged to use the toilet. However, if the patient is unable to walk they could be wheeled to the toilet on a stand-aid hoist. If the patient was unable to use the toilet then a bedpan or commode could be offered. Remember, whenever the patient uses toilet facilities or bedpan to offer facilities to wash their hands.

ACTIVITY 21-2 Burning on passing urine can be a sign of a urinary tract infection. Ensure the patient's observations are recorded, in particular her temperature. Ask the patient to collect midstream urine for testing. Observe the colour and amount of urine. Dipstick the urine and observe for signs of infection such as haematuria, white cells and protein. If there is clinical indication of infection send the urine sample for culture and sensitivity. Encourage the patient to drink plenty of water and, if she is able, to drink cranberry juice. Observe for further signs of pain on micturition. Inform doctor or senior nurse.

ACTIVITY 21-3 There are a number of reasons why you would not routinely catheterise patients. Catheterisation:

- is an invasive procedure that increases the risk of infection;
- is an undignified and embarrassing procedure;
- can cause patient discomfort;
- does not encourage continence.

REFERENCES

Baillie, L. and Arrowsmith, V. (2009) 'Meeting elimination needs', in Baillie, L. (ed.) *Developing practical nursing skills* (3rd edn), London: Hodder Arnold, 321–393.

Dixon, L., Dolan, L.M., Brown, K. and Hilton, P. (2010) 'RCT of urethral versus suprapubic catheterisation', *British Journal of Nursing* (Continence Care Supplement), 19(18), S7–S13.

Docherty, C. and McCallum, J. (2009) *Foundation clinical nursing Skills*, Oxford: Oxford University Press.

Dougherty, L. and Lister, S. (2004) *The Royal Marsden Hospital manual of clinical nursing procedures* (6th edn), Oxford: Wiley-Blackwell.

Farrell, M., Devine, K., Lancaster, G. and Judd, B. (2002) 'A method comparison study to assess the reliability of urine collection pads as a means of obtaining urine specimens from non-toilet-trained children for microbiological examination', *Journal of Advanced Nursing*, 37(4), 387–393.

Liaw, L.C.T., Nayar, D.M., Pedler, S.J. and Coulthard, M.G. (2000) 'Home collection of urine for culture from infants by three method: Survey of parents' preferences and bacterial contamination rates', *British Medical Journal*, 320, 1312–1313.

Macfarlane, P.I., Houghton, C. and Hughes, C. (1999) 'Pad urine collection for early childhood urinary-tract infections', *Lancet*, 354, 571.

NHS Choices (2008) *Preventing urinary tract infections*, available at **http://www.nhs.uk/Conditions/Urinary-tract-infection-adults/Pages/Prevention.aspx** (adults) and **http://www.nhs.uk/Conditions/Urinary-tract-infection-children/Pages/Prevention.aspx** (children) (accessed March 2011).

NMC (2010) *Standards for pre-registration nursing education*, London: NMC.

O'Donahue, D., Winsor, G., Gallagher, R., Maughan, J., Dooley, K. and Walsh, J. (2010) 'Issues for people living with long term urinary catheters in the community', *British Journal of Community Nursing*, 15(2), 65–70.

Pratt, R.J., Pellowe, C.M., Wilson, J.A., Loveday, H.P., Harper, P., Jones, S.R.L.J., McDougall, C. and Wilcox, M.H. (2007) Epic2: 'National evidence-based guidelines for preventing healthcare associated infections in NHS hospital in England', *Journal of Hospital Infection*, 655, S1–S64.

Richardson, M, (2003) 'The physiology of micturition', *Nursing Times*, 99(29), 40.

Schrier R.W. (2009) *Manual of nephrology* (7th edn), Philadelphia, PA: Lippincott Williams and Wilkins.

Simerville, J., Maxted, W. and Palura, J. (2005) 'Urinalysis: A comprehensive review', *American Family Physician*, 71(6), 1153–1162.

Stenson, A. and Danaher, T. (2005) 'Continence issues for people with learning disabilities', *Learning Disability Practice*, 8(9), 10–14.

Suvarna, R., Pirmohamed, M. and Henderson, L. (2003) 'Possible interaction between warfarin and cranberry juice', *British Medical Journal*, 327, 1454.

Wells, M. (2007) 'Urine testing', *Nursing Times*, available at **http://www.nursingtimes.net/nursing-practice-clinical-research/urine-testing/199377.article** (accessed 30 June 2011).

CHAPTER 22
BOWEL ELIMINATION

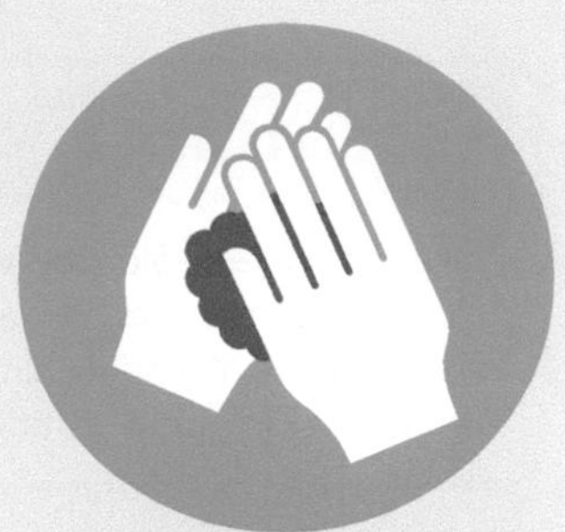

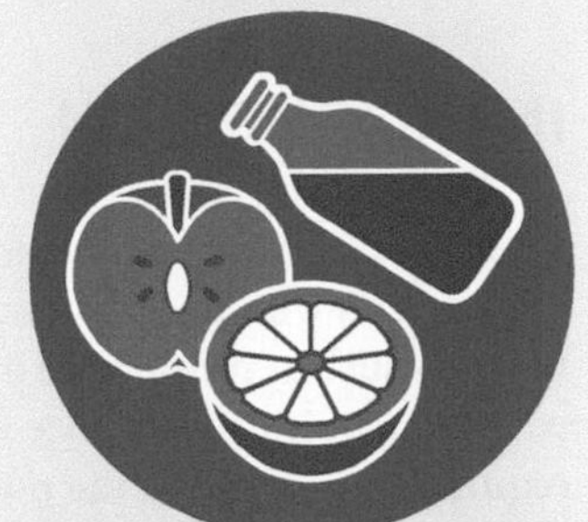

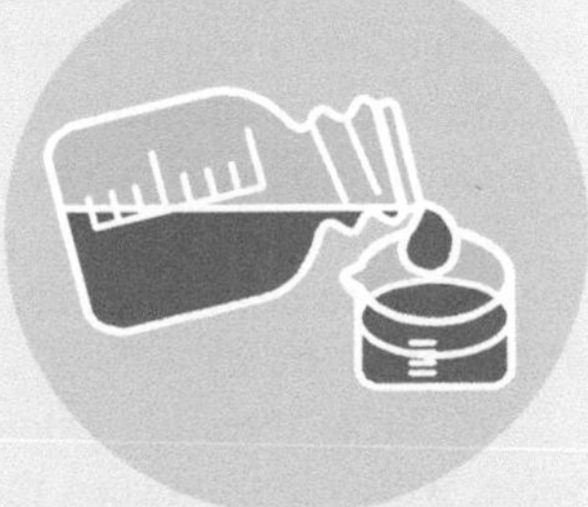

LEARNING OUTCOMES

After completing this chapter, you will be able to:

- Understand the physiology of defecation.
- Identify factors that influence bowel elimination.
- Distinguish normal from abnormal characteristics and constituents of faeces.
- Describe the assessment of bowel elimination.
- Identify common causes and effects of selected bowel elimination problems.
- Identify measures that maintain normal elimination patterns.
- Describe essentials of bowel stoma care for patients with ostomies.

After reading this chapter you will be able to discuss ways in which continence can be promoted and understand the process of defecation. This chapter relates to **Essential Skills Clusters (NMC, 2010) 1 to 11, 13, 14, 15, 16, 18, 22, 24, 26 and 36**, as appropriate for each progression point.

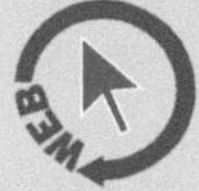

Ensure that you really understand this chapter by logging on to your complimentary **MyNursingKit** at **www.pearsoned.co.uk/kozier**. Complete the self-assessment tests to check your progress and utilise further activities to practise and confirm your understanding.

CASE STUDY

Jake, an 11-year-old boy with spinal injuries, has been discharged home. He has a care package that includes the district nurse attending him to manage a sacral pressure ulcer. You are in his home visiting him with the district nurse, when Jake's mother informs you that Jake hasn't had his bowels opened for 3 days but has noticed faecal leakage on his sheets and bed clothes.

INTRODUCTION

Bowel elimination is a fundamental function of humans. Assisting a person with this function requires the nurse to be sensitive to issues such as privacy and dignity. In order to provide care for patients requiring assistance with bowel elimination, the nurse requires knowledge of the normal function of the bowel along with the skills to manage problems with this function. Key to managing the care of a patient with bowel elimination problems is the holistic assessment of the person.

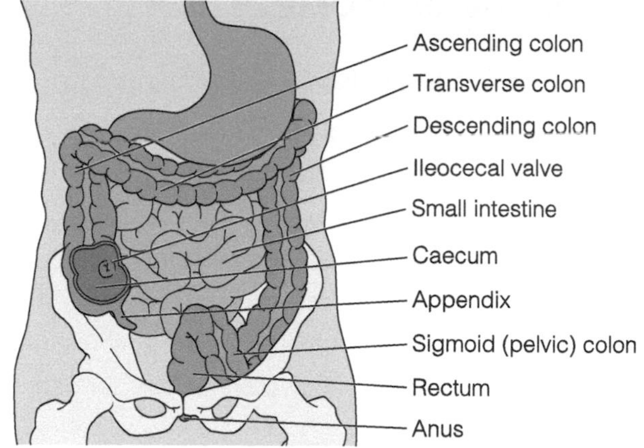

Figure 22-1 The large intestine and rectum.

PHYSIOLOGY OF DEFECATION

Elimination of waste products is a necessity for maintaining health and is a very personal, private and independent act (Pellatt, 2007). However, nurses are frequently consulted or involved in assisting patients with elimination problems. These problems can be embarrassing to patients and can cause considerable discomfort. Nurses need to have an understanding of the normal physiology of defecation and ways in which associated problems can be managed.

Elimination of the waste products of digestion from the body is essential to health. The excreted waste products are referred to as **faeces** or **stool**.

The large intestine extends from the ileocaecal (ileocolic) valve, which lies between the small and large intestines, to the anus. The colon (large intestine) in the adult is generally about 125–150cm (50–60 inches) long. It has seven parts: the caecum; ascending, transverse and descending colons; sigmoid colon; rectum; and anus (see Figure 22-1).

The large intestine is a muscular tube lined with mucous membrane. The muscle fibres are both circular and longitudinal, permitting the intestine to enlarge and contract in both width and length. The longitudinal muscles are shorter than the colon and therefore cause the large intestine to form pouches or **haustra**.

The colon's main functions are the absorption of water and nutrients, the mucal protection of the intestinal wall and bowel elimination. The contents of the colon normally represent foods ingested over the previous four days, although most of the waste products are excreted within 48 hours of ingestion (the act of taking food). The waste products leaving the stomach through the small intestine and then passing through the ileocaecal valve are called chyme. As much as 1,500ml of chyme passes into the large intestine daily, and all but about 100ml is reabsorbed in the proximal half of the colon. The 100ml of fluid is excreted in the faeces.

The colon also serves a protective function in that it secretes mucus. This mucus contains large amounts of bicarbonate ions and serves to protect the wall of the large intestine from trauma by the acids formed in the faeces, and it serves as an adherent for holding the faecal material together. Mucus also protects the intestinal wall from bacterial activity.

The products of digestion are flatus and faeces. Flatus is largely air and the by-products of the digestion of carbohydrates. Flatus and faeces are propelled along the intestines by wavelike movements produced by the circular and longitudinal muscle fibres of the intestinal walls, known as **peristalsis**.

The faeces and flatus pass along the intestine towards the rectum and anal canal. The rectum in the adult is usually 10–15cm long; the most distal portion, 2.5–5cm long, is the anal canal. In the rectum are folds that extend vertically. Each of the vertical folds contains a vein and an artery. It is believed that these folds help retain faeces within the rectum. When the veins become distended, as can occur with repeated pressure, a condition known as **haemorrhoids** occurs (see Figure 22-2).

The anal canal is bounded by an internal and an external sphincter muscle (see Figure 22-3). The internal sphincter is under involuntary control and the external sphincter normally is voluntarily controlled. The internal sphincter muscle is

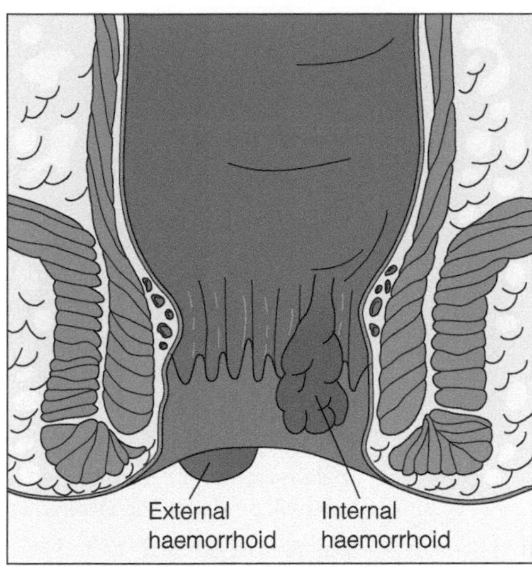

Figure 22-2 Internal and external haemorrhoids.

innervated by the autonomic nervous system; the external sphincter is innervated by the somatic nervous system.

The expulsion of faeces from the anal canal is known as defecation. It is also called a *bowel movement* or *motion*. The frequency of defecation is highly individual, varying from several times per day to two or three times per week. The amount defecated also varies from person to person. When peristaltic waves move the faeces into the sigmoid colon and the rectum, the sensory nerves in the rectum are stimulated and the individual becomes aware of the need to defecate.

When the internal anal sphincter relaxes, faeces move into the anal canal. After the individual is seated on a toilet or bedpan, the external anal sphincter is relaxed voluntarily. Expulsion of the faeces is assisted by contraction of the abdominal muscles and the diaphragm, which increases abdominal pressure, and by contraction of the muscles of the pelvic floor, which moves the faeces through the anal canal. Normal defecation is facilitated by (a) thigh flexion, which increases the pressure within the abdomen, and (b) a sitting position, which increases the downward pressure on the rectum.

If the defecation reflex is ignored, or if defecation is consciously inhibited by contracting the external sphincter muscle, the urge to defecate normally disappears for a few hours before occurring again. Repeated inhibition of the urge to defecate can result in expansion of the rectum to accommodate accumulated faeces and eventual loss of sensitivity to the need to defecate. Constipation can be the ultimate result.

The faeces that are expelled from the anal canal are made of about 75% water and 25% solid materials. They are soft but formed. If the faeces are propelled very quickly along the large intestine, there is not time for most of the water in the chyme to be reabsorbed and the faeces will be more fluid, containing perhaps 95% water. Normal faeces require a normal fluid intake; faeces that contain less water may be hard and difficult to expel.

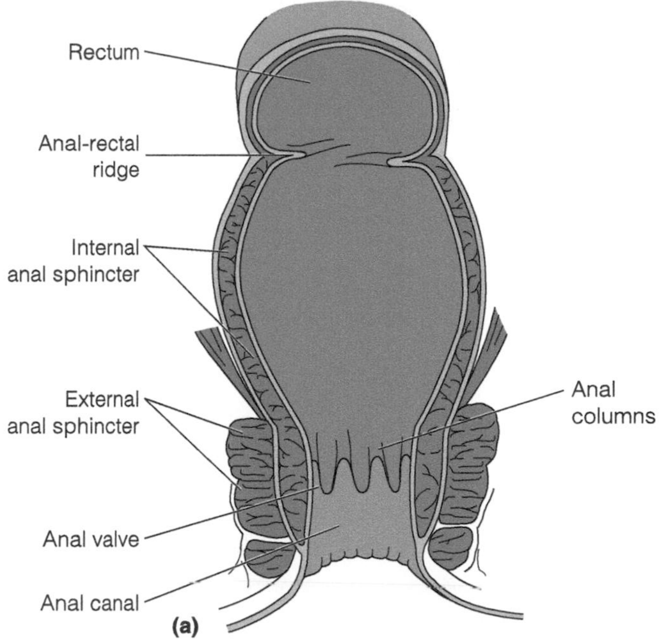

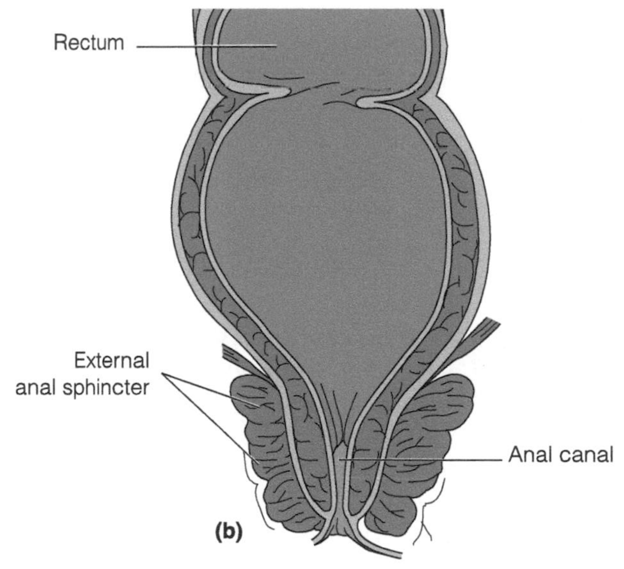

Figure 22-3 The rectum, anal canal and anal sphincters: (a) open; (b) closed.

Faeces are normally brown, chiefly due to the presence of stercobilin and urobilin, which are derived from bilirubin (a red pigment in bile). Another factor that affects faecal colour is the action of bacteria such as *Escherichia coli* or staphylococci, which are normally present in the large intestine. The action of micro-organisms on the chyme is also responsible for the odour of faeces. Table 22-1 lists the characteristics of normal and abnormal faeces.

An adult usually forms 7–10l of flatus (gas) in the large intestine every 24 hours. The gases include carbon dioxide, methane, hydrogen, oxygen and nitrogen. Some are swallowed

Table 22-1 Characteristics of Normal and Abnormal Faeces

Characteristic	Normal	Abnormal	Possible cause
Colour	Adult: brown	Clay or white	Absence of bile pigment (bile obstruction); diagnostic study using barium
	Infant: yellow	Black or tarry	Drug (e.g. iron); bleeding from upper gastrointestinal tract (e.g. stomach, small intestine); diet high in red meat and dark green vegetables (e.g. spinach)
		Red	Bleeding from lower gastrointestinal tract (e.g. rectum); some foods (e.g. beets)
		Pale	Malabsorption of fats; diet high in milk and milk products and low in meat
		Orange or green	Intestinal infection
Consistency	Formed, soft, semisolid, moist	Hard, dry	Dehydration; decreased intestinal motility resulting from lack of fibre in diet, lack of exercise, emotional upset, laxative abuse
		Diarrhoea	Increased intestinal motility (e.g. due to irritation of the colon by bacteria)
Shape	Cylindrical (contour of rectum) about 2.5cm (1 inch) in diameter in adults	Narrow, pencil-shaped, or string-like stool	Obstructive condition of the rectum
Amount	Varies with diet (about 100–400g per day)		
Odour	Aromatic: affected by ingested food and person's own bacterial flora	Pungent	Infection, blood
Constituents	Small amounts of undigested roughage, sloughed dead bacteria and epithelial cells, fat, protein, dried constituents of digestive juices (e.g. bile pigments, inorganic matter)	Pus Mucus Parasites Blood Large quantities of fat Foreign objects	Bacterial infection Inflammatory condition Gastrointestinal bleeding Malabsorption Accidental ingestion

with food and fluids taken by mouth, others are formed through the action of bacteria on the chyme in the large intestine, and other gas diffuses from the blood into the gastrointestinal tract.

FACTORS THAT AFFECT DEFECATION

There are a number of factors that can affect defecation. *Developmental stage* is a major factor for defecation as it dictates the stage of maturity of the intestine and the body's ability to cope with ageing. For example, some older adults suffer with constipation as a result of reduced activity levels, poor diet and fluid intake and muscle weakness whereas infants tend to have soft stools due to the immaturity of the intestine and the inability to reabsorb water.

Diet and fluid intake can also affect defecation, as a low fibre diet creates insufficient residue of waste products to stimulate the reflex of defecation and a reduced fluid intake leads to the chyme becoming drier than normal, both of which can cause constipation.

Activity stimulates peristalsis, thus facilitating the movement of chyme along the colon; therefore patients who are confined to bed often suffer with constipation.

The *psychological state* can also affect defecation. For example, some people who are anxious or angry experience increased peristaltic activity and subsequent nausea or diarrhoea, while people who are depressed may experience slowed intestinal motility, resulting in constipation.

Early bowel training may establish the habit of defecating at a regular time. Many people defecate after breakfast, when the gastrocolic reflex causes mass peristaltic waves in the large intestine. However, it should be recognised that each individual's bowel habits are different.

Some *medications* have side effects that can interfere with normal bowel elimination. Some cause diarrhoea; others, such as large doses of certain tranquillisers and repeated administration of morphine and codeine, cause constipation because they decrease gastrointestinal activity through their action on the central nervous system. Some medications are meant to directly affect bowel elimination (e.g. laxatives).

Patients who experience discomfort when defecating (e.g. following haemorrhoid surgery) often suppress the urge to defecate to avoid the pain. Such patients can experience constipation as a result.

ACTIVITY 22-1

What factors could affect a patient's normal bowel habits?

BOWEL ELIMINATION PROBLEMS

Four common problems are related to bowel elimination: constipation, diarrhoea, bowel incontinence and flatulence.

Constipation may be defined as fewer than three bowel movements per week. This implies the passage of dry, hard stool or the passage of no stool. It occurs when the movement of faeces through the large intestine is slow, thus allowing time for additional reabsorption of fluid from the large intestine. Relatively common in childhood, it affects up to 30% of children and young people in the UK (National Institute for Clinical Excellence (NICE), 2010). It is also the commonest digestive problem suffered by adults (Marsh and Sweeney, 2008). Many causes and factors contribute to constipation including insufficient fibre intake, insufficient fluid intake, inactivity or immobility and some medications.

RESEARCH NOTE

Researching the Management of Constipation in Long-Term Care

This action research study aimed to improve the management of constipation for residents in long-term care settings. The study was carried out in nine care homes, with a range of residents of varying ages and with a variety of chronic conditions. Initially questionnaires were used to provide baseline information on current practice used to manage constipation within the care homes. Staff within these care homes then attended a training session led by a trainer and a qualified representative from one of the drug companies specialising in bowel products. The action researchers then implemented a flow chart for the management of constipation amongst the residents. Staff were then asked to complete another questionnaire. The results showed that educating staff improves knowledge and practice in dealing with constipation with improved outcomes for the residents within the care homes.

Source: based on Grainger, M., Castledine, G., Wood, N. and Dilley, C. (2007) 'Researching the management of constipation in long-term care. Part 2', *British Journal of Nursing*, 16(19), 1212-1217.

Faecal impaction is a mass or collection of hardened faeces in the folds of the rectum. Impaction results from prolonged retention and accumulation of faecal material. In severe impactions the faeces accumulate and extend well up into the sigmoid colon and beyond. Faecal impaction can be recognised by the passage of liquid faecal seepage (diarrhoea) and no normal stool. The liquid portion of the faeces seeps out around the impacted mass. The causes of faecal impaction are usually poor defecation habits and constipation.

Diarrhoea refers to the passage of liquid faeces and an increased frequency of defecation. It is the opposite of constipation and results from rapid movement of faecal contents through the large intestine. Diarrhoea is generally the result of increased stool water content (Watson, 1999) and can be acute, chronic or iatrogenic, as with Clostridium difficile. Rapid passage of chyme reduces the time available for the large intestine to reabsorb water and electrolytes. Some people pass stool with increased frequency, but diarrhoea is not present unless the stool is relatively unformed and excessively liquid. The person with diarrhoea finds it difficult or impossible to control the urge to defecate for very long. Table 22-2 lists some of the major causes of diarrhoea and the physiologic responses of the body.

The nurse's role in managing patients with diarrhoea is to:

- obtain a stool specimen to identify if there are any infective causes for the diarrhoea;
- observe the stool for blood, or other abnormalities such as pale, offensive stools which indicate infection (Watson, 1999);
- take a history of onset, frequency and duration of diarrhoea;
- observe and assess for any other symptoms such as pain or nausea and vomiting;
- check past medical history including any medications;
- check hydration status (Dougherty and Lister, 2008).

Bowel incontinence, also called **faecal incontinence**, refers to the loss of voluntary ability to control faecal and flatus discharges through the anal sphincter (Watson, 1999). NICE (2007) estimate that between 1% and 10% of adults in the UK suffer faecal incontinence at some point in their lives, with approximately 0.5–1% experiencing regular faecal incontinence.

Table 22-2 Major Causes of Diarrhoea

Cause	Physiologic effect
Psychological stress (e.g. anxiety)	Increased intestinal motility and mucus secretion
Medications	
Antibiotics	Inflammation and infection of mucosa due to overgrowth of pathogenic intestinal micro-organisms
Iron	Irritation of intestinal mucosa
Cathartics	Irritation of intestinal mucosa
Allergy to food, fluid, drugs	Incomplete digestion of food or fluid
Intolerance of food or fluid	Increased intestinal motility and mucus secretion
Diseases of the colon (e.g. malabsorption syndrome Crohn's disease)	Reduced absorption of fluids Inflammation of the mucosa often leading to ulcer formation

However, Powell and Rigby (2000) suggest that this is probably an underestimation as the condition is embarrassing. Faecal incontinence is a sign or symptom but is not a diagnosis; therefore, it is important that the cause of the incontinence is diagnosed in order to initiate the correct interventions (NICE, 2007). Faecal incontinence may occur at specific times, such as after meals, or it may occur irregularly. It is generally associated with impaired functioning of the anal sphincter or its nerve supply, such as in some neuromuscular diseases, spinal cord trauma and tumours of the external anal sphincter muscle.

Faecal incontinence is an emotionally distressing problem that can have profound physical and emotional consequences for the patient which impact on nearly all aspects of the individual's life. The possible consequences of faecal incontinence include:

- stress, distress, anxiety, fear of public humiliation and feeling dirty;
- pain and soreness of skin;
- difficulty performing household chores;
- fear of using toilets in public places including in the work environment;
- fear of starting a new relationship or concealing symptoms from their partner;
- negative self-image;
- avoiding public places such as supermarkets;
- sexual avoidance or aversion.

Source: based on NICE (2007) CG49: *Faecal Incontinence. The management of faecal incontinence in adults*. London: NICE

Flatulence is the presence of excessive flatus in the intestines and leads to stretching and inflation of the intestines (intestinal distension). Flatulence can occur in the colon from a variety of causes, such as foods (e.g. cabbage, onions), abdominal surgery or narcotics. If the gas is propelled by increased colon activity before it can be absorbed, it may be expelled through the anus. If excessive gas cannot be expelled through the anus, it may be necessary to insert a rectal tube to remove it.

ACTIVITY 22-2

What do you think the possible consequences of altered bowel functioning would be the patient?

BOWEL DIVERSION OSTOMIES

Bowel diversion ostomies are openings from the gastrointestinal tract onto the skin surface. The purpose of bowel ostomies is to divert and drain faecal material and is often classified according to (a) their status as permanent or temporary, (b) their anatomic location, and (c) the construction of the **stoma**, the opening created in the abdominal wall by the ostomy.

Colostomies open into the colon and can be either temporary or permanent. Colostomies can be further classified according to anatomical position. An ascending colostomy empties from the ascending colon, a transverse colostomy from the transverse colon, a descending colostomy from the descending colon, and a sigmoidostomy from the sigmoid colon (see Figure 22-4).

The location of the colostomy influences the character of the faeces. Ascending colostomies tend to produce liquid stool which cannot be regulated. A transverse colostomy produces a malodorous, mushy drainage because some of the liquid has been reabsorbed which cannot usually be controlled. A descending colostomy produces increasingly solid faecal drainage and a sigmoidostomy produces faeces that are of normal or formed consistency, and the frequency of discharge can be regulated. People with a sigmoidostomy may not have to wear an appliance at all times, and odours can usually be controlled.

Temporary colostomies are generally performed for traumatic injuries or inflammatory conditions of the bowel. They allow the distal diseased portion of the bowel to rest and heal. Permanent colostomies are performed to provide a means of elimination when the rectum or anus is nonfunctional as a result of a birth defect or a disease such as cancer of the bowel.

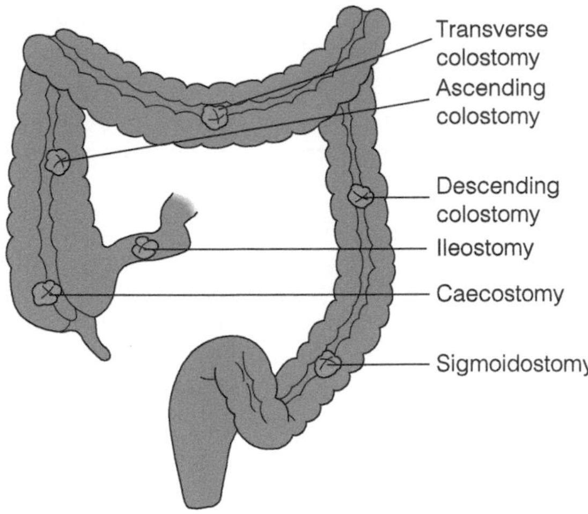

Figure 22-4 The locations of bowel diversion ostomies.

Ileostomies are openings into the ileum and generally empty from the distal end of the small intestine producing liquid faecal drainage. Drainage is constant and cannot be regulated. Ileostomy drainage contains some digestive enzymes, which are damaging to the skin. For this reason, ileostomy patients must wear an appliance continuously and take special precautions to prevent skin breakdown. Compared to colostomies, however, odour is minimal because fewer bacteria are present.

The length of time that an ostomy is in place also helps to determine the consistency of the stool, particularly with transverse and descending colostomies. Over time, the stool becomes more formed because the remaining functioning portions of the colon tend to compensate by increasing water reabsorption.

Colostomies are constructed by different techniques and are described as single, loop, divided or double-barrelled colostomies. The *single* stoma is created when one end of the bowel is brought out through an opening onto the anterior abdominal wall. This is referred to as an *end* or *terminal colostomy*; the stoma is permanent (see Figure 22-5).

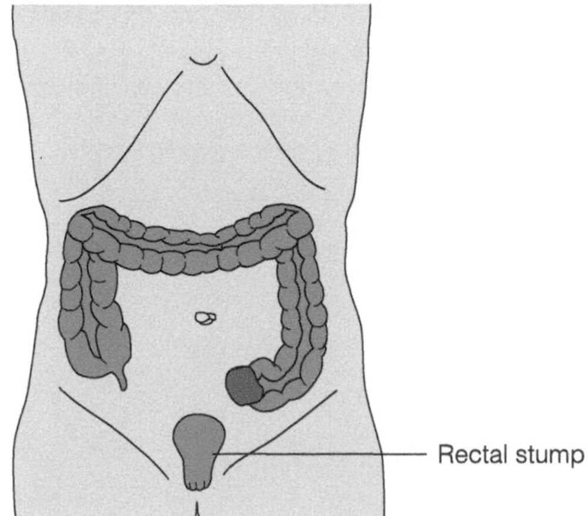

Figure 22-5 End colostomy: the diseased portion of bowel is removed and a rectal pouch remains.

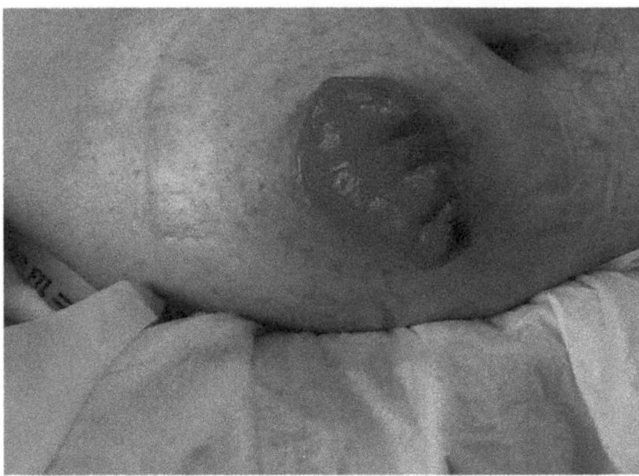

Figure 22-6 Loop colostomy.

Source: courtesy of Cory Patrick Hartley, San Ramon Regional Medical Center, San Ramon, CA.

In the *loop colostomy*, a loop of bowel is brought out onto the abdominal wall and supported by a plastic bridge, a glass rod or a piece of rubber tubing (see Figure 22-6). A loop stoma has two openings: the proximal or afferent end, which is active, and the distal or efferent end, which is inactive. The loop colostomy is usually performed in an emergency procedure and is often situated on the right transverse colon. It is a bulky stoma that is more difficult to manage than a single stoma.

The *divided colostomy* consists of two edges of bowel brought out onto the abdomen but separated from each other (see Figure 22-7). The opening from the digestive or proximal end is the colostomy. The distal end in this situation is often referred to as a mucous fistula, since this section of bowel continues to secrete mucus. The divided colostomy is often used in situations where spillage of faeces into the distal end of the bowel needs to be avoided.

The *double-barrelled colostomy* resembles a double-barrelled shotgun (see Figure 22-8). In this type of colostomy, the proximal and distal loops of bowel are sutured together for about 10cm (4 inches) and both ends are brought up onto the abdominal wall.

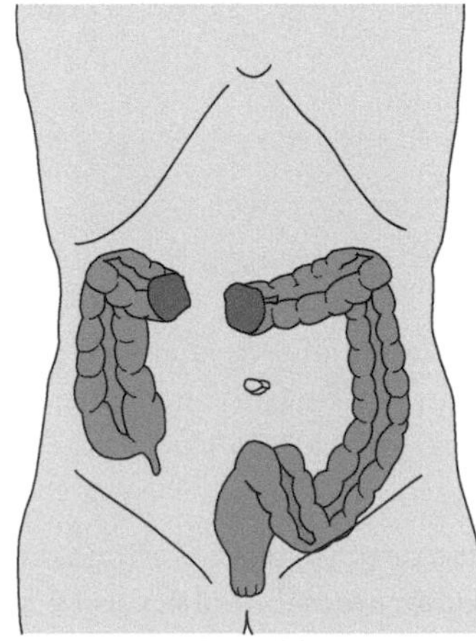

Figure 22-7 Divided colostomy with two separated stomas.

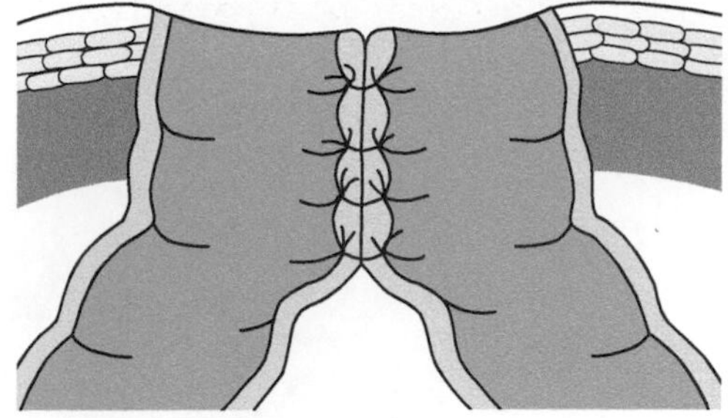

Figure 22-8 Double-barrelled colostomy.

ASSESSING BOWEL ELIMINATION

Assessment of bowel elimination includes taking a patient history; physically examining the patient; and inspecting the faeces. The nurse also should review any data obtained from relevant diagnostic tests.

Patient History

A patient history for bowel elimination helps the nurse ascertain the patient's normal pattern. The nurse elicits a description of usual faeces and any recent changes and collects information about any past or current problems with elimination, the presence of an ostomy and factors influencing the elimination pattern.

When obtaining information about the patient's defecation pattern, the nurse needs to understand that the time of defecation and the amount of faeces expelled are as individual as the frequency of defecation. Often, the patterns individuals follow depend largely on childhood training and on convenience.

Physical Examination

Physical examination of the abdomen in relation to bowel elimination problems includes inspection, listening for bowel sounds and palpation with specific reference to the intestinal tract. They should always listen for bowel sounds before palpation as palpation can alter peristalsis. Examination of the rectum and anus includes inspection and palpation; this may be done by medical staff or nursing staff who have been specifically trained in rectal examinations (see also Chapter 11).

Inspecting the Faeces

Observe the patient's stool for colour, consistency, shape, amount, odour and the presence of abnormal constituents. Table 22-1 on page 660 summarises normal and abnormal characteristics of stool and possible causes.

Diagnostic Studies

Diagnostic studies of the gastrointestinal tract include direct visualisation techniques, indirect visualisation techniques and laboratory tests for abnormal constituents (see Chapter 27).

COMMUNITY CARE CONSIDERATIONS

Assessment of Faecal Elimination in the Community Setting

Should include the assessment of:

- Bowel elimination problems, e.g. incontinence, constipation, diarrhoea
- Toilet facilities within the patient's home
- The ability of the patient to get to the toilet, manipulate clothing for toileting, to perform toilet hygiene and flush the toilet
- The requirement of aids such as walking aids and toileting aids
- Any physical barriers that could prevent the patient from accessing the toilet, e.g. cluttered pathway to bathroom
- Level of knowledge and understanding of condition, and planned bowel management
- Carer's willingness to promote normal bowel functioning

PLANNING

Following the assessment of the patient the nurse must identify any problems and plan realistic and achievable goals for the patient. The major goals for patients with bowel elimination problems are to:

- maintain or restore normal bowel elimination pattern;
- maintain or regain normal stool consistency;
- prevent associated risks such as fluid and electrolyte imbalance, skin breakdown, abdominal distention and pain.

Appropriate interventions need to be implemented in order to achieve these goals.

IMPLEMENTING

Promoting Regular Defecation

The nurse can help patients achieve regular defecation by (a) ensuring privacy, (b) offering toileting at specific times which are usually individual to the patient, for example after food,

(c) encouraging nutrition and fluids, (d) encouraging mobilisation and exercise, and (e) positioning appropriate for defecation (see the *Practice Guidelines* for use of bedpan). For advice on how patients can manage diarrhoea, see *Teaching: Patient Care*.

TEACHING: PATIENT CARE

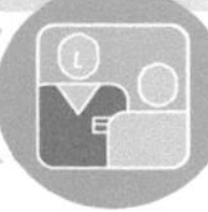

Managing Diarrhoea

- Drink at least eight glasses of water per day to prevent dehydration.
- Ingest foods with sodium and potassium. Most foods contain sodium. Potassium is found in meats, and many vegetables and fruits, especially tomatoes, potatoes, bananas, peaches and apricots.
- Increase foods containing soluble fibre, such as oatmeal and skinless fruits and potatoes.
- Avoid alcohol and beverages with caffeine, which aggravate the problem.
- Limit foods containing insoluble fibre, such as whole-wheat and whole-grain breads and cereals, and raw fruits and vegetables.
- Limit fatty foods.
- Thoroughly clean and dry the perineal area after passing stool to prevent skin irritation and breakdown. Use soft toilet tissue to clean and dry the area. Apply a moisture-barrier cream or ointment, such as zinc oxide or petrolatum, as needed.
- If possible, discontinue medications that cause diarrhoea.
- When diarrhoea has stopped, re-establish normal bowel flora by taking fermented dairy products, such as yoghurt or buttermilk.

Administering Enemas

An **enema** is a solution introduced into the rectum and large intestine. The action of an enema is to distend the intestine and sometimes to irritate the intestinal mucosa, thereby increasing peristalsis and the excretion of faeces and flatus. The most common type of enema used is the cleansing enema which is used to remove faeces and is given chiefly for constipation, or for bowel preparation prior to surgery or certain diagnostic tests. Instructions on how to administer an enema are given in *Procedure 22-1*.

PRACTICE GUIDELINES

Giving and Removing a Bedpan

- Provide privacy.
- Wear disposable gloves.
- If the bedpan is metal, warm it by rinsing it with warm water.
- Adjust the bed to a height appropriate to prevent back strain.
- Elevate the side rail on the opposite side to prevent the patient from falling out of bed.
- Ask the patient to assist by flexing the knees, resting the weight on the back and heels, and raising the buttocks, or by using a trapeze bar, if present.
- Help lift the patient as needed by placing one hand under the lower back, resting your elbow on the mattress, and using your forearm as a lever.
- Place a regular bedpan so that the patient's buttocks rest on the smooth, rounded rim. Place a slipper pan with the flat, low end under the patient's buttocks (see Figure 22-9).
- For the patient who cannot assist, obtain the assistance of another nurse to help move the patient onto the bedpan or place the patient on his or her side, place the bedpan against the buttocks (see Figure 22-10), and roll the patient back onto the bedpan.

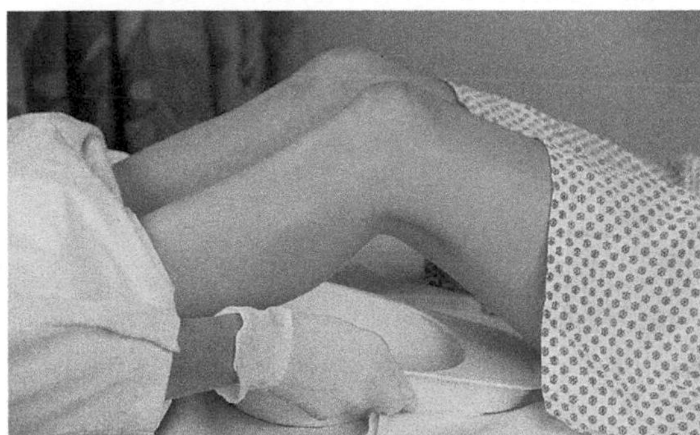

Figure 22-9 Placing a slipper pan under the buttocks.

- To provide a more normal position for the patient's lower back, elevate the patient's bed to a semi-Fowler's position, if permitted. If elevation is contraindicated, support the patient's back with pillows as needed to prevent hyperextension of the back.
- Cover the patient with bed linen to maintain comfort and self-dignity.

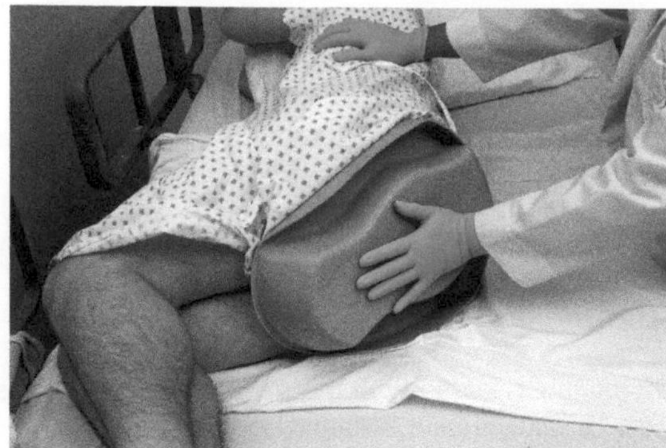

Figure 22-10 Placing a regular bedpan against the patient's buttocks.

- Provide toilet tissue, place the call light within reach, lower the bed to the low position, elevate the side rail if indicated, and leave the patient alone.
- Answer the call bell promptly.
- When removing the bedpan, return the bed to the position used when giving the bedpan, hold the bedpan steady to prevent spillage of its contents, cover the bedpan and place it on the adjacent chair.
- If the patient needs assistance, don gloves and wipe the patient's perineal area with several layers of toilet tissue. If a specimen is to be collected, discard the soiled tissue into a moisture-proof receptacle other than the bedpan. For female patients, clean from the urethra towards the anus to prevent transferring rectal micro-organisms into the urinary meatus.
- Wash the perineal area of dependent patients with soap and water as indicated and thoroughly dry the area.
- For all patients, offer warm water, soap, a washcloth and a towel to wash the hands.
- Assist the patient to a comfortable position, empty and clean the bedpan, and return it to the bedside.
- Remove and discard your gloves and wash your hands.
- Spray the room with air freshener as needed to control odour unless contraindicated because of respiratory problems or allergies.
- Document colour, odour, amount and consistency of urine and faeces, and the condition of the perineal area.

PROCEDURE 22-1 Administering an Enema

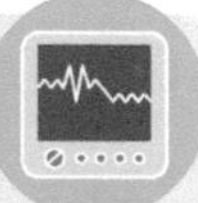

Purpose

To achieve one or more of the actions described above

Assessment

Assess

- When the patient last had a bowel movement and the amount, colour and consistency of the faeces
- Presence of abdominal distention (the distended abdomen appears swollen and feels firm rather than soft when palpated)
- Whether the patient has sphincter control
- Whether the patient can use a toilet or commode or must remain in bed and use a bedpan

Planning

Before administering an enema, determine whether the enema needs to be prescribed. Manufacturer's instruction should be read to ensure correct administration.

Equipment

- Incontinence sheet or pad
- Sheet
- Bedpan or commode
- Clean gloves
- Water-soluble lubricant if tubing not prelubricated
- Gauze swab
- Enema solution

Implementation

Preparation

- Warm the enema to body temperature to prevent intestinal cramping.
- Position the patient lying on the left-hand side as this eases the flow of the fluid into the rectum by following the anatomy of the colon (see Figure 22-11). The patient should flex their knees as this will aid the passage of the nozzle of the enema container through the anal canal.
- Place the incontinence sheet or pad under the buttocks.

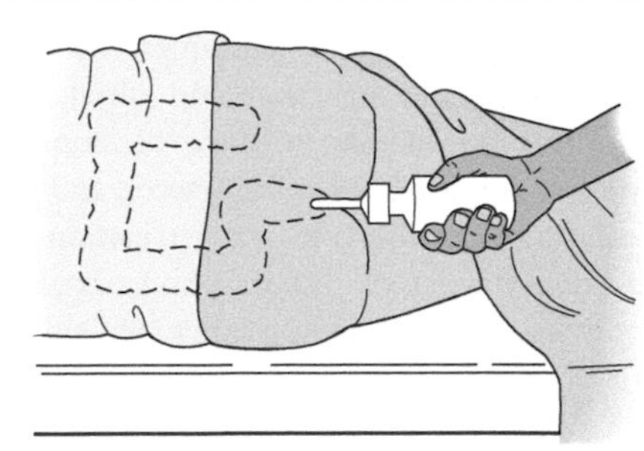

Figure 22-11 Assuming a left lateral position for an enema. Note the commercially prepared enema.

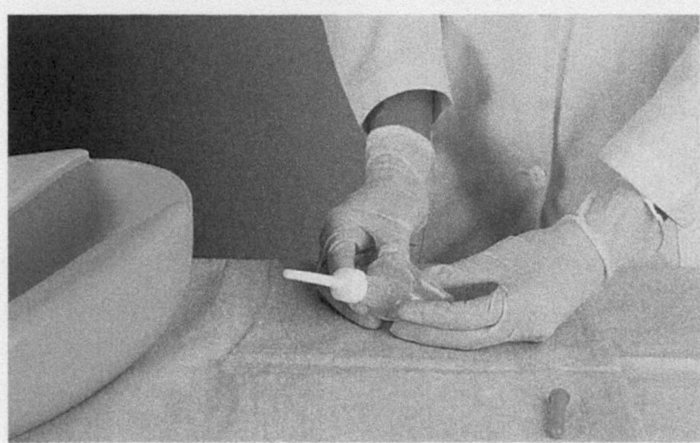

Figure 22-12 Rolling up a commercial enema container.

Performance

1 Follow local policy to ensure that you explain to the patient what you are going to do, why it is necessary and how they can cooperate. Obtain consent and maintain patient privacy and dignity and ensure that the appropriate local infection control procedures are observed.
2 Expel any air from the enema container. *To prevent the introduction of air into the colon which can cause distention and discomfort.*
3 Lubricate the tip of the container nozzle. *To aid insertion of the tip.*
4 Insert the tip smoothly and slowly into the rectum, directing it towards the umbilicus. *Slow insertion prevents spasm of the sphincter.*
5 If pain or resistance is felt at any time during the procedure, stop and seek medical advice.
6 Squeeze the fluid gently into the rectum from the base of the container to prevent back flow (see Figure 22-12).
7 Slowly withdraw the container nozzle. *To avoid reflux emptying of the rectum.*
8 Clean the perineal area and make the patient comfortable.
9 Ask the patient to retain the enema according to manufacturer's instructions.
10 The patient should remain lying down with access to a call bell.
11 Dispose of equipment, remove gloves and apron and wash hands thoroughly.
12 Document that the enema has been administered.
13 Monitor the patient and record the effects of the enema.
14 Offer handwashing facilities and perineal hygiene if the patient is unable to walk to the toilet.

Evaluation

Perform a detailed follow-up based on findings that deviated from expected or normal for the patient. Relate findings to previous assessment data if available. Report significant deviations to the doctor.

Digital Evacuation of Faeces

Digital evacuation of faeces is viewed as a last resort in the management of patients with constipation and is only used when all other methods for relief of constipation have failed. However, for some patients this procedure is a vital part of the bowel management (Royal College of Nursing (RCN), 2008). For example, patients with spinal cord injury may not be able to pass faeces without digital evacuation as they have lost sensation for defecation (Ash, 2005). It involves breaking up the faecal mass digitally and removing it in portions. Nurses should not attempt this without first receiving formal teaching as there is a risk of damage to the bowel mucosa.

Bowel Training Programmes

For patients who have chronic constipation, frequent impactions or faecal incontinence, some NHS trusts offer bowel training programmes. These programmes aim to establish normal defecation by implementing a range of interventions and techniques. These programmes generally consist of:

- A full assessment of the patient's usual bowel habits and factors that help and hinder normal defecation.
- Designing a plan with the patient that includes the following:
  - Fluid intake of about 2,500–3,000ml per day
  - Increase in fibre in the diet
  - Intake of hot drinks, especially just before the usual defecation time
  - Increase in exercise.
- Following a routine that includes the administration of a cathartic suppository (a capsule that is inserted into the rectum that aids evacuation of faeces); assisting the patient to the toilet, commode or onto a bedpan; providing the patient with privacy; educating the patient to lean forward at the hips and to apply pressure to the abdomen with the hands while defecating; and providing positive feedback when the patient successfully defecates.

Faecal Incontinence Pouch

To collect and contain large volumes of faeces, the nurse may place a faecal incontinence pouch (rectal pouch) around the anal area. The purpose of the pouch is to prevent progressive perineal skin irritation and breakdown and frequent linen changes necessitated by incontinence.

A rectal pouch is secured around the anal opening and may or may not be attached to drainage. Pouches are best applied before the perineal skin becomes excoriated. If perineal skin excoriation is present, the nurse either (a) applies a moisture-barrier cream to the skin to protect it from faeces until it heals and then applies the pouch or (b) applies a protective powder, skin barrier or hydrocolloid wafer such as Duoderm underneath the pouch to achieve the best possible seal.

Nursing responsibilities for patients with a rectal pouch include (a) regular assessment and documentation of the perineal skin status, (b) changing the bag every 72 hours or sooner if there is leakage, (c) maintaining the drainage system and (d) providing explanations and support to the patient and support people.

Some patients may be treated surgically for faecal incontinence with surgical repair of a damaged sphincter or an artificial bowel sphincter. The artificial sphincter consists of three parts: a cuff around the anal canal, a pressure-regulating balloon and a pump that inflates the cuff (see Figure 22-13). The cuff is inflated to close the sphincter, maintaining continence. To have a bowel movement, the patient deflates the cuff. The cuff automatically reinflates in 10 minutes.

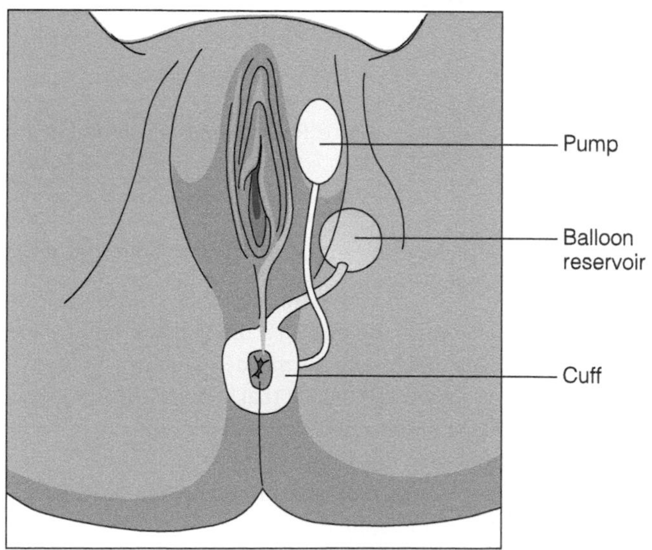

Figure 22-13 Inflatable artificial sphincter.

Ostomy Management

Patients with bowel diversions (ostomies) need considerable psychological support, instruction and physical care. However, here only physical interventions of stoma assessment, application of an appliance to collect faeces, and promotion of predictable evacuation with colostomy irrigation are discussed. Many NHS trusts have stoma nurses who work alongside other healthcare professionals, providing care to patients with stomas.

Stoma and Skin Care

Care of the stoma and skin is important for all patients who have ostomies. The faecal material from a colostomy or ileostomy is irritating to the peristomal skin. This is particularly true of ileal effluent, which contains digestive enzymes. It is important to assess the peristomal skin for irritation each time the appliance is changed. Any irritation or skin breakdown needs to be treated immediately. The skin is kept clean by washing with warm water and dried thoroughly. Specially formulated barrier creams and gels are available to protect the skin from excoriation. See *Procedure 22-2* for changing a bowel diversion ostomy appliance.

Colostomy Irrigation

Colostomy irrigation is a method of mechanically cleaning the colon of faeces by instilling water through the stoma. The water stimulates peristalsis resulting in evacuation of faeces. Colostomy irrigation aims to allow the patient some control over the evacuation of faeces from the stoma.

For most patients, a relatively small amount of fluid (300–500ml) stimulates evacuation. For others, up to 1,000ml may be needed because a colostomy has no sphincter and the fluid tends to return as it is instilled.

EVALUATING

The goals established during the planning phase are evaluated according to specific desired outcomes, also established in that phase. If outcomes are not achieved, the nurse should explore the reasons and modify the nursing care plan as appropriate.

Empathy and sensitivity are required when dealing with bowel elimination. Nurses need to be aware that patients may be embarrassed about their bowel habits and may be reluctant to discuss this with the nurse as it is considered 'dirty'. The nurse needs to effectively communicate with the patient in order to implement appropriate interventions and evaluate their effectiveness.

ACTIVITY 22-3

What interventions could you implement to help restore a patient's normal bowel functioning?

PROCEDURE 22-2 Changing a Bowel Diversion Ostomy Appliance

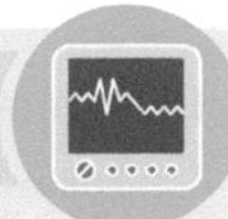

Purposes

- To assess and care for the peristomal skin
- To collect effluent for assessment of the amount and type of output
- To minimise odours for the patient's comfort and self-esteem

Assessment

Determine

- The kind of ostomy and its placement on the abdomen. Surgeons often draw diagrams when there are two stomas. If there is more than one stoma, it is important to confirm which is the functioning stoma.
- The type and size of appliance currently used and the special barrier substance applied to the skin, according to the nursing care plan.
- Any allergies.

Assess

- Stoma colour: the stoma should appear red, similar in colour to the mucosal lining of the inner cheek. Very pale or darker-coloured stomas with a bluish or purplish hue indicate impaired blood circulation to the area.
- Stoma size and shape: most stomas protrude slightly from the abdomen. New stomas normally appear swollen, but swelling generally decreases over two or three weeks or for as long as six weeks. Failure of swelling to recede may indicate a problem, for example, blockage.
- Stomal bleeding: Slight bleeding initially when the stoma is touched is normal, but other bleeding should be reported.
- Status of peristomal skin: Any redness and irritation of the peristomal skin - the 5-13cm of skin surrounding the stoma - should be noted. Transient redness after removal of adhesive is normal.
- Amount and type of faeces. Inspect for abnormalities, such as pus or blood.
- Complaints: complaints of burning sensation under the base plate may indicate skin breakdown. The presence of abdominal discomfort and/or distention also needs to be determined.
- The patient's and family members' learning needs regarding the ostomy and self-care.
- The patient's emotional status, especially strategies used to cope with the ostomy.

Planning

Review features of the appliance to ensure that all parts are present and function correctly.

Equipment

- Clean gloves
- Suitable container to empty appliance contents into
- Cleaning materials, including tissues, warm water, mild soap (optional), washcloth or cotton balls, towel
- Tissue or gauze pad
- Skin barrier (paste, powder, water or liquid skin sealant)
- Stoma measuring guide
- Pen or pencil and scissors
- Clean ostomy appliance
- Deodorant (liquid or tablet) for a nonodour-proof colostomy bag

Implementation

Preparation

1 Determine the need for an appliance change.
   - Assess the used appliance for leakage of effluent. *Effluent can irritate the peristomal skin.*
   - Ask the patient about any discomfort at or around the stoma. *A burning sensation may indicate breakdown beneath the faceplate of the pouch.*
   - Assess the fullness of the pouch. *The weight of an overly full bag may loosen the faceplate and separate it from the skin, causing the effluent to leak and irritate the peristomal skin.*

2 If there is pouch leakage or discomfort at or around the stoma, change the appliance.

3 Select an appropriate time to change the appliance.
   - Avoid times close to meal or visiting hours. *Ostomy odour and effluent may reduce appetite or embarrass the patient.*
   - Avoid times immediately after meals or the administration of any medications that may stimulate bowel evacuation. *It is best to change the pouch when drainage is least likely to occur.*

Performance

1. Follow local policy to ensure that you explain to the patient what you are going to do, why it is necessary and how they can cooperate. Obtain consent and maintain patient privacy and dignity and ensure that the appropriate local infection control procedures are observed.
2. Make the patient comfortable.
3. Empty and remove the ostomy appliance.
   - Empty the contents of the pouch through the bottom opening into a bedpan. *To prevent spillage of effluent onto the patient's skin.*
   - Assess the consistency and the amount of effluent.
   - The appliance is then gently removed from the top, using slight pressure with the fingers on the surrounding skin. *To ensure patient comfort and prevent pulling or tearing of the skin.*
   - If the appliance is disposable, discard according to local policy.
4. Clean and dry the peristomal skin and stoma.
   - Use toilet tissue to remove excess stool.
   - Use warm water, mild soap (optional) and soft tissues or wipes to clean the skin and stoma (see Figure 22-14).
   - Dry the area thoroughly by patting with soft tissues. *Excess rubbing can abrade the skin.*
5. Assess the stoma and peristomal skin.
   - Inspect the stoma for colour, size, shape and bleeding.
   - Inspect the peristomal skin for any redness, ulceration or irritation. Transient redness after the removal of adhesive is normal.
6. Apply skin barrier cream or gel if needed.
7. The stoma should be measured regularly using a guide (see Figure 22-15) and 3mm clearance allowed between the stoma edge and the appliance. *This allows space for the stoma to expand slightly when functioning and minimises the risk of effluent contacting peristomal skin.*

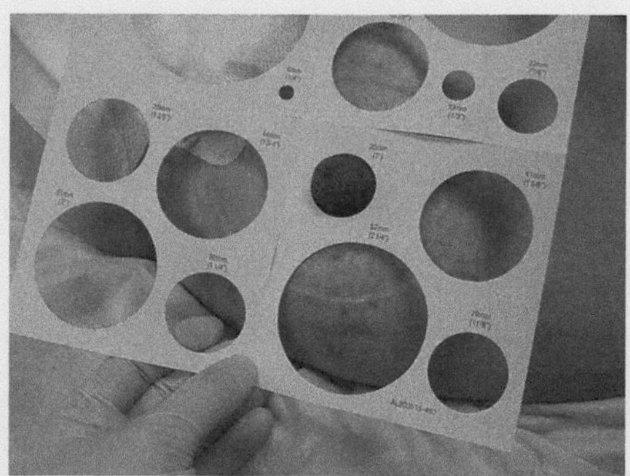

Figure 22-15 A guide for measuring the stoma. (Cory Patrick Hartley, San Ramon Regional Medical Center, San Ramon, CA. Reprinted with permission.)

8. If the stoma is irregular in shape or oval, the adhesive plate of some appliances can be cut to shape.
9. Cut out the traced stoma pattern to make an opening that is the appropriate size and shape.
10. Remove the backing to expose the sticky adhesive side.
11. Centre the skin barrier over the stoma, and gently press it onto the patient's skin, smoothing out any wrinkles or bubbles (see Figure 22-16).
12. Document the procedure in the patient record using forms or checklists supplemented by narrative notes when appropriate. Report and record the patient assessment and any interventions implemented. It is important that any changes in size, colour and skin irritation are documented. A change in stoma colour could be indicative of circulatory impairment and should be reported to the doctor immediately.

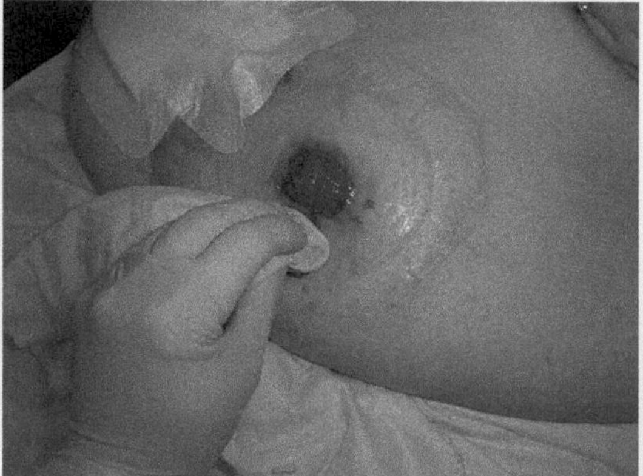

Figure 22-14 Cleaning the skin.
Source: Cory Patrick Hartley, San Ramon Regional Medical Center, San Ramon, CA.

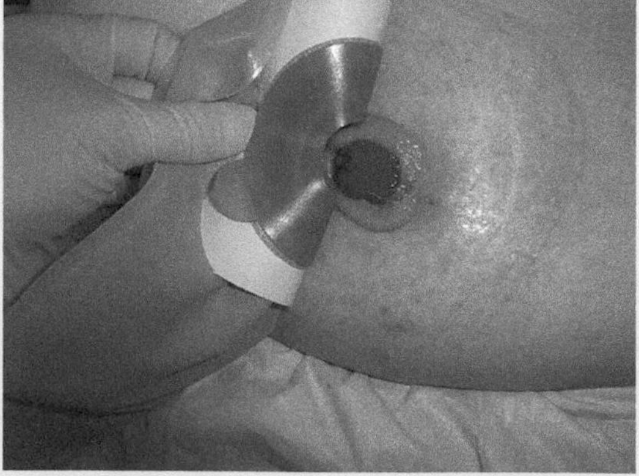

Figure 22-16 Centring the skin barrier over the stoma.
Source: Cory Patrick Hartley, San Ramon Regional Medical Center, San Ramon, CA.

Evaluation

- Relate findings to previous information if available. Adjust the nursing care plan as needed.
- Perform detailed follow-up based on findings if appropriate and report any significant changes to the doctor.

CRITICAL REFLECTION

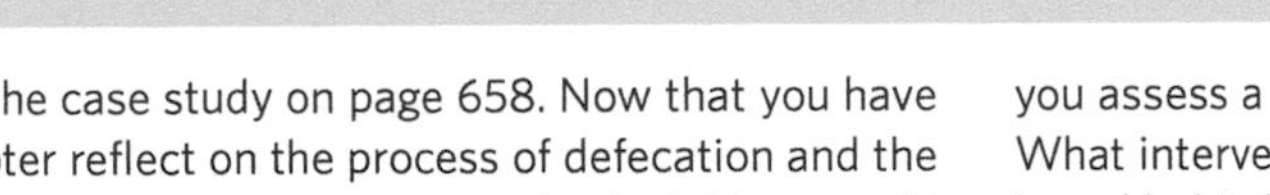

Let us revisit the case study on page 658. Now that you have read this chapter reflect on the process of defecation and the impact incontinence can have on the individual. How would you assess a patient with altered bowel functioning? What interventions would you implement to promote normal bowel habits?

CHAPTER HIGHLIGHTS

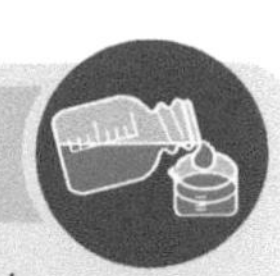

- Primary functions of the large intestine are the excretion of digestive waste products and the maintenance of fluid balance.
- Patterns of bowel elimination vary greatly among people, but a regular pattern of bowel elimination with formed, soft stools is essential to health and a sense of well-being.
- A variety of factors affects defecation: developmental level, diet, fluid intake, activity and exercise, psychological factors, medications and pathologic conditions.
- Normal defecation is often facilitated in both well and ill patients by providing privacy, teaching patients to attend to defecation urges promptly, assisting patients to normal sitting positions whenever possible, encouraging appropriate food and fluid intake, and scheduling regular exercise.
- Common bowel elimination problems include constipation, diarrhoea, bowel incontinence and flatulence.
- Lack of exercise, irregular defecation habits, low fibre diets and overuse of laxatives are all thought to contribute to constipation. Sufficient fluid and fibre intake are required to keep faeces soft.
- An adverse effect of prolonged diarrhoea is fluid and electrolyte imbalance.
- Assessment relative to bowel elimination includes a patient history; physical examination of the abdomen, rectum and anus; and in some situations, visualisation studies and inspection and analysis of stool for abnormal constituents such as blood.
- A patient history includes data about the patient's defecating pattern, description of faeces and any changes, problems associated with elimination, and data about possible factors altering bowel elimination.
- When inspecting the patient's stool, the nurse must observe its colour, consistency, shape, amount, odour and the presence of abnormal constituents.
- Nursing strategies include administering laxatives and antidiarrheals; administering cleansing enemas; applying protective skin agents; monitoring fluid and electrolyte balance; and instructing patients in ways to promote normal defecation.
- Manual evacuation can only be performed once the practitioner has received appropriate training.
- Patients who have bowel diversion ostomies require special care, with attention to psychological adjustment, diet, and stoma and skin care. A variety of stomal management methods is available to these patients, depending on the type and position of the ostomy.

ACTIVITY ANSWERS

ACTIVITY 22-1 Factors that could affect a patient's normal bowel habits could include:

- A change in normal diet
- A reduction in fluid intake
- Excessive fluid loss, e.g. sweating
- Reduced activity
- Low mood /depression
- Change in medication
- Suppression of the urge to defecate

ACTIVITY 22-2 The possible consequences of a change in bowel function for the patient could be:

- Embarrassment
- Low mood or depression
- May not want to interact with others
- Sexual avoidance or aversion
- Pain
- Distention of abdomen
- Increased flatus
- Excoriation of skin around the anus

→

ACTIVITY 22-3 A number of interventions can be implemented to restore a patient's normal bowel functioning. Any decisions need to include the patient and their carers. Interventions may include:

- Education to maintain normal bowel function and recognising changes in bowel functioning
- Advice on increasing dietary fibre
- Referral to dietician if needed
- Advice on increasing fluid intake
- Advise on increasing activity levels
- Management of underlying problem
- Administration of medication
- Referral to GP if there is low mood, self-esteem or altered body image

REFERENCES

Ash, D. (2005) 'Sustaining safe and acceptable bowel care in spinal cord injured patients', *Nursing Standard*, 20(8), 55–64.

Dougherty, L. and Lister, S. (2008) *The Royal Marsden Manual of clinical nursing procedures* (7th edn), Oxford: Wiley-Blackwell.

Grainger, M., Castledine, G., Wood, N. and Dilley, C. (2007) 'Researching the management of constipation in long-term care. Part 2', *British Journal of Nursing*, 16(19), 1212–1217.

Marsh, L. and Sweeney, J. (2008) 'Nurses' knowledge of constipation in people with learning disabilities', *British Journal of Nursing*, 17(4), S11–S16.

NICE (2007) *Faecal incontinence. The management of faecal incontinence in adults*, CG49, London: NICE.

NICE (2010) *Constipation in children and young people. Diagnosis and management of idiopathic childhood constipation in primary and secondary care*, CG99, London: NICE.

NMC (2010) *Standards for pre-registration nursing education*, London: NMC.

Pellatt, G.C. (2007) 'Clinical skills: Bowel elimination and management of complications', *British Journal of Nursing*, 16(6), 351–355.

Powell, M. and Rigby, D. (2000) 'Management of bowel dysfunction: Evacuation difficulties', *Nursing Standard*, 14(47), 47–54.

Royal College of Nursing (2008) *Bowel care, including digital rectal examination and manual removal of faeces: Guidance for nurses*, London: RCN.

Watson, A. (1999) 'Diarrhoea', in Jones, D. (ed.), *ABC of colorectal diseases*, London: BMJ Books.

CHAPTER 23
MEDICATION/DRUG ADMINISTRATION

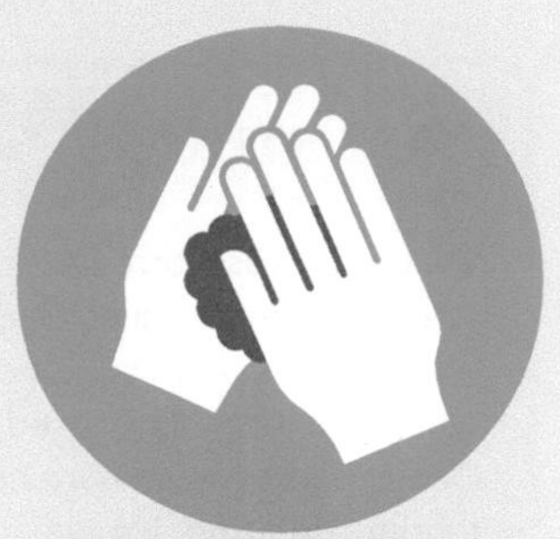

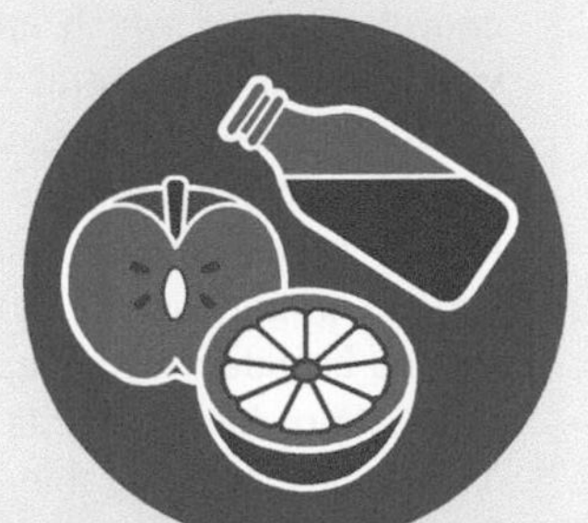

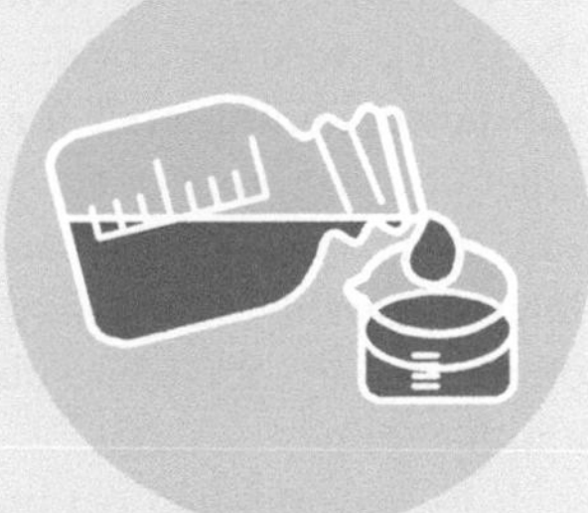

LEARNING OUTCOMES

After completing this chapter, you will be able to:

- Define selected terms related to the administration of medications.
- Describe legal aspects of administering medications.
- Describe various routes of medication administration.
- Recognise systems of measurement that are used in the administration of medications.
- List six essential steps to follow when administering medication.
- State the six 'rights' to accurate medication administration.
- Describe physiological changes in older adults that alter medication administration and effectiveness.
- Outline steps required to administer medications via various routes safely.

After reading this chapter you will be able to reflect on the nursing role in providing healthcare, the way care is organised and the ethical and moral issues to be considered when providing care. It relates to **Essential Skills Clusters (NMC, 2010) 1, 3, 4, 5, 6, 9, 10, 11, 18, 34, 35, 36**, as appropriate for each progression point.

Ensure that you really understand this chapter by logging on to your complimentary **MyNursingKit** at **www.pearsoned.co.uk/kozier**. Complete the self-assessment tests to check your progress and utilise further activities to practise and confirm your understanding.

CASE STUDY

When he was born, Daniel Richards, now six years old, suffered a form of muscle spasm and had his first convulsion within hours. He was cared for in the special care baby unit where he was diagnosed as suffering from cerebral palsy. Daniel had several more convulsions not associated with any febrile condition. He was prescribed a small dose of an anticonvulsant drug which appeared to stabilise his condition, was tube-fed and several days later began to put on weight.

During his early years, Daniels' parents were supported by social and health service professionals to help with caring for him. He developed significant spasticity of his left arm and leg and limited vision, particularly so in his right eye. By his second birthday, his epilepsy was effectively controlled with medication. Mrs Richards and her husband are recognised as showing considerable awareness and understanding of Daniel's needs, likes and dislikes and how to assist him best in his growth and development.

Even though his movement has always been limited, Daniel has showed aspects of his personality as receptive as well as temperamental, including consistent indications of liking some foods whilst disliking loud noises, some types of shoes (made of harder, stiffer materials) and some toys (similarly made of harder wood or materials). The physiotherapist helped the parents to promote Daniel's movement, for example by positioning him with aids so that he can raise his head or clap his hands. The first visit to a swimming pool met with great success as Daniel clearly enjoyed being in the water.

Two days ago Daniel developed an acute chest infection that required hospital admission. The unfamiliar hospital environment, coupled with his painful condition seems to have contributed to Daniel's anxieties. He has begun to refuse oral medication for his epilepsy and chest condition.

INTRODUCTION

The study of the effects of drugs within a living system is known as **pharmacology**. The term 'pharmaceutical' is derived from the Greek word for poison (Siler, 1982), while medication is a substance administered for the diagnosis, cure, treatment or relief of a symptom or for prevention of disease. In the healthcare context, the words medication and drug are generally used interchangeably. The term drug also has the potential meaning of an illegally obtained substance such as heroin, cocaine or amphetamines.

It is evident when reading the literature that the search for the treatment for illness has been recorded since the beginning of time and, indeed, according to Mahdi *et al.* (2006) the earliest prescription known is that written on a clay tablet by a Sumerian physician in 3000BC. It is interesting to note that opium tincture, a drug still used today, was first discovered in the 17th century with morphine developed in 1815. Insulin dates back to 1922. Drugs for the treatment of cancers came into use after the Second World War and, more recently, proton pump inhibitors in 2001. Pharmaceutical companies, government and other organisations constantly research and undertake clinical trials in order to improve knowledge and understanding and identify new drugs to improve the well-being of patients.

The Medicines Act 1968 and Prescription Only Medicines (Human Use) Order 1997 dictate the sale, use, production and prescribing of medication, with the Medicines and Healthcare Products Regulatory Agency (MHRA) regulating medicines within the UK. There are three main types of medicines within the UK:

- Prescription only medication (sold by appropriate practitioner)
- Pharmacy only medicines (sold under supervision of pharmacist)
- Medicines on the general sales list (over the counter medications)

Controlled drugs are governed by the Misuse of Drugs Act 1971 (refer to NMC (2006) for further information).

The written direction for the preparation and administration of a drug is called a prescription, and should be written in full (no abbreviations acceptable) in the generic/official name whenever possible. While many drugs will have trade names, these are not appropriate when prescribing as this can give rite to confusion and misinterpretation. When prescribing, it is important that nurses refer to the British National Formulary (BNF) or The Association of the British Pharmaceutical Industry data sheet compendium to check or confirm side-effects, contraindications, route and dosage.

Medications are often available in a variety of forms (see Table 23-1).

All drugs will have their own unique **pharmacodynamics**, the particular effect they have on the systems of the body. **Pharmacy** may be defined as the art of preparing, compounding and dispensing drugs. The word also refers to the place where drugs are prepared and dispensed. Prescription medication should only be prescribed by the appropriately qualified practitioner (doctor, dentist, pharmacist, nurse prescriber, paramedic, chiropodist and podiatrist (local anaesthetics)) which to some extent depends on the drug being prescribed.

The Cumberlege report (1986) followed by the Crown report (1989) proposed that community nurses should be able to

Table 23-1 Types of Drug Preparation

Type	Description
Aerosol spray or foam	A liquid, powder or foam deposited in a thin layer on the skin by air pressure
Aqueous solution	One or more drugs dissolved in water
Aqueous suspension	One or more drugs finely divided in a liquid such as water
Caplet	A solid form, shaped like a capsule, coated and easily swallowed
Capsule	A gelatinous container to hold a drug in powder, liquid or oil form
Cream	A non-greasy, semi-solid preparation used on the skin
Elixir	A sweetened and aromatic solution of alcohol used as a vehicle for medicinal agents
Extract	A concentrated form of a drug made from vegetables or animals
Gel or jelly	A clear or translucent semi-solid that liquefies when applied to the skin
Liniment	A medication mixed with alcohol, oil or soapy emollient and applied to the skin
Lotion	A medication in a liquid suspension applied to the skin
Lozenge	A flat, round or oval preparation that dissolves and releases a drug when held in the mouth
Ointment	A semi-solid preparation of one or more drugs used for application to the skin and mucous membrane
Paste	A preparation like an ointment, but thicker and stiff, that penetrates the skin less than an ointment
Pill	One or more drugs mixed with a cohesive material, in oval, round or flattened shapes
Powder	A finely ground drug or drugs; some are used internally, others externally
Suppository	One or several drugs mixed with a firm base such as gelatin and shaped for insertion into the body (e.g. the rectum); the base dissolves gradually at body temperature, releasing the drug
Syrup	An aqueous solution of sugar often used to disguise unpleasant-tasting drugs
Tablet	A powdered drug compressed into a hard small disc; some are readily broken along a scored line; others are enteric coated to prevent them from dissolving in the stomach
Tincture	An alcoholic or water-and-alcohol solution prepared from drugs derived from plants
Transdermal patch	A semi-permeable membrane shaped in the form of a disc or patch that contains a drug to be absorbed through the skin over a long period of time

prescribe from a limited formulary. In 1992 the Medicinal Products: Prescription by Nurses Act enabled district nurses to prescribe from a limited formulary. In May 2001 this list was further extended to include some prescription-only medicines. In 2006 the Nurse Prescribers' Extended Formulary was discontinued and replaced by Nurse Independent Prescribers (Department of Health, 2006). (Further information is available from hyperlink at the end of the chapter.) At the end of 2009, legislation was amended to allow nurse and midwife independent prescribers to prescribe unlicensed medicines for those in their care on the same basis as doctors, dentists and supplementary prescribers (NMC, 2010a).

Patient Group Directive (PGD) is a format by which a range of registered healthcare professionals can supply and administer a named licensed medicine for a defined clinical condition without referring to a doctor, e.g. child immunisation or family planning. These include:

- Registered nurses
- Midwives
- Health visitors
- Optometrists
- Pharmacists
- Chiropodists
- Radiographers
- Orthoptists
- Physiotherapists
- Paramedics
- Dieticians
- Occupational therapists
- Speech and language therapists
- Prosthetists and orthotists.

However, it is important to note that there are strict guidelines that have to be met and followed during this process.

Protocols have been used for a long time within hospitals and the community. They are different from Nurse Independent Prescribing as they do not allow the nurse to make independent choices in relation to the medication or treatment. They are often used in the community for immunisation. However, the nurse remains accountable and responsible for the medication administered (NMC, 2010b).

DRUG STANDARDS

Drugs may have natural (e.g. plant, mineral and animal) sources, or they may be synthesised in the laboratory. For example, digitalis and opium are plant derived, iron and sodium chloride are minerals, insulin and vaccines have animal or human sources, and the sulphonamides (trimethoprim an antibacterial drug) are the products of laboratory synthesis. Early drugs were derived from the three natural sources only. More and more drugs, however, are being produced synthetically.

Drugs vary in strength and activity. Drugs derived from plants, for example, vary in strength according to the age of the plant, the variety, the place in which it is grown and the method by which it is preserved. Drugs must be pure and of uniform strength if drug dosages are to be predictable in their effect. Drug standards have therefore been developed to ensure uniform quality.

CLINICAL ALERT

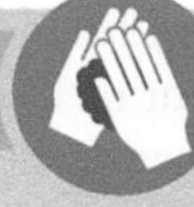

Whenever a nurse is administering any form of medicine it is essential that they are aware of the side-effects, contraindications, and the

- Right drug
- Right route
- Right dose
- Right patient
- Right time
- Right documentation.

LEGAL ASPECTS OF DRUG ADMINISTRATION

The administration of drugs is controlled by law. Key UK legislation relating to medicines and prescribing is as follows:

- *Medicines Act 1968* – the first comprehensive legislation on medicines in the UK. This is the primary legislation (including some other secondary legislation) that provides the legal framework for the manufacture, licensing, prescribing, supply and administration of medicines. The classification of the medicines is noted earlier in the chapter.
- *Misuse of Drugs Act (MDA) 1971* – provides the statutory framework for the control and regulation of controlled drugs. The MDA makes it unlawful to possess or supply a controlled drug unless an exception or exemption applies.
- *Misuse of Drugs Regulations (MDR) 2001* and *Misuse of Drugs Regulations Northern Ireland (NI) 2002*. The MDR classifies drugs into five schedules depending on the level of control required.
- *Misuse of Drugs (Safe Custody) Regulations 1973* and *Misuse of Drugs (Safe Custody) Regulations Northern Ireland 1973* – imposes controls on the storage of drugs.
- *Misuse of Drugs (Supply to Addicts) Regulations 1997* and *Misuse of Drugs (Notification and Supply to Addicts (Northern Ireland)) Regulations 1973* – prohibit doctors from prescribing, administering or supplying diamorphine, cocaine or dipipanone for the treatment of addiction or suspected addiction except under Home Office licence.
- *Amendment Order 2000* – forbids the sale of aspirin and paracetamol drugs in large quantities.
- *Professional Nurse Midwives and Health Visitors Act 1997* – extended nurse prescribing to additionally trained registered nurses other than community health specialists. It also allows midwives to possess and administer diamorphine, morphine, pethidine or pentazocine in the course of their work.
- *Health Act 2006* – key provisions:
  - All designated bodies such as healthcare organisations and independent hospitals required to appoint an accountable officer.
  - A duty of collaboration placed on responsible bodies, healthcare organisations and other local and national agencies including professional regulatory bodies, police forces, the Healthcare Commission and the Commission for Social Care inspection to share intelligence on controlled drug issues.
  - A power of entry and inspection for the police and other nominated people to enter premises to inspect stocks and records of controlled drugs.
- *Controlled Drugs (Supervision of Management and Use) Regulations 2006* – set out the requirements for certain NHS bodies and independent healthcare bodies to appoint an accountable officer, and describe the duties and responsibilities of accountable officers to improve the management and use of controlled drugs.

These regulations set out the requirements for certain NHS bodies and independent healthcare bodies to appoint an accountable officer, and describe the duties and responsibilities of accountable officers to improve the management and use of controlled drugs.

The Nursing Midwifery Council (NMC, 2010b) standards for medicines management have been amended from the 2007 publication. The standards inform and guide nurses in the correct procedure for ordering, storing, administering and, where applicable, prescribing medication, whether in the home or in a healthcare environment. The NMC (2010b) guidelines state that:

> *The clinical, cost-effective and safe use of medicines to ensure patients get the maximum benefit from the medicines they need, while at the same time minimising potential harm.* (MHRA, 2004, p. 1)

Nurses are accountable and responsible for their actions when administering drugs at each point of the process, before, during and after administration of the drug. As indicated above, there is a great deal of legislation and regulation governing both this process and the duties of the nurse. It is the responsibility of the nurse:

- To understand the drug and its properties and its effect on the patient, taking into account lifespan considerations.
- To ensure that the patient is aware of the reason for the medication being given and of any possible side-effects.
- To gain consent.

It is the responsibility of the nurse in charge to ensure that drugs are stored safely and that their administration is documented. The Medicines Act 1968, the Misuse of Drugs Act 1971 and all other regulation, including that specified by the Nursing and Midwifery governing body (NMC), govern the legal responsibilities of the nurse or midwife in areas such as:

- methods of supplying/administering medicines;
- dispensing;

- storage and transportation;
- standards for practice of administration of medicine;
- delegation;
- disposal of medicinal products;
- unlicensed medication;
- complementary and alternative therapies;
- management of adverse events (errors or incidents) in the administration of medicines;
- controlled drugs.

It is important that the nurse understands that while there are national guidelines in relation to administration of medicines there are also local policies that influence and guide practice. Controlled drugs, for example, should be checked and verified by two nurses prior to dispensing and again, e.g. at the bedside, when the drug is administered to the patient. Controlled drugs should also be checked on a daily basis for accuracy – local policies will dictate how this is managed – and log/records must be kept of this process. Included on the record are the controlled substances wasted during preparation. When a portion or all of a controlled substance dose is discarded, the nurse must ask a second registered nurse to witness the discarding. Both nurses must sign the control drug book or inventory record.

Despite all these legal and safety measures, errors occur. According to the National Patient Safety Organisation (2009) there were over 72,000 reported cases of drug errors made in 2007, and drug errors comprised the third highest group of incidents, after accidents and treatment procedures, with incidents occurring in acute care being the most common.

EFFECTS OF DRUGS

The therapeutic effect of a drug is the primary effect intended, and is the reason the drug is prescribed. For example, the therapeutic effect of morphine sulphate is analgesia (pain relief), and the therapeutic effect of diazepam is relief of anxiety. See Table 23-2 for kinds of therapeutic actions.

A side-effect, or secondary effect, of a drug is one that is unintended. Side-effects are usually predictable and may be either harmless or potentially harmful. For example, digitalis increases the strength of myocardial contractions (desired effect), but it can have the side-effect of inducing nausea and vomiting. Some side-effects are tolerated for the drug's therapeutic effect; more severe side-effects, also called adverse effects, may justify the discontinuation of a drug.

Drug toxicity (adverse effects of a drug on an organism or tissue) results from overdosage, ingestion of a drug intended for external use and build-up of the drug in the blood because of impaired metabolism or excretion (cumulative effect). Some toxic effects are apparent immediately; some are not apparent for weeks or months. Fortunately, most drug toxicity is avoidable if careful attention is paid to dosage and monitoring for toxicity. An example of a toxic effect is respiratory depression due to the cumulative effect of morphine sulphate in the body.

A drug allergy is an immunologic reaction to a drug. When a patient is first exposed to a foreign substance (antigen), the body may react by producing antibodies. A patient can react to a drug as to an antigen and thus develop symptoms of an allergic reaction.

Allergic reactions can be either mild or severe. A mild reaction has a variety of symptoms; from skin rashes to diarrhoea (see Table 23-3). An allergic reaction can occur any time from a few minutes to two weeks after the administration of the drug. A severe allergic reaction usually occurs immediately after the administration of the drug and is called an anaphylactic reaction. This response can be fatal if the symptoms are not noticed immediately and treatment is not obtained promptly. The earliest symptoms are acute shortness of breath, wheezing, rash, acute hypotension and tachycardia.

Drug tolerance exists in a person who has an unusually low physiological response to a drug and who requires increases in the dosage to maintain a given therapeutic effect. Drugs that commonly produce tolerance are opiates, barbiturates and tobacco. A cumulative effect is the increasing response to repeated doses of a drug that occurs when the rate of administration exceeds the rate of metabolism or excretion. As a result, the amount of the drug builds up in the patient's body unless the dosage is adjusted. Toxic symptoms may occur. An idiosyncratic effect is unexpected and individual. Under-response and

Table 23-2 Therapeutic Actions of Drugs

Drug type	Description	Examples
Palliative	Relieves the symptoms of a disease but does not affect the disease itself	Morphine sulphate, dexamethasone reduces oedema
Curative	Cures a disease or condition	Antibiotics for infection
Supportive	Supports body function until other treatments or the body's response can take over	Laxative for constipation
Substitutive	Replaces body fluids or substances	Thyroxine for hypothyroidism, insulin for diabetes mellitus
Chemotherapeutic	Destroys malignant cells	Melphalan for treatment of multiple myeloma
Restorative	Returns the body to health	Vitamin, mineral supplements

Table 23-3 Common Mild Allergic Responses

Symptom	Description/rationale
Skin rash	Either an intraepidermal vesicle rash or a rash typified by an urticarial wheal or macular eruption; rash is usually generalised over the body
Pruritus	Itching of the skin with or without a rash
Angioedema	Oedema due to increased permeability of the blood capillaries
Rhinitis	Excessive watery discharge from the nose
Lacrimal tearing	Excessive tearing
Nausea, vomiting	Stimulation of these centres in the brain
Wheezing and dyspnoea	Shortness of breath and wheezing on inhalation and exhalation due to accumulated fluids and swelling of the respiratory tissues
Diarrhoea/ abdominal pain	Irritation of the mucosa of the large intestine

over-response to a drug may be idiosyncratic. Also, the drug may have a completely different effect from the normal one or cause unpredictable and unexplainable symptoms in a particular patient.

A drug interaction occurs when the administration of one drug before, at the same time as, or after another drug alters the effect of one or both drugs. The effect of one or both drugs may be either increased (potentiating or synergistic effect) or decreased (inhibiting effect). Drug interactions may be beneficial or harmful. The use of aspirin with warfarin is contraindicated as they may enhance anticoagulant effect; however, depending on the diagnosis this is sometimes ignored.

Iatrogenic disease (disease caused unintentionally by medical therapy) can be due to drug therapy. Hepatic toxicity resulting in biliary obstruction, renal damage and malformations of the foetus as a result of specific drugs taken during pregnancy are examples.

DRUG MISUSE

Drug misuse is the improper use of common medications in ways that lead to acute and chronic toxicity. Both over-the-counter drugs and prescription drugs may be misused. Laxatives, antacids, vitamins, headache remedies and cough and cold medications are often self-prescribed and overused. Most people suffer no harmful effects from these drugs, but some people do. An irritable bowel may sometimes be ignored and may go undiagnosed as a possible polyp or a more serious condition.

Drug abuse is inappropriate intake of a substance, either continually or periodically. By definition, drug use is abusive when society considers it abusive. For example, the intake of alcohol at work may be considered alcohol abuse, but intake at a social gathering may not. Drug abuse has two main facets, drug dependence and habituation. Drug dependence is a person's reliance on or need to take a drug or substance. The two types of dependence, physiological and psychological, may occur separately or together. **Physiological** dependence is due to biochemical changes in body tissues, especially the nervous system. These tissues come to require the substance for normal functioning. A dependent person who stops using the drug experiences withdrawal symptoms. Psychological dependence is emotional reliance on a drug to maintain a sense of well-being, accompanied by feelings of need or cravings for that drug. There are varying degrees of psychological dependence, ranging from mild desire to craving and compulsive use of the drug.

Drug habituation denotes a mild form of psychological dependence. The individual develops the habit of taking the substance and feels better after taking it. The habituated individual tends to continue the habit even though it may be injurious to health.

Illicit drugs, also called street drugs, are those sold illegally. Illicit drugs are of two types: (a) drugs unavailable for purchase under any circumstances, such as cannabis, and (b) drugs normally available with prescriptions that are being obtained through illegal channels. Illicit drugs often are taken because of their mood-altering effect; that is, they make the person feel happy or relaxed.

ACTIONS OF DRUGS ON THE BODY

The action of a drug in the body can be described in terms of its half-life, the time interval required for the body's elimination processes to reduce the concentration of the drug in the body by one-half. For example, if a drug's half-life is eight hours, then the amount of drug in the body is as follows:

- initially: 100%
- after 8 hours: 50%
- after 16 hours: 25%
- after 24 hours: 12.5%
- after 32 hours: 6.25%.

Because the purpose of most drug therapy is to maintain a constant drug level in the body, repeated doses are required to maintain that level. When an orally administered drug is absorbed from the gastrointestinal tract into the blood plasma, its concentration in the plasma increases until the elimination rate equals the rate of absorption. This point is known as the peak plasma level (see Figure 23-1). Unless the patient receives another dose of the drug, the concentration steadily decreases. Key terms related to drug actions are as follows:

- *Onset of action*: the time after administration when the body initially responds to the drug.
- *Peak plasma level*: the highest plasma level achieved by a single dose when the elimination rate of a drug equals the absorption rate.

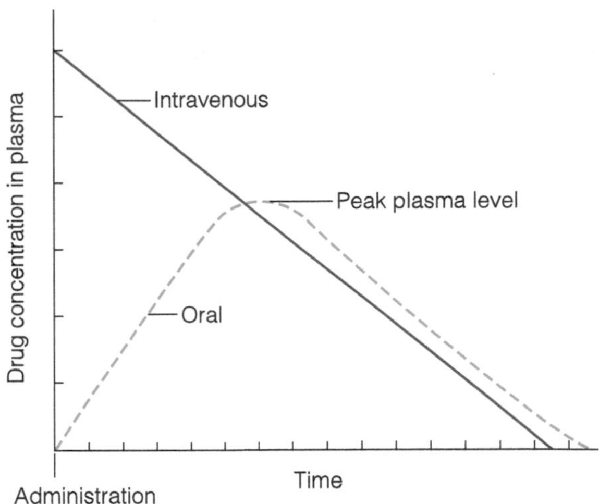

Figure 23-1 A graphic plot of drug concentration in the blood plasma following a single dose.

- *Drug half-life (elimination half-life)*: the time required for the elimination process to reduce the concentration of the drug to one-half what it was at initial administration.
- *Plateau*: a maintained concentration of a drug in the plasma during a series of scheduled doses.

Pharmacodynamics

Pharmacodynamics is the process by which a drug alters cell physiology. One of the mechanisms is the drug interaction with a cellular receptor to produce a response known as an agonist. Drugs that have no special pharmacological action of their own but that inhibit or prevent the action of an agonist are called specific antagonists. Drugs may also produce a response by stimulating enzyme activity or hormone production. They have a syngeristic effect.

Pharmacokinetics

Pharmacokinetics is the study of the absorption, distribution, biotransformation and excretion of drugs.

Absorption

Absorption is the process by which a drug passes into the bloodstream. Unless the drug is administered directly into the bloodstream, absorption is the first step in the movement of the drug through the body. For absorption to occur, the correct form of the drug must be given by the route intended.

The rate of absorption of a drug in the stomach is variable. Food, for example, can delay the dissolution and absorption of some drugs as well as their passage into the small intestine, where most drug absorption occurs. Food can also combine with molecules of certain drugs, thereby changing their molecular structure and subsequently inhibiting or preventing their absorption. Another factor that affects the absorption of some drugs is the acid medium in the stomach. Acidity can vary according to the time of day, foods ingested and the age of the patient. Some drugs do not dissolve or have limited ability to dissolve in the gastrointestinal guides, decreasing their absorption into the bloodstream. Some drugs are absorbed by tissues before they reach the stomach. For example, glyceryl trinitrate is administered under the tongue, where it is absorbed into the blood vessels that carry it directly to the heart, the intended site of action. If swallowed, this drug will be absorbed into the bloodstream and carried to the liver, where it will be destroyed.

A drug administered directly into the bloodstream, that is, intravenously, is immediately in the vascular system without having to be absorbed. This, then, is the route of choice for rapid action. Because subcutaneous tissue has a poorer blood supply than muscle tissue, absorption from subcutaneous tissue is slower. The rate of absorption of a drug can be accelerated by the application of heat, which increases blood flow to the area; conversely, absorption can be slowed by the application of cold. In addition, the injection of a vasoconstrictor drug such as epinephrine/adrenaline into the tissue can slow absorption of other drugs. Some drugs intended to be absorbed slowly are suspended in a low-solubility medium, such as oil. The absorption of drugs from the rectum into the bloodstream tends to be unpredictable. Therefore, this route is normally used when other routes are unavailable or when the intended action is localised to the rectum or sigmoid colon.

Distribution

Distribution is the transportation of a drug from its site of absorption to its site of action. When a drug enters the bloodstream, it is carried to the most vascular organs – that is, liver, kidneys and brain. Body areas with lower blood supply – that is, skin and muscles – receive the drug later. The chemical and physical properties of a drug largely determine the area of the body to which the drug will be attracted. For example, fat-soluble drugs will accumulate in fatty tissue, whereas other drugs may bind with plasma proteins.

Biotransformation

Biotransformation, also called detoxification or metabolism, is a process by which a drug is converted to a less active form. Most biotransformation takes place in the liver, where many drug-metabolising enzymes in the cells detoxify the drugs. The products of this process are called metabolites. There are two types of metabolites: active and inactive. An active metabolite has a pharmacological action itself, whereas an inactive metabolite does not.

Biotransformation may be impaired if a person is older or has an unhealthy liver. Nurses must be alert to the accumulation of the active drug in these patients and to subsequent toxicity.

Excretion

Excretion is the process by which metabolites and drugs are eliminated from the body. Most metabolites are eliminated by the kidneys in the urine; however, some are excreted in the faeces, the breath, perspiration, saliva and breast milk. Certain drugs, such as general anaesthetic agents, are excreted in an unchanged form via the respiratory tract. The efficiency with which the kidneys excrete drugs and metabolites diminishes with age. Older people may require smaller doses of a drug because the drug and its metabolites may accumulate in the body.

FACTORS AFFECTING MEDICATION ACTION

A number of factors other than the drug itself can affect its action. A person may not respond in the same manner to successive doses of a drug. In addition, the identical drug and dosage may affect different patients differently.

Developmental Factors

During pregnancy women must be very careful about taking medications. Drugs taken during pregnancy pose a risk throughout the pregnancy, but pose the highest risk during the first trimester, due to the formation of vital organs and functions of the foetus during this time. Most drugs are contraindicated because of the possible adverse effects on the foetus.

Infants usually require small dosages because of their body size and the immaturity of their organs, especially the liver and kidneys. They often do not have all of the enzymes required for drug metabolism and therefore may require different medications than adults. In adolescence or adulthood, allergic reactions may occur to drugs formerly tolerated.

Mature adults have different responses to medications due to physiological changes that accompany ageing. These changes include decreased liver and kidney function, which can result in the accumulation of the drug in the body. In addition, the older person may be on multiple drugs and incompatibilities may occur.

Mature adults often experience decreased gastric mobility and decreased gastric acid production and blood flow, which can impair drug absorption. Increased adipose tissue and decreased total body liquid proportionate to the body mass can increase the possibility of drug toxicity. Older adults may also experience a decreased number of protein-binding sites and changes in the blood–brain barrier. The latter permits fat-soluble drugs to move readily to the brain, often resulting in dizziness and confusion. This is particularly evident with beta blockers.

Gender

Differences in the way men and women respond to drugs are chiefly related to the distribution of body fat and liquid and hormonal differences. Because most drug research is done on men, more research on women is required to reflect the effects of hormonal changes on drug actions in women.

Cultural, Ethnic and Genetic Factors

A patient's response to a drug is influenced by age, gender, size and body composition. This variation in response is called drug polymorphism (Kumar and Clark, 2009). Research studies indicate that ethnicity may contribute to differences in responses to medication. This is called genetic polymorphism. Kumar and Clark (2009) state that the most common polymorphisms of the cytochrome P450 family of enzymes can affect the therapeutic and adverse response to drug treatment. A component of the herbal remedy St John's Wort (used to treat depression) is Hyperforin which carries a warning on its packaging reminding individuals that it may interact with other prescribed medication, due to the variability in the genes encoding drug-metabolising enzymes (Kumar and Clark, 2009).

Genes that control liver metabolism vary and some patients may have slow metabolism, whereas others are rapid metabolisers. Research has shown that certain medication may work well at usual therapeutic dosages for certain ethnic groups but be toxic for others.

Diet

Nutrients can affect the action of a medication. For example, vitamin K found in green leafy vegetables can counteract the effect of an anticoagulant such as warfarin.

Environment

The patient's environment can affect the action of drugs, particularly those used to alter behaviour and mood. Therefore, nurses assessing the effects of a drug need to consider the drug in the context of the patient's personality.

Environmental temperature may also affect drug activity. When environmental temperature is high the peripheral blood vessels dilate, thus intensifying the action of vasodilators. In contrast, a cold environment and the consequent vasoconstriction inhibit the action of vasodilators but enhance the action of vasoconstrictors. A patient who takes a sedative or analgesic in a busy, noisy environment may not benefit as fully as if the environment were quiet and peaceful.

Psychological Factors

A patient's expectations about what a drug can do can affect the response to the medication. For example, a patient who believes that codeine is ineffective as an analgesic may experience no relief from pain after it is given.

Illness and Disease

Illness and disease can also affect the action of drugs. For example, Paracetamol can reduce the body temperature of a feverish patient but has no effect on the body temperature of a patient without fever. Drug action is altered in patients with circulatory, liver or kidney dysfunction.

Time of Administration

The time of administration of oral medications affects the relative speed with which they act. Orally administered medications are absorbed more quickly if the stomach is empty. Thus oral medications taken two hours before meals, act faster than those taken after meals. However, some medications, for example iron preparations, irritate the gastrointestinal tract and need to be given after a meal, when they will be better tolerated. A patient's sleep/wake rhythm may affect the action of a drug. Circadian variations in urine output and blood circulation, for example, may affect a patient's response to a drug.

ROUTES OF ADMINISTRATION

Pharmaceutical preparations are generally designed for one or two specific routes of administration (see Table 23-4). The route of administration should be indicated when the drug is prescribed. When administering a drug, the nurse should ensure that the pharmaceutical preparation is appropriate for the route specified.

Oral

Oral administration is the most common, least expensive and most convenient route for most patients. In oral administration, the drug is swallowed. Because the skin is not broken as it is for an injection, oral administration is also a safe method.

The major disadvantages are possibly unpleasant taste of the drugs, irritation of the gastric mucosa, irregular absorption from the gastrointestinal tract, slow absorption and, in some cases, harm to the patient's teeth. For example, the liquid preparation of ferrous sulphate (iron) can stain the teeth.

Sublingual

In **sublingual** administration a drug is placed under the tongue, where it dissolves (see Figure 23-2). In a relatively short time, the drug is largely absorbed into the blood vessels on the underside of the tongue. The medication should not be swallowed. Glyceryl trinitrate is one example of a drug commonly given in this manner.

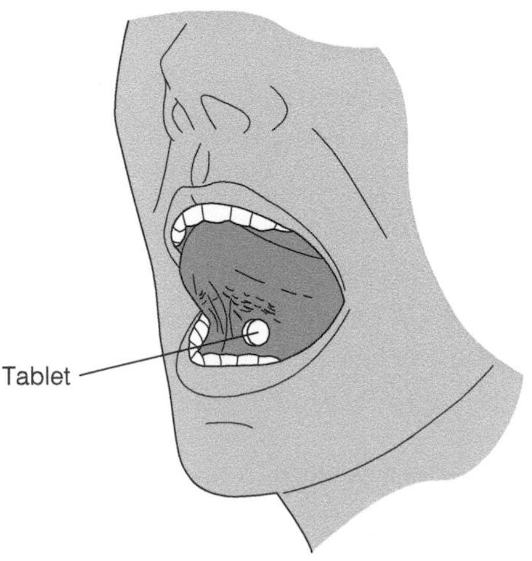

Figure 23-2 Sublingual administration of a tablet.

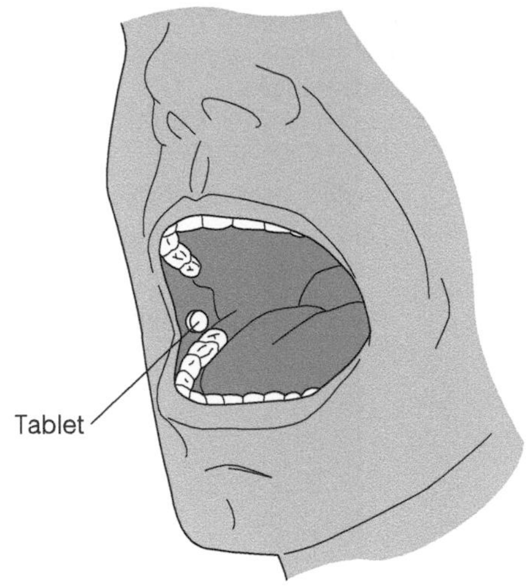

Figure 23-3 Buccal administration of a tablet.

Buccal

Buccal means 'pertaining to the cheek'. In buccal administration, a medication (e.g. a tablet) is held in the mouth against the mucous membranes of the cheek until the drug dissolves (see Figure 23-3). The drug may act locally on the mucous membranes of the mouth or systemically when it is swallowed in the saliva.

Parenteral

The **parenteral** route is defined as other than through the alimentary or respiratory tract; that is, by needle. The following are some of the more common routes for parenteral administration:

- subcutaneous – into the subcutaneous tissue, just below the skin;
- intramuscular – into a muscle;
- intradermal – under the epidermis (into the dermis);
- intravenous – into a vein.

Some of the less commonly used routes for parenteral administration are intra-arterial (into an artery), intracardiac (into the heart muscle), intraosseous (into a bone), intrathecal or intraspinal (into the spinal canal), intrapleural (into the pleural space), and intra-articular (into a joint). Sterile equipment and sterile drug solution are essential for all parenteral therapy. The main advantage is fast absorption. Epidural (into the epidural space) is one of the more common routes and has become increasingly more popular in the last decade. The epidural route is used as it provides improved 'postoperative analgesia and attenuation of the stress response to surgery' (Chanay, 2009). It is also the analgesia of choice for pregnant women during labour. However, this technique is not without its disadvantages, e.g. hypotension, respiratory depression, pruritus and nausea and vomiting (Chanay, 2009).

Table 23-4 Routes of Administration

Route	Advantages	Disadvantages
Oral	Most convenient.	Inappropriate for patients with nausea or vomiting.
	Usually least expensive.	Drug may have unpleasant taste or odour.
	Safe, does not break skin barrier.	Inappropriate when gastrointestinal tract has reduced motility.
	Administration usually does not cause stress.	Inappropriate if patient cannot swallow or is unconscious.
		Cannot be used before certain diagnostic tests or surgical procedures.
		Drug may discolour teeth, harm tooth enamel.
		Drug may irritate gastric mucosa.
		Drug can be aspirated by seriously ill patients.
Sublingual	Same as for oral, *plus*	If swallowed, drug may be inactivated by gastric juice.
	Drug can be administered for local effect.	Drug must remain under tongue until dissolved and absorbed.
	More potent than oral route because drug directly enters the blood and bypasses the liver.	Drug is rapidly absorbed into the bloodstream.
Buccal	Same as for sublingual.	Same as for sublingual.
Rectal	Can be used when drug has objectionable taste or odour.	Dose absorbed is unpredictable.
	Drug released at slow, steady rate.	
Vaginal	Provides a local therapeutic effect.	Limited use.
Topical	Provides a local effect.	May be messy and may soil clothes.
	Few side effects.	Drug can enter body through abrasions and cause systemic effects.
Transdermal	Prolonged systemic effect.	Leaves residue on the skin that may soil clothes.
	Few side effects.	
	Avoids gastrointestinal absorption problems.	
Subcutaneous	Onset of drug action faster than oral.	Must involve sterile technique because breaks skin barrier.
		More expensive than oral.
		Can administer only small volume.
		Slower than intramuscular administration.
		Some drugs can irritate tissues and cause pain.
		Can produce anxiety.
Intramuscular	Pain from irritating drugs is minimised.	Breaks skin barrier.
	Can administer larger volume than subcutaneous.	Can produce anxiety.
	Drug is rapidly absorbed.	
Intradermal	Absorption is slow (this is an advantage in testing for allergies).	Amount of drug administered must be small.
		Breaks skin barrier.
Intravenous	Rapid effect.	Limited to highly soluble drugs.
		Drug distribution inhibited by poor circulation.
Inhalation	Introduces drug throughout respiratory tract.	Drug intended for localised effect can have systemic effect.
	Rapid localised relief.	Of use only for the respiratory system.
	Drug can be administered to unconscious patient.	

Topical

Topical applications are those applied to a circumscribed surface area of the body. They affect only the area to which they are applied. Topical applications include the following:

- *dermatologic preparations* – applied to the skin;
- *instillations and irrigations* – applied into body cavities or orifices, such as the urinary bladder, eyes, ears, nose, rectum or vagina;
- *inhalations* – administered into the respiratory tract by a nebuliser or positive pressure breathing apparatus. Air, oxygen and vapour are generally used to carry the drug into the lungs.

MEDICATION PRESCRIPTIONS AND CHARTS

An appropriate qualified and experienced clinician (see earlier in chapter) usually determines the patient's medication requirements and prescribes the medication. Best practice is the written form; however, in some areas verbal and telephone orders are acceptable according to local policies. Confirmation of the request followed by written documentation (by nurse) supported as soon as possible after the event by the prescribing clinician is a legal requirement.

It is now a legal requirement that the generic or official name is printed on the prescription chart and abbreviations should NOT be used.

Types of Medication Prescriptions

Four common medication prescriptions are the stat, the single once only, the regular daily and the prn prescription.

- A stat prescription indicates that the medication is to be given immediately and only once (e.g. Dexamethasone 10mg stat prior to chemotherapy regime).
- The single or one once only is for medication to be given once at a specified time (e.g. Midazolam 0.5mg/kg oral premedication for children before minor operation).
- The routine daily medication may or may not have a termination date and is administered until the medication chart is reviewed.
- A prn or as needed prescription permits the nurse to give a medication when, in the nurse's judgement, the patient requires it (e.g. metoclopramide 10 mcgs for nausea twice daily for an infant up to one years of age). The nurse must use good judgement about when the medication is needed and when it can be safely administered.

Essential Parts of a Prescription Chart

The drug chart should be written legibly in black ink and signed by the person prescribing. There are seven essential parts:

1 full name and address of the patient;
2 patient's hospital/record/NHS number;
3 date and time the drug is written;
4 name of the drug to be administered;
5 dosage of the drug;
6 frequency of administration;
7 route of administration;
8 signature of the person prescribing.

In addition, unless it is a regular administration section it should state the number of doses or the number of days the drug is to be administered.

The patient's full name, that is, the first and last names and middle initials or names, should always be used to avoid confusion between two patients who have the same last name. Some hospitals imprint the patient's name, address, date of birth and identification number on all forms while some areas use stickers with similar information.

The name of the drug to be administered must be clearly written. In most settings only generic/official names are permitted.

The dosage of the drug includes the amount, the times or frequency of administration and, in many instances, the strength; for example, tetracycline 250mg (amount) four times a day (frequency); potassium chloride 10% (strength) 5ml (amount) three times a day with meals (time and frequency).

Also included on the chart is the route of administration of the drug. This part of the prescription, like other parts, is frequently abbreviated. It is not unusual for a drug to have several possible routes of administration; therefore, it is important that the route be included in the prescription.

The signature of the prescriber makes the drug chart a legal document. An unsigned chart has no validity, and the ordering prescriber needs to be notified if the chart is unsigned. Current practice with all inpatients (or as per local policy) is that a pharmacist will check all new admissions prescription charts to ensure that there are no contraindications within the prescribed medication. The pharmacist will also advise patients during their time in hospital of any new medication prescribed and offer advice in some cases (i.e. warfarin) and will re-check when dispensing medication for discharge.

Medication administration records (see Figure 23-4) vary in form, but all include the patient's name, identification number, clinical area name; drug name and dose; and times and method of administration.

The nurse should always question the prescriber about any chart that is ambiguous, unusual (e.g. an abnormally high dosage of a medication), contraindicated by the patient's condition or illegible. When the nurse judges a prescribed medication inappropriate, the following actions are required:

- Contact the prescriber and discuss the rationale for believing the medication or dosage to be inappropriate.
- Document in the patient notes the following: when the prescriber was notified, what was conveyed to the prescriber and how the prescriber responded.

IN-PATIENT MEDICATION ADMINISTRATION RECORD

NHS WALES GIG CYMRU

HOSPITAL ________________

WARD ________________

CONSULTANT ________________

MULTIPLE MEDICATION CHARTS

CHART .... OF ....

MEDICATION ON SUPPLEMENTARY CHARTS SHOULD BE RECORDED ON THE DRUG CHART.

DETAILS OF SUPPLEMENTARY CHARTS TICK APPROPRIATE BOX	
ANTICOAGULANT ☐	OXYGEN ☐
SUPPLEMENTARY INFUSION CHART ☐	PATIENT CONTROLLED ANALGESIA/EPIDURAL ☐
INSULIN ☐	SYRINGE DRIVER ☐
OTHER (PLEASE SPECIFY)	

PRESCRIPTION FOR ONCE-ONLY and PRE-ANAESTHETIC MEDICATION

DATE	MEDICINE (APPROVED NAME)	DOSE	ROUTE	TIME TO BE GIVEN	PRESCRIBER'S SIGNATURE	PHARMACY	DATE	TIME GIVEN	GIVEN BY	CHECKED BY
					bleep No.					
					bleep No.					
					bleep No.					
					bleep No.					
					bleep No.					
					bleep No.					
					bleep No.					
					bleep No.					
					bleep No.					
					bleep No.					
					bleep No.					
					bleep No.					
					bleep No.					
					bleep No.					

PHARMACY SECTION

MEDICATION HISTORY TAKEN

INITIALS .... DATE ....

OBTAINED FROM

PATIENT ☐ NH/RH ☐ CARER ☐

GP ☐ POD'S ☐ OTHER..............................

COMPLIANCE ISSUES IDENTIFIED?
(e.g. MDS, COMPLIANCE CARD)

SPECIFY ....

DISCHARGE PRESCRIPTION WRITTEN

SIGNATURE .... DATE ....

GP CONTACT DETAILS

COMMUNITY PHARMACY CONTACT DETAILS

COMMENTS / NOTES

IN-PATIENT MEDICATION ADMINISTRATION RECORD

Figure 23-4 Sample medication administration record.

- If the prescriber cannot be reached, document all attempts to contact the prescriber and the reason for withholding the medication.
- It may be appropriate for the nurse to contact a more senior doctor and/or pharmacist to advise and seek advice on whether the judgement made by the nurse is accurate and acceptable in line with his/her Professional Code of Conduct (NMC, 2008).
- If someone else gives the medication, document data about the patient's condition before and after the medication.
- If an incident report is indicated, clearly document factual information in accordance with local policy.

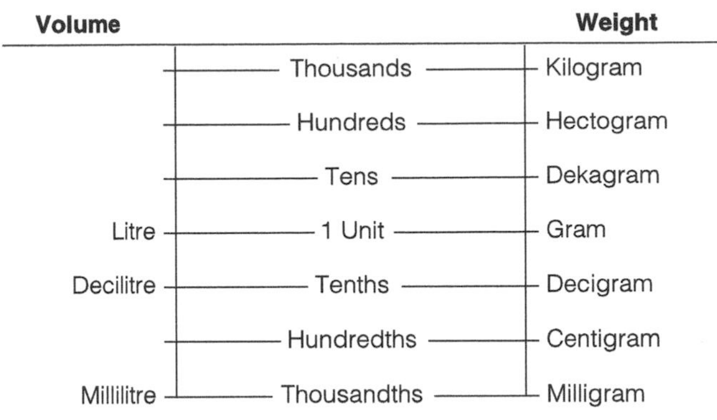

Figure 23-5 Basic metric measurements of volume and weight.

SYSTEMS OF MEASUREMENT: METRIC SYSTEM

The metric system, devised by the French in the latter part of the 18th century, is the system prescribed by law in most European countries. The metric system is logically organised into units of 10; it is a decimal system. Basic units can be multiplied or divided by 10 to form secondary units. Multiples are calculated by moving the decimal point to the right, and division is accomplished by moving the decimal point to the left.

Basic units of measurement are the metre, the litre and the gram. Prefixes derived from Latin designate subdivisions of the basic unit: deci (1/10 or 0.1), centi (1/100 or 0.01) and milli (1/1,000 or 0.001). Multiples of the basic unit are designated by prefixes derived from Greek: deka (10), hecto (100) and kilo (1,000). Only the measurements of volume (the litre) and of weight (the gram) are discussed in this chapter. These are the measures used in medication administration (see Figure 23-5). In nursing practice, the kilogram (kg) is the only multiple of the gram used, and the milligram (mg) and microgram (mcg or µg) are subdivisions. Fractional parts of the litre are usually expressed in millilitres (ml), for example, 600ml; multiples of the litre are usually expressed as litres or millilitres, for example, 2.5l or 2,500ml.

Converting Weights within the Metric System

It is relatively simple to arrive at equivalent units of weight within the metric system because the system is based on units of 10. Only three metric units of weight are used for drug dosages, the gram (g), milligram (mg) and microgram (mcg or µg): 1,000mg or 1,000,000 mcg equals 1g. Equivalents are computed by dividing or multiplying; for example, to change milligrams to grams, the nurse divides the number of milligrams by 1,000. The simplest way to divide by 1,000 is to move the decimal point three places to the left:

500mg = ? g

Move the decimal point three places to the *left*:

Answer = 0.5g

Conversely, to convert grams to milligrams, multiply the number of grams by 1,000 or move the decimal point three places to the right:

0.006g = ? mg

Move the decimal point three places to the *right*:

Answer = 6mg

Calculating Dosages

Several formulas can be used to calculate drug dosages. One formula uses ratios:

$$\frac{\text{Dose available}}{\text{Quantity available}} = \frac{\text{Desired dose}}{\text{Quantity desired } (x)}$$

For example, erythromycin 500mg is prescribed. It is supplied in a liquid form containing 250mg in 5ml. To calculate the dosage, the nurse uses the formula:

$$\frac{\text{Dose available (250mg)}}{\text{Quantity available (5ml)}} = \frac{\text{Desired dose (500mg)}}{\text{Quantity desired } (x)}$$

Then the nurse cross-multiplies:

$$250\,x = 5\text{ml} \times 500\text{mg}$$
$$x = \frac{5\text{ml} \times 500\text{mg}}{250\text{mg}}$$
$$x = 10\text{ml}$$

Therefore, the dose prescribed is 10ml. The nurse can also use this formula to calculate dosages:

$$\text{Amount to administer } (x) = \frac{\text{Desired dose}}{\text{Dose available}} \times \text{Quantity available}$$

For example, heparin sodium mucous is often distributed in vials in prepared dilutions of 10,000 units per millilitre. If 5,000 units is prescribed, the nurse can use the preceding formula to calculate

$$x = \frac{5{,}000}{10{,}000} \times 1 = 1/2\text{ml}$$

Therefore, the nurse injects 0.5ml for a 5,000-unit dose.

Dosages for Children

Although dosage is stated in the medication prescription, nurses must understand something about the safe dosage for children. Unlike adult dosages, children's dosages are not always standard. Body size significantly affects dosage.

Body surface area

Body surface area is determined by using a nomogram and the child's height and weight. This is considered to be the most accurate method of calculating a child's dose. Standard nomograms give a child's body surface area according to weight and height (see Figure 23-6). The formula is the ratio of the child's body surface area to the surface area of an average adult (1.7 square metres, or $1.7m^2$), multiplied by the normal adult dose of the drug:

$$\text{Child's dose} = \frac{\text{Surface area of child } (m^2)}{1.7m^2} \times \text{Normal adult dose}$$

For example, a child who weighs 10kg and is 50cm tall has a body surface area of $0.4m^2$. Therefore, the child's dose of tetracycline corresponding to an adult dose of 250mg would be as follows:

$$\text{Child's dose} = \frac{0.4m^2}{1.7m^2} \times 250\text{mg}$$
$$= 0.23 \times 250$$
$$= 58.82\text{mg}$$

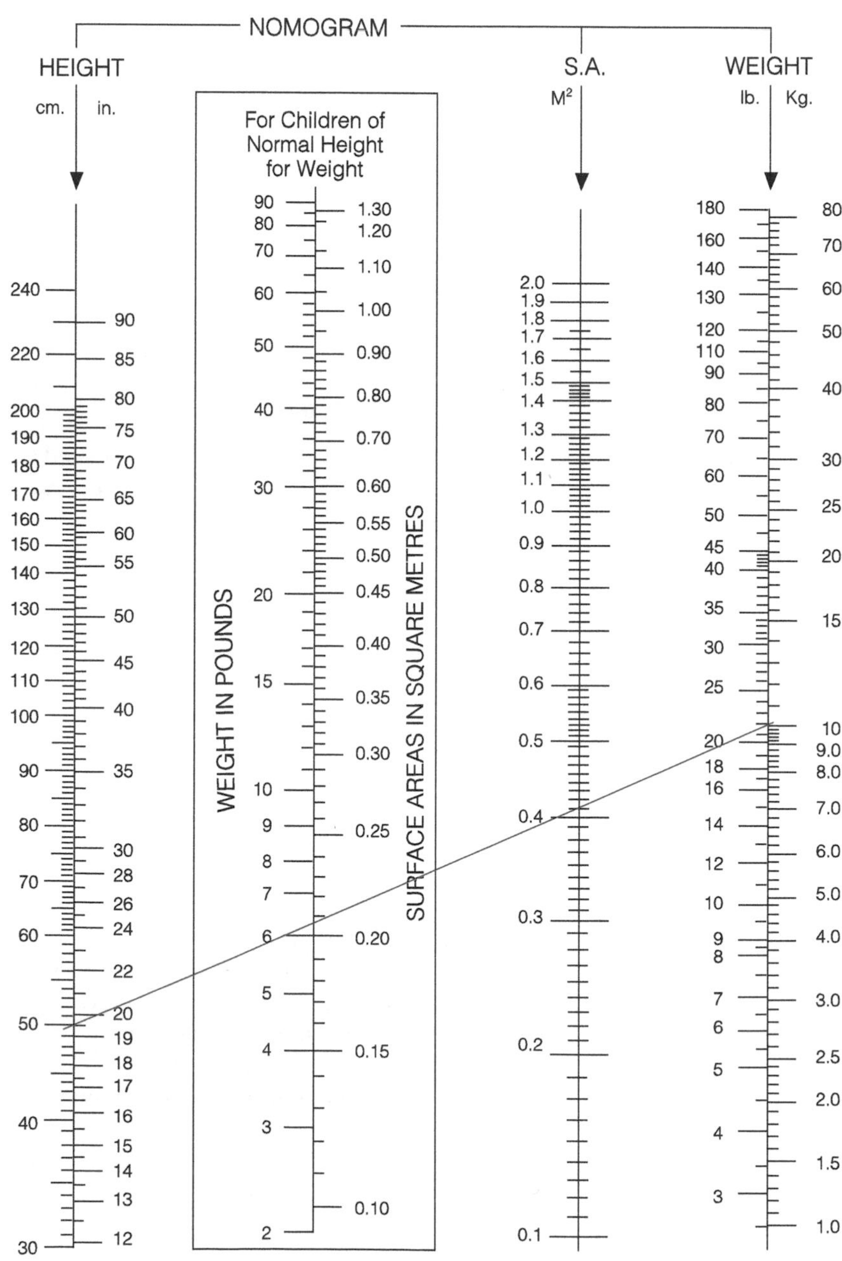

Figure 23-6 Nomogram with estimated body surface area. A straight line is drawn between the child's height (on the left) and the child's weight (on the right). The point at which the line intersects the surface area column is the estimated body surface area.

RESEARCH NOTE

Drug Errors

There were over 72,000 recorded drug errors in the UK in 2007 (NPA, 2009), which is a major concern for government. The introduction of bright tabards into some clinical areas and protected time are some measures that have been introduced into the clinical area to reduce these errors.

Many Higher Education organisations require a minimum mathematics qualification, e.g. a minimum grade C at GCSE level as an entry requirement, and also provide a pre-entry mathematics test at interview.

Many pre-registration nursing programmes support development of drug calculation skills, etc. throughout the student nurse's training and offer formative and summative tests and examinations to measure the student's knowledge and understanding of this important aspect of nursing.

ADMINISTERING MEDICATIONS SAFELY

The nurse should always assess a patient's health status and obtain a medication history prior to giving any medication. This may be done as part of the nursing process (see Chapter 10). The extent of the assessment depends on the patient's illness or current condition, the intended drug and the route of administration. For example, if a patient has dyspnoea, the nurse should assess respirations carefully before administering any medication that might affect breathing. It is important to determine whether the route of administration is suitable. For example, a patient who is nauseated may not be able to tolerate a drug taken orally. In general, the nurse assesses the patient prior to administering any medication to obtain baseline data by which to evaluate the effectiveness of the medication.

The medication history includes information about the drugs the patient is taking currently or has taken recently. This includes prescription drugs; over-the-counter drugs, such as antacids, alcohol and tobacco; and non-sanctioned drugs such as marijuana. Sometimes an incompatibility with one or more of these drugs affects the choice of a new medication.

Older adults often take vitamins, herbs, food supplements and/or use complementary remedies that they do not list in their medication history. Because many of these have unknown or unpredictable actions and side-effects, they need to be noted, with attention paid to possible incompatibilities with other prescribed medications.

An important part of the history is the patient's knowledge of their drug allergies. Some patients can tell a nurse, 'I am allergic to penicillin, adhesive tape and eggs.' Other patients may not be sure about allergic reactions. An illness occurring after a drug was taken may not be identified as an allergy, but the patient may associate the drug with an illness or unusual reaction. The patient's general practitioner can often give information about allergies. During the history, the nurse tries to elicit information about drug dependencies. How often drugs are taken and the patient's perceived need for them are measures of dependence.

Also included in the history are the patient's normal eating habits. Sometimes the medication regimen needs to be coordinated with mealtimes or the ingestion of foods. Where a medication must be taken with food on a specified timescale, patients can often adjust their mealtime or have a snack (e.g. with a bedtime medication). In addition, certain foods are incompatible with certain medications, for example, milk is incompatible with tetracycline.

Any problems the patient may have in self-administering a medication must also be identified. A patient with poor eyesight, for example, may require special labels for the medication container; elderly patients with unsteady hands may not be able to hold a syringe or to inject themselves or another person. Obtaining information as to how and where the patient stores their medications is also important. If the patient has difficulty opening certain containers, they may change containers but leave old labels on, which increases the risk of medication errors.

Socioeconomic factors need to be considered for all patients, but especially for older adults. Common problems include lack of transportation to obtain medications, although this is overcome by some community pharmacies arranging a home delivery service. If the nurse is aware of these problems, proper resources can be obtained for the patient. General advice on administering medications is given in the *Practice Guidelines*.

PRACTICE GUIDELINES

Administering Medications

- Nurses who administer medications are responsible for their own actions. Question any prescription that is illegible or that you consider incorrect. Call the person who prescribed the medication for clarification.
- Be knowledgeable about the medications you administer. You need to know why the patient is receiving the medication. Look up the necessary information if you are not familiar with the medication.
- Use only medications that are in a clearly labelled container.
- Do not use liquid medications that are cloudy or have changed colour.
- Calculate drug doses accurately. If you are uncertain, ask another nurse to double check your calculations.
- Administer only medications personally prepared.
- Before administering a medication, identify the patient correctly using the appropriate means of identification, such as checking the identification bracelet, asking a patient to state his or her name, or both.
- Do not leave medications at the bedside.
- If a patient vomits after taking an oral medication, report this to the nurse in charge and the doctor as a change of medication or route may be required. Document the information in the patient's notes.
- Take special precautions when administering certain medications, for example, have another nurse check the dosages of anticoagulants, insulin and certain IV preparations.
- When a medication is omitted for any reason, record the fact together with the reason.
- When a medication error is made, report it immediately to the nurse in charge, the medical staff, and follow local incident reporting policy.
- It is a legal requirement to correctly store controlled drugs and policies in the checking and administering of these drugs should be followed.
- Remembering and using the 6Rs would help with the process:
  - Right drug
  - Right dose
  - Right time and frequency
  - Right route
  - Right patient
  - Right documentation.

Process of Administering Medications

When administering any drug, regardless of the route of administration, the nurse must do the following:

- *Identify the patient.* Errors can and do occur, usually because one patient gets a drug intended for another. In hospitals, all patients wear some sort of identification, such as a wristband with name and hospital identification number. Before giving the patient any drug, always check the patient's identification band. As a double check, the nurse can ask the alert patient to state his or her name.
- *Inform the patient.* If the patient is unfamiliar with the medication, the nurse should explain the intended action as well as any side-effects or adverse effects that might occur.
- *Administer the drug.* Read medication charts and records carefully and check against the name on the medication package. Then administer the medication in the prescribed dosage, by the route indicated, at the correct time. There are six aspects of medication administration which are important for the nurse to check each time a medication is administered. These are referred to as the six 'rights' and are explained in the *Practice Guidelines.*
- *Provide adjunctive interventions as indicated.* Patients may need help when receiving medications. They may require physical assistance, for instance, in assuming positions for intramuscular injections, or they may need guidance about measures to enhance drug effectiveness and prevent complications, such as drinking fluids. Some patients convey fear about their medications. The nurse can allay fears by listening carefully to patients' concerns and giving correct information.
- *Record the drug administered.* The facts recorded on the chart in ink are name of the drug, dosage, method of administration, specific relevant data such as pulse rate (taken in most settings prior to the administration of digitalis) and any other pertinent information. The record should also include the exact time of administration and the signature of the nurse providing the medication. Often, medications that are given regularly are recorded on a special flow record. PRN (as needed) or stat (at once) medications are recorded separately.
- *Evaluate the patient's response to the drug.* The kinds of behaviour that reflect the action or lack of action of a drug and its untoward effects (both minor and major) are as variable as the purposes of the drugs themselves. The anxious patient may show the desired effects of a tranquilliser by behaviour that reflects a lowered stress level (e.g. slower speech or fewer random movements). The effectiveness of a sedative can often be measured by how well a patient slept, and the effectiveness of an antispasmodic by how much pain the patient feels. In all nursing activities, nurses need to be aware of the medications that a patient is taking and record their effectiveness as assessed by the patient and the nurse on the patient's chart.

PRACTICE GUIDELINES

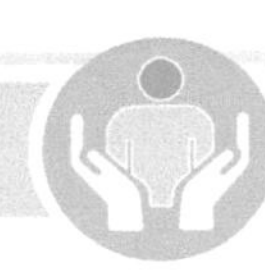

Six 'Rights' of Medication Administration

- Right medication
  - The medication given was the medication prescribed.
- Right dose
  - The dose prescribed is appropriate for the patient.
  - Give special attention if the calculation indicates multiple pills/tablets or a large quantity of a liquid medication.
  - Double check calculations that appear questionable.
  - Know the usual dosage range of the medication.
  - Question a dose outside of the usual dosage range.
- Right time
  - Give the medication at the right frequency and at the time prescribed according to local policy.
  - Medications given within 30 minutes before or after the scheduled time are considered to meet the right time standard.
- Right route
  - Give the medication by the prescribed route.
  - Make certain that the route is safe and appropriate for the patient.
- Right patient
  - Medication is given to the intended patient.
  - Check the patient's identification band with each administration of a medication.
  - Know the alert system appropriate to the clinical environment when patients with the same or similar last names are on the nursing unit. This may be a sticky label on the chart or a patient warning arm band.
- Right documentation
  - Document medication administration after giving it, not before.
  - If time of administration differs from prescribed time, note the time on the chart and explain reason and follow-through activities (e.g. pharmacy states medication will be available in two hours) in nursing notes.
  - If a medication is not given, follow local policy for documenting the reason why.

Developmental Considerations

It is important for the nurse to be aware of how growth and development impact administration of medications for all age groups, particularly the very young and the very old.

Infants and Children

Knowledge of growth and development is essential for the nurse administering medications to children. Oral medications for children are usually prepared in sweetened liquid form to make them more palatable. The parents may provide suggestions about what method is best for their child. Necessary foods such as milk or orange juice should not be used to mask the taste of medications, because the child may develop unpleasant associations and refuse that food in the future.

Children tend to fear any procedure in which a needle is used because they anticipate pain or because the procedure is unfamiliar and threatening. The nurse needs to acknowledge that the child will feel some pain; denying this fact only deepens the child's distrust. After the injection, the nurse (or the parent) can cuddle and speak softly to the infant and give the child a toy to dispel the child's association of the nurse only with pain.

Mature Adults

Mature adults can have specific problems, some of which relate to past experiences and established attitudes towards medications but most of which are concerned with physiological changes associated with ageing. These include:

- altered memory;
- less acute vision;
- decrease in renal function, resulting in slower elimination of drugs and higher drug concentrations in the bloodstream for longer periods;
- less complete and slower absorption from the gastrointestinal tract;
- increased proportion of fat to lean body mass, which facilitates retention of fat-soluble drugs and increases potential for toxicity;
- decreased liver function, which hinders biotransformation of drugs;
- decreased organ sensitivity, which means that the response to the same drug concentration in the vicinity of the target organ is less in older people than in the young;
- altered quality of organ responsiveness, resulting in adverse effects becoming pronounced before therapeutic effects are achieved;
- decrease in manual dexterity due to arthritis and/or decrease in flexibility.

Many of these changes enhance the possibility of cumulative effects and toxicity. For example, impaired circulation delays the action of medications given intramuscularly or subcutaneously. Digitalis, which is frequently taken by older adults, can accumulate to toxic levels and be lethal. It is not uncommon for older adults to take several different medications daily. The possibility of error increases with the number of medications taken, whether self-administered at home or administered in a hospital. The greater number of medications also compounds the problem of drug interactions. A general rule to follow is that older adults should take as few medications as possible.

Older adults usually require smaller dosages of drugs, especially sedatives and other central nervous system depressants. Reactions of older adults to medications, particularly sedatives, are unpredictable and often bizarre. It is not uncommon to see irritability, confusion, disorientation, restlessness and incontinence as a result of sedatives. Nurses therefore need to observe patients carefully for untoward reactions. Doctors often follow the unwritten rule to 'start low and go slow' when prescribing medications for older adults. The initial prescribed dosage will often be low and then be gradually increased with careful monitoring of actions and side-effects of the drug.

Attitudes of mature adults towards medical care and medications vary; they tend to believe in the wisdom of the consultant more readily than younger people. Some older people are bewildered by the prescription of several medications and may passively accept their medications from nurses but not swallow them, spitting out tablets or capsules after the nurse leaves the room. For this reason, the nurse is advised to stay with patients until they have swallowed the medications. Others may be suspicious of medications and actively refuse them.

Mature adults are capable of reasoning. Therefore, the nurse needs to explain the reasons for and the effects of medications. This education can prevent patients from continuing to take a medication long after there is a need for it or discontinuing a drug too quickly. For example, patients should know that diuretics will cause them to urinate more frequently and may reduce ankle oedema. Instructions about medications need to be given to all patients. These instructions should include when to take the drugs, what effects to expect, and when to seek further professional advice.

Because some patients are required to take several medications daily and because visual acuity and memory may be impaired, the nurse needs to develop simple, realistic plans for patients to follow at home. For example, remembering to take drugs can be difficult for most people, including the elderly. If medications are scheduled to be taken with meals or at bedtime, patients are not as likely to forget. However, there are many different types of pill dispenser packs available from pharmacies that enable the patient to maintain independence, e.g. from once a day pill dispensers to four times daily (weekly) pill dispensers. Furthermore there are, for example, eye drop dispensers which can aid the patient to apply their own eye drops.

ORAL MEDICATIONS

The oral route is the most common route by which medications are given. As long as a patient can swallow and retain the drug in the stomach, this is the route of choice (see *Procedure 23-1*). Oral medications are contraindicated when a patient is vomiting, has gastric or intestinal suction, or is unconscious and unable to swallow. Patients in this group are usually 'Nil by Mouth' (NBM).

PROCEDURE 23-1 Administering Oral Medications

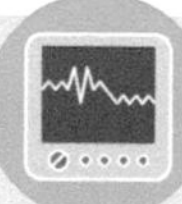

Purpose

To provide a medication that has systemic effects or local effects on the gastrointestinal tract or both (see specific drug action)

Assessment

Assess

- Allergies to medication(s)
- Patient's ability to swallow the medication
- Presence of vomiting or diarrhoea that would interfere with the ability to absorb the medication
- Specific drug action, side-effects, interactions and adverse reactions
- Patient's knowledge of and learning needs about the medication
- Perform appropriate assessments (e.g., vital signs, check laboratory results) specific to the medication.

Determine

- If the assessment data influence administration of the medication (i.e. is it appropriate to administer the medication or does the medication need to be withheld and the doctor notified?).

Planning

Equipment

- Medication trolley/key to bedside drug locker
- Disposable medication cups: small paper or plastic cups for tablets and capsules, plastic calibrated medication cups for liquids
- Prescription chart
- Pill crusher (only if recommended and supported by pharmacist or local and manufacturer's policy). Elixir (liquid) form should be ordered instead of tablet form
- Straws to administer medications that may discolour the teeth or to facilitate the ingestion of liquid medication for certain patients
- Drinking glass and water

Implementation

Preparation

- Determine why the patient is receiving the medication, the drug classification, contraindications, usual dosage range, side-effects and nursing considerations for administering and evaluating the intended outcomes for the medication.
- Check the medication prescription chart.
  - Check the chart for the drug name, dosage, frequency, route of administration and expiration date for administering the medication, if appropriate. *Certain medications (e.g. antibiotics) have a specified time frame at which they expire and need to be re-prescribed.*
  - If the chart is unclear or pertinent information is missing, report any discrepancies to the prescriber and withhold medication until issues are clarified.
- Verify the patient's ability to take medication orally.
  - Determine whether the patient can swallow, is NBM, is nauseated or vomiting or has gastric suction.

Performance

1 Follow local policy to ensure that you explain to the patient what you are going to do, why it is necessary and how they can cooperate. Obtain consent and maintain patient privacy and dignity and ensure that the appropriate local infection control procedures are observed.

2 Unlock the medication trolley/locker.

3 Obtain appropriate medication.
  - Read the medication chart and take the appropriate medication from the shelf or locker. The medication may be dispensed in a bottle, box or unit-dose package.
  - Check the label of the medication container or unit-dose package against the chart (see Figure 23-7). *This is a safety check to ensure that the right medication is given.* If these are not identical, recheck the patient's chart. If there is still a discrepancy, check with the nurse in charge or the pharmacist.
  - Check the expiration date of the medication. Return expired medications to the pharmacy. *Outdated medications are not safe to administer.*
  - Use only medications that have clear, legible labels *to ensure accuracy.*

4 Prepare the medication.
  - Calculate medication dosage accurately.
  - Prepare the correct amount of medication for the required dose, without contaminating the medication. *Aseptic technique maintains drug cleanliness (see Chapter 18).*
  - While preparing the medication, recheck each prepared drug and container with the chart again. *This second safety check reduces the chance of error.*

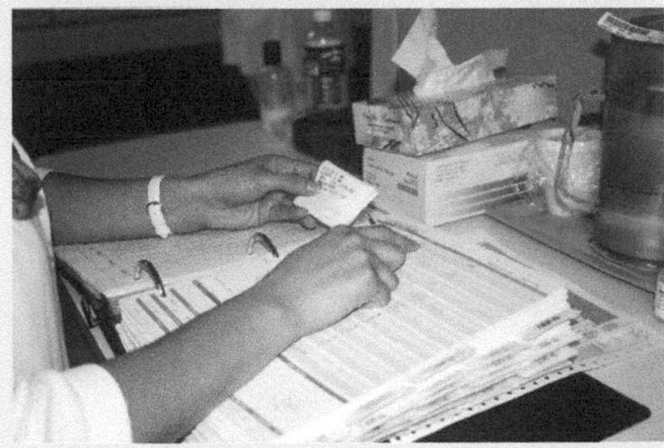

Figure 23-7 Compare the medication label to the medication chart.

Tablets or capsules

- Place packaged unit-dose capsules or tablets directly into the medicine cup.
- If using a stock container, pour the required number into the bottle cap, and then transfer the medication to the disposable cup without touching the tablets.
- Keep medications that require specific assessments, such as pulse measurements, respiratory rate or depth, or blood pressure, separate from the others. *This reminds the nurse to complete the needed assessment(s) in order to decide whether to give the medication or to withhold the medication if indicated.*

- Breaking scored tablets should only be undertaken on advice from pharmacist and recommendations of manufacturer.
- If the patient has difficulty swallowing, revise medication and request the prescriber to change the drug to an elixir form.

Liquid medication

- Shake the bottle containing the medication thoroughly before pouring. Discard any medication that has changed colour or turned cloudy.
- Remove the cap and place it upside down to avoid contaminating the inside of the cap.
- Hold the bottle so the label is next to your palm and pour the medication away from the label (see Figure 23-8). *This prevents the label from becoming soiled and illegible as a result of spilled liquids.*
- Hold the medication cup at eye level and fill it to the desired level, using the bottom of the meniscus (crescent-shaped upper surface of a column of liquid) to align with container scale (see Figure 23-9). *This method ensures accuracy of measurement.*
- Before capping the bottle, wipe the lip with appropriate wipe (as per local policy). *This prevents the cap from sticking.*
- When giving small amounts of liquids (e.g. < 5ml), prepare the medication in a sterile syringe without the needle.

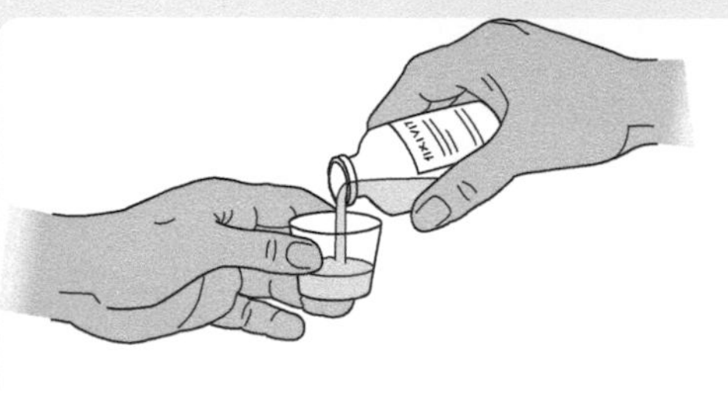

Figure 23-8 Pouring a liquid medication from a bottle.

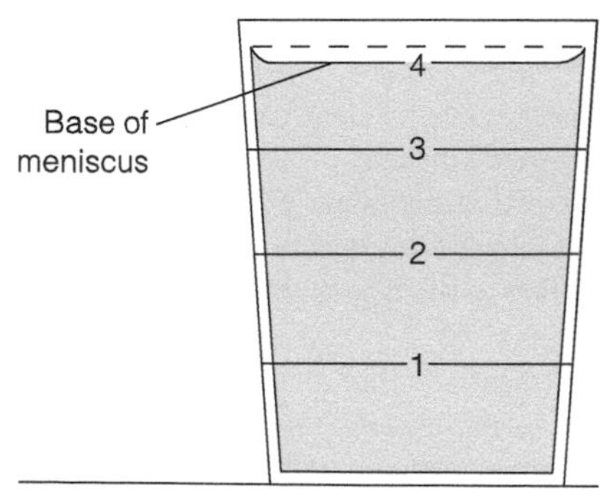

Figure 23-9 The *bottom* of the meniscus is the measuring guide.

- Keep unit-dose liquids in their package and open them at the bedside.

All medications

- Prepared medications should not be left unattended. *This precaution prevents potential mishandling errors.*
- Lock the medication trolley/locker before leaving a patient's room. This is a safety measure because medication stores are not to be left open when unattended.

5 Maintain patient dignity and privacy.

6 Prepare the patient.

- Obtain patient consent.
- Check the patient's identification band for name, address, date of birth and hospital number. Check this by also asking the patient to confirm his/her name and address. *This ensures that the right patient receives the medication.*
- Assist the patient to a sitting position or, if not possible, to a side-lying position. *These positions facilitate swallowing and prevent aspiration.*
- If not previously assessed, take the required assessment measures, such as pulse and respiratory rates or blood pressure. Take the apical pulse rate before administering digitalis preparations. Take blood pressure before giving antihypertensive drugs. Take the respiratory rate prior to administering narcotics. *Narcotics depress the respiratory centre.* If any of the findings are above or below the predetermined parameters, consult the physician before administering the medication.

7 Explain the purpose of the medication and how it will help, using language that the patient can understand. Include relevant information about effects; for example, tell the patient receiving a diuretic to expect an increase in urine output. *Information facilitates acceptance of and compliance with the therapy.*

8 Administer the medication at the correct time.

- Take the medication to the patient within the time frame of 30 minutes before or after the scheduled time.
- Give the patient sufficient water or preferred liquid to swallow the medication. Before using juice, check for any food and medication incompatibilities. *Fluids ease swallowing and facilitate absorption from the gastrointestinal tract.*
- If the patient is unable to hold the pill cup, use the pill cup to introduce the medication into the patient's mouth, and give only one tablet or capsule at a time. *Putting the cup to the patient's mouth maintains the cleanliness of the nurse's hands. Giving one medication at a time eases swallowing.*
- If an older child or adult has difficulty swallowing, ask the patient to place the medication on the back of the tongue before taking the water. *Stimulation of the back of the tongue produces the swallowing reflex.*

- If the medication has an objectionable taste, ask the patient to suck a few ice cubes beforehand, or give the medication with juice, if there are no contraindications. *The cold of the ice cubes will desensitise the taste buds, and juices can mask the taste of the medication.*
- If the patient says that the medication you are about to give is different from what the patient has been receiving, do not give the medication without first checking the original prescription. *Most patients are familiar with the appearance of medications taken previously. Unfamiliar medications may signal a possible error.*
- Stay with the patient until all medications have been swallowed. The nurse must see the patient swallow the medication before the drug administration can be recorded.

9 Document each medication given.
- Record the medication given, dosage, time, any complaints or assessments of the patient and your signature.
- If medication was refused or omitted, record this fact on the appropriate record; document the reason, when possible, and the nurse's actions according to local policy.

10 Dispose of all supplies appropriately.
- Replenish stock (e.g. medication cups).
- Discard used disposable supplies.

11 Evaluate the effects of the medication.
- Return to the patient when the medication is expected to take effect (usually 30 minutes) to evaluate the effects of the medication on the patient.

Evaluation

- Conduct appropriate follow-up:
  - desired effect (e.g. relief of pain or decrease in body temperature);
  - any adverse effects or side-effects (e.g. nausea, vomiting, skin rash, change in vital signs).
- Relate to previous findings, if available.
- Report significant deviations from normal to the physician.

LIFESPAN CONSIDERATIONS

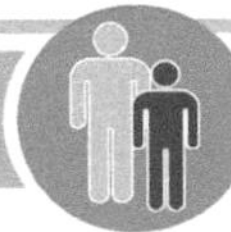

Administering Oral Medications

Infants

- The NMC (2008) advocates that wherever possible the medication should be given to the child by the parent.
- Care is needed with dosage as the dose is often directed by weight.
- It is important to appear confident and composed in front of the child.
- Allow the child as much control as possible.
- Use appropriate language that the child will understand.
- Discuss with the child what the medicine might taste like.
- Place small amounts of liquid along the side of the infant's mouth. To prevent aspiration or spitting out, wait for the infant to swallow before giving more (GOSH, 2008).
- If using a spoon, retrieve and re-feed medication that is thrust outward by the infant's tongue.

Children

- Knowledge of growth and development is essential for the nurse administering medications to children.
- Whenever possible, give children a choice between the use of a spoon or syringe.
- Dilute the oral medication, if indicated, with a small amount of water. Many oral medications are readily swallowed if they are diluted with a small amount of water. If large quantities of water are used, the child may refuse to drink the entire amount and receive only a portion of the medication.
- Oral medications for children are usually prepared in sweetened liquid form to make them more palatable.
- Present any altered medication to the child honestly and not as a food or treat.
- Place the young child or toddler on your lap or a parent's lap in a sitting position.
- Administer the medication slowly with a measuring spoon, plastic syringe or medicine cup.
- Follow medication with a drink of water, juice or a soft drink. This removes any unpleasant aftertaste.
- For children who take sweetened medications on a long-term basis, follow the medication administration with oral hygiene. These children are at high risk of dental caries.

Mature Adults

- The physiological changes associated with ageing influence medication administration and effectiveness. Examples include altered memory, less acute vision, decrease in renal function, less complete and slower absorption from the gastrointestinal tract, and decreased liver function. Many of these changes enhance the possibility of cumulative effects and toxicity.

- Mature adults usually require smaller dosages of drugs, especially sedatives and other central nervous system depressants.
- Mature adults are capable of reasoning. The nurse, therefore, needs to explain the reasons for and the effects of the patient's medications.
- Socioeconomic factors such as lack of transportation and decreased finances may influence obtaining medications when needed.
- An increase in marketing and availability of vitamins, herbs and supplements the nurse means that should include this information in a medication history.

CLINICAL ALERT

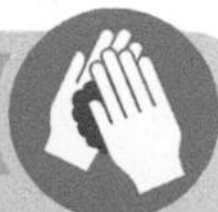

If using a syringe for administering oral medications it is important that the contents of the syringe is not squirted into the mouth, but dispensed slowly and carefully.

Fatalities have been reported when the oral medication via syringe has been given intravenously in error (McEwing and Kelsey, 2008).

COMMUNITY CARE CONSIDERATIONS

Administering Medications

Instruct the patient to:

- Learn the names of the medications as well as their actions and possible adverse effects.
- Keep all medications out of reach of children and pets.
- If using a syringe to administer the medication to an infant or child, remove and dispose of the plastic cap that fits on the end of the syringe. Infants and small children have been known to choke on these caps.
- Take the medications only as prescribed. Immediately consult the nurse, pharmacist or doctor about any problems with the medication.
- Always check the medication label to make sure the correct medication is being taken.
- Request labels printed with larger type on medication containers if there is difficulty reading the label.
- Check the expiry date and discard outdated medications.
- Ask the pharmacist to substitute childproof caps with ones that are more easily opened, as appropriate.
- If a dose or more is missed, do not take two or more doses; ask the pharmacist or physician for directions.
- Do not crush or cut a tablet or capsule without first checking with the physician or pharmacist. Doing so may affect the medication's absorption.
- Never stop taking the medication without the prescriber's permission.
- Always check with the pharmacist before taking any non-prescription medications. Some over-the-counter medications can interact with the prescribed medication.
- Set up a medication plan day schedule. Weekly pill containers (available at pharmacies) or a written plan may be helpful.

NASOGASTRIC AND GASTROSTOMY MEDICATIONS

For patients who cannot take anything by mouth (NBM) and have nasogastric tubes or a **gastrostomy** tube in place, an alternative route for administering medications is through the nasogastric or gastrostomy tube. A nasogastric (NG) tube is inserted by way of the nasopharynx and is placed into the patient's stomach for the purpose of feeding the patient or to remove gastric secretions. A gastrostomy tube is surgically placed directly into the patient's stomach and provides another route for administering medications and nutrition. Guidelines for administering medications by nasogastric tubes and gastrostomy tubes are shown in the *Practice Guidelines*.

PRACTICE GUIDELINES

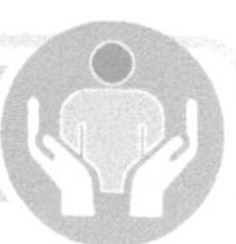

Administering Medications by Nasogastric or Gastrostomy Tube

- Always check with the pharmacist to see if the patient's medications come in a liquid form because these are less likely to cause tube obstruction.
- If medications do not come in liquid form, check to see if they may be crushed. (Note that enteric-coated, sustained action, **buccal** and **sublingual** medications should never be crushed.)
- Crush a tablet into a fine powder and dissolve in at least 30ml of warm water. Cold liquids may cause patient discomfort. Use only water for mixing and flushing.

- Read medication labels carefully before opening a capsule. Open capsules and mix the contents with water only with the pharmacist's advice.
- Do not administer whole or undissolved medications because they will clog the tube.

When administering the medication(s):

- If nasogastric or gastrostomy feed in process then stop the pump before commencing.
- Remove the plunger from the syringe and connect the syringe to a pinched or kinked tube. Pinching or kinking the tube prevents excess air from entering the stomach and causing distension.
- Put 15-30ml (5-10ml for children) of water into the syringe barrel to flush the tube before administering the first medication. Raise or lower the barrel of the syringe to adjust the flow as needed. Pinch or clamp the tubing before all the water is instilled to avoid excess air entering the stomach.
- Pour liquid or dissolved medication into syringe barrel and allow to flow by gravity into the enteral tube.
- If you are giving several medications, administer each one separately and flush with at least 15-30ml (5ml for children) of tap water between each medication.
- When you have finished administering all medications, flush with another 15-30ml (5-10ml for children) of warm water to clear the tube.
- If the tube is connected to suction, disconnect the suction and keep the tube clamped for 20-30 minutes after giving the medication to enhance absorption.
- Restart the pump following guidelines noted in Chapter 19.

PARENTERAL MEDICATIONS

Parenteral administration of medications is a common nursing procedure. Nurses give parenteral medications intradermally (ID), subcutaneously (SC), intramuscularly (IM) or intravenously (IV). Because these medications are absorbed more quickly than oral medications and are irretrievable once injected, the nurse must prepare and administer them carefully and accurately. Administering parenteral drugs requires the same nursing knowledge as for oral and topical drugs; however, because injections are invasive procedures, aseptic technique must be used to minimise the risk of infection.

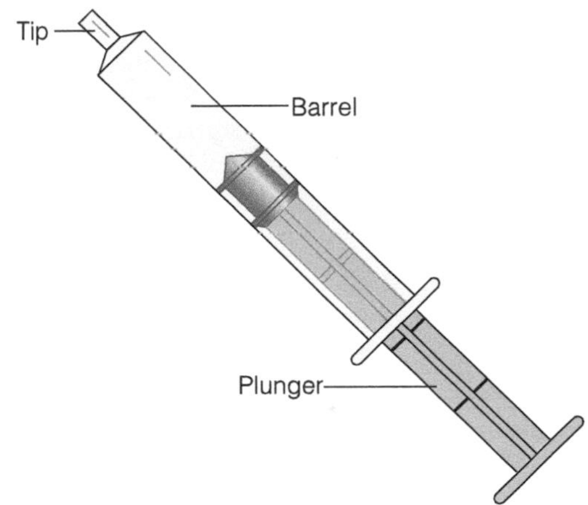

Figure 23-10 The three parts of a syringe.

Equipment

To administer parenteral medications, nurses use syringes and needles to withdraw medication from ampoules and vials.

Syringes

Syringes have three parts: the tip, which connects with the needle; the barrel, or outside part, on which the scales are printed; and the plunger, which fits inside the barrel (see Figure 23-10). When handling a syringe, the nurse may touch the outside of the barrel and the handle of the plunger; however, the nurse must *avoid letting any unsterile object contact the tip or inside of the barrel, the shaft of the plunger or the shaft or tip of the needle.*

There are several kinds of syringes, differing in size, shape and material. The three most commonly used types are the standard hypodermic syringe, the insulin syringe and the tuberculin syringe (see Figure 23-11). A hypodermic syringe comes in 2, 2.5 and 3ml sizes. The syringe usually has the millilitre scale or international units marked on it. The millilitre scale is the one normally used; the international unit scale is used for very small dosages.

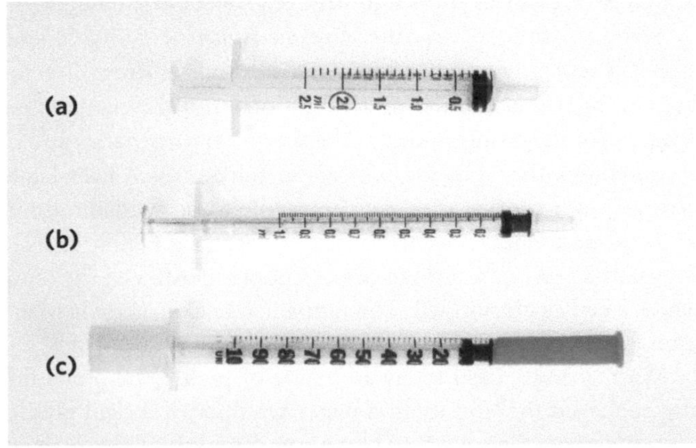

Figure 23-11 Three kinds of syringes: (a) hypodermic syringe marked in tenths (0.1) of millilitres and in minims; (b) insulin syringe marked in 100 units; (c) tuberculin syringe marked in tenths and hundredths (0.01) of cubic millimetres and in minims.

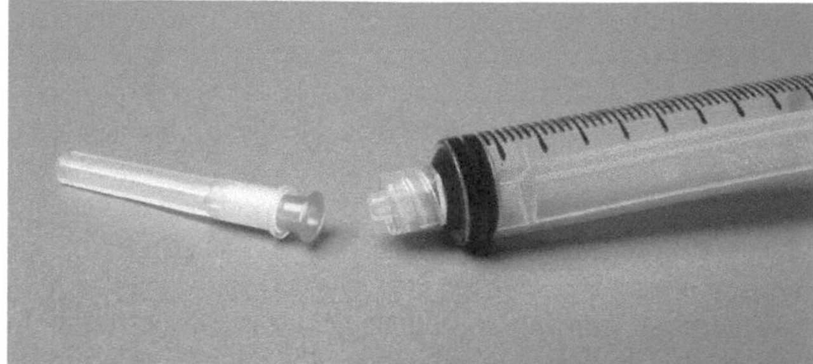

(a)

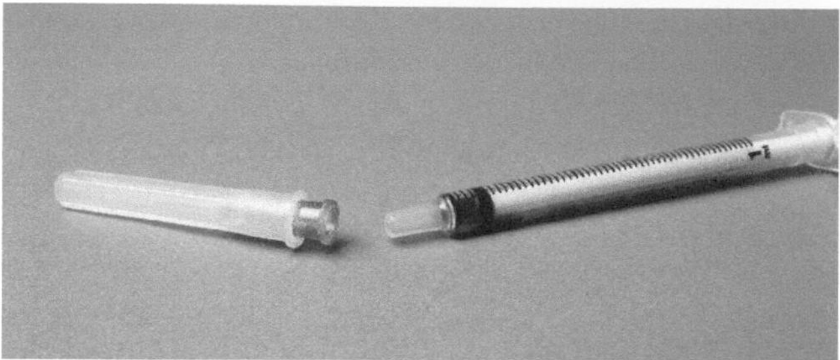

(b)

Figure 23-12 Tips of syringes: (a) Luer-Lok syringe (threaded tip); (b) non-Luer-Lok syringe (smooth graduated tip).

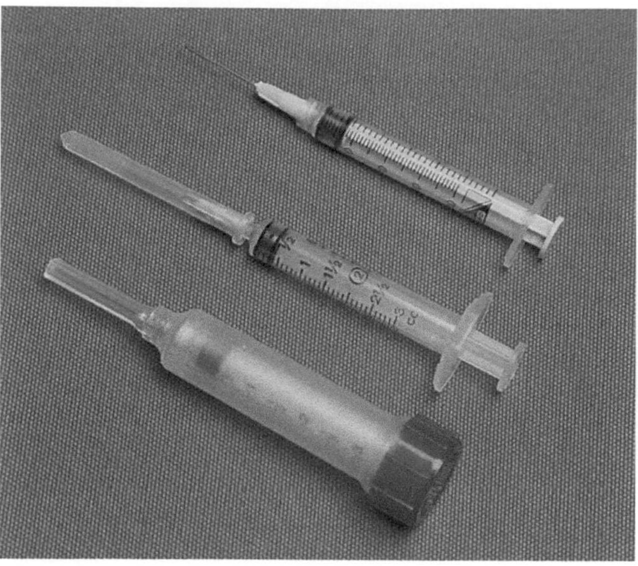

Figure 23-13 Disposable plastic syringes and needles: *Top*, with syringe and needle exposed; *Middle*, with plastic cap over the needle; *Bottom*, with plastic case over the needle and syringe.

An *insulin syringe* is similar to a hypodermic syringe, but the scale is specially designed for insulin: a 100-unit calibrated scale intended for use with U-100 insulin. Several low-dose insulin syringes are also available and frequently have a nonremovable needle. All insulin syringes are calibrated on the 100-unit scale. The correct choice of syringe is based on the amount of insulin required.

The *tuberculin syringe* was originally designed to administer tuberculin. It is a narrow syringe, calibrated in tenths and hundredths of a millilitre (up to 1ml). This type of syringe can also be useful in administering other drugs, particularly when small or precise measurement is indicated (e.g. paediatric dosages).

Syringes are made in other sizes as well (e.g. 5, 10, 20 and 50ml). These are not generally used to administer drugs directly but can be useful for adding medications to intravenous solutions or for irrigating wounds. The tip of a syringe varies and is classified as either a Luer-Lock or non-Luer-Lock. A Luer-Lock syringe has a tip that requires the needle to be twisted onto it to avoid accidental removal of the needle (see Figure 23-12). The non-Luer-Lock syringe has a smooth graduated tip onto which needles are slipped. The non-Luer-Lock syringe is often used for irrigation purposes (e.g. wounds, tubes).

Most syringes used today are made of plastic, are individually packaged for sterility in a paper wrapper or a rigid plastic container (see Figure 23-13), and are disposable. The syringe and needle may be packaged together or separately. Needleless systems are also available in which the needle is replaced by a plastic cannula.

Injectable medications are frequently supplied in disposable *prefilled unit-dose systems*. These are available as (a) prefilled syringes ready for use or (b) prefilled sterile cartridges and needles that require the attachment of a reusable holder (injection system) before use (see Figure 23-14). Examples of the latter system are the Clexane injection systems. The manufacturers provide specific directions for use. Because most pre-filled cartridges are overfilled, excess medication must be ejected before the injection to ensure the right dosage. Because the needle is fused to the syringe, the nurse cannot change the gauge or length of the needle.

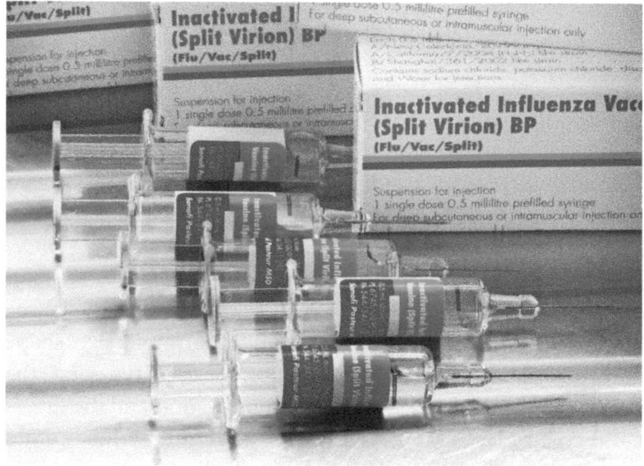

Figure 23-14 A prefillable syringe.
Source: Science Photo Library Ltd/Saturn Stills.

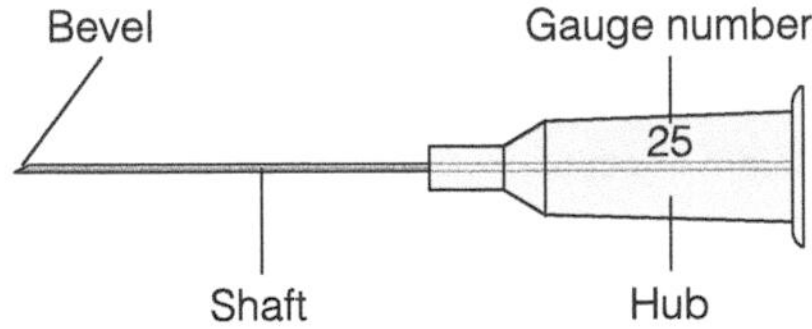

Figure 23-15 The parts of a needle.

Needles

Needles are made of stainless steel, and most are disposable. Reusable needles (e.g. for special procedures) need to be sharpened periodically before re-sterilisation because the points become dull with use and are occasionally damaged or acquire burrs on the tips. A dull or damaged needle should *never* be used.

A needle has three discernible parts: the hub, which fits onto the syringe; the **cannula** or shaft, which is attached to the hub; and the bevel, which is the slanted part at the tip of the needle (see Figure 23-15). A disposable needle has a plastic hub. Needles used for injections have three variable characteristics:

- *Slant or length of the bevel.* The bevel of the needle may be short or long. Longer bevels provide the sharpest needles and cause less discomfort. They are commonly used for subcutaneous and intramuscular injections. Short bevels are used for intradermal and intravenous injections because a long bevel can become occluded if it rests against the side of a blood vessel.
- *Length of the shaft.* The shaft length of commonly used needles varies from 1–5cm. The appropriate needle length is chosen according to the patient's muscle development, the patient's weight and the type of injection.
- *Gauge (or diameter) of the shaft.* The gauge varies from #18 to #28. The larger the gauge number, the smaller the diameter of the shaft. Smaller gauges produce less tissue trauma, but larger gauges are necessary for viscous medications, such as penicillin.

For an adult requiring a subcutaneous injection, it is appropriate to use a needle of #24–#26 gauge and 0.5–2cm long. Obese patients may require a 2.5cm needle. For intramuscular injections, a longer needle with a larger gauge (e.g. #20–#22 gauge) is used. Slender adults and children usually require a shorter needle. The nurse must assess the patient to determine the appropriate needle length.

Preventing Needlestick Injuries

One of the most potentially hazardous procedures that healthcare personnel face is using and disposing of needles and sharps. In England, Wales and Northern Ireland between 1997and 2007 there were nearly 4000 reported incidents of needlestick injuries in healthcare workers who were exposed to blood borne viruses (HPA, 2008). Needlestick injuries present a major risk for infection with hepatitis B virus, human immunodeficiency virus (HIV) and many other pathogens. The European Union has proposed legislation to protect healthcare workers and the Health and Safety Executive (HSE, 2011) recommend the following safety procedures relating to blood and body fluids, regardless of the source:

- Hand washing after each patient contact and after contact with blood or body fluids.
- Appropriate PPE (Personal Protective Equipment).
- Disposable gloves should be worn whenever working with blood or body fluids.
- Disposable plastic aprons/impermeable gowns should be worn when splashing with blood or body fluids may occur.
- Eye protection (visors, goggles or safety spectacles) should be worn when blood, body fluids or flying contaminated debris/tissue might splash into the face.
- Covering any cuts or abrasions with waterproof plasters.
- Immediate and safe disposal of sharps into appropriate, puncture-proof sharps bins.
- Not overfilling sharps containers and
- Never re-sheathing needles.

The Royal College of Nursing (RCN, 2009) state that according to a survey undertaken in 2008, 48% of nurses had had a needlestick injury. The World Health Organization, the European Agency of Occupational Safety, the Health Protection and the Health and Safety Executive all recognise the importance of education, training and support as important strategies to reduce or prevent needlestick injuries.

The Royal College of Nursing and the Department of Health (DH, 2004) have identified some key points to prevent needlestick injuries:

- Dispose of all sharps into appropriate containers at the point of use.
- Never overfill sharps containers.
- Avoid re-sheathing needles wherever possible.
- Avoid removing the needle from the syringe if possible. Dispose of them as single unit.
- Where the needle must be removed i.e. blood gas analysis, remove with extreme care (using needle forceps if possible) and attach a blind hub.

However, it is important to note that each individual Trust or health board will have a sharps policy which should be adhered to. If an accidental needlestick injury occurs, the nurse needs to follow specific steps outlined by local policy.

Safety syringes have been designed in recent years to protect healthcare workers. Safety devices are categorised as either *passive* or *active*. The nurse does not need to activate the passive safety device. For example, for some syringes, after injection, the needle retracts immediately into the barrel (see Figure 23-16). In contrast, the active safety device requires the nurse to manually activate the safety feature. For example, the nurse activates a mechanism to retract the needle into the syringe barrel or the nurse, after injection, manually pulls a plastic sheath or guard over the needle (see Figure 23-17).

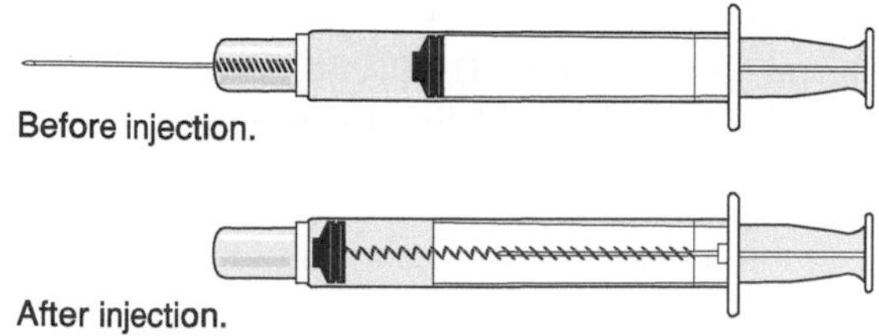

Figure 23-16 Passive safety device. The needle retracts immediately into the barrel after injection.

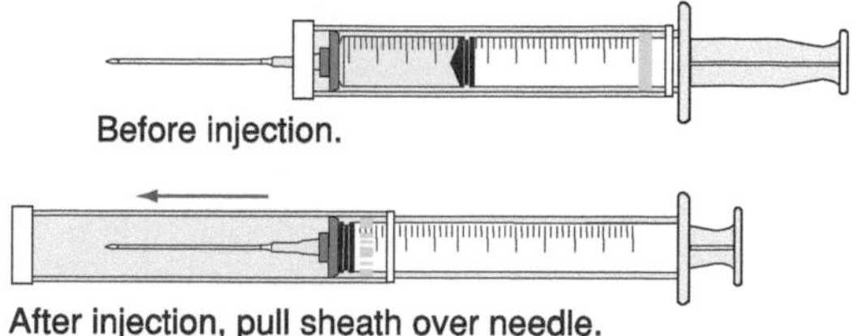

Figure 23-17 Active safety device. The nurse manually pulls the sheath or guard over the needle after injection.

COMMUNITY CARE CONSIDERATIONS

Disposal of Sharps

Smaller sharps boxes should be provided in the home and for the community nurse to dispose of 'sharps' safely. Appropriate collection or disposal can then be made as per local policy.

Preparing Injectable Medications

Injectable medications can be prepared by withdrawing the medication from an ampoule or vial into a sterile syringe, using prefilled syringes, or using needleless injection systems. Figure 23-18 shows an example of a needleless system used to access medication from a vial.

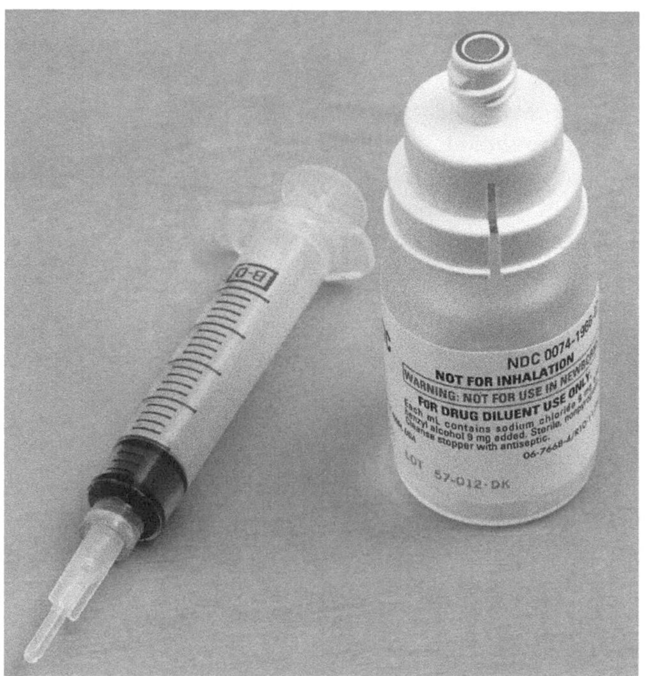

Figure 23-18 A needleless system can extract medication from a vial.
Source: Pearson Education Ltd.

Ampoules and Vials

Ampoules and vials (see Figure 23-19) are frequently used to package sterile parenteral medications. An **ampoule** is a glass container usually designed to hold a single dose of a drug. It is made of clear glass and has a distinctive shape with a constricted neck. Ampoules vary in size from 1–20ml or more. Most ampoule necks have coloured marks around them, indicating where they are pre-scored for easy opening.

To access the medication in an ampoule, the ampoule must be broken at its constricted neck. Ampoule openers are available that prevent injury from broken glass. The device consists of a plastic cap that fits over the top of an ampoule and a cutter within the cap that scores the neck of the ampoule when rotated. The head of the ampoule, when broken, remains inside the cap where it can then be ejected into a sharps container. If an ampoule opener is not available, the neck should be held with a small swab, and then broken off at that point or as per local policy. Once the ampoule is broken, the fluid is aspirated into a syringe using a small gauge needle. This prevents aspiration of any glass particles.

A vial is a small glass bottle with a sealed rubber cap. Vials come in different sizes, from single to multidose vials. They usually have a metal or plastic cap that protects the rubber seal. To access the medication in a vial, the vial must be pierced with a needle. In addition, air must be injected into a vial before the medication can be withdrawn. Failure to inject air before withdrawing the medication leaves a vacuum within the vial that makes withdrawal difficult.

Several drugs (e.g. penicillin) are dispensed as powders in vials. A liquid (solvent or diluent) must be added to a powdered medication before it can be injected. The technique of adding a solvent to a powdered drug to prepare it for administration is

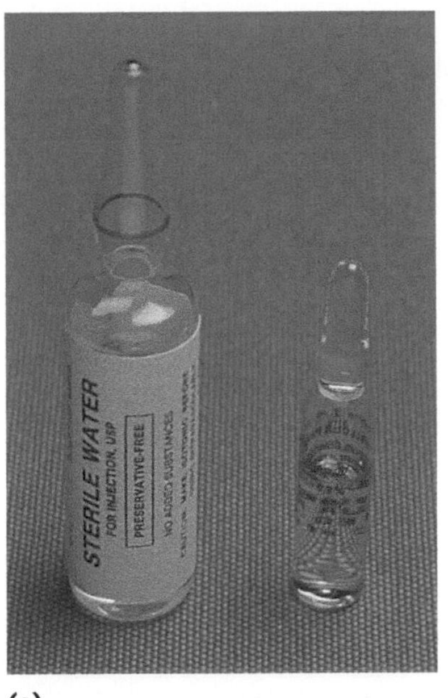

(a)

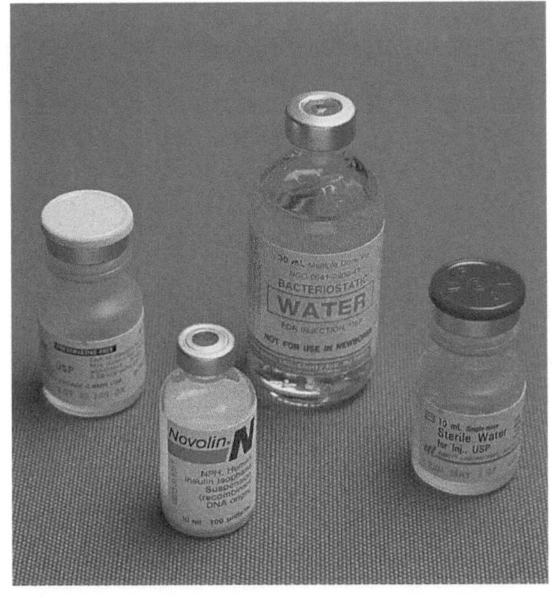

(b)

Figure 23-19 (a) ampoules; (b) vials.
Source: Pearson Education Ltd.

called reconstitution. Powdered drugs usually have printed instructions (enclosed with each packaged vial) that describe the amount and kind of solvent to be added. Commonly used solvents are sterile water or sterile normal saline. Some preparations are supplied in individual-dose vials; others come in multidose vials. Whether the drug reconstituted is for single or multidose, there are devices that can support nurses in the reconstitution to reduce and prevent contamination and/or needlestick injuries.

Whenever possible these devices should be used. While many Trusts and local health boards state that reconstructed medication should not be stored, individual Trust, local health board and manufacturer's guidelines should be adhered to.

The following are two examples of the preparation of powdered drugs:

- *Single-dose vial*: Instructions for preparing a single-dose vial direct that 1.5ml of sterile water be added to the sterile dry powder, thus providing a single dose of 2ml. The volume of the drug powder was 0.5ml. Therefore, the 1.5ml of water plus the 0.5ml of powder results in 2ml of solution. In other instances, the addition of a solution does not increase the volume. Therefore, it is important to follow the manufacturer's directions.
- *Multidose vial*: A dose of 750mg of a certain drug is ordered for a patient. Available is a 10g multidose vial. The directions for preparation read: 'Add 8.5ml of sterile water, and each millilitre will contain 1.0g or 1,000mg.' To determine the amount to inject, the nurse calculates as follows:

$$1\text{ml} = 1{,}000\text{mg}$$
$$x\text{ml} = 750\text{mg}$$
(cross multiply)
$$x = \frac{750 \times 1}{1{,}000}$$
$$= 0.75$$

The nurse will thus give 0.75ml of the medication.

Glass and rubber particulate have been found in medications withdrawn from ampoules and vials using a regular needle. As a result, it is strongly recommended that the nurse use a small gauge needle when withdrawing medications from ampoules and vials to prevent withdrawing glass and rubber particles. After drawing the medication into the syringe, the filter needle is replaced with the regular needle for injection. This prevents tracking of the medication through the patient's tissues during the insertion of the needle, which minimises discomfort.

Procedures 23-2 and *23-3* describe how to prepare medications from ampoules and vials. Additionally, it is important to remember that when powdered drugs have been reconstituted, the date and time should be written on the label of the vial. Many of these drugs have to be used immediately, so nurses need to know the expiration time after it has been reconstituted.

PROCEDURE 23-2 Preparing Medications from Ampoules

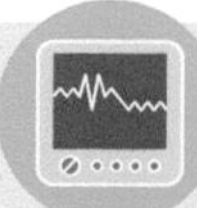

Planning

Aseptic technique should be used at all times to prevent cross-contamination.

Equipment

- Medication chart
- Ampoule of sterile medication
- Ampoule opener or, if it is not scored, small gauze square (as per local policy)
- Antiseptic swabs
- Needle and syringe
- Filler needle
- Gloves

Implementation

Preparation

- Check the medication administration chart.
  - Check the label on the ampoule carefully against the chart to make sure that the correct medication is being prepared.
  - Follow the three checks for administering medications. Read the label on the medication (1) when it is taken from the medication store, (2) before withdrawing the medication and (3) after withdrawing the medication.
- Organise the equipment.

Performance

1 Follow local policy to ensure that you explain to the patient what you are going to do, why it is necessary and how they can cooperate. Obtain consent and maintain patient privacy and dignity and ensure that the appropriate local infection control procedures are observed.

2 Prepare the medication ampoule for drug withdrawal.
- Flick the upper stem of the ampoule several times with a fingernail or, holding the upper stem of the ampoule, shake the ampoule similar to shaking down a mercury thermometer. *This will bring all medication down to the main portion of the ampoule.*
- Attach ampoule opener and open ampoule as instructed.
- If local policy supports: partially file the neck of the ampoule, if necessary, to start a clean break.
- Place a piece of sterile gauze between your thumb and the ampoule neck or around the ampoule neck, and break off the top by bending it towards you (see Figure 23-20). *The sterile gauze protects the fingers from the broken glass and any glass fragments will spray away from the nurse.*

or
- Place the antiseptic wipe packet over the top of the ampoule before breaking off the top. This method ensures that all glass fragments fall into the packet and reduces the risk of cuts.
- Dispose of the top of the ampoule in the sharps container.

3 Withdraw the medication.
- Place the ampoule on a flat surface.
- Using a filter needle to withdraw the medication, disconnect the regular needle, leaving its cap on, and attach the filter needle to the syringe. *The filter needle prevents glass particles from being withdrawn with the medication.*
- Remove the cap from the filter needle and insert the needle into the centre of the ampoule. Do not touch the rim of the ampoule with the needle tip or shaft. *This will keep the needle sterile.* Withdraw the amount of drug required for the dosage.
- With a single-dose ampoule, hold the ampoule slightly on its side, if necessary, to obtain all medication (see Figure 23-21).
- Replace the filter needle with a regular needle and tighten the cap at the hub of the needle before injecting the patient.

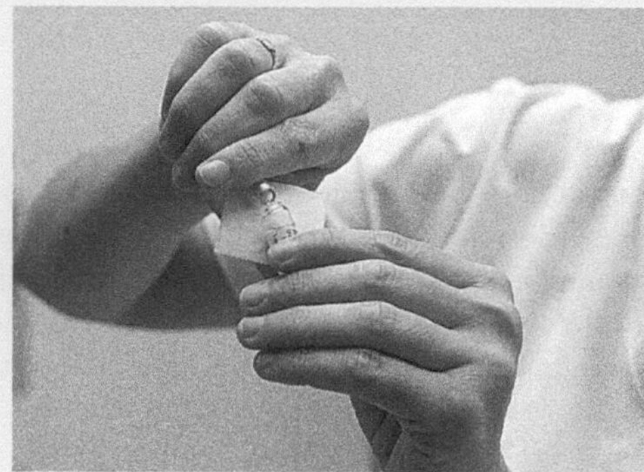

Figure 23-20 Breaking the neck of an ampoule.

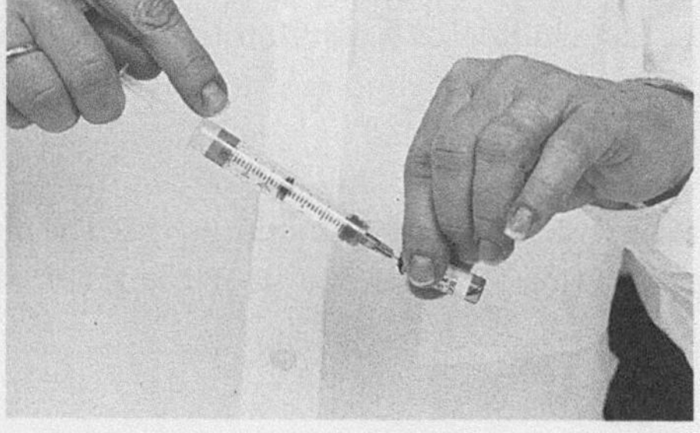

Figure 23-21 Withdrawing a medication from an ampoule.

PROCEDURE 23-3 Preparing Medications from Vials

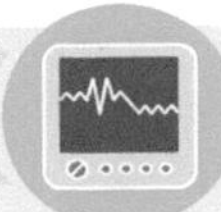

Planning

Aseptic technique should be used at all times to prevent cross-contamination.

Equipment

- Medication chart
- Vial of sterile medication
- Antiseptic swabs
- Needle and syringe
- Filter needle (as per local policy)
- Sterile water or 0.9% saline, if drug is in powdered form
- Gloves

Implementation

Preparation

As for Procedure 23-2.

Performance

1 Follow local policy to ensure that you explain to the patient what you are going to do, why it is necessary and how they can cooperate. Obtain consent and maintain patient privacy and dignity and ensure that the appropriate local infection control procedures are observed.

2 Prepare the medication vial for drug withdrawal.
   - Mix the solution, if necessary, by rotating the vial between the palms of the hands, not by shaking. Some vials contain aqueous suspensions, which settle when they stand. In some instances, shaking is contraindicated because it may cause the mixture to foam.
   - Remove the protective cap.
   - Withdraw the medication.
   - Attach a filter needle, as per local policy dictates, to draw up pre-mixed liquid medications from multidose vials. *Using the filter needle prevents any solid particles from being drawn up through the needle.*
   - Ensure that the needle is firmly attached to the syringe.
   - Remove the cap from the needle, then draw up into the syringe the amount of air equal to the volume of the medication to be withdrawn, i.e. if 5ml of medication is to be withdrawn then insert 5ml of air prior to removal of medication.
   - Carefully insert the needle into the upright vial through the centre of the rubber cap, maintaining the sterility of the needle.
   - Inject the air into the vial, keeping the bevel of the needle above the surface of the medication (see Figure 23-22). The air will allow the medication to be drawn out easily because negative pressure will not be created inside the vial. The bevel is kept above the medication to avoid creating bubbles in the medication.
   - Withdraw the prescribed amount of medication using either of the following methods:
     (a) Hold the vial down (i.e. with the base lower than the top), move the needle tip so that it is below the fluid level, and withdraw the medication (see Figure 23-23). Avoid drawing up the last drops of

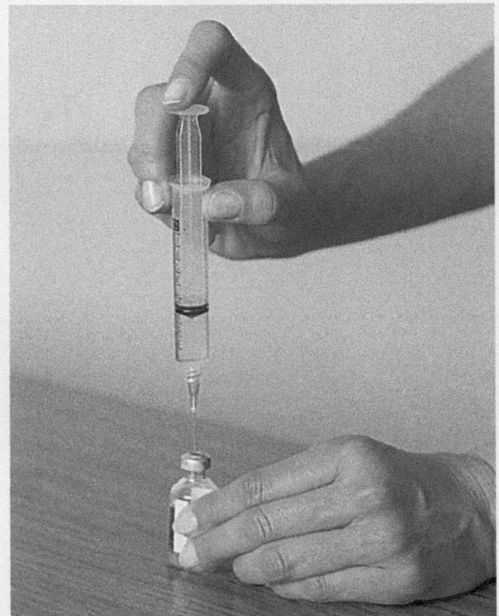

Figure 23-22 Injecting air into a vial.
Source: Pearson Education Ltd.

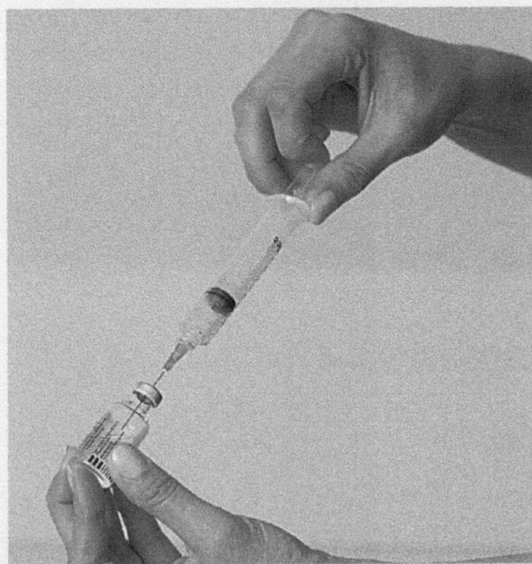

Figure 23-23 Withdrawing a medication from a vial that is held with the base down.
Source: Pearson Education Ltd.

the vial. *Proponents of this method say that keeping the vial in the upright position while withdrawing the medication allows particulate matter to precipitate out of the solution. Leaving the last few drops reduces the chance of withdrawing foreign particles.*

or

(b) Invert the vial; ensure the needle tip is *below* the fluid level; and gradually withdraw the medication (see Figure 23-24). *Keeping the tip of the needle below the fluid level prevents air from being drawn into the syringe.*

- Hold the syringe and vial at eye level to determine that the correct dosage of drug is drawn into the syringe. Eject air remaining at the top of the syringe into the vial.
- When the correct volume of medication is obtained, withdraw the needle from the vial, and replace the cap over the needle using the scoop method, thus maintaining its sterility.
- If necessary, tap the syringe barrel to dislodge any air bubbles present in the syringe. The tapping motion will cause the air bubbles to rise to the top of the syringe where they can be ejected out of the syringe.
- Replace the filter needle, if used, with a regular needle and cover of the correct gauge and length before injecting the patient.

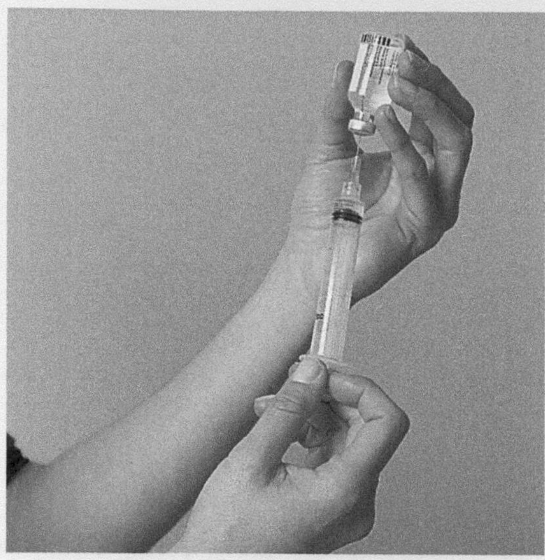

Figure 23-24 Withdrawing a medication from an inverted vial.
Source: Pearson Education Ltd.

Variation: Preparing and using multidose vials

- Read the manufacturer's directions.
- Withdraw an equivalent amount of air from the vial before adding the dilution, unless otherwise indicated by the directions.
- Add the amount of sterile water or saline indicated in the directions.
- If a multidose vial is reconstituted, label the vial with the date and time it was prepared, the amount of drug contained in each millilitre of solution and your initials. *Time is an important factor to consider in the expiration of these medications.*
- Once the medication is reconstituted, store it in a refrigerator or as recommended by the manufacturer.

Mixing Medications in One Syringe

Frequently, patients need more than one drug injected at the same time. To spare the patient the experience of being injected twice, two drugs (if compatible) are often mixed in one syringe and given as one injection (see *Procedure 23-4*). It is common, for instance, to combine diamorphine hydrochloride and cyclizine for palliative care patients. Drugs can also be mixed in intravenous solutions. When uncertain about drug compatibilities, the nurse should consult a pharmacist or check a compatibility chart before mixing the drugs.

PROCEDURE 23-4 Mixing Medications Using One Syringe

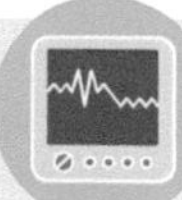

Planning

Equipment

- Medication chart
- Two vials of medication; one vial and one ampoule; two ampoules; or one vial or ampoule and one cartridge
- Antiseptic swabs
- Sterile hypodermic needle
- Additional sterile subcutaneous or intramuscular needle (optional)
- Gloves

Implementation

Preparation

- Check the medication chart.
  - Check the label on the medications carefully against the medication chart to make sure that the correct medication is being prepared.
  - Follow the three checks for administering medications. Read the label on the medication (1) when it is taken from the medication store, (2) before withdrawing the medication and (3) after withdrawing the medication.
  - Before preparing and combining the medications, ensure that the total volume of the injection is appropriate for the injection site.
- Organise the equipment.

Performance

1 Follow local policy to ensure that you explain to the patient what you are going to do, why it is necessary and how they can cooperate. Obtain consent and maintain patient privacy and dignity and ensure that the appropriate local infection control procedures are observed.

2 Prepare the medication ampoule or vial for drug withdrawal.
- See Procedure 23-2 (ampoule) or Procedure 23-3 (vial).
- Inspect the appearance of the medication for clarity. Some medications are always cloudy. *Preparations that have changed in appearance should be discarded.*
- Clean the tops of the vials with antiseptic swabs.

3 Withdraw the medications.

Mixing medications from two vials

- Take the syringe and draw up a volume of air equal to the volume of medications to be withdrawn from both vials A *and* B.
- Inject a volume of air equal to the volume of medication to be withdrawn into vial A. Make sure the needle does not touch the solution. *This prevents cross-contamination of the medications.*
- Withdraw the needle from vial A and inject the remaining air into vial B.
- Withdraw the required amount of medication from vial B. The same needle is used to inject air into and withdraw medication from the second vial. It must not be contaminated with the medication in vial A.
- Using a newly attached sterile needle, withdraw the required amount of medication from vial A. Avoid pushing the plunger as that will introduce medication B into vial A. If using a syringe with a fused needle, withdraw the medication from vial A. The syringe now contains a mixture of medications from vials A and B. *With this method, neither vial is contaminated by micro-organisms or by medication from the other vial.* Be careful to withdraw only the ordered amount and to not create air bubbles. *The syringe now contains two medications and an excess amount cannot be returned to the vial.*

Mixing medications from one vial and one ampoule

- First prepare and withdraw the medication from the vial. Ampoules do not require the addition of air prior to withdrawal of the drug.
- Then withdraw the required amount of medication from the ampoule.

Mixing medications from one cartridge and one vial or ampoule

- First ensure that the correct dose of the medication is in the cartridge. Discard any excess medication and air.
- Draw up the required medication from a vial or ampoule into the cartridge. Note that when withdrawing medication from a vial, an equal amount of air must first be injected into the vial.
- If the total volume to be injected exceeds the capacity of the cartridge, use a syringe with sufficient capacity to withdraw the desired amount of medication from the vial or ampoule, and transfer the required amount from the cartridge to the syringe.

Intradermal Injections

An intradermal (ID) injection is the administration of a drug into the dermal layer of the skin just beneath the epidermis. Usually only a small amount of liquid is used, for example, 0.1ml. This method of administration is frequently used for allergy testing, antibody and tuberculosis (TB) screening. Common sites for intradermal injections are the inner lower arm, the upper chest and the back beneath the scapulae (see Figure 23-25). The left arm is commonly used for TB screening and the right arm is used for all other tests. The steps for administering an intradermal are described in *Procedure 23-5.*

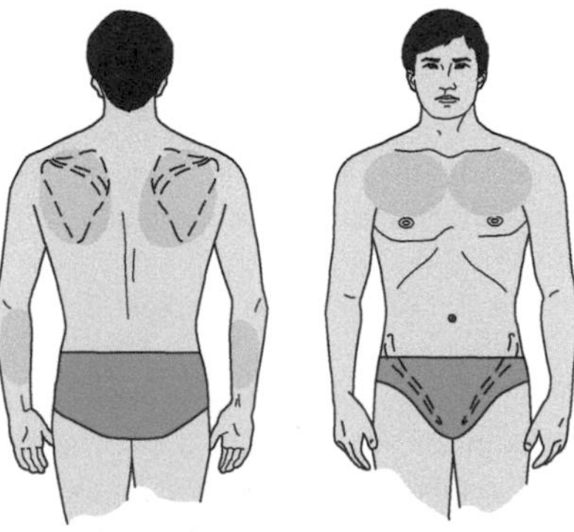

Figure 23-25 Body sites commonly used for intradermal injections.

PROCEDURE 23-5 Administering an Intradermal Injection

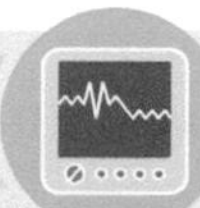

Purpose

- To provide a medication that the patient requires for allergy testing, antibody and TB screening

Assessment

Assess

- Appearance of injection site
- Specific drug action and expected response
- Patient's knowledge of drug action and response

Check local protocol about sites to use for skin tests.

Planning

Equipment

- Vial or ampoule of the correct medication
- Sterile 1ml syringe calibrated into hundredths of a millilitre (i.e. tuberculin syringe) and a # 25- to # 27-gauge needle
- Alcohol swabs
- 5cm × 5cm sterile gauze square (optional)
- Clean gloves (according to local protocol)
- Dressing (optional)
- Epinephrine/adrenaline (a bronchodilator and antihistamine) on hand for allergic reactions. As per local policy.

Implementation

Preparation

- Check the medication chart.
  - Check the label on the medication carefully against the chart to make sure that the correct medication is being prepared.
  - Follow the three checks for administering medications. Read the label on the medication (1) when it is taken from the medication store, (2) before withdrawing the medication and (3) after withdrawing the medication.
- Organise the equipment.

Performance

1 Follow local policy to ensure that you explain to the patient what you are going to do, why it is necessary and how they can cooperate. Obtain consent and maintain patient privacy and dignity and ensure that the appropriate local infection control procedures are observed.

2 Prepare the medication from the vial or ampoule for drug withdrawal.
- See Procedures 23-2 (ampoule) or 23-3 (vial).

3 Prepare the patient.
- Check the patient's identification band for name, address, date of birth and hospital number. Check this by also asking the patient to confirm his/her name and address. *This ensures that the right patient receives the medication.*

4 Explain to the patient that the medication will produce a small weal/swelling. A *weal* is a small raised area, like a blister. The patient will feel a slight prick as the needle enters the skin. Some medications are absorbed slowly through the capillaries into the general circulation, and the swelling gradually disappears. Other drugs remain in the area and interact with the body tissues to produce redness and induration (hardening), which will need to be interpreted at a particular time (e.g. in 24 or 48 hours). This reaction will also gradually disappear. *Information facilitates acceptance of and compliance with the therapy.*

5 Select and clean the site.
- Select a site (e.g. the forearm about a hand's width above the wrist and three or four fingerwidths below the antecubital space).
- Avoid using sites that are tender, inflamed or swollen and those that have lesions.
- Put on clean gloves as per local policy.
- Cleanse the skin at the site using a firm circular motion starting at the centre and widening the circle outward. Allow the area to dry thoroughly.

6 Prepare the syringe for the injection.
- Remove the needle cap while waiting for the antiseptic to dry.
- Expel any air bubbles from the syringe. Small bubbles that adhere to the plunger are of no consequence. *A small amount of air will not harm the tissues.*

- Grasp the syringe in your dominant hand, holding it between thumb and forefinger. Hold the needle almost parallel to the skin surface, with the bevel of the needle up. *The possibility of the medication entering the subcutaneous tissue increases when using an angle greater than 15 degrees or if the bevel is down.*

7 Inject the fluid.

- With the non-dominant hand, pull the skin at the site until it is taut. For example, if using the ventral forearm, grasp the patient's dorsal forearm and gently pull it to tighten the ventral skin. *Taut skin allows for easier entry of the needle and less discomfort for the patient.*
- Insert the tip of the needle far enough to place the bevel through the epidermis into the dermis (see Figure 23-26(a)). The outline of the bevel should be visible under the skin surface.
- Stabilise the syringe and needle, inject the medication carefully and slowly so that it produces a small weal on the skin (see Figure 23-26(b-c)). *This verifies that the medication entered the dermis.*
- Withdraw the needle quickly at the same angle at which it was inserted. Apply a dressing if indicated.
- Do not massage the area. Massage can disperse the medication into the tissue or out through the needle insertion site.
- Dispose of the syringe and needle safely. Do not recap the needle in order to prevent needlestick injuries.
- Remove gloves.
- Mark the circumference of the injection site with appropriate marker to observe for redness or induration (hardening), as per local policy if indicated.

8 Document all relevant information.

- Record the testing material given, the time, dosage, route and site.

(a)

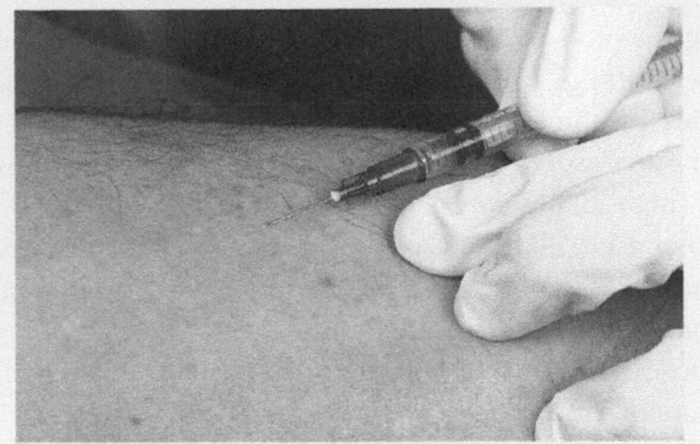

(b)

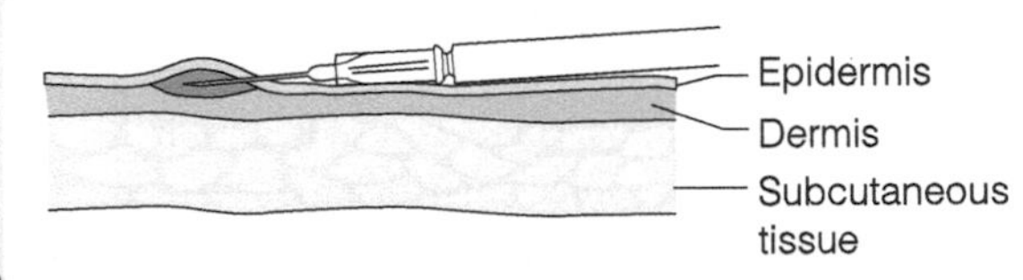

(c)

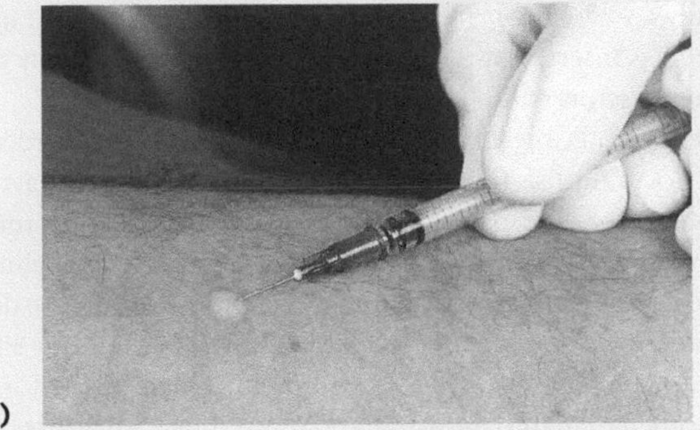

Figure 23-26 For an intradermal injection: (a) the needle enters the skin at a 5- to 15-degree angle; (b-c) the medication forms a bleb under the epidermis.
Source: Pearson Education Ltd.

Evaluation

- Evaluate the patient's response to the testing substance. *Some medications used in testing may cause allergic reactions.* An antidote drug (e.g. epinephrine) may need to be used.
- Evaluate the condition of the site in 24 or 48 hours, depending on the test. Measure the area of redness and induration in millimetres at the largest diameter and document findings.

LIFESPAN CONSIDERATIONS

Administering an Intradermal Injection

Children

- A small child or infant will need to be well prepared and possibly sit in the parent or carer's lap during the procedure. *This prevents injury from sudden movement.*
- Make sure the child understands that the procedure is not a punishment.
- Ask the child not to rub or scratch the injection site. Place a stockinet or gauze dressing over the site if needed. *Rubbing the site can interfere with test results by irritating the underlying tissue.*

Subcutaneous Injections

Among the many kinds of drugs administered subcutaneously (just beneath the skin) are vaccines, pre-operative medications, narcotics, insulin and heparin. Common sites for SC injections are the outer aspect of the upper arms and the anterior aspect of the thighs. These areas are convenient and normally have good blood circulation. Other areas that can be used are the abdomen, the scapular areas of the upper back and the upper ventrogluteal and dorsogluteal areas (see Figure 23-27). Only small doses (0.5–1ml) of medication are usually injected via the subcutaneous route.

The type of syringe used for subcutaneous injections depends on the medication to be given. Generally a 2ml syringe is used for most SC injections. However, if insulin is being administered, an insulin syringe is used; and if heparin is being administered, a pre-filled cartridge may be used.

Needle sizes and lengths are selected based on the patient's body mass, the intended angle of insertion and the planned site. Generally a #25-gauge is used for adults of normal weight and the needle is inserted at the recommended angle advised by the drug manufacturer and local policy.

Subcutaneous injection sites need to be rotated in an orderly fashion to minimise tissue damage, aid absorption and avoid discomfort. This is especially important for patients who must receive repeated injections, such as diabetics. Because insulin is absorbed at different rates at different parts of the body, the diabetic patient's blood glucose levels can vary when various sites are used. Insulin is absorbed more quickly when injected into the abdomen than into the arms, and more slowly when injected into the thighs and buttocks.

Nurses have traditionally been taught to aspirate by pulling back on the plunger after inserting the needle and before injecting the medication. The nurse could then determine whether the needle had entered a blood vessel. Absence of blood was believed to indicate that the needle was in subcutaneous tissue and not in the more vascular muscular tissue. According to medical experts aspirating is no longer necessary for SC injections.

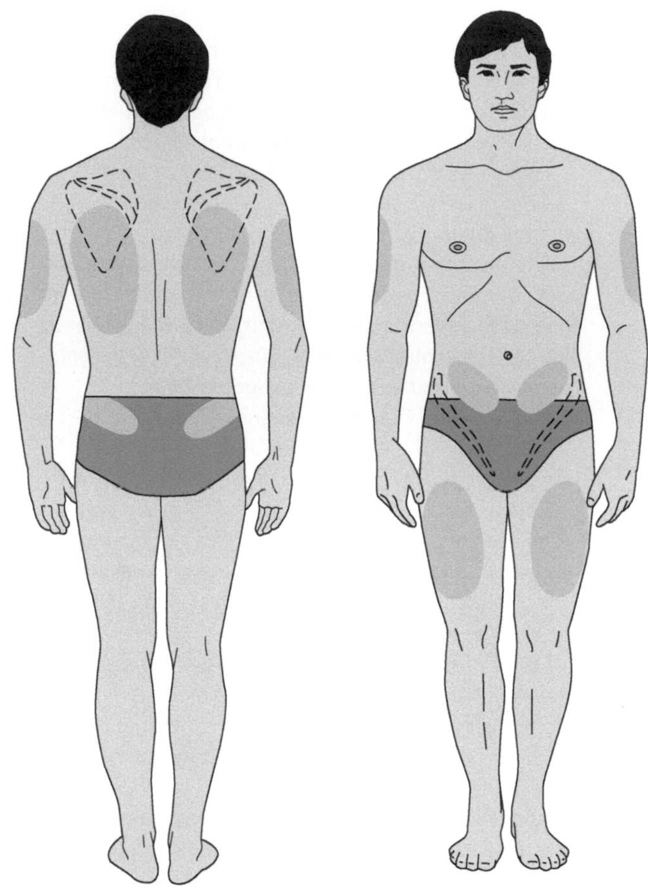

Figure 23-27 Body sites commonly used for subcutaneous injections.

The steps for administering a subcutaneous injection are described in *Procedure 23-6*.

PROCEDURE 23-6 Administering a Subcutaneous Injection

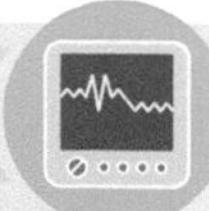

Purposes

- To provide a medication the patient requires (see specific drug action)
- To allow slower absorption of a medication compared with either the intramuscular or intravenous route

Assessment

Assess

- Allergies to medication
- Specific drug action, side-effects and adverse reactions
- Patient's knowledge and learning needs about the medication
- Status and appearance of subcutaneous site for lesions, erythemia, swelling, ecchymosis, inflammation and tissue damage from previous injections
- Ability of patient to cooperate during the injection
- Previous injection sites used

Planning

Equipment

- Patient medication prescription chart
- Vial or ampoule of the correct sterile medication
- Syringe and needle (e.g. 2ml syringe, #25-gauge needle)
- Antiseptic swabs
- Ampoule opener
- Dry sterile gauze for opening an ampoule (optional)
- Clean gloves

Implementation

Preparation

- Check the medication chart.
  - Check the label on the medication carefully against the chart to make sure that the correct medication is being prepared.
  - Follow the three checks for administering medications. Read the label on the medication (1) when it is taken from the medication store, (2) before withdrawing the medication and (3) after withdrawing the medication.
- Organise the equipment.

Performance

1 Follow local policy to ensure that you explain to the patient what you are going to do, why it is necessary and how they can cooperate. Obtain consent and maintain patient privacy and dignity and ensure that the appropriate local infection control procedures are observed.

2 Prepare the medication from the ampoule or vial for drug withdrawal.
  - See Procedure 23-2 (ampoule) or 23-3 (vial).

3 Prepare the patient.
  - Check the patient's identification band for name, address, date of birth and hospital number. Check this by also asking the patient to confirm his/her name and address. *This ensures that the right patient receives the medication.*
  - Assist the patient to a position in which the arm, leg or abdomen can be relaxed, depending on the site to be used. *A relaxed position of the site minimises discomfort.*
  - Obtain assistance in holding an uncooperative patient. *This prevents injury due to sudden movement after needle insertion.*

4 Explain the purpose of the medication and how it will help, using language that the patient can understand. Include relevant information about effects of the medication. *Information facilitates acceptance of and compliance with the therapy.*

5 Select and clean the site.
  - Select a site free of tenderness, hardness, swelling, scarring, itching, burning or localised inflammation. Select a site that has not been used frequently. *These conditions could hinder the absorption of the medication and also increase the likelihood of injury and discomfort at the injection site.*
  - Put on fresh clean gloves as per local policy.
  - As local policy indicates, clean the site with an antiseptic swab. Start at the centre of the site and clean in a widening circle to about 5cm. Allow the area to dry thoroughly. *The mechanical action of swabbing removes skin secretions, which contain micro-organisms.*
  - Place and hold the swab between the third and fourth fingers of the nondominant hand, or position the swab on the patient's skin above the intended site. *Using this technique keeps the swab readily accessible when the needle is withdrawn.*

6 Prepare the syringe for injection.
  - Remove the needle cap while waiting for the antiseptic to dry. Pull the cap straight off to avoid contaminating the needle by the outside edge of the cap. *The needle will become contaminated if it touches anything but the inside of the cap, which is sterile.*

7 Inject the medication.
  - Grasp the syringe in your dominant hand by holding it between your thumb and fingers. With palm facing to the side or upward for a 45-degree angle insertion, or with the palm downward for a 90-degree angle insertion, prepare to inject (see Figure 23-28).
  - Using the nondominant hand, spread the skin at the site, and insert the needle using the dominant hand and a firm steady push (see Figure 23-29).
  - Recommendations vary about whether to pinch or spread the skin and at what angle to administer

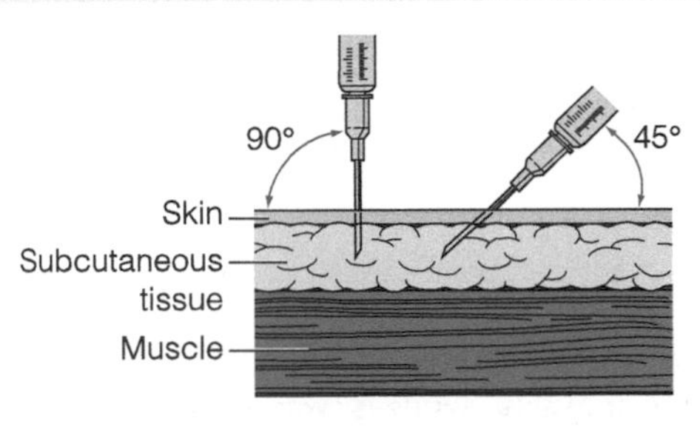

Figure 23-28 Inserting a needle into the subcutaneous tissue using 90- and 45-degree angles.

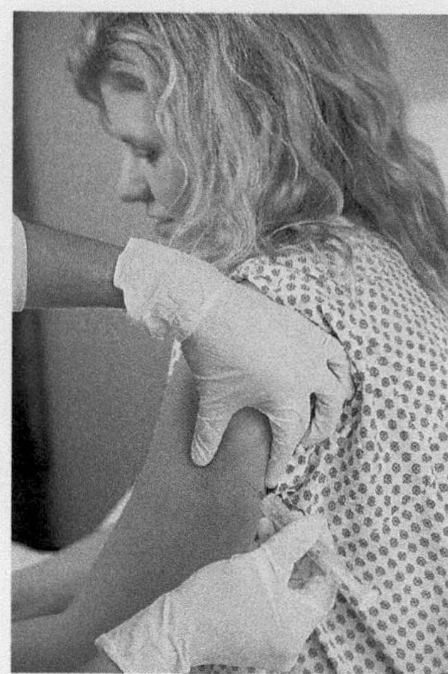

Figure 23-29 Administering a subcutaneous injection into pinched tissue.

subcutaneous injections and the nurse needs to refer to the drug manufacturer and local policy guidelines for each drug as they vary. The most important consideration is the depth of the subcutaneous tissue in the area to be injected.

- When the needle is inserted, move your nondominant hand to the end of the plunger. Some nurses find it easier to move the nondominant hand to the barrel of the syringe and the dominant hand to the end of the plunger.
- Inject the medication by holding the syringe steady and depressing the plunger with a slow, even pressure. *Holding the syringe steady and injecting the medication at an even pressure minimises discomfort for the patient.*

8 Remove the needle.
   - Remove the needle slowly and smoothly, pulling along the line of insertion while depressing the skin with your nondominant hand. *Depressing the skin places countertraction on it and minimises the patient's discomfort when the needle is withdrawn.*
   - If bleeding occurs, apply pressure to the site with dry sterile gauze until it stops. *Bleeding rarely occurs after subcutaneous injection.*

9 Dispose of supplies appropriately.
   - Discard the uncapped needle as per local policy.
   - Remove gloves. Wash hands.

10 Document all relevant information.
   - Document the medication given, dosage, time, route and any assessments.

11 Assess the effectiveness of the medication at the time it is expected to act.

Variation: Administering a heparin injection

The subcutaneous administration of heparin requires special precautions because of the drug's anticoagulant properties.

- Select a site on the abdomen 3-5cm away from the umbilicus and above the level of the iliac crests. Some clinical areas support the practice of subcutaneous injection of heparin in the thighs or arms as alternate sites to the abdomen.
- Alternate the sites of subsequent injections.

Evaluation

- Conduct appropriate follow-up such as desired effect (e.g. relief of pain, sedation, lowered blood sugar, a prothrombin time within pre-established limits), any adverse effects (e.g. nausea, vomiting, skin rash), and clinical signs of side-effects.
- Relate to previous findings if available.
- Report deviations from normal to the physician.

COMMUNITY CARE CONSIDERATIONS

Subcutaneous Injections

- Ensure that there is safe and appropriate storage for the medication, e.g. refrigerator.
- For frequent injections, develop a plan for site rotation with the patient.
- For cost-saving measures, teach able patients to safely reuse disposable syringes where appropriate. Diabetic patients in the home can safely use disposable syringes until the needles become dull, which can vary from 2-10 times (Fleming, 1999).
- For insulin-dependent patients, ensure that at least one knowledgeable relative/friend can correctly inject insulin in an emergency situation and recognise and treat hypoglycaemia.
- Supply patient with appropriate sharp disposable boxes and inform patient of where the sharps boxes can be collected or taken to for safe disposal.

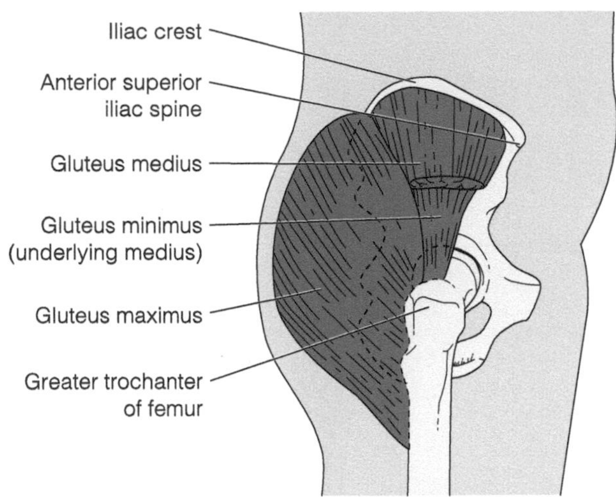

Figure 23-30 Lateral view of the right buttock showing the three gluteal muscles used for intramuscular injections.

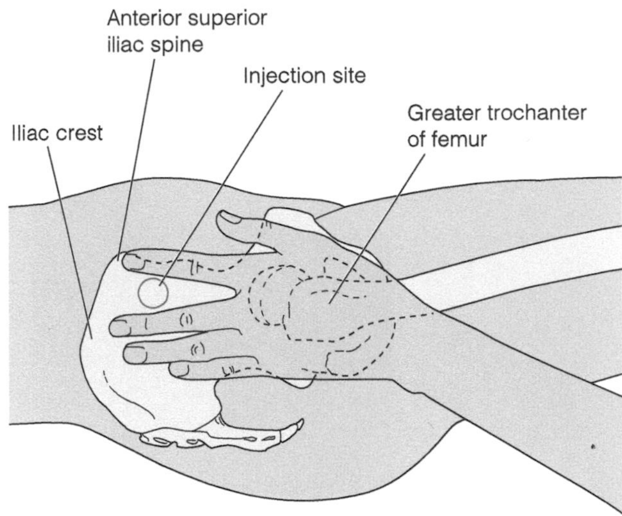

Figure 23-31 Landmarks for the ventrogluteal site for an intramuscular injection.

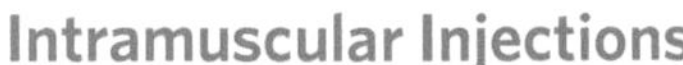

Intramuscular Injections

Injections into muscle tissue, or intramuscular (IM) injections, are absorbed more quickly than subcutaneous injections because of the greater blood supply to the body muscles. Muscles can also take a larger volume of fluid without discomfort than subcutaneous tissues can, although the amount varies among individuals, chiefly with muscle size and condition and with the site used. An adult with well-developed muscles can usually safely tolerate up to 5ml of medication in the gluteus medius and gluteus maximus muscles (see Figure 23-30). A volume of 1–2ml is usually recommended for adults with less developed muscles. In the deltoid muscle, volumes of 0.5–1ml are recommended.

Usually a 2–5ml syringe is needed. The size of syringe used depends on the amount of medication being administered. The standard pre-packaged intramuscular needle is 3cm and #21 or #22 gauge. Several factors indicate the size and length of the needle to be used:

- the muscle;
- the type of solution;
- the amount of adipose tissue covering the muscle;
- the age of the patient.

For example, a smaller needle such as a #23- to #25-gauge needle is commonly used for the deltoid muscle. More viscous solutions require a larger gauge (e.g. #20 gauge). Very obese patients may require a needle longer than 4cm and emaciated patients may require a shorter needle (e.g. 2cm).

A major consideration in the administration of intramuscular injections is the selection of a safe site located away from large blood vessels, nerves and bone. Several body sites can be used for intramuscular injections. These sites are discussed in detail next. Contraindications for using a specific site include tissue injury and the presence of nodules, lumps, abscesses, tenderness or other pathology.

Ventrogluteal Site

The ventrogluteal site is in the gluteus medius muscle, which lies over the gluteus minimus (see Figure 23-31). The ventrogluteal site is the *preferred* site for intramuscular injections because the area:

- contains no large nerves or blood vessels;
- provides the greatest thickness of gluteal muscle consisting of both the gluteus medius and gluteus minimus;
- is sealed off by bone;
- contains consistently less fat than the buttock area, thus eliminating the need to determine the depth of subcutaneous fat.

This site is suitable for children over seven months and adults. The patient position for the injection can be a back, prone or side-lying position. The side-lying position, however, helps locate the ventrogluteal site more easily. Position the patient on his or her side with the knee bent and raised slightly towards the chest. The trochanter will protrude, which facilitates locating the ventrogluteal site. To establish the exact site, the nurse places the heel of the hand on the patient's greater trochanter, with the fingers pointing towards the patient's head. The right hand is used for the left hip, and the left hand for the right hip. With the index finger on the patient's anterior superior iliac spine, the nurse stretches the middle finger dorsally (towards the buttocks), palpating the crest of the ilium and then pressing below it. The triangle formed by the index finger, the third finger and the crest of the ileum is the injection site (see Figures 23-31 and 23-32).

Vastus Lateralis Site

The vastus lateralis muscle is usually thick and well developed in both adults and children. It is recommended as the site of choice for intramuscular injections for infants seven months and younger. Because there are no major blood vessels or nerves in

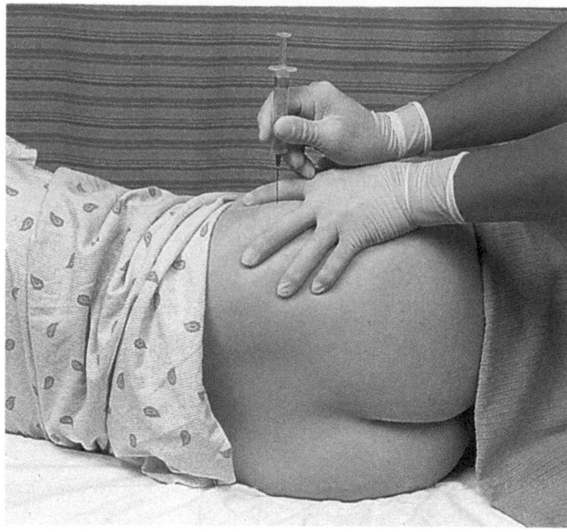

Figure 23-32 Administering an intramuscular injection into the ventrogluteal site.
Source: Pearson Education Ltd.

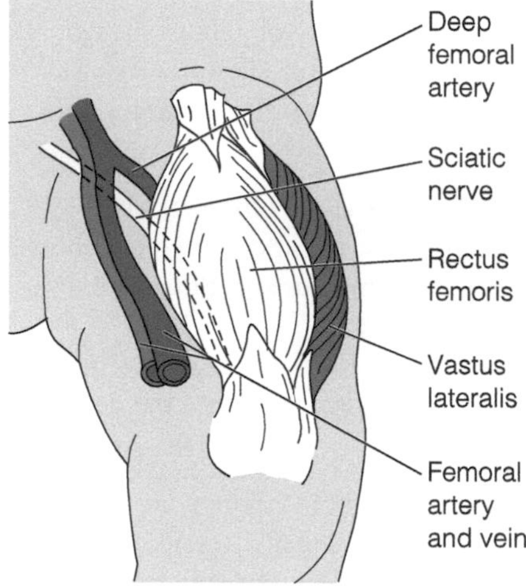

Figure 23-33 The vastus lateralis muscle of an infant's upper thigh, used for intramuscular injections.

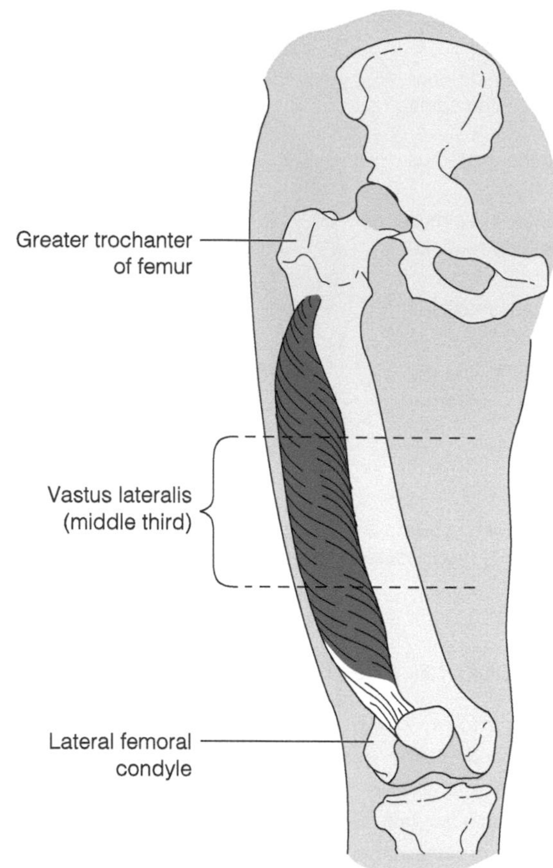

Figure 23-34 Landmarks for the vastus lateralis site of an adult's right thigh, used for an intramuscular injection.

the area, it is desirable for infants whose gluteal muscles are poorly developed. It is situated on the anterior lateral aspect of the infant's thigh (see Figure 23-33). The middle third of the muscle is suggested as the site. In the adult, the landmark is established by dividing the area between the greater trochanter of the femur and the lateral femoral condyle into thirds and selecting the middle third (see Figures 23-34 and 23-35). The patient can assume a back-lying or a sitting position for an injection into this site.

Dorsogluteal Site

The dorsogluteal site is composed of the thick gluteal muscles of the buttocks (see Figure 23-30 on page 709). The dorsogluteal site can be used for adults and for children with well-developed gluteal muscles. Because these muscles are developed by walking, this site should not be used for children under three unless the child has been walking for at least a year. The nurse must choose the injection site carefully to avoid striking the sciatic nerve, major blood vessels or bone.

The nurse palpates the posterior superior iliac spine, and then draws an imaginary line to the greater trochanter of the femur. This line is lateral to and parallel to the sciatic nerve. The injection site is lateral and superior to this line (see Figure 23-36). Palpating the ilium and the trochanter is important; visual calculations alone can result in an injection that is placed too low and injures other structures.

The patient needs to assume a prone position with the toes pointed inward or a side-lying position with the upper knee flexed and in front of the lower leg. These positions promote muscle relaxation and therefore minimise discomfort from the injection.

Deltoid Site

The deltoid muscle is found on the lateral aspect of the upper arm. Care is needed when using the deltoid muscle for intramuscular injections because it is a relatively small muscle and is very close to the radial nerve and radial artery. It is sometimes considered for use in adults because of rapid absorption from the deltoid area, but no more than 1ml of solution can be

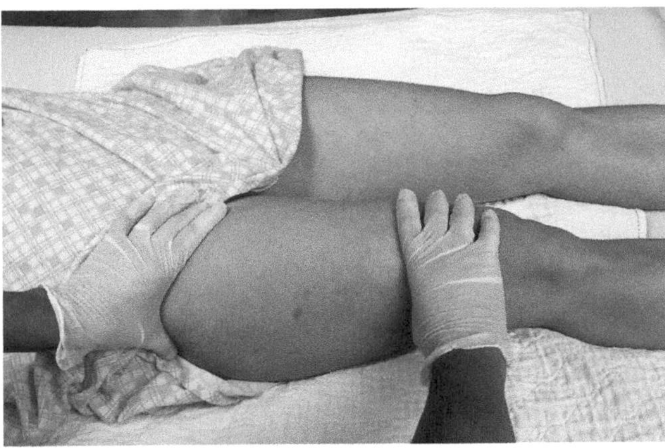

(a)

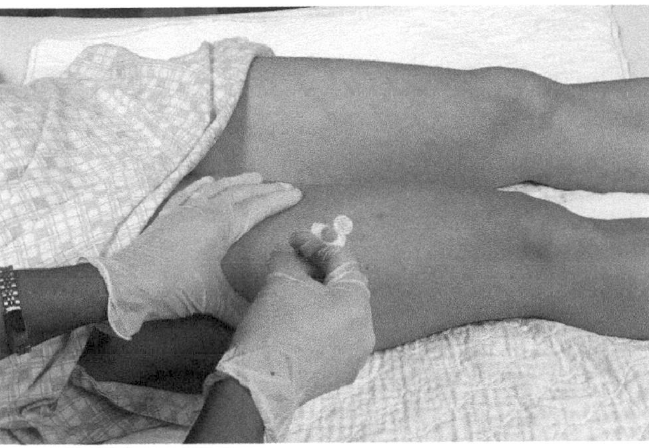

(b)

Figure 23-35 (a) Determining landmarks and (b) Administering an intramuscular injection into the vastus lateralis site.

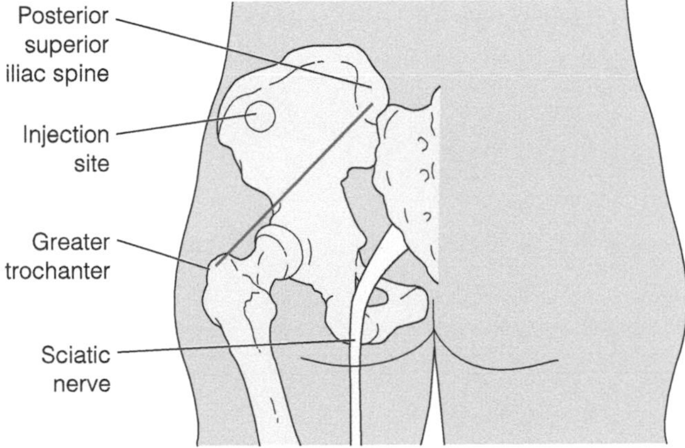

Figure 23-36 Landmarks for the dorsogluteal site for an intramuscular injection.

administered. This site is recommended for the administration of hepatitis B vaccine in adults.

The upper landmark for the deltoid site is located by the nurse placing four fingers across the deltoid muscle with the first finger on the acromion process. The top of the axilla is the line

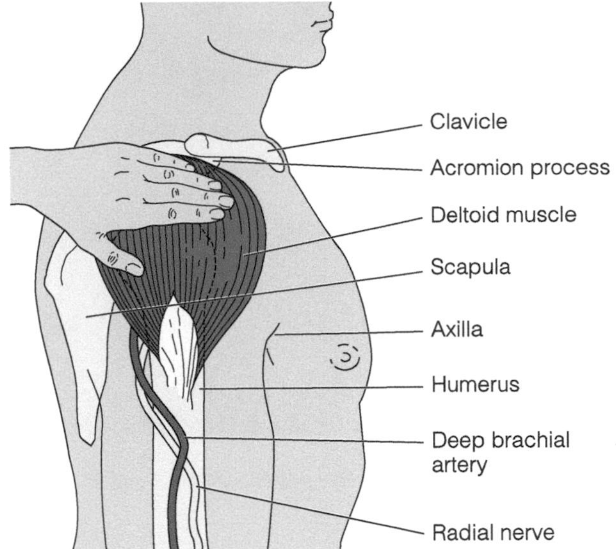

Figure 23-37 A method of establishing the deltoid muscle site for an intramuscular injection.

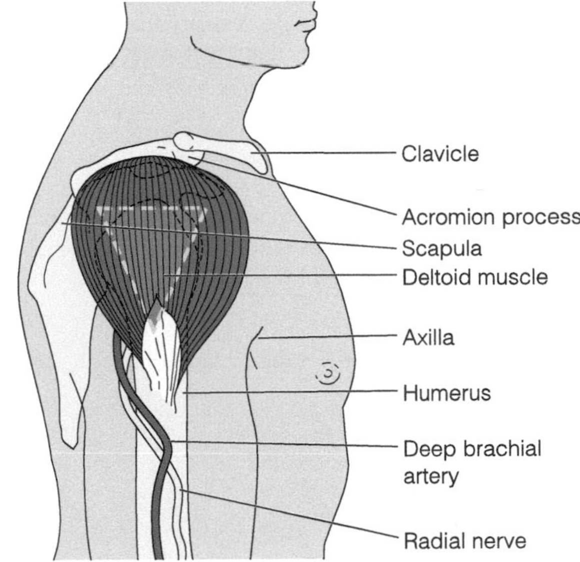

Figure 23-38 Landmarks for the deltoid muscle of the upper arm, used for intramuscular injections.

that marks the lower border landmark (see Figure 23-37). A triangle within these boundaries indicates the deltoid muscle about 5cm below the acromion process (see Figures 23-38 and 23-39).

The use of a pinch-grasp technique can reduce the discomfort of an IM injection into the deltoid muscle. This technique involves grasping the muscle, pulling it about 2–3cm towards the nurse, and applying a pinching pressure hard enough to cause mild discomfort. The injection is given at a 90-degree angle (McCaffery and Pasero, 1999). It is important for the nurse to inform the patient about pinching the skin and explain the purpose.

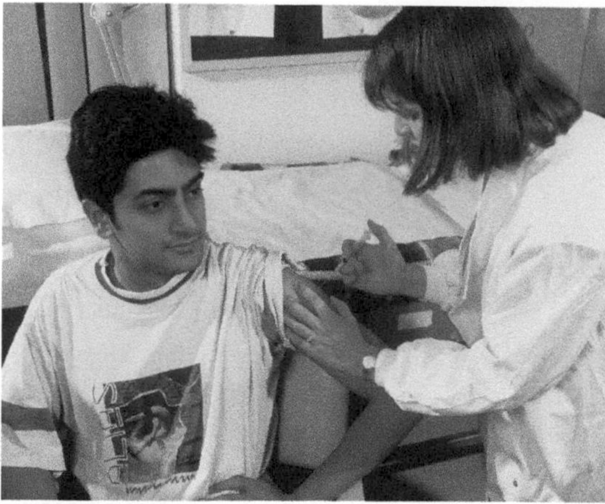

Figure 23-39 Administering an intramuscular injection into the deltoid site.

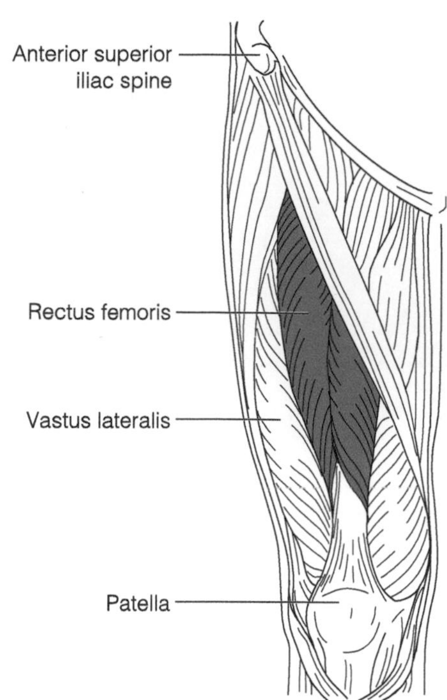

Figure 23-40 Landmarks for the rectus femoris muscle of the upper right thigh, used for intramuscular injections.

Rectus Femoris Site

The rectus femoris muscle, which belongs to the quadriceps muscle group, is used only occasionally for intramuscular injections. It is situated on the anterior aspect of the thigh (see Figure 23-40). Its chief advantage is that patients who administer their own injections can reach this site easily. Its main disadvantage is that an injection here may cause considerable discomfort for some people.

IM Injection Technique

Procedure 23-7 describes how to administer an intramuscular injection using the Z-track technique, which is recommended for any intramuscular injection:

- Follow Procedure 23-7.
- Pulling the skin and the subcutaneous layer 2–3cm away from the injection site.
- Hold the needle at 90° angle.
- Follow procedure for injection giving.
- Withdraw needle same angle as it went in.
- Hold the skin back for a few seconds and then release.

The Z-track method has been found to be less painful than the traditional injection technique. This prevents any of the administered drugs leaking from the site through the track the needle originally took (McCaffery and Pasero, 1999).

PROCEDURE 23-7 Administering an Intramuscular Injection

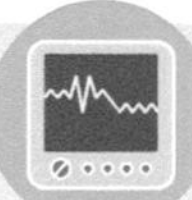

Purpose

- To provide a medication the patient requires (see specific drug action)

Assessment

Assess

- Patient allergies to medication(s)
- Specific drug action, side-effects and adverse reactions
- Patient's knowledge of and learning needs about the medication
- Tissue integrity of the selected site
- Patient's age and weight to determine site and needle size
- Patient's ability or willingness to cooperate

Determine

Determine whether the size of the muscle is appropriate to the amount of medication to be injected. An average adult's deltoid muscle can usually absorb 0.5-1ml of medication, although some authorities believe 1-2ml can be absorbed by a well-developed deltoid muscle. The gluteus medius muscle can often absorb 1-4ml, although 4ml may be very painful.

Planning

Equipment

- Medication chart
- Sterile medication (usually provided in an ampoule or vial)
- Syringe and needle of a size appropriate for the amount of solution to be administered
- Antiseptic swabs
- Clean gloves

Implementation

Preparation

- Check the prescription chart.
  - Check the label on the medication carefully against the chart to make sure that the correct medication is being prepared.
  - Follow the three checks for administering the medication and dose. Read the label on the medication (1) when it is taken from the medication store, (2) before withdrawing the medication and (3) after withdrawing the medication.
  - Confirm that the dose is correct.
- Organise the equipment.

Performance

1 Follow local policy to ensure that you explain to the patient what you are going to do, why it is necessary and how they can cooperate. Obtain consent and maintain patient privacy and dignity and ensure that the appropriate local infection control procedures are observed.

2 Prepare the medication from the ampoule or vial for drug withdrawal.
  - See Procedure 23-2 (ampoule) or 23-3 (vial).
  - Whenever feasible, change the needle on the syringe before the injection. Because the outside of a new needle is free of medication, it does not irritate subcutaneous tissues as it passes into the muscle.
  - Invert the syringe needle uppermost and expel all excess air.

3 Prepare the patient.
  - Check the patient's identification band for name, address, date of birth and hospital number. Check this by also asking the patient to confirm his/her name and address. *This ensures that the right patient receives the medication.*
  - Assist the patient to a supine, lateral, prone or sitting position, depending on the chosen site. If the target muscle is the gluteus medius (ventrogluteal site), have the patient in the supine position flex the knee(s); in the lateral position, flex the upper leg; and in the prone position, toe in. *Appropriate positioning promotes relaxation of the target muscle.*

4 Explain the purpose of the medication and how it will help, using language that the patient can understand. Include relevant information about effects of the medication. *Information facilitates acceptance of and compliance with the therapy.*

5 Select, locate and clean the site.
  - Select a site free of skin lesions, tenderness, swelling, hardness or localised inflammation and one that has not been used frequently.
  - If injections are to be frequent, alternate sites. Avoid using the same site twice in a row, or consider discussing an alternative route with the patient and doctor. *This is to reduce the discomfort of intramuscular injections.* If necessary, discuss with the prescriber an alternative method of providing the medication.
  - Locate the exact site for the injection.
  - Put on clean gloves as per local policy.
  - Clean the site with an antiseptic swab. Using a circular motion, start at the centre and move outward about 5cm.
  - Transfer and hold the swab between the third and fourth fingers of your nondominant hand in readiness for needle withdrawal, or position the swab on the patient's skin above the intended site. Allow skin to dry prior to injecting medication *because this will help reduce the discomfort of the injection.*

6 Prepare the syringe for injection.
  - Remove the needle cover without contaminating the needle.
  - If using a pre-filled unit-dose medication, take caution to avoid dripping medication on the needle prior to injection. If this does occur, wipe the medication off the needle with a sterile gauze. *Medication left on the needle can cause pain when it is tracked through the subcutaneous tissue.*

7 Inject the medication using a Z-track technique.
  - Use the ulnar side of the nondominant hand to pull the skin approximately 2.5cm to the side (see Figure 23-41). Under some circumstances, such as for an emaciated patient or an infant, the muscle may be pinched. *Pulling the skin and subcutaneous tissue or pinching the muscle makes it firmer and facilitates needle insertion.*
  - Holding the syringe between the thumb and forefinger (as if holding a pencil), pierce the skin quickly and smoothly at a 90-degree angle (see Figure 23-32 on

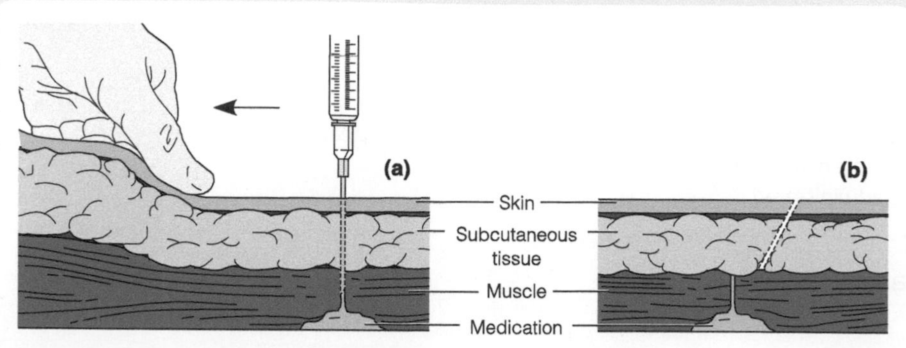

Figure 23-41 Inserting an intramuscular needle at a 90-degree angle using the Z-track method: (a) skin pulled to the side; (b) skin released. *Note:* When the skin returns to its normal position after the needle is withdrawn, a seal is formed over the intramuscular site. This prevents seepage of the medication into the subcutaneous tissues and subsequent discomfort.

page 710), and insert the needle into the muscle. *Using a quick motion lessens the patient's discomfort.*

- Hold the barrel of the syringe steady with your nondominant hand and aspirate by pulling back on the plunger with your dominant hand. Aspirate for 5 seconds. *If the needle is in a small blood vessel, it takes time for the blood to appear.* If blood appears in the syringe, withdraw the needle, discard the syringe and prepare a new injection. *This step determines whether the needle has been inserted into a blood vessel.*
- If blood does not appear, inject the medication steadily and slowly (approximately 10 seconds per millilitre) while holding the syringe steady. *Injecting medication slowly promotes comfort and allows time for tissue to expand and begin absorption of the medication. Holding the syringe steady minimises discomfort.*
- After injection, wait 10 seconds to permit the medication to disperse into the muscle tissue, thus decreasing the patient's discomfort.

8 Withdraw the needle.
   - Withdraw the needle smoothly at the same angle of insertion. *This minimises tissue injury.*
   - Apply gentle pressure at the site with dry gauze. Do not massage the site. *Massaging the site can increase discomfort of the injection and can result in tissue irritation.*
   - If bleeding occurs, apply pressure with dry sterile gauze until it stops.

9 Discard the uncapped needle and attached syringe into the sharps box.
   - Remove gloves. Wash hands.

10 Document all relevant information.
   - Include the time of administration, drug name, dose and route.

Assess effectiveness of the medication at the time it is expected to act.

Evaluation

- Conduct appropriate follow-up, such as:
  - desired effect (e.g. relief of pain or vomiting);
  - any adverse reactions or side-effects;
  - local skin or tissue reactions at injection site (e.g. redness, swelling, pain or other evidence of tissue damage).
- Relate to previous findings, if available.
- Report significant deviation from normal to medical staff.

ACTIVITY 23-1

A patient has returned from theatre and has not been prescribed analgesia via a patient controlled analgesia (PCA) pump. You note on the prescription chart that she has been prescribed diamorphine hydrochloride injection intramuscularly. What are the key aspects you need to consider before, during and after administering the drug?

LIFESPAN CONSIDERATIONS

Intramuscular Injections

Infants

- The ventrogluteal site cannot be used for children under seven months.
- The vastus lateralis site is recommended as the site of choice for intramuscular injections for infants seven months and younger. Because there are no major blood vessels or nerves in the area, it is desirable for infants whose gluteal muscles are poorly developed. It is situated on the anterior lateral aspect of the thigh (see Figure 23-35 on page 703).
- The parent may hold the infant or young child in their lap. This prevents accidental injury during the procedure.

Children

- Infants and young children usually require smaller, shorter needles (#22- to #25- gauge) for intramuscular injection.
- The gluteal muscles are developed by walking. Therefore, the dorsogluteal site should not be used for children under three unless the child has been walking for at least a year.

Mature Adults

- Mature patients may have a decreased muscle mass or muscle atrophy. A shorter needle may be needed. Assessment of appropriate injection site is critical. Absorption of medication may occur more quickly than expected.

Intravenous Medications

Intravenous (IV) medications enter the patient's bloodstream directly by way of a vein. They are appropriate when a rapid effect is required. This route is also appropriate when medications are too irritating to tissues to be given by other routes. When an intravenous line is already established, this route is desirable because it avoids the discomfort of other parenteral routes. Medications are administered intravenously by the following methods:

- large-volume infusion of intravenous fluid;
- intermittent intravenous infusion (piggyback or tandem setups);
- volume-controlled infusion (often used for children);
- intravenous bolus;
- intermittent injection ports (device).

In all of these methods, the patent has an existing intravenous line or an IV access site, e.g. IV cannula with wings, with or without injection ports, tunneled catheter or a peripheral intravenous central catheter (PICC). There are strict policies in relation to administration via invasive devices and all nurses should be aware of these.

With all IV medication administration, it is very important to observe patients closely for signs of adverse reactions. Because the drug enters the bloodstream directly and acts immediately, there is no way it can be withdrawn or its action terminated. Therefore, the nurse must take special care to avoid any errors in the preparation of the drug and the calculation of the dosage. When the drug being administered is particularly potent, an antidote to the drug should be available. In addition, the vital signs are assessed before, during and after infusion of the drug.

Before adding any medications to an existing intravenous infusion, the nurse must check for the six 'rights' and check compatibility of the drug and the existing intravenous fluid. Be aware of any incompatibilities of the drug and the fluid that is infusing.

Large-Volume Infusions

Mixing a medication into a large-volume IV fluid bag is the safest and easiest way to administer a drug intravenously. The drugs are diluted in volumes of 1,000ml or 500ml of compatible fluids or as per directions. See *Procedure 23-8*.

The main danger of infusing a large volume of fluid is circulatory overload (hypervolaemia).

The medication should be added to the fluid container before it is attached and infusing.

PROCEDURE 23-8 Adding Medications to Intravenous Fluid Containers

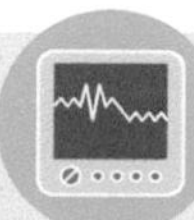

Purposes

- To provide and maintain a constant level of a medication in the blood
- To administer well-diluted medications at a continuous and slow rate

Assessment

- Inspect and palpate the intravenous insertion site for signs of infection, infiltration or a dislocated cannula.
- Inspect the surrounding skin for redness, pallor or swelling.
- Palpate the surrounding tissues for coldness and the presence of oedema, which could indicate leakage of the IV fluid into the tissues.
- Take vital signs for baseline data if the medication being administered is particularly potent.
- Determine if the patient has allergies to the medication(s).
- Check the compatibility of the medication(s) and IV fluid.

Planning

Equipment

- Prescription chart
- Correct sterile medication
- Dilutent solvent for medication in powdered form (see manufacturer's instructions)
- Correct solution container, if a new one is to be attached
- Antiseptic or alcohol swabs
- Sterile syringe of appropriate size (e.g. 5 or 10ml) and a #20- or #21-gauge sterile needle or equivalent from needleless system
- IV additive label
- Gloves

Implementation

Preparation

- Check the medication chart.
  - Check the label on the medication carefully against the medication chart to make sure that the correct medication is being prepared.
  - Follow the three checks for administering medications. Read the label on the medication (1) when it is taken from the medication store, (2) before withdrawing the medication and (3) after withdrawing the medication.
  - Confirm that the dosage and route is correct.
  - Verify which infusion solution is to be used with the medication.
  - Consult a pharmacist, if required, to confirm compatibility of the drugs and solutions being mixed.
- Organise the equipment.

Performance

1 Follow local policy to ensure that you explain to the patient what you are going to do, why it is necessary and how they can cooperate. Obtain consent and maintain patient privacy and dignity and ensure that the appropriate local infection control procedures are observed.

2 Prepare the medication ampoule or vial for drug withdrawal.
  - See Procedure 23-2 (ampoule) or 23-3 (vial).

3 Check the patient's identification band for name, address, date of birth and hospital number. Check this by also asking the patient to confirm his/her name and address. *This ensures that the right patient receives the medication.*

4 Add the medication.

To new IV container/fluid bag

- Locate the injection port and carefully remove its cover. Asepsis should be maintained at all times.

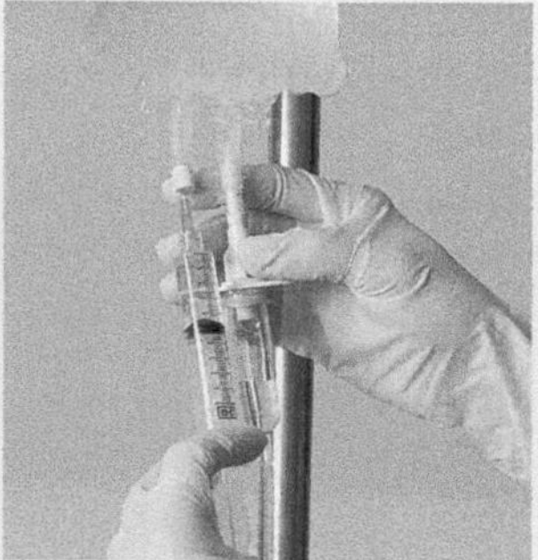

Figure 23-42 Inserting a medication through the injection port of an infusing container.

- Remove the needle cap from the syringe, insert the needle through the centre of the injection port, and inject the medication into the bag or bottle (see Figure 23-42).

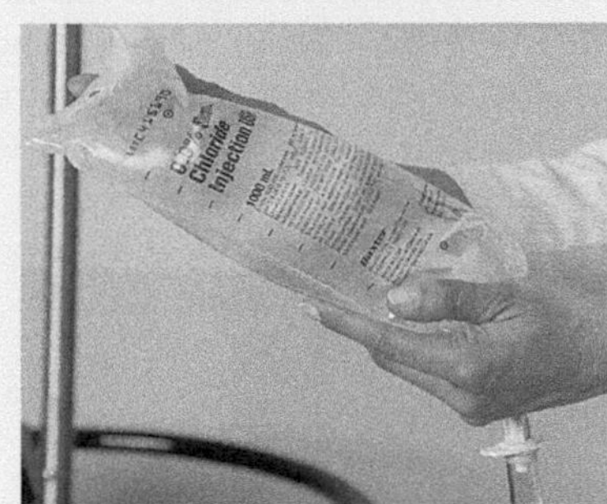

Figure 23-43 Rotating an intravenous bag to distribute a medication.
Source: Pearson Education Ltd.

- Mix the medication and solution by gently rotating the bag or bottle (see Figure 23-43). *This should disperse the medication throughout the solution.*
- Complete the IV additive label with name and dose of medication, date, time and nurse's initials. Attach it upside down on the bag or bottle (see Figure 23-44). *This documents that medication has been added to the solution. When the label is attached upside down, it is easily read when the bag is hanging up.*

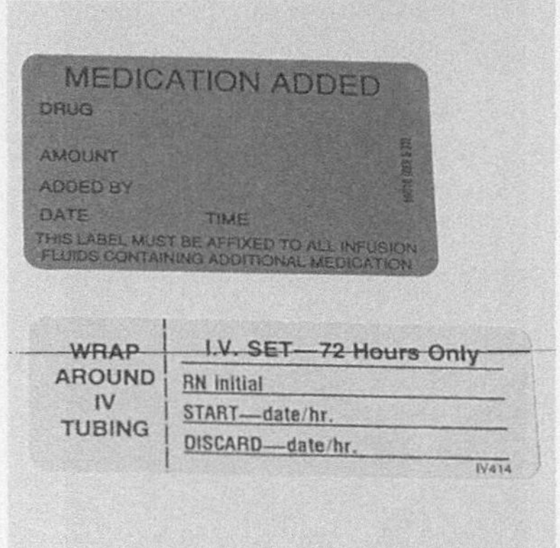

Figure 23-44 *Top*, label indicating a medication added to an IV infusion; *Bottom*, label indicating time for IV tubing change.
Source: Pearson Education Ltd.

- Clamp the IV tubing. Spike the bag or bottle with IV administration set and hang the fluid. *Clamping prevents rapid infusion of the solution.*
- Regulate infusion rate via pump as prescribed.

Evaluation

- Check bag for any cloudiness or abnormal colouring.
- Ensure all documentation is up to date (treatment charts, etc.)
- Maintain and observe patency of infusion site.
- Monitor condition of patient and report any changes.

Intermittent Intravenous Infusions

An intermittent infusion is a method of administering a medication mixed in a small amount of IV solution, such as 50 or 100ml (see Figure 23-45). The drug is administered at regular intervals, such as every four hours, with the drug being infused for a short period of time such as 30–60 minutes. Two commonly used additive or secondary IV setups are the *tandem* and the *piggyback*.

Another method of intermittently administering an IV medication is by a syringe pump. The medication is mixed in a syringe that is connected to an intravenous cannula and administered at a controlled administration rate (see Figure 23-46).

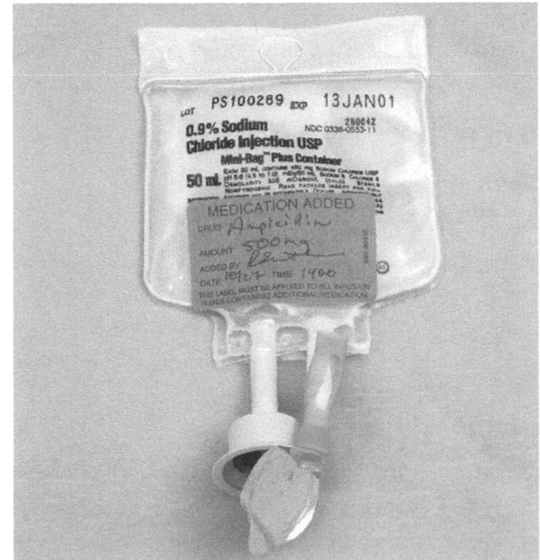

Figure 23-45 Medication in a labelled infusion bag.
Source: Pearson Education Ltd.

Intravenous Bolus

Intravenous bolus is the intravenous administration of a drug directly into the systemic circulation. It is used when a medication is not diluted or in an emergency. An IV bolus can be introduced directly into a vein by venipuncture or into an existing IV line through an existing access site, e.g. cannula.

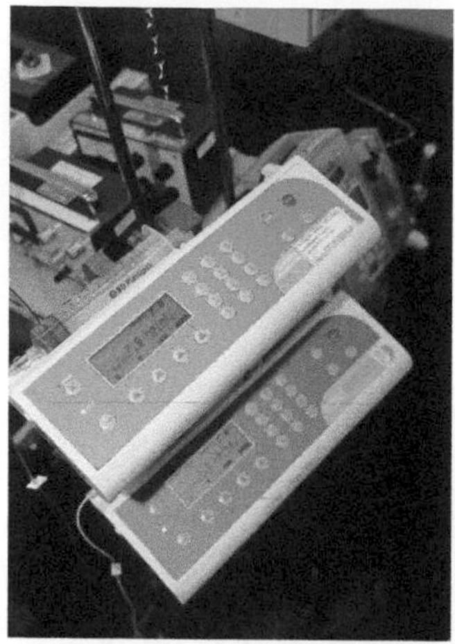

Figure 23-46 Syringe pump or mini-infuser for administration of IV medications.

Source: Science Photo Ltd/Antonia Reeve.

There are two major disadvantages to this method of drug administration: any error in administration cannot be corrected after the drug has entered the patient, and the drug may be irritating to the lining of the blood vessels. Before administering a bolus, the nurse should look up the maximum concentration recommended for the particular drug and the rate of administration. The administered medication takes effect immediately (see *Procedure 23-9*).

CLINICAL ALERT

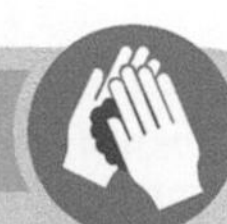

Some medication cannot be given as an intravenous bolus in the same dose as orally, e.g. 80mg of Furosemide can be tolerated orally but, if given as an IV bolus, may cause deafness and other side-effects.

PROCEDURE 23-9 Administering Intravenous Medications Using IV Bolus

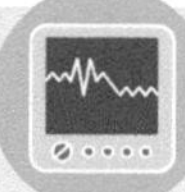

Purpose

To achieve immediate and maximum effects of a medication

Assessment

- Inspect and palpate the IV insertion site for signs of infection, infiltration or a dislocated cannula.
- Inspect the surrounding skin for redness, pallor or swelling.
- Palpate the surrounding tissues for coldness and the presence of oedema, which could indicate leakage of the IV fluid into the tissues.
- Take vital signs for baseline data if the medication being administered is particularly potent.
- Determine if the patient has allergies to the medication(s).
- Check the compatibility of the medication(s) and IV fluid.
- Determine specific drug action, side-effects, normal dosage, recommended administration time and peak action time.
- Check patency of IV line by assessing flow rate.

Planning

Equipment

IV bolus for an existing line

- Medication in a vial or ampoule
- Sterile syringe (size dependent upon volume of drug) (to prepare the medication) × 3 (including flush)
- Sterile needles #21- to #25-gauge, 2.5cm or equivalent from a needleless system
- Antiseptic swabs
- Watch with a digital readout or second hand
- 5ml 0.9% saline or 5ml heparin as per local policy
- Clean gloves

Implementation

Preparation

- Check the medication chart.
    - Check the label on the medication carefully against the chart to make sure that the correct medication is being prepared.
    - Follow the three checks for correct medication and dose. Read the label on the medication (1) when it is taken from the medication store, (2) before withdrawing the medication and (3) after withdrawing the medication.
    - Calculate medication dosage accurately.
    - Confirm that the route is correct.
- Organise the equipment.

Performance

1 Follow local policy to ensure that you explain to the patient what you are going to do, why it is necessary and how they can cooperate. Obtain consent and maintain patient privacy and dignity and ensure that the appropriate local infection control procedures are observed.
2 Prepare the medication.
   - Prepare the medication according to the manufacturer's direction. *It is important to have the correct dose and the correct dilution.*

   (a) Flushing with saline
   - Prepare two syringes, each with 2.5ml of sterile normal saline.

   (b) Flushing with heparin and saline
   - Prepare one syringe with 2.5ml of heparin flush solution.
   - Prepare two syringes with 2.5ml each of sterile, 0.9% saline.
3 Draw up the medication into a syringe.
4 Put a small-gauge needle on the syringe if using a needle system through a bung.
5 Wash hands and put on clean gloves. *This reduces the transmission of micro-organisms and reduces the likelihood of the nurse's hands contacting the patient's blood.*
6 Prepare the patient.
   - Check the patient's identification band for name, address, date of birth and hospital number. Check this by also asking the patient to confirm his/her name and address. *This ensures that the right patient receives the medication.*
   - If not previously assessed, take the appropriate assessment measures necessary for the medication. If any of the findings are above or below the predetermined parameters, consult the prescriber before administering the medication.
7 Explain the purpose of the medication and how it will help, using language that the patient can understand. Include relevant information about the effects of the medication.
8 Administer the medication by IV bolus slowly in accordance with manufacturer advice for rate of adminstration.

IV cannula

- Remove the protective cap from the cannula port.
- Insert syringe containing 0.9% saline into the lock.
- Flush the lock with 2.5ml sterile saline. *This clears the lock of blood.*
- Remove the syringe.
- Insert the syringe containing the medication into the valve of the cannula.
- Inject the medication following the precautions described previously.
- Withdraw the syringe.
- Repeat injection of 2.5ml of saline.
- Replace cap on cannula.

9 Dispose of equipment according to local policy. *This reduces needlestick injuries and spread of micro-organisms.*
10 Remove and dispose of gloves. Wash hands.
11 Observe the patient closely for adverse reactions.
12 Document all relevant information.
   - Record the date, time, drug, dose and route; patient response; and assessments of infusion or cannula site if appropriate.

Variation: existing line

1 Ensure compatibility of drug with infusion.
2 Identify the appropriate injection port.
3 Clean the port as per local policy.
4 Stop the IV infusion and pinch the tubing above the injection port. *This will prevent air bubbles and back flow.*
5 Insert the needle and syringe containing flush (dilutant) into the injection port.
6 Flush the line with appropriate dilutant, i.e. 0.9% saline or heparin.
7 Disconnect the syringe from the needle and attach the syringe containing the drug.
8 Administer the drug slowly as per manufacturer's instruction taking care to monitor the time on a watch.
9 Observe the patient, the site of the infusion and injection for any abnormal signs.
10 Disconnect the empty syringe from the needle and attach the second dilutant (flush).
11 Flush the drug and remove the needle and syringe from the injection port, then attach a new sterile cap to the port.
12 Remove the clamp *to avoid kinking of the tube.*
13 Recommence the infusion ensuring the rate, time, etc. are correct.
14 Dispose of all sharps in the sharps box (as per hospital policy).
15 Remove and dispose of gloves.
16 Document all relevant information.

Evaluation

- Conduct appropriate follow-up such as desired effect of medication, any adverse reactions or side-effects, or change in vital signs.
- Reassess status of IV cannula site and patency of IV infusion, if running.
- Relate to previous findings, if available.
- Report significant deviations from normal.

Topical Medications

A topical medication is applied locally to the skin or to mucous membranes in areas such as the eye, external ear canal, nose, vagina and rectum. Most topical applications used therapeutically are not absorbed well, completely or predictably when applied to intact skin because the skin's thick outer layer serves as a natural barrier to drug diffusion. This route of absorption through the skin, called percutaneous, can be increased if the skin is altered by a laceration, burn or some other problem. However, if high concentrations or large amounts of a topical medication are applied to the skin, especially if it is done repeatedly, sufficient amounts of the drug can enter the bloodstream to cause systemic effects, usually undesirable ones.

A particular type of topical or dermatologic medication delivery system is the transdermal patch. This system administers sustained-action medications (e.g. nitroglycerin, oestrogen, fentanyl and nicotine) via multilayered films containing the drug and an adhesive layer. The rate of delivery of the drug is controlled and varies with each product (e.g. from 12 hours to one week). Generally, the patch is applied to a hairless, clean area of skin that is not subject to excessive movement or wrinkling (i.e. the trunk or lower abdomen). It may also be applied on the side, lower back or buttocks. Patches should not be applied to areas with cuts, burns or abrasions, or on distal parts of extremities (e.g. the forearms). If hair is likely to interfere with patch adhesion or removal, clipping may be necessary before application.

Reddening of the skin with or without mild local itching or burning, as well as allergic contact dermatitis, may occasionally occur. Upon removal of the patch, any slight reddening of the skin usually disappears within a few hours. All applications should be changed regularly to prevent local irritation, and each successive application should be placed on a different site. All patients need to be assessed for allergies to the drug and to materials in the patch before the patch is applied. If a patient has a transdermal patch on and develops a fever, the medication may be absorbed and metabolise at a faster rate than normal. The patient will need to be monitored for changes in effects of the medication.

When transdermal patches are removed, care needs to be taken as to how and where they are discarded. In the home environment, if they are simply discarded into normal refuse, pets or children can be exposed to them, causing effects from any drug remaining on the patch. When removed, they should be folded with the medication side to the inside, put into a closed container and kept out of reach of children and pets.

CLINICAL ALERT

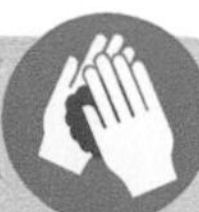

The nurse should always wear gloves when applying a transdermal patch to avoid getting any of the medication on their skin, which can result in receiving the effect of the medication.

Skin Applications

Topical skin or dermatologic preparations include ointments, pastes, creams, lotions, powders, sprays and patches (see Table 23-1 on page 690). See *Practice Guidelines* for applying topical medications. Before applying a dermatologic preparation, thoroughly clean the area as per guidelines (soap may not always be appropriate) and allow it to dry. Skin encrustations harbour micro-organisms and these as well as previously applied applications can prevent the medication from coming in contact with the area to be treated. Nurses should wear gloves when administering skin applications and always use surgical asepsis when an open wound is present.

Ophthalmic Medications

Medications may be administered to the eye using irrigations or instillations. Eye irrigation is administered to wash out the conjunctival sac to remove secretions or foreign bodies or to remove chemicals that may injure the eye. Medications for the eyes, called ophthalmic medications, are instilled in the form of liquids or ointments. Eye drops are packaged in single drip plastic containers that are used to administer the preparation. Ointments are usually supplied in small tubes. All containers must state that the medication is for ophthalmic use. Sterile preparations and sterile technique are indicated. Prescribed liquids are usually dilute, for example, less than 1% strength.

Procedure 23-10 illustrates how to administer ophthalmic instillations.

PRACTICE GUIDELINES

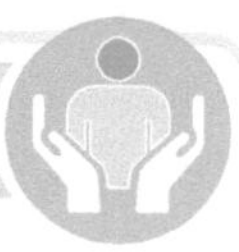

Applying Skin Preparations

Powder

Make sure the skin surface is dry. Spread apart any skin folds, and sprinkle the site until the area is covered with a fine *thin* layer. Cover the site with a dressing if ordered.

Suspension-based Lotion

Shake the container before use to distribute suspended particles. Put a little lotion on a small gauze dressing or pad, and apply the lotion to the skin by stroking it evenly in the direction of the hair growth.

Creams, Ointments, Pastes and Oil-based Lotions

Warm and soften the preparation in gloved hands to make it easier to apply and to prevent chilling (if a large area is to be treated). Smear it evenly over the skin using long strokes that follow the direction of the hair growth. Explain that the skin may feel somewhat greasy after application. Only apply a sterile dressing if necessary or recommended by drug manufacturer.

Aerosol Spray

Shake the container well to mix the contents. Hold the spray container at the recommended distance from the area (usually about 15-30cm (check the label)). Cover the patient's face with a towel if the upper chest or neck is to be sprayed. Spray the medication over the specified area.

Transdermal Patches

Select a clean, dry area that is free of hair and matches the manufacturer's recommendations. Remove the patch from its protective covering, holding it without touching the adhesive edges, and apply it by pressing firmly with the palm of the hand for about 10 seconds. Advise the patient to avoid using a heating pad over the area to prevent an increase in circulation and the rate of absorption. Remove the patch at the appropriate time, folding the medicated side to the inside so it is covered.

PROCEDURE 23-10 Administering Ophthalmic Instillations

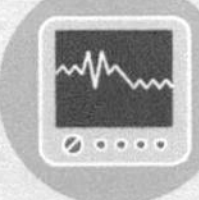

Purpose

To provide an eye medication the patient requires (e.g. an antibiotic) to treat an infection or for other reasons (see specific drug action)

Assessment

In addition to the assessment performed by the nurse related to the administration of any medication, prior to applying ophthalmic medications, **assess**:

- Appearance of eye and surrounding structures for lesions, exudate, erythema or swelling
- The location and nature of any discharge, lacrimation, and swelling of the eyelids or of the lacrimal gland
- Patient complaints (e.g. itching, burning pain, blurred vision and photophobia)
- Patient behaviour (e.g. squinting, blinking excessively, frowning or rubbing the eyes)

Determine if assessment data influence administration of the medication.

Planning

Equipment

- Clean gloves
- Sterile absorbent gauze soaked in sterile 0.9% saline
- Medication
- Sterile eye dressing (pad) as needed and paper eye tape to secure it

For irrigation, add:

- Irrigating solution (e.g. 0.9% saline) and irrigating syringe or tubing

- Dry sterile gauze swabs
- Moisture-resistant towel
- Basin (e.g. kidney basin)
- Anaesthetic drops (if required)
- Plastic cape
- pH check test strip (specific eye test strip) (as per local policy)

Implementation

Preparation

- Check the prescription chart.
  - Check the chart for the drug name, dose and strength. Also confirm the prescribed frequency of the instillation and which eye is to be treated.
- Know the reason why the patient is receiving the medication, the drug classification, contraindications, usual dose range, side-effects and nursing considerations for administering and evaluating the intended outcomes of the medication.

Performance

1. Follow local policy to ensure that you explain to the patient what you are going to do, that it is not painful, why it is necessary and how they can cooperate. Obtain consent and maintain patient privacy and dignity and ensure that the appropriate local infection control procedures are observed. Ointments are often soothing to the eye, but some liquid preparations may sting initially. Discuss how the results will be used in planning further care or treatments.
2. Check the label on the medication tube or bottle and compare with the prescription chart and also check the expiration date.
3. If necessary, calculate the medication dosage.
4. Prepare the patient.
   - Check the patient's identification band for name, address, date of birth and hospital number. Check this by also asking the patient to confirm his/her name and address. *This ensures that the right patient receives the medication.*
   - Ask the patient to remove contact lenses if worn.
   - Assist the patient to a comfortable position, either sitting or lying.
5. Clean the eyelid and the eyelashes.
   - Put on clean gloves.
   - Use sterile gauze moistened with sterile irrigating solution or sterile normal saline, and wipe from the inner canthus to the outer canthus. *If not removed, material on the eyelid and lashes can be washed into the eye. Cleaning towards the outer canthus prevents contamination of the other eye and the lacrimal duct.*
6. Administer the eye medication.
   - Check the ophthalmic preparation for the name, strength and number of drops if a liquid is used. Draw the correct number of drops into the shaft of the dropper if a dropper is used. If ointment is used, discard the first bead. *The first bead of ointment from a tube is considered to be contaminated.*
   - Instruct the patient to look up to the ceiling. Give the patient dry sterile absorbent gauze. The person is less likely to blink if looking up. While the patient looks up, the cornea is partially protected by the upper eyelid. A gauze swab is needed to press on the nasolacrimal duct after a liquid instillation or to wipe excess ointment from the eyelashes after an ointment is instilled.
   - Expose the lower conjunctival sac by placing the thumb or fingers of your nondominant hand on the patient's cheekbone just below the eye and gently drawing down the skin on the cheek. If the tissues are oedematous, handle the tissues carefully to avoid damaging them. *Placing the fingers on the cheekbone minimises the possibility of touching the cornea, avoids putting any pressure on the eyeball, and prevents the person from blinking or squinting.*
   - Approach the eye from the side and instill the correct number of drops onto the outer third of the lower conjunctival sac. Hold the dropper 1-2cm above the sac (see Figure 23-47). *The patient is less likely to blink if a side approach is used. When instilled into the conjunctival sac, drops will not harm the cornea as they might if dropped directly on it. The dropper must not touch the sac or the cornea.*

   or

   - Holding the tube above the lower conjunctival sac, squeeze 2cm of ointment from the tube into the lower conjunctival sac from the inner canthus outward (see Figure 23-48).
   - Instruct the patient to close the eyelids but not to squeeze them shut. *Closing the eye spreads the medication over the eyeball. Squeezing can injure the eye and push out the medication.*

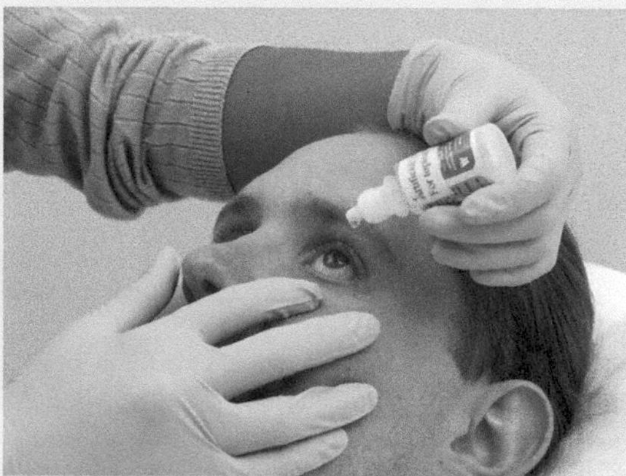

Figure 23-47 Instilling an eyedrop into the lower conjunctival sac.

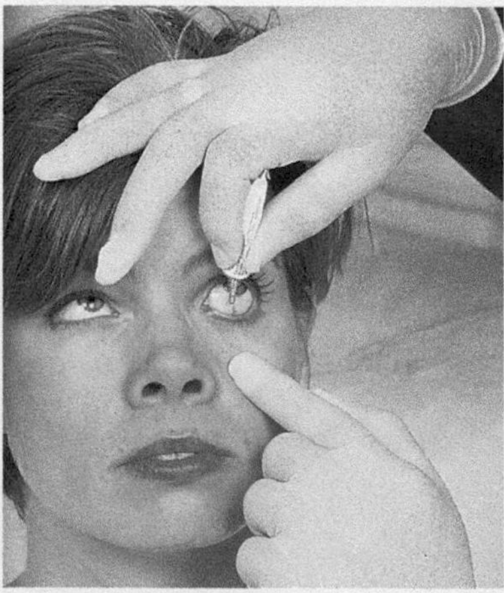

Figure 23-48 Instilling an eye ointment into the lower conjunctival sac.
Source: Jenny Thomas.

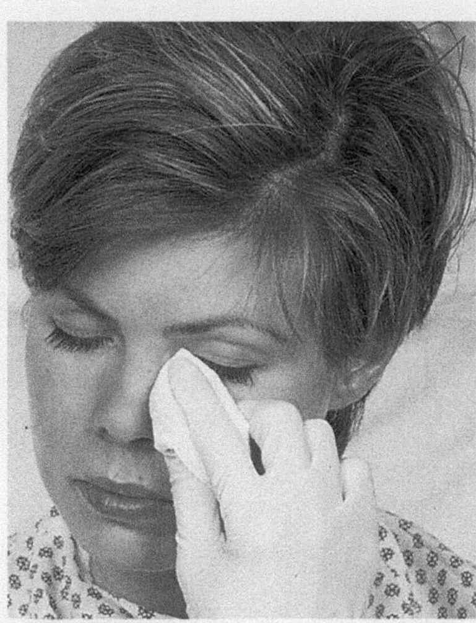

Figure 23-49 Pressing on the nasolacrimal duct.
Source: Jenny Thomas.

- For liquid medications, press firmly or have the patient press firmly on the nasolacrimal duct for at least 30 seconds (see Figure 23-49). *Pressing on the nasolacrimal duct prevents the medication from running out of the eye and down the duct.*

Variation: irrigation

- Check ph level prior to treatment (to determine if an acid or alkaline corrosive substance is present) as per local policy and again 20 minutes after procedure to check for chemical injury (as per local policy).
- Place absorbent pads under the head, neck and shoulders. Place a kidney basin next to the eye to catch drainage. Patient could be asked to hold the kidney basin secure. Some eye medications cause systemic reactions such as confusion or a decrease in heart rate and blood pressure if the eye drops go down the nasolacrimal duct and get into the systemic circulation.
- Administer anaesthetic drop if required.
- Expose the lower conjunctival sac. Or, to irrigate in stages, first hold the lower lid down, then hold the upper lid up. Exert pressure on the bony prominences of the cheekbone and beneath the eyebrow when holding the eyelids. *Separating the lids prevents reflex blinking. Exerting pressure on the bony prominences minimises the possibility of pressing the eyeball and causing discomfort.*
- Fill and hold the eye irrigator about 2.5cm above the eye. *At this height the pressure of the solution will not damage the eye tissue, and the irrigator will not touch the eye.*
- Inform patient that irrigation is about to start.
- Ask patient to look up and down and from side to side during irrigation.
- Irrigate the eye, directing the solution onto the lower conjunctival sac and from the inner canthus to the outer canthus. *Directing the solution in this way prevents possible injury to the cornea and prevents fluid and contaminants from flowing down the nasolacrimal duct.*
- Irrigate until the solution leaving the eye is clear (no discharge is present) or until all the solution has been used and pH is normal 7-5–8.0 (as per local policy).
- Instruct the patient to close and move the eye periodically. Eye closure and movement help to move secretions from the upper to the lower conjunctival sac.

7 Clean and dry the eyelids as needed. Wipe the eyelids gently from the inner to the outer canthus to collect excess medication.

8 Apply an eye pad if needed, and secure it with paper eye tape.

9 Assess the patient's response immediately after the instillation or irrigation and again after the medication should have acted.

10 Document all relevant assessments and interventions. Include the name of the drug or irrigating solution, the strength, the number of drops if a liquid medication, the time, and the response of the patient.

Evaluation

- Perform follow-up based on findings of the effectiveness of the administration or outcomes that deviated from expected or normal for the patient.
- Relate findings to previous data if available.

LIFESPAN CONSIDERATIONS

Administering Ophthalmic Medications

Infants/Children

- Explain the technique to the parents of an infant or child.
- For a young child or infant, obtain assistance either from a colleague or a parent. Nursing the infant or young child may prevent the child moving during the procedure. *This prevents accidental injury during medication administration.*
- For a young child, use a doll to demonstrate the procedure. *This facilitates cooperation and decreases anxiety.*
- An IV bag and tubing may be used to deliver irrigating fluid to the eye (see Figure 23-50).

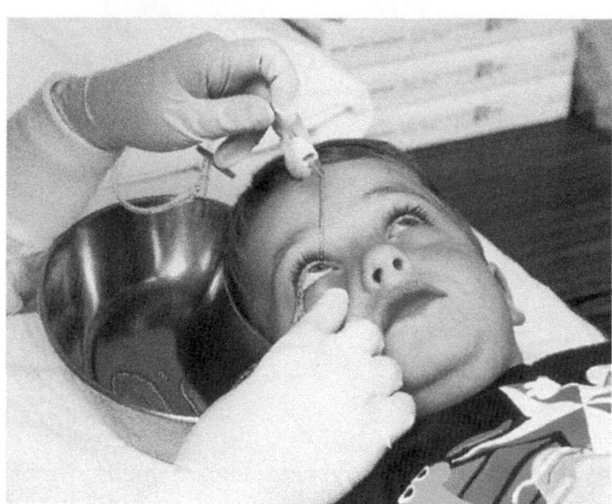

Figure 23-50 Eye irrigation using IV tubing.
Source: Jenny Thomas.

Otic Medications

Instillations or irrigations of the external auditory canal are referred to as **otic** and are generally carried out for cleaning purposes. Sometimes applications of heat and antiseptic solutions are prescribed. Irrigations performed in a hospital require aseptic technique so that micro-organisms will not be introduced into the ear. Sterile technique is used if the eardrum is perforated. The position of the external auditory canal varies with age. In the child under three, it is directed upward. In the adult, the external auditory canal is an S-shaped structure about 2.5cm long.

CLINICAL ALERT

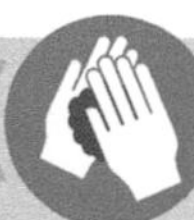

This procedure is only to be carried out by a doctor, trained nurse or audiologist.

Irrigation should not cause pain, if the patient complains of pain the procedure should be stopped immediately.

Procedure 23-11 explains how to administer otic instillations.

PROCEDURE 23-11 Administering Otic Instillations

Purpose

- To soften earwax so that it can be readily removed at a later time
- To provide local therapy to reduce inflammation, destroy infective organisms in the external ear canal, or both
- To relieve pain

Assessment

In addition to the assessment performed by the nurse related to the administration of any medications, prior to applying otic medications, **assess**:

- Appearance of the pinna of the ear and **meatus** for signs of redness and abrasions
- Type and amount of any discharge

Determine if assessment data influence administration of the medication.

Planning

Equipment

- Clean gloves
- Correct medication bottle with a dropper
- Flexible rubber tip (optional) for the end of the dropper, which prevents injury from sudden motion, for example, by a disoriented patient
- Cotton wool

For irrigation, add:

- Protective cape
- Basin (e.g. kidney basin)
- Irrigating solution at the appropriate temperature, about 500ml (container for the irrigating solution)

Implementation

Preparation

- Check the medication chart.
  - Check the chart for the drug name, strength, number of drops and prescribed frequency.
  - If the chart is unclear or pertinent information is missing check with the prescriber.
- Know the reason why the patient is receiving the medication, the drug classification, contraindications, usual dose range, side effects and nursing considerations for administering and evaluating the intended outcomes of the medication.

Performance

1 Follow local policy to ensure that you explain to the patient what you are going to do, that it is not painful, why it is necessary and how they can cooperate. Obtain consent and maintain patient privacy and dignity and ensure that the appropriate local infection control procedures are observed.

2 Compare the label on the medication container with the medication chart and check the expiration date.

3 If necessary, calculate the medication dosage.

4 Prepare the patient.
  - Check the patient's identification band for name, address, date of birth and hospital number. Check this by also asking the patient to confirm his/her name and address. *This ensures that the right patient receives the medication.*
  - Assist the patient to a comfortable position for eardrops, lying with the ear being treated uppermost.

5 Clean the pinna of the ear and the meatus of the ear canal.
  - Put on gloves if infection is suspected.
  - Use a gauze swab and solution to wipe the pinna and auditory meatus. *This removes any discharge present before the instillation so that it won't be washed into the ear canal.*

6 Administer the ear medication.
  - Warm the medication container in your hand, or place it in warm water for a short time. *This promotes patient comfort.*
  - Partially fill the ear dropper with medication.
  - Straighten the auditory canal. Pull the pinna upward and backward (see Figure 23-51). *The auditory canal is straightened so that the solution can flow the entire length of the canal.*
  - Instill the correct number of drops along the side of the ear canal (see Figure 23-52).

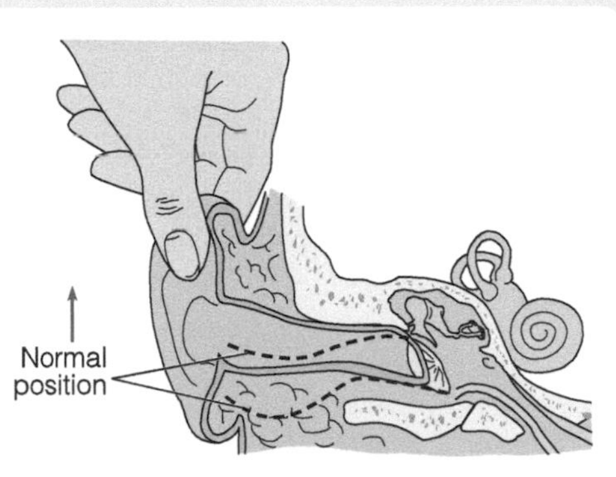

Figure 23-51 Straightening the adult ear canal by pulling pinna upward and backward.

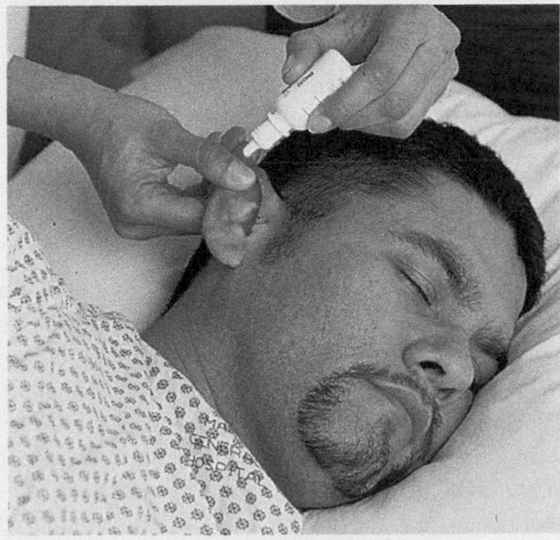

Figure 23-52 Instilling eardrops.
Source: Jenny Thomas.

- Press gently but firmly a few times on the tragus of the ear (the cartilaginous projection in front of the exterior meatus of the ear). *Pressing on the tragus assists the flow of medication into the ear canal.*
- Ask the patient to remain in the side-lying position for about five minutes. *This prevents the drops from escaping and allows the medication to reach all sides of the canal cavity.*
- Insert a small piece of cotton wool loosely at the meatus of the auditory canal for 15–20 minutes. Do not press it into the canal. *The cotton helps retain the medication when the patient is up. If pressed tightly into the canal, the cotton would interfere with the action of the drug and the outward movement of normal secretions.*

Variation: ear irrigation

- Check with the patient if they have had this procedure previously, or if there are any contraindications to the patient having the treatment.
- Explain that the patient may experience a feeling of fullness, warmth and, occasionally, discomfort when the fluid comes in contact with the tympanic membrane.
- Assist the patient to a sitting or lying position with head turned towards the affected ear. *The solution can then flow from the ear canal to a basin.*
- Place the protective cape around the patient's shoulder under the ear to be irrigated, and place the basin under the ear to be irrigated.

or

- Hang up the irrigating container, and run solution through the tubing and the nozzle. *Solution is run through to remove air from the tubing and nozzle.*
- Straighten the ear canal.
- Insert the tip of the syringe into the auditory meatus, and direct the solution gently upward against the top of the canal. The solution will flow around the entire canal and out at the bottom. *The solution is instilled gently because strong pressure from the fluid can cause discomfort and damage the tympanic membrane.*
- Continue instilling the fluid until all the solution is used or until the canal is cleaned, depending on the purpose of the irrigation. Take care not to block the outward flow of the solution with the syringe.
- Assist the patient to a side-lying position on the affected side. *Lying with the affected side down helps drain the excess fluid by gravity.*
- Place a cotton wool in the auditory meatus to absorb the excess fluid.

7 Assess the patient's response and the character and amount of discharge, appearance of the canal, discomfort, and so on, immediately after the instillation and again when the medication is expected to act. Inspect the cotton wool for any drainage.

8 Document all nursing assessments and interventions relative to the procedure. Include the name of the drug or irrigating solution, the strength, the number of drops if a liquid medication, the time, and the response of the patient.

Evaluation

- Perform follow-up based on findings of the effectiveness of the administration or outcomes that deviated from expected or normal for the patient.
- Relate findings to previous data if available.

LIFESPAN CONSIDERATIONS

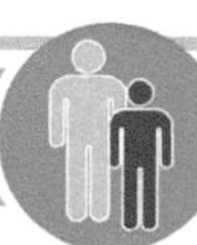

Administering Otic Medications

Infants/Children

- Obtain assistance to ensure that the infant or young child doesn't make any sudden movements. This prevents accidental injury due to sudden movement during the procedure. The infant or child could sit in parent or carer's lap.
- For a child older than three, pull the pinna upward and backward similar to the procedure with an adult (see Figure 23-51). In infants and children under three, because the ear canal is directed upward and backward, the pinna should be pulled gently down and back (see Figure 23-53).

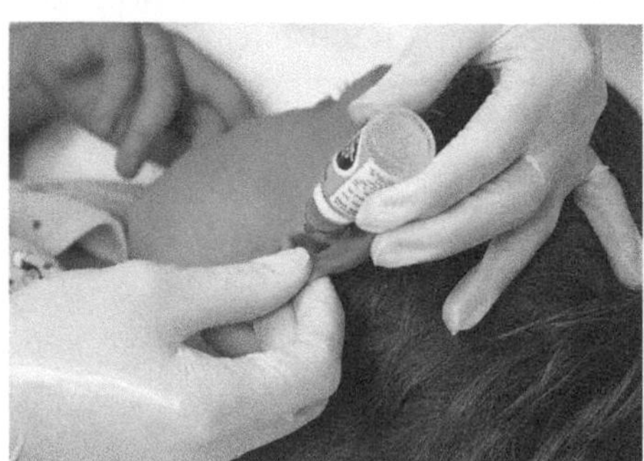

Figure 23-53 Straightening the ear canal of a child by pulling the pinna down and back.
Source: Jenny Thomas.

Nasal Medications

Nasal instillations (nose drops and sprays) are usually instilled for their astringent effect (to shrink swollen mucous membranes), to loosen secretions and facilitate drainage or to treat infections of the nasal cavity or sinuses. Nasal decongestants are the most common nasal instillations. Many of these products are available without a prescription. Patients need to be taught to use these agents with caution. Chronic use of nasal decongestants may lead to a rebound effect, that is, an increase in nasal congestion. If excess decongestant solution is swallowed, serious systemic effects may also develop, especially in children. Saline drops are safer as a decongestant for children.

Usually patients self-administer sprays. In the supine position with the head tilted back, the patient holds the tip of the container just inside the nares and inhales as the spray enters the nasal passages. For patients who use nasal sprays repeatedly, the nares need to be assessed for irritation. In children, nasal sprays are given with the head in an upright position to prevent excess spray from being swallowed.

Nasal drops are used to treat sinus infections. Patients need to learn ways to position themselves to effectively treat the affected sinus:

- To treat the ethmoid and sphenoid sinuses, instruct the patient to lie back with the head over the edge of the bed or a pillow under the shoulders so that the head is tipped backward (see Figure 23-54).
- To treat the maxillary and frontal sinuses, instruct the patient to assume the same back-lying position, with the head turned towards the side to be treated (see Figure 23-55). The patient should also be instructed to (a) breathe through the mouth to prevent aspiration of medication into the trachea and bronchi, (b) remain in a back-lying position for at least a minute so that the solution will come into contact with the entire nasal surface, and (c) avoid blowing the nose for several minutes. The 6R's of safe administration of medication should be used.

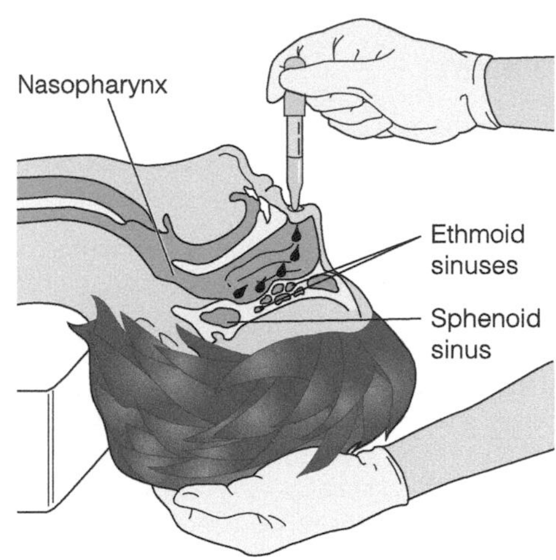

Figure 23-54 Position of the head to instill drops into the ethmoid and sphenoid sinuses.

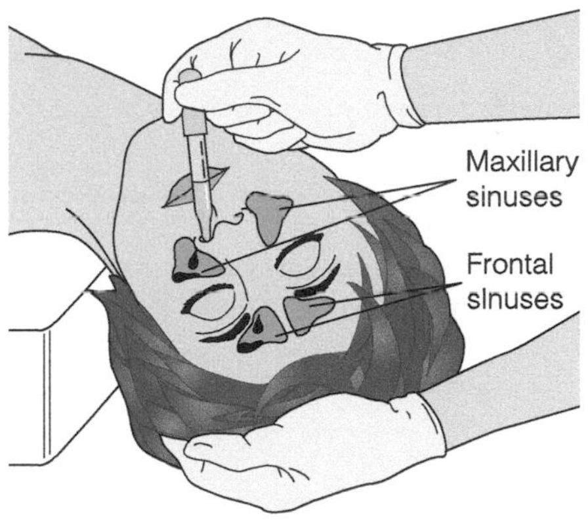

Figure 23-55 Position of the head to instill drops into the maxillary and frontal sinuses.

Vaginal Medications

Vaginal medications or instillations, are inserted as creams, jellies, foams or pessaries to treat infection or to relieve vaginal discomfort (e.g. itching or pain). Medical aseptic technique is usually used. Vaginal creams, jellies and foams are applied by using a tubular applicator with a plunger. Suppositories are inserted with the index finger of a gloved hand. Suppositories are designed to melt at body temperature, so they are generally stored in the refrigerator to keep them firm for insertion. See *Procedure 23-12* for administering vaginal instillations.

PROCEDURE 23-12 Administering Vaginal Instillations

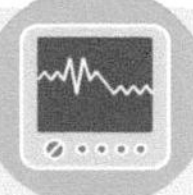

Purpose

- To treat or prevent infection
- To reduce inflammation
- To relieve vaginal discomfort

Assessment

In addition to the assessment performed by the nurse related to the administration of any medications, prior to applying vaginal medications, **assess**:

- The vaginal orifice for inflammation; amount, character and odour of vaginal discharge
- For complaints of vaginal discomfort (e.g. burning or itching)

Determine if assessment data influence administration of the medication (i.e. is it appropriate to administer the medication or does the medication need to be reviewed).

Planning

Equipment

- Drape/patient bed sheet
- Correct vaginal suppository or cream
- Applicator for vaginal cream
- Clean gloves
- Lubricant for a suppository
- Disposable towel
- Clean perineal pad

For an irrigation, add:

- Moisture-proof pad
- Vaginal irrigation set (these are often disposable) containing a nozzle, tubing and a clamp, and a container for the solution
- IV drip stand
- Irrigating solution

Implementation

Preparation

- Check the prescription chart.
  - Check the chart for the drug name, strength and prescribed frequency.
- Determine the reason why the patient is receiving the medication, the drug classification, contraindications, usual dose range, side effects and nursing considerations for administering and evaluating the intended outcomes of the medication.

Performance

1 Follow local policy to ensure that you explain to the patient what you are going to do, why it is necessary and how they can cooperate. Obtain consent and maintain patient privacy and dignity and ensure that the appropriate local infection control procedures are observed. Explain to the patient that a vaginal instillation is normally a painless procedure, and in fact may bring relief from itching and burning if an infection is present. Many people feel embarrassed about this procedure, and some may prefer to perform the procedure themselves if instruction is provided. Discuss how the results will be used in planning further care or treatments.

2 Check the label on the medication container against the medication chart and check the expiration date.

3 If necessary, calculate the medication dosage.

4 Prepare the patient.
  - Check the patient's identification band for name, address, date of birth and hospital number. Check this by also asking the patient to confirm his/her name and address. *This ensures that the right patient receives the medication.*
  - Ask the patient to void urine. *If the bladder is empty, the patient will have less discomfort during the treatment, and the possibility of injuring the vaginal lining is decreased.*
  - Assist the patient to a back-lying position with the knees flexed and the hips rotated laterally.
  - Cover the patient appropriately so that only the perineal area is exposed.

5 Prepare the equipment.
  - Unwrap the suppository, and put it on the opened wrapper

  or
  - Fill the applicator with the prescribed cream, jelly or foam. Directions are provided with the manufacturer's applicator.

6 Assess and clean (according to local policy) the perineal area.
  - Put on gloves. *Gloves prevent contamination of the nurse's hands from vaginal and perineal micro-organisms.*
  - Inspect the vaginal orifice, note any odour of discharge from the vagina and ask about any vaginal discomfort.
  - Provide perineal care to remove micro-organisms. *This decreases the chance of moving micro-organisms into the vagina.*

7 Administer the vaginal suppository, cream, foam, jelly or irrigation.

Suppository

- Lubricate the end of the suppository that is to be inserted first (check manufacturer's guidelines). *Lubrication facilitates insertion.*

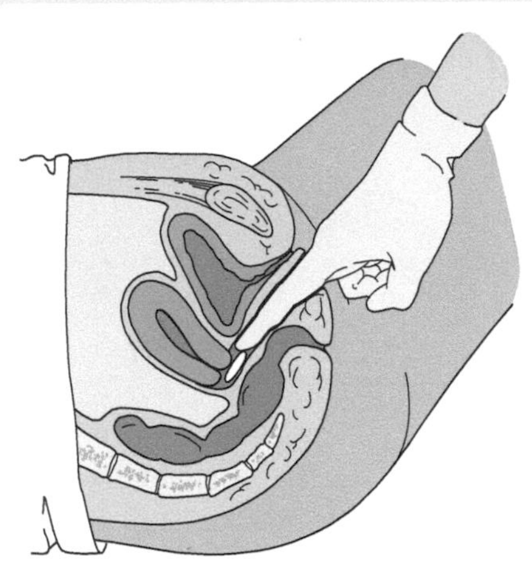

Figure 23-56 Instilling a vaginal suppository.

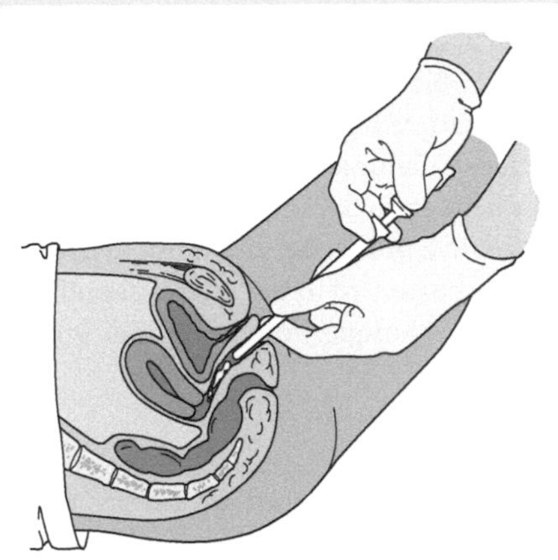

Figure 23-57 Using an applicator to instill a vaginal cream.

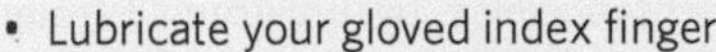

- Lubricate your gloved index finger.
- Expose the vaginal orifice by separating the labia with your nondominant hand.
- Insert the suppository about 8-10cm along the posterior wall of the vagina, or as far as it will go (see Figure 23-56). The posterior wall of the vagina is about 2.5cm longer than the anterior wall because the cervix protrudes into the uppermost portion of the anterior wall.
- Ask the patient to remain lying in the supine position for 5-10 minutes following insertion. The hips may also be elevated on a pillow. *This position allows the medication to flow into the posterior fornix after it has melted.*
- This procedure is best late evening as the patient is less likely to get out of bed.

Vaginal cream, jelly or foam

- Gently insert the applicator about 5cm.
- Slowly push the plunger until the applicator is empty (see Figure 23-57).
- Remove the applicator and place it on the towel. *The applicator is put on the towel to prevent the spread of micro-organisms.*
- Discard the applicator if disposable or clean it according to the manufacturer's directions.
- Ask the patient to remain lying in the supine position for 5-10 minutes following the insertion.

Irrigation

- Place the patient on a bedpan.
- Clamp the tubing. Hang the irrigating container on the IV drip stand so that the base is about 30cm above the vagina. *At this height, the pressure of the solution should not be great enough to injure the vaginal lining.*
- Run fluid through the tubing and nozzle into the bedpan. *Fluid is run through the tubing to remove air and to moisten the nozzle.*
- Insert the nozzle carefully into the vagina. Direct the nozzle towards the sacrum, following the direction of the vagina.
- Insert the nozzle about 7-10cm, start the flow and rotate the nozzle several times. *Rotating the nozzle irrigates all parts of the vagina.*
- Use all of the irrigating solution, permitting it to flow out freely into the bedpan.
- Remove the nozzle from the vagina.
- Assist the patient to a sitting position on the bedpan. *Sitting on the bedpan will help drain the remaining fluid by gravity.*

8 Ensure patient comfort.
   - Dry the perineum with tissues as required.
   - Apply a clean perineal pad if there is excessive drainage.

9 Document all nursing assessments and interventions relative to the procedure. Include the name of the drug or irrigating solution, the strength, the time, and the response of the patient.

Evaluation

- Perform follow-up based on findings of the effectiveness of the administration or outcomes that deviated from expected or normal for the patient.
- Relate findings to previous data if available.

A vaginal irrigation (douche) is the washing of the vagina by a liquid at a low pressure. Vaginal irrigations are not necessary for ordinary female hygiene but are used to prevent infection by applying an antimicrobial solution that discourages the growth of micro-organisms, to remove an offensive or irritating discharge, and to reduce inflammation or prevent haemorrhage by the application of heat or cold. In hospitals, sterile supplies and equipment are used; in a home, sterility is not usually necessary because people are accustomed to the micro-organisms in their environments. Sterile technique, however, is indicated if there is an open wound.

Rectal Medications

Insertion of medications into the rectum in the form of suppositories is a frequent practice. Rectal administration is a convenient and safe method of giving certain medications. Advantages include the following:

- It avoids irritation of the upper gastrointestinal tract in patients who encounter this problem.
- It is advantageous when the medication has an objectionable taste or odour.
- The drug is released at a slow but steady rate.
- Rectal suppositories are thought to provide higher bloodstream levels (titres) of medication because the venous blood from the lower rectum is not transported through the liver.

To insert a rectal suppository:

- Assist the patient to a left lateral position, with the upper leg flexed or supine with the knees drawn up and legs apart.
- Fold back the top bedclothes to expose the buttocks.
- Put on a glove on the hand used to insert the suppository.
- Unwrap the suppository and lubricate the appropriate end (see manufacturer's instructions) to be inserted first. A lubricant reduces irritation of the mucosa.

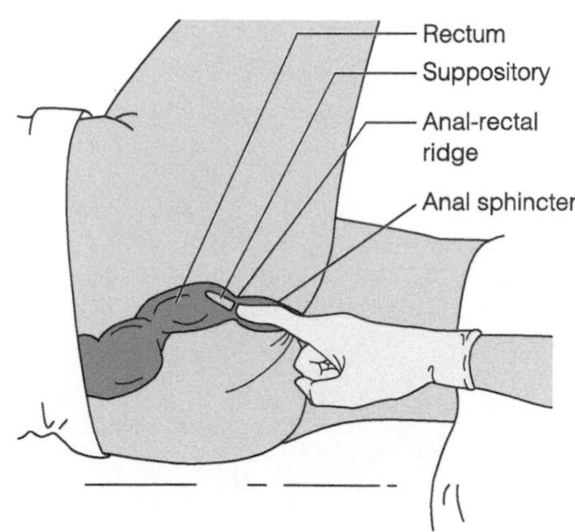

Figure 23-58 Inserting a rectal suppository beyond the internal sphincter and along the rectal wall.

- Lubricate the gloved index finger.
- Encourage the patient to relax by breathing through the mouth. This usually relaxes the external anal sphincter.
- Insert the suppository gently into the anal canal, rounded end first (or according to manufacturer's instructions), along the rectal wall using the gloved index finger. For an adult, insert the suppository beyond the internal sphincter (i.e. 10cm) (see Figure 23-58).
- Avoid embedding the suppository in faeces in order for the suppository to be absorbed effectively.
- Press the patient's buttocks together for a few minutes.
- Ask the patient to remain in the left lateral or supine position for at least 5 minutes to help retain the suppository. The suppository should be retained for at least 30–40 minutes or according to manufacturer's instructions.

LIFESPAN CONSIDERATIONS

Administering Rectal Medications

Infants/Children

- Obtain assistance to support the child and prevent any unexpected movements from the infant or young child. This prevents accidental injury during the procedure.
- For a child or infant, insert a suppository 5cm or less. Rectal medication is not routinely administered to children other routes are used in preference.

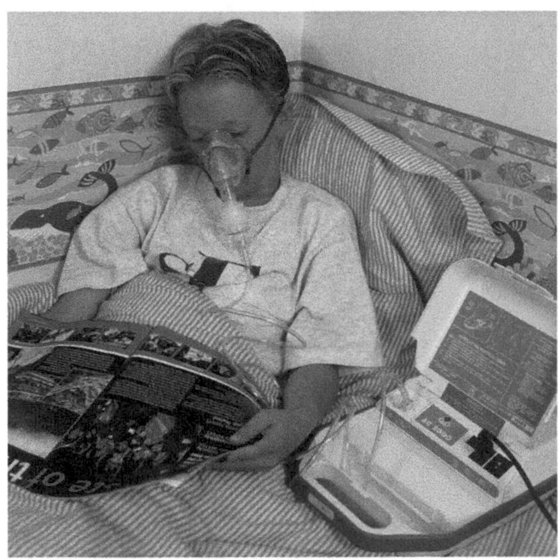

Figure 23-59 Compressor or Ultrasonic nebuliser.
Source: Science Photo Library Ltd/Mark Clarke.

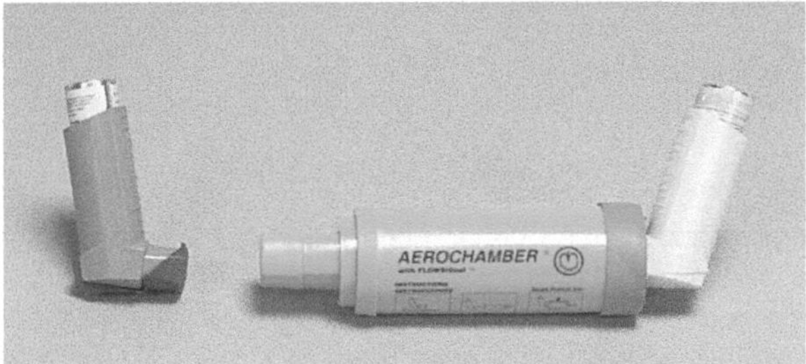

Figure 23-60 Metred-dose inhaler.
Source: Pearson Education Ltd.

RESPIRATORY INHALATION

The purpose of respiratory inhalation is to deliver one or a combination of medication to the lower part of the respiratory system. There are predominantly two techniques of delivering the medication: nebulisation and aerolisation.

A nebuliser is used to deliver a fine spray (fog or mist) of medication or moisture to a patient, which is inhaled via a face mask or tracheostomy mask. Antibiotics have been known to be administered in this way. A large-volume nebuliser can provide a heated or cool mist. It is used for long-term therapy, such as that following a tracheostomy. The ultrasonic nebuliser (see Figure 23-59) provides 100% humidity and can provide particles small enough to be inhaled deeply into the respiratory tract.

In aerosolisation, the droplets are suspended in a gas, such as oxygen. The smaller the droplets, the further they can be inhaled into the respiratory tract. When a medication is intended for the nasal mucosa, it is inhaled through the nose; when it is intended for the trachea, bronchi and/or lungs, it is inhaled through the mouth either by metered-dose inhaler or dry powder.

The *metered-dose inhaler (MDI)*, a handheld nebuliser/aerosol (see Figure 23-60) is a pressurised container of medication that can be used by the patient to release the medication through a nosepiece or mouthpiece. The force with which the air moves through the nebuliser causes the large particles of medicated solution to break up into finer particles, forming a mist or fine spray.

A dry-powdered inhaler releases a fine dry powder when the mouth is wrapped around the inhaler and a breath is taken. Breath-actuated inhalers automatically dispense medication when the patient takes a deep breath. However, there is no need to coordinate breathing as there is no release button and a spacer is not required. Breath-actuated aerosols are the preferred method of delivery of medication in young children and adults.

To ensure correct delivery of the prescribed medication by MDIs, nurses need to instruct patients to use aerosol inhalers correctly. The patient compresses the medication canister by hand to release medication through a mouthpiece. An extender or spacer may be attached to the mouthpiece to facilitate medication absorption for better results (see Figure 23-61). Spacers are holding chambers into which the medication is fired and from which the patient inhales, so that the dose is not lost by exhalation. *Teaching: Patient Care* provides instructions for patients about using an MDI. Newer breath-activated MDIs are being produced in which inhalation triggers the release of a premeasured dose of medication.

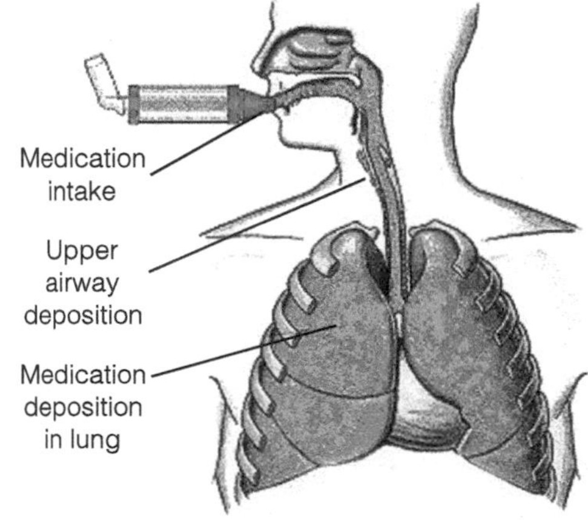

Figure 23-61 Delivery of medication to the lungs using a metered-dose inhaler extender.
Source: courtesy of Trudell Medical International.

TEACHING: PATIENT CARE

Using a Metered-Dose Inhaler

- Reinforce the 6R's of administration of medication.
- Make sure the canister is firmly and fully inserted into the inhaler.
- Remove the mouthpiece cap and, holding the inhaler upright, shake the inhaler vigorously for 3–5 seconds to mix the medication evenly.
- Exhale comfortably (as in a normal full breath).
- Hold the canister upside down.
- Put the mouthpiece far enough into the mouth with its opening towards the throat. Close the lips tightly around the mouthpiece. An MDI with a spacer or extender is always placed in the mouth (see Figure 23-62).

Administering the Medication

- Press down *once* on the MDI canister (which releases the dose) and inhale slowly and deeply through the mouth.
- Hold the breath for 10 seconds. This allows the aerosol to reach deeper airways.
- Remove the inhaler from or away from the mouth.
- Exhale slowly through pursed lips. Controlled exhalation keeps the small airways open during exhalation.
- Repeat the inhalation if ordered. Wait 20–30 seconds between inhalations of bronchodilator medications *so the first inhalation has a chance to work and the subsequent dose reaches deeper into the lungs.*
- After the inhalation is completed, rinse mouth with tap water to remove any remaining medication and reduce irritation and risk of infection.
- Clean the MDI mouthpiece after each use. Use mild soap and water, rinse it, and let it air dry before replacing it on the device.
- Store the canister at room temperature. Avoid extremes of temperature.
- Report adverse reactions such as restlessness, palpitations, nervousness or rash to the prescriber.

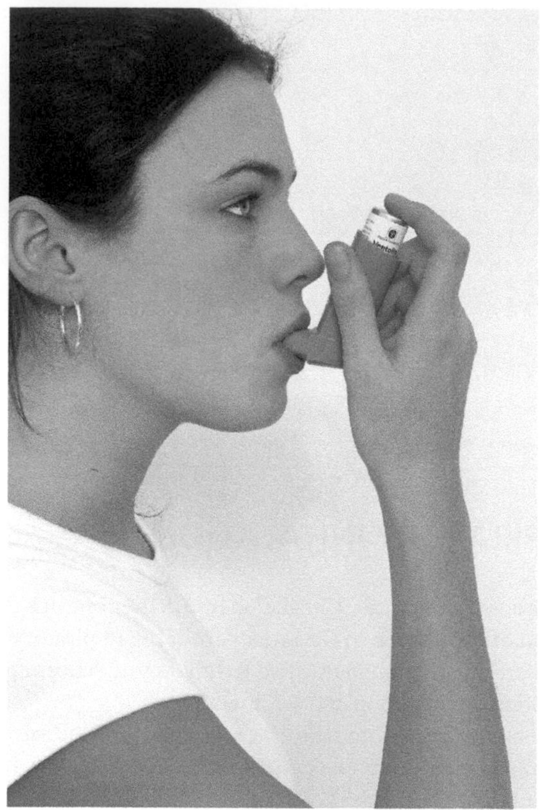

Figure 23-62 Inhaler positioned away from the open mouth.
Source: Pearson Education Ltd.

- Many MDIs contain steroids for an anti-inflammatory effect. Prolonged use increases the risk of fungal infections in the mouth.

LIFESPAN CONSIDERATIONS

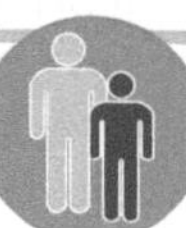

Children

Metered-dose inhalers are not suitable for children under 5 as they require good hand coordination and frequently spacers are used. Dry powder inhalers may be better for children over five.

Breath actuated inhalers may be more suitable for the older child.

Mature Adults

Breath actuated inhalers may be more suitable for the mature adult.

SUMMARY

Administration of medication is one of the important aspect of a nurse's role. The development and complexities of medicines, the different routes, the contraindications and side-effects and the lifespan considerations can make this complicated. Extreme care is therefore needed as drug errors are an everyday occurrence. Systems and strategies are in place to minimise these. Government and the regulatory body the Nursing Midwifery Council work together with other organisations to develop guidelines, policies, standards, etc. to reduce and prevent such errors and to ensure the well-being of the individual when receiving medication.

CRITICAL REFLECTION

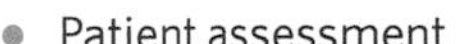

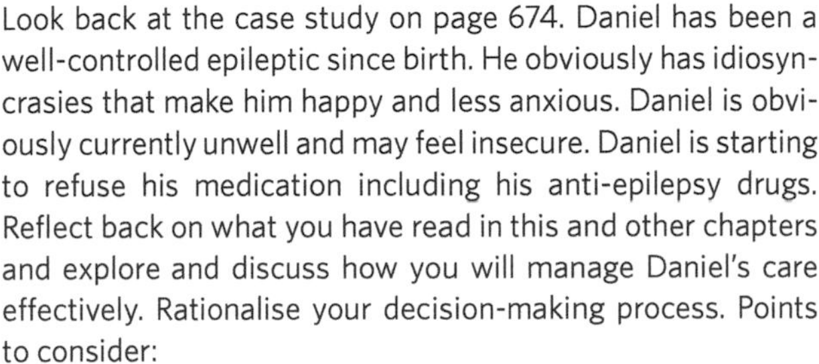

Look back at the case study on page 674. Daniel has been a well-controlled epileptic since birth. He obviously has idiosyncrasies that make him happy and less anxious. Daniel is obviously currently unwell and may feel insecure. Daniel is starting to refuse his medication including his anti-epilepsy drugs. Reflect back on what you have read in this and other chapters and explore and discuss how you will manage Daniel's care effectively. Rationalise your decision-making process. Points to consider:

- Communication
- Maintaining patient safety
- Patient assessment
- Route of analgesia
- Type of analgesia
- Type of medication
- 6 R's
- Responsibility
- Respect and dignity
- Patient autonomy
- Mental Health Act
- Human Rights Act

CHAPTER HIGHLIGHTS

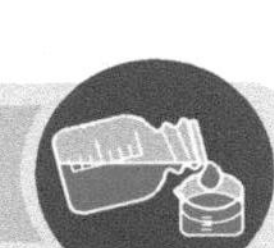

- Nurses need to know the generic and trade names of a medication and be aware of both its therapeutic and side-effects.
- Adverse effects of medications include drug toxicity, drug allergy, drug tolerance, idiosyncratic effect and drug interactions.
- Various routes are used to administer medications: oral, sublingual, buccal, parenteral, topical or via a nasogastric or gastrostomy tube. When administering a medication, the nurse must ensure that it is appropriate for the route specified.
- Nurses must always assess a patient's physical status before giving any medication and obtain a medication history.
- When administering medications the nurse observes the six rights to ensure accurate administration. When preparing medications, the nurse checks the medication container label against the prescription chart.
- The nurse who prepares the medication administers it and must never leave a prepared medication unattended.
- The nurse always identifies the patient appropriately before administering a medication and stays with the patient until the medication is taken.
- Medications, once given, are documented as soon as possible after administration.
- Medications given parenterally act more quickly than those given orally or topically and must be prepared using sterile technique.
- Proper site selection is essential for an intramuscular injection to prevent tissue, bone and nerve damage. The nurse should always palpate anatomic landmarks when selecting a site.
- The Z-track method for intramuscular injection is recommended to prevent discomfort caused by seepage of the medication into subcutaneous tissues.
- Patients receiving a series of injections should have the injection sites rotated or an alternative route should be considered for those who are having long-term injections.
- After use, needles should not be recapped but must be placed in puncture-resistant containers.
- Topical medications are applied to the skin and mucous membranes primarily for their local effects, although some systemic effects may occur.
- A metered-dose inhaler (MDI) is a handheld nebuliser that can be used by patients to self-administer measured doses of an aerosol medication. To ensure correct delivery of the prescribed medication by MDIs, nurses need to instruct patients to use aerosol inhalers correctly.

ACTIVITY ANSWERS

ACTIVITY 23-1 There are many methods, routes and types of drugs that manage pain following theatre. The fundamental nursing requirement is to establish what analgesic was given last and when it was given, e.g. in theatre or recovery, before the patient is delivered into your care. In view of this, the following points should be considered when nursing a patient and providing analgesia:

- Maintaining a safe environment
- Effective communication
- Hospital policy
- The 6R's
- Drug allergy
- Skin integrity
- Time when the patient last received the analgesia
- The right site
- The right position for the patient
- The technique
- Routine observations
- Medical conditions
- Breathing
- Antiemetic

Reflecting on the activity should provide the rationale for each of the above points.

REFERENCES

Chanay, M. (2009) 'Thoracic epidural anaesthesia in cardiac surgery – the current standing', *Annals of Cardiac Anaesthetics*, 12(1), 1–3.

Department of Health (2006) *Improving patient's access to medicines: A guide to implementing nurse and pharmacist independent prescribing within the NHS in England*, London: Department of Health.

Department of Health (2004) *Building a safer NHS for patients: Improving medication safety*, London: Department of Health.

Department of Health (2006) *Medicine matters*, London: Department of Health.

Fleming, D.R. (1999) 'Challenging traditional insulin injection practices', *American Journal of Nursing*, 99(2), 72–74.

GOSH (2008) *Giving your child medicines: How to give your child liquid medicines using an oral syringe*, London: Great Ormond Street Hospital Trust.

HSE (2011) *Needlestick Injuries*, Bootle: HSE, available at http://www.hse.gov.uk/healthservices/needlesticks/ (accessed March 2011).

HPA (2008) *Health professionals still at risk of blood borne viruses through work*, London: HPA.

Kelsey, J. and McEwing, G. (2008) cited Adcock (2001) in *Clinical skills in child health practice*. Elsevier, 163.

Kumar, P. and Clark, M. (2009) *Clinical medicine* (7th edn), London: Elsevier.

Mahdi, J.G., Mahdi, A.J., and Bowen, I.D. (2002) 'The historical analysis of aspirin discovery, its relation to the willow tree and antiproliferative and anticancer potential', *Cell Proliferation*, 39(2), 147–155.

McCaffery, M. and Pasero, C. (1999) *Pain Clinical Manual* (2nd edn), St Louis, MO: Mosby.

National Patient Safety Organisation (2009) *Safety in doses. Improving the use of medicines in the NHS*, London: National Patient Safety Agency.

NMC (2008) *The Code – standards of conduct, performance and ethics for nurses*, London: NMC.

NMC (2010) *Standards for pre-registration nursing education*, London: NMC.

NMC (2010a) *Nurse and midwife independent prescribing of unlicensed medicines*, Circular 04/2010, London: NMC, available at http://www.nmc-uk.org/Documents/Circulars/2010circulars/NMCcircular04_2010.pdf (accessed March 2011).

NMC (2010b) *Standards for medicine management*, London: Nursing Midwifery Council.

RCN (2009) *Needlestick injuries the point of prevention*, London: Royal College of Nursing.

Siler, W.A. (1982) *Death by Prescription* (revised 2nd edn), Tallahassee, FL: Health Care Projects.

USEFUL WEBLINKS

For the full text of Acts and Regulations mentioned in this chapter see:
www.legislation.hmso.gov.uk

Nurse Independent Prescribers:
http://www.scotland.gov.uk/Home
http://www.wales.gov.uk/
http://www.dhsspsni.gov.uk/

CHAPTER 24
PAIN MANAGEMENT

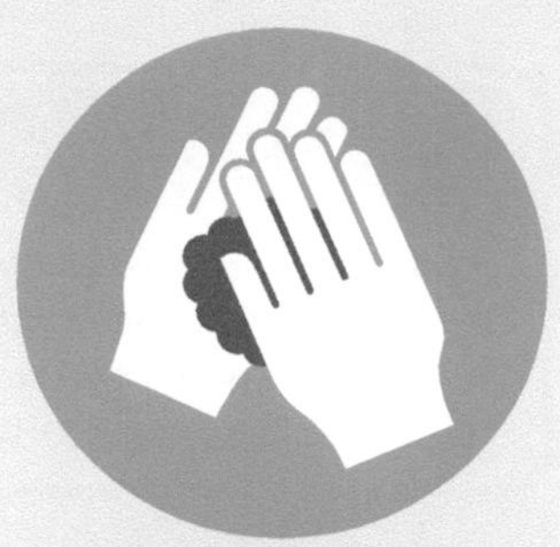

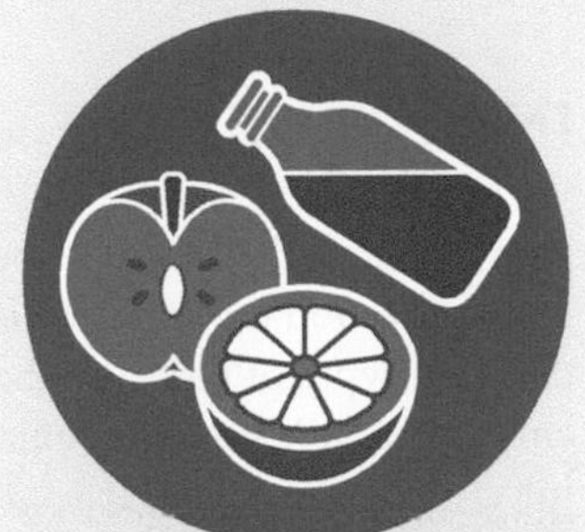

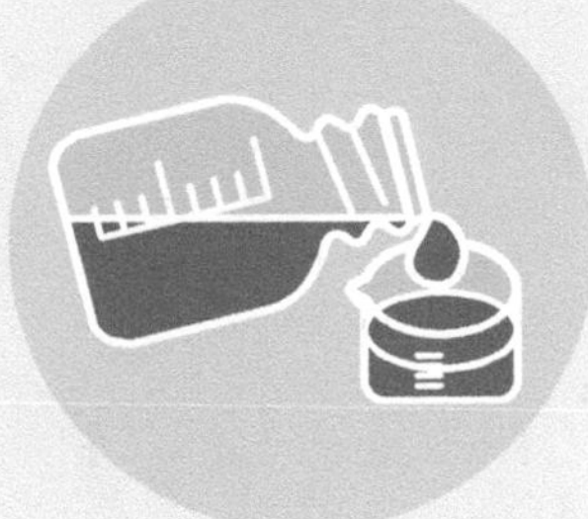

LEARNING OUTCOMES

After completing this chapter, you will be able to:

- Identify types and categories of pain according to location, aetiology and duration.
- Differentiate pain threshold from pain tolerance.
- Describe the four processes involved in nociception and how pain interventions can work during each process.
- Outline the gate control theory and its application to nursing care.
- Identify subjective and objective data to collect and analyse when assessing pain.
- Identify barriers to effective pain management.
- Describe pharmacological interventions for pain.
- Describe the World Health Organization's ladder step approach to cancer pain.
- Identify rationales for using various analgesic delivery routes.
- Describe nonpharmacological pain control interventions.

After reading this chapter you will be able to reflect on the nursing role in providing healthcare and effective care and pain management. It relates to **Essential Skills Clusters (NMC, 2010) 1, 3, 4, 5, 6, 9, 35, 36**, as appropriate for each progression point.

Ensure that you really understand this chapter by logging on to your complimentary **MyNursingKit** at **www.pearsoned.co.uk/kozier**. Complete the self-assessment tests to check your progress and utilise further activities to practise and confirm your understanding.

CASE STUDY

John is a 45-year-old gentleman who has been on step one of the WHO pain ladder for the last 5 years to manage his pain. Recently, his visits to the health centre have increased as his pain management is not effective. Prior to reading this chapter, you should explore and make notes of ways that as a nurse you could assess and plan effective pain management for John.

INTRODUCTION

Pain is a sensation that is experienced by most individuals, and it is a sensation that cannot be shared by others. There are many different types of pain and they are often referred to as acute or chronic pain. Acute or chronic pain can be broken down further into terms such as superficial or referred pain (see Figure 24-1 for referred pain). Pain is one of the first reasons why patients seek healthcare. Interestingly, the theory that pain is subjective and includes both a physiological and psychological component was only introduced with the Gate Control Theory developed by Melzack and Wall in 1965. Melzack and Wall (1965) recognised that the psychophysiological phenomenon resulting from the interaction between physiological and psychological influences was just as important as the mechanisms governing the transmission and modulation of **nociceptive** signals of pain (Main and Spanswick, 2000). However, McCaffery and Pasero (1999) suggest that there are four processes involved in **nociception** (no-si-sep-shon), a term used to describe the point at which an individual becomes conscious of pain: (1) **transduction**, (2) **transmission**, (3) perception and (4) **modulation** (Paice, 2002) (see Figure 24-2).

GATE CONTROL THEORY

Melzack and Wall (1965) proposed an alternative notion for the perception and treatment of pain. Their theory is based on the fact that pain impulses are normally carried to the spinal cord from the peripheries in small nerve fibres. Large nerve fibres, on the other hand, carry non-nociceptive stimuli such as touch, warmth, massage, vibration, etc. According to Melzack and Wall (1965) impulses travelling through the large fibres can block the impulses travelling through the small fibres at a 'gate', which is

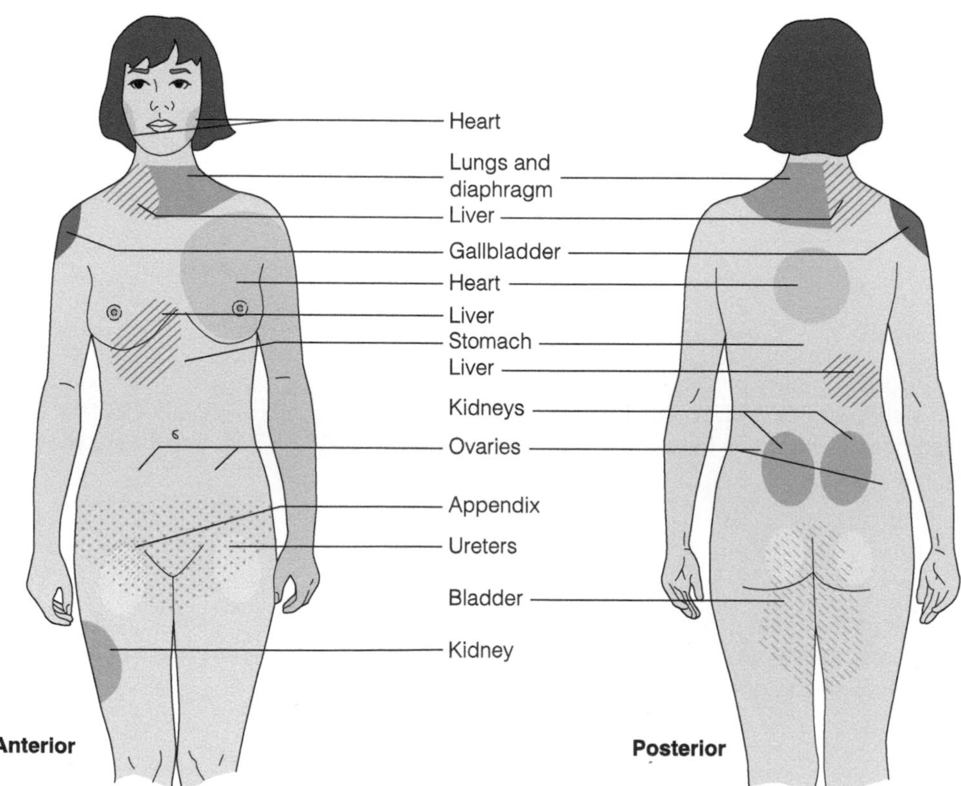

Figure 24-1 Common sites of referred pain from various body organs.

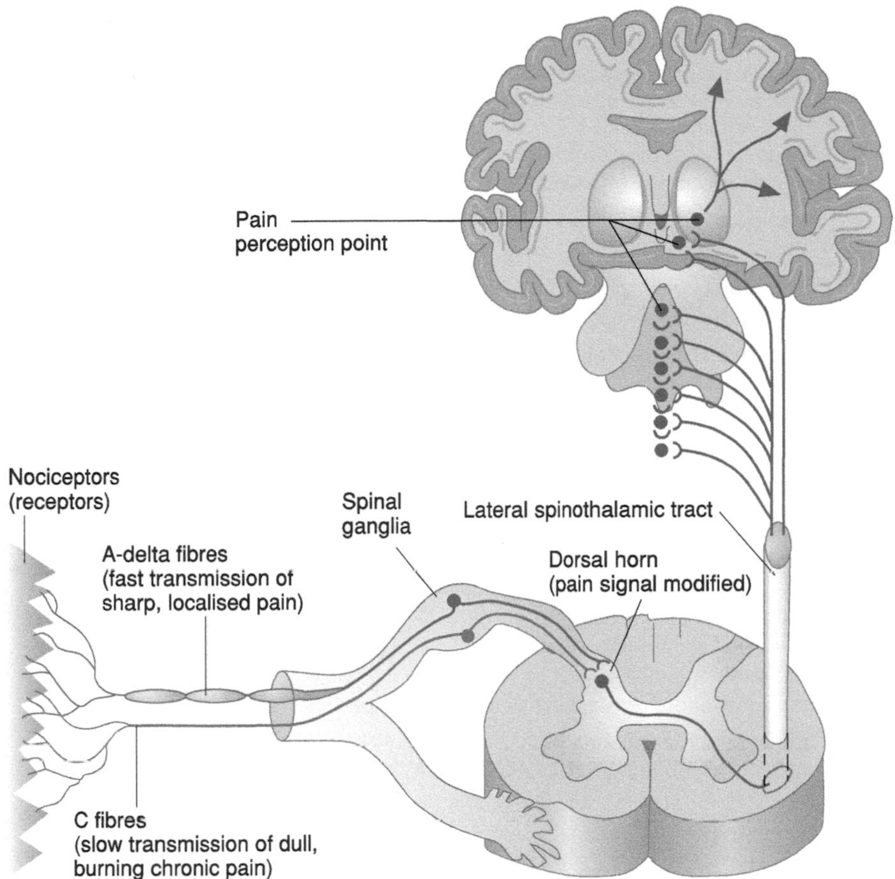

Figure 24-2 Physiology of pain perception.

situated at the spinal cord (see Figure 24-3). They therefore suggest that skin stimulation following injury can block the pain impulses from the injury. For example, if you bang your head what is the first thing you do? You rub it.

Transduction

Transduction is the first process whereby stimuli detected in receptor cells are converted to electrical impulses that are then transported by the nervous system – e.g., jamming a finger in the door – as the injury is sensed by **nociceptors** (the nerve endings that sense pain) and transferred to the spinal cord (see Table 24-1). They work by triggering the release of chemical substances (e.g. prostaglandins, bradykinin, serotonin, histamine, substance P, see Figure 24-2). Certain analgesics (e.g. ibuprofen) can work effectively in this phase to block off production of prostaglandin or by decreasing the movement of ions across the cell membrane.

Transmission

The second process of nociception, transmission of pain, includes three segments (McCaffery and Pasero, 1999):

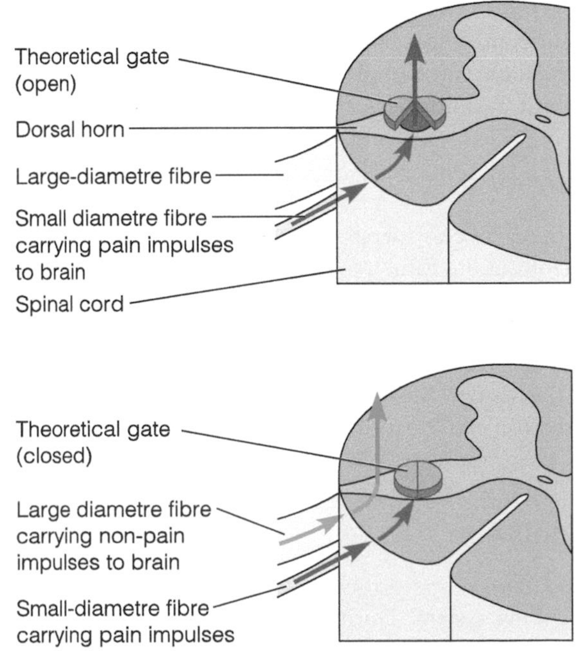

Figure 24-3 A schematic illustration of the gate control theory.

Table 24-1 Types of Pain Stimuli

Stimulus type	Physiological basis of pain
Mechanical	
Trauma to body tissues (e.g. surgery)	Tissue damage; direct irritation of the pain receptors; inflammation
Alterations in body tissues (e.g. oedema)	Pressure on pain receptors
Blockage of a body duct	Distention (swelling) of the lumen (hole) of the duct
Tumour	Pressure on pain receptors; irritation of nerve endings
Muscle spasm	Stimulation of pain receptors (also see chemical stimuli)
Thermal	
Extreme heat or cold (e.g. burns)	Tissue destruction; stimulation of thermo-sensitive pain receptors
Chemical	
Tissue ischemia (e.g. blocked coronary artery)	Stimulation of pain receptors because of accumulated lactic acid (and other chemicals, such as bradykinin and enzymes) in tissues
Muscle spasm	Tissue ischemia secondary to mechanical stimulation (see above)

1 The pain impulse travels from the peripheral nerve fibres to the spinal cord.
2 Transmission of the signals and ascension via spinothalmic tracts (spinal cord), to the brain stem and thalamus (see Figure 24-2 on page 737).
3 Transmission of pain signals between the thalamus and the somatic sensory cortex where pain perception occurs.

Pain control can take place during the second segment of transmission. For example, opioids (morphine) block the release of neurotransmitters which stops the pain at the spinal level.

Perception

The third process, perception, is when the patient becomes conscious of the pain. It is known that pharmacological stimulation of certain regions in the midbrain produces pain relief, and it is believed that perception of pain occurs in the cortical structures. Effective behavioural and cognitive strategies support this theory. Music and relaxation therapies, for example, can redirect the focus of the individual thereby reducing pain (McCaffery and Pasero, 1999).

Modulation

The fourth process – modulation – is often described as the 'descending system'. During this process, nerves in the brain stem send signals back down the dorsal horn of the spinal cord (Paice, 2002: 75). These returning signals release substances such as endorphins and serotonin. However, the lifespan of these substances is limited, which limits their analgesic usefulness (McCaffrey and Pasero, 1999). Patients with chronic pain may be prescribed medications such as tricyclic antidepressants which inhibit (stop) the body from absorbing the endorphins and serotonin, thus extending the modulation phase that hampers painful stimuli.

TYPES OF PAIN

There are many different classifications and types of pain (see Table 24-2). It is important to identify these as, according to Warren (2010), different types of pain respond to different management strategies. Pathophysiological pain is referred to as nocicpetive and neuropathic. Some classification systems refer to types of pain as either:

- acute
- chronic (non-malignant) or
- cancer (malignant).

While others classify pain by location, i.e.

- superficial
- deep or
- referred.

Pain is a warning, alerts the individual to actual tissue damage. It is a means of protecting the individual from life-threatening injury. People experience and react to pain differently. As nurses, we cannot feel what the patient feels, yet we have a duty to maintain the individual's dignity and, where possible, relieve their pain and promote comfort. Indeed, pain management is an important aspect of nursing care. Nurses need to understand the difference between acute and chronic (mechanisms of) pain (see Table 24-3), the different types of pain and the management strategy for each type of pain to promote the well-being of the patient.

CONCEPTS ASSOCIATED WITH PAIN

A number of terms are used in relation to pain: One of these is pain threshold, which refers to the amount of painful stimulation that an individual requires in order to feel pain. A number of research studies have looked at this concept over the past six decades. The study by Hardy *et al.* (1943) suggested that everyone perceives the same intensity of pain from the same stimuli, meaning that we all have the same pain threshold. However, later studies have proved that this is not the case (Beecher, 1956). Indeed, pain threshold and intensity varies from person to person as in the case of someone with hyperalgesia who is extremely sensitive to pain compared to another person with congenital analgesia who feels no pain.

Another common term heard in nursing is pain tolerance. Pain tolerance is the maximum amount and duration of pain that an individual is willing to endure. Some patients are unable to tolerate even the slightest pain, whereas others are willing to endure severe pain rather than be treated for it. Like pain

Table 24-2 Types of Pain

Type of pain	Location/severity/duration	Sensation	Examples
Nociceptive	Results from injury to the skin, mucous membranes, bones, muscles or organs of the body. Short or long lasting. Mild to severe depending on cause. Can be acute, chronic, superficial, deep or referred in nature.	Sharp, burning, pricking, aching pains noted.	Sprains, fractures, inflammation (such as arthritis) and obstructions.
Neuropathic	Caused by injury or malfunction of the peripheral or central nervous system.	Sharp, burning, pricking, aching pains noted.	Post-herpetic zoster pain (pain felt after having shingles), phantom pain following amputation of a limb.
Acute	Anywhere in the body. Sudden onset and foreseeable end. Mild to severe pain depending on cause. Relatively short duration. The patient will display fight or flight responses (see Table 24-3 below). Can be superficial, deep, referred or nociceptive in nature.	Sharp, burning, pricking, aching pains noted.	Pain following surgery.
Chronic	Anywhere in the body. Usually lasts longer than six months. Moderate to severe pain depending on the cause.	Sharp, burning, pricking, aching pains noted.	Arthritis, back pain.
Cancer	Anywhere in the body. Usually increases as disease progresses.	A compression of peripheral nerves or meninges or from the damage to these structures following surgery, chemotherapy, radiation or tumor growth and infiltration.	Bone metastasis, neuropathic pain, lymphodema.
Superficial	Skin and mucous membranes. Short duration, mild to severe pain depending on cause. Can be acute, chronic, nociceptive or neuropathic in nature.	Burning or pricking sensation.	First degree burn (superficial burn minimal damage to skin).
Deep	Muscles, joints and body organs. Short to long lasting depending on cause. Mild to severe pain depending on cause. Can be acute, chronic, nociceptive or neuropathic in nature.	Aching, not easily localised.	Sprain, bowel obstruction.
Referred	Felt at a site other than the injured site. Mild to severe pain depending on cause. Usually short duration. Usually acute or nociceptive in nature.	Aching pain.	Pain in left arm during myocardial infarction (heart attack). 'Brain freeze' – when cold food hits the roof of the mouth the vagus nerve is chilled and causes referred pain in the forehead. See Figure 24-1 on page 736 for common sites for referred pain.

Table 24-3 Comparison of Acute and Chronic Pain

Acute pain	Chronic pain
Mild to severe	Mild to severe
Sympathetic nervous system responses: Increased pulse rate Increased respiratory rate Elevated blood pressure Diaphoresis Dilated pupils	Parasympathetic nervous system responses: Vital signs normal Dry, warm skin Pupils normal or dilated
Related to tissue injury; resolves with healing	Continues beyond healing
Patient appears restless and anxious	Patient appears depressed and withdrawn
Patient reports pain	Patient often does not mention pain unless asked
Patient exhibits behaviour indicative of pain: crying, rubbing area, holding area	Pain behaviour often absent

threshold, pain tolerance varies from person to person and is widely influenced by psychological and sociocultural factors.

RESPONSES TO PAIN

The body's response to pain is a complex process incorporating physiological and psychosocial aspects. When pain is initially felt, the sympathetic nervous system responds, resulting in the fight or flight response. As pain continues, the body adapts as the parasympathetic nervous system takes over. This adaptation to pain occurs after several hours or days of pain. The actual pain receptors adapt very little and continue to transmit the pain message. The person may learn to cope with the pain through cognitive and behavioural activities, such as diversions, imagery and excessive sleeping.

CLINICAL ALERT

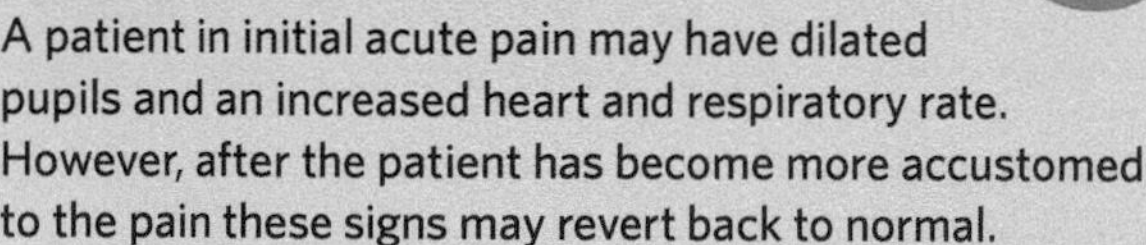

A patient in initial acute pain may have dilated pupils and an increased heart and respiratory rate. However, after the patient has become more accustomed to the pain these signs may revert back to normal.

A proprioceptive reflex also occurs with the stimulation of pain receptors. Impulses travel along sensory pain fibres to the spinal cord. There they synapse with motor neurons, and the impulses travel back via motor fibres to a muscle near the site of the pain. The muscle then contracts in a protective action. For example, when a person touches a hot stove the hand reflexively draws back from the heat even before the person is aware of the pain.

FACTORS AFFECTING THE PAIN EXPERIENCE

Numerous factors can affect a person's perception of and reaction to pain. These include ethnic and cultural values, developmental stage, environment and support persons, past pain experiences, the meaning attached to the pain, as well as anxiety and stress.

Ethnic and Cultural Values

Ethnic background and cultural heritage have long been recognised as factors that influence both a person's reaction to pain and the expression of that pain. Behaviour related to pain is a part of the socialisation process. For example, individuals in one culture may have learned to be expressive about pain (shouting and waving of hands), whereas individuals from another culture may have learned to keep those feelings to themselves and not bother others (British stiff upper lip).

Although there appears to be little variation in pain threshold, cultural background can affect the level of pain that an individual is willing to tolerate. In some Middle Eastern and African cultures, self-infliction of pain is a sign of mourning or grief. In other groups, pain may be anticipated as part of the ritualistic practices, and therefore tolerance of pain signifies strength and endurance. Additionally, there are significant variations in the expression of pain. Studies have shown that individuals of northern European descent tend to be more stoic and less expressive of their pain than individuals from southern European backgrounds.

A study carried out by Andrews and Boyle in 2003 identified that healthcare has been dominated by white Anglo-Saxon Protestants whose values and beliefs were built on silent suffering and self-control in pain management. It is important that nurses recognise the importance of cultural values and beliefs in pain management, and deliver care in a non-judgemental effective manner.

Developmental Stage

The age and developmental stage of a patient is an important variable that will influence both the reaction to and the expression of pain. Age variations and related nursing interventions are presented in Table 24-4.

The field of pain management for infants and children has grown significantly. It is now accepted that anatomic, physiological and biochemical elements necessary for pain transmission are present in newborns, regardless of their gestational age. Physiological indicators may vary in infants, so behavioural observation is recommended for pain assessment (Ball and Bindler, 2003). Children may be less able than an adult to articulate their experience or needs related to pain, which may result in their pain being under treated.

Mature adults constitute a major portion of the individuals within the healthcare system. The prevalence of pain in the older population is generally higher due to both acute and chronic disease conditions. Pain threshold does not appear to change with ageing, although the effect of analgesics may increase due to physiological changes related to drug metabolism and excretion (Eliopoulos, 2001).

Environmental Factors and Support Persons

Any environmental changes can compound pain, such as a different nurse, admission to hospital or moving to another ward. A mature adult who lives alone with little support may perceive pain as severe, whereas an individual who is surrounded by supportive family and friends may perceive less pain.

Expectations of significant others can affect a person's perceptions of and responses to pain. In some situations, for example, girls may be permitted to express pain more openly than boys. Family role can also affect how a person perceives or responds to pain. For instance, a single mother supporting three children may ignore pain because of her need to stay on the job.

Table 24-4 Age Variations in the Pain Experience

Age group	Pain perception and behaviour	Selected nursing interventions
Infant	Perceives pain. Responds to pain with increased sensitivity. Older infant tries to avoid pain; for example, turns away and physically resists.	Use tactile stimulation. Play music or tapes of a heartbeat.
Toddler and preschooler	Develops the ability to describe pain and its intensity and location. Often responds with crying and anger because child perceives pain as a threat to security. Reasoning with child at this stage is not always successful. May consider pain a punishment. Feels sad. Tends to hold someone accountable for the pain.	Distract the child with toys, books, pictures. Involve the child in blowing bubbles as a way of 'blowing away the pain'. Appeal to the child's belief in magic by using a 'magic' blanket or glove to take away pain. Hold the child to provide comfort. Explore misconceptions about pain.
School-age child	Tries to be brave when facing pain. Rationalises in an attempt to explain the pain. Responsive to explanations. Can usually identify the location and describe the pain. With persistent pain, may regress to an earlier stage of development.	Use imagery to turn off 'pain switches'. Provide a behavioural rehearsal of what to expect and how it will look and feel. Provide support and nurturing.
Adolescent	May be slow to acknowledge pain. Recognising pain or 'giving in' may be considered weakness. Wants to appear brave in front of peers and not report pain.	Provide opportunities to discuss pain. Provide privacy. Present choices for dealing with pain. Encourage music or TV for distraction.
Adult	Behaviours exhibited when experiencing pain may be gender-based behaviours learned as a child. May ignore pain because to admit it is perceived as a sign of weakness or failure. Fear of what pain means may prevent some adults from taking action.	Deal with any misconceptions about pain. Focus on the patient's control in dealing with the pain. Allay fears and anxiety when possible.
Mature adult	May have multiple conditions presenting with vague symptoms. May perceive pain as part of the ageing process. May have decreased sensations or perceptions of the pain. Lethargy, anorexia and fatigue may be indicators of pain. May withhold complaints of pain because of fear of the treatment, of any lifestyle changes that may be involved, or of becoming dependent. May describe pain differently, that is, as 'ache', 'hurt' or 'discomfort'. May consider it unacceptable to admit or show pain.	Thorough history and assessment is essential. Spend time with the patient and listen carefully. Clarify misconceptions. Encourage independence whenever possible.

Past Pain Experiences

Previous pain experiences alter a patient's sensitivity to pain. People who have personally experienced pain or who have been exposed to the suffering of someone close are often more threatened by anticipated pain than people without a pain experience. In addition, the success or lack of success of pain relief measures influences a person's expectations for relief. For example, a person who has tried several pain relief measures without success may have little hope about the helpfulness of nursing interventions.

The Patient's Perception of the Meaning of Pain

Some patients may accept pain more readily than others, depending on the circumstances and the patient's interpretation of its significance. A patient who associates the pain with a positive outcome may withstand the pain amazingly well. For example, a woman giving birth to a child or an athlete undergoing knee surgery to prolong his or her career may tolerate pain better because of the benefit associated with it. These patients may view the pain as a temporary inconvenience rather than a potential threat or disruption to daily life.

By contrast, patients with unrelenting chronic pain may suffer more intensely. They may respond with despair, anxiety and depression because they cannot attach a positive significance or purpose to the pain. In this situation, the pain may be looked on as a threat to body image or lifestyle and as a sign of possible impending death.

Fundamental to carrying out an accurate pain assessment of the patient is the nurse asking the appropriate questions to elicit the information and the ability of the patient to express in their own words how they view the pain and the situation. This will help the nurse understand what the pain means to the patient and how the patient is coping with it. Each person's pain experience is unique and the patient is the best interpreter of the pain experience.

Anxiety and Stress

Anxiety often accompanies pain. The threat of the unknown and the inability to control the pain or the events surrounding it often augment the pain perception. Fatigue also reduces a person's ability to cope, thereby increasing pain perception. When pain interferes with sleep, fatigue and muscle tension often result and increase the pain; thus a cycle of pain–fatigue–pain develops. People in pain who believe that they have control of their pain have decreased fear and anxiety, which decreases their pain perception. A perception of lacking control or a sense of helplessness tends to increase pain perception. Patients who are able to express pain to an attentive listener and participate in pain management decisions can increase a sense of control and decrease pain perception.

ASSESSING PAIN

The British Pain Society (2007) state that the fifth vital sign, alongside recording blood pressure, pulse, temperature and respiratory rate, is the assessment of pain. Accurate pain assessment is essential for effective pain management. Pain is subjective and experienced uniquely by each individual; nurses need to assess all factors affecting the pain experience – physiological, psychological, behavioural, emotional and sociocultural.

The extent and frequency of the pain assessment varies according to the situation. For patients experiencing acute or severe pain, the nurse may focus only on location and radiation, quality, onset and duration, severity and early intervention. Patients with less severe or chronic pain can usually provide a more detailed description of the experience. Frequency of pain assessment usually depends on the pain control measures being used and the clinical circumstances. Following pain management interventions, pain intensity should be reassessed at an interval appropriate for the intervention. For example, following the intravenous administration of morphine, the severity of pain should be reassessed in 20–30 minutes.

Because it has been found that many people will not voice their pain unless asked about it, pain assessments must be initiated by the nurse. It is also essential that nurses listen to and rely on the patient's perceptions of pain. Believing the person experiencing and conveying the perceptions is crucial in establishing a sense of trust. Amongst the reasons why patients may be reluctant to report pain are the following:

- unwillingness to trouble staff who are perceived as busy;
- fear of the injectable route of analgesic administration;
- belief that pain is to be expected as part of the recovery process;
- belief that pain is a normal part of ageing or a necessary part of life – older adults in particular;
- belief that expressions of pain reveal weakness;
- difficulty expressing personal discomfort;
- concern about risks associated with opioid drugs (e.g. addiction);
- fear about the cause of pain;
- concern about unwanted side-effects, especially of opioid drugs;
- concern that use of drugs now will render the drug inefficient if or when the pain becomes worse;
- belief that they have already had optimum pain relief and don't want to have a negative response to their request.

Pain assessments consist of two major components: (a) a history of the pain to obtain facts from the patient and (b) direct observation of behavioural and physiological responses of the patient. The goal of assessment is to gain an objective understanding of a subjective experience, and mnemonics can be a useful and to achieving this:

- OLDCART mnemonic
  - O – onset
  - L – location
  - D – duration
  - C – characteristic
  - A – aggravating factors
  - R – radiation
  - T – treatment (what was previously ineffective and what has alleviated the pain)
- PQRST mnemonic
  - P – provoked (what brought about pain)
  - Q – quality
  - R – region/radiation
  - S – severity
  - T – timing

Source: From 'Undertreated pain: Could it land you in court?' by S. LaDuke (2002), *Nursing, 32*, p. 18. Reprinted with permission.

Pain History

When taking a pain history from a patient, the questions asked should be geared to the specific patient: for example, questions asked of an accident victim would be different from those asked of a post-operative patient or one suffering from chronic pain. The initial pain assessment for someone in severe acute pain may consist of only a few questions before intervention occurs. In addition, the nurse may focus on the following:

- previous pain treatment and effectiveness;
- when and what analgesics were last taken;
- other medications being taken;
- allergies to medications.

For the patient with chronic pain, the nurse should discuss past pain experiences and should seek to gain an understanding of the patient's individual perception of the meaning of the pain. The effectiveness of current pain management strategies should be assessed. A pain history should also include information on pain location, intensity/severity, quality, patterns, precipitating factors, alleviating factors, associated symptoms, effect on activities of daily living (ADLs), coping mechanisms and psychological responses.

Location

To ascertain the specific location of the pain, the individual can be asked to point to the site of the discomfort. The patient can also identify or mark the location of the pain on a chart consisting of drawings of the body. This tool can be especially effective with patients who have more than one source of pain.

When assessing the location of a child's pain, the nurse needs to understand the child's vocabulary. For example, *tummy* might refer either to the abdomen or to part of the chest. Asking the child to point to the pain helps clarify where the pain is located. Again, the use of figure drawings can assist in identifying pain locations. Parents can also be helpful in interpreting the meaning of a child's words.

Intensity/severity

The single most important indicator of the existence and intensity of pain is the patient's report of pain. In practice, however, McCaffery *et al.* (2000) found that nurses tend to use less reliable measures for assessing pain. The top factors used to identify the level of pain in a patient were facial expressions, verbalisation (what the patient reports) and request for pain relief. In addition, studies have shown that healthcare professionals may underrate or overrate the pain intensity (Bergh and Sjostrom, 1999). The use of pain assessment tools is an easy and reliable method of determining the patient's pain intensity. Such scales provide consistency for nurses to communicate with the patient and other healthcare providers. Most scales use either a 0–5 or 0–10 range with 0 indicating 'no pain' (numerical rating scale – NRS) and/or the highest number indicating the 'worst pain possible' for that individual (visual analogue scale – VAS – see Figure 24-4). A 10-point rating scale is shown in Figure 24-5. Word modifiers are used in these scales such as 'no pain' or 'severe pain' which enable those patients who find it difficult to apply a number level to their pain to express their pain level effectively.

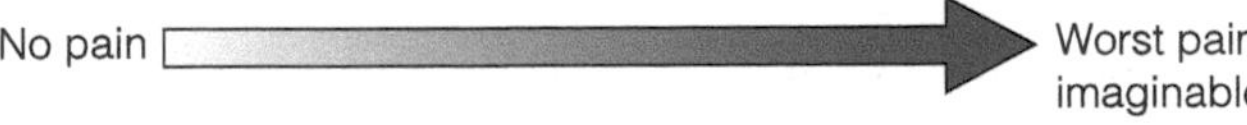

Figure 24-4 A visual analogue scale (VAS).

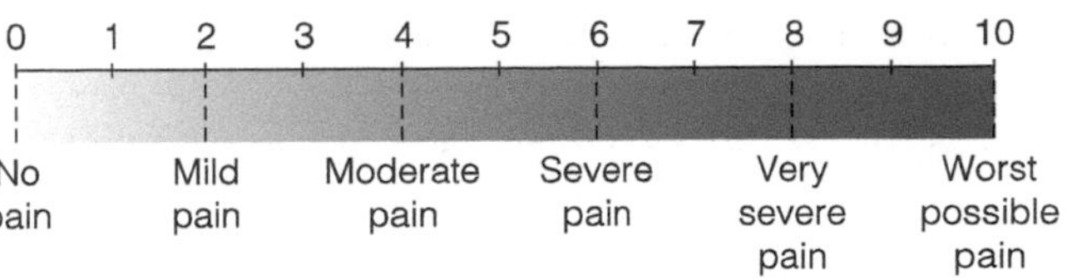

Figure 24-5 A 10-point pain intensity scale with word modifiers.

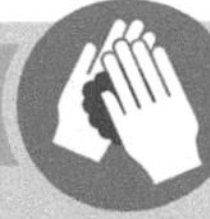

CLINICAL ALERT

Pain is whatever the experiencing person says it is, existing whenever s/he says it does (McCaffery and Pasero, 1999).

When noting pain intensity, it is important to determine any related factors that may be affecting the pain. If there is a change in the intensity of the pain, the nurse needs to consider possible causes. Several factors affect the perception of intensity: (1) the amount of distraction or the patient's concentration on another event; (2) the patient's state of consciousness; (3) the level of activity; and (4) the patient's expectations.

Not all patients can understand or relate to numerical pain intensity scales. These include children who are unable to communicate discomfort verbally, older patients with impairments in cognition or communication, and people who do not speak English. For these patients, the Wong–Baker FACES Rating Scale (see Figure 24-6) may be easier to use (Hockenberry-Eaton and Wilson, 2009). The face scale includes a number scale in relation to each expression so that the pain intensity can be documented. When it is not possible to use any kind of rating scale with a patient, the nurse must rely on observation of behaviour and any physiological cues discussed later in this section. The input of the patient's significant others, such as parents or caregivers, can assist the nurse in interpreting the observations. An objective description of the patient's behaviour and any physiological observations such as an increase in blood pressure should then be documented.

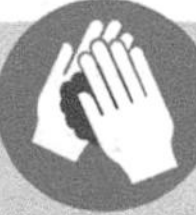

CLINICAL ALERT

A guideline based on studies: on a scale of 0–10, a pain rating of 3 or greater signals a need to revise the pain treatment plan (e.g. higher dose or different analgesia). A rating of 6 or more demands immediate attention (McCaffery and Pasero, 1999: 74–75).

Pain Quality

Descriptive adjectives help people communicate the quality of pain. A headache may be described as 'hammerlike' or an

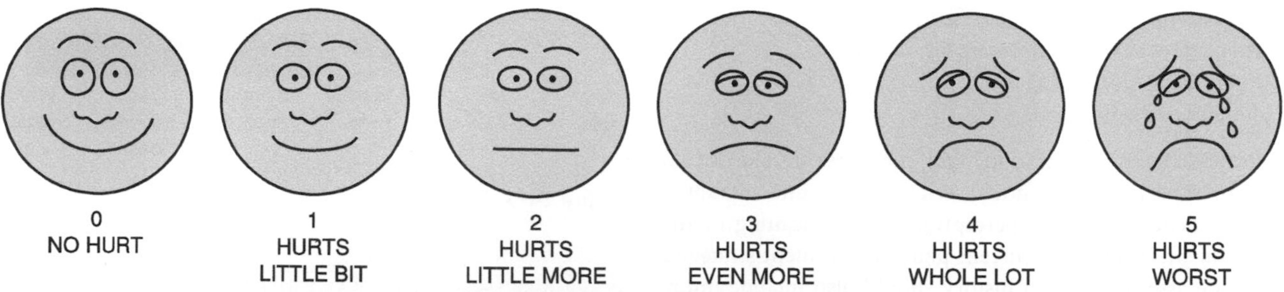

Explain to the person that each face is for a person who feels happy because he has no pain (hurt) or sad because he has some or a lot of pain. Face 0 is very happy because he doesn't hurt at all. Face 1 hurts just a little bit. Face 2 hurts a little more. Face 3 hurts even more. Face 4 hurts a whole lot. Face 5 hurts as much as you can imagine, although you don't have to be crying to feel this bad. Ask the person to choose the face that best describes how he is feeling.

Rating scale is recommended for persons age 3 years and older.

Brief word instructions: Point to each face using the words to describe the pain intensity. Ask the child to choose the face that best describes own pain and record the appropriate number.

Figure 24-6 The Wong-Baker FACES Pain Rating Scale.
Source: from Hockenberry, M.J., Wilson, D.: *Wong's Essentials of pediatric Nursing*, ed. 8, St Louis, 2009, Mosby. Used with permission. Copyright Mosby.

abdominal pain as 'piercing like a knife'. Sometimes patients have difficulty describing pain because they have never experienced any sensation like it. Some of the terms commonly used to describe pain are listed in Table 24-5.

Nurses need to record the exact words patients use to describe pain. A patient's words are more accurate and descriptive than an interpretation in the nurse's words. Identifying the cause of pain, diagnosing and treating it are supported by the information gathered from the patient.

Patterns

The pattern of pain includes time of onset, duration and recurrence or intervals without pain. The nurse therefore determines when the pain began; how long the pain lasts; whether it recurs and, if so, the length of the interval without pain; and when the pain last occurred.

Precipitating Factors

Certain activities sometimes precede pain. For example, physical exertion may precede chest pain or abdominal pain may occur after eating. These observations can help prevent pain and determine its cause.

Environmental factors such as extreme cold or heat and extremes of humidity can affect some types of pain. For example, sudden exercise on a hot day can cause muscle spasm.

Physical and emotional stressors can also precipitate pain. Emotional tension frequently brings on a migraine headache. Intense fear or physical exertion can cause angina.

Alleviating Factors

Nurses must ask patients to describe anything that they have done to alleviate the pain (e.g. home remedies such as herbal teas, medications, rest, applications of heat or cold, prayer or distractions like TV). It is important to explore the effect any of these measures had on the pain, whether or not relief was obtained, or whether the pain became worse.

Table 24-5 Commonly Used Pain Descriptors

Term	Sensory words	Affective words
Pain	Searing	Unbearable
	Scalding	Killing
	Sharp	Intense
	Piercing	Torturing
	Drilling	Agonising
	Wrenching	Terrifying
	Shooting	Exhausting
	Burning	Suffocating
	Crushing	Frightful
	Penetrating	Punishing
		Miserable
Hurt	Hurting	Heavy
	Pricking	
	Pressing	
	Tender	Throbbing
Ache	Numb	Annoying
	Cold	Nagging
	Flickering	Tiring
	Radiating	Troublesome
	Dull	Gnawing
	Sore	Uncomfortable
	Aching	Sickening
	Cramping	Tender

Associated Symptoms

Also included in the clinical appraisal of pain are associated symptoms such as nausea, vomiting, dizziness and diarrhoea. These symptoms may relate to the onset of the pain or they may result from the presence of the pain.

Effect on Activities of Daily Living (ADLs)

Knowing how ADLs are affected by chronic pain helps the nurse understand the patient's perspective on the pain's severity. The pain assessment should therefore be incorporated into the activities of daily living.

Coping Mechanisms

Each individual will exhibit personal ways of coping with pain. Strategies may relate to earlier pain experiences or the specific meaning of the pain; some may reflect religious or cultural influences. Nurses can encourage and support the patient's use of methods known to have helped in alleviating or reducing the pain. Strategies may include withdrawal, distraction, prayer or other religious practices, and support from significant others.

Psychological Responses

Psychological responses vary according to the situation, the degree and duration of pain, the patient's interpretation of it and many other factors. The nurse needs to explore the patient's feelings of anxiety, fear, exhaustion, depression or a sense of failure. Because many people with chronic pain become depressed and potentially suicidal, it may also be necessary to assess the patient's suicide risk.

Observation of Behavioural and Physiological Responses

There are wide variations in nonverbal responses to pain. For patients who are very young, **aphasic**, confused or disoriented, nonverbal expressions may be the only means of communicating pain. Facial expression is often the first indication of pain and it may be the only one. Clenched teeth, tightly shut eyes, biting of the lower lip and other facial grimaces may be indicative of pain. Moaning, groaning, crying or screaming are also associated with pain.

Immobilising the body or a part of the body may also indicate pain. The patient with chest pain often holds the left arm across the chest. A person with abdominal pain may assume the position of greatest comfort, often with the knees and hips hexed, and moves reluctantly. Purposeless body movements can also indicate pain – for example, tossing and turning in bed or flinging the arms about.

Rhythmic body movements or rubbing may indicate pain. An adult or child may assume a foetal position and rock back and forth when experiencing abdominal pain. During labour a woman may massage her abdomen rhythmically with her hands.

It is important to note that behavioural responses can be controlled and so may not be very revealing.

CLINICAL ALERT

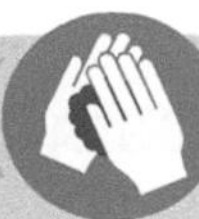

Patients with chronic pain often do not present with visual signs of pain as their own coping strategies manage and sometimes mask distress and discomfort.

Physiological responses vary with the origin and duration of the pain. Early in the onset of acute pain, the sympathetic nervous system is stimulated, resulting in increased blood pressure, pulse rate, respiratory rate, pallor, diaphoresis and pupil dilation. The body does not sustain the increased sympathetic function over a prolonged period of time and, therefore, the sympathetic nervous system adapts, making the physiological responses less evident or even absent. Physiological responses are most likely to be absent in people with chronic pain because the central nervous system (CNS) adapts to the pain. Thus, it is important that the nurse assess more than only physiological responses, because they may be poor indicators of pain.

Daily Pain Diary

For patients who experience chronic pain, a daily diary may help the patient and nurse identify pain patterns and factors that exacerbate or mediate the pain experience. In the community, the family or other carer can be taught to complete the diary. The record can include:

- time or onset of pain;
- activity before pain;
- pain-related positions or behaviours;
- pain intensity level;
- use of analgesics or other relief measures;
- duration of pain;
- time spent in relief activities.

Recorded data can provide the basis for developing or modifying the plan of care and aid the nurse in the decision making process. For this tool to be effective, it is important that the nurse educate the patient and family about the value and use of the diary in achieving effective pain control. Determining the patient's abilities to use the diary is essential.

ACTIVITY 24-1

Reflect on what you have read and discuss and explore your understanding of acute and chronic pain, and how this may impact on patient care.

PLANNING

The established goals for the patient will vary according to the diagnosis and its defining characteristics. Specific nursing interventions can be selected to meet the individual needs of the patient (see *Practice Guidelines*).

PRACTICE GUIDELINES

Individualising Care for Patients with Pain

- Establish a trusting relationship through effective communication.
- Consider the patient's ability and willingness to participate actively in pain relief measures. Some patients who are excessively fatigued are sedated; those who have altered levels of consciousness are less able to participate actively.
- Use a variety of pain relief measures. It is thought that using more than one measure has an additive effect in relieving pain.
- Provide measures to relieve pain before it becomes severe. For example, providing an analgesic before the onset of pain is preferable to waiting for the patient to complain of pain, when a larger dose may be required, or for example, 20–40 minutes prior to a wound dressing change.
- Use pain-relieving measures that the patient believes are effective unless it is known to be harmful.
- Base the choice of pain relief measure on the patient's report of the severity of the pain.
- If a pain relief measure is ineffective, encourage the patient to try it once or twice more before abandoning it. Anxiety may diminish the effects of a pain measure, and some approaches, such as distraction strategies, require practice before they are effective.
- Maintain an open mind about what may relieve the pain. New ways to relieve pain are continually being developed. It is not always possible to explain pain relief measures; however, measures should be supported unless they are harmful.
- Keep trying. Do not ignore a patient because pain persists in spite of measures. In these circumstances, reassess the pain, and consider other means as relieving pain.
- Prevent harm to the patient. Pain therapy should not increase discomfort or harm the patient. Some pain relief measures may have adverse effects, such as drowsiness, but they should not disable the patient.
- Educate the patient and support persons about pain. Patients and their families need to be informed about possible causes of pain, precipitating and alleviating factors, and alternatives to drug therapy. Misconceptions also need to be corrected.

Planning Independent of Setting

When planning, nurses need to choose pain relieving measures appropriate for the patient, based on the assessment. Nursing interventions may include a variety of pharmacological and nonpharmacological interventions. Developing a plan that incorporates a wide range of strategies is usually most effective. Whether in acute care or in the community, it is important for everyone involved in pain management to understand the plan of care.

IMPLEMENTING

Pain management is the alleviation of pain or a reduction in pain to a level of comfort that is acceptable to the patient. It includes two basic types of nursing interventions: pharmacological and nonpharmacological. Good effective teamwork is essential in the effective management of pain.

Generally speaking, a combination of strategies is best for the patient in pain. Sometimes strategies need to be tried and changed until the patient obtains effective pain relief. See the *Practice Guidelines* above for individualising care for patients with pain.

Barriers to Pain Management

Misconceptions and biases can affect pain management. These may involve attitudes of the nurse or the patient as well as knowledge deficits. Patients respond to pain experiences based on their culture, personal experiences and the meaning the pain has for them. For many people, pain is expected and accepted as a normal aspect of illness. Patients and their families may lack knowledge of the effects of pain and the use of analgesia. Common misconceptions are shown in Table 24-6.

Table 24-6 Common Misconceptions about Pain

Misconception	Correction
Patients experience severe pain only when they have had major surgery.	Even after minor surgery, patients can experience intense pain.
The nurse or other healthcare professionals are the authorities on a patient's pain.	The person who experiences the pain is the only authority on its existence and nature.
Administering analgesia regularly for pain will lead to addiction.	Patients are unlikely to become addicted to analgesia provided to treat pain.
The amount of tissue damage is directly related to the amount of pain.	Pain is a subjective experience, and the intensity and duration of pain vary considerably among individuals.
Visible physiological or behavioural signs accompany pain and can be used to verify its existence.	Even with severe pain, periods of physiologic and behavioural adaptation can occur.

Key Factors in Pain Management

Acknowledging and accepting the patient's pain are key factors, alongside assisting relatives and carers, reducing misconceptions about pain, reducing fear and anxiety and preventing pain, in managing and reducing pain.

Acknowledging and Accepting Patient's Pain

Basic to all strategies for reducing pain is that nurses convey to patients that they believe the patient is experiencing pain. Simple ways of doing this are:

- Verbally acknowledging the presence of the pain, for example, 'I understand your leg is very painful. How do you feel about the pain?'
- Listening attentively to what the patient says about the pain.
- Conveying that you are assessing the patient's pain to understand it better, not to determine whether the pain is real, for example, 'How does your pain feel now?' or 'Tell me how it feels compared to an hour ago.'
- Attending to the patient's needs promptly.

Assisting Family and Friends

Family and friends of the patient often need assistance to respond positively to the patient experiencing pain. Nurses can help by giving them accurate information about the pain and providing opportunities for them to discuss their emotional reactions, which may include anger, fear, frustration and feelings of inadequacy. Enlisting the aid of family members in providing pain relief to the patient, such as massaging the patient's back, may diminish their feelings of helplessness and foster a more positive attitude towards the patient's pain experience.

Reducing Misconceptions about Pain

Reducing a patient's misconceptions about the pain and its treatment will often avoid intensifying the pain. The nurse should explain to the patient that pain is a highly individual experience and that it is only the patient who really experiences the pain, although others can understand and empathise. Misconceptions are also dealt with when nurse and patient discuss why the pain has increased or decreased at certain times. For example, a patient whose pain increases in the evening may mistakenly think this is the result of eating dinner rather than fatigue.

Reducing Fear and Anxiety

It is important to help relieve the emotional component, that is, anxiety or fear, associated with the pain. When patients have no opportunity to talk about their pain and associated fears, their perceptions and reactions to the pain can be intensified. The patient may become angry or complain about the nurse's care when the problem really is a belief that the pain is not being treated. If the nurse is honest and sincere and promptly attends to the patient's needs, the patient is much more likely to know that the nurse does believe the patient is in pain.

By providing accurate information, the nurse can also reduce many of the patient's fears, such as a fear of addiction or a fear that the pain will always be present. It also helps many patients to have privacy when they are experiencing pain.

Preventing Pain

A preventive approach to pain management involves the provision of measures to treat the pain before it occurs or before it becomes severe. Pre-emptive analgesia is the administration of analgesics prior to an invasive or operative procedure in order to treat pain before it occurs. For example, treating patients preoperatively with local infiltration of an anaesthetic or parenteral administration of an opioid can reduce post-operative pain. Nurses can also use a pre-emptive approach by providing an analgesic around the clock (ATC), rather than as needed (prn).

Pharmacological Pain Management

Pharmacological pain management involves the use of opioids (narcotics), nonopioids/nonsteroidal anti-inflammatory drugs (NSAIDS), and adjuvants, or coanalgesic drugs (see Table 24-7).

Opioid Analgesia

Opioid analgesia uses opium derivatives, such as morphine and codeine, to relieve pain and provide a sense of euphoria. Changes in mood and attitude and feelings of well-being make the person feel more comfortable even though the pain persists.

When administering any analgesia, the nurse must review side-effects. All opioids result in some initial drowsiness when first administered but, with regular administration, this side-effect tends to decrease. Opioids also may cause nausea, vomiting, constipation and respiratory depression. Opioids must be used cautiously in patients with respiratory problems.

Table 24-7 Categories and Examples of Analgesics

Generic name	Brand name
Opioid analgesics	
Codeine phosphate	Promethazine HCl
Diamorphine hydrochloride	Diamorphine
Fentanyl	Durogesic
Hydromorphone hydrochloride	Palladone
Methadone hydrochloride	Physepotone
Morphine	Sevredol
Oxycodone hydrochloride	OxyContin
Nonopioid analgesics/NSAIDs	
Paracetamol	
Acetylsalicylic acid	aspirin
Diclofenac sodium	Voltarol
Ibuprofen	Brufen
Naproxen	Naprosyn
Piroxicam	Feldene
Adjuvant analgesics	
Amitriptyline	Triptafen
Chlorpromazine	Chloractil
Diazepam	Rimapam
Hydroxyzine	Atarax

CLINICAL ALERT

Constipation is an almost universal adverse effect of opioid use and, as such, all patients receiving opioids should receive laxatives, unless contraindicated. Inform patients about the following options to prevent constipation: increasing fibre intake, using a mild laxative (e.g. milk of magnesia) regularly, taking oral laxatives at bedtime, and using rectal suppositories if absolutely necessary.

If the patient experiences significant respiratory depression or is overly sedated, the dosage is excessive. The nurse needs to assess a patient's level of alertness and respiratory rate for baseline data before administering opioid analgesia. An increasing sedation level can be an early warning sign of impending respiratory depression (Pasero and McCaffery, 2002). The nurse should assess and document the patient's level of sedation at the same time respiratory status is checked. Early recognition of an increasing level of sedation or respiratory depression will enable the nurse to implement appropriate measures promptly (e.g. reducing the opioid dosage).

CLINICAL ALERT

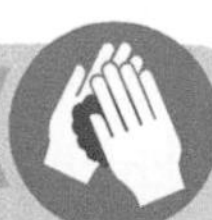

Assessing for sedation and respiratory status is critical during the first 12–24 hours after starting opioid therapy. The longer the patient receives opioids, the wider the safety margin as the patient develops a tolerance to the sedative and respiratory depressive effects of the drug.

Older patients are particularly sensitive to the analgesic properties of opioids and often require less medication than younger patients. This sensitivity may be related to reduced excretion of the drug in elderly patients. Advice on managing side-effects of opiod analgesics is given in the *Practice Guidelines*.

PRACTICE GUIDELINES

Managing Side-Effects of Opioid Analgesia

Constipation

- Increase fluid intake (e.g. 6–8 glasses daily).
- Increase fibre and bulk-forming agents to the diet (e.g. fresh fruits and vegetables).
- Increase exercise regimen.
- Administer stool softeners and if necessary provide a mild laxative.

Nausea and vomiting

- Inform patient that tolerance to this emetic effect generally develops after several days of opiate therapy.
- Provide an antiemetic as required.
- Change the analgesic as indicated.

Sedation

- Inform patient that tolerance usually develops over 3–5 days.
- Administer a stimulant each morning to patients who receive opiate therapy for chronic pain and do not develop tolerance (if necessary and prescribed).

Respiratory depression

- Administer an opioid antagonist, such as naloxone hydrochloride (Narcan) until respirations return to an acceptable rate. Administer the medication slowly by intravenous route with 10ml of saline. Monitor the patient, and repeat the procedure as required.
- If the patient is receiving intravenous patient-controlled analgesia, stop or slow the infusion.

Pruritus (proo-RY-tuss - itching).

- Apply cool packs, lotion and diversional activity.
- Administer an antihistamine (e.g. diphenhydramine hydrochloride (Benadryl)).
- Inform the patient that tolerance also develops to pruritus.

Urinary retention

- May need to catheterise patient.
- Administer narcotic antagonist (naloxone hydrochloride (Narcan)).

Nonopioids/NSAIDs

Nonopioids include paracetamol and **nonsteroidal anti-inflammatory drugs (NSAIDs)** such as ibuprofen. NSAIDs have anti-inflammatory, analgesic and antipyretic effects, whereas acetaminophen has only analgesic and antipyretic effects.

The most common side-effect of nonopioid analgesics is gastrointestinal, such as heartburn or indigestion. Patients should be taught to take NSAIDs with food or a glass of water. Most NSAIDs also interfere with platelet aggregation. Paracetamol, on the other hand, does not affect platelet function and rarely causes gastrointestinal distress. It can, however, cause hepatotoxicity (liver toxicity) and should be used cautiously in patients with liver problems.

The NSAIDs reduce the dose of opioids needed when the drugs are given together and provide better pain relief than use of either type separately. There are advantages to giving combination drugs such as NSAIDS and opioids for pain management, but close attention must be paid to the amount that the patient takes in a 24-hour period. Opioids have no ceiling, so the codeine could be gradually increased as needed for pain management. A change in medication or dosage may be needed to provide pain relief while maintaining safe, nontoxic levels.

Pharmacological management of mild to moderate pain should begin with NSAIDs, unless there is a septic contraindication. NSAIDs are contraindicated, for example, in patients diagnosed asthmatic, in patients with impaired blood clotting or those on warfarin, in patients at risk of gastrointestinal bleeding or ulcer or with renal disease or thrombocytopenia, and in any case where infection is possible. Table 24-8 lists common misconceptions about nonopioids. However, some NSAIDs have also been linked to an increased risk of coronary heart disease (Antman *et al.*, 2007).

Table 24-8 Misconceptions about Nonopioids

Misconception	Correction
Regular daily use of NSAIDs is much safer than taking opioids.	Side-effects from long-term use of NSAIDs are considerably more severe and life threatening than the side-effects from daily doses of oral morphine or other opioids. The most common side-effect from long-term use of opioids is constipation, whereas NSAIDs can cause gastric ulcers, increased bleeding time and renal insufficiency. Paracetamol can cause hepatotoxicity.
A nonopioid should not be given at the same time as an opioid.	It is safe to administer a nonopioid and opioid at the same time. Giving a dose of nonopioid at the same time as a dose of opioid poses no more danger than giving the doses at different times.
Administering antacids with NSAIDs is an effective method of reducing gastric distress.	Administering antacids with NSAIDs can lessen distress but may be counterproductive. Antacids reduce the absorption and therefore the effectiveness of the NSAID by releasing the drug in the stomach rather than in the small intestine where absorption occurs.
Nonopioids are not useful analgesics for severe pain.	Nonopioids alone are rarely sufficient to relieve severe pain, but they are an important part in achieving pain relief. One of the basic principles of analgesic therapy is: whenever pain is severe enough to require an opioid, adding a nonopioid should be considered.
Gastric distress (e.g. abdominal pain) is indicative of NSAID-induced gastric ulceration.	Most patients with gastric lesions have no symptoms until bleeding or perforation occurs.

Source: *Pain: Clinical Manual*, 2nd edn, by M. McCaffery and C. Pasero, 1999, St Louis, MO: Mosby. Reprinted with permission from Elsevier Science.

CLINICAL ALERT

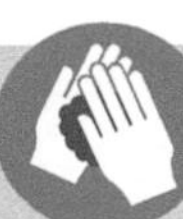

Patient with known heart disease should only take NSAIDs on Doctor's advice.

CLINICAL ALERT

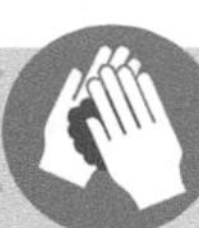

Any degree of worsening of asthma may be related to the ingestion of NSAIDs, either prescribed or (in the case of ibuprofen and others) purchased over the counter (BNF, 2011).

Adjuvant Analgesics

An adjuvant analgesic is a medication that was developed for a use other than analgesia but has been found to reduce chronic pain and sometimes acute pain, in addition to its primary action. For example, mild sedatives or tranquillisers may help reduce anxiety, stress and tension so that the patient can obtain a good night's sleep. Antidepressants are used to treat underlying depression or mood disorders but may also enhance other pain strategies. Anticonvulsants, usually prescribed to treat seizures (fits), can be useful in controlling painful neuropathies (abnormal functioning of the nerves) such as herpes zoster (shingles) and diabetic neuropathies.

WHO Three-Step Ladder Approach

The World Health Organization (WHO) recommends a three-step ladder approach to the management of chronic cancer pain (see Figure 24-7). This approach focuses on the intensity of the pain, and patients do not necessarily progress through the three steps. Step 1 of the analgesic ladder suggests a nonopioid analgesic and the possibility of an adjuvant analgesic. If the patient receives the maximum recommended dose of nonopioids and continues to experience pain, step 2 recommends adding an opioid. It appears that there is no difference between steps 2 and 3; however, in practice, the difference is in the choice of analgesic. For example, opioid analgesics at step 3 should be available by a variety of routes (e.g. oral, rectal, subcutaneous). They should also have a short half-life in order to increase the dosage for severe, escalating (increasing) pain (McCaffery and Pasero, 1999: 117).

However, over 20 years since the introduction of the three-step ladder approach, there have been several modifications to the ladder with one modification omitting step two of the ladder completely. Interesting to note is that Vargas-Schaffer (2010) suggests adding a fourth step to the ladder for the treatment of crisis chronic pain. According to Vargas-Schaffer (2010) the fourth step should consider e.g. nerve blocks, epidurals and spinal stimulators.

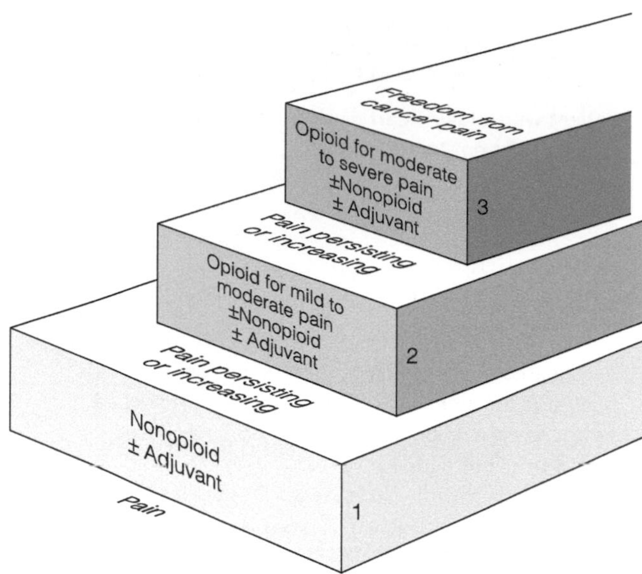

Figure 24-7 The WHO three-step analgesic ladder.

Source: *Cancer Pain Relief*, 2nd edn, by World Health Organization, 1996, Geneva: Author. Reprinted with permission.

Routes for Opiate Delivery

Opioids have traditionally been administered by oral, subcutaneous, intramuscular, intravenous infusions, transdermal drug therapy (patches), continuous subcutaneous infusions and epidural infusion.

Oral

Oral administration of opiates remains the preferred route of delivery because of ease of administration. Patients prefer oral medication as it is less invasive. Long acting or sustained relief medication can be prescribed, and until the required dose is established e.g. oramorph solution or fentanyl lozenges can be prescribed for break through pain.

Transdermal

Transdermal drug therapy is advantageous in that it delivers a relatively stable plasma drug level and is non-invasive. Fentanyl is an opioid frequently used as a skin patch with various dosages. It provides drug delivery for up to 72 hours.

Rectal

Several opiates are now available in suppository form. The rectal route is particularly useful for patients who have dysphagia (difficulty swallowing) or nausea and vomiting.

Subcutaneous

Although the subcutaneous (SC) route has been used extensively to deliver opioids, another technique uses subcutaneous catheters and infusion pumps to provide continuous subcutaneous infusion (CSCI) of narcotics. CSCI is particularly helpful for patients (a) whose pain is poorly controlled by oral medications, (b) who are experiencing dysphagia or gastrointestinal obstruction or (c) who have a need for prolonged use of parenteral narcotics. CSCI involves the use of a small, light, battery-operated pump that administers the drug through a #23- or #25-gauge butterfly needle. The needle can be inserted into the anterior chest, the subclavicular region, the abdominal wall, the outer aspects of the upper arms or the thighs. This method via a syringe driver is often the preferred choice for end stage cancer pain management.

Intramuscular

The intramuscular (IM) route is the least desirable route for opioid administration because of variable absorption, pain involved with administration and the need to repeat administration every 3–4 hours.

Intravenous

The intravenous (IV) route provides rapid and effective pain relief with few side-effects. The analgesic can be administered by IV bolus or by continuous infusion controlled by the patient using a patient-controlled analgesia (PCA) machine at the bedside (see the discussion of PCA later in this chapter).

Intraspinal

An increasingly popular method of delivery is the infusion of opiates into the epidural or intrathecal (subarachnoid) space (see Figure 24-8). Intraspinal analgesia acts directly on opiate receptors in the dorsal horn of the spinal cord. Two commonly used medications are morphine sulphate and fentanyl. The major benefit of intraspinal drug therapy is that it exerts a lesser sedative effect compared to systemic opiates. The epidural space is most commonly used because the dura mater acts as a protective barrier against infection, including meningitis. Because the epidural catheter is in a space and not a blood vessel, a continuous epidural infusion may be stopped for hours and restarted without concern that the catheter has become occluded (blocked) (McCaffery and Pasero, 1999: 37).

Intraspinal analgesia can be administered by three methods:

1 *Bolus.* For some surgical procedures (e.g. caesarean section), a single bolus may provide sufficient pain control for up to 24 hours. After this time, the patient may be given oral or IV analgesia.
2 *Continuous infusion administered by pump.* The pump may be external (for acute or chronic pain) or implanted (for chronic pain).
3 *Patient-controlled epidural analgesia (PCEA).* Patient-controlled epidural analgesia is administered by the patient using a pump. This is similar to patient-controlled analgesia: a basal rate may meet the patient's analgesic needs but, if not, the patient can push a button to deliver a preset dose. PCEA is often used to manage acute post-operative pain, chronic pain and intractable cancer pain.

Temporary catheters, used for short-term acute pain management, are usually placed at the lumbar or thoracic vertebral level and often removed after 2–4 days. Permanent catheters, for patients with chronic pain, may be tunnelled subcutaneously through the skin and exit at the patient's side. Tunnelling of the catheter reduces the risk of infection and displacement of the catheter. After the catheter is inserted, the nurse is responsible for monitoring the infusion and assessing the patient.

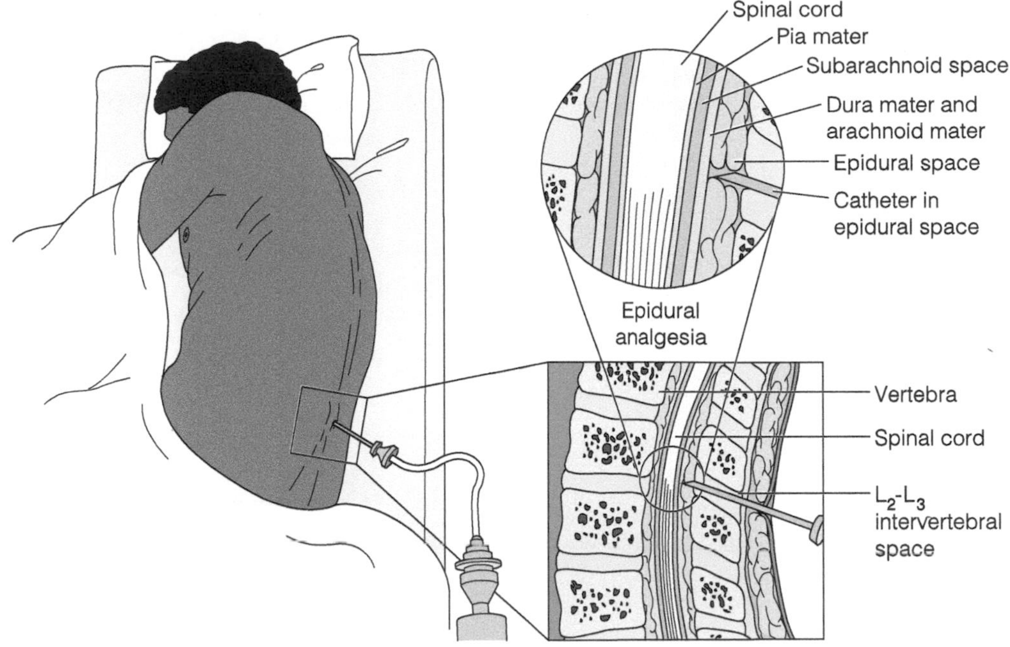

Figure 24-8 Placement of intraspinal catheter in the epidural space.

> **CLINICAL ALERT**
>
> As a precaution, have naloxone, sodium chloride 0.9% diluent, and injection equipment on hand for each patient receiving an opioid-containing epidural infusion (Cox, 2001), as this will reverse the effects of the opioid.

Continuous Local Anaesthetics

Continuous subcutaneous administration of long-acting local anaesthetics into or near the surgical site is a technique being used to provide post-operative pain control. This technique is being used for a variety of surgical procedures including knee arthroplasty, abdominal hysterectomy, hernia repair and mastectomy (Pasero, 2000: 22).

The surgeon inserts a catheter under the subcutaneous tissue and on top of the muscle near or in the surgical wound site. A transparent dressing secures the catheter. The patient is given a loading dose of local anaesthetic before the continuous infusion is started. The catheter is connected to an infusion pump that is set at the rate specified in the prescription.

Nursing interventions for the patient with infusion of a continuous local anaesthetic include:

- Conduct pain assessment and documentation every 2–4 hours while the patient is awake.
- Check the dressing every shift for intactness. The dressing is not usually changed in order to avoid dislodging the catheter.
- Check the site of the catheter. It should be clean and dry.
- Assess the patient for signs of local anaesthetic toxicity (e.g. dizziness; ringing in the ears; a metallic taste; tingling or numbness of the lips, gums or tongue) (Pasero, 2000: 22–23) and notify the doctor if any of the signs are noted.

Patient-Controlled Analgesia

Patient-controlled analgesia (PCA) is an interactive method of pain management that permits patients to treat their pain by self-administering analgesia (McCaffery and Pasero, 1999). The oral route for PCA is most common, but the subcutaneous, intravenous and epidural routes are increasingly being used. The PCA mode of therapy minimises the roller-coaster effect of peaks of sedation and valleys of pain that occur with the traditional method of 'as required' dosing. With the parenteral routes, the patient administers a predetermined dose of an opioid by an electronic infusion pump. This allows the patient to maintain a more constant level of relief yet need less medication for pain relief. Patient-controlled analgesia can be effectively used for patients with acute pain related to a surgical incision, traumatic injury, or labour and delivery, and for chronic pain as with cancer.

While the nurse is responsible for the initial instruction regarding use of the PCA and for the ongoing monitoring of the therapy, many Trusts or Health Boards have specific policies in relation to the initial setting up of the pump. The increasing popularity of the use of PCA has led to increased errors due, for example, to mistakes with the decimal point in converting between milliliters and milligrams or bolus and basal rate, etc. (D'Arcy, 2008). The patient's pain must be assessed at regular intervals and the use of the analgesia should be documented in the patient's record.

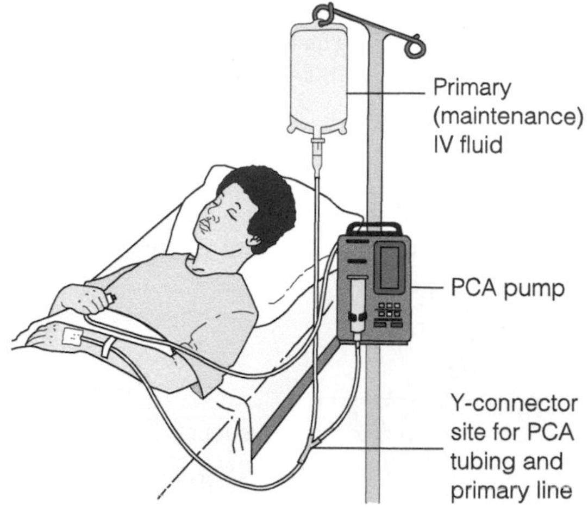

Figure 24-9 PCA line introduced into the injection port of a primary line.

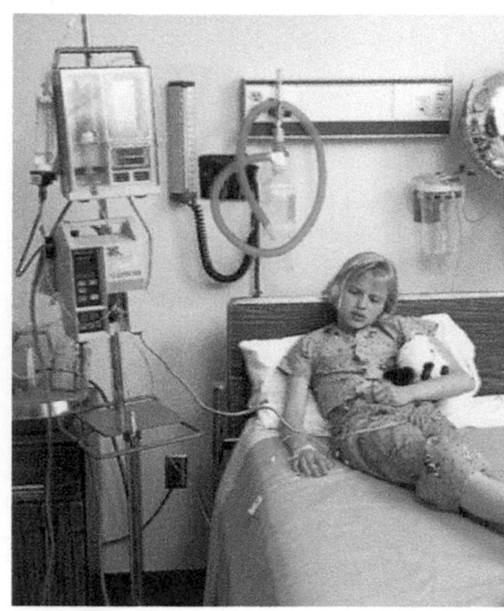

Figure 24-10 The older child is able to regulate a PCA pump.
Source: Pearson Education Ltd.

Patient-controlled analgesia pumps are designed with built-in safety mechanisms to prevent patient overdosage, abusive use and narcotic theft. The most significant adverse effects are respiratory depression and hypotension; however, they occur rarely. Although PCA pumps vary in design, they all have the same protective features. The line of the PCA pump, a syringe-type pump, is usually introduced into the injection port of a primary IV fluid line (see Figure 24-9). When patients want a dose of analgesia, they can push a button attached to the infusion pump and the preset dose is delivered (see Figure 24-10). A programmable lockout interval (usually 10–15 minutes) follows the dose, when an additional dose cannot be given even if the patient activates the button. It is also possible to programme the maximum dose that can be delivered over a period of hours. Many pumps are capable of delivering a low continuous infusion, to provide sustained analgesia during times of rest and sleep. It is imperative that careful selection and accurate assessment of the patient is undertaken prior to PCA selection and that the patient is instructed in the care of the equipment (see *Teaching: Patient Care*).

TEACHING: PATIENT CARE

Patient Self-Management of Pain

Choose a time to teach the patient about pain management when the pain is controlled so that the patient is able to focus on the teaching.

Teaching the patient about self-management of pain can include the following:

- Demonstrate the operation of the PCA pump and explain that the patient can safely push the button without fear of overmedicating.
- Describe the use of the pain scale and encourage the patient to respond in order to demonstrate understanding.
- Explain to the patient the need to notify staff when ambulation is desired (e.g. for bathroom use).

LIFESPAN CONSIDERATIONS

PCA Pump

Children

- Include the parents in teaching.
- Assess the child's ability to use the patient control button.

Mature Adults

- Carefully monitor for drug side-effects.
- Use cautiously for individuals with impaired pulmonary or renal function.
- Assess the patient's cognitive and physical ability to use the patient control button.

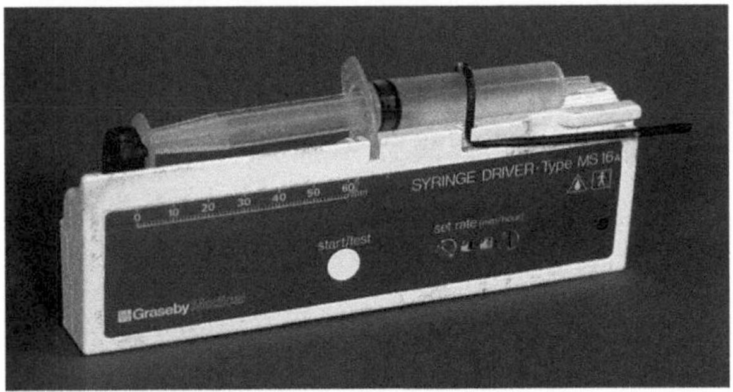

Figure 24-11 Graseby MS16A Syringe Driver.
Source: Wellcome Images, Wellcome Library, London.

Syringe drivers

A syringe driver (see Figure 24-11) or pump is often the preferred choice to administer analgesia and combinations of drugs when managing pain for patients diagnosed with cancer and is often used in coronary care and with neonates. A syringe driver is a battery operated pump infusion device that delivers a predetermined dose via a parental route. Subcutaneous administration is often used in palliative care.

According to Dougherty and Lister (2008) there are many advantages to using this device:

- Combination of drugs administered together.
- Reduces amount of cannulation or needle siting.
- Improves independence.
- Rate and dose can be easily changed.

However, there are some disadvantages which Dougherty and Lister (2008) list as:

- dependency;
- inflammation and/or infection;
- care is needed as different models can be confusing and drug errors are a possibility;
- alarm systems can be problematic.

Nonpharmacological Pain Management

Nonpharmacological pain management consists of a variety of physical and cognitive-behavioural pain management strategies. Physical interventions include cutaneous stimulation, immobilisation, transcutaneous electrical nerve stimulation (TENS) (see Figure 24-12) and acupuncture. Mind–body (cognitive-behavioural) interventions include distraction activities, relaxation techniques, imagery, meditation, hypnosis and therapeutic touch.

Physical Interventions

The goals of physical intervention include providing comfort, altering physiological responses and reducing fears associated with pain-related immobility or activity restriction.

Cutaneous stimulation

Cutaneous stimulation can provide effective temporary pain relief. It distracts the patient and focuses attention on the tactile stimulation and away from the painful sensations, thus reducing pain perception. Cutaneous stimulation techniques include the following:

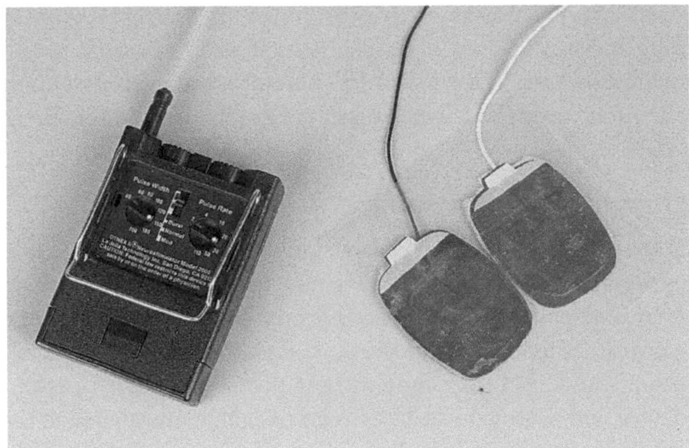

Figure 24-12 A transcutaneous electric nerve stimulator.
Source: Jenny Thomas.

- massage;
- application of heat or cold;
- acupressure.

Cutaneous stimulation can be applied directly to the painful area, proximal (near) to the pain, distal (away from) to the pain and contralateral (opposite side) to the pain. Cutaneous stimulation is contraindicated in areas of skin breakdown.

Massage

Massage is a comfort measure that can aid relaxation, decrease muscle tension and may ease anxiety because the physical contact communicates caring. It can also decrease pain intensity by increasing superficial circulation to the area. Massage can involve the back and neck, hands and arms, or feet. The use of ointments or liniments may provide localised pain relief with joint or muscle pain. Massage is contraindicated in areas of skin breakdown.

Heat and cold applications

A warm bath, heating pads, ice bags, ice massage, hot or cold compresses and warm or cold baths in general relieve pain and promote healing of injured tissues.

Acupressure

Acupressure developed from the ancient Chinese healing system of acupuncture. The therapist applies finger pressure to points that correspond to many of the points used in acupuncture. While using the same areas as acupuncture, acupressure does not involve the use of needles.

Immobilisation

Immobilising or restricting the movement of a painful body part (e.g. arthritic joint, traumatised limb) may help to manage episodes of acute pain. Splints or supportive devices should hold joints in the position of optimal function and should be removed regularly in accordance with agency protocol to provide range-of-motion exercises. Prolonged immobilisation can result in joint contracture (distortion), muscle atrophy (shrinking) and cardiovascular problems such as an increased risk of thrombosis (clot formation). Therefore, patients should be encouraged to participate in self-care activities and remain as active as possible.

Transcutaneous electrical nerve stimulation

Transcutaneous electrical nerve stimulation (TENS) is a method of applying low-voltage electrical stimulation directly over identified pain areas, at an acupressure point, along peripheral nerve areas that innervate the pain area or along the spinal column. The TENS unit consists of a portable, battery-operated device with lead wire and electrode pads that are applied to the chosen area of skin (see Figure 24-12). Cutaneous stimulation from the TENS unit is thought to activate large-diameter fibres and close the pain 'gate', resulting in pain relief. The use of TENS is contraindicated for patients with pacemakers, arrhythmias or in areas of skin breakdown.

Distraction

Distraction draws the person's attention away from the pain and lessens the perception of pain. In some instances, distraction can make a patient completely unaware of pain. For example, a patient recovering from surgery may feel no pain while watching a football game on television, yet feel pain again when the game is over. Different types of distraction include:

- Visual distraction
  - reading or watching TV;
  - watching a football match;
  - guided imagery (using imagination).
- Auditory distraction
  - humour;
  - listening to music.
- Tactile distraction
  - slow, rhythmic breathing;
  - massage;
  - holding or stroking a pet or toy.
- Intellectual distraction
  - crossword puzzles;
  - sudoku;
  - card games (e.g. bridge);
  - hobbies (e.g. stamp collecting, writing a story).

Nonpharmacological Invasive Therapies

A nerve block is a chemical interruption of a nerve pathway, effected by injecting a local anaesthetic into the nerve. Nerve blocks are widely used during dental work. The injected drug blocks nerve pathways from the painful tooth, thus stopping the transmission of pain impulses to the brain. Nerve blocks are often used to relieve the pain of whiplash injury, lower back disorders and cancer.

COMMUNITY CARE CONSIDERATIONS

Pain Management at Home

- Teach patient to keep a pain diary to monitor pain onset, activity before pain, pain intensity, use of analgesia or other relief measures, and so on.
- Instruct patient to contact a healthcare professional if planned pain control measures are ineffective.
- Teach the use of preferred and selected nonpharmacological techniques such as relaxation, guided imagery, distraction, music therapy, massage, and so on.
- Instruct the patient to use pain control measures before the pain becomes severe.
- Inform the patient of the effects of untreated pain.
- Provide appropriate information about how to access community resources, home care agencies, and associations that offer self-help groups and educational materials.

EVALUATING

The goals established in the planning phase are evaluated according to a specific desired outcome. To assist in the evaluation process, nurse documentation or a patient diary may be helpful.

If outcomes are not achieved, the nurse and patient need to explore the reasons before modifying the care plan. The nurse might consider the following questions:

- Is adequate analgesia being given? Would the patient benefit from a change in dose or in the time interval between doses?
- Were the patient's beliefs and values about pain therapy considered?
- Did the patient understate the pain experience for some reason?
- Were appropriate instructions provided to allay misconceptions about pain management?
- Did the patient and their family understand the instructions about pain management techniques?
- Is the patient receiving adequate support from significant others?
- Has the patient's physical condition changed, necessitating modifications in interventions?
- Should selected intervention strategies be reevaluated?

CRITICAL REFLECTION

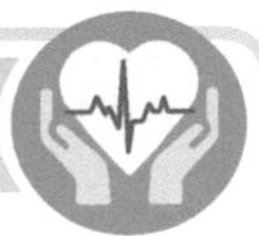

Returning to the case study on page 736 and reflecting on the new knowledge gained from reading the chapter, identify any changes that you would now consider when assessing and managing John's care. Consider the different types of pain, i.e. acute, chronic (non-malignant) and cancer pain (malignant), and identify which is the most applicable to John. Also consider the key issues that are pertinent to managing John's care effectively and explore the barriers for John when managing his pain. Points to consider:

- Psychological and physical assessment
- Acute, chronic (non-malignant) and cancer pain (malignant)
- Pain history
- Prevention of pain
- Culture
- Pain diary
- Understanding of pain management
- Compliance with medication

CHAPTER HIGHLIGHTS

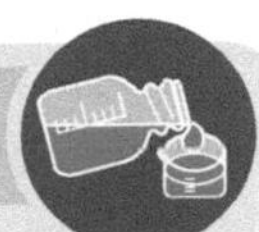

- Pain is a subjective sensation to which no two people respond in the same way. It can directly impair health and prolong recovery from surgery, disease and trauma.
- Pain can be categorised according to its origin - as superfical, deep or referred - or according to its duration - as acute pain or chronic pain.
- Pain threshold is generally similar in all people, but pain tolerance and response vary considerably.
- For pain to be perceived, nociceptors must be stimulated. Three types of pain stimuli are mechanical, thermal and chemical.
- Nociception comprises the physiological processes related to pain perception. It involves four processes: transduction, transmission, perception and modulation.
- According to the gate control theory, small nerve fibres which carry pain impulses to the spinal cord can be blocked by stimulation of the large nerve fibres at a 'gate'.
- Numerous factors influence a person's perception and reaction to pain: ethnic and cultural values, developmental stage, environmental factors and support persons, earlier pain experiences, meaning of pain, and anxiety and stress.
- Pain is subjective, and the most reliable indicator of the presence or intensity of pain is the patient's self-report. Assessment of a patient who is experiencing pain should include a comprehensive pain history.
- Overall patient goals include preventing, modifying or eliminating pain so that the patient is able to partly or completely resume usual daily activities and to cope more effectively with the pain experience.
- When planning, nurses need to choose pain relief measures appropriate for the patient.
- Pain management includes two basic types of nursing interventions: pharmacological and nonpharmacological.
- Scheduling measures to prevent pain is far more supportive of the patient than trying to deal with pain once it is established.
- Major nursing strategies for all patients are to acknowledge and convey belief in the patient's pain, assist family, reduce misconceptions about pain, prevent pain and reduce fear and anxiety associated with the pain.
- Pharmacological interventions, prescribed by the doctor, include the use of opioids, nonopioids/NSAIDs and adjuvant drugs.
- The World Health Organization recommends a three-step ladder approach to the management of chronic cancer pain.
- Analgesic medication can be delivered through a variety of routes and methods to meet the specific needs of the patient. These routes include oral, rectal, transdermal, topical, subcutaneous or intravenous with a continuous infusion or a bolus dose, and intraspinal.
- Patient-controlled analgesia enables the patient to exercise control and treat the pain by self-administering doses of analgesics.
- Physical nonpharmacological pain interventions include such cutaneous stimulation as hot and cold applications, massage and acupressure; transcutaneous electrical nerve stimulation; immobilisation; and acupuncture.
- Cognitive-behavioural interventions include distraction techniques, relaxation techniques, guided imagery, therapeutic touch and hypnosis.

ACTIVITY ANSWERS

ACTIVITY 24-1 There are significant types of pain which are managed differently. In order to provide holistic care to an individual an understanding of these is essential. Reflecting back, you may wish to reflect on patients that you have nursed and consider how their care was managed in relation to the information provided in this chapter. Points to consider are as follows:

- Patient's perception of pain.
- Patient's understanding of pain.
- Patient's acceptance of pain.
- How chronic pain presents itself.
- Symptoms.

REFERENCES

Andrews, M.M. and Boyle, J.S. (2003) *Transcultural concepts in nursing care* (4th edn), Philadelphia, PA: Lippincott, Williams and Wilkins.

Antman, E.M., Bennett, J.S., Daugherty, A., Furberg, C., Roberts, H. and Taubert, K.A.; American Heart Association (2007) 'Use of nonsteroidal anti-inflammatory drugs: An update for clinicians: A scientific statement from the American Heart Association', *Circulation*, 115(12), 1634–1642.

Ball, J.W. and Bindler, R.C. (2003) *Pediatric nursing: Caring for children* (3rd edn), Upper Saddle River, NJ: Prentice Hall.

Beecher, H.K. (1956) 'Limiting factors in experimental pain', *Journal of Chronic Disease*, 4, 11–22.

Bergh, I. and Sjostrom, B. (1999) 'A comparative study of nurses' and elderly patients' ratings of pain and pain tolerance', *Journal of Gerontological Nursing*, 25(5), 30–36.

BNF (2011) *BNF61*, London: BNF.

British Pain Society (2007) *Pain News*, London: The British Pain Society.

Cox, F. (2001) 'Clinical care of patients with epidural infusions', *The Professional Nurse*, 16, 1429–1432.

D'Arcy, Y. (2008) 'Keeping your patient safe during PCA', *Nursing*, 38(1), 50–55.

Dougherty, L. and Lister, S. (2008) *The Royal Marsden Manual of clinical nursing procedures* (7th edn), Oxford: Wiley-Blackwell.

Eliopoulos, C. (2001) *Gerontological nursing* (5th edn), Philadelphia, PA: Lippincott, Williams and Wilkins.

Hardy, J.D., Wolff, H.G. and Goodell, H. (1943) 'Pain threshold in man', *Association of Research into Nervous Mental Diseases*, 23, 1–15.

Hockenberry-Eaton, M. and Wilson, D. (2009) *Wong's essentials of paediatric nursing* (8th edn), St Louis, MO: Mosby.

LaDuke, S. (2002) 'Undertreated pain: Could it land you in court?', *Nursing*, 32, 18.

Main, C. J. and Spanswick, C. C. (2000) *Pain management: An interdisciplinary approach*, Edinburgh: Churchill Livingstone.

McCaffery, M., Ferrell, B.R. and Pasero, C. (2000) 'Nurses' personal opinions about patients' pain and their effect on recorded assessments and titration of opioid doses', *Pain Management Nursing*, 1(3), 79–87.

McCaffery, M. and Pasero, C. (1999) *Pain: Clinical manual* (2nd edn), St Louis, MO: Mosby.

Melzack, R. and Wall, P.D. (1965) 'Pain mechanisms: A new theory', *Science*, 150, 971–979.

NMC (2010) *Standards for pre-registration nursing education*, London: NMC.

Paice, J.A. (2002) 'Controlling pain. Understanding nociceptive pain', *Nursing*, 32(3), 74–75.

Pasero, C. (2000) 'Continuous local anaesthetics', *American Journal of Nursing*, 100(8), 22–23.

Pasero, C. and McCaffery, M. (2002) 'Pain control: Monitoring sedation', *American Journal of Nursing*, 102(2), 67–68.

Vargas-Schaffer, G. (2010) 'Is the WHO analgesic ladder still valid?' *Canadian Family Physician*, 56(6), 514.

Warren, E. (2010) 'Pain: types, theories and therapies', *Practice Nurse*, 39(8), 19–22.

WHO (1996) *Cancer pain relief* (2nd edn), Geneva: WHO.

CHAPTER 25
EMERGENCY MANAGEMENT OF AN ACUTELY ILL PATIENT

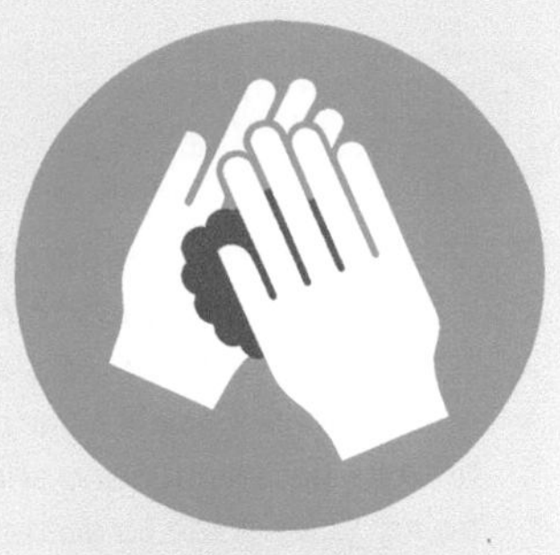

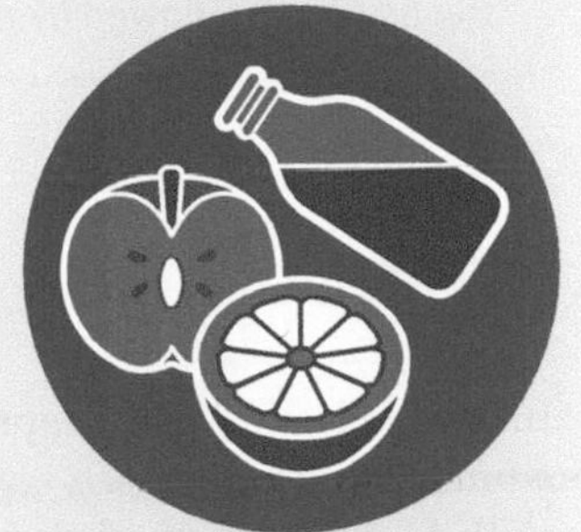

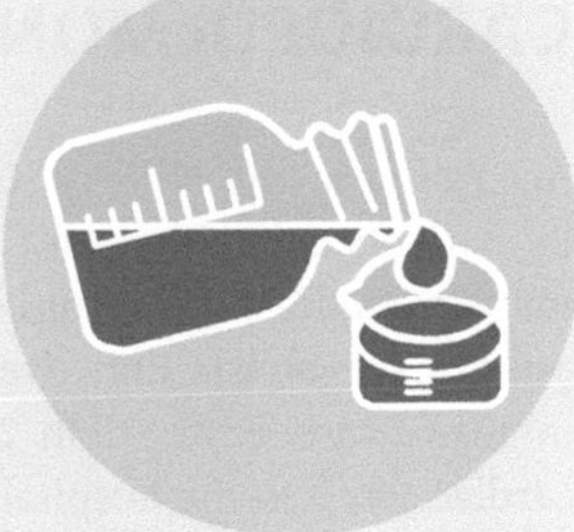

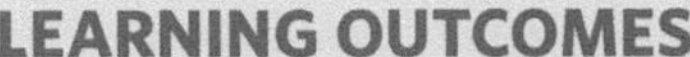

LEARNING OUTCOMES

After completing this chapter, you will be able to:

- Discuss the assessment of the acutely ill patient.
- Explain the initial management of a patient who has become acutely ill.
- Describe the possible causes of cardiac arrest.
- Identify the different ways in which the patient's airway can be protected.
- Describe the systematic procedure for resuscitating an infant, child and adult.
- Discuss the possible reversible causes of cardiac arrest and the range of drugs used in a cardiac arrest.

After reading this chapter you will be able to discuss how to recognise and respond to a patient who is deteriorating and discuss the management of the patient who has suffered cardiac arrest. The chapter relates to **Essential Skills Cluster (NMC, 2010) 9**, as appropriate for each progression point.

Ensure that you really understand this chapter by logging on to your complimentary **MyNursingKit** at **www.pearsoned.co.uk/kozier**. Complete the self-assessment tests to check your progress and utilise further activities to practise and confirm your understanding.

CASE STUDY

Mrs Jacobs is a 72-year-old woman who has been to theatre following an operation to repair a fractured neck of femur. On return from theatre, Mrs Jacobs appears stable; BP 140/70, heart rate is 79 beats per minute (bpm), respiratory rate is 12 breaths per minute and she is alert but sleepy. As per hospital policy you decide to do her observations every 15 minutes for the first hour, followed by every 30 minutes for the next hour.

When you return to Mrs Jacobs to do her second set of observations you note that she is less responsive, only responding when you tell her to open her eyes, her BP is 100/70, heart rate is 115 bpm, and her respiratory rate is 22 breaths per minute. You decide to Fast bleep Mrs Jacobs' medical team. While you are waiting for the doctors to arrive you note that Mrs Jacobs becomes unresponsive.

INTRODUCTION

In England and Wales, approximately 13 million people are admitted to hospital each year (National Patient Safety Agency (NPSA), 2007), many of whom are or become acutely ill. A large proportion of patients who deteriorate and suffer cardiopulmonary arrest show signs of deterioration up to 24 hours before the arrest (Andrews and Waterman, 2005). Therefore early recognition and management of the acutely ill patient can prevent **cardiopulmonary arrest** and reduce mortality (NPSA, 2007) (see Figure 25-1).

EARLY RECOGNITION OF THE ACUTELY ILL PATIENT TO PREVENT CARDIOPULMONARY ARREST

According to the NPSA (2007), there is evidence that acutely ill patients are either not identified or are inappropriately managed in hospital, resulting in up to 23,000 avoidable cardiopulmonary arrests and over 20,000 avoidable admissions to intensive care. Fewer than 20% of adult patients who suffer a cardiac arrest in the hospital environment are discharged home (Peberdy *et al.*, 2003). In order to improve these statistics, the NHS Modernisation Agency (2003) suggested that all staff providing acute care should be able to 'recognise basic signs of deterioration and appreciate the necessity of obtaining timely and appropriate help' (p. 5).

To aid identification of patients at risk of deteriorating, NICE (2007) recommends the use of physiological 'track and trigger' systems to monitor all adults in acute hospital settings. 'Track and trigger' systems are used to detect abnormal physiological parameters in the patient and 'trigger' an appropriate response to those abnormalities based on an aggregate weighted score.

Although widely used with adult patients, the use of 'track and trigger' systems is more sporadic in paediatrics (Monaghan, 2005). One review suggested that 61% of paediatric cardiac arrests were caused by **respiratory failure** and 29% were caused by **shock**, both of which are potentially reversible (Reis *et al.*, 2002). Therefore early recognition and appropriate management of acutely ill paediatric patients may equally prevent cardiopulmonary arrest and reduce mortality (Monaghan, 2005).

A number of different 'track and trigger' systems are in use in the United Kingdom including the patient at risk scoring (PARS) (see Figure 25-2) and the modified early warning systems (MEWS). NICE (2007) do not specify the type of track and trigger system to be used but recommend that the following physiological parameters should be included:

- heart rate;
- respiratory rate;
- systolic blood pressure;
- level of consciousness;
- oxygen saturation;
- temperature.

In specific circumstances the following parameters should be considered:

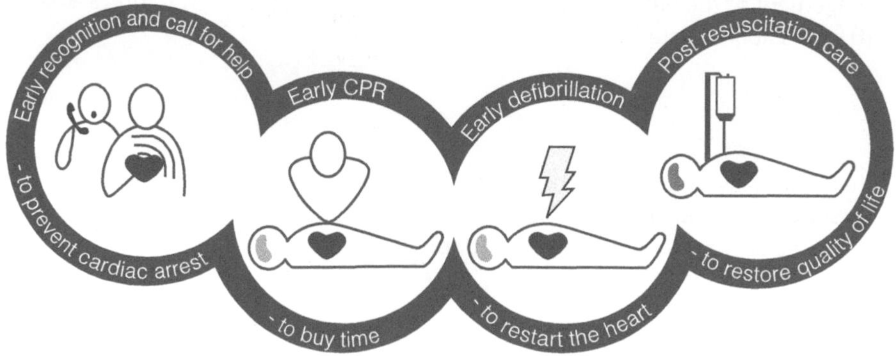

Figure 25-1 Chain of survival.
Source: http://www.beatresponders.org/chainofsurvival.html.

	4	2	1	0	1	2	4
Resp Rate per min	<10			10–14	15–20	21–29	>30
Altered Conscious level				Alert	Confused Or Agitated	Drowsy	Unresponsive Or To pain only
Heart rate per min	<50			50–90	91–110	111–129	>130
Systolic blood pressure (mmHg)	<90	90–110		110–150	150–200		>200
Age				<70	>70		

IF THE TOTAL SCORE FOR YOUR PATIENT >10?

Call Medical Emergency Team 2222

IS THE SCORE >7–10?

Fast bleep the Patient's Team's SHO/SpR
AND FOLLOW PROCEDURES

IS THE SCORE >4–6?

1. Inform the Senior Nurse on the ward/Nurse Practitioner and
2. Inform the Patient's Team or on call Team's SHO/HO and ask them to attend.
3. If unable to attend in <30 mins, call the SpR
4. After a further 30 mins the Patients SpR is unable to attend, then call the Consultant/on call Consultant.

IN THE MEANTIME

MONITOR – RR, O_2 Saturations BP, Pulse
OXYGEN – Administrate 100% oxygen score >7 40% score >4
VENOUS – Prepare Venflons. Blood bottles. Fluids
ECG – Have ready in case needed

Referral to the intensive Therapy Unit is at the discretion of clinical staff. Early referral is encouraged in appropriate patients with high scores or patients whose scores are not improving.

THIS SCORING SYSTEM MUST BE USED AS AN ADJUNCT TO CLINICAL EXPERIENCE AND PROFESSIONAL JUDGEMENT. IT DOES NOT REPLACE COMMON SENSE.

Figure 25-2 Patient at risk (PAR) scoring system.

- hourly urine output;
- biochemical analysis, such as **lactate**, blood glucose, **base deficit**, arterial **pH**;
- pain assessment.

ACTIVITY 25-1

Using the PARS (see Figure 25-2), calculate the following patient's score and state the correct course of action for him.

Mr Jones is a 75-year-old gentleman who has been admitted to the medical ward after collapsing at home. You need to do his observations and the following is noted:

- blood pressure 90/45;
- heart rate 110 bpm;
- respiratory rate 22 breaths per min;
- oxygen saturations 95%;
- he looks very pale and is drowsy.

With children, however, some of these parameters are wholly unsuitable in the early detection of deterioration; for example, blood pressure is a late indicator of shock. Paediatric 'track and trigger' systems have therefore needed to be adapted. The Royal Alexandra Hospital for Sick Children in Brighton have developed a 'track and trigger' system based on three parameters (Monaghan, 2005) (see Figure 25-3):

- behaviour;
- cardiovascular;
- respiratory.

Calling for Assistance

Each organisation should have the necessary arrangements to deal with an emergency clinical situation. Many hospitals have **medical emergency teams** (MET) or **outreach teams** who are alerted by ward staff when a patient shows signs of deterioration. These teams are made up of doctors, anaesthetists and nurses, and are responsible for the effective and safe management of the acutely ill patient.

	0	1	2	3	Score
Behaviour	Playing/ appropriate	Sleeping	Irritable	**Lethargic/confused Reduced response to pain**	
Cardiovascular	Pink or capillary refill 1–2 seconds	Pale or capillary refill 3 seconds	Grey or capillary refill 4 seconds. Tachycardia of 20 above normal rate	**Grey and mottled or capillary refill 5 seconds or above. Tachycardia of 30 above normal rate or bradycardia.**	
Respiratory	Within normal parameters, no recession or tracheal tug	>10 above normal parameters, using accessory muscles, 30+ % Fi02 or 4+ litres/min	>20 above normal parameters recessing, tracheal tug. 40+% Fi02 or 6+ litres/min	**5 below normal parameters with sternal recession, tracheal tug or grunting. 50% Fi02 or 8+ litres/min**	
Score 2 extra for 1/4 hourly nebulisers or persistent vomiting following surgery					

Figure 25-3 Paediatric early warning score.
Source: Royal Alexandra Hospital for Children.

Recognising the Acutely Ill Patient - A Primary Survey

Deteriorating patients may display common physiological signs of failing respiratory, cardiovascular and neurological status. Systematic assessment of the patient will ensure appropriate prioritisation of care. The A–B–C–D–E framework (Resuscitation Council (UK) (2005)) ensures a swift assessment of the acutely ill patient's needs (see Table 25-1).

Table 25-1 A-B-C-D-E Framework

Framework	Assessment	How to assess
A	Airway	Is the patient responsive and talking? YES: Are there abnormal breathing sounds? **Stridor**, wheeze, crackling or gurgling sounds. NO: Follow **cardiopulmonary resuscitation** guidelines.
B	Breathing	Is the patient responsive and talking? YES: Check rate, depth, rhythm and symmetry of breathing (see Chapter 15) and document. NO: Look, listen and feel for breathing (see cardiopulmonary resuscitation guidelines). If no breathing or only occasional gasps, call for MET or cardiac arrest team. Follow cardiopulmonary resuscitation guidelines.
C	Circulation	Is the patient responsive and talking? YES: Check patient's pulse and blood pressure NO: Follow cardiopulmonary resuscitation guidelines.
D	Disability	Is the patient responsive and talking? YES: Assess if patient is orientated to time, day and place. NO: Assess consciousness level using AVPU scale (see cardiopulmonary resuscitation guidelines). Assess using Glasgow Coma Scale (GCS) (see Chapter 11). Assess blood glucose levels.
E	Exposure	Perform a visual top-to-toe assessment of the patient. Are there signs of: • bleeding • haematomas • fractures • rashes/**oedema** (swelling)

CARDIOPULMONARY RESUSCITATION

Resuscitation as a concept has been described since 3000BC with both Mayan and Peruvian Incas using **rectal fumigation** as a means of resuscitation (Hart First Response, 2010). However, it was not until 1891 that closed chest cardiopulmonary resuscitation (CPR), as we know it today, was used in humans (Hart First Response, 2010). Then in the early 1960s training courses were developed in the United States for both healthcare professionals and the general public (Hart First Response, 2010).

Cardiopulmonary resuscitation is an emergency procedure which attempts to restore breathing and spontaneous circulation in a person who has suffered a cardiopulmonary arrest, by external **chest compression**, artificial **ventilation** of the lungs, **defibrillation** and the injection of drugs (BMA, 2007). In order to standardise the assessment and management of patients in cardiopulmonary arrest, the Resuscitation Council (UK) have developed a number of protocols.

- The Resuscitation Council (UK), formed in 1981, reviews and encourages research into the protocols for basic, advanced, paediatric and newborn resuscitation and works closely with the European Resuscitation Council (ERC). Its main objective is to facilitate the education of healthcare professionals and lay persons in the most effective methods of resuscitation.
- The ERC are represented within the International Liaison Committee on Resuscitation (ILCOR) along with the American Heart Association (AHA), the Heart and Stroke Foundation of Canada (HSFC), the Australia and New Zealand Committee on Resuscitation (ANZCOR), the Resuscitation Councils of Southern Africa (RCSA) and the Inter American Heart Foundation (IAHF). ILCOR's sole purpose is to identify and review worldwide international science and knowledge relevant to CPR, as well as to offer consensus on treatment recommendations.

Decisions Related to Cardiopulmonary Resuscitation

The primary goal of healthcare is to maintain and restore patients' health until such point as treatment ceases to work or benefit patients or until the patient refuses any further intervention. Prolonging someone's life is not always appropriate. Quality of life and potential harm that treatments can cause patients need to be considered. Like any treatment, cardiopulmonary resuscitation should only be considered if it will be of benefit to the patient.

Cardiopulmonary resuscitation is an invasive medical treatment that can cause more harm than good in some patients. It is not always successful; in fact, the survival rate after suffering a cardiopulmonary arrest is relatively low (BMA, 2007). Cardiopulmonary resuscitation can cause rib and **sternum** fractures, hepatic and splenic rupture, and can result in a prolonged recovery usually in intensive care, as well as brain damage and permanent disability (BMA, 2007).

The decision to initiate cardiopulmonary resuscitation is, therefore, one that needs to be considered carefully and, if possible, discussed with the patient and their family before the event. Nurses have an important role to play in discussing these delicate issues with patients and their families. Indeed, BMA (2007) suggests that helping patients to come to a decision regarding cardiopulmonary resuscitation is good practice. Currently it is the doctor's responsibility to document Do Not Attempt Resuscitation (DNAR) or Not For Resuscitation (NFR) orders, although nurses can act as the patient's advocate in such decisions. A decision not to resuscitate should be clearly communicated to the patient, family and healthcare professionals and should be reviewed regularly.

In some cases, deciding not to initiate cardiopulmonary resuscitation is clinically relatively straightforward. If there is doubt as to whether resuscitation would benefit the patient, or if there is thought to be little chance that the heart can be restarted, resuscitation need not be commenced. The BMA, RCN and Resuscitation Council (2007) set out guidance regarding decisions related to cardiopulmonary resuscitation (see *Practice Guidelines*).

PRACTICE GUIDELINES

Decisions Related to Cardiopulmonary Resuscitation. Guidance from BMA (2007: p. 3)

- Decisions about CPR must be made on the basis of an individual assessment of each patient's case.
- Advance care planning, including making decisions about CPR, is an important part of good clinical care for those at risk of **cardiorespiratory arrest**.
- Communication and the provision of information are essential parts of good quality care.
- It is not necessary to initiate discussion about CPR with a patient if there is no reason to believe that the patient is likely to suffer a cardiorespiratory arrest.
- Where no explicit decision has been made in advance there should be an initial presumption in favour of CPR.
- If CPR would not re-start the heart and breathing, it should not be attempted.
- When the expected benefit of attempted CPR may be outweighed by the burdens, the patient's informed views are of paramount importance. If the patient lacks capacity, those close to the patient should be involved in discussions to explore the patient's wishes, feelings, beliefs and values.
- If a patient with capacity refuses CPR or a patient lacking capacity has a valid and applicable advance decision refusing CPR, this should be respected.
- A Do Not Attempt Resuscitation (DNAR) decision does not override clinical judgement in the unlikely event of a reversible cause of the patient's respiratory or cardiac arrest that does not match the circumstances envisaged.
- DNAR decisions apply only to CPR and not to any other aspects of treatment.

Early Cardiopulmonary Resuscitation (CPR)

In order to maximise the chance of a patient surviving a cardiopulmonary arrest, it is essential that the four steps of resuscitation or the chain of survival are followed promptly (Resuscitation Council (UK), 2010) (see Figure 25-1 on page 758). The first link in the chain of survival is the early recognition of cardiac arrest and the prompt summoning of help. For in-hospital patient resuscitation, the Resuscitation Council (UK) published a simple algorithm to follow (see Figure 25-4).

The assessment of a collapsed person should be systematic and logical:

- D Danger
- R Response
- S Shout for help (do not leave the patient)
- A Airway
- B Breathing/signs of life
- C Circulation/compressions

When initially approaching a patient who is acutely ill or collapsed, it is important that the nurse assess for danger. The patient, bystanders and nurse should be safe before proceeding to assess the patient. Dangers frequently associated with cardiopulmonary arrest include electrocution, slipping, aggression and infection.

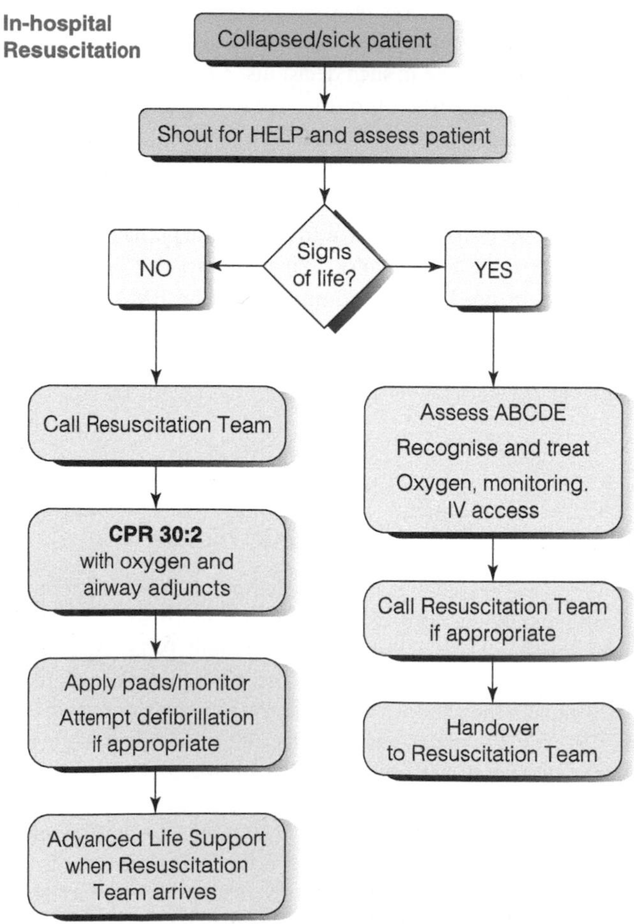

Figure 25-4 Flow chart for in-hospital resuscitation.

Source: Resuscitation Council (UK) 2010. Reproduced with the kind permission of the Resuscitation Council (UK).

Once it is safe to approach the patient, the patient's response needs to be assessed. One of the simplest methods of assessing level of consciousness or responsiveness is the AVPU **scale** (Jevon, 2008):

- Alert – spontaneous eye opening and awareness of surroundings.
- Voice – responds to commands only.
- Pain – responds only to painful stimulus.
- Unresponsive – does not respond to voice or pain.

First, is the patient awake and alert? If so, continue with other methods of assessing the patient's condition (see Chapter 11). If the patient is not awake, check if they respond to your voice. Ask the patient a question, 'Hello, are you alright?'; then give a command, 'Open your eyes!'. If there is no response to voice, administer a painful stimulus.

Painful stimulus assesses the brain's ability to recognise that something is hurting and elicit a response from the patient (Waterhouse, 2005). Over the years, a number of painful stimuli have been used to establish patients' level of consciousness including rubbing the sternum, touching the cornea and pinching the patient; however, many of these cause temporary or permanent injury to the patient. Only acceptable painful stimuli should be used. The trapezium squeeze or pinch is acceptable for both adults and children (Advanced Life Support Group, 2005; Lister and Dougherty, 2008). To administer a trapezium squeeze, squeeze the muscle between the thumb and two fingers where the neck meets the shoulder firmly (see Figure 25-5).

According to the Resuscitation Council (UK) (2010) guidelines, if the patient responds to voice or pain, they should undergo a medical assessment urgently. Depending on local protocol this assessment could be done by the medical emergency or resuscitation team. While waiting for the medical emergency team the patient should be assessed using the A–B–C–D–E framework (see Table 25-1 on page 760). This should include assessment of any injuries or wounds, blood glucose levels, and any other factors that could account for the patient's deterioration or collapse. The patient should be given oxygen (according to local

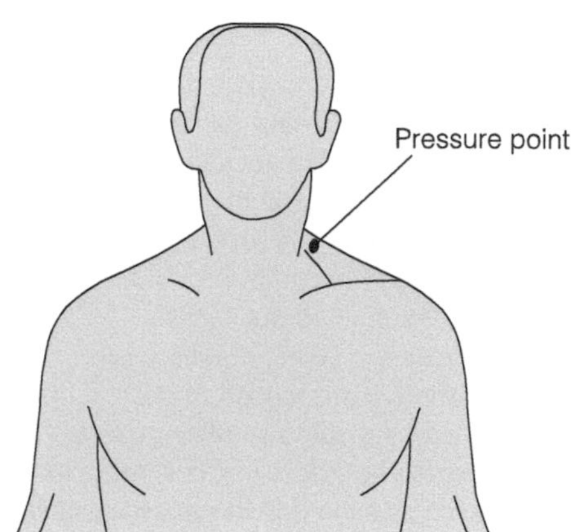

Figure 25-5 The pressure point used when performing a trapezius pinch.

policy), a cardiac monitor should be attached and vital signs recorded. If possible, venous access should be obtained.

If the patient is unresponsive to voice or pain this means that the patient is acutely ill and, as such, help is required immediately. Help should be summoned immediately by shouting or pulling the emergency buzzer if in the hospital setting. If there are two or more responders, one person should stay with the patient while the others seek help. Once help has been summoned, the responder should continue with the assessment of the patient's airway, breathing and circulation.

Assessing the Airway

In order to assess the patient fully, they must be turned onto their back. In the unconscious patient, the tongue and soft palate can cause airway obstruction; therefore manual techniques should be used to open the patient's airway (see Figures 25-6 and 25-7). If there is no risk of cervical spine injury the head-tilt/chin-lift technique should be used (see Figure 25-6). This technique is achieved by placing one hand on the patient's forehead and two fingers under the chin and tilting the head backwards. It is important not to push on the soft tissue of the neck as this could cause airway obstruction, particularly in infants and children.

If there is a risk of cervical spine injury, the **jaw thrust** technique should be used (see Figure 25-7). This is achieved by placing the flat of the hand and thumbs on the cheeks whilst hooking the fingers under the angle of the lower mandible. The lower mandible should be lifted and the head tilted a small amount at a time until the airway is open. It is important that no pressure is placed downwards on the patient's face as this could cause injury. However, it is important to note that a patent airway takes priority over any potential injury to the patient (Resuscitation Council (UK), 2010).

Once the airway is open, any visible foreign bodies or debris that could cause airway obstruction should be removed. Loose fitting dentures, food stuff, vomit and secretions can all cause airway obstruction and should be removed if at all possible. However, well-fitting dentures should remain in place as they can maintain the shape of the patient's face. In the clinical setting, the best way to remove debris from the airway is with suction. If suction equipment is not available then forceps can be used with extreme caution as these can cause injury or push the obstruction further into the airway. Alternative postural manoeuvres can be used to remove debris. Simply turning the head to the side can allow liquid debris to run from the airway. Finger sweeps should not be used as the patient may regain some level of consciousness and bite.

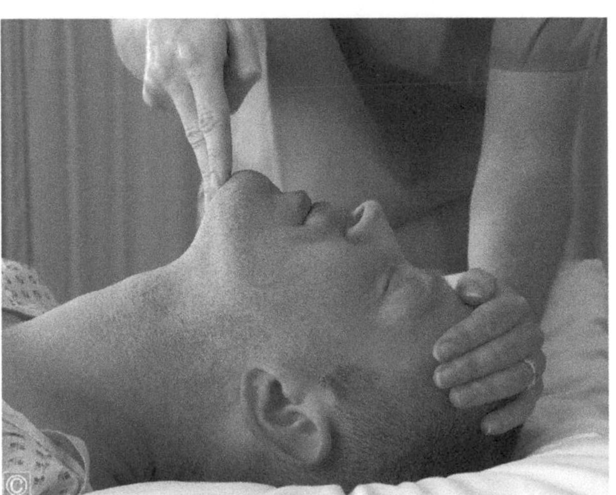

Figure 25-6 Opening the airway using **head tilt chin lift** technique.
Source: reproduced with kind permission by Michael Scott and the Resuscitation Council (UK).

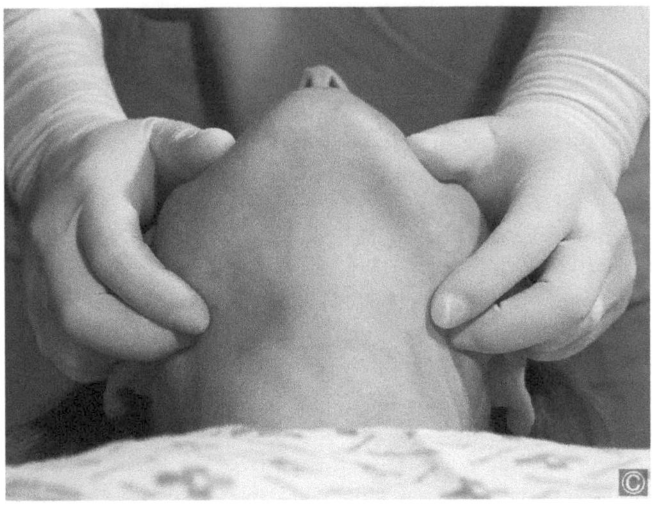

(a)

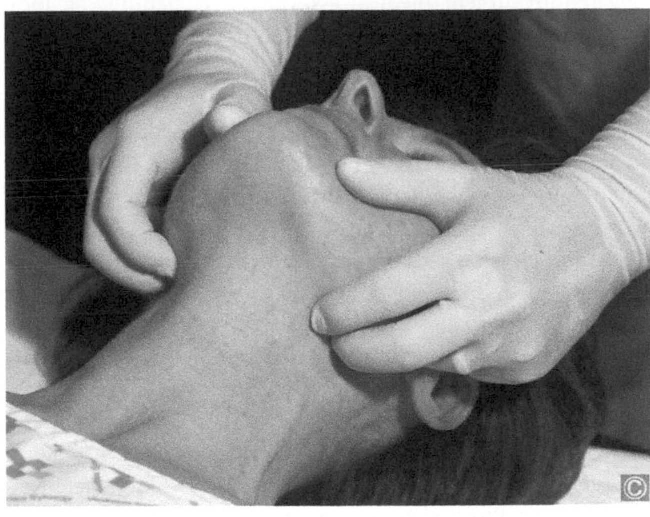

(b)

Figure 25-7 Jaw thrust.
Source: reproduced with kind permission by Michael Scott and the Resuscitation Council (UK).

Assessing for Signs of Life

Once the airway is clear and open, the patient should be assessed to see if there are any signs of life. This is done by simultaneously listening for breath sounds, looking for chest movement and feeling for air on your cheek – Look, Listen and Feel. This should be done for not more than 10 seconds. Occasional gasps or slow, laboured or noisy breathing (**agonal** breathing) should be ignored as this can be the early signs of a cardiac arrest.

Other signs of life include a palpable carotid pulse, swallowing, eye flickering/blinking (visible when eyes are closed) and any movements. Some practitioners may choose to check the carotid pulse for no more than 10 seconds. However, checking a carotid pulse in an emergency situation can be difficult so should be left to experienced practitioners (Resuscitation Council (UK), 2010).

The carotid pulse is located by placing the first and second fingers over the carotid artery. The carotid artery location can be found approximately 2cm either side of the trachea and requires only gentle pressure. It is important to check the carotid on the same side as the nurse; otherwise, damage could be caused to underlying structures or it could be perceived by bystanders that you are strangling the patient.

If the patient is showing signs of life or has a carotid pulse they require urgent medical assessment. Depending on local protocol, this assessment could be done by the medical emergency or resuscitation team. While waiting for the medical emergency team the patient should be assessed using the A–B–C–D–E framework (see Table 25-1). This should include assessment of any injuries or wounds, blood glucose levels, and any other factors that could account for the patient's deterioration or collapse. The patient should be given oxygen (according to local policy), a cardiac monitor should be attached and vital signs recorded. If possible, venous access should be obtained.

If the patient is not showing signs of life then CPR or basic life support (BLS) should be immediately initiated. If the resuscitation team has not already been summoned, they should be called immediately. If there are two or more responders to the collapsed patient, one responder should call the medical emergency team and collect the resuscitation equipment and defibrillator while the others begin CPR (Resuscitation Council (UK), 2010).

Performing Adult CPR

If there are no signs of life, the patient should be given 30 chest compressions, followed by two breaths. Interruptions in the sequence should be minimised and high quality compressions should be maintained at all times (Resuscitation Council (UK), 2010).

In order to perform chest compressions, the heel of one hand should be placed in the middle of the lower half of the sternum (mid nipple line in an average male). The other hand should be placed on top with the fingers interlocked (see Figure 25-8). Pressure should be applied to the sternum through the heel of the hand. Arms should be kept straight and pressure applied from the upper body. Chest compressions should be performed at a rate of at least 100 per minute but no more than 120 compressions a minute, at a depth of one third of the chest (at least 5cm but no more than 6cm) (Resuscitation Council (UK), 2010). The person performing compressions should be changed every 2 minutes to ensure high quality chest compressions (Resuscitation Council (UK), 2010).

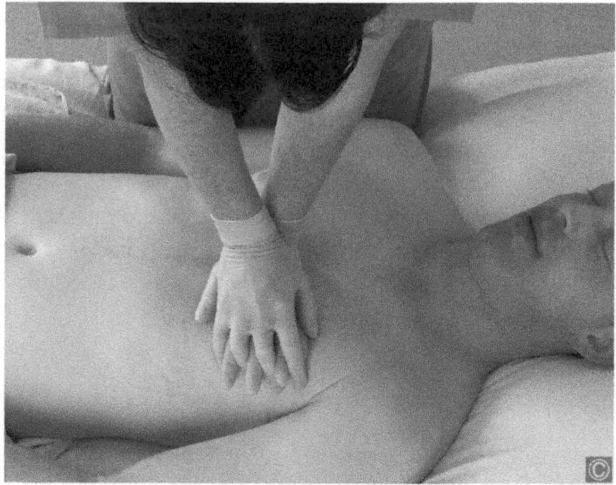

Figure 25-8 Hand position for chest compressions.
Source: reproduced with kind permission by Michael Scott and the Resuscitation Council (UK).

Following the first 30 compressions, two ventilations should be given. The responder should aim for an inspiratory time of 1 second and give enough volume to produce a normal chest rise.

A number of techniques can be used to administer ventilations; mouth to mouth, mouth to **pocket mask** (see Figure 25-9), **bag valve mask device** (see Figure 25-10) or **ventilator**. In the clinical environment, there should be no need to perform mouth to mouth as resuscitation trolleys have the necessary equipment to effectively give ventilations to patients. In order to improve oxygenation, when using a device such as a pocket mask or bag valve mask device, supplemental oxygen should be used at 15L/min.

The bag valve mask device is an effective means of ventilating patients; however, it requires two people to use the device; one to hold the mask on the patient's face and the other to squeeze

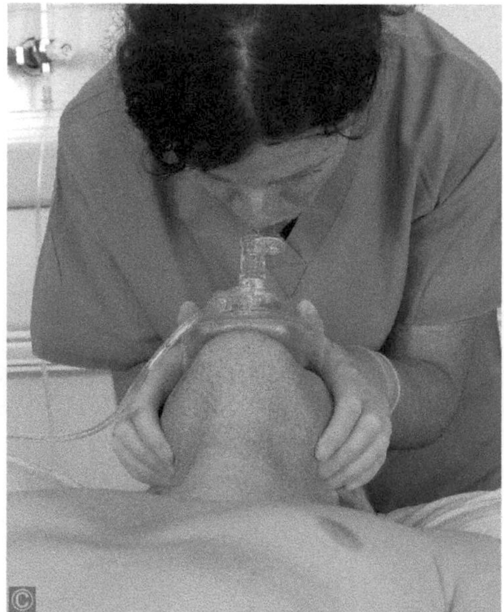

Figure 25-9 Using a pocket mask.
Source: reproduced with kind permission by Michael Scott and the Resuscitation Council (UK).

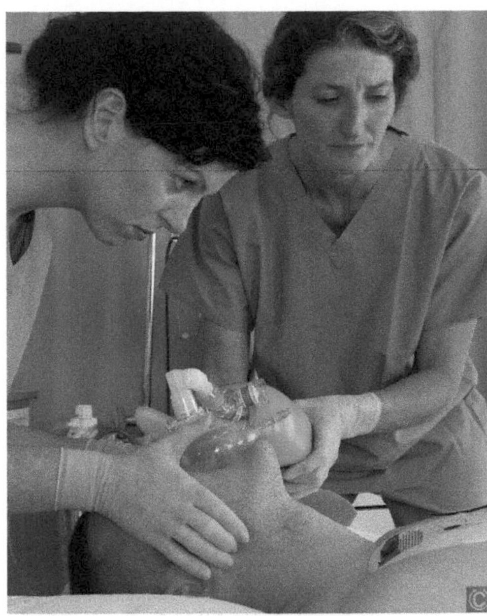

Figure 25-10 Using a bag valve mask device.
Source: reproduced with kind permission by Michael Scott and the Resuscitation Council (UK).

the bag (ventilate the patient). Practitioners experienced at using the bag valve mask may use the device alone. Bag valve mask devices come in a range of sizes for adult, child and neonate lung volumes. The appropriate sized device must be used. With a **reservoir bag** with supplemental oxygen at 15L/min, the patient can receive approximately 80% oxygen. If used without a reservoir bag but attached to high flow oxygen, the patient can receive approximately 40% oxygen and on room air alone 21% oxygen. With any breathing technique, it is important to maintain a good seal around the mouth and nose and not to force air/oxygen into the patient as this can lead to air being forced into the stomach which can result in the patient vomiting.

If an appropriately trained practitioner such as an anaesthetist is available, tracheal intubation should be attempted. Waveform capnography should be used to monitor the quality of CPR in the arrested patient (Resuscitation Council (UK), 2010). Once the airway is secured by tracheal intubation or supraglottic airway device, compressions should be performed uninterrupted at a rate of 100 per minute.

When the defibrillator arrives, it should be immediately attached to the patient with minimal disruption to CPR. Defibrillation can only be attempted by appropriately trained staff, however, the defibrillator can be attached and turned on by untrained personnel.

ACTIVITY 25-2

A patient you are caring for suffers a cardiac arrest. You assess her using D-R-S-A-B-C. What ratio of compressions to ventilations would you use? What would be the most effective way of ventilating the patient?

Performing Paediatric CPR

For the purposes of resuscitation an infant is a child under the age of 1 year and a child is an individual between 1 year and the onset of puberty. A child or infant should be assessed in the same way as an adult, i.e. D–R–S–A–B–C.

Paediatric life support differs from adult life support. Adult cardiac arrests are commonly associated with problems within the heart or circulation, e.g. **myocardial infarction** or **pulmonary embolus**; however, cardiac arrest in children is usually, but not exclusively, associated with airway or breathing problems, e.g. drowning or **asthma**. As a result, if a child or infant is found collapsed, five rescue breaths should be given. While performing these rescue breaths, it is important to note any cough or gag as this will add to your assessment of the signs of life (see Figure 25-11).

In order to give a child over the age of 1 year rescue breaths, ensure head tilt and chin lift, and ventilate the patient. For an infant under the age of 1 year, ensure a neutral position of the head and apply chin lift. If using a pocket mask or bag valve mask, ensure that it is the correct size for child. If using mouth to mouth on an infant, place your mouth over the infant's mouth and nasal apertures. Create an effective seal around the child's mouth/nose and blow steadily into the mouth for about 1–1.15 seconds watching for the chest to rise. Repeat this five

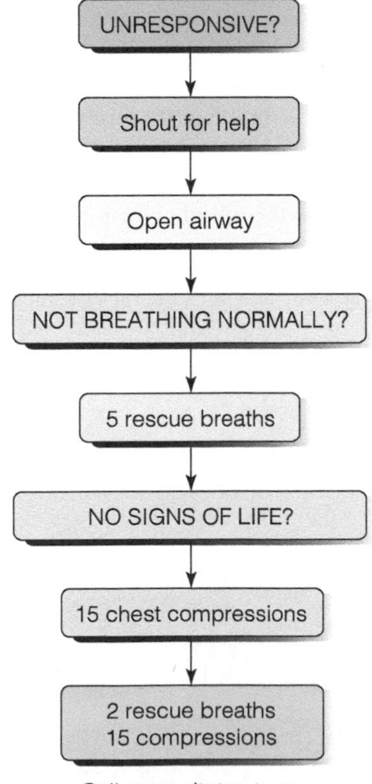

Figure 25-11 Paediatric basic life support flow chart.
Source: Resuscitation Council (UK), 2010. Reproduced with the kind permission of the Resuscitation Council (UK).

times. Make five attempts to achieve effective breaths, otherwise move on to do chest compressions.

If there are signs of life but no effective breathing, continue with rescue breaths and call for assistance. If, however, there are no signs of life, no pulse or a pulse of less than 60 beats per minute and poor perfusion, compressions should be started immediately. Both infants and children should be given 15 chest compressions at a rate of 100–120 per minute followed by two breaths (15:2 ratio). So as to avoid compressing the abdomen, locate the **xiphisternum** and compress the sternum one finger's breadth above this. The compression should be sufficient to depress the sternum by approximately one third of the depth of the chest. In infants this could be achieved by compressing with two fingers while for young children one hand can be used to depress the chest.

Resuscitation should continue until the child shows signs of life, help arrives from the medical emergency (resuscitation) team or paramedics or you become exhausted.

LIFESPAN CONSIDERATIONS

Cardiopulmonary Arrest

Children

Cardiopulmonary arrest in children is uncommon and the aetiology differs from that of adults. Causes of cardiopulmonary arrest in children are usually associated with respiratory problems, sepsis, dehydration and **hypovolaemia**.

AIRWAY ADJUNCTS

Using manual techniques to maintain a patent airway can make ventilation difficult; therefore, airway adjuncts should be used (see Figure 25-12).

The most common form of airway adjunct is the oropharyngeal airway (OPA), and there are readily available in a range of sizes on the resuscitation trolley. An OPA should only be used if the patient is unconscious and has no gag reflex. In order to choose the most appropriate size for the patient, place the OPA from the corner of the mouth at the level of the incisor teeth to the angle of the jaw (see Figure 25-13). To insert the OPA in an adult or child over the age of 8 years, turn the OPA upside down and insert gently into the mouth; when it is approximately one third into the mouth, rotate the OPA and advance the airway until the flange rests on the lips (see Figure 25-14). In infants and children under the age of 8 years, the rotation method should not be used as there is a chance of injury to the soft palate. Insert the OPA the right way up and follow the curvature of the tongue. A tongue depressor can be used to press the tongue down and ease insertion (Cameron *et al.*, 2006). Removal of the OPA, in adults and children, should be done by pulling the OPA out following the curvature of the tongue (down towards the patient's feet). The OPA should be removed if the patient's consciousness level improves or they gag or vomit.

Nasopharyngeal airways (NPA) are used widely in medical and specialist clinical settings. It is an effective way of managing patients' airways where the patient is unable to expectorate

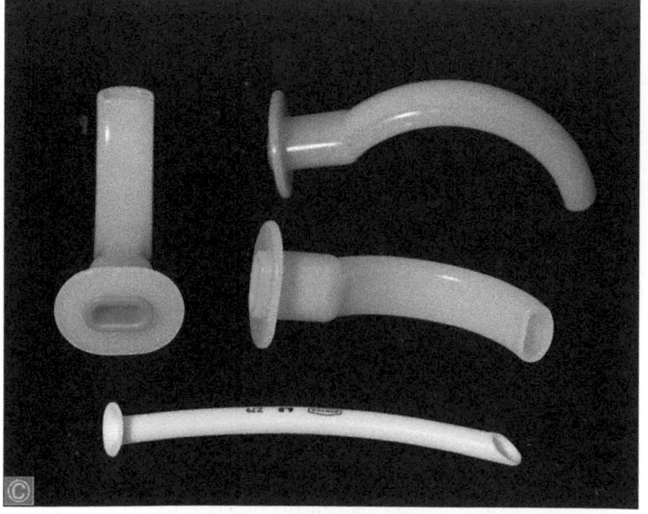

(a)

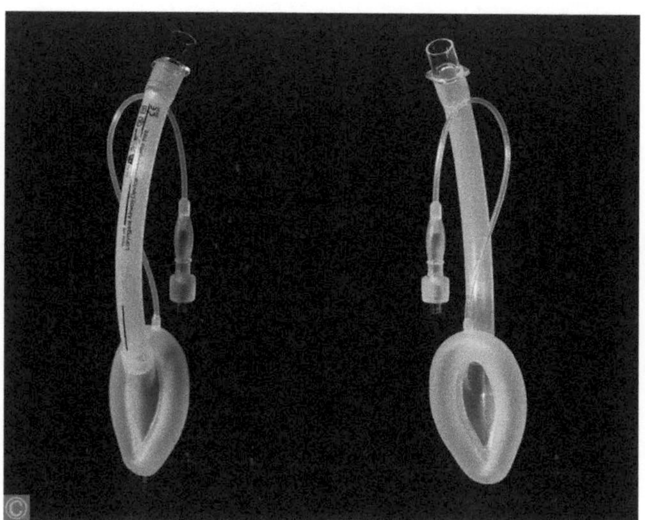

(b)

Figure 25-12 Oropharyngeal airways, nasopharyngeal airways and laryngeal mask airways.
Source: reproduced with kind permission by Michael Scott and the Resuscitation Council (UK).

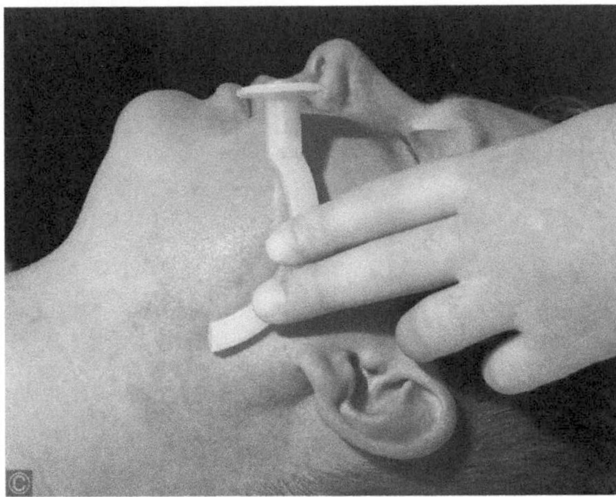

(a)

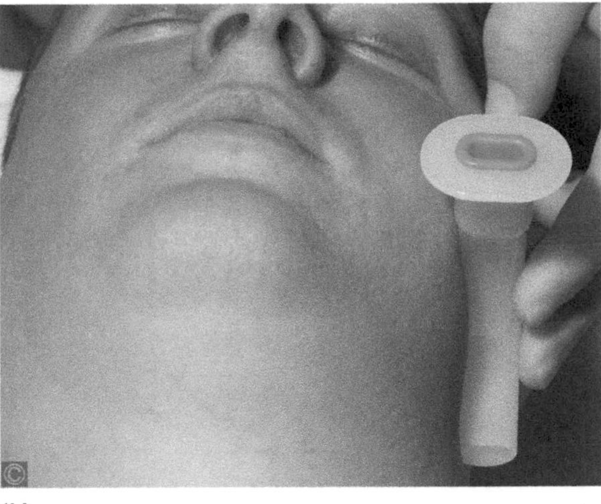

(b)

Figure 25-13 Sizing an oropharyngeal airway.

Source: reproduced with kind permission by Michael Scott and the Resuscitation Council (UK).

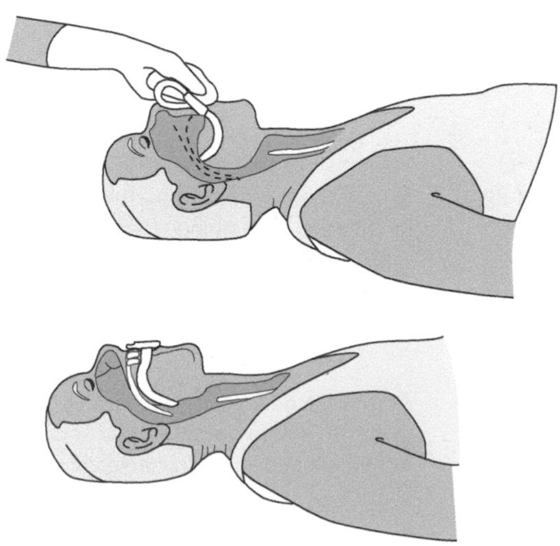

Figure 25-14 Inserting an oropharyngeal airway.

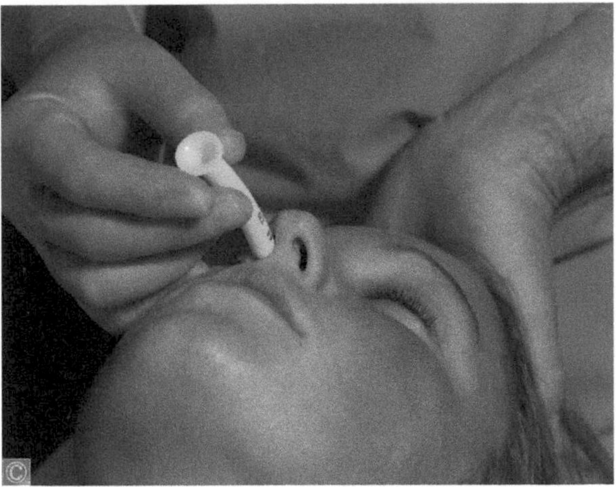

Figure 25-15 Inserting an nasopharangeal airway.

Source: reproduced with kind permission by Michael Scott and the Resuscitation Council (UK).

sputum or has difficulty breathing through the mouth. NPAs are rarely used in cardiopulmonary resuscitation; however, they can be found on most resuscitation trolleys. There are a number of contraindications for the use of NPAs. NPAs should not be used on children or infants, or where there is an actual or potential fracture to the base of the skull, in patients who have facial trauma, maxillofacial surgery or have a broken nose.

Both the internal diameter and length must be considered when choosing an appropriate NPA: too long and it will enter the oesophagus causing **distension** and **hypoventilation**; too short or too narrow and it will be ineffective; too large and it will cause trauma to the nasal passages. Usually a size 6mm is used for female patients and a size 7mm for males. Certain NPAs need to be prepared prior to use. Some manufacturers pack the item sterile with a safety pin to be placed through the end. This needs to be placed through the end of the airway near the flange in order to prevent the airway from going too far into the nostril (the safety pin only goes through the airway and not the patient's nostril), although caution should be exercised when using with a patient with mental health problems.

To insert the NPA, it should be lubricated with a water-based gel and gently inserted into the chosen nostril. The NPA should then be rotated gently and passed slowly down the nasal passage until the end of the NPA is at the anterior nares (see Figure 25-15).

EARLY DEFIBRILLATION

Defibrillation is the application of an electric current to the heart to stop fibrillation of the heart and restore the normal rhythm. Defibrillation is the only treatment for patients presenting with **ventricular fibrillation** (VF) and **pulseless ventricular tachycardia** (VT). With every one minute delay in defibrillation, for patients in VF or VT, their chance of survival decreases by approximately 7–10% (Resuscitation Council (UK), 2010). Therefore, when a patient collapses with suspected cardiac arrest the defibrillator must be brought to the patient's side as

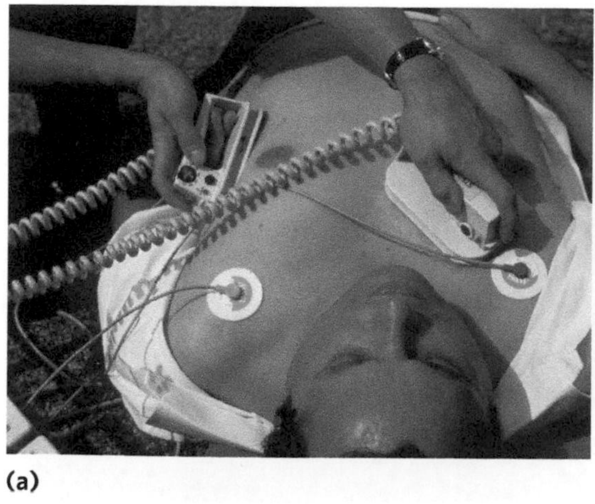
(a)

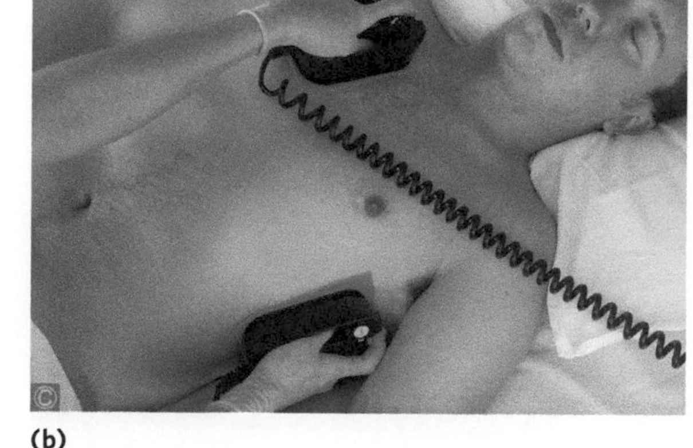
(b)

Figure 25-16 Defibrillator electrode positions.
Source: Science Photo Library Ltd/Adam Hart-Davis.

a matter of urgency. However, it is important to note that only those that have received appropriate training should attempt to use the defibrillator.

The electrical current or shock applied to the heart is delivered from two electrodes or paddles placed on the chest. The electrodes are placed on the ride side of the chest below the right clavicle and in the mid axilla line at the level of the base of the heart on the lower ribs (see Figure 25-16). The shock stops the heart instantaneously, which may allow the pacemaker centres within the heart to take control.

Defibrillation is an integral component of the universal cardiac treatment algorithm (see Figure 25-17). One shock is given followed by two minutes of CPR. During the two minutes of CPR, appropriately trained persons will administer drugs (see Table 25-2) and explore and treat the possible reversible causes of the arrest (see Table 25-3).

Table 25-2 Commonly Used Drugs in Cardiopulmonary Resuscitation

Drug	Adult dose and route	Child dose and route	Action
Epinephrine (Adrenaline)	1mg (10ml of 1:10000) intravenously (IV) or intraosseusly (IO) after the third round of defibrillation and every 3-5 minutes thereafter.	10mcg/kg IV/IO every 3-5 minutes.	Adrenaline is the first-line cardiac arrest drug. It causes vasoconstriction, increased systemic vascular resistance and increases cerebral and coronary perfusion. It also increases myocardial excitability, when the myocardium is hypoxic or ischaemic.
Amiodarone	300mg IV/IO (if not pre-diluted, it must be diluted in 5% dextrose to 20ml). Ideally should be given via a central line, but in an emergency can be given peripherally. A further 150mg can be given followed by an infusion of 900mg over 24 hours.	5mg/kg IV/IO.	Administered for refractory VF/VT, haemodynamically stable VT and other resistant tachyarrhythmias.
Magnesium sulphate	2g (4ml of 50% magnesium sulphate) IV/IO over 1-2 minutes. This dose can be repeated after 10-15 minutes.	25-50mg/kg IV/IO (to a maximum of 2g).	Administered for refractory VF when hypomagnesaemia is possible or ventricular tachyarrhythmias when hypomagnesaemia is possible.
Lidocaine	1mg/kg	Use only if amiodarone unavailable. 1mg/kg IV/IO.	Administered for refractory VF/pulseless VT (when amiodarone is unavailable).
Sodium bicarbonate	50mmol (50ml of 8.4% solution).	1-2ml/kg of 8.4% solution.	Administered for tricyclic antidepressant overdose and **hyperkalaemia**. Should not be routinely used in cardiac arrests.
Calcium chloride	10ml of 10% calcium chloride IV repeated according to blood results.	0.2ml/kg of 10% calcium chloride IV.	Administered for cardiac arrest caused by hyperkalaemia, hypocalcaemia or an overdose of calcium channel-blocking drugs.

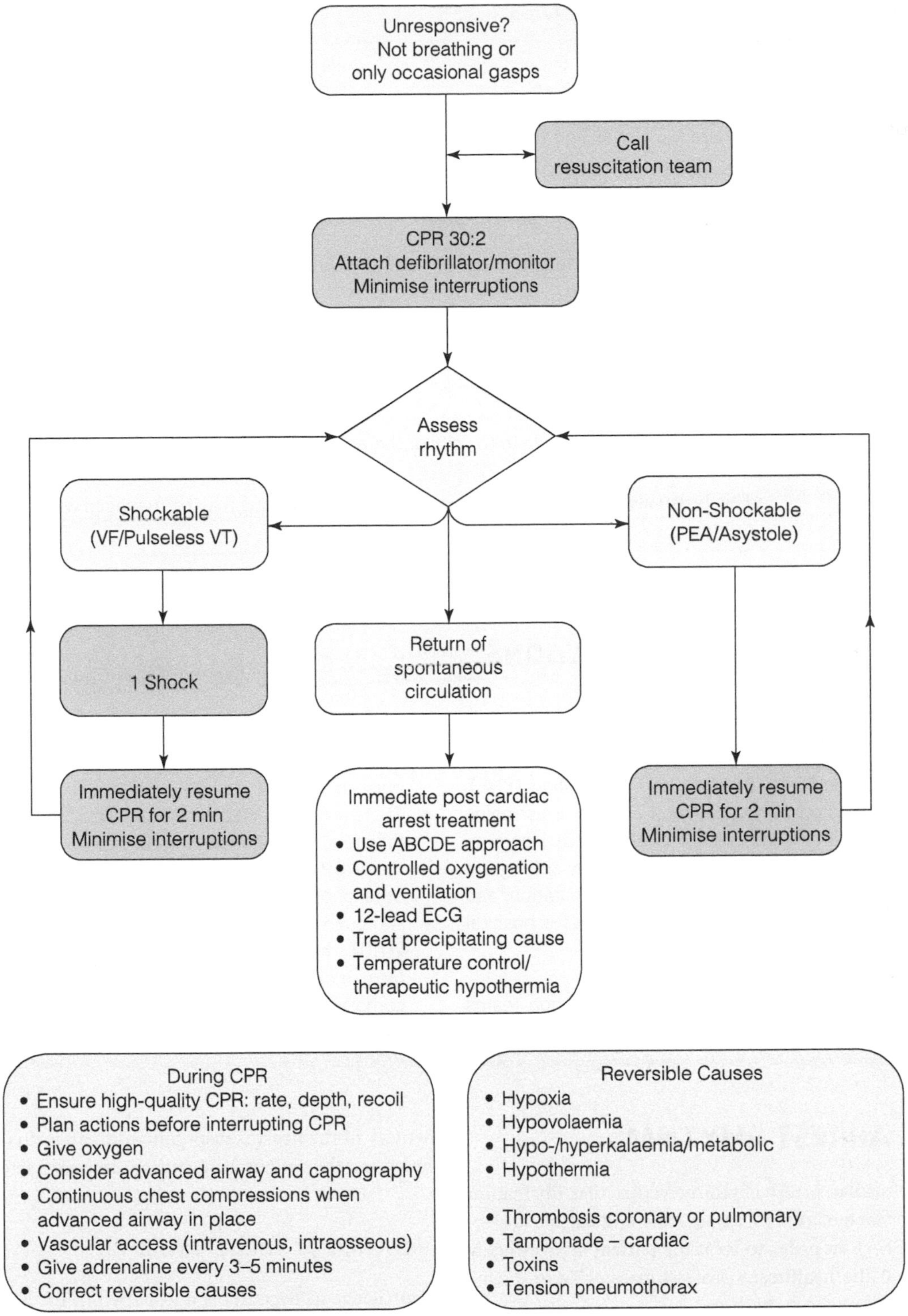

Unresponsive?
Not breathing or
only occasional gasps

Call
resuscitation team

CPR 30:2
Attach defibrillator/monitor
Minimise interruptions

Assess
rhythm

Shockable
(VF/Pulseless VT)

1 Shock

Immediately resume
CPR for 2 min
Minimise interruptions

Return of
spontaneous
circulation

Immediate post cardiac
arrest treatment
- Use ABCDE approach
- Controlled oxygenation and ventilation
- 12-lead ECG
- Treat precipitating cause
- Temperature control/ therapeutic hypothermia

Non-Shockable
(PEA/Asystole)

Immediately resume
CPR for 2 min
Minimise interruptions

During CPR
- Ensure high-quality CPR: rate, depth, recoil
- Plan actions before interrupting CPR
- Give oxygen
- Consider advanced airway and capnography
- Continuous chest compressions when advanced airway in place
- Vascular access (intravenous, intraosseous)
- Give adrenaline every 3–5 minutes
- Correct reversible causes

Reversible Causes
- Hypoxia
- Hypovolaemia
- Hypo-/hyperkalaemia/metabolic
- Hypothermia

- Thrombosis coronary or pulmonary
- Tamponade – cardiac
- Toxins
- Tension pneumothorax

Figure 25-17 Adult advanced life support algorithm.

Source: Resuscitation Council (UK), 2010. Reproduced with the kind permission of the Resuscitation Council (UK).

CLINICAL ALERT

When any drug is administered in a cardiac arrest the cannula that it is given through should always be flushed with a minimum of 20ml of fluid.

Table 25-3 Potentially Reversible Causes of Cardiac Arrest

Cause	Treatment
Four H's	
Hypoxia	Secure the airway and ventilate the lungs with oxygen at the highest concentration ideally 100%.
Hypovolaemia	Ensure intravenous access and give intravenous fluid if hypovolaemia is suspected.
Hyper/**H**ypokalaemia and metabolic disturbances	Take an arterial blood gas sample to monitor electrolytes and administer appropriate treatment as necessary.
Hypothermia	Maintain core body temperature within normal limits by using warming blankets and warmed intravenous fluids.
Four T's	
Tension pneumothorax	Insert chest drain or large bore intravenous cannula to allow the collapsed lung to reinflate.
Tamponade	Usually relieved by emergency surgery or aspiration of the fluid with a large needle by an experienced healthcare practitioner.
Toxic/**T**herapeutic disturbances	Patient history may allude to toxicity or therapeutic disturbances. Administer appropriate treatment as necessary.
Thrombo-embolic	This is usually as a result of a clot in the heart or lung. This may be managed with **thrombolytic** drugs.

COMMUNITY CARE CONSIDERATIONS

Resuscitation in the Community

The survival rate for people who suffer a cardiac arrest out of hospital is less than 10% (British Heart Foundation (BHF), 2010) with the most common cause of cardiac arrest being ventricular fibrillation (Jevon and Halliwell, 2006). However, the principles of resuscitation in the community setting are fundamentally the same as for in-hospital resuscitation, and community staff are trained to the same standards as hospital staff. However, there are some differences:

- There are no medical emergency or resuscitation teams available in the community. Therefore expert help should be sought from paramedics/ambulance personnel by telephoning 999.
- There may be limited access to advanced care such as defibrillators, resuscitation drugs and airway adjuncts. However, many GP surgeries, shopping centres, train stations and other public places now have defibrillators readily available.
- Although mouth-to-mouth ventilations are ideal (BHF, 2010), the practitioner may be unwilling/unable to perform mouth-to-mouth therefore they can just perform compressions at a rate of 100–120 compressions a minute (Resuscitation Council (UK), 2010).

CARDIAC ARREST RHYTHMS

There are four cardiac arrest rhythms: ventricular fibrillation (VF), **ventricular tachycardia** (VT), **asystole** and **pulseless electrical activity** (PEA). In order to treat the patient appropriately it is essential that the healthcare professional is able to distinguish between each of these rhythms.

Ventricular Fibrillation

Ventricular fibrillation is the single largest cause of sudden cardiac death in the Western world (Ten Tusscher *et al.*, 2007). It is a fatal, chaotic rhythm that results in uncoordinated contraction of the ventricles (see Figure 25-18). As the electrical activity of the heart is disorganised there is no output from the heart and the patient is in cardiopulmonary arrest.

Ventricular Tachycardia

Ventricular tachycardia is a fast rhythm of the heart that does not allow the atria and ventricles to fill and empty effectively (see Figure 25-19). VT can be pulsed or pulseless. If a patient presents in VT and has a pulse, this is a medical emergency and could lead to a pulseless VT. Pulseless VT is treated in the same way as VF. Both VF and VT require defibrillation. The most common cause of VF and VT is myocardial infarction or other cardiac event.

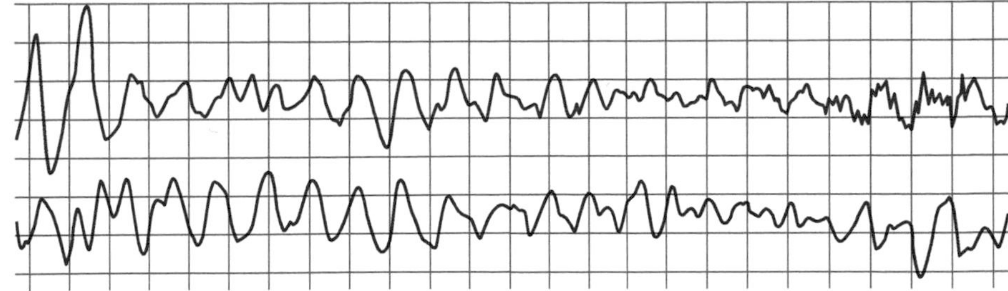

Figure 25-18 Ventricular fibrillation (VF).

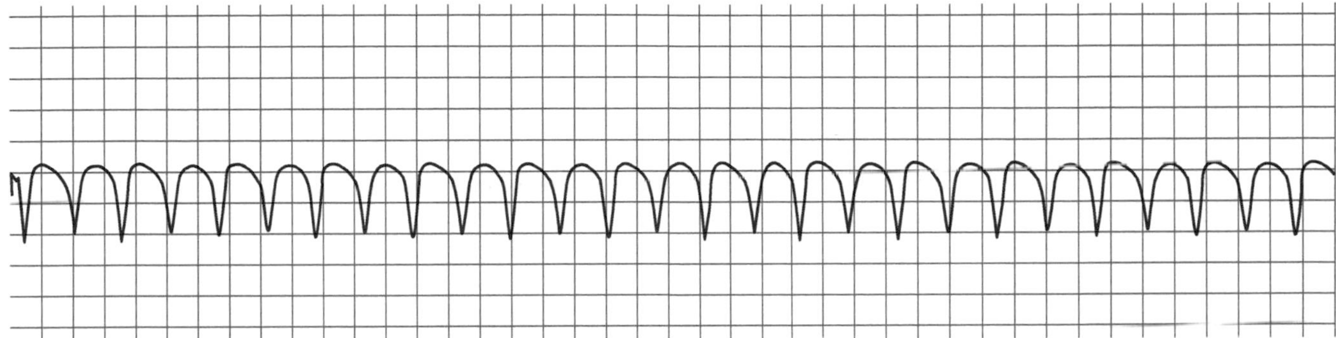

Figure 25-19 Ventricular tachycardia (VT).

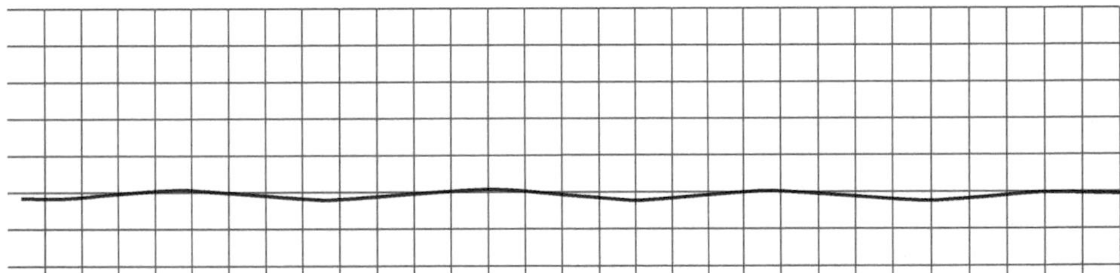

Figure 25-20 Asystole.

Asystole

Asystole is the absence of electrical activity within the heart (see Figure 25-20). Although described as a 'flat line', it is in fact represented as an undulating line on an **electrocardiogram (ECG)**.

Pulseless Electrical Activity

Pulseless electrical activity, on the other hand, is a term used to describe a cardiac arrest with normal or life-sustaining electrical activity (see Figure 25-21). Asystole and PEA are the commonest rhythms associated with in-hospital cardiac arrests and have the poorest prognosis as these rhythms will not respond to defibrillation.

ACTIVITY 25-3

You attach a defibrillator to a collapsed patient and note that she is in asystole. Does this rhythm require defibrillation? How would you manage this type of cardiac arrest?

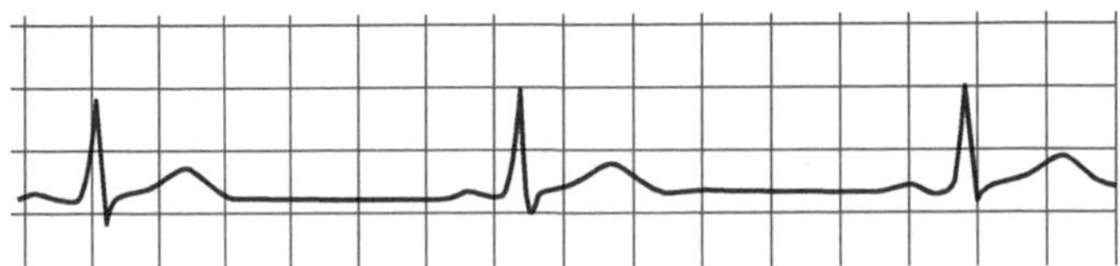

Figure 25-21 Pulseless electrical activity (PEA).

RESEARCH NOTE

Immediate Life Support (ILS) Training Impact in a Primary Care Setting?

This quasi-experimental and qualitative study aimed to evaluate immediate life support (ILS) training in the primary care setting. Data was collected by feedback forms, pre/post course knowledge and skills tests and by focus group interview from 170 healthcare professionals in Devon and Cornwall. The findings from the study showed that knowledge and skill retention following the ILS course was significantly higher than in basic life support (BLS) courses indicating the added value of ILS. The researchers felt that skill decline in those who are not updated regularly is significant and that the issues with funding and staff resources needed to be addressed.

Source: Based on Cooper, S., Johnston, E. and Priscott, D. (2007) 'Immediate life support (ILS) training impact in a primary care setting?' *Resuscitation*, 72, 92–99.

POST-RESUSCITATION CARE

Following successful resuscitation, the patient requires expert post-resuscitation care. This is usually undertaken in a critical care environment, where the patient will be monitored closely by experienced healthcare practitioners. If the patient's consciousness level is compromised or they are unable to breathe post-resuscitation, they may require endotracheal intubation and artificial ventilation. They may also have circulatory problems such as arrhythmias or low blood pressure/**cardiac output** which may require the administration of specialised medications. Post-resuscitation care will involve further investigations for the surviving patient:

- 12 lead ECG to detect any post-resuscitation arrhythmias/cardiac **ischaemia**.
- Full blood count to detect infection/anaemia.
- Urea and electrolytes to detect electrolyte imbalances/blood glucose levels/renal impairment/check cardiac enzymes.
- Arterial blood gas to check adequate oxygenation and acid–base balance.
- Chest X-ray to check position of endotracheal tube and central line and to exclude **pneumothorax/pulmonary aspiration/pulmonary oedema**/fractures.

It is important to note that therapeutic hypothermia can be of benefit to the comatosed patient who has experienced either a non-shockable or shockable cardiac arrest (Resuscitation Guidelines (UK), 2010).

CRITICAL REFLECTION

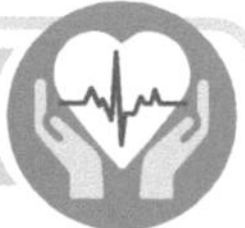

Let us revisit the case study on page 758. Now you have read this chapter, what were the signs of deterioration in Mrs Jacobs? What was Mrs Jacobs patient at risk (PAR) score? Was Mrs Jacobs appropriately managed? What would you include in the assessment of a collapsed patient?

CHAPTER HIGHLIGHTS

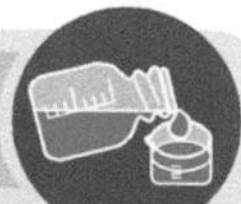

- The systematic assessment of the acutely ill patient is essential.
- Early recognition of the acutely ill patient can prevent a cardiac arrest from occurring.
- A number of patient at risk scoring systems have been developed in order to detect deterioration in the patient.
- Patient at risk scoring systems consider a variety of physicological parameters, e.g. blood pressure, to predict the risk of deterioration.
- Prompt assessment and early access to expert help are essential to the patient's chance of survival.
- Prompt CPR, defibrillation and advanced care can improve the outcome of the cardiac arrest.
- Airway adjuncts and ventilation devices may also be used as part of the management of the patient being resuscitated.
- A number of drugs are available to assist in the management of a patient in cardiac arrest.
- Identification and treatment of the potentially reversible causes of cardiac arrest (four H's and four T's) can improve the outcome of the arrest.

ACTIVITY ANSWERS

ACTIVITY 25-1 The patient's PAR score is 8. The correct course of action would be to fast bleep the patient's SHO/SpR and monitor the patient.

ACTIVITY 25-2 The ratio of compressions to ventilations is 30:2. Compressions should be performed at a rate of at least 100 per minute at a depth of 5-6cm. Inspiratory time of ventilations should be 1 second with enough volume given to produce normal chest rise. Ideally we would want to maintain a clear airway and allow for effective ventilations through tracheal intubation and use of a bag valve device.

ACTIVITY 25-3 Asystole does not require defibrillation as there is no electrical activity within the heart to organise. Therefore, the management of this patient would be CPR and trying to find out the cause of the arrest by going through the 4Hs and 4Ts. Adrenaline can be given every 3-5 minutes and electrolyte would be resolved by administering appropriate drugs, e.g. calcium.

REFERENCES

Advanced Life Support Group (2005) *Advanced paediatric life support: The practical approach* (4th edn), London: Blackwell.

Andrews, T. and Waterman, H. (2005) 'Packaging: A grounded theory of how to report physiological deterioriation effectively', *Journal of Advanced Nursing*, 52(5), 473–81.

British Heart Foundation (2010) *'Chest compressions and mouth-to-mouth skill 'ideal' says new UK guidance'*, London: BHF available at http://www.bhf.org.uk/default.aspx?page=12416 (accessed 1st July 2011).

BMA (2007) 'A joint statement from the British Medical Association, the Resuscitation Council (UK) and the Royal College of Nursing: Decisions relating to cardiopulmonary resuscitation', London: BMA, available at http://www.bma.org.uk/ethics/cardiopulmonary-resuscitation/CPR Decisions 07.jsp (accessed 1st July 2011).

Cameron, P., Jelinek, G., Everitt, I., Browne, G. and Raftos, J. (2006) *Textbook of paediatric emergency medicine*, Edinburgh: Churchill Livingstone.

Cooper, S., Johnston, E. and Priscott, D. (2007) 'Immediate life support (ILS) training impact in a primary care setting?' *Resuscitation*, 72, 92–99.

Hart First Response (2010) *Quick history of resuscitation*, Fleet: Hart First Response, available at http://www.hartfirstresponse.org.uk/CPRhistory2.html (accessed 1st July 2011).

Jevon, P. (2008) 'Neurological assessment. Part 1 – assessing level of consciousness', *Nursing Times*, 104(27), 26–27.

Jevon, P. and Halliwell, D. (2006) 'Principles of resuscitation in primary care', *Nursing Times.net*, available at http://www.nursingtimes.net/nursing-practice-clinical-research/principles-of-resuscitation-in-primary-care/201582.article (accessed 1st July 2011).

Lister, S. and Dougherty, L. (2008) *The Royal Marsden Hospital manual of clinical nursing procedures*. Oxford: Wiley-Blackwell.

Monaghan, A. (2005) 'Detecting and managing deterioration in children', *Paediatric Nursing*, 17(1), 32–35.

NHS Modernisation Agency (2003) *Critical Care Outreach 2003: Progress in developing services*, London: DH, available at www.dh.gov.uk/en/Publicationsandstatistics/Publications/PublicationsPolicyAndGuidance/DH_4091873 (accessed 1st July 2011).

NICE (2007) *Acutely ill patients in hospital: Recognition of and response to acute illness in adults in hospital*, CGSO, London: NICE.

NMC (2010) *Standards for pre-registration nursing education*, London: NMC.

NPSA (2007) *The fifth report from the Patient Safety Observatory. Safer care for the acutely ill patient: Learning from serious incidents*, London: NPSA.

Peberdy, M.A., Kaye, W., Ornato, J.P., Larkin, G.L., Nadkarni, V., Mancini, M.E., Berg, R.A. and Lane-Trultt, N.T. (2003) 'Cardiopulmonary resuscitation of adults in the hospital: A report of 14720 cardiac arrests from the National Registry of Cardiopulmonary Resuscitation', *Resuscitation*, 58, 297–308.

Reis, A.G., Nadkarni, V., Perondi, M.B., Grisi, S. and Berg, R.A. (2002) 'A prospective investigation into the epidemiology of in-hospital Paediatric cardiopulmonary resuscitation using the International Utstein reporting style', *Paediatrics*, 109, 200–209.

Resuscitation Council (UK) (2010) *Resuscitation Guidelines 2010*, London: RC (UK), available at http://www.resus.org.uk/pages/guide.htm (accessed 1st July 2011).

Ten Tusscher, K.H.W.J., Hren, R. and Panfilov, A.V. (2007) 'Organisation of ventricular fibrillation in the human heart', *Circulation Research*, 100, 87–101.

Waterhouse, C. (2005) 'The Glasgow Coma Scale and other neurological observations', *Nursing Standard*, 19(33), 56–64.

Williams, M.A. and Rushton, C.H. (2009) 'Justified use of painful stimuli in the coma examination: a neurological and ethical rationale', *Neurocritical Care*, 10, 408–413.

CHAPTER 26
PRE- AND POST-OPERATIVE CARE

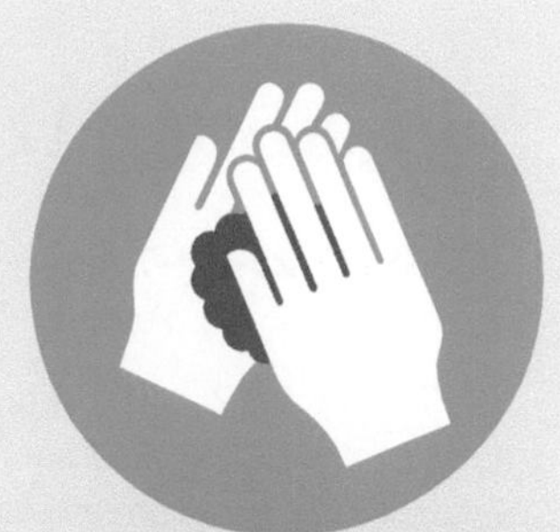

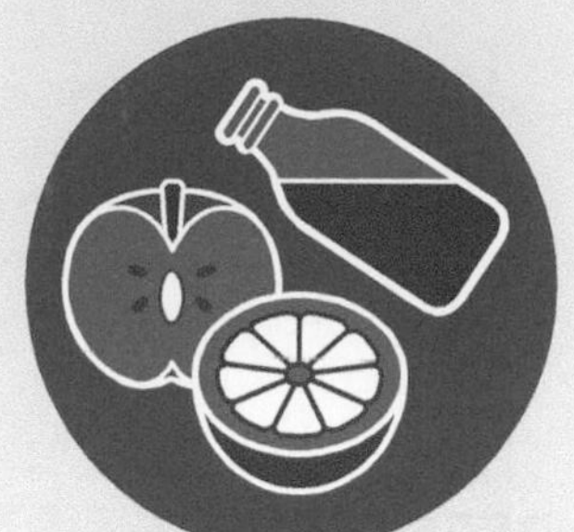

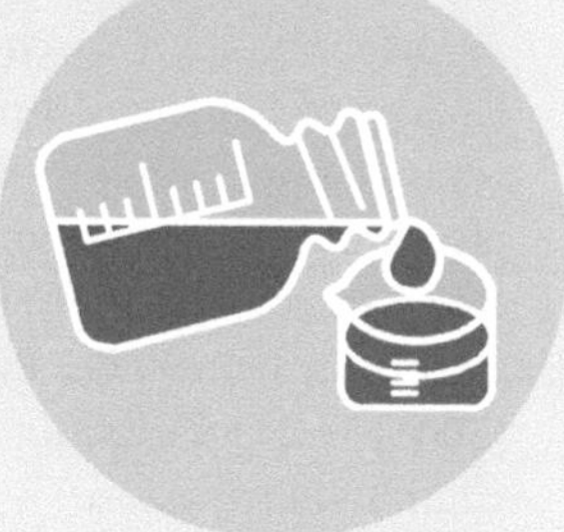

LEARNING OUTCOMES

After completing this chapter, you will be able to:

- Describe the phases of surgery.
- Discuss various types of surgery according to degree of urgency, degree of risk and purpose.
- Identify essential aspects of pre-operative assessment.
- Identify nursing responsibilities in planning pre- and post-operative nursing care.
- Describe essential pre-operative teaching, including pain control, moving, leg exercises and coughing and deep-breathing exercises.
- Describe essential aspects of preparing a patient for surgery, including skin preparation.
- Identify essential nursing assessments and interventions during the immediate post-anaesthetic phase.
- Demonstrate ongoing nursing assessments, interventions and evaluation of the care provided to the post-operative patient.
- Identify potential post-operative complications and describe nursing interventions to prevent them.
- Describe appropriate wound care for a post-operative patient.

After reading this chapter you will be able to demonstrate appropriate care for the patient in both the pre- and post-operative settings. It relates to **all of the Essential Skills Clusters (NMC, 2010)**, as appropriate for each progression point.

Ensure that you really understand this chapter by logging on to your complimentary **MyNursingKit** at **www.pearsoned.co.uk/kozier**. Complete the self-assessment tests to check your progress and utilise further activities to practise and confirm your understanding.

CASE STUDY

Mr Teng is a 77-year-old man with a history of chronic obstructive pulmonary disease (COPD). Currently, his respiratory condition is being controlled with medications and he is free of infection. He has just been transferred to the recovery unit following the repair of an uncomplicated hernia performed under spinal anaesthesia. His blood pressure is 132/88, pulse 84, respirations 28 and tympanic temperature 36.5°C (97.8°F). He is awake and stable.

After reading this chapter you will be able to identify the factors that place Mr Teng at increased risk of complications during and after surgery and understand why he was given a spinal anaesthesia as opposed to a general anaesthesia.

INTRODUCTION

Mr Teng's decision to undergo a surgical procedure was probably not taken lightly as it can be a terrifying thought. But imagine the prospect of having surgery before the advent of modern anaesthesia and pain relief. Well, that is what faced people living in the Middle Ages. In those days, surgery was a crude practice and not considered to be a skilled trade as it is today. Yet they still performed complex operations such as amputations, setting of broken bones and replacing dislocations. If the patient was lucky when undergoing these surgical procedures they were given opium as an anaesthetic which merely served to dull the pain.

You may think that surgery was only performed by trained physicians, but this was not the case in the Middle Ages. In fact, physicians, who were well educated, felt it was beneath them to actually perform surgery but chose to diagnose their patients by examining and treating the outside of the body. The forerunners of medicine and surgery were in fact barbers. The 'Barber Surgeons', as they became known, were extremely versatile and innovative characters acting not only as barbers but also as local doctors and dentists. The most well-known barber surgeon from the 16th century, Frenchman Ambroise Paré, is said to be the founder of modern surgery as he developed a number of surgical techniques that are still used today, in particular the ligating or tying off of blood vessels to control bleeding during surgery.

Despite these developments, death following surgery was extremely common, particularly for those undergoing amputations. In fact, the most common cause of death post-surgery was infection and this remained so until the mid-19th century when the French chemist Louis Pasteur discovered that the death of body tissue was caused by bacteria in the air. Simultaneously, a Hungarian physician, Ignaz Semmelweiss, demonstrated that the transmission of infectious diseases could be reduced by hand washing. With this knowledge, in 1865, Joseph Lister, a renowned British surgeon, developed antiseptic techniques, including the use of carbolic acid, to kill bacteria in his operating theatres.

Modern day surgery has benefited from these and other pioneers. In particular it has benefited from the development of effective anaesthesia in the 1840s. Ether and chloroform, the first anaesthetic agents to be used, helped to alleviate patient suffering. Effective anaesthesia meant that more intricate operations could be performed to the internal organs of the body. This advanced knowledge of both the human body and surgical techniques.

Today, surgery is much more advanced and less traumatic for patients as a result of these developments. In fact, it has become a commonplace occurrence in hospitals, with over nine million patients undergoing procedures or interventions each year (Hospital Episode Statistics, 2009). The types of surgery available to patients have become progressively more sophisticated over the past 20–30 years with the advent of less invasive techniques such as keyhole surgery and a number of different types of surgery are available. Advancing techniques, an increase in surgical workload and increasing pressure to reduce waiting lists have led to more and more minor operations being performed in community hospitals and general practitioner practices. This has obviously had an impact on nursing provision within these environments as there must be adequate care for patients undergoing surgery.

CLASSIFICATION OF SURGERY

Surgery is classified according to its purpose, whether it is urgent or not and the degree of risk associated with the surgery.

Purpose

Surgical procedures may be categorised according to their purpose:

- *Diagnostic* – confirms or establishes a diagnosis, for example biopsy of a mass in a breast.
- *Palliative* – relieves or reduces pain or symptoms of a disease; it does not cure, for example, resection of nerve roots.
- *Ablative* – removes a diseased body part, for example removal of a gallbladder (cholecystectomy).
- *Constructive* – restores function or appearance that has been lost or reduced, for example breast implant.
- *Transplant* – replaces malfunctioning structures, for example hip replacement.

Degree of Urgency

Surgery is classified by its urgency and necessity to preserve the patient's life, body part or body function. Emergency surgery is performed immediately to preserve function or the life of the patient. Surgeries to control internal haemorrhage or repair a fracture are examples of emergency surgeries. Elective surgery is performed when surgical intervention is the preferred treatment for a condition that is not imminently life threatening (but may ultimately threaten life or well-being) or to improve the patient's life. Examples of elective surgeries include cholecystectomy for chronic gallbladder disease, hip replacement surgery and plastic surgery procedures such as breast reduction surgery.

Degree of Risk

Surgery is also classified as major or minor according to the degree of risk to the patient. Major surgery involves a high degree of risk, for a variety of reasons: it may be complicated or prolonged; large losses of blood may occur; vital organs may be involved; or post-operative complications may be likely. Examples are organ transplant, open heart surgery and removal of a kidney. In contrast, minor surgery normally involves little risk, produces few complications and is often performed in a 'day surgery'. Examples are breast biopsy, removal of tonsils and knee surgery.

The degree of risk involved in a surgical procedure is affected by the patient's age, general health, nutritional status, use of medications and mental status. There are particular health problems that increase surgical risk:

- **Malnutrition** – can lead to delayed wound healing, infection and reduced energy. Protein and vitamins are needed for wound healing; vitamin K is essential for blood clotting.
- **Obesity** – leads to hypertension, impaired cardiac function and impaired respiratory ventilation. Obese patients are also more likely to have delayed wound healing and wound infection because adipose tissue impedes blood circulation and its delivery of nutrients, antibodies and enzymes required for wound healing.
- **Cardiac conditions** – such as angina pectoris, recent myocardial infarction, hypertension and heart failure weaken the heart. Well-controlled cardiac problems generally pose minimal operative risk.
- **Blood coagulation disorders** – may lead to severe bleeding, haemorrhage and subsequent shock.
- **Upper respiratory tract infections or chronic obstructive lung diseases** – can adversely affect pulmonary function, especially when renal disease impairs regulation of the body's fluids and electrolytes and excretion of drugs and other toxins.
- **Diabetes mellitus** – predisposes the patient to wound infection and delayed healing.
- **Liver disease (e.g. cirrhosis)** – impairs the liver's abilities to detoxify medications used during surgery, produce the prothrombin necessary for blood clotting and metabolise nutrients essential for healing.
- **Uncontrolled neurological disease such as epilepsy** – may result in seizures during surgery or recovery.

Although there may be different types of surgery each surgical procedure will have three distinct phases: pre-operative, intra-operative and post-operative. Together these make up the total management of a patient undergoing surgery.

The *pre-operative phase* begins when the decision to have surgery is made and ends when the patient is transferred to the operating table. The nursing activities associated with this phase include assessing the patient, identifying potential or actual health problems, planning specific care based on the individual's needs, and providing pre-operative teaching for the patient and their family and friends.

The *intra-operative phase* begins when the patient is transferred to the operating table and ends when the patient is admitted to the recovery unit. The nursing activities related to this phase include a variety of specialised procedures designed to create and maintain a safe therapeutic environment for the patient and the healthcare personnel.

The *post-operative phase* begins with the admission of the patient to the recovery unit and ends when healing is complete. During the post-operative phase, nursing activities include assessing the patient's physiological and psychological response to surgery, performing interventions to facilitate healing and prevent complications, teaching and providing support to the patient and their family and friends, and planning for their discharge. The goal is to assist the patient to achieve the most optimal health status possible following surgery.

Regardless of the type of surgery a patient is to undergo, all will go through this process. What will differ is the length of each phase. For instance, a person who has been in a road traffic accident who requires emergency surgery will have a short pre-operative phase while a patient who has a chronic condition may have a longer pre-operative phase in order to ensure they are at their optimum health status before surgery.

PRE-OPERATIVE PHASE

Pre-operative care is the psychological and physical preparation of the patient for surgery and involves a number of nursing interventions. It must be said that the psychological preparation of the patient is equally as important as their physical preparation as inadequate psychological preparation and anxiety can have a negative impact on post-operative recovery (Kagan and Bar-Tal, 2008). In fact it has been found that the more anxious patients are, the more pain they experience post-operatively (Vaughn *et al.*, 2007). Psychological preparation involves informing and obtaining written consent for the procedure and allaying any unnecessary fears that the patient may have.

Most hospitals have policies and protocols for the physical preparation of patients for surgery. These usually involve:

- A thorough assessment of the patient including the patient's surgical and anaesthetic background, and risk factors such as impaired healing, drug or alcohol abuse, malnutrition.
- Pre-operative investigations such as blood tests and x-rays.
- Preparation of the patient, such as improving nutritional status, administration of bowel preparations to clear the bowels, skin preparation such as shaving.

The type of physical and psychological preparation required depends on a number of factors, such as the type of surgery and the individual patient. Regardless of the type of surgery and preparation required, all patients will be required to give their consent to the procedure.

Informed Consent

Prior to any nursing, surgical or medical intervention, the patient should give their consent to the intervention. Indeed the Nursing and Midwifery Council (NMC, 2008) states that nurses have a professional responsibility to ensure that patients in their care consent to these interventions.

But what is **informed consent**? According to UK law, patients have the right to **self-determination** or the right to choose their own fate voluntarily, which basically means they have their own free will. The law also states that healthcare professionals have a duty to provide the patient with sufficient information in order for the patient to make informed choices.

In the clinical environment this means that the health professional needs to gain consent before continuing with the desired intervention. As far as surgical procedures are concerned, the surgeon is responsible for ensuring that valid consent is obtained from the patient, but the nurse may be involved in the clarification of certain aspects of the procedure. If it is not clear that the patient understands and consents to the surgery, the nurse should contact the surgeon before surgery proceeds.

Pre-operative informed consent should include:

- nature and intention of the surgery;
- name and qualifications of the person performing the surgery;
- risks, including tissue damage, disfigurement or even death;
- chances of success;
- possible alternative measures;
- the right of the patient to refuse consent or later withdraw consent.

Informed consent is only possible when the patient understands the information being provided, that is, speaks the language and is conscious, mentally competent and not sedated. As far as the treatment of children is concerned, they may be able to give their consent to surgery depending on whether they have sufficient understanding and intelligence to be able to make up their own mind. This is known as the **Gillick principle** which stems from a judgment made in the House of Lords in 1985 which held that a doctor could lawfully prescribe contraception to a girl under the age of 16 without the consent of her parents. (See Chapter 4 for further details on informed consent and the Gillick principle.)

PRE-OPERATIVE ASSESSMENT

Pre-operative assessment should include the gathering of information from the patient, their medical and nursing notes to establish what their physical, psychological and social needs are both pre-operatively and post-operatively. The most essential pre-operative information that should be gathered is summarised in the *Practice Guidelines*.

Physical Assessment

Pre-operatively, the nurse will perform a brief physical assessment. This will form baseline information that can be used to evaluate the patient post-operatively. For example, the nurse will assess the patient's mental status by recording their Glasgow Coma and establishing if they are orientated to time and place and have the ability to understand what is happening. This information will then be used to establish the patient's mental status and alertness after surgery. Also the nurse will perform respiratory and cardiovascular assessments, not only to provide baseline data for evaluating the patient's post-operative status but also to alert the nurse to any underlying problem (e.g. a respiratory infection or irregular pulse rate) that may affect the patient's response to surgery and anaesthesia. Other systems (gastrointestinal, genitourinary and musculoskeletal) may also be examined to provide baseline data (see Chapter 11). However, it is important to note that it is not only the nurse that will assess the patient pre-operatively; the patient will also be assessed by the surgeon and the anaesthetist.

Routine investigations and tests are given in Table 26-1.

Table 26-1 Routine Pre-operative Investigations and Tests

Test	Rationale
Full blood count (FBC)	Red blood cells (RBC), haemoglobin (Hb) and haematocrit (Hct) are important to the oxygen-carrying capacity of the blood; white blood cells (WBC) can indicate infection.
Blood grouping and cross-matching	Determined in case blood transfusion is required during or after surgery.
Serum electrolytes (sodium, potassium, calcium, magnesium, chloride, bicarbonate)	To evaluate fluid and electrolyte status.
Fasting blood glucose	High levels may indicate undiagnosed diabetes mellitus.
Blood urea nitrogen (BUN) and creatinine	To evaluate renal function.
Alanine aminotransferase (ALT), aspartarte aminotransferase (AST) and bilirubin	To evaluate liver function.
Serum albumin and total protein	To evaluate nutritional status.
Urinalysis	To determine urine composition and possible abnormal components (e.g. protein or glucose) or infection.
Chest x-ray	To evaluate respiratory status and heart size.
Electrocardiogram (ECG)	To identify pre-existing cardiac problems or disease.

PRACTICE GUIDELINES

Pre-operative Assessment

- *Current health.* What is the patient's general health like at the present time? Does the patient have any chronic diseases, such as diabetes or asthma, that may affect the patient's response to surgery or anaesthesia? Any physical limitations that may affect the patient's mobility or ability to communicate after surgery should be noted, as well as any prostheses such as hearing aids or contact lenses.
- *Allergies.* Include allergies to prescription and non-prescription drugs, food allergies, and allergies to tape, latex, soaps or antiseptic agents. Some food allergies may indicate a potential reaction to drugs or substances used during surgery or diagnostic procedures; for example, an allergy to seafood alerts the nurse to a potential allergy to iodine-based dyes commonly used in radiological procedures.
- *Medications.* List all current medications. It may be vital to maintain a blood level of some medications (e.g. anticonvulsants) throughout the surgical experience; others, such as anticoagulants or aspirin, increase the risks of surgery and anaesthesia and may need to be discontinued several days prior to surgery. It is important to include in the list any herbal remedies the patient currently takes as these can interact with some medications.
- *Previous surgeries.* Previous surgery may influence the patient's physical and psychological responses to surgery or may reveal unexpected responses to anaesthesia.
- *Activities of daily living.* The patient's abilities to meet their activities of daily living in order to establish a baseline for the recovery process (see Chapter 9 for ADLs).
- *Mental status.* The patient's mental status and ability to understand and respond appropriately can affect the whole surgical process. Any developmental disabilities, mental illness, dementia or excessive anxiety need to be noted.
- *Understanding of the surgical procedure and anaesthesia.* The patient should have a good understanding of the planned procedure and what to expect during and after surgery as well as the expected outcome of the procedure.
- *Smoking.* Smokers may have more difficulty clearing respiratory secretions after surgery, increasing the risk of post-operative complications such as pneumonia and atelectasis (collapse of part of the lung).
- *Alcohol and substance abuse.* Use of substances that affect the central nervous system, liver or other body systems can affect the patient's response to anaesthesia and surgery, and post-operative recovery.
- *Coping mechanisms.* Patients who use appropriate coping mechanisms such as talking with the family may be better able to deal with the stress of surgery.
- *Social support.* Determine the availability of family or other caregivers as they are important to the patient's recovery, particularly for the patient undergoing day surgery.
- *Religious and cultural considerations.* Religion and culture can influence the patient's response to surgery; respecting religious and cultural beliefs and practices can reduce pre-operative anxiety and improve recovery.

Pre-operative Investigations and Tests

It is usually the surgeon that orders specific investigations or test pre-operatively. However, the National Institute for Health and Clinical Excellence (NICE, 2003) suggest which tests should be performed according to the patient's age, the type of surgery and whether the patient has any underlying health problems such as diabetes or ischaemic heart disease. If abnormalities are detected from these tests they may need to be treated prior to surgery.

These tests should be carried out and the results obtained and brought to the surgeon's attention prior to surgery. In addition to these routine tests, diagnostic tests directly related to the patient's disease are usually appropriate (e.g. gastroscopy to clarify the condition before gastric surgery).

PLANNING

The overall goal in the pre-operative period is to ensure that the patient is mentally and physically prepared for surgery. Planning should involve the patient and their family and friends. The length of the pre-operative period affects pre-operative care and planning. When the patient is admitted several days before surgery, a nursing care plan is compiled during this period. However, it is becoming more common for patients to attend pre-operative assessment clinics before or even on the day of surgery.

Planning for Discharge

For the surgical patient, discharge planning should begin on or before admission for the planned procedure. Early planning to meet the discharge needs of the patient is particularly important for the day-surgery patient who is to be discharged soon after recovering from anaesthesia. Care pathways are a useful way to plan care for surgical patients. Care pathways are structured multidisciplinary care plans that map the expected recovery of patient's undergoing specific procedures (see Chapter 9).

Discharge planning usually incorporates an assessment of the patient's and their family's resources for caring for the patient at home, including their financial status, and assesses the need for referral to other agencies (e.g. to the district nurse or social services). However, the extent of discharge planning will vary significantly for patients having different types of surgery.

IMPLEMENTING

One of the most important nursing interventions to prepare the patient for surgery is pre-operative teaching.

Pre-operative Teaching

Pre-operative teaching is a vital part of nursing care. Studies have shown that pre-operative teaching reduces patients' anxiety and post-operative complications and increases their satisfaction with the surgical experience (Vaughn *et al.*, 2007). Good pre-operative teaching also facilitates the patient's return to work and other activities of daily living.

Pre-operative teaching involves:

- Giving the patient information about what will happen to them and when, and what they will experience such as expected sensations and discomfort.
- Psychosocial support to reduce anxiety.
- Teaching patients ways of improving their recovery, such as how to move, deep breathing and coughing exercises, how to splint incisions to ease pain when moving or coughing, and leg exercises to reduce the risk of clots forming in the veins in the legs (deep vein thrombosis – DVT). *Procedure 26-1* discusses teaching patients specific exercises to improve their recovery.

If the patient is having day surgery, pre-operative teaching is often provided before the day of surgery in pre-admission or pre-assessment clinics, using some combination of videos and verbal and written instructions. Information may then be reinforced on admission where any concerns that the patient or their family have may be discussed. This is particularly vital if the patient is a child, as both the child and the parents need to know what to expect and be able to express their concerns. Indeed, some consider the parents as part of the team caring for the child and, as such, they should actively participate in as much of the care as possible.

PROCEDURE 26-1 Teaching Moving, Leg Exercises, Deep Breathing and Coughing

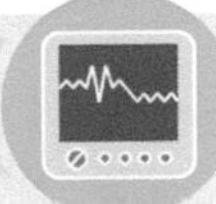

Surgery, although meant to benefit the patient, can cause serious complications post-operatively (see Table 26-2 on page 788). In order to prevent post-operative complications and assist the patient's recovery, the nurse needs to teach the patient techniques that will aid this process regardless of the type of surgery the patient has undergone.

Purposes

Moving

Following surgery, most patients are encouraged to move early on in the recovery period: for example, patients who have undergone coronary artery bypass grafts (a treatment for coronary heart disease) are encouraged to sit out in a chair and walk around within 26 hours of surgery, to reduce the risk of post-operative complications.

Moving:

- Maintains blood circulation and prevents the formation of clots (thrombi)
- Stimulates respiratory function
- Increases gut motility
- Facilitates early mobilisation

Leg exercises

Intra-operatively and post-operatively, patients usually have reduced mobility, and this causes blood to pool in the veins in the legs (venous stasis) resulting in the formation of clots (deep vein thrombosis). Blood clots in the veins are a very serious complication as the clots can travel back to the heart and then to the lungs (pulmonary emboli) resulting in serious illness or even death. Patients should therefore be encouraged to perform leg exercises to reduce the risk of blood clots forming.

Deep breathing and coughing

Chest infection is a common complication associated with surgery. If the patient is immobile or is not able to take deep breaths, the sputum that would normally be coughed up (expectorated) stays in the lungs and becomes the focus of infection. This can be prevented by encouraging the patient to perform deep breathing exercises. Following major surgery such as joint replacements or coronary artery bypass grafts, the physiotherapist may be involved in encouraging deep breathing and coughing exercises.

Deep breathing and coughing facilitates lung expansion for patients with known respiratory (breathing) problems, thereby preventing collapse of the lung (atelectasis) and pneumonia.

Assessment

Assess

- Vital signs
- Discomfort/pain
- Temperature and colour of feet and legs
- Breath sounds
- Presence of dyspnoea (shortness of breath) or cough
- Learning needs of the patient
- Anxiety level of the patient
- Patient experience with previous surgeries and anaesthesia

Planning

Before beginning to teach moving, leg exercises, deep-breathing exercises and coughing, the nurse needs to determine:

- The type of surgery
- The time of the surgery
- The name of the surgeon and their individual pre-operative orders
- The hospital's protocols regarding pre-operative care

Equipment

- Pillow or rolled up towel
- Teaching materials (e.g. videotape, written materials) if available

Implementation

Preparation

Ensure that there is as little distraction as possible (e.g. TV, visitors) and that the patient is not in pain as this too can distract them. If appropriate, the nurse can include the patient's family and friends if the patient so wishes.

Performance

1 Follow local policy to ensure that you explain to the patient what you are going to do, why it is necessary and how they can cooperate. Obtain consent and maintain patient privacy and dignity and ensure that the appropriate local infection control procedures are observed. Discuss how the patient's participation in the exercises they are going to be taught pre-operatively will be helpful during the post-operative recovery. *To promote concordance.*

2 Show the patient ways to turn in bed and to get out of bed.
- Patients with right-sided abdominal or chest incisions should be taught to get out of bed on the left side while patients with left-sided incisions should be taught to get out of bed on the right side. Rolling on the unaffected side will help them rise to a sitting position on the edge of the bed. *To promote comfort and ease of movement.*
- In order for the patient to sit up before getting out of bed the patient should be instructed to:
  (a) Bend their knees.
  (b) Splint the wound by holding a small pillow or rolled up towel against the incision. *To support the wound and promote comfort.*
  (c) Turn onto their unaffected side by pushing with their opposite foot.
  (d) Come to a sitting position on the side of the bed by using the affected side's arm and hand to push down against the mattress and swinging the feet over the edge of the bed.
- For patients with orthopaedic surgery (e.g. hip surgery), use special aids, such as a monkey pole (see Figure 26-1), to assist with movement.

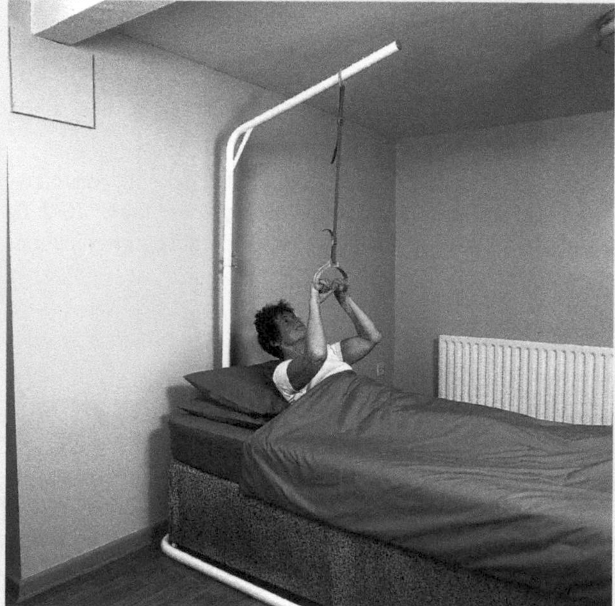

Figure 26-1 Monkey pole.
Source: Homecraft Rdyan Ltd.

3 Teach the patient the following three leg exercises - *to ensure circulation of blood back to the heart:*
- Alternate dorsiflexion and plantar flexion of the feet. This exercise is sometimes referred to as calf pumping (see Figure 26-2). *To contract and relax the calf muscle and increase circulation.*
- Flex and extend the knees, and press the backs of the knees into the bed while dorsiflexing the feet (see Figure 26-3). Instruct patients who cannot raise their legs to do **isometric** exercises that contract and relax the muscles.
- Raise and lower the legs alternately from the surface of the bed. Flex the knee of the stable leg and extend the knee of the moving leg (see Figure 26-4). *To contract and relax the quadriceps muscles in the thighs.*

4 Demonstrate deep-breathing (diaphragmatic) exercises as follows - *to facilitate lung expansion and reduce the risk of infection or lung collapse:*

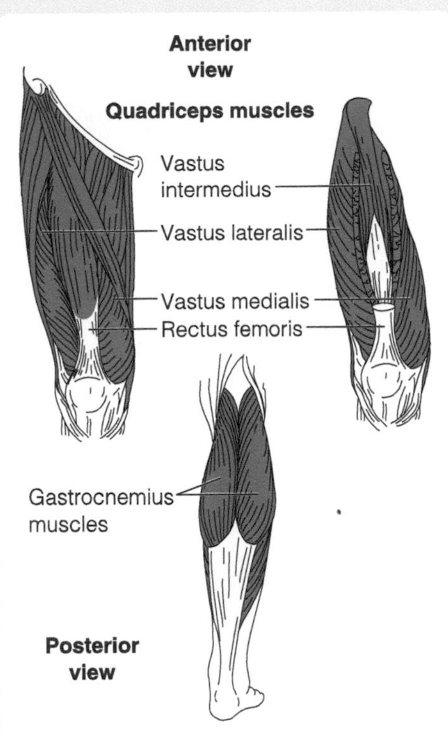

Figure 26-2 Leg muscles: anterior and posterior views.

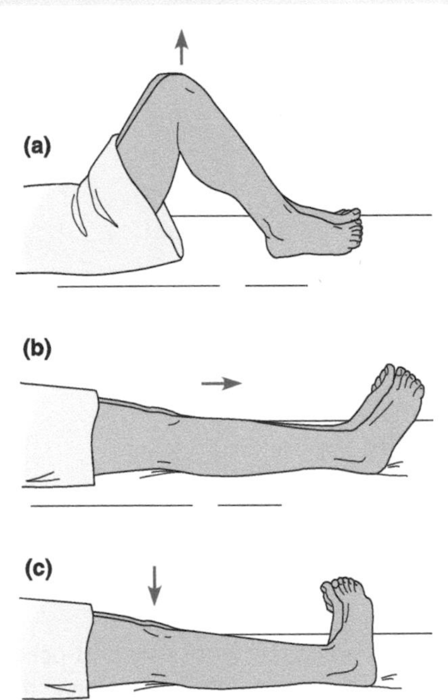

Figure 26-3 Flexing and extending the knees.

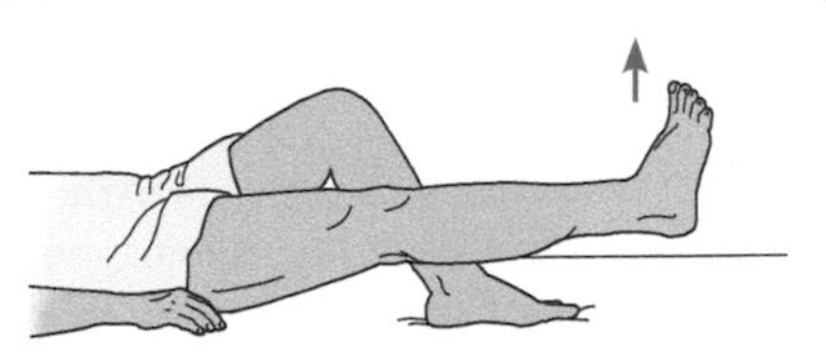

Figure 26-4 Raising and lowering the legs.

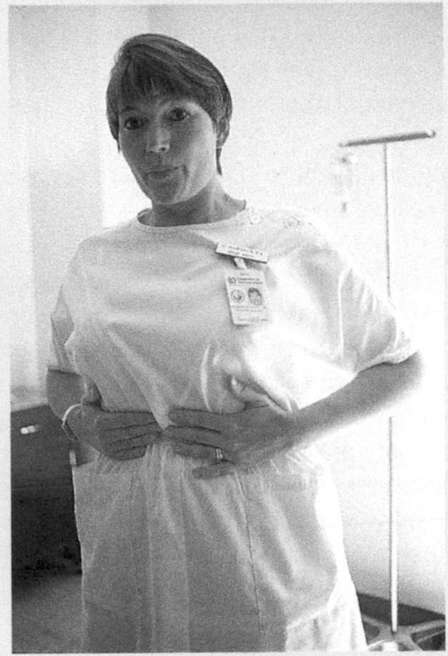

Figure 26-5 Demonstrating deep breathing.
Source: Elena Dorfmann.

- Place your hands palms down on the border of your rib cage, and inhale slowly and evenly through the nose until the greatest chest expansion is achieved (Figure 26-5).
- Hold your breath for 2–3 seconds.
- Then exhale slowly through the mouth.
- Continue exhalation until maximum chest contraction has been achieved.

5 Help the patient perform deep-breathing exercises.
- Ask the patient to assume a sitting position. *To ensure full lung expansion.*
- Place the palms of your hands on the border of the patient's rib cage. *To assess respiratory depth.*
- Ask the patient to perform deep breathing, as described in step 6.

6 Instruct the patient to cough voluntarily after a few deep inhalations.
- Ask the patient to inhale deeply, hold the breath for a few seconds, and then cough once or twice.
- Ensure that the patient coughs deeply and does not just clear the throat.

7 If the incision is painful when the patient coughs, demonstrate techniques to splint the incision.
- Show the patient how to support the incision by placing the palms of the hands on either side of the incision site or directly over the incision site, holding the palm of one hand over the other. Coughing uses the abdominal and other accessory respiratory muscles. *Splinting the incision may reduce pain while coughing if the incision is near any of these muscles.*
- Show the patient how to splint the incision with clasped hands and a firmly rolled pillow or towel held against the patient's wound (see Figure 26-6).

8 Inform the patient about the expected frequency of these exercises.
- Instruct the patient to start the exercises as soon after surgery as possible.
- Encourage patients with abdominal or chest surgery to carry out deep breathing and coughing at least every two hours, taking a minimum of five breaths at each session. Note, however, that the number of breaths and frequency of deep breathing varies with the patient's condition. People who are susceptible to pulmonary problems may need deep-breathing exercises every hour. People with chronic respiratory disease may need special breathing exercises (e.g. pursed-lip breathing, abdominal breathing, exercises using various kinds of incentive spirometers). See Chapter 16.

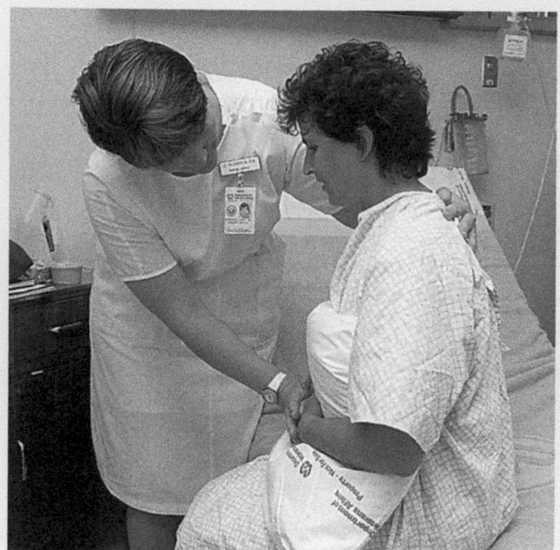

Figure 26-6 Splinting an incision with a pillow while coughing.
Source: Elena Dorfmann.

9 Document the teaching and all assessments.

Evaluation

Conduct appropriate follow-up such as:
- Evaluate the patient's ability to perform the exercises and reiterate the teaching if needed.
- Ask the patient to verbally recap the key information given.

LIFESPAN CONSIDERATIONS

Pre-operative Teaching

Children

- Parents need to know what to expect and to be able to express their concerns.
- Separation from parents often is the child's greatest fear; the time of separation should be minimised and parents allowed to interact with the child both immediately before and after surgery.
- Teaching of children should be appropriate for their age and development.
- Use simple terms to help the child understand (e.g. 'You will have a sore tummy').
- Play is an effective teaching tool with children; the child can put a bandage on an incision on a doll.

Mature Adults

- Assess hearing ability to ensure the patient hears the necessary information.
- Assess short-term memory. Presenting one focused idea at a time and repeating or reinforcing information may be necessary.
- Mature adults are at greater risk for post-operative complications, such as pneumonia. Reinforce moving and deep-breathing and coughing exercises.
- Assess potential post-operative needs. The patient may need to be referred to occupational therapy for equipment such as raised toilet seats.
- Assess the patient for risk of pressure ulcer development post-operatively.

Physical Preparation of the Patient

Pre-operative physical preparation of the patient ensures that they are in the best condition prior to surgery. This includes that the patient is adequately nourished and hydrated, that there are no elimination problems, that appropriate medication has been discontinued, that prostheses are removed or notified to the surgeon or anaesthetist and that there is appropriate preparation of the skin. Most hospitals utilise pre-operative checklists to ensure that all aspects of pre-operative care are addressed.

Nutrition and Fluids

Adequate hydration and nutrition promote healing. Nurses need to record any signs of malnutrition or fluid imbalance. If the patient is on intravenous fluids or on measured fluid intake, nurses must ensure that the fluids are carefully measured.

The order 'nil by mouth (NBM) from midnight' is a long-standing tradition as it was believed that anaesthetics depress gastrointestinal functioning and there was a danger that the patient could vomit and aspirate during the administration of a general anaesthetic. However, the recent Royal College of Nursing (RCN, 2005) guidelines state that healthy adult and child patients can drink clear fluids up to two hours before surgery while solid foods including milk can be eaten up to six hours before surgery. According to this guideline, higher risk patients should be assessed on an individual basis but could follow the same regimen as healthy patients.

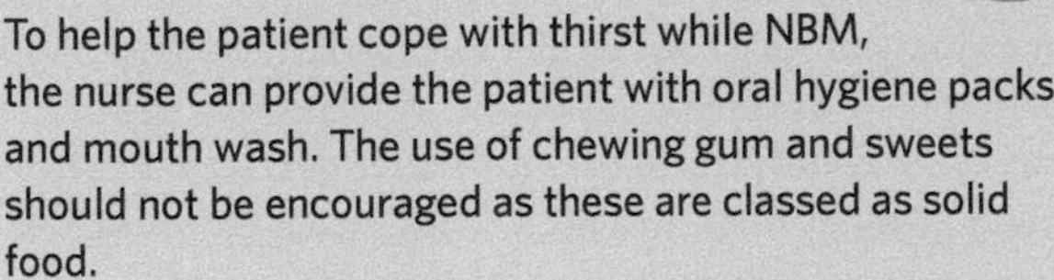

CLINICAL ALERT

To help the patient cope with thirst while NBM, the nurse can provide the patient with oral hygiene packs and mouth wash. The use of chewing gum and sweets should not be encouraged as these are classed as solid food.

Elimination

Some surgery requires that the bowels or the bladder are empty. Therefore it is the nurse's responsibility to ensure that this preparation is carried out. Enemas may be administered or osmotic laxatives such as sodium picosulfate (Picolax) to empty the bowel while a urinary catheter could be ordered to ensure that the bladder remains empty. If the patient does not have a catheter, it is important to empty the bladder prior to receiving pre-operative medications as patients can be unsteady on their feet after taking medication such as diazepam or temazepam.

Medications

The anaesthetist or surgeon may temporarily discontinue routinely taken medications, such as aspirin, the day of surgery or a few days before surgery in order to prevent intra-operative and post-operative complications such as bleeding. In some settings, pre-operative medications are given to patients for a number of reasons:

- *sedatives and tranquillisers* such as diazepam to reduce anxiety and ease anaesthetic induction;
- *narcotic analgesics* such as morphine to sedate the patient and reduce the amount of anaesthetic required;
- *anticholinergics* such as atropine to reduce oral and pulmonary secretions and prevent laryngospasm (closing of the larynx);
- *histamine-receptor antihistamines* such as ranitidine to reduce gastric fluid volume and gastric acidity.

Pre-operative medications must be given at a scheduled time or when the operating theatre notifies the nurse to give the medication.

Rest and Sleep

Nurses should do everything to help the patient sleep the night before surgery as this helps the patient manage the stress of surgery and helps healing. If the patient is having difficulty sleeping, the surgeon may prescribe a sedative.

Prostheses

All prostheses (artificial body parts, such as partial or complete dentures, contact lenses, artificial eyes and artificial limbs) and eyeglasses, wigs and false eyelashes must be removed before surgery. Hearing aids are often left in place and the operating theatre staff notified.

As well as dentures, the nurse should check if the patient has capped, crowned or loose teeth as these can become dislodged and aspirated during anaesthesia.

Skin Preparation

Some types of surgery require preparation of the skin pre-operatively. Often patients are asked to bathe or shower the evening or morning of surgery (or both) in a specific antiseptic solution (e.g. chlorhexidine). The purpose of this is to reduce the risk of wound infection post-operatively. Some hospitals and surgeons also ask for patients to shave the part of the body that is to be operated on before surgery, again to minimise the risk of infection. However, this is a controversial subject as some research has shown that shaving actually increases the risk of infection rather than minimising it (Dizer *et al.*, 2009).

All nail polish and makeup should be removed prior to surgery so that the nail beds, skin and lips are visible for circulation to be assessed during and following surgery. Also any hair grips or pins should be removed from the hair as they may cause pressure ulcers while the patient is unconscious.

As part of the physical preparation of the patient pre-operatively, the patient may require the use of antiembolic stockings. This is particularly important for patients who will have long recovery periods or will have reduced mobility post-operatively. Antiembolic (elastic) stockings compress the veins of the legs and thereby facilitate the return of venous blood to the heart. This helps to prevent or reduce oedema (swelling) of the feet and lower legs and helps to reduce the formation of clots (deep vein thrombosis) in the lower legs. These stockings are frequently applied pre-operatively as well as post-operatively.

LIFESPAN CONSIDERATIONS

Antiembolic Stockings

Children

- Antiembolic stockings are infrequently used on children.

Mature Adults

- As the elastic is quite strong in antiembolic stockings, the older adult may need assistance with putting on the stockings. Patients with arthritis may need to have another person put the stockings on for them.
- Stockings should be removed once every 24 hours or more often if required, so that a thorough assessment can be made of legs and feet. Redness and skin breakdown on the heels can occur quickly and go undetected if not thoroughly assessed on a regular basis.

ACTIVITY 26-1

Consider a pre-operative patient you have recently cared for. What specific pre-operative care did you give him/her?

INTRA-OPERATIVE PHASE

The intra-operative nurse is a vital member of the surgical team, acting as the patient advocate, maintaining safety, and continually assessing the needs of the patient and the team. There are a number of nursing roles within the theatre, including anaesthetics, scrub and circulating nurses.

Anaesthetic Nurses

The anaesthetic nurse works closely with the anaesthetist, giving assistance from induction to the immediate recovery of the patient. The main functions of the anaesthetic nurse include:

- The provision of a safe environment, which includes preparing equipment, medicines and fluids, checking monitors and apparatus, ensuring adequate stock and ensuring a clean environment and equipment.
- Administration, which includes arranging to send for the patient, ensuring correct patient for correct procedure, recording patient details on departmental records and ensuring appropriate information accompanies the patient, e.g. case notes and x rays.
- Communication with the patient, other healthcare professionals in theatre and ward staff.
- Assisting with induction of anaesthesia and airway management.
- Assisting with local anaesthetic blocks.
- Assisting with positioning of the patient.
- Observing the patient's condition.
- Monitoring for any adverse effects of the anaesthesia.
- Monitoring the maintenance of fluids and medications.
- Ensuring that safe systems of work are being employed at all times.

Part of the role of the anaesthetic nurse is the induction of the patient using anaesthetics. Therefore, the nurse needs to have a comprehensive knowledge of the types of anaesthetics used.

Types of Anaesthesia

There are two common types of anaesthesia, namely general and local. Anaesthetic agents are normally administered by an anaesthetist or nurse anaesthetist. *General anaesthesia* is the loss of all sensation and consciousness. Under general anaesthesia, protective reflexes such as cough and gag reflexes are lost. A general anaesthetic acts by blocking awareness centres in the brain so that amnesia (loss of memory), analgesia (insensibility to pain), hypnosis (artificial sleep) and relaxation (rendering a part of the body less tense) occur. General anaesthetics are usually administered by intravenous infusion or by inhalation of gases through a mask or through an endotracheal tube inserted into the trachea.

General anaesthesia has certain advantages such as the relatively easy regulation of the patient's respirations and cardiac function because the patient is unconscious and therefore is not anxious. General anaesthesia can be adjusted according to the patient's age, their physical status and the length and type of operation. The main disadvantage with general anaesthetic is that it depresses the respiratory function. This means that the patient is unable to maintain their own airway and cannot ventilate their lungs themselves. In order to maintain the patient's airway and provide ventilation to the patient the anaesthetist will usually introduce a tube into the patient's airway and attach this to a ventilator which helps to aerate the patient's lungs.

Patients are often fearful of general anaesthetic more than surgery, possibly as a result of the lack of control over their body and others. Local anaesthesia, on the other hand, only anaesthetises the local area (e.g. a hand) by temporarily interrupting the transmission of nerve impulses to and from that area or region. The patient loses sensation in an area of the body but remains conscious. Several techniques are used.

- *Topical (surface) anaesthesia* is applied directly to the skin and mucous membranes, open skin surfaces, wounds and burns. The most commonly used topical agents are lidocaine (Xylocaine) and benzocaine. These are particularly useful for numbing a child's hand to introduce an intravenous catheter. However, it is very important that the topical agent is given time to numb the area before proceeding.
- *Local anaesthesia* (infiltration) is injected into a specific area and is used for minor surgical procedures such as suturing a small wound or performing a biopsy. Lidocaine 0.1% may be used for this purpose.
- A *nerve block* is a technique in which the anaesthetic agent is injected into and around a nerve or small nerve group that supplies sensation to a small area of the body. Major blocks involve multiple nerves or a plexus (e.g. the brachial plexus anesthetises the arm); minor blocks involve a single nerve (e.g. a facial nerve).
- An *intravenous block (Bier block)* is used most often for procedures involving the arm, wrist and hand. An occlusion tourniquet is applied to the extremity to prevent infiltration and absorption of the injected intravenous agent beyond the involved extremity.
- *Spinal anaesthesia* requires a lumbar puncture through one of the interspaces between lumbar disc 2 (L_2) and the sacrum (S_1) and the introduction of an anaesthetic agent into the cerebrospinal fluid (CSF). Spinal anaesthesia is often categorised as a low, mid or high spinal. Low spinals (saddle or caudal blocks) are primarily used for surgeries involving the perineal or rectal areas. Mid spinals (below the level of the umbilicus – T_{10}) can be used for hernia repairs or appendectomies, and high spinals (reaching the nipple line – T_4) can be used for surgeries such as caesarean sections. Spinal anaesthesia is usually chosen as it reduces the effects on the respiratory system and recovery is much quicker than general anaesthesia.
- *Epidural anaesthesia* is an injection of an anaesthetic agent into the epidural space, the area inside the spinal column but outside the dura mater.

Some types of surgery may require that the patient has conscious sedation as well as the local anaesthetic for patient comfort and safety. *Conscious sedation* refers to minimal depression of the level of consciousness in which the patient retains the ability to maintain a patent airway and respond appropriately to commands (Kost, 1999). Intravenous narcotics such as morphine or fentanyl and anti-anxiety agents such as diazepam or midazolam are commonly used to induce and maintain conscious sedation. Conscious sedation increases the patient's pain threshold and induces a degree of amnesia but allows for prompt reversal of its effects and a rapid return to normal activities of daily living. Procedures such as endoscopies, incision and drainage of abscesses, and even balloon angioplasty may be performed under conscious sedation.

As well as assisting the anaesthetist with the administration of anaesthesia, the anaesthetic nurse may also assist in the intubation (the procedure for inserting a tube into the trachea of a patient who is not able to breathe) and ventilation (movement of oxygen and air into and out of a patient's lungs) of the patient. Nurse anaesthetists have a more extended role than anaesthetic nurses and may be able to cannulate (insert intravenous catheters) into patients, intubate patients and administer anaesthesia themselves.

Anaesthetic nurses, however, are only part of the theatre team of nurses. Surgery would not be able to take place if there were no scrub nurses or circulating nurses.

ACTIVITY 26-2

Consider why a patient with chronic obstructive pulmonary disease would be offered a spinal anaesthetic for elective, constructive surgery?

Scrub Nurses

The scrub nurse performs a vital function in any operation theatre, ensuring that all the appropriate instruments and equipment are available and sterile. The scrub nurse works closely with the surgeon and needs to have the knowledge and expertise to anticipate the instruments that are needed by the surgeon. They wear sterile gowns, gloves, caps, and so on. Their main responsibilities include draping the patient with sterile drapes and handling sterile instruments and supplies. They also account for used sponges, needles and instruments. In some surgical settings, a surgeon does not close, that is, suture an incision, until the scrub nurse can account for all sponges and instruments. This precaution avoids leaving any surgical materials inside the patient.

Circulating Nurse

The circulating nurse, or 'runner' as they are colloquially called, assists the scrub nurses and surgeons by ensuring that the operating theatre is adequately stocked with supplies. They help position the patient for the operation and often position any needed equipment such as cameras or lighting.

INTRA-OPERATIVE ASSESSMENT

On admission to theatre or surgical suite, the anaesthetic nurse confirms the patient's identity and assesses the patient's psychological and physical state. The nurse verifies the information on the pre-operative checklist and evaluates the patient's knowledge about the surgery and events to follow. The patient's response to pre-operative medications is assessed, as well as the placement and patency of any tubes such as IV lines, nasogastric tubes and urinary catheters.

Assessment continues throughout surgery, as the nurse and the anaesthetist continuously monitor the patient's vital signs (including blood pressure, heart rate, respiratory rate and temperature), ECG and oxygen saturation. Fluid intake and urinary output are monitored throughout surgery, and blood loss is estimated. Depending on the complexity of the surgery and the status of the patient other health parameters may be monitored such as haemoglobin and haematocrit (components of the blood), blood glucose and electrolytes within the blood. A more accurate way of monitoring the patient's oxygen and carbon dioxide levels can be achieved by taking regular arterial blood gases. Continual assessment is necessary to rapidly identify adverse responses to surgery or anaesthesia and intervene promptly to prevent complications.

PLANNING

The overall goals of care in the intra-operative period are to maintain the patient's safety and to maintain homoeostasis (stability). Examples of nursing activities to achieve these goals include the following:

- Position the patient appropriately for surgery.
- Perform pre-operative skin preparation.
- Assist in preparing and maintaining the sterile field.
- Open and dispense sterile supplies during surgery.
- Provide medications and solutions for the sterile field.
- Monitor and maintain a safe, aseptic environment.
- Manage catheters, tubes, drains and specimens.
- Perform sponge, sharp and instrument counts.
- Document nursing care provided and the patient's response to interventions.

IMPLEMENTING

Surgical Skin Preparation

Even though the patient may have been asked to wash in antiseptic solution and shave appropriate parts of their body before surgery, while in theatre, the surgeon may insist that the skin be further prepared. This involves cleaning the surgical site with an antiseptic solution such as Betadine, which helps to reduce the risk of post-operative wound infection.

Positioning

Proper positioning of the patient during surgery is an important responsibility shared by the nurse, surgeon and anaesthetist. The ideal intra-operative patient position provides:

- Optimal visualisation of and access to the surgical site.
- Optimal access for assessing and maintaining anaesthesia and vital functions (vital signs, respirations, cardiovascular function).
- Protection of the patient from harm.

Positioning is performed after anaesthesia is induced and before surgical draping of the patient. The patient is manoeuvred into position in such a manner as to prevent shearing forces on the skin. The exact position for the patient depends on the operation; that is, the surgical approach. For example, a lithotomy position (lying on back with legs apart and feet supported in stirrups) is usually used for vaginal surgery.

Positions on the operating table are maintained by straps, and body prominences are frequently padded.

CLINICAL ALERT

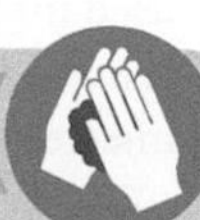

Be especially aware of the intra-operative position required for older adults as they are vulnerable to pressure ulcer formation. Check the appropriate pressure points of that surgical position on the patient.

EVALUATING

This is performed by considering whether the goals set out in the planning stage have been met (e.g. maintain patient safety).

Documentation

Throughout the intra-operative phase the nurse documents patient care activities such as IV fluid infusions, positioning, gastric suction and urinary catheterisation.

POST-OPERATIVE PHASE

Nursing during the post-operative phase is especially important for the patient's recovery. Patients who have undergone surgery under general or local anaesthetic are at risk of compromise to their airway, breathing and circulation. Therefore it is important that post-operative patients are closely monitored.

Immediate Post-anaesthetic Phase

Recovery nurses have specialised skills to care for patients recovering from anaesthesia and surgery (see Figure 26-7). Once the patient is stabilised, they can be returned to the ward or unit from which they came from. It is the recovery nurse's role to stabilise the patient before transfer by continuously monitoring and treating them. Assessment of the patient in the immediate post-anaesthetic period is summarised in the *Practice Guidelines*.

The return of the patient's reflexes, such as swallowing and gagging, usually indicates that the anaesthetic is wearing off. Recovery time from anaesthesia varies according to the type of anaesthetic used, its dosage and the patient's response to it. Nurses should arouse patients by calling them by name, and in

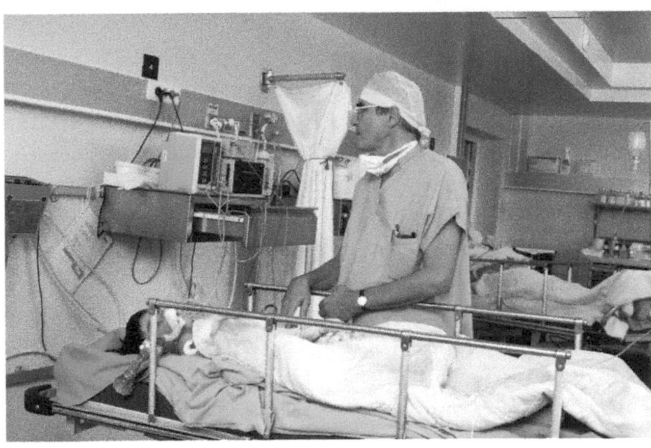

Figure 26-7 Recovery room nurse provides constant assessment and care for patients recovering from anaesthesia and surgery.

a normal tone of voice repeatedly telling them that the surgery is over and that they are in the recovery room.

Once the patient's condition is stabilised, they are returned to the ward or unit. However, there are strict transfer criteria that the patient has to meet before they can be discharged from the recovery room. The patient must:

- Be conscious and oriented.
- Be able to maintain a clear airway and deep breathe and cough freely.
- Have stable vital signs that are consistent with their pre-operative vital signs for at least 30 minutes.
- Have active protective reflexes (e.g. gag, swallowing).
- Be able to move their limbs.
- Have adequate intake and urinary output (at least 30ml/hr).
- Have dry and intact dressings. Any drains that may be in place should not have excessive drainage for the type of operation.

PRACTICE GUIDELINES

Clinical Assessment

- Adequacy of airway
- Oxygen saturation
- Adequacy of ventilation
- Respiratory rate, rhythm and depth
- Use of accessory muscles
- Breath sounds
- Cardiovascular status
- Heart rate and rhythm
- Peripheral pulse amplitude and equality
- Blood pressure
- Capillary filling
- Level of consciousness
- Not responding
- Arousable with verbal stimuli
- Fully awake
- Oriented to time, person and place
- Presence of protective reflexes (e.g. gag, cough)
- Activity, ability to move extremities
- Skin colour (pink, pale, dusky, blotchy, cyanotic, jaundiced)
- Fluid status
- Intake and output
- Status of IV infusions (type of fluid, rate, amount in container, patency of tubing)
- Signs of dehydration or fluid overload
- Condition of operative site
- Status of dressing
- Drainage (amount, type and colour)
- Patency of and character and amount of drainage from catheters, tubes and drains
- Discomfort (i.e. pain) (type, location and severity), nausea, vomiting
- Safety (i.e. necessity for side rails, call bell within reach)

Once the immediate recovery period is over and the patient is stable, they can be transferred back to the ward or unit. It is usual for the recovery nurse to inform the ward nurse that the patient is ready for collection from the recovery room. The ward nurse will then take over from the recovery nurse and ensure themselves that the patient is stable before transferring them back to the ward or unit. It is important to note that, if the ward nurse feels that the patient does not meet the criteria for discharge, they must voice this to the recovery nurse and delay transfer until they are happy with the patient's condition.

POST-OPERATIVE ASSESSMENT

As soon as the patient returns to the ward or unit, the nurse conducts an initial assessment. Once the nurse has performed the initial assessment, the specific orders set out by the surgeon, such as the intake of fluids and food, any intravenous solutions and medications that need to be administered, the position that they should be nursed in, and any further tests that may be required, need to be considered.

The nurse also checks the theatre notes to establish:

- Operation performed
- Presence and location of any drains
- Anaesthetic used
- Post-operative diagnosis
- Estimated blood loss
- Medications administered in the recovery room.

Many hospitals have post-operative protocols for regular assessment of patients. Some protocols require that assessments are made every 15 minutes until vital signs stabilise, every hour for the next four hours, then every four hours for the next two days. It is important that the assessments be made as often as the patient's condition requires. The nurse assesses the following:

- *Level of consciousness.* Assess orientation to time, place and person. Most patients are fully conscious but drowsy when returned to their unit. Assess reaction to verbal stimuli and ability to move extremities.
- *Vital signs.* Take the patient's vital signs (pulse, respiration, blood pressure and oxygen saturation level) every 15 minutes until stable or in accordance with the hospital's policy. These should be compared with the initial findings in the recovery room and with the patient's pre-operative vital signs. In addition, assess the patient's lung sounds and assess for signs of common circulatory problems such as post-operative hypotension, haemorrhage or shock. Hypovolaemia due to fluid losses during surgery is a common cause of post-operative hypotension. Haemorrhage can result from insecure ligation of blood vessels or disruption of sutures. Massive haemorrhage or cardiac insufficiency can lead to shock post-operatively. Common post-operative complications with their manifestations and preventive measures are listed in Table 26-2.
- *Skin colour and temperature*, particularly that of the lips and nail beds. The colour of the lips and nail beds is an indicator of tissue perfusion (passage of blood through the vessels). Pale, cyanotic, cool and moist skin may be a sign of circulatory problems.

Table 26-2 Potential Post-operative Problems

Problem	Description	Cause	Clinical signs	Preventive interventions
Respiratory				
Pneumonia	Inflammation of the alveoli	Infection, toxins or irritants causing inflammatory process	Elevated temperature, cough, expectoration of blood-tinged or purulent sputum, dyspnoea, chest pain	Deep-breathing exercises and coughing, moving in bed, early ambulation
Infectious pneumonia	May be limited to one or more lobes (lobar) or occur as scattered patches throughout the lungs (bronchial); also can involve interstitial tissues of lungs	Common organisms include *Streptococcus pneumoniae, Haemophilus influenzae* and *Staphylococcus aureus*	Same as above	Same as above
Hypostatic pneumonia		Immobility and impaired ventilation result in atelectasis and promote growth of pathogens	Same as above	Same as above
Aspiration pneumonia	Inflammatory process caused by irritation of lung tissue by aspirated material, particularly hydrochloric acid (HCl) from the stomach	Aspiration of gastric contents, food or other substances; often related to loss of gag reflex	Same as above	Same as above
Atelectasis	A condition in which alveoli collapse and are not ventilated	Mucous plugs blocking bronchial passageways, inadequate lung expansion, analgesics, immobility	Dyspnoea, tachypnoea, tachycardia; diaphoresis, anxiety; pleural pain, decreased chest wall movement; dull or absent breath sounds; decreased oxygen saturation (SaO_2)	Deep-breathing exercises and coughing, moving in bed, early ambulation
Pulmonary embolism	Blood clot that has moved to the lungs and blocks a pulmonary artery, thus obstructing blood flow to a portion of the lung	Stasis of venous blood from immobility, venous injury from fractures or during surgery, use of oral contraceptives high in oestrogen, pre-existing coagulation or circulatory disorder	Sudden chest pain, shortness of breath, cyanosis, shock (tachycardia, low blood pressure)	Turning, ambulation, antiembolic stockings, sequential compression devices

Table 26-2 *(continued)*

Problem	Description	Cause	Clinical signs	Preventive interventions
Circulatory				
Hypovolaemia	Inadequate circulating blood volume	Fluid deficit, haemorrhage	Tachycardia, decreased urine output, decreased blood pressure	Early detection of signs; fluid and/or blood replacement
Haemorrhage	Internal or external bleeding	Disruption of sutures, insecure ligation of blood vessels	Overt bleeding (dressings saturated with bright blood; bright, free-flowing blood in drains or chest tubes), increased pain, increasing abdominal girth, swelling or bruising around incision	Early detection of signs
Hypovolaemic shock	Inadequate tissue perfusion resulting from markedly reduced circulating blood volume	Severe hypovolaemia from fluid deficit or haemorrhage	Rapid weak pulse, dyspnoea, tachypnoea; restlessness and anxiety; urine output less than 30ml/hr; decreased blood pressure; cool, clammy skin, thirst, pallor	Maintain blood volume through adequate fluid replacement, prevent haemorrhage; early detection of signs
Thrombophlebitis	Inflammation of the veins, usually of the legs and associated with a blood clot	Slowed venous blood flow due to immobility or prolonged sitting; trauma to vein, resulting in inflammation and increased blood coagulability	Aching, cramping pain; affected area is swollen, red and hot to touch; vein feels hard; discomfort in calf when foot is dorsiflexed or when patient walks (Homans' sign)	Early ambulation, leg exercises, antiembolic stockings, adequate fluid intake
Thrombus	Blood clot attached to wall of vein or artery (most commonly the leg veins)	As for thrombophlebitis for venous thrombi; disruption or inflammation of arterial wall for arterial thrombi	*Venous*: same as thrombophlebitis *Arterial*: pain and pallor of affected extremity; decreased or absent peripheral pulses	*Venous*: same as thrombophlebitis *Arterial*: maintain prescribed position; early detection of signs
Embolus	Foreign body or clot that has moved from its site of formation to another area of the body (e.g. the lungs, heart or brain)	Venous or arterial thrombus; broken intravenous catheter, fat or amniotic fluid	In venous system, usually becomes a pulmonary embolus (see pulmonary embolism); signs of arterial emboli may depend on the location	As for thrombophlebitis or thrombus; careful maintenance of IV catheters
Urinary				
Urinary retention	Inability to empty the bladder, with excessive accumulation of urine in the bladder	Depressed bladder muscle tone from narcotics and anaesthetics; handling of tissues during surgery on adjacent organs (rectum, vagina)	Fluid intake larger than output; inability to void or frequent voiding of small amounts, bladder distention, suprapubic discomfort, restlessness	Monitoring of fluid intake and output, interventions to facilitate voiding, urinary catheterisation as needed

Table 26-2 *(continued)*

Problem	Description	Cause	Clinical signs	Preventive interventions
Urinary tract infection	Inflammation of the bladder, ureters or urethra	Immobilisation and limited fluid intake, instrumentation of the urinary tract	Burning sensation when voiding, urgency, cloudy urine, lower abdominal pain	Adequate fluid intake, early ambulation, aseptic straight catheterisation only as necessary, good perineal hygiene
Gastrointestinal				
Nausea and vomiting		Pain, abdominal distention, ingesting food or fluids before return of peristalsis, certain medications, anxiety	Complaints of feeling sick to the stomach, retching or gagging	IV fluids until peristalsis returns; then clear fluids, full fluids and regular diet; antiemetic drugs if ordered; analgesics for pain
Constipation	Infrequent or no stool passage for abnormal length of time (e.g. within 48 hours after solid diet started)	Lack of dietary roughage, analgesics (decreased intestinal motility), immobility	Absence of stool elimination, abdominal distention and discomfort	Adequate fluid intake, high-fibre diet, early ambulation
Tympanites	Retention of gases within the intestines	Slowed motility of the intestines due to handling of the bowel during surgery and the effects of anaesthesia	Obvious abdominal distention, abdominal discomfort (gas pains), absence of bowel sounds	Early ambulation; avoid using a straw, provide ice chips or water at room temperature
Post-operative ileus	Intestinal obstruction characterised by lack of peristaltic activity	Handling the bowel during surgery, anaesthesia, electrolyte imbalance, wound infection	Abdominal pain and distention; constipation; absent bowel sounds; vomiting	
Wound				
Wound infection	Inflammation and infection of incision or drain site	Poor aseptic technique; laboratory analysis of wound swab identifies causative micro-organism	Purulent exudate, redness, tenderness, elevated body temperature, wound odour	Keep wound clean and dry, use surgical aseptic technique when changing dressings
Wound dehiscence	Rupture or splitting open of a wound	Malnutrition (emaciation, obesity), poor circulation, excessive strain on suture line	Increased incision drainage, tissues underlying skin become visible along parts of the incision	Adequate nutrition, appropriate incisional support and avoidance of strain
Wound evisceration	Exposure of the internal organs and tissues through a wound	Same as for wound dehiscence	Opening of incision and visible protrusion of organs	Same as for wound dehiscence
Psychological				
Post-operative depression	Mental disorder characterised by altered mood	Weakness, surprise nature of emergency surgery, news of malignancy, severely altered body image, other personal matter; may be a physiologic response to some surgeries	Anorexia, tearfulness, loss of ambition, withdrawal, rejection of others, feelings of dejection, sleep disturbances (insomnia or excessive sleeping)	Adequate rest, physical activity, opportunity to express anger and other negative feelings

CLINICAL ALERT

Older adults may not show the classic signs of infection (e.g. fever, tachycardia, increased WBC) as the defence mechanisms of the body tend to reduce as a person ages (e.g. ageing reduces the number of antibodies produced). However, infection in the older adult can cause them to become confused, disorientated and agitated as the brain tolerates infection less with ageing.

- *Comfort.* Assess pain with the patient's vital signs and, as needed, between vital sign measurements. Assess the location and intensity of the pain. Do not assume that reported pain is incisional; other causes may include muscle strains, flatus and angina. Ask the patient to rate pain on a scale of 0–10, with 0 being no pain and 10 the worst pain imaginable. Evaluate the patient for objective indicators of pain: pallor, perspiration, muscle tension and reluctance to cough, move or ambulate. Determine when and what analgesics were last administered, and assess the patient for any side-effects of medication such as nausea and vomiting.
- *Fluid balance.* Assess the type and amount of intravenous fluids, flow rate and infusion site. Monitor the patient's fluid intake and output. In addition to watching for shock, assess the patient for signs of circulatory overload and monitor serum electrolytes. Anaesthetics and surgery affect the hormones regulating fluid and electrolyte balance (aldosterone and antidiuretic hormone in particular), placing the patient at risk for decreased urine output and fluid and electrolyte imbalances.
- *Dressing and bedclothes.* Inspect the patient's dressings and bedclothes underneath the patient. Excessive bloody drainage on dressings or on bedclothes, often appearing underneath the patient, can indicate haemorrhage. The amount of drainage on dressings is recorded by describing the diameter of the stains or by denoting the number and type of dressings saturated with drainage.
- *Drains and tubes.* Determine colour, consistency and amount of drainage from all tubes and drains. All tubes should be patent, and tubes and suction equipment should be functioning. Drainage bags must be hanging properly.

Document the patient's time of arrival and all assessments. The frequency of assessment should be altered according to the patient's condition. If a patient is showing signs of deterioration, assessments may need to be performed much more regularly.

PLANNING

Post-operative care planning and discharge planning begin in the pre-operative phase when pre-operative teaching is implemented.

Planning for Discharge

In order to provide continuity of care for the surgical patient after discharge from the hospital, the nurse needs to consider what type of assistance the patient requires in the home setting according to their individual needs. Discharge planning for both the day-surgery patient and the patient who has been hospitalised for several days following surgery incorporates an assessment of the patient's ability to self-care and the family's abilities to support the patient's physical and psychological needs after discharge. The nurse may feel that the patient may require further assistance from the district nurse, social services or private care agencies. This is discussed fully with the patient and family and a package of care is established.

IMPLEMENTING

The main aim of post-operative care is prevention, early identification and treatment of post-operative complications, in order for the patient to be safely discharged home. Some of the nursing interventions that promote recovery and prevent complications, in most cases, will have been introduced to the patient pre-operatively, such as deep-breathing and coughing exercises, leg exercises and moving (see *Procedure 26-1 on page 779*). However, there are a number of other nursing interventions used to help the patient recover, including pain management, positioning, incentive spirometry, hydration, nutrition and wound care.

Pain Management

Pain is a natural response to injury and serves to alert us to harm and initiate responses to minimise harm. Pain is both a sensory and emotional experience that can hinder a patient's recovery after surgery. In fact, surgical pain can be severely detrimental to the patient leading to tachycardia (heart rate over 100 beats per minute), shallow breathing, atelectasis (lung collapse), altered gas exchanged, immobility and immunosuppression (Van Keuren and Eland, 1997). Chapter 24 provides a more in-depth discussion of pain and pain management.

Pain is usually greatest 12–36 hours after surgery, decreasing after the second or third post-operative day. During the initial post-operative period, patient-controlled analgesia (PCA) or continuous analgesic administration through an intravenous or epidural catheter may be prescribed. The nurse monitors the infusion or amount of analgesic administered by PCA, assesses the patient's pain relief, and notifies the doctor or anaesthetist if the patient is experiencing unacceptable side-effects or inadequate pain relief. Analgesia that is prescribed as required (PRN) should be administered on a routine basis for the first 26–36 hours. Once the patient's pain is more controlled then routine pain relief need only be administered before moving or dressing changes.

Alongside pharmacological analgesia, the nurse may implement other forms of pain relief. These include ensuring that the patient is warm and providing back rubs, position changes, diversional activities such as a book or television, and adjunctive measures such as imagery (using the person's imagination to relieve the pain).

Positioning

The positioning of the patient may be governed by the type of surgery the patient has undergone and the type of anaesthetic they have received. For instance, patients who have had a laminectomy (surgical removal of part of the vertebra in the spine) must be nursed on their back. In order for them to eat and drink the patient must have an appropriate bed that can be positioned so that the patient's back is not bent. Likewise, patients who have had spinal anaesthetics usually lie flat for 8–12 hours. On the other hand, an unconscious or semi-conscious patient is placed on one side with the head slightly elevated, if possible, or in a position that allows fluids to drain from the mouth. If, however, there are no specific orders for the patient, they should be positioned so that they are comfortable.

Incentive Spirometry

Following surgery and a period of immobility, sputum can collect in the lungs and lead to chest infection. Incentive spirometry is often used to encourage deep breathing following surgery to reduce the risk of chest infections. This device measures the flow of air inhaled through a mouthpiece (see Chapter 16). The patient is instructed to breathe in through the mouthpiece until a certain level is achieved (usually measured by a ball within an enclosed chamber). Inhalation and ventilation are enhanced using the incentive spirometer.

Hydration

Initially, post-operative hydration is usually maintained by intravenous infusions, in order to replace body fluids lost either before or during surgery. If oral intake of fluids is not contraindicated, it is wise for the nurse to only offer sips of water to the patient initially as large amounts of water can induce vomiting. If the patient is unable to take fluid orally it is important that the nurse provides mouth care and offers mouthwashes to the patient. Post-operative patients often complain of thirst and a dry sticky mouth. These symptoms are a sign of dehydration due to pre-operative fasting, medications and loss of body fluid.

If the patient is receiving intravenous fluids post-operatively, it is important to measure the patient's fluid intake and output. Adequate hydration is important as it keeps the respiratory mucous membranes and secretions moist and maintains cardiovascular and renal function.

Nutrition

Depending on the extent of surgery and the organs involved, the patient may be allowed nothing by mouth for several days or may be able to resume oral intake when nausea is no longer present. If the surgeon states that the patient can have 'diet as tolerated', the nurse should begin by offering clear fluids. If the patient tolerates these with no nausea, the diet can often progress to full liquids and then to a regular diet, provided that gastrointestinal functioning is normal. Assess the return of peristalsis by auscultating the abdomen. Gurgling and rumbling sounds indicate peristalsis. Anaesthetic agents, narcotics, handling of the intestines during abdominal surgery, fasting and inactivity all inhibit peristalsis. Therefore, bowel sounds should be carefully assessed every 4–6 hours. Oral fluids and food are usually started after the return of peristalsis. It is important that the nurse documents the patient's food tolerance and the passage of flatus or abdominal distention.

Wound Care

Most patients return from surgery with a sutured wound covered by a dressing, although in some cases the wound may be left unsutured. Dressings are inspected regularly to ensure that they are clean, dry and intact. Excessive drainage may indicate haemorrhage, infection or an open wound.

When dressings are changed, the nurse assesses the wound for appearance, size, drainage, swelling, pain and the status of a drain or tubes. Details about these assessments are outlined in the *Practice Guidelines*.

PRACTICE GUIDELINES

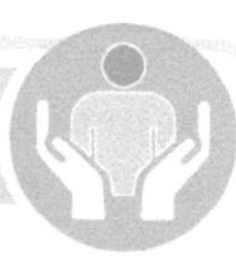

Assessing Surgical Wounds

Appearance

- Inspect colour of wound and surrounding area and approximation of wound edges.

Size

- Note size and location of dehiscence, if present.

Drainage

- Observe location, colour, consistency, odour and degree of saturation of dressings. Note number of gauzes saturated or diameter of drainage on gauze.

Swelling

- Observe the amount of swelling; minimal to moderate swelling is normal in early stages of wound healing.

Pain

- Expect severe to moderate post-operative pain for 3-5 days; persistent severe pain or sudden onset of severe pain may indicate internal haemorrhaging or infection.

Drains or Tubes

- Inspect drain security and placement, amount and character of drainage, and functioning of collecting apparatus, if present.

Because surgical incisions heal by **primary intention** (see Chapter 18), the nurse can expect the following signs of healing:

1 *Absence of bleeding and the appearance of a clot binding the wound edges.* The wound edges are well approximated and bound by fibrin in the clot within the first few hours after surgical closure.
2 *Inflammation (redness and swelling) at the wound edges for 1–3 days.*
3 *Reduction in inflammation when the clot diminishes,* as granulation tissue starts to bridge the area. The wound is bridged and closed within 7–10 days. Increased inflammation associated with fever and drainage is indicative of wound infection; the wound edges then appear brightly inflamed and swollen.
4 *Scar formation.* Collagen synthesis starts four days after injury and continues for six months or longer.
5 *Diminished scar size over a period of months or years.* An increase in scar size indicates keloid formation (excessive tissue forming on a scar).

CLINICAL ALERT

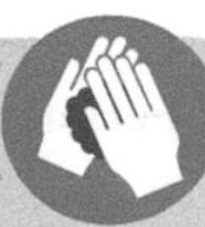

Assess the patient immediately if they report a 'giving' or 'popping' sensation in the incisional area. The patient may be experiencing dehiscence (splitting) or evisceration (contents of body cavity spilling out) of the wound.

Surgical Dressings

Dressings are applied to the incision while the patient is in theatre. If there are no signs of bleeding or excessive drainage on the dressing it should be left for at least 24 hours. Too many dressing changes can cool the wound, open the wound to microorganisms and ultimately delay healing. However, if there is drainage on the dressing the wound needs to be inspected to ensure that there are no signs of haemorrhage or infection. Cleaning a wound and applying a sterile dressing are detailed in *Procedure 26-2.*

PROCEDURE 26-2 Cleaning a Sutured Wound and Applying a Sterile Dressing

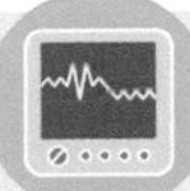

Purposes

- To promote wound healing by primary intention
- To prevent infection
- To assess the healing process
- To protect the wound from mechanical trauma

Assessment

Assess

- Patient allergies to wound cleaning agents
- The appearance and size of the wound
- The amount and character of exudates (liquid discharge)
- Patient complains of discomfort
- The time of the last pain medication
- Signs of systemic infection (e.g. elevated body temperature, diaphoresis, malaise, leukocytosis)

Planning

Before changing a dressing, determine any specific orders about the wound or dressing.

Equipment

- Sterile dressing pack
- Clean gloves
- Sterile gloves
- Sterile saline
- Dressings
- Surgical tape
- Clinical waste bag

Implementation

Preparation

Prepare the patient and assemble the equipment.

- If the patient is confused or restless then acquire assistance to change the dressing. *The person might move and contaminate the sterile field or the wound.*
- Assist the patient to a comfortable position in which the wound can be readily exposed. Expose only the wound area, using a sheet to cover the rest of the patient. *Undue exposure is physically and psychologically distressing to most people.*
- Place the clinical waste bag close to the wound. *Placement of the bag within reach prevents the nurse from reaching across the sterile field and the wound and potentially contaminating these areas.*

Performance

1. Follow local policy to ensure that you explain to the patient what you are going to do, why it is necessary and how they can cooperate. Obtain consent and maintain patient privacy and dignity and ensure that the appropriate local infection control procedures are observed.
2. With clean gloves on loosen the dressing, holding down the skin and pulling the dressing gently but firmly towards the wound. Pressing down on the skin provides counter traction against the pulling motion. *To prevent strain on the sutures or wound.*
3. Remove and dispose of soiled dressings in the clinical waste bag, remove gloves and wash hands.
4. Assess the location, type (colour, consistency) and odour of any wound drainage. Assess the wound, size, wound closure, signs of infection.
5. Set up the sterile supplies.
   - Open the sterile dressing pack, using aseptic technique.
   - Place the sterile towel beside the wound.
   - Open the sterile cleaning solution and pour it over the gauze sponges in the plastic container.
   - Put on sterile gloves.
6. Clean the wound, only if visibly soiled.
   - Clean the wound, using your gloved hands or forceps and gauze swabs moistened with cleaning solution.
   - Use the cleaning methods illustrated and described in Figure 26-8.
   - Use a separate swab for each stroke and discard each swab after use. *To prevent the introduction of micro-organisms to other wound areas.*
   - If a drain is present, clean it next, taking care to avoid reaching across the cleaned incision. Clean the skin around the drain site by swabbing in half or full circles from around the drain site outward, using separate swabs for each wipe (see Figure 26-8(c)).
   - Support and hold the drain erect with a sterile swab while cleaning around it. Clean as many times as necessary to remove the drainage.
   - Dry the surrounding skin with dry gauze swabs as required. Do not dry the incision or wound itself. *To promote wound healing.*
7. Apply dressings to the drain site and the incision (see Figure 26-9).
8. Remove gloves and dispose of all equipment used in the clinical waste.
9. Document the procedure and all nursing assessments.

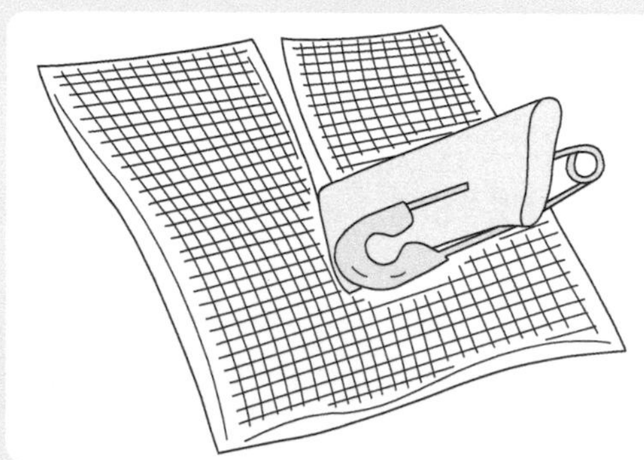

Figure 26-9 Pre-cut gauze in place around a drain.

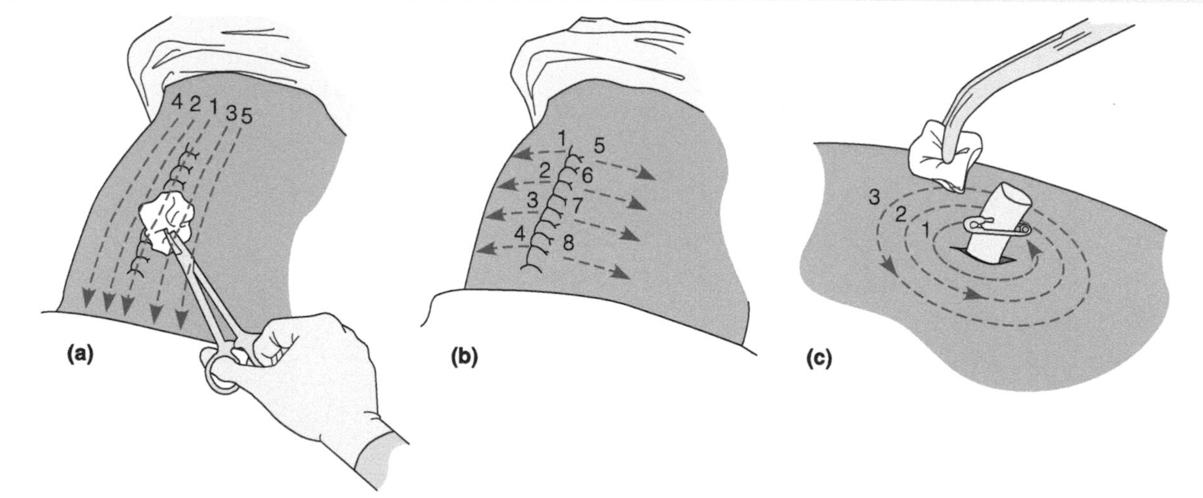

Figure 26-8 Methods of cleaning surgical wounds: (a) cleaning the wound from top to bottom, starting at the centre; (b) cleaning a wound outward from the incision; (c) cleaning around a Penrose drain site. For all methods, a clean sterile swab is used for each stroke.

Evaluation

- Evaluate the choice of dressings by relating assessment to previous assessment of the wound.
- Report any significant changes to a tissue viability nurse, wound care nurse or doctor.

Wound Drains and Suction

Surgical drains are inserted to permit the drainage of excessive serosanguineous (light red liquid) fluid and purulent material and to promote healing of underlying tissues. These drains may be inserted and sutured through the incision line, but they are most commonly inserted through stab wounds a few centimetres away from the incision line so that the incision itself may be kept dry. Without a drain, some wounds would heal on the surface and trap the discharge inside, and an abscess might form.

Drains vary in length and width. The length can be 25–22cm, and the width 1.2–4cm. If the drainage is minimal, the surgeon may ask the nurse to remove the drain. The wound where the drain was will usually heal in a day or two.

A suction drainage system consists of a drain connected to either an electric suction or portable drainage suction (see Figure 26-10). The closed system reduces the possible entry of micro-organisms into the wound through the drain. The drainage tubes are sutured in place and connected to a reservoir, this allows for accurate measurement of the drainage.

When emptying the container of the closed-wound drainage systems, the nurse should adhere to standard precautions wearing gloves, apron and even goggles.

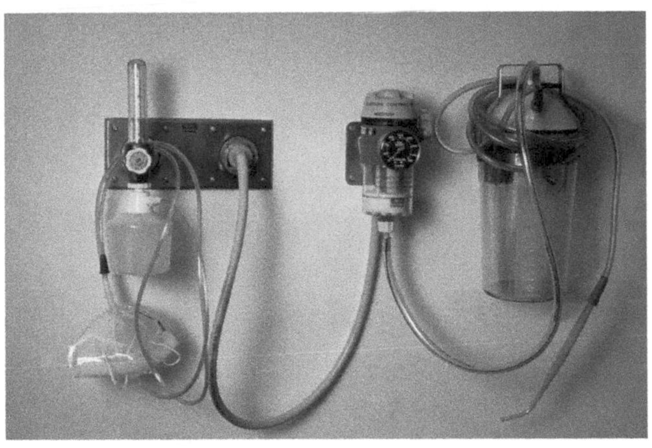

Figure 26-10 Suction drainage system.

Sutures

A suture is a thread used to sew body tissues together. Sutures used to attach tissues beneath the skin are often made of an absorbable material that disappears in several days. Skin sutures, by contrast, are made of a variety of nonabsorbable materials, such as silk, cotton, linen, wire, nylon and Dacron (polyester fibre). Silver wire clips or staples are also available. Usually skin sutures are removed 7–10 days after surgery.

There are various methods of suturing. Skin sutures can be broadly categorised as either interrupted (each stitch is tied and knotted separately) or continuous (one thread runs in a series of stitches and is tied only at the beginning and at the end of the run). Common methods of suturing are illustrated in Figure 26-11.

Retention sutures are very large sutures used in addition to skin sutures for some incisions (see Figure 26-12). They attach

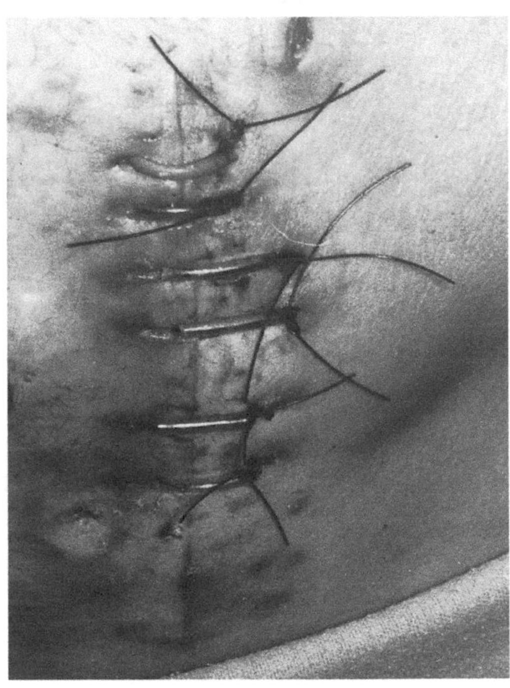

Figure 26-12 A surgical incision with retention sutures.
Source: Jenny Thomas.

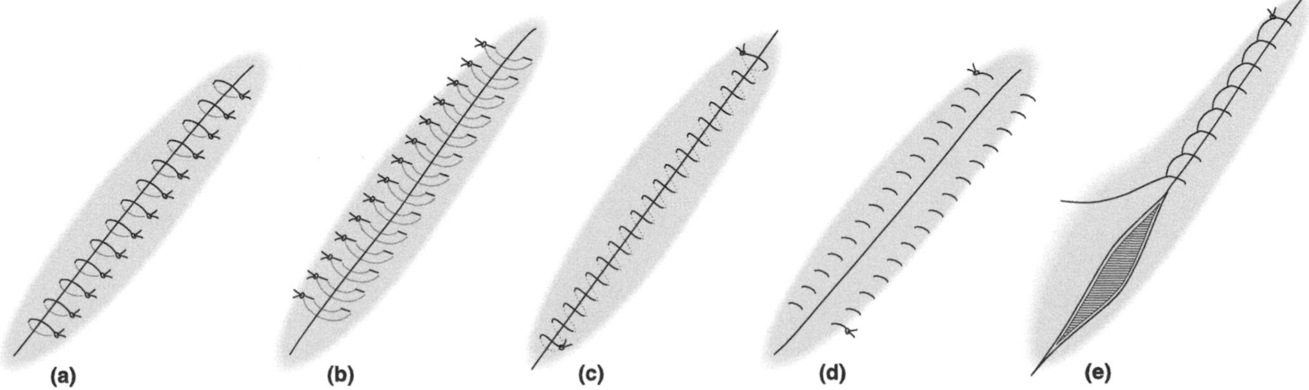

Figure 26-11 Common sutures: (a) plain interrupted; (b) mattress interrupted; (c) plain continuous; (d) mattress continuous; (e) blanket continuous.

underlying tissues of fat and muscle as well as skin and are used to support incisions in obese individuals or when healing may be prolonged. They are frequently left in place longer than skin sutures (14–21 days) but in some instances are removed at the same time as the skin sutures. To prevent these large sutures from irritating the incision, the surgeon may place rubber tubing over them or a roll of gauze under them extending down the incision line.

Usually the surgeon will inform the nurse when the sutures are to be removed. Sterile technique and special suture cutters are used in suture removal. Suture cutters have a short, curved blade that readily slides under the suture (see Figure 26-13).

Wire clips or staples are removed with a special instrument that squeezes the centre of the clip to remove it from the skin (see Figure 26-14). Guidelines for removing sutures and staples are as follows:

1 Before removing skin sutures, verify (a) the orders for suture removal (in many instances, only *alternate* interrupted sutures are removed one day, and the remaining sutures are removed a day or two later) and (b) whether a dressing is to be applied following the suture removal. Some surgeons prefer no dressing; others prefer small, light gauze dressing to prevent friction by clothing.
2 Inform the patient that suture removal may produce slight discomfort, such as a pulling or stinging sensation, but should not be painful.
3 Remove dressings and clean the incision if necessary.
4 Put on sterile gloves.
5 Remove plain interrupted sutures as follows:
   - Grasp the suture at the knot with a pair of forceps.
   - Place the curved tip of the suture cutter under the suture as close to the skin as possible, either on the side opposite the knot (see Figure 26-15) or directly under the knot. Cut the suture. Sutures are cut as close to the skin as possible on one side of the visible part because the suture material that is visible to the eye is in contact with resident bacteria of the skin and must not be pulled beneath the skin during removal. Suture material that is beneath the skin is considered free from bacteria.
   - With the forceps, pull the suture out in one piece. Inspect the suture carefully to make sure that all suture material is removed. Suture material left beneath the skin acts as a foreign body and causes inflammation.

Figure 26-13 Suture or stitch cutters.

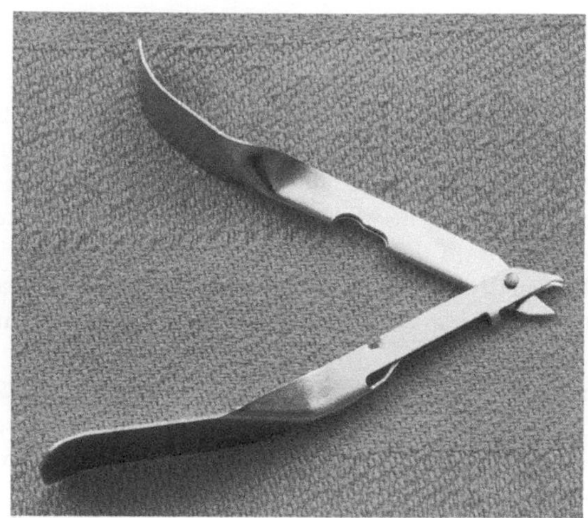

Figure 26-14 Staple remover.

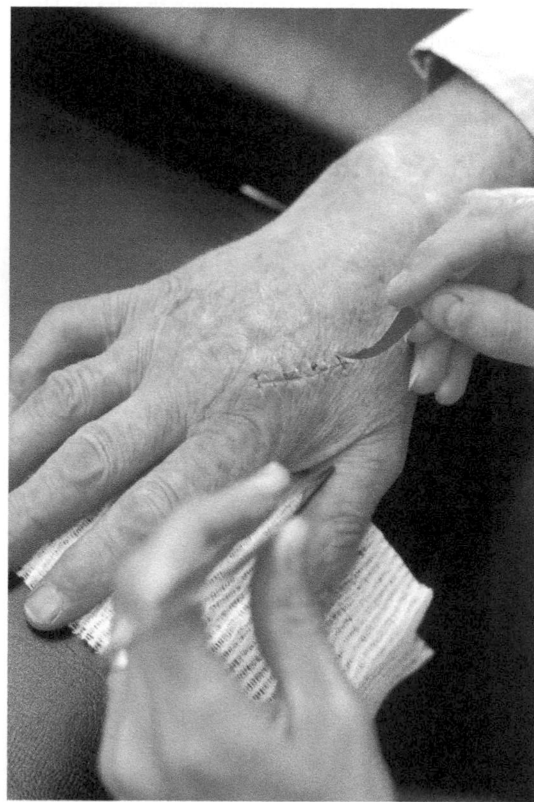

Figure 26-15 Removing a plain interrupted skin suture.

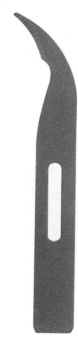

6 Discard the suture onto a piece of sterile gauze or into a clinical waste bag, being careful not to contaminate the forceps tips.

7 Continue to remove alternate sutures, that is, the third, fifth, seventh, and so forth. Alternate sutures are removed first so that remaining sutures keep the skin edges in close approximation and prevent any dehiscence from becoming large.

8 If no dehiscence occurs, remove the remaining sutures. If dehiscence does occur, do not remove the remaining sutures, and report the dehiscence to the nurse in charge.

9 Reapply a dressing, if indicated.

10 Document the suture removal; number of sutures removed; appearance of the incision; application of a dressing, patient teaching; and patient tolerance of the procedure.

11 Remove staples as follows:
- Remove dressings and clean the incision if necessary.
- Place the lower tips of a sterile staple remover under the staple.
- Squeeze the handles together until they are completely closed (see Figure 26-16). Pressing the handles together causes the staple to bend in the middle and pulls the edges of the staple out of the skin. Do not lift the staple remover when squeezing the handles.
- When both ends of the staple are visible, gently move the staple away from the incision site.
- Hold the staple remover over a disposable container, release the staple remover handles and release the staple.

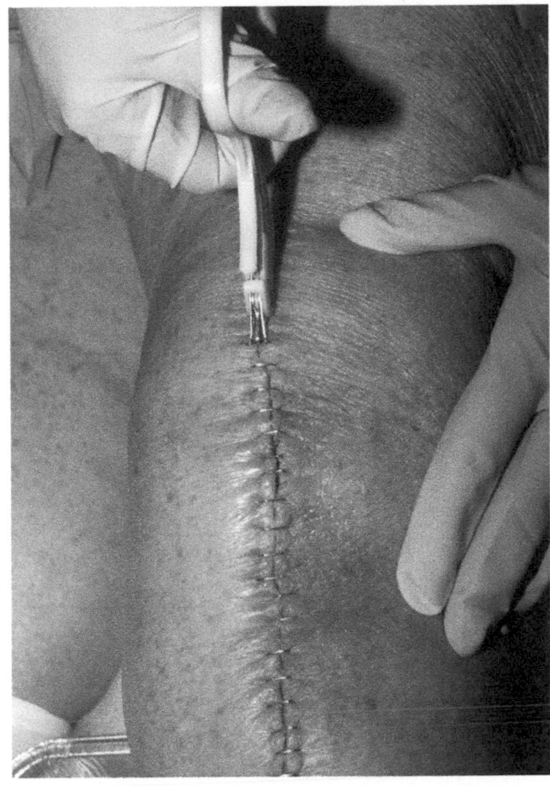

Figure 26-16 Removing surgical clips or staple.

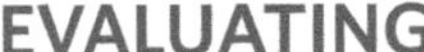

EVALUATING

Using the goals developed during the planning stage, the nurse collects data to evaluate whether the identified goals and desired outcomes have been achieved. If the desired outcomes are not achieved, the nurse, patient and family need to explore the reasons before modifying the care plan. For example, if the outcome 'Pain control' is not met, questions to be considered include:

- What is the patient's perception of the problem?
- Does the patient understand how to use PCA (patient controlled analgesia)?
- Is the prescribed analgesic dose adequate for the patient?
- Is the patient allowing pain to become intense prior to requesting medication or using PCA?
- Where is the patient's pain? Could it be due to a problem unrelated to surgery (e.g. chronic arthritis, anginal pain)?
- Is there evidence of a complication that could cause increased pain (an infection, abscess or **haematoma**)?

RESEARCH NOTE

Rapid Recovery Following Cardiac Surgery

Fast-track or rapid-recovery pathways for cardiac surgery patients are commonplace in order to maximise the use of scarce resources. However, there are no nationally agreed protocols to guide this practice. In order to evaluate the safety of this practice in a London teaching hospital, a nursing audit was undertaken. It considered length of hospital stay and incidences of post-operative complications as well as the patient's views of rapid recovery. One hundred and four patients who followed the rapid-recovery pathway were included in this study alongside a comparison group of forty-eight patients who followed the conventional recovery pathway. The results showed that length of stay was the same for both groups; however, there was significantly less post-operative complications in the patients who followed the rapid-recovery pathway. They concluded that rapid recovery is safe for carefully selected cardiac surgical patients, but barriers to rapid recovery, such as resources, need to be explored.

Source: Naughton, C. Cheek, L. and O'Hara, K. (2005) 'Rapid recovery following cardiac surgery: a nursing perspective', *British Journal of Nursing*, 14(4), 214–219.

ACTIVITY 26-3

What are the priorities of care for a patient in the immediate post-operative phase?

CRITICAL REFLECTION

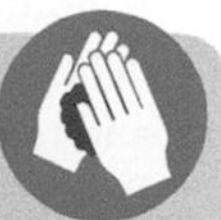

Let us revisit the case study on page 775. Now that you have finished reading this chapter, what are the factors that placed Mr Teng at increased risk of complications during and after surgery and why do you think he was given spinal anaesthesia as opposed to general anaesthesia.

CHAPTER HIGHLIGHTS

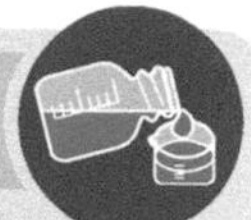

- Surgery is a unique experience that creates stress that requires the patient to make necessary physical and psychological changes.
- There are three phases: pre-operative, intra-operative and post-operative.
- Surgical procedures are categorised by degree of urgency, purpose and degree of risk.
- Factors such as age, general health, nutritional status, medication use and mental status affect a patient's risk during surgery.
- Patients must agree to surgery and sign an informed consent.
- Pre-operative physical and psychological assessment can provide important information for planning pre-operative and post-operative care.
- The overall goal of nursing care during the pre-operative phase is to prepare the patient mentally and physically for surgery.
- Pre-operative teaching includes situational information and psychosocial support, the role of the patient, expected sensations and discomfort, and training for the post-operative period.
- Pre-operative teaching should include moving, leg exercises and coughing and deep-breathing exercises. Many aspects of pre-operative teaching are intended to prevent post-operative complications.
- Physical preparation includes the following areas: nutrition and fluids, elimination, rest, medications, care prostheses and skin preparation.
- A pre-operative checklist provides a guide to and documentation of a patient's preparation before surgery.
- Maintaining the patient's safety is the overall goal of nursing care during the intra-operative phase.
- Anaesthesia may be general or local.
- Positioning of the patient during surgery is important to reduce the risk of tissue and nerve damage.
- Immediate post-anaesthetic care focuses on assessment and monitoring parameters to prevent complications from anaesthesia or surgery.
- Initial and ongoing assessment of the post-operative patient includes level of consciousness, vital signs, oxygen saturation, skin colour and temperature, comfort, fluid balance, dressings, drains and tubes.
- The overall goals of nursing care during the post-operative period are to promote comfort and healing, restore the highest possible level of wellness, and prevent associated risks such as infection or respiratory and cardiovascular complications.
- Ongoing post-operative nursing interventions include (a) managing pain (see Chapter 24), (b) appropriate positioning, (c) encouraging incentive spirometry and deep-breathing and coughing exercises, (d) promoting leg exercises and early ambulation, (e) maintaining adequate hydration and nutritional status, (f) promoting urinary elimination, (g) continuing gastrointestinal suction and (h) providing wound care.
- Aseptic technique (sterile technique) is used when changing dressings on surgical wounds to promote healing and reduce the risk of infection.
- Sutures, wire clips or staples are used to approximate skin and underlying tissues after surgery. These are generally removed 7–10 days after surgery.

ACTIVITY ANSWERS

ACTIVITY 26-1 The pre-operative care that you would have given your patient would be quite specific. However, some fundamental care he would have received would have included:

- A full physical assessment
- Pre-operative investigations - blood tests, chest x-ray, abdominal x-ray, ECG, arterial blood gases to establish respiratory status
- Social care assessment - to establish the patient's care requirements on discharge
- Teaching - breathing techniques and exercises and mobilising
- Nutritional assessment - to assess his nutritional status
- Medication - to record his current medication and establish if any pre-operative medications are required
- Preparation of the patient - physical preparation, e.g. skin preparation, and psychological preparation

ACTIVITY 26-2 Spinal anaesthetic is often offered to patients with underlying conditions such as COPD in order to reduce the risk of intra-operative and post-operative complications and encourage a swift recovery.

ACTIVITY 26-3 The priorities of care for a patient in the immediate post-operative phase would be:

- *Airway.* Is he able to maintain his airway. What is his consciousness level?
- *Breathing.* Respiratory rate, depth, any signs of respiratory collapse. His central and peripheral colour. Oxygen saturations.
- *Circulation.* Blood pressure and pulse.
- *Pain.* Assess pain and administer analgesia as prescribed.
- *Wound.* Where is the wound? Any drains? Any soiling to dressing? What type of dressing?
- *Other.* Surgeons orders regarding recovery period, e.g. medication positioning, mobilising, etc.

REFERENCES

Dizer, B., Hatipoglu, S., Kaymakcioglu, N., Tufan, T., Yav, A., Iyigun, E. and Senses, Z. (2009) 'The effect of nurse-performed pre-operative skin preparation on postoperative surgical site infections in abdominal surgery', *Journal of Clinical Nursing*, 18, 3325–3332.

Hospital Episode Statistics (2009) *Headline figures 2008–09*, London: Department of Health, available at http://www.hesonline.nhs.uk/ (accessed 30 June 2011).

Kagan, I. and Bar-Tal, Y. (2008) 'The effect of pre-operative uncertainty and anxiety on short-term recover after elective arthroplasty', *Journal of Clinical Nursing*, 17, 576–583.

Kost, M. (1999) 'Conscious sedation: Guarding your patient against complications', *Nursing*, 29(4), 34–39.

Naughton, C., Cheek, L. and O'Hara, K. (2005) 'Rapid recovery following cardiac surgery: A nursing perspective', *British Journal of Nursing*, 14(4), 214–219.

NICE (2003) *Pre-operative tests: The use of routine pre-operative tests for elective surgery*, CG3, London: NICE.

NMC (2008) *The Code: Standards of conduct, performance and ethics for nurses and midwives*, London: NMC.

NMC (2010) *Standards for pre-registration nursing education*, London: NMC.

RCN (2005) *Perioperative fasting in adults and children*, London: RCN.

Van Keuren, K. and Eland, J.A. (1997) 'Perioperative pain management in children', *Nursing Clinics of North America*, **32**(1), 31–44.

Vaughn, F., Wichowski, H. and Bosworth, G. (2007) 'Does pre-operative anxiety level predict post-operative pain?' *Association of perioperative Registered Nurses (AORN) Journal*, 85, 589–604.

CHAPTER 27
DIAGNOSTIC TESTING

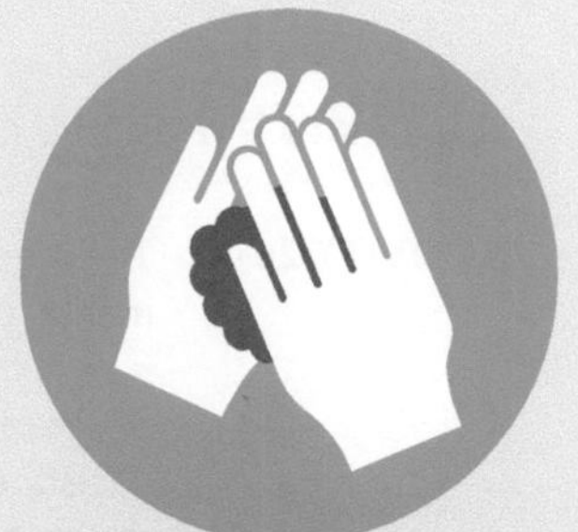

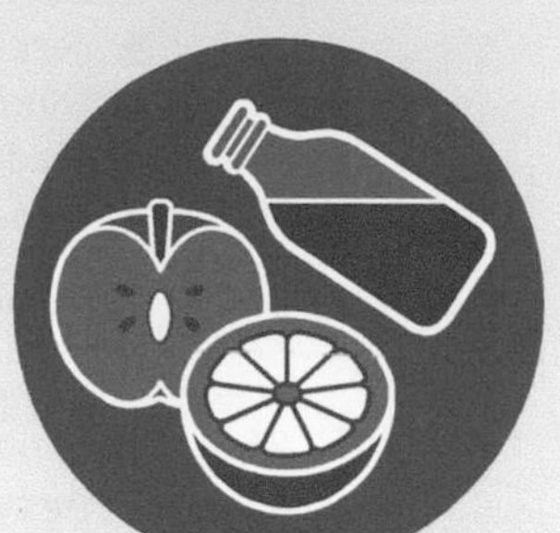

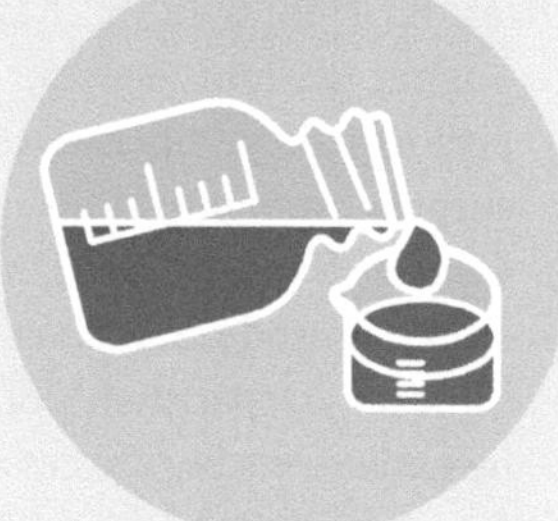

LEARNING OUTCOMES

After completing this chapter, you will be able to:

- Describe the nurse's role for each of the phases involved in diagnostic testing.
- List common blood tests.
- Discuss the nursing responsibilities for specimen collection.
- Explain the rationale for the collection of each type of specimen.
- Collect and test stool specimens.
- Compare and contrast the different types of urine specimens.
- Collect sputum and throat specimens.
- Describe how you would prepare a patient for procedures that may be used for the patient with gastrointestinal, urinary and cardiopulmonary changes.
- Compare and contrast computed tomography (CT), magnetic resonance imaging (MRI) and nuclear imaging studies.
- Describe the nurse's role in caring for patients undergoing aspiration/biopsy procedures.

After reading this chapter you will be able to reflect on the nursing role in providing healthcare, the way care is organised and effective care management. It relates to **Essential Skills Clusters (NMC, 2010) 1, 2, 3, 4, 5, 6, 7, 8, 9, 10, 11, 14, 19**, as appropriate for each progression point.

Ensure that you really understand this chapter by logging on to your complimentary **MyNursingKit** at **www.pearsoned.co.uk/kozier**. Complete the self-assessment tests to check your progress and utilise further activities to practise and confirm your understanding.

CASE STUDY

John is a 72-year-old gentleman who has been in and out of hospital for many years with a bipolar disorder (manic depression). Three years ago, John was admitted to an acute medical ward and was diagnosed with squamous cell carcinoma of the lung (a slow developing cancer). At the time of diagnosis John was relatively well. He refused all advice and treatment offered to him in relation to his current medical condition, refused to speak to the psychiatrist looking after him and took his own discharge from hospital.

During the course of your morning shift John has been admitted into your care. He is obviously breathless, anxious and vulnerable. The doctor has ordered a chest x-ray and a CT scan of the lungs and abdomen and a sputum specimen is required. The doctor has also advised John that he may need a bronchoscope.

INTRODUCTION

Diagnostic and laboratory tests (commonly called lab tests) are tools that provide information about the patient. Tests may be used as basic screening as part of a wellness check. Frequently tests are used to help confirm a diagnosis, monitor an illness and provide valuable information about the patient's response to treatment. Nurses need knowledge of the most common lab and diagnostic tests because one primary role of the nurse is to teach the patient, family and/or carer how to prepare for the test and the care that may be required following the test. Nurses must also know the implications of the test results in order to provide the patient with the appropriate information and nursing care.

Diagnostic testing occurs in many environments. The traditional sites include hospitals, clinics and the community, for example the home, workplace, shopping centres and mobile units. The more complex diagnostic tests are performed at diagnostic centres specifically built for those tests.

DIAGNOSTIC TESTING

Diagnostic testing involves three phases: pre-test, peri-test and post-test.

Pre-test

The major focus of the pre-test phase is patient preparation. A thorough assessment and data collection (e.g. biological, psychological, sociological, cultural and spiritual) using effective communication skills assists the nurse to guide patient care and inform the patient.

The nurse also needs to know what equipment and supplies are needed for the specific test. Common questions include these:

- What type of sample will be needed and how will it be collected?
- Does the patient need to stop oral intake for a certain number of hours prior to the test?
- Does the test include administration of dye (contrast media) and, if so, is it injected or swallowed?
- Are fluids restricted or forced?
- Are medications given or withheld?
- How long is the test?

Gathering and assessing this information will aid the nurse in making an effective decision to enhance the well-being of the patient.

Peri-test

This phase focuses on specimen collection and performing or assisting with certain diagnostic testing. The nurse uses standard precautions and sterile technique as appropriate. During the procedure, the nurse provides emotional and physical support while monitoring the patient as needed (e.g., vital signs, pulse oximetry, ECG). The nurse ensures correct labelling, storage and transportation of the specimen to avoid invalid test results.

Post-test

The focus of this phase is on nursing care of the patient and follow-up activities and observations. It is the responsibility of the nurse to observe and undertake any vital sign reading as appropriate to maintain the safety of the patient. The nurse will also compare the previous (if applicable) and current test results and modify nursing interventions as needed. The nurse also reports the results to doctor.

BLOOD TESTS

Blood tests are one of the most commonly used diagnostic tests and can provide valuable information about the haematologic system and many other body systems. A venepuncture (puncture of a vein for collection of a blood specimen) can be performed by various members of the healthcare team. Usually a phlebotomist, a person from a laboratory who performs venepuncture, collects the blood specimen for the tests ordered by the doctor. Many nurses have now taken on this extended role following training, and are also able to take bloods from patients.

Table 27-1 Normal Values (approx.) of Some Full Blood Counts

Age	Haemoglobin Hb (g/dl)	MCV (fl) Mean Cell Volume	WBC (×10 9/1)	Platelets (×10 9/1)
Birth	14.5-21.5	100-135	10-26	150-450 for all ages
2 weeks	13.4-19.8	88-120	6-21	
2 months	9.4-13.0	84-105	6-18	
1 year	11.3-14.1	71-85	6-17.5	
2-6 years	11.5-13.5	75-87	5-17	
6-12 years	11.5-15.5	77-95	4.5-14.5	
12-18 years	10.0-15.5	78-100	4.5-13	
Adult Male	13.0-16.0	78-95	4.5-13	
Adult Female	12.0-16.0	78-95	4.5-13	

Full Blood Count

Specimens of venous blood are taken for a full blood count (FBC), which includes haemoglobin and haematocrit measurements, erythrocyte (red blood cell – RBC) count, leukocyte (white blood cell – WBC) count, RBC indices and a differential white cell count. The FBC is a basic screening test and one of the most frequently ordered blood tests (see Table 27-1).

The **haemoglobin** is a measure of the total amount of haemoglobin in the blood. The **haematocrit** measures the percentage of red blood cells in the total blood volume. Normal values for both haemoglobin and haematocrit vary, with males having higher levels than females. Haemoglobin and haematocrit increase with dehydration as the blood becomes more concentrated, and decrease with hypervolaemia and resulting haemodilution. Both the haemoglobin and haematocrit are related to the RBC count, the number of RBCs per cubic millimetre of whole blood. It also varies by gender and age. Low RBC counts are indicative of anaemia. Patients with chronic hypoxia may develop higher than normal counts, a condition known as **polycythaemia**. Red blood cell (RBC) indices may be performed as part of the FBC to evaluate the size, weight and haemoglobin concentration of RBCs. The leukocyte or white blood cell (WBC) count determines the number of circulating WBCs per cubic millimetre of whole blood. High WBC counts are often seen in the presence of a bacterial infection; by contrast, WBC counts may be low if a viral infection is present. In the WBC differential, leukocytes are identified by type, and the percentage of each type is determined. This information is useful in diagnosing certain disorders that have characteristic patterns of distribution.

Urea and Electrolytes

Urea and electrolytes are often routinely ordered for any patient admitted to a hospital as a screening test for urea and electrolyte imbalances. Such tests are often requested, for example for patients in the community who are being treated for hypertension and have been prescribed a diuretic, to assess the electrolyte balance. The most commonly ordered urea and electrolyte tests are for sodium, potassium chloride, bicarbonate ions, urea and creatinine. Normal values of urea and electrolytes are seen in Table 27-2.

Table 27-2 Normal Ranges for some Urea and Electrolyte Counts.

Blood Component	Normal Range
Sodium	13.5-14.5mmol/l
Potassium	3.5-5.2mmol/l
Bicarbonate	22-28mmol/l
Urea	2.5-6.5mmol/l
Creatinine	55-105mmol/l
Calcium	4.5-5.5mmol/l
Chloride	95-105mmol/l
Magnesium	1.5-2.5mmol/l
Phosphate	1.8-2.6mmol/l

Blood levels of two metabolically produced substances, urea and creatinine, are routinely used to evaluate renal function. The kidneys, through filtration and tubular secretion, normally eliminate both. Urea, the end product of protein metabolism, is measured as blood urea nitrogen (BUN). **Creatinine** is produced in relatively constant quantities by the muscles and is excreted by the kidneys. Thus, the amount of creatinine in the blood relates to renal excretory function.

Drug Monitoring

Therapeutic drug monitoring is often conducted when a client is taking a medication with a narrow therapeutic range (e.g. digoxin). This monitoring includes drawing blood samples for peak and trough levels to determine if the blood serum levels of a specific drug are at a therapeutic level and not a sub-therapeutic or toxic level. The peak level indicates the highest concentration of the drug in the blood serum and the trough level represents the lowest concentration. Ideally, a patient's peak and trough levels fall within the therapeutic range.

Arterial Blood Gases

Measurement of **arterial blood gases** is another important diagnostic procedure (see Chapter 16). Specialty nurses or medical technicians normally take specimens of arterial blood from the radial, brachial or femoral arteries. Because of the relatively great pressure of the blood in these arteries, it is important to prevent haemorrhaging by applying pressure to the puncture side for about 5–10 minutes after removing the needle.

Blood Cultures

A blood culture is taken when the doctor suspects that there is an infection (bacterial) or yeast in the bloodstream (septicaemia or sepsis). A doctor may order blood cultures when a patient presents with symptoms such as chills, fever, nausea, rapid breathing, confusion or low urine output. Sepsis can be a life-threatening infection and can spread rapidly throughout the body and into the joints. The immune system works very hard to try and fight the infections. However, patients who are already immunocompromised, such as those having chemotherapy, are more at risk. Blood cultures are normally taken by the doctor or those who have been trained in taking the sample.

Blood Chemistry

A number of other tests may be performed on blood serum (the liquid portion of the blood). These are often referred to as a blood chemistry. In addition to serum electrolytes, common chemistry examinations include determining certain enzymes that may be present (including lactic dehydrogenase [LDH], creatine kinase [CK], aspartate aminotransferase [AST] and alanine aminotransferase [ALT]), serum glucose, hormones such as thyroid hormone and other substances such as cholesterol and triglycerides. These tests provide valuable diagnostic cues. For example, cardiac markers (e.g., CPK-MB, myoglobin, troponin T and troponin I) are released into the blood during a myocardial infarction (MI, or heart attack). Elevated levels of these markers in the venous blood can help differentiate between an MI and chest pain from a different cause such as angina or pleuritic pain.

A common lab test is the glycosylated haemoglobin or haemoglobin A1C (HbA1C), which is a measurement of blood glucose that is bound to haemoglobin. Haemoglobin A1C is a reflection of how well blood glucose levels have been controlled during the prior 3–4 months. An elevated HbA1C reflects hyperglycemia in diabetics.

Capillary Blood Glucose

A capillary blood specimen is often taken to measure blood glucose when frequent tests to monitor blood glucose levels are required. This technique is less painful than a venipuncture and easily performed. Hence, patients can perform this technique on themselves.

Capillary blood specimens are commonly obtained from the lateral aspect or side of the finger in adults. This site avoids the nerve endings and calloused areas at the fingertip. The earlobe may be used if the patient is in shock or the fingers are oedematous. Capillary blood tests are not always undertaken by student nurses as they haven't received appropriate training in the monitoring machines available. Prior to undertaking this procedure student nurses should check local policy.

SPECIMEN COLLECTION

Laboratory examination of specimens such as urine, blood, stool, sputum and wound drainage provides important adjunct information for diagnosing healthcare problems and also provides a measure of the responses to therapy. It is the nurse's responsibility to collect specimens of body fluid.

While nurses often have the responsibility for specimen collection, depending on the type of specimen and skill required, the nurse may be able to delegate this task to healthcare support worker (HCSW).

Nursing responsibilities associated with specimen collection include the following:

- Explain the purpose of the specimen collection and the procedure for obtaining the specimen and the impending results.
- Provide patient with privacy, dignity, comfort and safety at all times.
- Obtain consent.
- Use aseptic technique and follow local policy in carrying out the procedure for obtaining a specimen or ensure that the patient follows the correct procedure.
- Note that the relevant information on the laboratory request form is included, e.g. medications that the patient is taking that may affect the results.
- Transport the specimen to the laboratory promptly. Fresh specimens provide more accurate results.
- Report abnormal laboratory findings to the doctor.
- Document procedure and findings when available.

Stool Specimens

Analysis of stool specimens can provide information about a patient's health condition. Some of the reasons for testing faeces include the following:

- To determine the presence of **occult** (hidden) blood. Bleeding can occur as a result of ulcers, inflammatory disease or tumours.
- To analyse for dietary products and digestive secretions. For example, an excessive amount of fat in the stool (steatorrhea) can indicate faulty absorption of fat from the small intestine. A decreased amount of bile can indicate obstruction of bile flow from the liver and gallbladder into the intestine. For these kinds of tests, the nurse needs to collect and send the total quantity of stool expelled at one time instead of a small sample.
- To detect the presence of ova and parasites. When collecting specimens for parasites, it is important that the sample be

transported immediately to the lab while it is still warm. Usually three stool specimens are evaluated to confirm the presence of and to identify the organism so that appropriate treatment can be ordered, but this needs to be confirmed as per local policy (Kee, 2002).

- To detect the presence of bacteria or viruses. Only a small amount of faeces is required because the specimen will be cultured.
- Collection containers or tubes must be sterile and aseptic technique used during collection. Stools need to be sent immediately to the laboratory. The nurse needs to note on the lab requisition if the patient is receiving any antibiotics.

Collecting Stool Specimens

The nurse is responsible for collecting stool specimens ordered for laboratory analysis. Before obtaining a specimen, the nurse needs to determine the reason for collecting the stool specimen and the correct method of obtaining and handling (i.e. how much stool to obtain, whether a preservative needs to be added to the stool, and whether it needs to be sent immediately to the laboratory). It may be necessary to confirm this information by checking with the laboratory. In many situations only a single specimen is required; in others, timed specimens are necessary, and every stool passed is collected within a designated time period.

HCSW may obtain and collect stool specimen(s). The nurse, however, needs to consider the collection process before delegating this task. For example, a random stool specimen collected in a specimen container may be delegated, but a stool culture requiring a sterile swab in a test tube should be done by the nurse. An incorrect collection technique can cause inaccurate test results.

Obtaining and testing a stool specimen for occult blood may be performed by HCSW; however, it is important that the nurse instruct the HCSW to tell the nurse if blood is detected and/or whether the test is positive. In addition, the stool specimen should be saved to allow the nurse to repeat the test.

Nurses need to give patients the following instructions:

- Defecate in a clean bedpan or bedside commode.
- Do not contaminate the specimen, if possible, with urine or menstrual discharge. Void before the specimen collection.
- Do not place toilet tissue in the bedpan after defecation. Contents of the paper can affect the laboratory analysis.
- Notify the nurse as soon as possible after defecation, particularly for specimens that need to be sent to the laboratory immediately.

When obtaining stool samples, that is, when handling the patient's bedpan, when transferring the stool sample to a specimen container and when disposing of the bedpan contents, the nurse should:

- Follow aseptic technique procedure.
- Wear disposable gloves to prevent hand contamination and take care not to contaminate the outside of the specimen container.
- Use one or two clean tongue blades to transfer the specimen to the container and then wrap them in a paper towel before disposing of them (as per local policy).

The amount of stool to be sent depends on the purpose for which the specimen is collected. Usually about 2.5cm (1in.) of formed stool or 15–30mL of liquid stool is adequate. For some timed specimens, however, the entire stool passed may need to be sent. Visible pus, mucus or blood should be included in sample specimens. For a stool culture, the nurse dips a sterile swab into the specimen, preferably where purulent faecal matter is present and, using sterile technique, places the swab in a sterile test tube.

Ensure that the specimen label and the laboratory request form have the correct information on them and are securely attached to the specimen container. Inappropriate identification of the specimen risks errors of diagnosis or therapy for the patient.

Because fresh specimens provide the most accurate results, the nurse sends the specimen to the laboratory immediately. Document all relevant information. Record the collection of the specimen on the patient's chart and on the nursing care plan.

Include in the recording the date and time of the collection and all nursing assessments (e.g. colour, odour, consistency and amount of faeces); presence of abnormal constituents, such as blood or mucus; results of test for occult blood if obtained; discomfort during or after defecation; status of perianal skin; and any bleeding from the anus after defecation.

LIFESPAN CONSIDERATIONS

Stool Specimen

Infants

- To collect a stool specimen for an infant, the stool is scraped from the nappy.

Children

- A child who is toilet trained should be able to provide a faecal specimen, but may prefer being assisted by a parent.
- When explaining the procedure to the child, use words appropriate for the child's age rather than medical terms. Ask the parent what words the family normally uses to describe a bowel movement.

Mature Adults

- Mature adults may need assistance if serial stool specimens are required.

COMMUNITY CARE CONSIDERATIONS

Stool Specimen

- Ask the patient or caregiver to call when the stool specimen is obtained. If a laboratory test is needed, the nurse can pick up the specimen or a family member may take it to the laboratory.
- Place the stool specimen inside a plastic biohazard bag. Carry the bag in a sealed container marked 'biohazard' and take it to the laboratory promptly. Do not expose the specimen to extreme temperatures in the car.

Urine Specimens

The nurse is responsible for collecting urine specimens for a number of tests: clean voided specimens for routine urinalysis, clean-catch or midstream urine specimens for urine culture, and timed urine specimens for a variety of tests that depend on the patient's specific health problem. Urine specimen collection may require collection via straight catheter insertion. If this is necessary, refer to Chapter 21.

Clean Voided Urine Specimen

A clean voided specimen is usually adequate for routine examination. Many patients are able to collect a clean voided specimen and provide the specimen independently with minimal instructions. Male patients generally are able to void directly into the specimen container, and female patients usually sit or squat over the toilet, holding the container between their legs during voiding. Routine urine examination is usually done on the first voided specimen in the morning because it tends to have a higher, more uniform concentration and a more acidic pH than specimens later in the day. At least 10mL of urine is generally sufficient for a routine urinalysis. Patients who are seriously ill, physically incapacitated or disoriented may need to use a bedpan or urinal in bed; others may require supervision or assistance in the bathroom. Whatever the situation, clear and specific directions are required:

- The specimen must be free of faecal contamination, so urine must be kept separate from faeces.
- Female patients should discard the toilet tissue in the toilet or in a waste bag rather than in the bedpan because tissue in the specimen makes laboratory analysis more difficult.
- Put the lid tightly on the container to prevent spillage of the urine and contamination of other objects.
- If the outside of the container has been contaminated by urine, clean it with appropriate solution (as per local policy).
- The nurse must:
  - make sure that the specimen label and the laboratory request form carry the correct information

  and
  - attach them securely to the specimen. Inappropriate identification of the specimen can lead to errors of diagnosis or treatment for the patient.

HCSW may be assigned to collect a routine urine specimen. Provide the HCSW with clear directions on how to instruct the patient to collect his or her own urine specimen or how to correctly collect the specimen for the client who may need to use a bedpan or urinal.

Midstream Urine Specimen

Midstream voided specimens are collected when a urine culture is ordered to identify micro-organisms causing urinary tract infection. Although some contamination by skin bacteria may occur with a clean-catch specimen, the risk of introducing micro-organisms into the urinary tract through catheterisation is more significant. Care is taken to ensure that the specimen is as free as possible from contamination by micro-organisms around the urinary meatus. Midstream urine specimens are collected into a sterile specimen container with a lid (see Figure 27-1).

Procedure 27-1 explains how to collect a midstream specimen for culture and sensitivity.

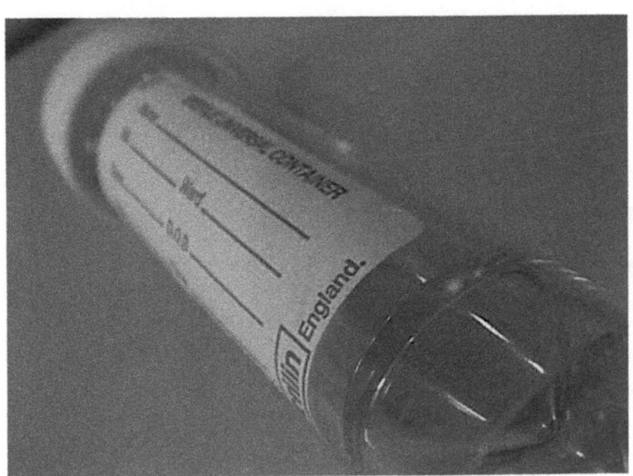

Figure 27-1 Urine sample collection container.
Source: E M Clements Photography.

PROCEDURE 27-1 Collecting a Midstream Urine Specimen for Culture and Sensitivity

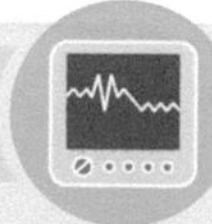

Purposes

- To collect a sample of urine for diagnostic purposes
- To identify bacteria present in the urine and any sensitivity the patient may have to antibiotics

Assessment

Assess

- The ability of the patient to provide the specimen.
- The colour, odour, and consistency of the urine and the presence of clinical signs of urinary tract infection (e.g., frequency, urgency, dysuria, haematuria, flank pain, cloudy urine with foul odour).
- Whether the procedure can be delegated to a HCSW. A HCSW may perform the collection of a clean-catch or midstream urine specimen. It is important, however, that the nurse inform the HCSW about how to instruct the patient in the correct process for obtaining the specimen. Proper cleansing of the urethra should be emphasised to avoid contaminating the urine specimen.

Delegation

HCSW may perform the collection of a clean-catch or midstream urine specimen. It is important, however, that the nurse inform the HCSW about how to instruct the patient in the correct process for obtaining the specimen. Proper cleansing of the urethra should be emphasised to avoid contaminating the urine specimen.

Planning

Equipment

Equipment used varies from organisation to organisation. Some organisations use commercially prepared disposable midstream urine kits. Others use organisation-prepared sterile trays. Both prepared trays and kits generally contain the following items:

- Clean gloves
- Clean wipes
- 0.9% saline
- Sterile cotton balls or 2 × 2 gauze pads
- Sterile specimen container
- Specimen identification label

In addition the nurse needs to obtain:

- Completed laboratory requisition form
- Urine receptacle, if the patient is not ambulatory
- Basin of warm water, soap or cleansing agent as per local policy, wipe and towel for the nonambulatory patient

Implementation

Preparation

Gather the necessary equipment needed for the collection of the specimen. Use visual aids, if available, to assist the patient to understand the midstream collection technique.

Performance

1 Follow local policy to ensure that you explain to the patient what you are going to do, why it is necessary and how they can cooperate. Obtain consent and maintain patient privacy and dignity and ensure that the appropriate local infection control procedures are observed.

2 Provide for patient dignity and privacy.

3 For an ambulatory patient who is able to follow directions, instruct the patient on how to collect the specimen.
   - Direct or assist the patient to the bathroom.
   - Ask the patient to wash and dry the genitals and perineal area with soap or cleansing agent and water. *Washing the perineal area reduces the number of skin and transient bacteria, decreasing the risk of contaminating the urine specimen.*
   - Instruct the patient on how to clean the urinary meatus with appropriate wipes.

For female patients *(Dougherty and Lister, 2008)*

- Use each wipe only once. Clean the perineal area from front to back using the 0.9% saline and discard the wipes as per hospital policy. *Cleaning from front to back cleans the area that is least contaminated to the area of greatest contamination* (Figure 27-2).

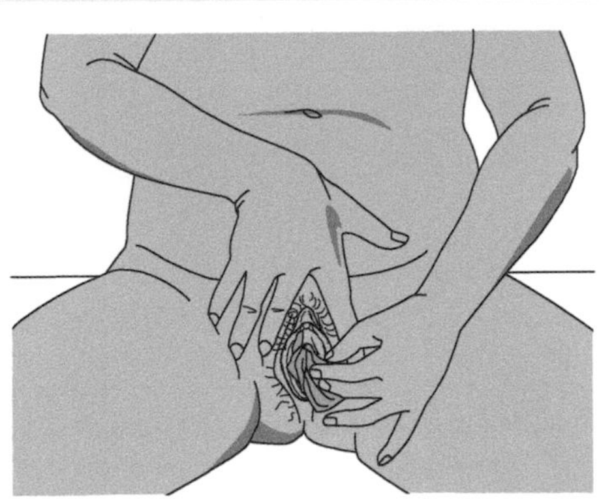

Figure 27-2 Cleaning the female urinary meatus.

- Ask the female patient to micturate into a bedpan or toilet while spreading the labia with one hand while micturating.
- Place the receiver under the stream of urine and remove before micturation finishes.
- Transfer the specimen into a sterile container.

For male patients *(Dougherty and Lister, 2008)*

- If uncircumcised, retract the foreskin slightly to expose the urinary meatus.
- Using a circular motion, clean the urinary meatus and the distal portion of the penis with 0.9% saline. Use each wipe only once, then discard as per hospital policy.
- Clean several inches down the shaft of the penis. *This cleans from the area of least contamination to the area of greatest contamination* (Figure 27-3).
- Ask the patient to direct the first and last part of his stream into the urinal or toilet but to collect the mid part of his stream into the container.
- Transfer the specimen into the sterile container.

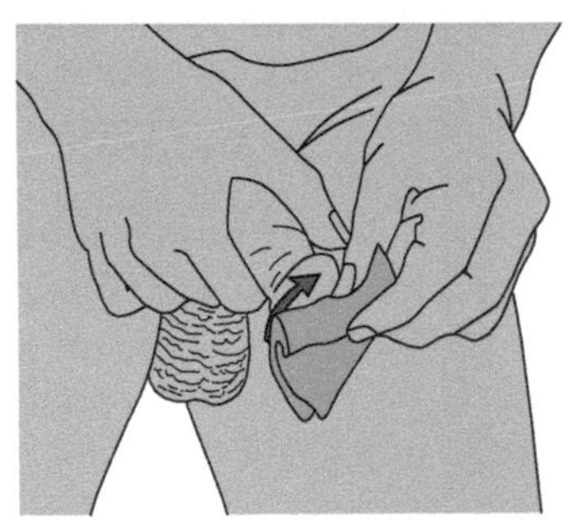

Figure 27-3 Cleansing the male urinary meatus.

For a patient who requires assistance

Prepare the patient and equipment.

- Wash the perineal area with soap or appropriate cleansing agent and water, rinse and dry.
- Assist the patient onto a clean commode or bedpan. If using a bedpan or urinal, position the patient as upright as allowed or tolerated. *Assuming a normal anatomic position for voiding facilitates urination.*
- When handling the sterile receiver, care is needed so as not to contaminate the inside of the specimen container or lid. *It is important to maintain sterility of the specimen container to prevent contamination of the specimen.*
  (a) Put on clean gloves.
  (b) Maintain local and national infection control standards.
  (c) Maintain patient privacy and dignity.
- Clean the urinary meatus and perineal area as described in step 4.
- Collect the specimen from a nonambulatory patient or instruct an ambulatory patient on how to collect it.
- Instruct the patient to start voiding. *Bacteria in the distal urethra and at the urinary meatus are cleared by the first few millilitres of urine expelled.*
- Place the specimen container into the stream of urine and collect the specimen, taking care not to touch the container to the perineum or penis. *It is important to avoid contaminating the interior of the specimen container and the specimen itself.*
- Collect 30–60mL of urine in the container.

4 Cap the container tightly, touching only the outside of the container and the cap. *This prevents contamination or spilling of the specimen.*
  - If necessary, clean the outside of the specimen container as per local policy.

5 Label the specimen and transport it to the laboratory.
  - Ensure that the specimen label and the laboratory request form carry the correct information. Attach them securely to the specimen. *Inaccurate identification or information on the specimen container risks errors in diagnosis or treatment.*
  - Arrange for the specimen to be sent to the laboratory immediately.

6 Document pertinent data.
  - Record collection of the specimen, any pertinent observations of the urine such as colour, odour or consistency, and any difficulty in voiding that the patient experienced.
  - Indicate on the lab slip if the patient is taking any current antibiotic therapy or if the patient is menstruating.

Evaluation

- Report lab results to the doctor.
- Discuss findings of the laboratory test with doctor and the patient.
- Conduct appropriate follow-up nursing interventions as needed, such as vital sign monitoring bed rest, administering ordered medications and patient information.
- Document procedure and findings.

LIFESPAN CONSIDERATIONS

Urine Specimen

Infants

- The process for cleaning the perineal area and the urethral opening is similar to the process for an adult. A specimen bag, however, is used to collect the urine specimen. The specimen bag has an adhesive backing that attaches to the skin. After the infant has voided a desired amount, gently remove the bag from the skin.
- If you are having trouble obtaining a bagged urine specimen from an infant, try cutting a hole in the nappy (front for a boy and middle for a girl) and pulling part of the bag through. You can see when urine is collected without having to untape the nappy (Lindemann, 2000).

Children

- When collecting a routine urine specimen, explain the procedure in simple nonmedical terms to the child and ask the child to void using a potty chair or a bedpan placed inside the toilet.
- Give the child a clean specimen container to play with.
- Allow a parent to assist the child, if possible. The child may feel more comfortable with a parent present.

Mature Adults

- For a midstream urine specimen, mature adults may have difficulty controlling the stream of urine.
- Mature women with arthritis may have difficulty holding the labia apart during the collection of midstream urine.

COMMUNITY CARE CONSIDERATIONS

Taking Urine Specimen in the Home

- Assess the patient's ability and willingness to collect a timed urine specimen. If poor eyesight or hand tremors are a problem, suggest using a clean funnel to pour the urine into the container.
- Always wash hands well with warm, soapy water before and after collecting urine samples.
- Always wear gloves if handling another person's urine.
- Return the specimen to the laboratory as soon as possible.

Timed Urine Specimen

Some urine examinations require collection of all urine produced and voided over a specific period of time, ranging from 1–2 hours to 24 hours. Timed specimens generally contain a preservative to prevent bacterial growth or decomposition of urine components. Each voiding of urine is collected in a small, clean container and then emptied immediately into the large or carton. Some of the tests performed on timed urine specimens include the following:

- to assess the ability of the kidney to concentrate and dilute urine;
- to determine disorders of glucose metabolism, for example, diabetes mellitus;
- to determine levels of specific constituents, for example, albumin, amylase, creatinine, urobilinogen, certain hormones (e.g. corticosteroids) in the urine.

To collect a timed urine specimen, follow these steps:

1. Explain the procedure and its impending results to the patient.
2. Obtain consent.
3. Maintain patient dignity and privacy.
4. Obtain a specimen container with preservative (if indicated) from the laboratory. Label the container with identifying information for the patient, the test to be performed, time started and time of completion.
5. Provide a clean receptacle to collect urine (bedpan, commode or toilet collection device).
6. Inform all staff regarding need to save all urine during the specified time.
7. At the start of the collection period, have the patient void and discard this urine and start collection from then.
8. Save all urine produced during the timed collection period in the container provided. Avoid contaminating the urine with toilet paper or faeces.
9. At the end of the collection period, instruct the patient to completely empty the bladder and save this voiding as part of the specimen. Take the entire amount of urine collected to the laboratory with the completed request form.
10. Record collection of the specimen, time started and completed and any pertinent observations of the urine on appropriate records.

CLINICAL ALERT

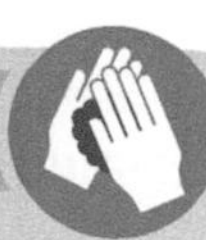

If the patient or staff forget and discard the patient's urine during a timed collection, the procedure must be restarted from the beginning.

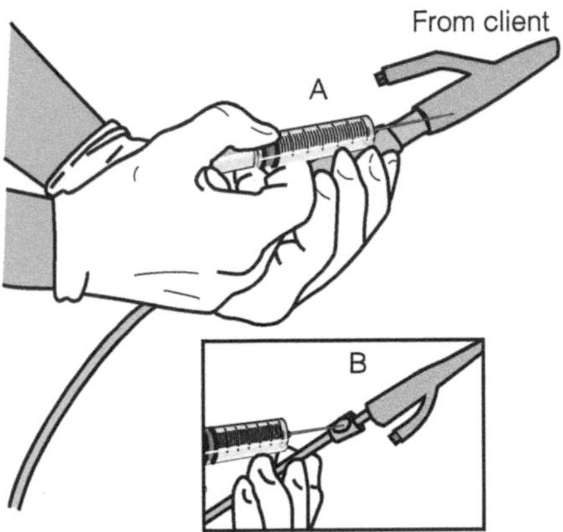

Figure 27-4 Obtaining a urine sample from a urinary catheter.

Indwelling Catheter Specimen

Sterile urine specimens can be obtained from closed drainage systems by inserting a sterile needle attached to a syringe through a drainage port in the tubing. Aspiration of urine from catheters can be done only with self-sealing rubber catheters – not plastic, silicone or Silastic catheters. When self-sealing rubber catheters are used, the needle is inserted just above the location where the catheter is attached to the drainage tubing.

The area from which to obtain urine may be marked by a patch on the catheter (see Figure 27-4).

To collect a specimen from a Foley catheter or a drainage tube, follow these steps:

1. Explain the procedure to the patient and the implications of the test.
2. Obtain consent.
3. Put on disposable gloves.
4. If there is no urine in the catheter, clamp the drainage tubing for about 30 minutes. *This allows fresh urine to collect in the catheter.*
5. Wipe the area where the needle will be inserted with a disinfectant swab. The site should be distal to the tube leading to the balloon to avoid puncturing this tube. *Sanitising the needle insertion site removes any micro-organisms on the surface of the catheter, thereby avoiding contamination of the needle and the entrance of micro-organisms into the catheter.*
6. Insert the needle at a 30- to 45-degree angle (Figure 27-4). *This angle of entrance facilitates self-sealing of the rubber.*
7. Unclamp the catheter.
8. Withdraw the required amount of urine, for example, 3mL for a urine culture or 30mL for a routine urinalysis.
9. Transfer the urine to the specimen container. If a sterile culture tube is used, make sure the needle does not touch the outside of the container.
10. Without recapping the needle, discard the syringe and needle in an appropriate sharps container (as per local policy).
11. Cap the container.
12. Remove gloves and discard appropriately.
13. Label the container, and send the urine to the laboratory.
14. Record collection of the specimen and any pertinent observations of the urine on the appropriate records.

Note that this procedure can be followed if needleless port systems are being used.

Ileal Conduit or Urostomy

An ileal conduit is a surgical intervention that uses part of the gut to create an artificial bladder when the bladder is removed from the body. The end of the ileum is brought out through an opening (stoma) in the abdominal wall to excrete urine. See *Procedure 27-2* for the collection of a urine sample from an ileal conduit or urostomy.

PROCEDURE 27-2 Collection of a Sample from an Ileal Conduit or Urostomy

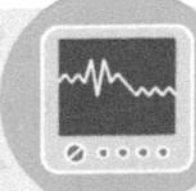

Purpose

- As per Procedure 27-1.

Assessment

Assess the condition of the patient and the ilealostomy site.

Planning

Equipment

- Sterile dressing pack
- Soft catheter
- Specimen container
- Cleansing agent (as per local policy)
- Stoma bag and fixative
- Gloves

Implementation

Preparation

Gather the necessary equipment needed for the collection of the specimen.

Performance

1 Follow points 1-5 as for Procedure 27-1.
2 Ensure the patient is in a comfortable position.
3 Prepare an aseptic trolley and take it to the patient's bedside, *to prevent the risk of infection*.
4 Prepare the necessary sterile field ready to start the procedure.
5 Put on gloves.
6 Remove the appliance from the patient's stoma and cover the stoma with a clean topical swab.
7 Clean hands as per local policy and put on sterile gloves.
8 Remove sterile gauze with forceps.
9 Arrange an absorbent towel around the stoma site to absorb spillage.
10 Apply gentle skin traction to facilitate entry of the catheter and to observe the site for any abnormalities. Insert the catheter tip to a depth of 2.5-5cm and allow urine to drain into a sterile container.
11 Remove the catheter and replace a clean bag over the stoma.
12 Transfer the urine sample into the container.
13 Wipe (as per local policy) the side of the container if there is any overspill.
14 Label the container with patient's name, number, etc. as per local policy.
15 Send the specimen to the laboratory for processing as soon as possible.
16 Ensure the patient is comfortable.
17 Dispose of all equipment as per local policy.
18 Clean the trolley as per infection control policy.

Source: Dougherty and Lister (2008).

Evaluation

- Document procedure and results (when received) in patient's notes.
- Inform doctor.
- Carry out appropriate nursing observations, change of medications and plan of care as appropriate.

Urine Testing

Several simple urine tests are often done by nurses on the nursing units. These include tests for specific gravity, pH and the presence of abnormal constituents such as glucose, ketones, protein and occult blood. Nurses in a healthcare facility or patients in the home setting can use many commercially prepared kits to test abnormal constituents in the urine. These kits contain the required equipment and an appropriate reagent (substance used in a chemical reaction to detect a specific substance). Reagents may be in the form of a tablet, fluid or paper test strips or, more often, dipsticks. When the urine contacts the reagent, a chemical reaction occurs, causing a colour change that is then compared with a chart to interpret the significance of the colour (Figure 27-5). Specific directions for the amount of urine needed, the time required for the chemical reaction and the meaning of the colours produced vary among manufacturers. Thus it is essential that nurses and patients read and follow directions supplied by each manufacturer.

In addition, testing materials need to be checked to ascertain that they are not outdated. Urine testing may be performed by HCSW, but it is important that the HCSW understands the specific specimen collection procedure and reports the results of the test to the nurse. Inform the HCSW to save the urine sample to allow the nurse to repeat the test if necessary.

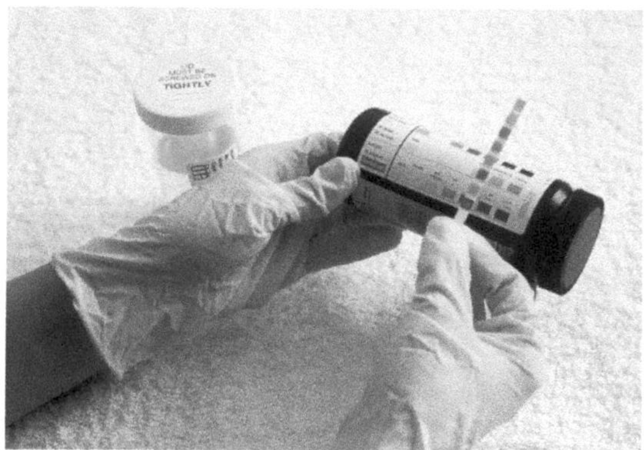

Figure 27-5 Urine dipsticks.
Source: Science Photo Library Ltd/Faye Norman.

Urinary pH

Urinary pH is measured to determine the relative acidity or alkalinity of urine and assess the patient's acid–base status. Quantitative measurements of urine pH can be performed in the laboratory, but dipsticks are often used on nursing units or in clinics to obtain less precise pH measurements. Urine is normally slightly acidic, with an average pH of 6 (7 is neutral, less than 7 is acidic, greater than 7 is alkaline). Because the kidneys play a critical role in regulating acid–base balance, assessment of urine pH can be useful in determining whether the kidneys are responding appropriately to acid–base imbalances. In metabolic acidosis, urine pH should decrease as the kidneys excrete hydrogen ions; in metabolic alkalosis, the pH should increase.

CLINICAL ALERT

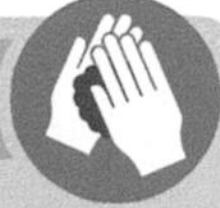

The appearance of blood in the urine is one of the early indications of renal disease. If blood is found in the urine the test should be retaken and the doctor informed.

Glucose

Urine is tested for glucose to screen patients for diabetes mellitus and to assess patients during pregnancy for abnormal glucose tolerance. Normally, the amount of glucose in the urine is negligible, although individuals who have ingested large amounts of sugar may show small amounts of glucose in their urine.

Ketones

Ketone bodies, a product of the breakdown of fatty acids, are normally not present in the urine. They may, however, be found in the urine of patients with poorly controlled diabetes. Urine ketone testing with a dipstick is also used to evaluate ketoacidosis in patients who are alcoholic, fasting, starving or consuming high-protein diets.

Protein

Protein molecules are normally too large to escape from glomerular capillaries into the filtrate. If the glomerular membrane has been damaged, however (e.g. because of an inflammatory process such as glomerulonephritis), the presence of proteins in the urine will aid confirmation of this. Urine testing for the presence of protein is generally done with a dipstick.

Sputum Specimens

Sputum is the mucous secretion from the lungs, bronchi and trachea. It is important to differentiate it from saliva, the clear liquid secreted by the salivary glands in the mouth, sometimes referred to as 'spit.' Healthy individuals do not produce sputum. Patients need to cough to bring sputum up from the lungs, bronchi, and trachea into the mouth in order to expectorate it into a collecting container.

A HCSW can obtain a sputum specimen that is expectorated by a patient. It is important to instruct the HCSW on when to collect the specimen, how to position the patient and how to correctly collect the specimen. Obtaining a sputum specimen by use of pharyngeal suctioning, however, should be performed by a trained nurse because it is an invasive, sterile process and requires knowledge application and problem solving. A 'sputum trap' is used when the specimen is obtained by suctioning (see Chapter 16). Sputum specimens are usually collected for one or more of the following reasons:

- For culture and sensitivity to identify a specific micro-organism and its drug sensitivities.
- For cytology to identify the origin, structure, function and pathology of cells, specimens for cytology often require serial collection of three early-morning specimens and are tested to identify cancer in the lung and its specific cell type.
- For acid-fast bacillus (AFB), which also requires serial collection, often for 3 consecutive days, to identify the presence of tuberculosis (TB).
- To assess the effectiveness of therapy.

Sputum specimens are often collected in the morning. Upon awakening, the patient can cough up the secretions that have accumulated during the night. Sometimes specimens are collected during postural drainage, when the patient can usually produce sputum. When a patient cannot cough, the nurse must sometimes use pharyngeal suctioning to obtain a specimen.

To collect a sputum specimen, the nurse follows these steps:

1. Explain the procedure to the patient and what the test is for.
2. Obtain consent.
3. Maintain patient dignity and privacy.
4. Put on gloves and prepare sterile container.
5. Follow local policy if tuberculosis is suspected.
6. Ask the patient to breathe deeply and then cough up 1–2 tablespoons, or 15–30mL (4–8 fluid drams), of sputum.
7. Ask the patient to **expectorate** (spit out) the sputum into the specimen container. Make sure the sputum does not contact the outside of the container. If the outside of the container does become contaminated, clean it as per local policy.
8. Close the cap.
9. Following sputum collection, offer mouthwash to remove any unpleasant taste.
10. Label and transport the specimen to the laboratory. Ensure that the specimen label and the laboratory request form contain the correct information.
11. Arrange for the specimen to be sent to the laboratory immediately.
12. Document the collection of the sputum specimen on the patient's chart. Include the amount, colour, odour, consistency (thick, tenacious, watery), presence of haemoptysis (blood in the sputum), odour of the sputum, any measures needed to obtain the specimen (e.g. postural drainage) and any discomfort experienced by the patient.

Throat Culture

A throat culture sample is collected from the mucosa of the oropharynx and tonsillar regions using a culture swab. The sample is then cultured and examined for the presence of disease-producing micro-organisms. Obtaining a throat culture is an invasive procedure that requires the application of scientific knowledge and potential problem-solving to ensure patient safety. Thus, it is best for the trained nurse to perform this procedure (or as per local policy).

To obtain a throat culture swab, the nurse puts on clean gloves, depresses the patient's tongue with a spatula then inserts the swab into the oropharynx and runs the swab along the tonsils and areas on the pharynx that are reddened or contain exudate. The gag reflex, active in some patients, may be decreased by having the patient sit upright if health permits, open the mouth, extend the tongue and say 'ah,' and by taking the specimen quickly. The sitting position and extension of the tongue help expose the pharynx; saying 'ah' relaxes the throat muscles and helps minimise contraction of the constrictor muscle of the pharynx (the gag reflex). Touching the sides of the mouth or tongue should be avoided.

ACTIVITY 27-1

You are working on a paediatric ward and a 4-week-old baby girl has been admitted to your care. During the consultant's ward round the baby was about to be discharged but the consultant required a urine sample prior to discharge to test for culture and sensitivity. Your mentor has asked you to organise, collect and deliver the sample to the laboratory, What are the key issues you need to consider and how would you collect the sample.

LIFESPAN CONSIDERATION

Sputum and Throat Specimens

Infants

- Avoid occluding an infant's nose because infants normally breathe only through the nose.

Children

- The young child will need to be restrained gently while the throat specimen is collected. Allow the parents to assist and explain that the procedure will be over quickly.
- Observe for signs of an ear infection (e.g. rubbing the ears). A child's short respiratory tract allows bacteria to migrate easily to the ears.

Mature Adults

- Mature adults may need encouragement to cough because a decreased cough reflex occurs with ageing.
- Allow time for mature adults to rest and recover between coughs when obtaining a sputum specimen.

Wound Swab

Wound swabs should be taken if the nurse suspects an infection in the wound. This procedure should be undertaken by the trained nurse when the wound dressing is being changed. This is in order to reduce the risk of infection or further infection due to exposure. As previously noted within this chapter, all infection control policies and other local policies should be adhered to when taking any swab. The patient should be informed and consent obtained. Patient dignity and privacy should be maintained at all times and the nurse should be non-judgemental when providing care and taking a wound swab. Wound swabs should be taken before any cleaning procedure begins, and the wound swab should be rotated gently over the site.

COMMUNITY CARE CONSIDERATIONS

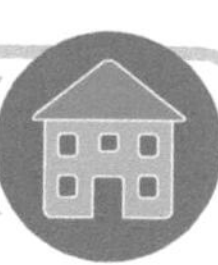

Specimen Collection

- If specimen collection is done on an outpatient basis or in the home, the nurse teaches the patient how to obtain the specimens. Provide written instructions and specimen containers to ensure correct and safe performance of the procedure.
- Ensure that the laboratory knows where to send the test results.

INVASIVE AND NONINVASIVE TECHNIQUES

Patients with Gastrointestinal Changes

Techniques such as a proctoscopy, the viewing of the rectum, sigmoidoscopy (flexible), the viewing of the rectum up to the sigmoid colon, and colonoscopy, the viewing of the large intestine, are carried out with the use of a microscope. While indirect techniques such as x-rays of the gastrointestinal tract can detect strictures, obstructions, tumours, ulcers, inflammatory disease or other structural changes such as hiatus hernias, visualisation of the tract is enhanced by the introduction of a radiopaque substance such as barium. Many consultants prefer the bowel to be empty prior to the investigations and prescribe a laxative to help with this (depending on the medical condition and presentation of the patient).

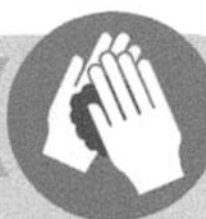

CLINICAL ALERT

Bowel preparation may be contraindicated with some medical conditions.

For examination of the upper gastrointestinal tract or small bowel, the patient drinks the barium sulfate. This examination is often referred to as a *barium swallow.* For examination of the lower gastrointestinal tract, the patient is given an enema containing the barium. This examination is commonly referred to as a *barium enema.* These x-rays include fluoroscopic examination; that is, projection of the x-ray films onto a screen, which permits continuous observation of the flow of barium.

Patients with Urinary Changes

An x-ray of the kidneys/ureters/bladder is commonly referred to as a *KUB. Intravenous pyelography (IVP)* and *retrograde pyelography* also are radiographic studies used to evaluate the urinary tract. In an intravenous pyelogram, contrast medium is injected intravenously; during retrograde pyelography, the contrast medium is instilled directly into the kidney pelvis via the urethra, bladder and ureters. Following injection or instillation of the contrast medium, x-rays are taken to evaluate urinary tract structures. Renal *ultrasonography* is a noninvasive test that uses reflected sound waves to visualise the kidneys. During a *cystoscopy*, the bladder, ureteral orifices and urethra can be directly seen using a cystoscope, a lighted instrument inserted through the urethra. Nurses are responsible for preparing patients before these studies and for follow-up care.

Patients with Cardiopulmonary Changes

There are a number of procedures which can be done to examine the cardiovascular system and respiratory tract.

Electrocardiography provides a graphic recording of the heart's electrical activity. Electrodes placed on the skin transmit the electrical impulses to an oscilloscope or graphic recorder. With the wave forms recorded, the electrocardiogram or ECG can then be examined to detect dysrhythmias and alterations in conduction indicative of myocardial damage, enlargement of the heart or drug effects.

Stress electrocardiography uses ECGs to assess the patient's response to an increased cardiac workload during exercise. As the body's demand for oxygen increases with exercising, the cardiac workload increases, as does the oxygen demand of the heart muscle itself. Patients with coronary artery disease may develop chest pain and characteristic ECG changes during exercise.

Angiography is an invasive procedure requiring informed consent of the patient. A radiopaque dye is injected into the vessels to be examined. Using fluoroscopy and x-rays, the flow through the vessels is assessed and areas of narrowing or blockage can be observed. Coronary angiography is performed to evaluate the extent of coronary artery disease; pulmonary angiography may be performed to assess the pulmonary vascular system, particularly if pulmonary emboli are suspected. Other vessels that may be studied include the carotid and cerebral arteries, the renal arteries and the vessels of the lower extremities.

An *echocardiogram* is a noninvasive test that uses ultrasound to observe structures of the heart and evaluate left ventricular function. Images produced as ultrasound waves reflect back to a transducer after striking cardiac structures. The nurse should tell the patient that this test causes no discomfort, although the conductive gel used may be cold. X-ray examination of the chest is done both to diagnose disease and to assess the progress of a disease. For an x-ray examination, the nurse needs to inform the patient that jewellery and clothing from the waist up must be removed.

A *lung scan*, also known as a V/Q (ventilation/perfusion) scan, records the emissions from radioisotopes that indicate how well gas and blood are travelling through the lungs. The *perfusion scan* is used to assess blood flow through the pulmonary vascular system. For this, the radioisotope is injected intravenously and measured as it circulates through the lung.

Laryngoscopy and **bronchoscopy** are sterile procedures that are conducted with a laryngoscope and bronchoscope, respectively. Tissue samples may also be taken for biopsy. A local anaesthetic is usually sprayed on the patient's pharynx before the examination to prevent gagging and to anesthetise the throat. The bronchoscope is then inserted to examine the larynx or bronchi. Informed consent is required for these procedures.

Ultrasound

An *ultrasound* is a noninvasive technique that uses sound waves to create images of organs and structures inside the body. The sound wave travels through fluids and soft tissue and throws back a high pitched sound when it comes up against a dense surface (as for an echocardiogram).

An ultrasound is used for diagnosing, treating and screening for disease, and is used to routinely monitor progression of pregnancy. Cold jelly is spread over the area to be scanned prior to the procedure. This can be cold and a discomfort to the patient.

A *Doppler ultrasound* is used to assess the peripheral vascular system. By moving a handheld tranducer over a limb or the neck it evaluates the blood flow in major arteries and veins in the arms, legs and neck. The Doppler ultrasound is used both in the care environment and in the home and is often used to help diagnose a thrombus (clot).

Computed Tomography

Computed tomography (CT), also called *CT scanning, computerised tomography* or *computerised axial tomography (CAT),* is a painless, noninvasive x-ray procedure that has the unique capability of distinguishing minor differences in the density of tissues. The CT produces a three-dimensional image of the organ or structure making it more sensitive than the x-ray machine.

Magnetic Resonance Imaging

Magnetic resonance imaging (MRI) is a noninvasive diagnostic scanning technique in which the patient is placed in a magnetic field. Patients with implanted metal devices (e.g. pacemaker, metal hip prosthesis) cannot undergo an MRI because of the strong magnetic field. There is no exposure to radiation. If a contrast media is injected during the procedure, it is not an iodine contrast. Another advantage to the MRI is that it provides a better contrast between normal and abnormal tissue than the CT scan. It is, however, more costly.

The MRI is commonly used for visualisation of the brain, spine, limbs and joints, heart, blood vessels, abdomen and pelvis. The procedure involves the patient lying on a platform that moves into either a narrow, closed, high-magnet scanner, or into an open, low-magnet scanner. The patient must lie very still. A two-way communication system is used to monitor the patient's response and to help relieve feelings of claustrophobia. Earplugs are offered to the patient to reduce the discomfort from the loud noises that occur during the test. The procedure lasts between 60 and 90 minutes.

Nuclear Imaging Studies

Nuclear scans study the 'physiology or function' of an organ system in contrast to other studies (e.g. CT, MRI, x-ray) which examine 'anatomic' structures. A *radiopharmaceutical*, a pharmaceutical (targeted to a specific organ) labelled with a radioisotope, is administered through various routes for the test. Patients retain the radioisotope for a relatively short time with the most common radiopharmaceutical having a half-life of 6 hours. A gamma camera is placed over the part of the body under study. The camera, which is networked with a computer, converts the emission of the radioisotope and forms a detailed image. An equal distribution of colour is normal; however, darker spots ('hot' spots) indicate hyperfunction and lighter areas ('cold' spots) indicate hypofunction.

Positron emission tomography (PET) is a noninvasive radiologic study that involves the injection or inhalation of a radioisotope. Images are created as the radioisotope is distributed in the body. This allows study of various aspects of organ function and may, for example, include evaluation of blood flow and tumour growth.

ASPIRATION/BIOPSY

Aspiration is the withdrawal of fluid that has abnormally collected (e.g. pleural cavity, abdominal cavity) or to obtain a specimen (e.g., cerebral spinal fluid). A biopsy is the removal and examination of tissue. Usually the biopsy is performed to determine a diagnosis or to detect malignancy. Both aspiration and biopsy are invasive procedures and require strict sterile technique.

Lumbar Puncture

In a lumbar puncture (LP, or spinal tap), cerebrospinal fluid (CSF) is withdrawn through a needle inserted into the subarachnoid space of the spinal canal between the third and fourth lumbar vertebrae or between the fourth and fifth lumbar vertebrae. At this level, the needle avoids damaging the spinal cord and major nerve roots. The patient is positioned laterally with the head bent towards the chest, the knees flexed onto the abdomen and the back at the edge of the bed or examining table (Figure 27-6(a) for an adult and Figure 27-6(b) for a child). In this position, the back is arched, increasing the spaces between the vertebrae so that the spinal needle can be inserted readily. During a lumbar puncture, the doctor frequently takes CSF pressure readings using a manometer, a glass or plastic tube calibrated in millimetres. It is the doctor's duty to carry out a lumbar puncture, but it is the nurse's role to provide support for both the patient and the doctor (see *Procedure 27-3*).

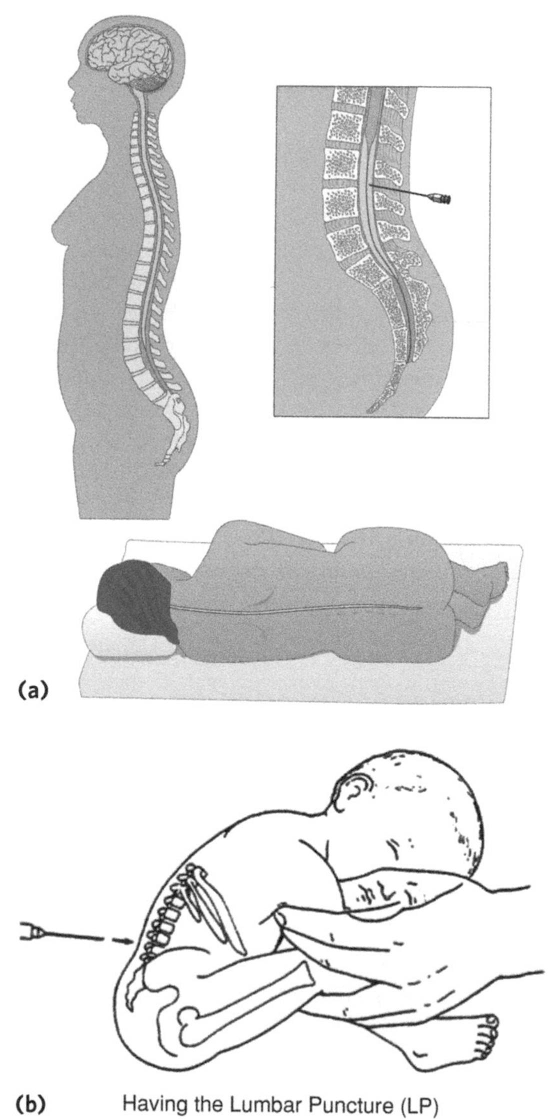

Figure 27-6 (a) Position for lumbar puncture in adult. (b) Position for lumbar puncture in child.

Source: (a) Science Photo Library Ltd/Pete Gardiner; (b) http://www.chkd.org

PROCEDURE 27-3 Assisting with a Lumbar puncture

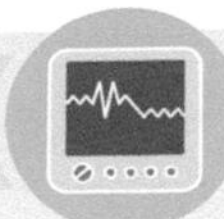

Purposes

- To obtain a sample of cerebrospinal fluid (CSF) to aid diagnosis
- To introduce therapeutic agents e.g. chemotherapy
- For administration of spinal anaesthetic
- For administration of radioopaque contrast medium

Assessment

Assess

- The ability of the patient to undergo the procedure
- How much support the patient will need during the procedure
- Whether the patient is fully informed prior to the procedure
- If there are any contraindications to the procedure.

Planning

Gather the appropriate equipment prior to the procedure including sterile containers for the samples obtained.

Equipment

- Antiseptic skin-cleaning agents, e.g. 0.5% chlorhexidine in 70% alcohol
- Lumbar puncture pack
- Selection of needles (not always included in pack)
- Local anaesthetic (as per local policy)
- Sterile gloves
- Sterile dressing pack
- Manometer
- Three sterile containers for specimen (should be labelled 1–3)
- Dressing as per local policy

Implementation

Preparation

- Have the patient empty the bladder and bowels prior to the procedure to prevent unnecessary discomfort.
- Prepare aseptic trolley.
- Position and drape the patient.
- Maintain infection control policy throughout.
- Open the lumbar puncture set.

Performance

1. Follow local policy to ensure that you explain to the patient what you are going to do, why it is necessary and how they can cooperate. Obtain consent and maintain patient privacy and dignity and ensure that the appropriate local infection control procedures are observed.
    - Explain when and where the procedure will occur (e.g. the bedside or in a treatment room) and who will be present (e.g. the doctor and the nurse).
    - Explain that it will be necessary to lie in a certain position without moving for about 15 minutes.
    - A local anaesthetic will be given to minimise discomfort.
    - Advise the patient that a slight pinprick will be felt when the local anaesthetic is injected and a sensation of pressure as the spinal needle is inserted.
2. Assist the patient into the appropriate position (see Figure 27-6(a) or (b) earlier).
3. Support the patient and be the patient's advocate throughout procedure.
4. Assist the doctor as required.
5. Label and provide the sterile containers as appropriate to the doctor, in order of sequence.
6. When the needle is withdrawn apply pressure over the lumbar puncture using sterile dressing, *in order to prevent further or prolonged bleeding.*
7. When all fluid oozing from the site has stopped apply appropriate dressing as per local policy, *maintaining aseptic technique to prevent infection.*
8. Give prescribed analgesia if required.
9. Make the patient comfortable, ensure call bell is close at hand as the patient has to lie flat for a minimum of 4 hours or as per hospital policy.
10. Dispose of the equipment as per local policy and infection control policy.
11. Monitoring of the patient's condition is essential to observe for oozing from the wound, headache or backache or any abnormal vital or neurological signs, e.g. tingling or numbness in hands or feet.

Evaluation

- Document the procedure and the samples taken in the patient's notes.
- Send off samples to laboratory.
- Inform doctor or results immediately when received.

LIFESPAN CONSIDERATIONS

Lumbar Puncture

Children

- Briefly explain the procedure to the child in the language that they can understand. Allow time to answer questions.
- One member of the healthcare team should maintain eye contact with the young patient and provide reassurance during the procedure.

Mature Adults

- Some patients need help maintaining the flexed position due to arthritis, weakness or tremors.
- Provide an extra blanket to keep the patient warm during the procedure. Mature adults have a decreased metabolism and less subcutaneous fat.
- If the patient has a hearing loss, speak slowly and distinctly, especially when unable to make eye contact.

Abdominal Paracentesis

Normally the body creates just enough peritoneal fluid for lubrication. The fluid is continuously formed and absorbed into the lymphatic system. However, in some disease processes, a large amount of fluid accumulates in the abdominal cavity; this condition is called **ascites**. Normal ascitic fluid is serous, clear and light yellow in colour.

An *abdominal paracentesis* is carried out to obtain a fluid specimen for laboratory study and to relieve pressure on the abdominal organs due to the presence of excess fluid. A doctor performs the procedure with the assistance of a nurse, and strict sterile technique is followed. A common site for abdominal paracentesis is midway between the umbilicus and the symphysis pubis on the midline (Figure 27-7).

The doctor makes a small incision with a scalpel, inserts the trocar (a sharp, pointed instrument) and **cannula** (tube), and then withdraws the trocar, which is inside the cannula (Figure 27-8). Tubing is attached to the cannula and the fluid flows through the tubing into a receptacle. If the purpose of the paracentesis is to obtain a specimen, the doctor may use a long aspirating needle attached to a syringe rather than making an incision and using a trocar and cannula. Normally, about 1,500mL is the maximum amount of fluid drained at one time to avoid hypovolemic shock. The fluid is drained very slowly for the same reason. Some fluid is placed in the specimen container before the cannula is withdrawn.

The small incision may or may not be sutured; in either case, it is covered with a small sterile dressing. The doctor will carry out the procedure but it is the nurse's responsibility to support the patient and the doctor during the procedure (see *Procedure 27-4*).

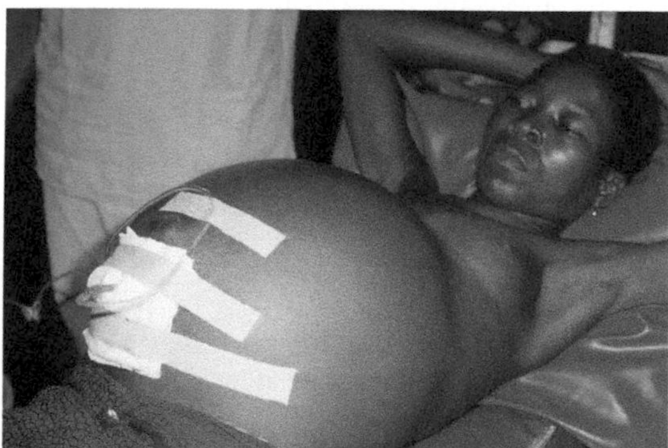

Figure 27-7 Abdominal paracentesis.
Source: Science Photo Library Ltd/Scott Camazine.

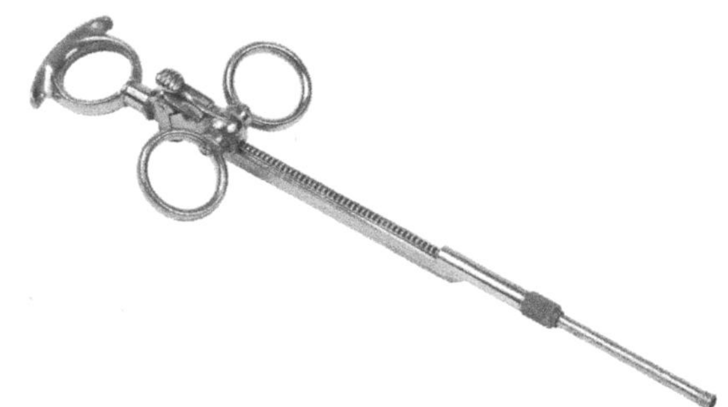

Figure 27-8 Trocar needle.
Source: Thinkstock/Hemera Technologies.

PROCEDURE 27-4 Assisting with an Abdominal Paracentesis

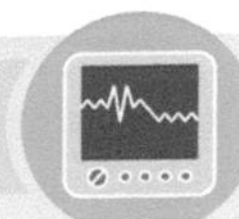

Purposes

- To obtain a sample of fluid to aid diagnosis
- For pain relief
- For administration of substances or other agents into the peritoneal cavity

Assessment

Assess

- The ability of the patient to undergo the procedure
- How much support the patient will need during the procedure
- Whether the patient is fully informed prior to the procedure
- If there are any contraindications to the procedure

Planning

Gather the appropriate equipment prior to the procedure including sterile containers for the samples obtained.

Equipment

- Antiseptic skin-cleaning agents, e.g. 0.5% chlorhexidine in 70% alcohol
- Abdominal paracentesis set
- Selection of needles and various sized syringes
- Local anaesthetic (as per local policy)
- Sterile gloves
- Sterile dressing pack
- Sterile container for specimen
- Drainage bag or container with tap and connector to attach to cannula
- Gate clamps
- Tape measure
- Dressing as per local policy

Implementation

Preparation

- Have the patient void just before the paracentesis to reduce the possibility of puncturing the urinary bladder.
- Prepare aseptic trolley.
- Weigh patient before and after procedure.

Performance

1 Follow local policy to ensure that you explain to the patient what you are going to do, why it is necessary and how they can cooperate. Obtain consent and maintain patient privacy and dignity and ensure that the appropriate local infection control procedures are observed. Explain that obtaining the specimen usually takes about 15 minutes. Emphasise the importance of remaining still during the procedure.

2 Help the patient assume a supine position in bed with the head raised 45–50cm.

3 Support and be patient advocate throughout the procedure.

4 Assist the doctor as required.
  - Aid the doctor in transferring the ascetic fluid into the appropriate sterile container and prepare for sending for cytology.

5 Label the sterile containers and attach to the request form. Send off to laboratory as soon as possible.

6 Care of closed drainage system (if attached to the cannula) is required.

7 Apply dressing as per local policy.

8 Measure patient's girth.

9 Monitor vital signs and fluid balance and observe for hypovolaemic shock.

10 Clamp the tubing if drainage is in excess of local policy.

11 Dispose of equipment as per local policy and infection control policy.

Evaluation

- Document the procedure and the samples taken in the patient's notes.
- Send off samples to laboratory.
- Inform doctor or results immediately when received.

LIFESPAN CONSIDERATIONS

Abdominal Paracentesis

Mature Adults

- Provide pillows and blankets to help mature adults remain comfortable during the procedure.
- Ask the patient to empty the bladder just before the procedure. Mature adults may need to void more frequently and in smaller amounts.
- Remove ascitic fluid slowly and monitor the patient for signs of hypovolaemia. Mature adults have less tolerance for fluid loss and may develop hypovolaemia if a large volume of fluid is drained rapidly.

Bone Marrow Biopsy

Another type of diagnostic study is the *biopsy.* A biopsy is a procedure whereby tissue is obtained for examination. Biopsies are performed on many different types of tissues, for example, bone marrow, liver, breast, lymph nodes and lung.

A bone marrow biopsy is the removal of a specimen of bone marrow for laboratory study. The biopsy is used to detect specific diseases of the blood, such as pernicious anaemia and leukaemia. The bones of the body commonly used for a bone marrow biopsy are the sternum, iliac crests, anterior or posterior iliac spines and proximal tibia in children (Pagana and Pagana, 2009). *The posterior superior iliac crest* is the preferred site with the patient placed prone or on the side (Figure 27-9).

After injecting a local anaesthetic, a small incision may be made with a scalpel to avoid tearing the skin or pushing skin into the bone marrow with a needle. The doctor then introduces a bone marrow needle with stylet into the red marrow of the spongy bone.

Once the needle is in the marrow space, the stylet is removed and a 10ml syringe is attached to the needle. The plunger is withdrawn until 1–2ml of marrow has been obtained. The doctor replaces the stylet in the needle, withdraws the needle and places the specimen in test tubes and/or on glass slides. While it is the doctor who carries out the procedure, it is the nurse's responsibility to support the patient and the doctor (see *Procedure 27-5*).

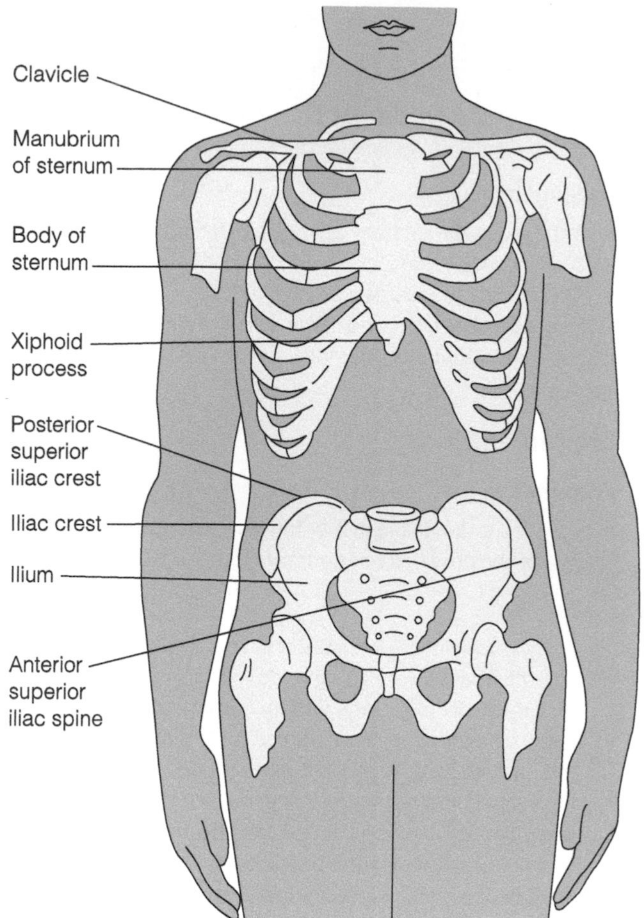

Figure 27-9 Sites for a bone marrow biopsy.

PROCEDURE 27-5 Assisting with a Bone Marrow Biopsy

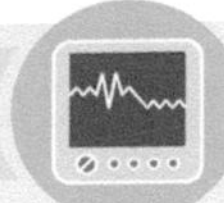

Purposes

- To obtain a sample of fluid to aid diagnosis
- For harvesting

Assessment

Assess

- The ability of the patient to undergo the procedure
- How much support the patient will need during the procedure
- Whether the patient is fully informed prior to the procedure
- If there are any contraindications to the procedure

Planning

Gather the appropriate equipment prior to the procedure including sterile containers for the samples obtained.

Equipment

- Antiseptic skin-cleaning agents, e.g. 0.5% chlorhexidine in 70% alcohol
- Bone marrow aspiration set
- Microscope slides and coverslip or fixative lotion (as per hospital policy)
- Local anaesthetic (as per local policy) with appropriate needles and syringes
- Sterile gloves
- Sterile dressing pack
- Sterile container for specimen
- Dressing as per local policy

Implementation

Preparation

- Advise the patient that they may experience pain during the procedure and they may hear a crunching sound when the needle is pushed through the cortex of the bone.
- Administer analgesia if required.
- Prepare aseptic trolley.
- Maintain the patient's privacy and dignity at all times and provide blankets for warmth.

Performance

1. Follow local policy to ensure that you explain to the patient what you are going to do, why it is necessary and how they can cooperate. Obtain consent and maintain patient privacy and dignity and ensure that the appropriate local infection control procedures are observed. Explain that obtaining the specimen usually takes about 15-30 minutes. (Bone marrow harvests are performed under general anaesthetic as the procedure may last up to an hour.) Emphasise the importance of remaining still during the procedure.
2. Help the patient assume a supine position in bed with one pillow (if the sternum is used) or the prone position for a biopsy if iliac crest is used.
3. Support and be patient advocate throughout procedure.
4. Assist the doctor as required.
   - Once the doctor has removed the needle apply pressure over the puncture site using a sterile dressing. Once the bleeding has stopped apply dressing as per local policy.
5. Monitor vital signs.
6. Make the patient comfortable.
7. Label the slides and attach to the request form. Send off to laboratory as soon as possible.
8. Dispose of equipment as per local policy and infection control policy.

Evaluation

- Document the procedure and the samples taken in the patient's notes.
- Send off samples to laboratory.
- Inform doctor or results immediately when received.

CLINICAL ALERT

The posterior iliac crest may be less painful for the patients than the anterior iliac crest.

Source: Hermandez-Garcia *et al.* (2008).

LIFESPAN CONSIDERATIONS

Bone Marrow Biopsy

Children

- Children need emotional support due to the pain and pressure associated with this procedure.
- Children may require their parents to hold them to prevent movement during the procedure.

Mature Adults

- Mature adults with osteoporosis will experience less needle pressure.
- Ask the patient to empty the bladder for comfort before the procedure.
- Provide pillows and blankets to help mature adults remain comfortable during the procedure.

Liver Biopsy

A liver biopsy is a short procedure, generally performed at the patient's bedside, in which a sample of liver tissue is aspirated. A doctor inserts a needle in the intercostal space between two of the right lower ribs and into the liver or through the abdomen below the right rib cage (subcostally). The patient exhales and stops breathing while the doctor inserts the biopsy needle, injects a small amount of sterile normal saline to clear the needle of blood or particles of tissue picked up during insertion, and aspirates liver tissue by drawing back on the plunger of the syringe. After the needle is withdrawn, the nurse applies pressure to the site to prevent bleeding.

Because many patients with liver disease have blood clotting defects and are prone to bleeding, prothrombin time and platelet count are normally taken well in advance of the test. If the test results are abnormal, the biopsy may be contraindicated. *Procedure 27-6* describes how the nurse assists with a liver biopsy.

PROCEDURE 27-6 Assisting with a Liver Biopsy

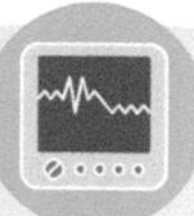

Purpose

To obtain a sample to aid diagnosis

Assessment

Assess

- The ability of the patient to undergo the procedure
- How much support the patient will need during the procedure
- Whether the patient is fully informed prior to the procedure
- If there are any contraindications to the procedure

Planning

Gather the appropriate equipment prior to the procedure including sterile containers for the samples obtained.

Equipment

- Antiseptic skin-cleaning agents, e.g. 0.5% chlorhexidine in 70% alcohol
- Liver biopsy set
- Selection of needles and various sized syringes
- Local anaesthetic (as per local policy)
- Sterile gloves
- Sterile dressing pack
- Sterile container for specimen
- Dressing as per local policy
- Pre-medication (if required)
- Ultrasound if required

Implementation

Preparation

- Ensure patient fasts for 2 hours before the procedure.
- Prepare aseptic trolley.
- Administer prescribed medication, e.g. Vitamin K may be given several days before the biopsy to reduce the risk of haemorrhage and/or appropriate sedative 30 minutes before procedure.

Performance

1 Follow local policy to ensure that you explain to the patient what you are going to do, why it is necessary and how they can cooperate. Obtain consent and maintain patient privacy and dignity and ensure that the appropriate local infection control procedures are observed. Explain that obtaining the specimen usually takes about 15 minutes. Emphasise the importance of remaining still during the procedure.

2 Help the patient assume a supine position in bed with the upper right quadrant of the abdomen exposed.

3 Support and be patient advocate throughout procedure. Instruct the patient to take a few deep breaths in and out and to hold his or her breath when the needle is being inserted, the biopsy being obtained and the needle withdrawn. *Holding the breath after exhalation immobilises the chest wall and liver and keeps the diaphragm in its highest position, avoiding injury to the lung and laceration of the liver.*

4 Assist the doctor as required.
   - Apply pressure to the site of the puncture once the needle has been removed. Apply dressing as per local policy
   - Aid the doctor in transferring the biopsy into the appropriate sterile container.
   - Label the sterile containers and attach to the request form. Send off to laboratory as soon as possible.
   - Ensure the patient is comfortable and monitor vital signs every 15 minutes for 1 hour after the procedure. Observe for signs of bleeding from the site.
   - Dispose of equipment as per local policy and infection control policy.

Evaluation

- Document the procedure and the samples taken in the patient's notes.
- Send off samples to laboratory.
- Inform doctor of results immediately when received.

LIFESPAN CONSIDERATIONS

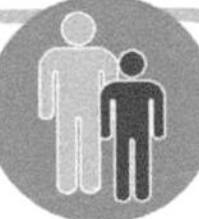

Liver Biopsy

Mature Adults

- Observe for skin irritation from tape applied to the sterile dressing. Mature adults often have fragile skin.
- Ask the patient to empty the bladder before the procedure. Mature adults may need to void more often and in smaller amounts.

CLINICAL ALERT

- Abnormalities of the liver may reduce the ability of the liver to clot. It is important that the appropriate blood tests are carried out before the procedure to identify blood clotting times.
- Medication such as Vitamin K should be prescribed if there are any abnormal clotting times prior to the procedure.

LIFESPAN CONSIDERATIONS

General Considerations

Mature Adults

In mature adults, homeostatic mechanisms are not as efficient as in the younger person. When undergoing diagnostic tests that challenge these functions, care must be taken to accurately monitor functions and note any changes. Examples:

- Dehydration can occur from laxative preps given before bowel diagnostic tests, such as a colonoscopy.
- Fluid restrictions can lead to electrolyte imbalances.
- Many dye contrasts used for x-rays and scans can cause renal damage (especially in diabetics).
- Sedation used for certain procedures may require a longer recovery time for older patients.
- Having several tests at a time or for several days compounds these potential problems.

Interventions should focus on ensuring that the patient is hydrated during and after these diagnostic tests, monitoring intake and output and vital signs frequently and accurately, and noting any mental status changes that might suggest electrolyte imbalance. Identification of patients at risk (persons with diabetes, kidney disease or on certain medications) will help initiate measures to prevent injuries or complications from diagnostic tests.

CRITICAL REFLECTION

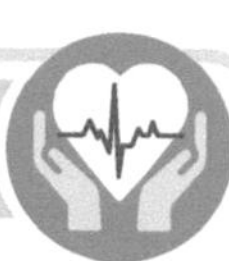

This chapter has explored some aspects of diagnostic testing and the procedures involved. In view of this, can you reflect back on this chapter and other earlier chapters and, by consolidating your new knowledge, discuss the key issues in relation to John in the case study. Ideally the nursing theory should be explored, the nursing process, the human rights act, care management, care delivery psychosocial aspects of care and many other aspects should be considered e.g.

- Effective communication
  - Informing the patient
  - Reduce anxiety and provide support
  - Maintain patient privacy and dignity
  - Manic Depression (mood swings)
- Breathing
  - Oxygen (or no oxygen
  - Positioning
  - Airflow
  - Limited conversation
- Maintaining patient safety
  - Informed decision
  - Consent
  - Manic depression (safety aspect)
  - Preparing for procedures
  - Collecting, and processing specimen samples.

CHAPTER HIGHLIGHTS

- Diagnostic testing involves three phases. Patient preparation is the focus during the pre-test phase. During the peritest phase, the nurse performs or assists with the diagnostic test and collects the specimen. Providing nursing care of the patient and follow-up activities and observations are the role of the nurse during the post-test phase.
- Blood tests are one of the most commonly used diagnostic tests. Routinely ordered blood tests can include full blood count (FBC) and urea and electrolytes.
- Nursing responsibilities associated with specimen collection include (a) providing patient comfort, privacy and safety; (b) explaining the purpose of and procedure for the specimen collection; (c) using correct procedure for obtaining the specimen; (d) noting relevant information on the laboratory request slip; (e) transporting the specimen promptly; and (f) reporting abnormal findings.
- Patients may need assistance to obtain stool specimens for laboratory analysis. In many organisations, nurses test the stool for occult blood.
- Nurses collect urine specimens for a number of tests. A midstream urine specimen is used for routine examination. A midstream voided specimen is collected when a urine

culture is ordered to identify micro-organisms. Timed urine specimens are collected for a variety of tests depending on the patient's health problem. Nurses can complete some simple urine tests (e.g. pH, ketones, protein) at the bedside.

- Sputum and throat culture specimens help determine the presence of disease-producing organisms.
- Invasive and noninvasive procedures include indirect examination noninvasive and direct examination invasive techniques for examining body organs and system functions. Examples of invasive procedures include colonoscopy, barium enema, intravenous pyelography and angiography. Noninvasive procedures include lung scan, echocardiogram, electrocardiography, x-ray, CT and MRI.
- Examples of aspiration/biopsy tests include lumbar puncture, abdominal paracentesis, thoracentesis, bone marrow biopsy, and liver biopsy. These tests are invasive procedures and require strict sterile technique. After the procedure, the nurse assesses the patient for possible complications and provides appropriate nursing interventions as needed.

ACTIVITY ANSWER

ACTIVITY 27-1 It is evident from the activity that sample collection depends greatly on age, gender, compliance and many other aspects. In relation to a child, there are added considerations necessary prior to collecting the sample and ensuring that due protocol and procedure have been followed. Points to consider:

- Inform parent or carer and obtain consent.
- Explain the procedure to the parent or carer.
- Ensure the baby has had bowel movement prior to testing.
- Wash the area as per policy.
- Gently stick the bag to the baby.
- Cut a hole in the middle section of the nappy.
- Collect the urine sample and transfer into sterile container.
- Label the container and check and confirm details on the request form. Send sample to path lab.
- Document procedure in baby's notes.
- When results are obtained alter baby's care as appropriate.

On reflection, discuss the points raised and rationalise the protocols and procedures followed. As an added activity read local policies and procedures to identify if there are any differences to those discussed within the chapter, and if so identify why?

REFERENCES

Dougherty, L. and Lister, S. (2008) *The Royal Marsden Hospital manual of clinical nursing procedures* (7th edn), Oxford: Wiley-Blackwell.

Hernández-García, M.T., Hernández-Nieto, L., Pérez-González, E. and Brito-Barroso, M. (2008) 'Bone marrow trephine biopsy: Anterior superior iliac spine versus posterior superior iliac spine', *Clinical and Laboratory Haematology*, 15(1), 15–19.

Kee, J.L. (2002) *Laboratory and diagnostic tests with nursing implications*, Harlow: Prentice Hall.

Lindemann, M. (2000) 'Tips and timesavers', *Nursing*, 30(3), 70.

NMC (2010) *Standards for pre-registration nursing education*, London: NMC.

Pagana, K.D. and Pagana, T.J. (2009) *Manual of diagnostic and laboratory tests* (4th edn), St Louis, MO: Mosby's Elsevier.

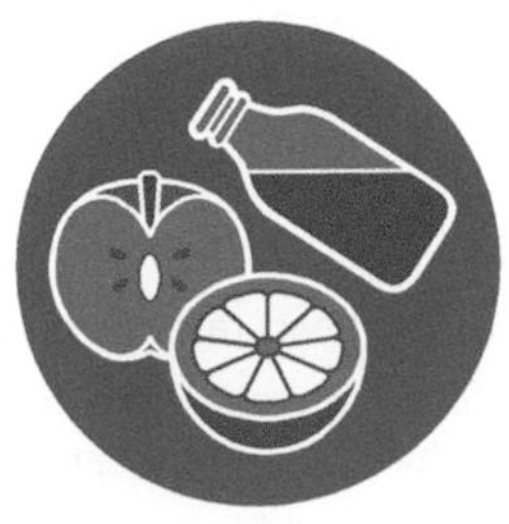
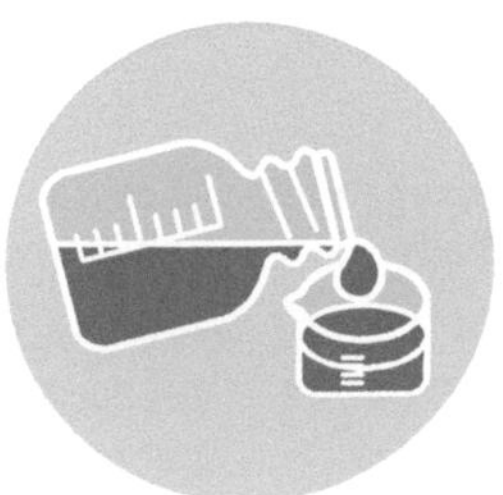
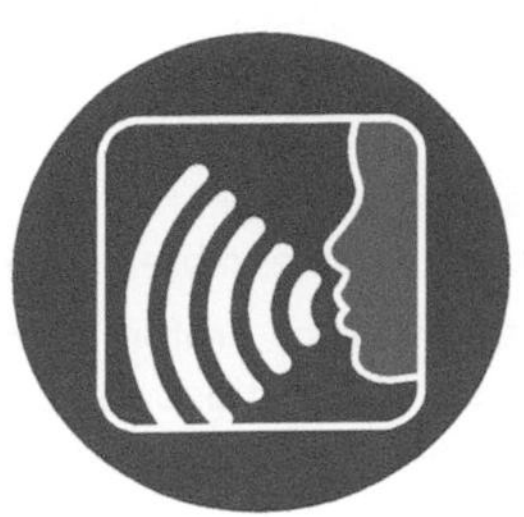
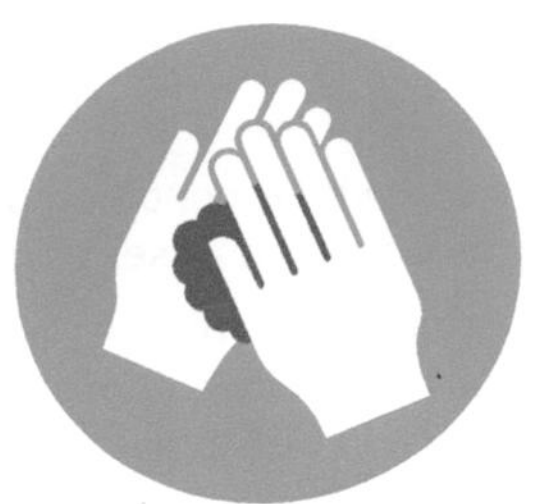

GLOSSARY

Abduction The movement of a body part away from the midline.

Accountability The obligation of being answerable for one's actions and omissions.

Acetylcholine A *neurotransmitter* associated with attention, memory and sleep. It also activates muscles.

Acid Any chemical compound that, when dissolved in water, gives a solution with a hydrogen ion activity greater than in pure water, i.e. a pH less than 7.0.

Acid-base balance The normal equilibrium between *acids* and alkalis within the body.

Acidosis Abnormally high acidity (excess hydrogen ion concentration) of the blood and other body tissues.

Active transport Transport of a substance (e.g. a protein or drug) across a cell membrane against the concentration gradient; requires an expenditure of energy.

Activities of daily living Routine activities performed every day.

Acute A *disease* or condition of rapid onset, severe symptoms and brief duration.

Addiction A physical dependence resulting from changes in the body chemistry. Associated with substances such as alcohol, nicotine and many drugs.

Adduction The movement of a body part towards the midline.

Adjustment disorder A *reactive depression*, i.e. a response to circumstances. Also called *exogenous depression*.

Advanced paediatric life support Advanced management of an infant or child who has suffered a *cardiac arrest*.

Advocacy Pleading for, or to support.

Advocate To promote and safeguard the well-being and interests of the patient or client.

Aetiology The study of the causes of a *disease*.

Affective disorder A disorder of mood, e.g. depression or *mania*.

Agonal Pertaining to death. Agonal breaths are occasional gasps.

Alkalosis Abnormally high alkalinity (low hydrogen ion concentration) of the blood and other body tissues.

Alogia Poverty of speech – one of the negative symptoms of *schizophrenia*.

Alzheimer's disease A degenerative brain disorder characterised by premature senility and *dementia*.

Amino acids Organic compounds that combine to form proteins.

Ampoule A small sealed vial. It is used primarily to store solutions that are to be administered by injection.

Anaemia Reduced concentration of *haemoglobin* or red blood cells. May be as a result of decreased production or increased destruction of red blood cells, and is accompanied by symptoms of *pallor* and breathlessness. Examples are iron deficiency anaemia and sickle cell anaemia.

Anankastic Any behaviour relating to a compulsion. Generally refers to behaviours in OCD or when responding to voices in *schizophrenia*.

Anhedonia An inability to experience pleasure. A symptom of depression and one of the negative symptoms of *schizophrenia*.

Anorexia A physical disorder, resulting in inability to eat or a loss of appetite. Often confused with *anorexia nervosa*.

Anorexia nervosa A psychological disorder characterised by an aversion to, or avoidance of, food.

Anoxia A condition in which tissues are severely or totally deprived of oxygen.

Anterior Relating to the front.

Anti-dementia medication Medication that is used to slow down the progress of *Alzheimer's disease*. Also called *drugs for dementia*.

Antigen Any substance that causes the immune system to produce antibodies.

Anuria Failure of the kidneys to produce urine.

Anxiety An extreme, prolonged, or abnormal response and psychological reaction to stress.

Aphasic Inability to use or understand language.

Apical pulse Central *pulse* located at the apex of the heart.

Apnoea Absence of breathing.

Appetitive Something for which one has an intense craving, or an insatiable appetite. Similar to an *addiction* but with a psychological rather than physical dependence.

Arrhythmia An irregular heartbeat.

Arterial blood gas A blood test taken from the artery. Provides information about oxygenation and pH.

Arteriosclerosis The loss of ability of the arteries to constrict and dilate. The most common type is *atherosclerosis*.

Ascites Accumulation of *serous* fluid in the peritoneal cavity. Most common cause is cirrhosis of the liver; other causes include congestive heart failure and kidney failure.

Asociality A lack of ability to form social relationships – one of the negative symptoms of *schizophrenia*. Also called *autism*.

Asphyxia A condition of severely deficient supply of oxygen to the body that arises from being unable to breathe normally.

Assessment tool A questionnaire or proforma to aid assessment, usually comprising a set of questions which carry a score which in turn can identify the severity of symptoms.

Asthma *Chronic* respiratory disorder characterised by wheezing. Muscles in the walls of the airways tighten, the airways become narrow and inflamed, making expiration and inspiration difficult.

Asystole *Cardiac arrest* rhythm associated with the absence of electrical activity within the heart.

Atelectasis Collapse of portion of lung.

Atherosclerosis Hardening or thickening of the arteries, limiting the blood supply. Symptoms occur when blood flow becomes restricted or blocked.

Auscultation Listening to sounds produced by the body, usually using a stethoscope.

Autism A lack of ability to form social relationships - one of the negative symptoms of *schizophrenia*. Also called *asociality*.

Autoantigen *Antigen* to self. An *endogenous* (from within) substance that provokes an immune response.

Autonomy The right of personal freedom of action.

Autosomes A *chromosome* not involved in sex determination. Of the 23 pairs of chromosomes, 22 pairs are autosomes.

Avolition A lack of motivation - one of the negative symptoms of *schizophrenia*.

Bacteraemia The presence of bacteria in the blood.

Bacteriocins A protein substance that is produced by a specific type of bacteria and which kills closely related strains.

Bag valve mask device Handheld device used to provide positive pressure *ventilation*.

Base A substance in chemistry that neutralises acid. Alkali is a soluble base.

Base deficit Decrease in the amount of alkali in the body.

Beneficence 'Doing good'.

Benzodiazepines A group of psychoactive drugs sometimes called minor tranquilisers. Used in *anxiety*, depression, etc. They include diazepam, temazepam, etc.

Beta amyloid A protein that may be deposited outside and around *neurons* resulting in the formation of *neuritic plaques*, a possible cause of *Alzheimer's disease*.

Binge drinking In men drinking more than the recommended 3-4 units of alcohol a day in a single session. For women more than 2-3 units in a single session.

Bio-psycho-social model A theory and tradition of healing that promotes treatment of the whole person. The approach of taking into consideration the whole body and environment when offering treatment. See *whole-person approach, holistic approach, complex needs*.

Bizarre delusions Fixed beliefs about events that could never realistically occur.

Body mass index (BMI) Scale that divides the weight of a person in kilograms by the square of the person's height in metres.

Bolam test Derives from a legal case. It is used to determine whether the care provided by a medical practitioner meets acceptable standards that would be expected of a person in a similar position.

Bradycardia A low heart rate (below 60 bpm).

Bradypnoea Slow *respirations*. Defined as fewer than 12 breaths per minute in adults under 50 years.

Bronchoscopy Method for investigating the airways. An instrument called a bronchoscope, which may be rigid or flexible, is inserted into the airways via the nose, mouth or a tracheostomy, and the airways can be examined for abnormalities or foreign bodies.

Buccal Relating to cheek or mouth cavity.

Buffer An ionic compound that resists changes in its *pH*.

Calorie A unit of heat energy.

Cannula A tube inserted into the body. Intravenous cannulation can be into a vein (to administer fluids or medicine or to withdraw blood) or an artery (to draw repeated samples). Nasal cannulation can be used to deliver gases, e.g. oxygen. A tracheostomy cannula is inserted into the trachea to aid *ventilation*.

Capacity The ability to make a decision or enter into a contract.

Cardiac arrest The abrupt cessation of normal circulation of the blood owing to failure of the heart to contract effectively during systole.

Cardiac output Amount of blood ejected from the heart in one minute. It is calculated by multiplying the stroke volume (amount of blood ejected per beat) by the number of beats in one minute.

Cardiac rehabilitation programme Exercise and information sessions that provide sufferers of heart attacks or surgery to understand their condition, to recover, to make lifestyle changes that will improve the condition of their heart and reduce the chances of a heart attack.

Cardiopulmonary arrest See *cardiac arrest*.

Cardiopulmonary resuscitation An invasive medical procedure that involves compressing the chest and ventilating the lungs of a patient in a bid to restore spontaneous circulation/breathing.

Cardiorespiratory arrest See *cardiac arrest*.

Care pathway A formal plan that specifies the nursing care for patients.

Care Programme Approach The 1991 initiative which places person-centred care and the rights of the individual at the forefront of services.

Cataract Clouding of the lens of the eye.

Central venous catheter A *cannula* that is inserted into a large (central) vein, e.g. internal jugular.

Cerea flexibilitas A symptom of catatonic *schizophrenia* where individuals can be manipulated into shapes or positions which they will hold for hours. Also known as *waxy flexibility*.

Cerebral cortex The outer region of the brain concerned with memory, language, reasoning and judgement. More commonly called the *cortex*, or even 'grey matter'.

Cerebral palsy A loss or deficiency of motor control with involuntary spasms caused by permanent brain damage present at birth.

Cerebro-vascular accident (CVA) See *stroke*.

Challenging behaviours Those behaviours associated with restlessness or aggression in individuals with e.g. *dementia*.

Chemotherapy The prevention or treatment of a *disease* by use of chemical substances.

Chest compression Compression of the chest wall to produce a change in pressure within the thorax, which in turn fills and empties the heart.

Chickenpox A highly contagious illness caused by primary infection with varicella zoster virus.

Child protection A set of usually government-run services designed to protect children and young people.

Chlorpromazine The first anti-psychotic medication, developed in France in the 1950s. Known as Largactil in Europe and as Thorazine in the USA.

Cholesterol Steroid metabolite used in body to make cell membranes, to insulate nerve fibres and to make hormones and bile acids. Although cholesterol is vital for normal functioning, too much can lead to *atherosclerosis*, heart attack and *stroke*.

CHRE Council for Healthcare Regulatory Excellence. Promotes the health and well-being of patients and the public. The CHRE scrutinises and oversees the work of the nine regulatory bodies that set standards for training and conduct of health professionals.

Chromosome An organised structure of DNA and protein that is found in cells. Human cells contain 46 chromosomes (gametes contain only 23). Chromosomes vary in size, and are estimated to contain between roughly 400 and just over 4000 genes each.

Chronic A disease or condition with gradual onset and long duration. Common chronic conditions include *asthma*, *epilepsy*, *diabetes*, among many others.

Circadian rhythm Physical, mental and behavioural changes that follow a roughly 24-hour cycle.

Civil actions Law suits between private parties to redress private rights.

Civil law Deals with disputes between individuals and/or organisations.

Cleft lip A congenital cleft in the middle of the upper lip.

Clubbing A deformity of the nail (the normal angle of <165° between the nail and the nail bed is lost).

Coccyx The lowermost part of the spine.

Cognition The process of thought. Sometimes applied to the process of understanding, although strictly speaking they are different concepts.

Cognitive behavioural therapy A technique that helps clients to identify their thoughts (cognitive) and actions (behavioural). The therapy involves proposing healthier alternatives and discussing these so that the client can consider change.

Collagen Protein that makes up skin, bone, cartilage and ligaments.

Colonisation Colonisation is a state where there are micro-organisms present but no associated signs of infection.

Command hallucinations Voices instructing the individual to undertake an activity or task. Usually of an unpleasant nature.

Common law The body of law evolved by judges from precedent and custom.

Communicable disease An infectious *disease* that can spread from person to person.

Complex needs A theory and tradition of healing that promotes treatment of the whole person. The approach of taking into consideration the whole body and environment when offering treatment. See *bio-psycho-social model*, *whole-person approach*, *holistic approach*.

Conceptual framework A group of related ideas, statements, concepts.

Concordance A joint understanding between client and practitioner to undertake a therapy or course of treatment such as medication.

Conduction Transfer of heat from one molecule to a molecule of lower temperature. Takes place in solids.

Congenital Present at birth but not necessarily hereditary.

Congruent delusions Fixed beliefs in keeping with *affect* or mood.

Constipation Irregular, infrequent and/or difficult evacuation of *faeces*.

Convection Type of heat transfer in liquids and gases. A heated fluid becomes less dense and rises, and colder fluid moves in to take its place. Body heat can be dispersed by convection currents.

Core temperature Temperature of the deep tissue of the body. This is the temperature at which enzymatic reactions occur, and it is important that this is maintained within a narrow range. The gold standard for measurement of core temperature is via the rectum.

Cortex The outer region of the brain concerned with memory, language, reasoning and judgement. Properly known as *cerebral cortex*, more commonly called 'grey matter'.

Creatinine A waste product of skeletal muscle metabolism. Renal function can be measured by measuring clearance of creatinine from the plasma.

Cri-du-chat syndrome A rare genetic disorder identified by the catlike cry of the infant.

Criminal law The body of law dealing with crimes and their punishment.

Critical analysis To examine, for example, someone's work and look at it as a whole to explore the content both positively and negatively.

Critical thinking To reflect and purposely consider the evidence provided to make a valid decision.

Cyanosis Bluish discoloration of the skin and mucous membranes. Results from reduced oxygen in the blood. Associated with cold temperatures, heart failure, lung diseases and smothering.

Cyclothymia A disorder of *affect* characterised by minor highs and lows rather than dramatic swings toward *mania* or depression seen in bipolar disorder.

Cystoscopy Examination of the bladder using a cystoscope (a lighted flexible tube; an image is carried to the viewing end) inserted through the *urethra*.

Cytomegalovirus Any of a group of herpes viruses that enlarge epithelial cells and can cause birth defects.

Dandruff (seborrhea) A skin inflammation of the scalp.

Decontamination The removal of infective material through cleaning, disinfection and sterilisation.

Deductive reasoning Deductive reasoning moves from a general premise to a more specific conclusion.

Defibrillation Treatment for life-threatening *arrhythmias* of the heart, usually by electric shock using a machine called a defibrillator.

Dehiscence Splitting open of a sutured wound. Risk factors include age, obesity, strain and trauma to the wound, and *diabetes*, among others.

Delusions Fixed belief or beliefs that are false, fanciful or derived from deception.

Dementia Literally meaning 'deprived of mind' refers to chronic organic brain disorders such as *Alzheimer's disease*, etc.

Dementia praecox Literally *dementia* of the young. The original term applied to the disorder now known as *schizophrenia*.

Dental caries Tooth decay or cavities. Bacteria in the mouth convert sugary carbohydrates on teeth into acid, which then demineralises the hard substances (such as dentine and enamel) of the tooth, leaving holes which are called cavities.

Deontology The worth of an action is determined by its conformity to some binding rule.

Deprivation of Liberty Safeguards (DoLS) A set of responsibilities and legal duties on registered care, homes and hospital inpatient services that introduce protection for people in hospitals and care homes who may need to be deprived of their liberty to protect them from serious harm.

Dermis The layer of skin under the *epidermis*. The dermis contains blood and *lymph* vessels, hair follicles and sweat glands. It produces *sebum*.

Detrusor muscle Muscle of the bladder. The detrusor muscle relaxes to allow bladder filling, and contracts to expel urine from the bladder.

Diabetes A metabolic disorder in which blood glucose is unregulated. This is either because the pancreas cannot produce insulin or because the insulin that is produced does not work properly (insulin resistance). Glucose builds up in the blood and the body tries to reduce this, leading to symptoms such as frequent urination, increased thirst and extreme tiredness, weight loss and reduced wound healing ability, among many others.

Diarrhoea Frequent and watery bowel movements.

Diastolic pressure The pressure of blood when the ventricles are at rest and the heart is filling with blood. It is the latter of the values given in a blood pressure reading, e.g. 110/*70*, and is lower than the *systolic pressure*.

Diffusion Movement of a substance from an area of high concentration of that substance to an area of lower concentration. *Osmosis* is the diffusion of water.

Disability Any impairment (physical or mental) that can make routine tasks more difficult or impossible.

Disability Rights Commission Commission charged with being responsible for the civil rights of disabled people. It has now been replaced by the Equality and Human Rights Commission.

Disaccharides Two *monosaccharides* joined together. Examples are lactose and sucrose.

Disease A scientifically detectable alteration in body functions resulting in a reduction of capacities or a shortening of the normal lifespan.

Distension Swelling of the stomach and intestine caused by excessive amounts of gas.

Diuresis Increased secretion of urine from the kidneys.

Diuretics Increase the amount of urine that the kidneys produce. They are used in *pulmonary oedema* and chronic heart failure. Furosemide is a commonly used diuretic.

Diurnal enuresis Incontinence during the day.

Diurnal variation Literally means change during the day. When applied to *affect* it means that the mood worsens as the day progresses.

Dopamine A *neurotransmitter* associated with fine motor movements and the positive symptoms of *schizophrenia* and also with 'excitable' and 'pleasurable' behaviours. Depletion of dopamine results in Parkinson's disease.

Dorsal Relating to the back of the body or organ.

Down's syndrome Delayed physical and mental development caused by a genetic disorder, *trisomy 21*.

Drive A compulsion to undertake, or avoid, an act. This may be an internal mechanism or a response to external stimuli. Also known as a *motive*, *impulse* or *volition*.

Drugs for dementia Acetylcholinesterase inhibitors or ACE inhibitors such as donepezil, galantamine and rivastigmine used to slow down the progress of *Alzheimer's disease*. Also called *anti-dementia medication*.

Dyscopia A failure to cope. This can be a physical or psychological condition. In psychological terms it refers to an individual who displays stress reactions in non-threatening situations.

Early warning signs A unique pattern of psychological changes often occurring in a predictable sequence, indicating a potential further psychotic episode. Also called *relapse signature*.

Edwards syndrome A genetic disorder caused by the presence of all or part of an extra 18th *chromosome*. It is named after John H. Edwards, who first described the syndrome in 1960.

Egocentric Self-centred or focussing on self. In personality disorders it refers to behaviours associated with self-need or self-gratification.

Egosyntonic A belief that one's own perceptions are true and that those of others are not. It involves congruence of mood and behaviour and an absence of empathy.

Electrocardiogram Non-invasive diagnostic test that captures the electrical activity of the heart.

Electro convulsive therapy (ECT) Sometimes called 'shock therapy', a controversial treatment for depression, and occasionally *schizophrenia*, where an electric current is passed through the brain to induce an epileptic fit.

Electrolytes Substances in the blood (such as sodium, magnesium, potassium, calcium and chloride ions) that affect the water balance and blood acidity. Electrolytes are lost in fluid by sweating and *diarrhoea*, and it is important that they are replaced.

Emollient Topical treatment that reduces water loss from the *epidermis* by covering it with a protective film. Also known as moisturisers.

Emphysema A progressive disease of the lungs. Over-inflation of the alveoli.

Encephalitis An acute inflammation of the brain, often due to infection. Symptoms may be fever, headache, nausea and vomiting, and may progress to confusion, drowsiness, disorientation and seizures.

Endogenous In relation to *infection* means that the infection has come from the person's own microbial flora.

Endogenous depression A depression that comes from within, i.e. without a cause.

Endoscopy Examining the inside of the body. This is done using an endoscope, a long, thin, flexible tube with a light at the end. This is inserted into the body and images are passed to a screen.

Endotracheal intubation Placement of a tube into the trachea to aid *ventilation* of the lungs.

Enduring Persistent and long lasting. Also known as *chronic*.

Enema Administration of a liquid into the rectum to stimulate evacuation of *faeces*.

Engagement The working relationship between a nurse (therapist) and a patient (client). Sometimes called the *therapeutic relationship*, the working alliance or a helpful relationship. What Peplau described as the 'proper focus of nursing'.

Enhanced observations A structured method of observing individuals to reduce risk. Normally it involves a set of criteria that must be met, such as who, what, where, when, why, how, etc. Reporting and documentation will form a part of the process.

Enteral Pertaining to the small intestine.

Epicanthic fold A fold of skin of the upper eyelid that partially covers the inner corner of the eye.

Epidermis The uppermost layer of the skin.

Epilepsy A group of disorders resulting in recurrent seizures. These seizures are caused by temporary and sudden bursts of electrical activity in the brain that disrupt the normal passing of messages between brain cells.

Epithelialisation Wound healing by the growth of *granulation tissue*.

Erythema Redness of the skin.

Eschar Black, leathery necrotic tissue.

Eustress Good stress, the pressure that makes some individuals perform.

Euthanasia The act of killing someone painlessly to relieve suffering.

Excoriation Destruction of the surface of the skin.

Exogenous In relation to *infection*, means that the infection stems from an outside source, including other people, the environment, animals and equipment.

Expectorate Cough up and spit out.

Extended family A family consisting of the *nuclear family* and their blood relatives.

Extra-pyramidal side-effects (EPSE) Side-effects associated with certain drugs, notably major tranquilisers, which resemble symptoms of Parkinson's disease.

Exudate A liquid containing proteins and white cells that has filtered out of a tissue or capillaries due to injury or inflammation.

Faecal impaction A solid, immobile mass of *faeces* that forms as a result of chronic *constipation*.

Faecal incontinence Involuntary egestion of faeces.

Faeces Solid excretory product evacuated from the bowels. Comprises undigestable material, bacteria, mucosal cells and mucus.

Familial tendency A preponderance of a condition within a family. It does not necessarily indicate a genetic link as it could be caused by environment, diet, lifestyle, etc.

Family-centred care Functional approach to care within acute care settings for children.

Fatty acids Molecules that are long chains of lipid-carboxylic acids found in fats and oils and in cell membranes.

Fibrin Forms the basis of a blood clot.

Flange Projection used for strength or for attaching to another object.

Flashbacks Pervasive thoughts forcing themselves into consciousness against one's will when awake, a symptom of *post-traumatic stress disorder*.

Flexion Bending movement that decreases the angle between two parts.

Fowler's position A bed position when the head and trunk are raised by 45–90°.

Fragile X syndrome A faulty gene on the X *chromosome*.

Functional nursing Task- and activity-orientated form of assigning nursing tasks. Tasks that need to be done during a shift are identified and assigned to different members of the team, who concentrate on completing the assigned task.

Galactosaemia Rare genetic metabolic disorder that affects an individual's ability to metabolise the sugar galactose properly.

Gametes A cell (sperm or egg) that fuses with another gamete during fertilisation (conception) in organisms that reproduce sexually.

Gastroenteritis Inflammation of the stomach and intestines.

Gastrostomy A surgical opening in the stomach.

Genes The basic unit of heredity in a living organism. A gene is a portion of DNA that codes for a protein.

German measles Or *rubella* – viral *disease* that may cause foetal malformation if contracted during the first trimester of pregnancy.

Gillick competent A child under 16 is said to be Gillick competent if he or she is assessed to have full understanding of the implications and effects of his or her medical treatment.

Gillick principle Referring to whether children under 16 have the maturity and understanding to make their own decisions with regard to their own medical treatment, and whether they are able to understand the implications of those decisions. The name derives from a legal case.

Gingiva Connective tissue that lines the base of the teeth.

Glaucoma The disturbance of the circulation of the aqueous fluid in the eye. Leads to an increase in pressure within the eye that can damage the structure or function.

Global functioning Refers to all aspects of daily living: personal, occupational, social, psychological, etc.

Glomerulus The network of capillaries within the *nephron*. Substances are filtered out of the blood in the glomerulus into the Bowman's capsule of the *nephron*.

Glutamate A *neurotransmitter* associated with thinking and memory. Interruptions to its function or supply may be a cause of *Alzheimer's disease*.

Gluteal fold A fold that marks the upper limit of the thigh.

Granulation tissue Formation of multicellular tissue in response to injury. It is perfused with blood from new capillaries, and grows from the base of the wound. It is light red/pink in colour and is soft, moist and bumpy.

Guardianship Enables patients to receive compulsory care in the community under Section 7 of the Mental Health Act 2003.

Haematocrit The proportion of red blood cells in blood.

Haematoma Localised swelling filled with blood (a bruise).

Haemoglobin Carries oxygen around the body (in the blood).

Haemorrhoids Swelling and inflammation of the veins in the rectum.

Haemostasis The arrest of bleeding.

Haemothorax A collection of blood within the pleural cavity.

Hallucinations A perception whilst conscious and awake in the absence of an external stimulus. It may involve any of the five senses.

Haustra Small pouches in the colon that give it its segmented appearance.

Head tilt chin lift Manual manoeuvre to maintain a patent airway.

Health promotion A set of strategies to promote an individual's physical, mental and emotional health.

Heart disease An umbrella term for a variety of different diseases affecting the heart. It includes conditions such as coronary heart disease, angina, *arteriosclerosis*, *myocardial infarction*, valvular disease and others.

High Court Deals with higher level civil disputes in England and Wales.

Holistic approach Concerned with the whole. The approach of taking into consideration the whole body and environment when offering treatment. See *bio-psycho-social model*, *whole-person approach*, *complex needs*.

Hospice An institution that specialises in the care of terminally ill patients.

HPC Health Professions Council. The HPC is a regulator set up to protect the public. This is done in part by keeping a register of health professionals.

Humanist and humanistic An approach to care that focuses on the positive image of what it means to be human. Humanistic care focuses on allowing fulfilment of potential.

Hunter syndrome Rare metabolic disorder characterised by a deficiency of an enzyme that breaks down nutrients.

Hurler syndrome Rare genetic disorder caused by the deficiency of an enzyme, resulting in the inability to break down complex carbohydrates.

Hydrocephalus Abnormal increase in the amount of cerebrospinal fluid within the ventricles of the brain.

Hypercalcaemia High serum calcium.

Hypercarbia (hypercapnia) Too much carbon dioxide circulating in the blood.

Hyperchloraemia High serum chloride.

Hyperkalaemia High serum potassium.

Hypermagnesaemia High serum magnesium.

Hypermania A severe form of *mania* in which the individual is highly disordered.

Hypernatraemia High serum sodium.

Hyperphosphataemia High serum phosphate.

Hypertension A blood pressure that is above the normal range (140/90 mmHg). Hypertension is a risk factor for *stroke*, *myocardial infarction*, heart failure and kidney failure.

Hypertonic A solution with a higher salt concentration than inside a cell.

Hyperventilation Deep, rapid *respirations*. Often a reaction to anxiety or fear. Results in too little circulating carbon dioxide, and produces symptoms of palpitations, dizziness and faintness.

Hypnagogic A misperception in an individual just entering sleep who mistakes stimuli that are familiar to them.

Hypnopompic A misperception in an individual just awakening from sleep who mistakes stimuli that are familiar to them.

Hypocalcaemia Low serum calcium.

Hypochloraemia Low serum chloride.

Hypoglycaemia Low blood glucose levels. Can be a result of *diabetes*. Produces symptoms of headache, tremor, sweating, faintness, convulsions and coma.

Hypokalaemia Low serum potassium.

Hypomagnesaemia Low serum magnesium.

Hypomania An elevated or 'high' mood that does not quite equate to a full blown *mania*.

Hyponatraemia Low serum sodium.

Hypophosphataemia Low serum phosphates.

Hypoproteinaemia Decrease in the amount of protein in the blood.

Hypotension A blood pressure that is constantly below the normal range (below 90/60 mmHg). Can be accompanied by dizziness and fainting.

Hypothyroidism An underactive thyroid gland. Results in a slowed metabolic rate, sluggishness, lethargy, *pallor* and menstrual disorders. A goitre may be visible.

Hypotonic A solution with a lower salt concentration than inside a cell.

Hypoventilation Reduced *ventilation* of the lungs. Normal oxygen and carbon dioxide levels cannot be maintained, leading to headache, drowsiness and confusion.

Hypovolaemia Reduced volume of circulating blood. Can be a result of dehydration or haemorrhage.

Hypoxaemia Reduced oxygen concentration in arterial blood.

Hypoxia Inadequate oxygen supply to tissues.

Immunity Increased resistance to harmful agents. Provided by leukocytes.

Immunosuppression Suppression of the immune response. Is a common side-effect of chemotherapy for cancer.

Impulse A compulsion to undertake, or avoid, an act. This may be an internal mechanism or a response to external stimuli. Also known as a *motive, drive* or *volition*.

Incapacity The lack of a capacity; an inability.

Incongruent delusions Fixed beliefs not in keeping with *affect* or mood.

Inductive reasoning Reasoning from a specific fact to a general conclusion.

Infarct A collection of dead cells or dead tissue owing to oxygen depletion.

Infarction An interruption to the blood supply causing an *infarct*.

Infection The invasion of body tissue by micro-organisms, their subsequent growth and associated host response.

Informed consent A legal procedure to ensure that a patient knows all of the risks and carts involved in a treatment.

Insensible fluid loss Fluid loss usually through perspiration and *respiration*.

Insight The capacity to fully understand a situation. The ability to perceive the true inner nature fully. To recognise one's illness for what it is and the symptoms for what they are.

Insult A disease, injury or trauma which causes harm to the organism. Includes lesions, bruising, inflammation, etc. May be caused by force, heat/cold, poison, etc.

Intrusive thoughts Unwelcome, involuntary thoughts or memories forcing themselves into consciousness against your will. Also known as *pervasive thoughts*.

Ischaemia Inadequate flow of blood to a body part or organ.

Isokinetic Muscle contraction against resistance.

Isometric A change in muscle tension but not in muscle length.

Isotonic When referring to exercise, muscular contraction in which the muscle remains in constant tension while its length changes.

Jaundice Yellow discoloration of the skin and mucous membranes resulting from too much of the pigment bilirubin in the blood.

Jaw thrust Manual manoeuvre to maintain a patent airway. Used if there is any indication of head or neck injury.

Jejunostomy An artificial opening of the jejunum.

Keloid Overproduction of collagen in response to an injury.

Klinefelter syndrome Syndrome in males that is characterised by small testes, long legs, enlarged breasts and reduced sperm production and mental retardation. The syndrome is associated with at least one extra X *chromosome*.

Korsakoff's psychosis A type of *dementia* associated with excessive alcohol consumption.

Lactate A salt or ester of lactic acid. To secrete.

Laryngoscopy A visual examination of the vocal folds and glottis.

Lateral Situated to the side of an organ or the body.

Limited self-disclosure The conscious, or sometimes unconscious, act of withholding information (thoughts, feelings) of a personal nature.

Lipoprotein A complex of lipid and protein.

Locus of control The belief that individuals have high or low control over events.

Lymph A colourless, watery, bodily fluid carried by the lymphatic system, that consists mainly of white blood cells.

Maceration Softening of a solid by leaving it immersed in a liquid that may contain acid or enzymes.

Malleolus Protuberances at the side of the ankle.

Malnutrition An imbalance between the amount of food the body needs and the amount of food that it receives. It can be a result of problems with digestion or absorption as a result of certain medical conditions. It may result from lack of a single component of the diet, e.g. a vitamin.

Mania Excessively elevated but unstable mood. Symptoms include hyperactivity and mental overactivity.

Maple-syrup disease An inherited disorder in which the body is unable to process certain protein building blocks (*amino acids*) properly.

Meatus Passage or opening.

Medial Situated to the centre of the body or organ.

Medical emergency team Team of doctors, nurses and anaesthetists that attend medical emergencies.

Medical model A model that emphasises the need to identify and treat illness.

Melanocytes Cells in skin, hair and eye that produce melanin, a brown pigment that protects against harmful ultraviolet radiation.

Meningitis Inflammation of the meninges, the three membranes (dura, arachnoid and pia mater) that surround the brain and spinal cord.

Mental Capacity Act (2005) Provides a statutory framework to empower and protect vulnerable people who 'lack *capacity*', i.e. are not able to make their own decisions.

Mental disorder A significant impairment of an individual's cognitive, affective and/or relational abilities which may require intervention and may be a recognised, medically diagnosable illness or disorder.

Mental health A state of wellness or well-being in which persons are able to function to the optimum level of their own innate ability, achieving their own life goals and thus realising their full potential.

Mental Health Act (1983) Revision of the 1959 act. Provides a statutory framework to allow compulsory detention and treatment of those with *mental disorder*.

Metabolic acidosis Increased production of H^+ by the body or the inability of the body to form bicarbonate ($HCO3^-$) in the kidney.

Metabolic alkalosis Alkalosis resulting from hydrogen ion loss or excessive intake of alkaline substances.

Metabolism Physical and chemical processes in the body that produce or use energy. Catabolism breaks down substances, e.g. food, to produce energy, while anabolism uses energy to construct substances, e.g. proteins and nucleic acids.

Metacommunication A form of communication that indicates the meaning behind the spoken word.

Metatarsals Five bones of the foot that connect the ankle to the toes.

Micturition To pass urine.

Modulation Returning the signal and releasing substances that act as natural painkillers.

Monosaccharides Single sugar, the simplest form of carbohydrates. The most important monosaccharide is glucose.

Morbidity The state of being diseased. The incidence of *disease* in a given population.

Mortality The incidence of death in a given population.

Mosaicism syndrome A developmental learning disability caused by an additional third chromosome in the 14th pair. Also known as *trisomy 14*.

Motive A compulsion to undertake, or avoid, an act. This may be an internal mechanism or a response to external stimuli. Also known as a *drive*, *impulse* or *volition*.

Myocardial infarction Commonly known as heart attack. Occurs when a clot occludes one or more of the coronary arteries.

National Institute for Health and Clinical Excellence (NICE) The NHS body established in 1999 to provide guidance, set quality standards and manage a national database to improve people's health and prevent and treat ill health.

National Service Frameworks National healthcare standards.

Negative symptoms The 4 A's of *schizophrenia* - *avolition*, *anhedonia*, *asociality/autism*, *alogia*.

Nephron The active unit of excretion in the kidney. Nephrons filter the blood in the *glomerulus*, and then reabsorb some of the constituents from the filtrate in the loop of Henle.

Neuritic plaques Deposits of the protein *beta amyloid* on neurons, a possible cause of *Alzheimer's disease*.

Neuro-fibrillary tangles The formation of twists and tangles in the tiny fibres, or tubules, connecting *neurons*. A possible cause of *Alzheimer's disease*.

Neurofibromatosis Characterised by numerous neurofibromas and by spots on the skin and often by developmental abnormalities.

Neuroleptic malignant syndrome (NMS) A rare but potentially fatal side-effect to phenothiazines. Characterised by fever, muscle clonicity, altered mental status and autonomic instability.

Neurons Nerve cells which process and transmit messages through an electrochemical process. The human brain has approximately 100 billion neurons.

Neuroses A term now largely redundant in contemporary psychiatry. A class of functional mental disorders involving distress but an absence of illusions and hallucinations. Insight remains intact; there is depression, *anxiety*, etc.

Neurotransmitters Chemicals which carry messages from one *neuron* to another. They create a bridge between neurons, filling the synaptic gap (the gap between synapses). Examples include dopamine, serotonin and noradrenaline.

Night terrors Pervasive thoughts forcing themselves into consciousness against your will when asleep. Can be a symptom of *post traumatic stress disorder*.

Nihilism Negative thoughts and beliefs. A perception that nothing is worthwhile and that everything is hopeless.

NMC Nursing and Midwifery Council. Regulatory body for nursing and midwifery in England, Wales, Scotland, Northern Island and the islands. The NMC sets standards for nursing and midwifery education, training and conduct, and is a key tool in safeguarding the health and well-being of the public

Nociception Sense of pain.

Nociceptive Sensitivity to stimuli capable of eliciting pain.

Nociceptors Sense organs that respond to stimuli that threaten or produce tissue damage, e.g. pain receptors.

Nocturia Passage of urine at night.

Nocturnal enuresis Involuntary passage of urine at night.

Non-bizarre delusions Fixed beliefs about events that could realistically occur.

Nonmaleficence 'Do no harm'.

Nuclear family A structure made up of parents and their offspring.

Nursing process A systematic, method of planning and providing individualised nursing care.

Occult Not apparent to the naked eye, or not easily detected.

Oedema Swelling.

Oliguria Production of abnormally small volumes of urine.

Organic brain disease/disorder Any disorder where the change in personality, mood or behaviour is as a result of injury to the brain.

Orthopnoeic position Sitting either in bed or on the side of the bed with an over bed table across the lap.

Orthostatic hypotension Falling blood pressure when patients stand or sit.

Osmolality A measurement of *solute* concentration of the blood.

Osmosis Diffusion of water molecules through a semipermeable membrane from a place of higher concentration to a place of lower concentration until the concentration on both sides is equal.

Ostomy Formation of a *stoma* opening.

Otic Relating to the ear.

Otoscope A scope that is used to examine the ear.

Outreach team Usually made up of critical care staff who attend patients who are at risk of deteriorating condition.

Oxyhaemoglobin The bright red compound formed when oxygen and *haemoglobin* combine in the blood.

Palliative care A multidisciplinary approach which aims to improve the quality of life of patients with life-threatening illness. Covers physical, emotional, spiritual and social difficulties.

Pallor A pale colour, caused by lack of *oxyhaemoglobin* in the skin or mucous membranes. Can also be caused by lack of melanin.

Palpation Using touch to examine the body. Palpation may be used to locate the position of anatomical landmarks, and to assess tenderness and swelling.

Paradigm Theory/idea.

Parasomnias Behaviours that interfere with sleep. Include nightmares, *night terrors*, sleepwalking and bedwetting.

Parasuicide Literally meaning 'near suicide'. Refers to acts of deliberate self-harm where harm is significant but not necessarily intended to result in death. Also known as a '*suicidal gesture*'.

Parenteral A route that involves piercing the skin or mucous membrane.

Paronychia A skin infection around the nails.

Pathogenicity Ability of a micro-organism to cause *disease*.

Pediculosis Infestation of lice. The crawling stages feed on human blood, resulting in itching. Head lice are usually located on the scalp, crab lice in the pubic area and body lice along the seams of clothing.

Peer review Practice of being evaluated by colleague or equal (professional).

Percussion Tapping or striking the body.

Percutaneous Through the skin.

Periodontal disease Gum *disease*.

Peripheral pulse *Pulse* located away from the heart. Examples are radial, brachial and femoral pulses.

Peristalsis The wave-like muscular contraction of the alimentary canal.

Pervasive thoughts Unwelcome, involuntary thoughts or memories forcing themselves into consciousness against your will. Also known as *intrusive thoughts*.

PES Problem(P), *Aetiology* (E), Signs and Symptoms (S).

pH The measure of acidity or alkalinity of a solution. A pH of 7 is neutral, less than 7 is acidic, and more than 7 is alkaline.

Phagocytosis The engulfing and digestion of bacteria and foreign material by white blood cells.

Phalange Toes and fingers.

Pharmacodynamics The *physiological* effects of drugs on the body.

Pharmacological interventions Care approaches that focus on the prescribing, administering and monitoring of drugs.

Pharmacology Study of drugs, including their origin, preparation, isolation, chemistry, effects and uses.

Pharmacy A place where drugs are prepared, made up and dispensed. Pharmacy also refers to the practice of ensuring the safe and effective use of pharmaceutical drugs.

Phenylalanine An essential *amino acid* found in proteins and needed for growth of children and for protein *metabolism* in children and adults.

Phenylketonuria An inherited disease in which the body cannot metabolise *phenylalanine*. It is a genetic disorder that is screened for at birth. Sufferers require a diet that is low in phenylalanine. If left untreated, phenylketonuria leads to mental retardation, brain damage and seizures.

Phobia An *anxiety* disorder which differs from general anxiety disorder in that it is focussed on a specific issue rather than being global in nature. A phobia may be described as an irrational fear.

Physiological Consistent with the normal functioning of an organism.

Physiotherapy Therapy that uses physical agents: exercise and massage and other modalities.

Pitting oedema Swelling that when pressed leaves an indentation.

PKU See *phenylketonuria*.

Plantar Sole of the foot.

Plantar wart Caused by a virus; is more commonly known as a verruca.

Plasma The colorless watery fluid of the blood and *lymph* that contains no cells.

Pneumothorax Collapse of one or both lungs. This is caused by air in the space around the lung(s), which means that the lung(s) cannot inflate when the person inhales.

Pocket mask A device used to safely deliver rescue breaths during a *cardiac arrest*.

Polycythaemia An increased number of red blood cells, and often white blood cells and platelets, in blood.

Polysaccharide A carbohydrate that, on hydrolysis, produces *monosaccharides*.

Polyuria Over-production of urine.

Positive symptoms In *schizophrenia*, the symptoms of delusions, hallucinations, thought insertion, etc.

Posterior Relating to the back of the body or organ.

Post-traumatic stress disorder (PTSD) A delayed, possibly pervasive and enduring reaction to a stressful event occurring at a later date.

Prader-Willi syndrome Caused by deletion of part of *chromosome* 15, and manifested by mental retardation and other problems.

Precordium The area of the chest overlying the heart.

Premorbid Before or preceding a disease or disorder.

Pre-psychotic changes Subtle changes in mood or behaviour which may precipitate a breakdown in *schizophrenia*. More commonly referred to as *prodromes* or *prodromal changes*.

Pressure ulcer Ulcerated area of skin usually caused by continuous pressure. Range in severity from discolored skin to open wounds that expose the bone. They are caused by disruption of bloodflow, and are more common in the elderly and those with *type 2 diabetes*.

Primary intention Healing that occurs when the surface of the skin has been closed.

Primary nursing A method of organising nursing care where one nurse is responsible for the care of a patient.

Private law Private law (civil law) is that part of a legal system that involves relationships between individuals without the intervention of the state or government. See also *public law*.

Problem solving A cognitive process of identifying, clarifying and finding solutions.

Prodromal changes Subtle changes in mood or behaviour which may precipitate a breakdown in *schizophrenia*. Also known as *prodromes* or occasionally *pre-psychotic changes*.

Prodromes Subtle changes in mood or behaviour which may precipitate a breakdown in *schizophrenia*. Also known as *prodromal changes* or occasionally *pre-psychotic changes*.

Pronation Moving the bones of, for example, the forearm so that the palm of the hand faces downward when held in front of the body. Also the inward roll of the foot.

Prone Position in which the patient is positioned lying on their front.

Prophylaxis A measure to prevent a *disease* or condition, e.g. medication to stabilise mood to prevent *mania* or depression in bipolar disorder.

Protein energy malnutrition Develops in those who do not ingest sufficient calories from protein to satisfy the body's metabolic requirements. It is the leading cause of death in children in developing countries.

Proximal Close to the origin, the attached end, the midline or the centre.

Psychoanalysis An approach to psychotherapy which involves structured questioning of the individual with the purpose of uncovering and interpreting unconscious thoughts or emotions. Sometimes called 'Mind Investigation'.

Psycho-education A means of helping a person or group to learn about and to develop new skills or new behaviours to allow them to manage their own care.

Psychological Affecting the human mind, or mental process.

Psychomotor Relating to the function of muscles under the control of the mind. Includes the production of voluntary movement and seizures giving rise to sensory auras.

Psychoneurological Applies to psychology (the mind) and neurology (the structure and function of the nervous system).

Psychopathy Being a psychopath. An outdated term now replaced by 'personality disorder'.

Psychoses A term now largely redundant in contemporary psychiatry. A severe functional mental disorder such as *schizophrenia* or bipolar disorder in which skills, cognition, emotions and behaviours are impaired to a degree which limits a person's capacity to meet the demands of normal life. There is usually an absence of *insight*.

Psychosocial interventions Any care approach that does not involve drugs. Generally it refers to the establishment of a *therapeutic relationship* and applying *talking therapies*.

Public law A law affecting the public at large. It governs the relationships between individuals and the state.

Puerperal psychosis Postpartum or postnatal psychosis. Common symptoms are *delusions* and *hallucinations*.

Pulmonary aspiration Entry of foreign body or secretions into the trachea and lungs. Usually associated with contents of the stomach entering the lungs.

Pulmonary embolus A clot on the lung.

Pulmonary oedema Fluid accumulation in the lungs usually as the result of heart failure.

Pulse Wave of blood created by the contraction of the left ventricle of the heart.

Pulseless electrical activity *Cardiac arrest* rhythm associated with normal or life-sustaining electrical activity within the heart without any corresponding *cardiac output*.

Pulseless ventricular tachycardia A *cardiac arrest* rhythm resulting from normal electrical conduction but no mechanical function of the heart.

Pulse oximeter A device that measures a patient's arterial blood oxygen saturation.

Purulent *Pus*-like.

Pus *Exudate* comprised of leukocytes, cell debris and protein-rich fluid. Is usually produced as a response to infections caused by bacteria or other micro-organisms.

Pyrexia A body temperature above the usual range.

Radiation Thermal or infrared radiation. Heat transfer using the medium of waves, so heat can be transferred in a vacuum.

Reactive depression A depression as a response to circumstances. Also called *exogenous depression* or *adjustment disorder*.

Reactive hyperaemia A process in which extra blood floods to an area to compensate for the preceding period of impeded blood flow.

Reality orientation (RO) Assisting the individual's orientation in terms of time, place and person. A therapy applied in care of persons with *dementia*.

Reciprocity Responding in a similar manner, reciprocating. In communication it means that if an individual is open and honest with another then this should be returned.

Rectal fumigation A core rewarming practice from the past.

Recurrent depression Second or subsequent episodes of depression.

Reflux Backflow of liquid.

Rehabilitation Any therapeutic process intended to assist a Person to return to their own habitat or home. Usually taken to mean a return to their previous life/lifestyle.

Relapse Generally refers to a period when people experience a recurrence of symptoms that they have previously had. Literally it means 'falling back' and refers to a return to a previous condition after experiencing a partial recovery.

Relapse signature A unique pattern of psychological changes often occurring in a predictable sequence, indicating a potential further psychotic episode. Also called *early warning signs*.

Relaxation therapy A technique that helps the patient to be able to relax, usually by undertaking a series of exercises designed to control breathing and heart rate.

Reminiscence therapy A technique used in treating persons with *dementia* that involves stimulating the memories of previous events in the long-term memory in the belief that the current short-term memory may be maintained or improved.

Research process Formalised, logical systematic approach to solving problems.

Reservoir Places where micro-organisms maintain a presence are known as reservoirs (these may be humans, animals or inanimate objects).

Reservoir bag Bag attached to oxygen mask or *bag valve mask device* to allow accumulation of oxygen. Enables the device to deliver higher concentrations of oxygen.

Resident flora Micro-organisms that live naturally within the skin's normal flora. They are not easily transferred to patients.

Residual urine Urine remaining in the bladder after *micturition*.

Respiration The act of breathing. Respiration rate is the number of breaths taken per minute.

Respiratory acidosis *Acidosis* caused by retention of carbon dioxide. The blood *pH* can fall to below 7.35 owing to the build up of carbonic acid.

Respiratory alkalosis *Alkalosis* caused by low carbon dioxide levels. This can be as a result of *hyperventilation*. The blood *pH* can rise above 7.45.

Respiratory failure Failure of the lungs either in their capacity to oxygenate the blood (*hypoxaemia*) or to remove carbon dioxide (*hypercapnia*) from the blood. This may be acute or chronic.

Respiratory membrane The alveolar and capillary walls form the respiratory membrane. It is extremely thin (less than 0.5 mm).

Rhesus One of the blood group systems. It is the most important after ABO. Individuals can be Rhesus positive (indicating that they have the Rhesus factor - an antigen - on the surface of their red blood cells) or Rhesus negative (indicating that they do not have the antigen).

Rubella Or *German measles.* Mildly contagious viral disease usually affecting children aged 5 to 15 years. Symptoms commonly include fever, tender lymph nodes and rash.

Schema/schemata The collective term for a group, or family, of related thoughts or beliefs. Schemata can be used to organise patterns of thinking and to provide a framework to store knowledge and to help future understanding.

Schism A division or split. Used in serious mental disorders to describe the division between thoughts and behaviours.

Schizophrenia Major mental illness characterised by deterioration of the personality. Sufferers withdraw from reality and may suffer delusions and hallucinations.

Sebum Oily substance responsible for keeping the skin and hair moisturised.

Secondary intention Healing which occurs when the wound is too extensive for the edges to be closed.

Selective serotonin reuptake inhibitors (SSRIs) A class of antidepressants that act on *serotonin*, the *neurotransmitter* responsible for managing mood, e.g. citalopram, fluoxetine, etc.

Selectively permeable A membrane that will allow certain molecules or ions to pass through it by *diffusion*.

Self-determination The freedom to be in charge of your own destiny. The right to choose.

Sequelae A *chronic* condition emerging as a complication to an *acute* condition. Commonly, symptoms may first appear during the acute phase.

Serotonin A *neurotransmitter* controlling various functions, including appetite, sleep, memory, mood and behaviour.

Serous Clear/straw-like exudate.

Shock Clinical syndrome characterised by low blood pressure, poor peripheral perfusion and mental dulling. There are many types of shock, including hypovolaemic shock (loss of circulating blood volume), cardiogenic shock (arising from impaired myocardial function) and neurogenic shock (arising from increased activity of the sympathetic nervous system).

Sleep apnoea A periodic cessation of breathing during sleep. The relaxed walls of the oropharynx obstruct inspiration. Risk factors include obesity, smoking, *diabetes* and age. Symptoms include loud snoring, restless sleep and fatigue during the day.

Slough Yellowy-white necrotic tissue.

Social model Changing or adapting the lifestyle of the individual or of society at large to reduce 'problems' or their impact on society.

Social readjustment rating Stressful events that typically would precede the advent of illness.

Social role valorisation The name given to an analysis of human relationships and human services.

Sociopathy Being a sociopath. An outdated term now replaced by 'personality disorder'.

Solute Substance dissolved in solution.

Somatic Affecting the body rather than the psyche, i.e. physical not psychological.

Somatic passivity phenomena (SPP) A positive symptom of *schizophrenia* where the individual believes they are a passive recipient of physical sensations from an external source.

Spastic diplegia A form of *cerebral palsy* in which the legs are mostly affected.

Spatial relationship The connection between oneself and the environment or between two or more objects outside of oneself.

Specific gravity A *urinalysis* parameter commonly used in the evaluation of kidney function.

Spina bifida A developmental birth defect caused by the incomplete closure of the embryonic neural tube.

Sternum Breast bone.

Stoma A deliberate artificial opening into the body. Can be temporary or permanent. Types of stoma include colostomy, ileostomy, tracheostomy and urostomy.

Stool See *faeces*.

Stress A normal physical and psychological response of the body to demands placed upon it. A stress reaction is characterised by shortness of breath, increased heart rate, palpitations, etc.

Stridor A high-pitched sound resulting from turbulent air flow in the upper airway. May be caused by laryngeal obstruction.

Stroke A *cerebro-vascular accident*. A sudden attack of weakness affecting one side of the body, resulting from an interruption to the flow of blood to the brain owing to *ischaemia* or *haemorrhage*.

Sturge-Weber syndrome *Congenital disease* characterised by three major symptoms including excessive blood vessel growth, intracranial calcification and seizures.

Sub-cortex The layer beneath the *cortex* of the brain comprising brainstem, midbrain and forebrain. Also known as 'white matter'.

Sublingual Under the tongue.

Suicidal gesture Acts of deliberate self-harm where harm is significant but not necessarily intended to result in death. Also known as a *parasuicide*.

Supination Moving the bones of, for example, the forearm so that the hand faces upward when held in front of the body.

Supine Position where the patient is positioned lying on their back.

Supreme Court The highest judicial body within that jurisdiction's court system.

Surfactant A *lipoprotein*. It is present in the fluid lining the alveoli of the lungs, and helps to prevent collapse and aids reinflation of deflated alveoli.

Syndactyly Birth defect in which there is partial or total webbing connecting two or more fingers or toes.

Systolic pressure The pressure of the blood as a result of the contraction of the ventricles. A person's blood pressure is usually expressed as systolic pressure over *diastolic pressure*, in mmHg, e.g. 130/80.

Tachycardia Fast heart rate, e.g. over 100 bpm in an adult. It can occur in the atria or the ventricles, and results in inefficient pumping of oxygen to the body.

Tachypnoea Rapid breathing, e.g. greater than 20 breaths per minute.

Talking therapies A range of psychosocial interventions which mainly involve sharing emotions, thoughts, etc. with a trained counsellor, e.g. *cognitive behavioural therapy*, counselling, *psycho-education*, etc.

Tamponade Collection of fluid around the heart, that can lead to reduced *cardiac output* and *cardiac arrest*.

Tay-Sachs disease A hereditary disorder of lipid *metabolism*.

Team nursing A method of organising nursing care in which a team of nurses is responsible for the care of a patient.

Telecare Remote care of the vulnerable, offering support and reassurance so that people can continue to live in their own homes. Telecare can work by a phone that has a connection to a monitoring centre, through which the user can raise the alarm.

Telehealth A wider form of *telemedicine*, encompassing preventive and curative aspects.

Telemedicine The use of the telephone or internet to diagnose and treat patients.

Tension pneumothorax Life-threatening condition in which air within the chest cannot escape, leading to a build up of pressure within the thorax.

Therapeutic relationship The working relationship between a nurse (therapist) and a patient (client). Sometimes called *engagement*, the working alliance or a helpful relationship. What Peplau described as the 'proper focus of nursing'.

Thought disorder A positive symptom of *schizophrenia* where the individual believes thoughts are being shared, that they can read the minds of others and/or that others can read their thoughts.

Thrombo-embolic Occlusion of a vessel by a blood clot.

Thrombolytic Drugs that dissolve blood clots - 'clot busting' drugs.

Tonicity Tone of an organ/structure/muscle.

Topical Applied to the body surface.

Transdermal Through the skin.

Transduction The first sensing of pain and trigger to release chemical substances.

Transient Passing or short lived. Similar to, and sometimes used to mean, *acute*.

Transient flora These are micro-organisms that are picked up from the environment, equipment or during patient contact. They can then be transferred from the hands to other people, surfaces and equipment.

Transient ischaemic attack A temporary (*transient*) reduction to blood/oxygen supply (*ischaemia*) to part of the brain. Sometimes called a 'mini stroke' - symptoms last less than 24 hours.

Transmission The journey from the pain impulse to the spinal cord.

Transpersonal psychology The psychology of health and human potential.

Trapezius Flat triangular muscles of the shoulder and upper back that are involved in moving the shoulders and arms.

Tricyclic antidepressants Older original antidepressants such as amitriptyline, lofepramine, etc. Largely replaced by *selective serotonin reuptake inhibitors* which have similar benefits but fewer side-effects.

Triglycerides The major form of fat stored by the body. Consist of glycerol and three fatty acids.

Trigone Triangular area of tissue, e.g. in the bladder.

Triple X syndrome A form of chromosomal variation characterised by the presence of an extra X *chromosome* in each cell of a human female.

Trisomy An additional third *chromosome* in some individuals instead of having a pair of chromosomes as is normal. Individuals have 47 chromosomes in cells rather than the normal 46. Disorders that result from trisomies are *Down's syndrome, Edwards syndrome* and *mosaicism syndrome*.

Trisomy 14 An additional third *chromosome* in the 14th pair. The genetic cause of *mosaicism syndrome*.

Trisomy 21 An additional third *chromosome* in the 21st pair. The genetic cause of *Down's syndrome*.

Tuberous sclerosis A rare, multi-system genetic disease that causes benign tumours to grow in the brain and on other vital organs such as the kidneys, heart, eyes, lungs and skin.

Turner syndrome A genetic disorder in females that results from a *chromosome* abnormality. There is only one X chromosome in all or some cells. Sufferers may have short stature and have incomplete sexual development, which may result in sterility.

Type 2 diabetes Non-insulin-dependent diabetes. Adult onset, usually after age 40. Often associated with obesity.

Urea A toxic nitrogen-containing substance normally cleared from the blood by the kidney into the urine. Produced in liver from breakdown of proteins.

Ureter Tubule passing from the kidney to the bladder.

Urethra Tubule passing from the bladder to outside the body.

Urgency A desire to pass urine urgently.

Urinalysis Laboratory examination of urine. Urine is evaluated for colour, concentration, pH, and the presence of chemicals such as sugar, protein and blood.

Urinary hesitancy A hesitancy to pass urine.

Urinary incontinence The involuntary passage of urine.

Urinary retention Inability to pass urine that is held in the bladder.

Validation therapy A technique that involves confirmation and affirmation rather than confrontation. Validation therapy involves 'validating' the individual's conversation by acknowledging the underlying meaning.

Vaporisation Continuous evaporation of moisture from the respiratory tract and the mucosa of the mouth and the skin.

Vasodilation Dilation (widening) of the blood vessels.

Ventilation The intentional movement of air/oxygen from outside the body to the lungs.

Ventilator A machine that supports breathing. It moves breatheable air into and out of the lungs mechanically in patients who are unable to breathe for themselves.

Ventricular fibrillation Uncoordinated contractions of the cardiac muscle of the ventricles. Fibrillation is twitching, and blood is not ejected from the ventricles, leading to *cardiac arrest*.

Ventricular tachycardia A condition in which the ventricles cause a very fast heartbeat. Can cause *cardiac arrest*.

Vicarious liability A legal principle in which one person can be held liable for the actions or non-actions of another with whom the person has a special relationship, e.g. employer and employee.

Virulence The disease-producing capacity of any infectious agent.

Visual acuity The ability to distinguish details and shapes (eyes).

Visual field The total area in which objects can be seen in the peripheral vision when the subject focuses on a central point.

Vital signs *Physiological* measures that nurses record in clinical situations. They include body temperature, *pulse*, *respirations* and blood pressure.

Vitiligo Disorder of the skin. Leads to patchy loss of pigmentation.

Voiding Passing of urine.

Volition A compulsion to undertake, or avoid, an act. This may be an internal mechanism or a response to external stimuli. Also known as a *motive*, *drive* or *impulse*.

Volume expander Fluid that will stay in circulation longer than crystalloid fluids.

Waxy flexibility A symptom of catatonic *schizophrenia* where individuals can be manipulated into shapes or positions which they will hold for hours. Also known as *cerea flexibilitas*.

Wernicke's encephalitis A type of *dementia* associated with excessive alcohol consumption.

Whole-person approach A theory and tradition of healing that promotes treatment of the whole person. The approach of taking into consideration the whole body and environment when offering treatment. See *bio-psycho-social model*, *holistic approach*, *complex needs*.

Xiphisternum A small cartilaginous extension to the lower part of the sternum.

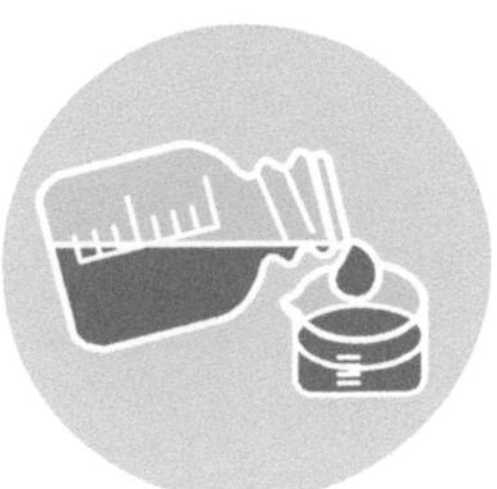
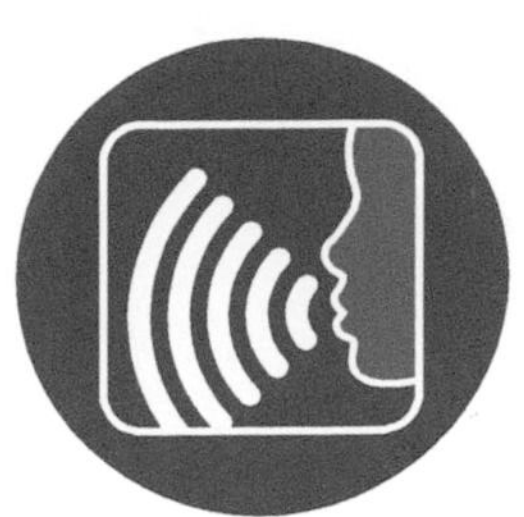

INDEX

Note: Boxes, Case Studies, Clinical Alerts, Figures, Guidelines and Tables are indicated by *italic page numbers*; and Glossary by **emboldened numbers.**

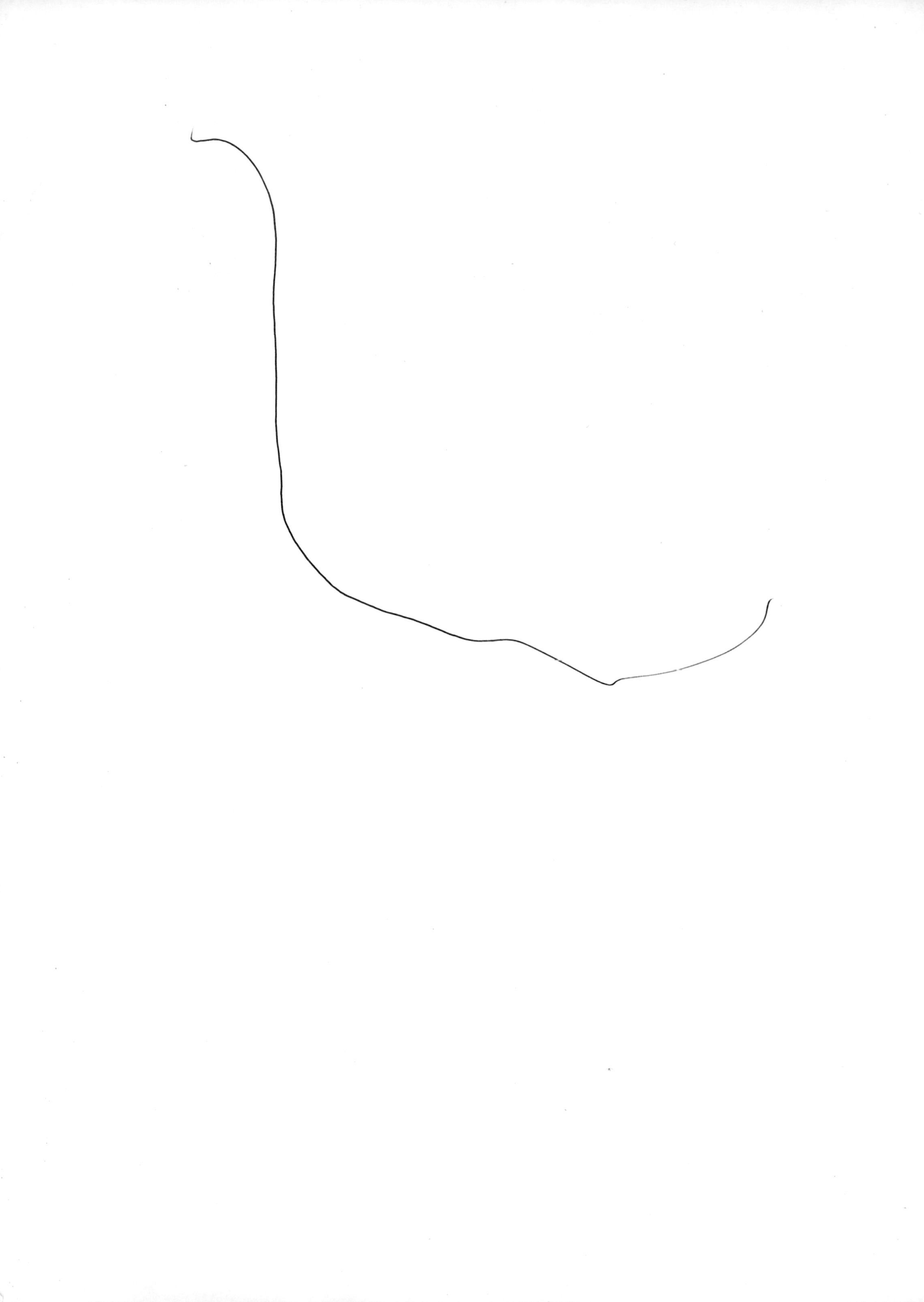

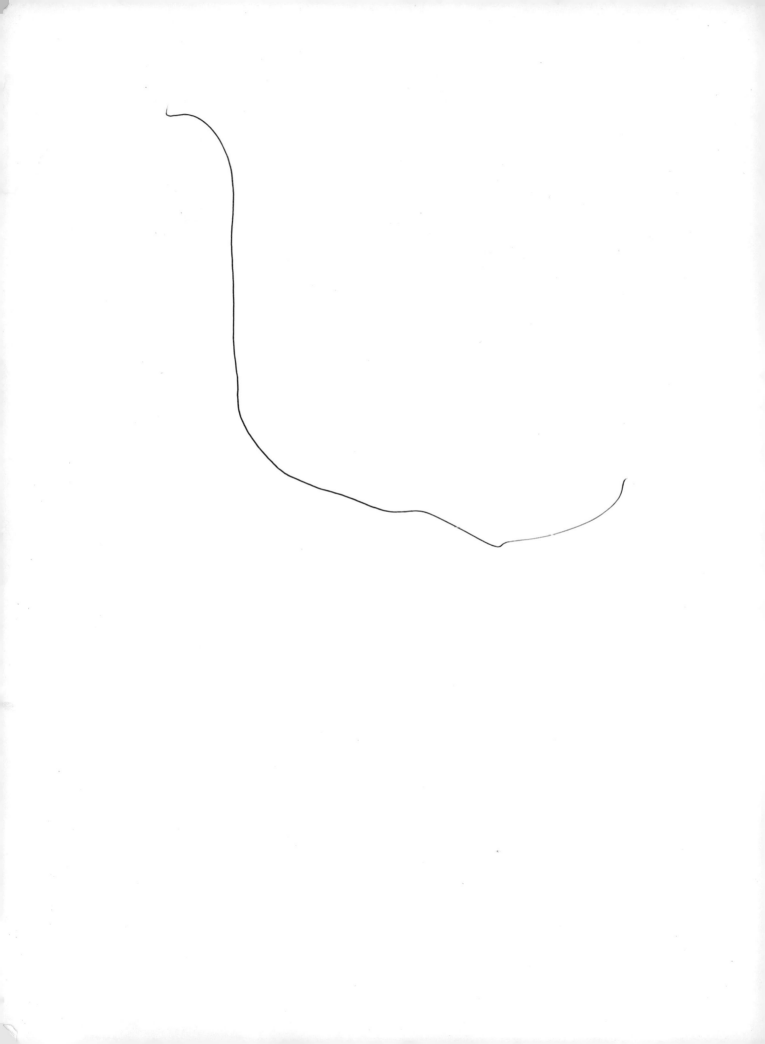

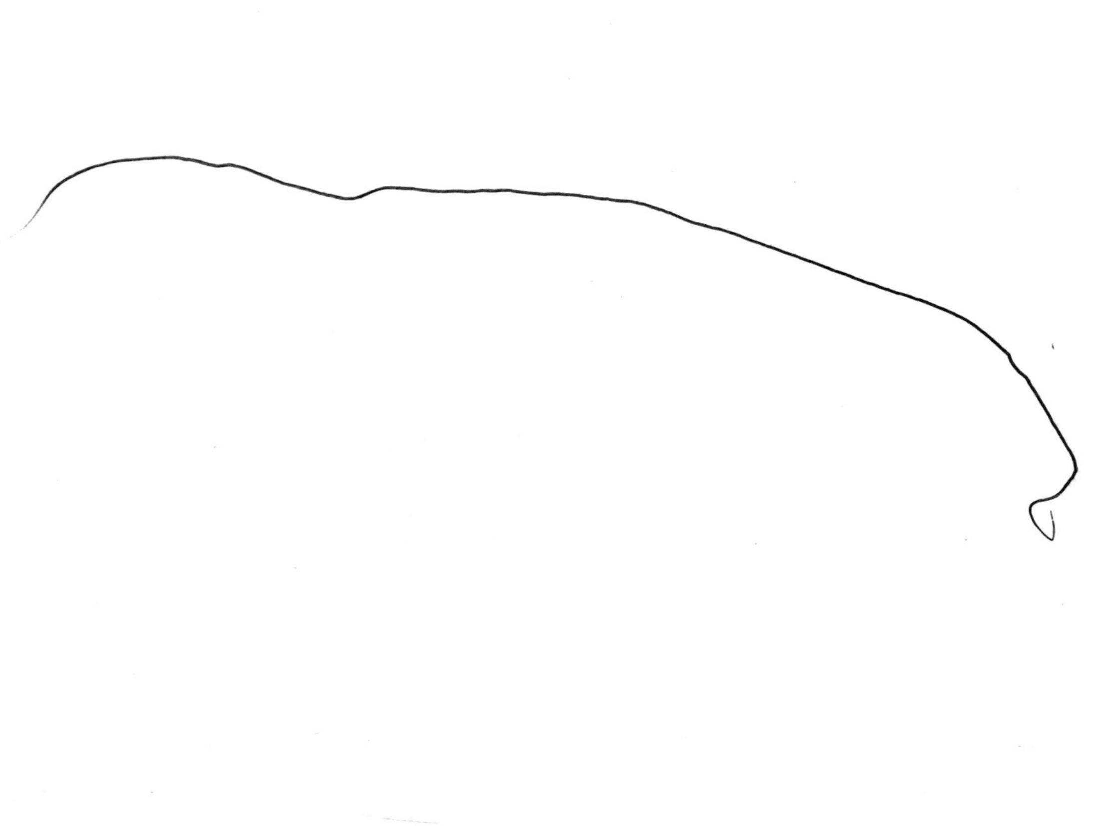

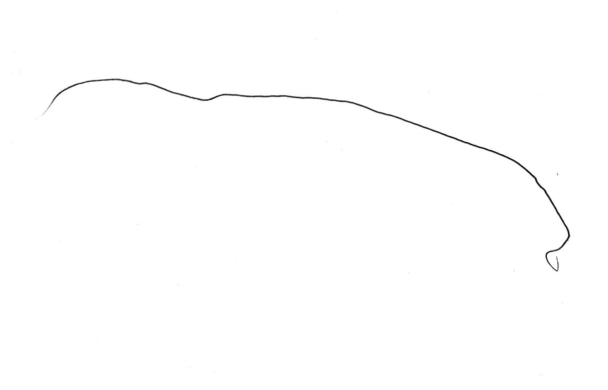

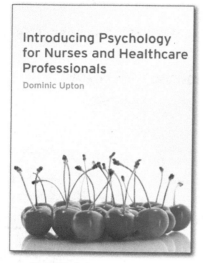

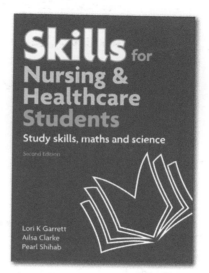

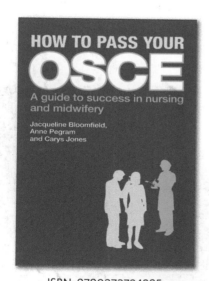

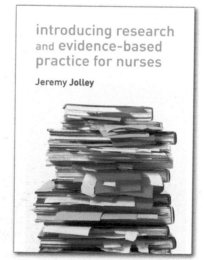

F[illegible]ent[illegible]
NURSING

Visit the *Fundamentals of Nursing*, Second Edition **MyNursingKit** at **www.pearsoned.co.uk/kozier** to find valuable **student** learning material including:

- Diagnostic Tests to confirm your understanding
- Interactive Scenario Simulations allowing you to practise skills safely and to confirm your knowledge and abilities
- Skills Videos
- An Integrated Customisable eText
- Useful Websites for further research
- Additional Short Answer Case Studies
- Flashcards to test your knowledge
- A fully searchable Glossary.

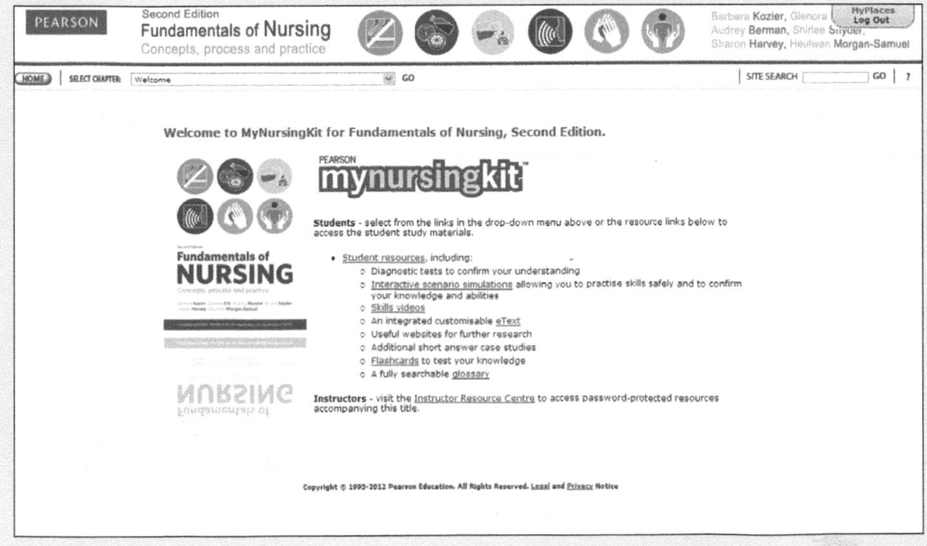